a LANGE medical book

CURRENT
Diagnosis & Treatment
Rheumatology

Third Edition

Editors

John B. Imboden, MD
Alice Betts Endowed Chair for Research in Arthritis
Professor of Medicine
University of California, San Francisco
Chief, Division of Rheumatology
San Francisco General Hospital

David B. Hellmann, MD, MACP
Aliki Perroti Professor of Medicine
Vice Dean for Bayview
Johns Hopkins university School of Medicine
Chairman, Department of Medicine
Johns Hopkins Bayview Medical Center

John H. Stone, MD, MPH
Professor of Medicine
Harvard Medical School
Director, Clinical Rheumatology
Massachusetts General Hospital

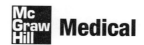

New York   Chicago   San Francisco   Lisbon   London   Madrid   Mexico City
Milan   New Delhi   San Juan   Seoul   Singapore   Sydney   Toronto

The McGraw-Hill Companies

Current Diagnosis & Treatment: Rheumatology, Third Edition

2 3 4 5 6 7 8 9 0   DOC/DOC   17 16 15 14 13

ISBN 978-0-07-163805-0
MHID 0-07-163805-9
ISSN 1547-8998

Notice

Medicine is an ever-changing science. As new research and clinical experience broaden our knowledge, changes in treatment and drug therapy are required. The authors and the publisher of this work have checked with sources believed to be reliable in their efforts to provide information that is complete and generally in accord with the standards accepted at the time of publication. However, in view of the possibility of human error or changes in medical sciences, neither the authors nor the publisher nor any other party who has been involved in the preparation or publication of this work warrants that the information contained herein is in every respect accurate or complete, and they disclaim all responsibility for any errors or omissions or for the results obtained from use of the information contained in this work. Readers are encouraged to confirm the information contained herein with other sources. For example and in particular, readers are advised to check the product information sheet included in the package of each drug they plan to administer to be certain that the information contained in this work is accurate and that changes have not been made in the recommended dose or in the contraindications for administration. This recommendation is of particular importance in connection with new or infrequently used drugs.

This book was set in Minion by Thomson Digital.
The editors were Christine Diedrich and Harriet Lebowitz.
The production supervisor was Sherri Souffrance.
Project Management was provided by Charu Bansal, Thomson Digital.
RR Donnelley was the printer and binder.

This book is printed on acid-free paper.

McGraw-Hill books are available at special quantity discounts to use as premiums and sales promotions, or for use in corporate training programs. To contact a representative please e-mail us at bulksales@mcgraw-hill.com.

With love, admiration, and gratitude, we remember and
dedicate this book to our three physician-fathers: Dr. John B. Imboden (1925-2008),
Dr. Jack K. Hellmann (1925-1999), and Dr. John H. Stone, III (1936-2008).
Their examples inspired us in our professional work and their
influence continues to guide us in our lives.

Contents

---

*Deceased.

Color insert appears between pages 40 and 41.

Contributors

Jeffrey S. Alderman, MD
Associate Professor
Department of Internal Medicine
University of Oklahoma School of Community Medicine
Tulsa, Oklahoma
Pseudogout: Calcium Pyrophosphate Dihydrate Crystal Deposition Disease

Johnathan A. Bernard, MD
Resident, Department of Orthopaedic Surgery
Johns Hopkins Medical Institutions
Baltimore, Maryland
Approach to the Patient with Shoulder Pain

Clifton O. Bingham III, MD
Associate Professor of Medicine
Director, Johns Hopkins Arthritis Center
Division of Rheumatology and Allergy and
    Clinical Immunology
Johns Hopkins University School of Medicine
Baltimore, Maryland
Reactive Arthritis; Psoriatic Arthritis

Linda K. Bockenstedt, MD
Harold W. Jockers Professor of Medicine/Rheumatology
Department of Medicine
Yale University School of Medicine
New Haven, Connecticut
Lyme Disease

David Borenstein, MD
Clinical Professor of Medicine
Department of Medicine
The George Washington University Medical Center
Washington, District of Columbia
Approach to the Patient with Neck Pain

Pilar Brito-Zerón, MD, PhD
Department of Systemic Autoimmune Diseases
Hospital Clinic
Barcelona, Spain
Primary Sjögren Syndrome

Calvin R. Brown Jr., MD
Professor of Medicine
Division of Rheumatology
Northwestern University Feinberg School of Medicine
Chicago, Illinois
Common Injuries from Running

Christopher Burns, MD
Assistant Professor, Section of Rheumatology
Department of Medicine
Geisel School of Medicine at Dartmouth
Lebanon, New Hampshire
Gout

Henry F. Chambers, MD
Professor
Division of Infectious Diseases
Department of Medicine
University of California, San Francisco
San Francisco, California
Mycobacterial & Fungal Infections of Bone & Joints

Edward S. Chen, MD
Assistant Professor,
Division of Pulmonary and Critical Care Medicine
Department of Medicine
Johns Hopkins University School of Medicine
Baltimore, Maryland
Sarcoidosis

Ernest H. S. Choy, MD, FRCP
Professor and Head of Rheumatology
Department of Medicine
Cardiff University School of Medicine,
    Cardiff University
Cardiff, United Kingdom
The Patient with Diffuse Pain

Lisa Christopher-Stine, MD, MPH
Co-Director, Johns Hopkins Myositis Center
Assistant Professor of Medicine and Neurology
Johns Hopkins University School of Medicine
Baltimore, Maryland
Dermatomyositis, Polymyositis, & Immune-Mediated Necrotizing Myopathy

Megan E. B. Clowse, MD, MPH
Assistant Professor of Medicine
Division of Rheumatology and Immunology
Duke University Medical Center
Durham, North Carolina
Pregnancy & Rheumatic Diseases

Harold R. Collard, MD
Associate Professor of Medicine
Director, Interstitial Lung Disease Program
University of California, San Francisco
San Francisco, California
*Connective Tissue Disease–Associated Interstitial
  Lung Disease*

Gaye Cunnane, MB, PhD, FRCPI
Clinical Professor of Rheumatology
Trinity College Dublin
Consultant Rheumatologist
St. James's Hospital
Dublin, Ireland
Whipple Disease

Maria Dall'Era, MD
Associate Professor of Medicine
University of California, San Francisco
San Francisco, California
*Systemic Lupus Erythematosus; Treatment of Systemic
  Lupus Erythematosus*

Richard J. de Asla, MD
Orthopedic Surgery
Instructor, Harvard Medical School
Boston, Massachusetts
Approach to the Patient with Foot & Ankle Pain

E. Gene Deune, MD
Department of Orthopedic Surgery
Co-Director, Division of Hand Surgery
Johns Hopkins Medical Center
Baltimore, Maryland
Approach to the Patient with Hand, Wrist, or Elbow Pain

Rajiv K. Dixit, MD
Clinical Professor of Medicine
University of California, San Francisco
Director, Northern California Arthritis Center
Walnut Creek, California
Approach to the Patient with Low Back Pain

Geetha Duvuru, MD, MRCP
Johns Hopkins Medical Center
Baltimore, Maryland
Microscopic Polyangiitis; Henoch-Schönlein Purpura

David T. Felson, MD, MPH
Professor of Medicine and Epidemiology
Clinical Epidemiology Research and Training Unit
Boston University School of Medicine
Boston, Massachusetts
Osteoarthritis

John A. Flynn, MD, MBA
Professor, Division of Rheumatology
  & Department of Medicine
Johns Hopkins University School of Medicine
Baltimore, Maryland
*Ankylosing Spondylitis & the Arthritis of
  Inflammatory Bowel Disease*

Howard W. Francis, MD, MBA
Associate Professor
Vice Department Director,
Residency Program Director,
Department of Otolaryngology- Head and Neck Surgery
Johns Hopkins University School of Medicine
Baltimore, Maryland
*Sensorineural Hearing Loss (Immune-mediated
  Inner Ear Disease)*

Michael T. Freehill, MD
Assistant Professor
Department of Orthopedic Surgery
Wake Forest University
Winston-Salem, North Carolina
Approach to the Patient with Shoulder Pain

Andrew A. Freiberg, MD
Associate Professor, Harvard Medical School
Arthroplasty Service Chief and Vice Chair
Department of Orthopedic Surgery
Massachusetts General Hospital
Boston, Massachusetts
Approach to the Patient with a Painful Prosthetic Hip or Knee

Kenneth H. Fye, MD
Deceased, formerly from the Division of Rheumatology
University of California
San Francisco
Joint Aspiration & Injection

Monica Gandhi, MD, MPH
Associate Professor, Division of HIV/AIDS
Department of Medicine
University of California, San Francisco
San Francisco, California
Septic Arthritis

Kelly A. Gebo, MD, MPH
Associate Professor of Medicine,
Division of Infectious Diseases
Johns Hopkins University School of Medicine
Director, Undergraduate Public Health Studies Program
Johns Hopkins University Krieger School of Arts and Sciences
Baltimore, Maryland
Evaluation of Rheumatic Complaints in Patients with HIV

Lianne S. Gensler, MD
Assistant Clinical Professor of Medicine
Division of Rheumatology
Department of Medicine
University of California
San Francisco, California
Osteonecrosis

Morie Gertz, MD, MACP
Roland Seidler, Jr.
Professor and Chair
Department of Medicine
College of Medicine
Consultant, Division of Hematology
Mayo Distinguished Clinician, Mayo Clinic
Rochester, Minnesota
Amyloidosis

Khalil G. Ghanem, MD, PhD
Associate Professor of Medicine
Johns Hopkins University School of Medicine
Baltimore, Maryland
*Disseminated Gonococcal Infection; Evaluation of Rheumatic
    Complaints in Patients with HIV*

Reda E. Girgis, MB, BCh
Medical Director, Lung Transplantation
Richard DeVos Heart and Lung Transplant Program
    Spectrum Health
Grand Rapids, Michigan
Pulmonary Hypertension

Jonathan Graf, MD
Associate Professor of Clinical Medicine
University of California, San Francisco
San Francisco General Hospital
San Francisco, California
*Antiphospholipid Antibody Syndrome; Endocrine
    & Metabolic Disorders*

Sarah Beckman Gratton, MD
Fellow, Division of Rheumatology
Department of Medicine
University of California
San Francisco, California
Endocrine & Metabolic Disorders

Andrew Gross, MD
Associate Clinical Professor
Clinical Director, Rheumatology
University of California
San Francisco, California
Approach to the Patient with Knee Pain

Anan Haija, MD
AtlantiCare Regional Medical Center
Atlantic City, New Jersey
Physician Advisor
Executive Health Resources
Newton Square, Pennsylvania
Complementary & Alternative Therapies

Kristen Hayward, MD, MA
Assistant Professor, Department of Pediatrics
Division of Rheumatology
Seattle Children's Hospital and University of Washington
Seattle, Washington
Juvenile Idiopathic Arthritis

David B. Hellmann, MD, MACP
Aliki Perroti Professor of Medicine
Vice Dean for Bayview
Johns Hopkins university School of Medicine
Chairman, Department of Medicine
Johns Hopkins Bayview Medical Center
Baltimore, Maryland
*Introduction to Vasculitis: Classification & Clinical Clues;
    Giant Cell Arteritis & Polymyalgia Rheumatica; Takayasu
    Arteritis; Behçet Disease; Vasculitis of the Central Nervous
    System; Common Rheumatologic Problems Encountered by
    the Hospitalist: Pearls & Myths*

Laura K. Hummers, MD
Assistant Professor of Medicine
Division of Rheumatology
Johns Hopkins University School of Medicine
Baltimore, Maryland
Scleroderma

John B. Imboden, MD
Alice Betts Endowed Chair for Research in Arthritis
Professor of Medicine
University of California, San Francisco
Chief, Division of Rheumatology
San Francisco General Hospital
San Francisco, California
*Joint Aspiration & Injection; Laboratory Diagnosis;
    Approach to the Patient with Arthritis; Rheumatoid
    Arthritis; Adult-Onset Still Disease; Mycobacterial
    & Fungal Infections of Bone & Joints; Rheumatic
    Manifestations of Malignancy; Common
    Rheumatologic Problems Encountered by the
    Hospitalist: Pearls & Myths*

Richard A. Jacobs, MD, PhD
Emeritus Clinical Professor of Medicine
Division of Infectious Diseases
Department of Medicine
University of California
San Francisco, California
Septic Arthritis

Preeti Jaggi, MD
Assistant Professor of Clinical Pediatrics
The Ohio State University College of Medicine
Nationwide Children's Hospital
Ohio State University
Columbus, Ohio
Rheumatic Fever

James C. Johnston, MD
Maine General Health System
    Augusta Orthopaedics
Augusta, Maine
Approach to the Patient with Hand,
    Wrist, or Elbow Pain

Ravi S. Kamath, MD, PhD
Muscoskeletal Radiologist
Fairfax Radiological Consultants, PC
Fairfax, Virginia
Musculoskeletal Magnetic Resonance Imaging

Susan V. Kattapuram, MD
Associate Professor
Harvard Medical School
Boston, Massachusetts
Musculoskeletal Magnetic Resonance Imaging

Chris E. Keh, MD
MSP Physician
Department of Medicine
Division of Infectious Diseases
University of California, San Francisco
San Francisco, California
Septic Arthritis

Eunice J. Kim, MD
Fellow, Pulmonary & Critical Care Division
Department of Medicine
University of California, San Francisco
Pulmonary and Critical Care Medicine
Palo Alto Medical Foundation
Santa Cruz, California
Connective Tissue Disease–Associated
    Interstitial Lung Disease

Sharon L. Kolasinski, MD
Professor of Medicine
Cooper Medical School of Rowan University
Head, Division of Rheumatology
Cooper University Hospital
Camden, New Jersey
Complementary & Alternative Therapies

Young-Min Kwon, MD, PhD
Assistant Professor of Orthopaedic Surgery
Harvard Medical School
Director, Center for Metal-on-Metal Hip Replacements
Department of Orthopaedic Surgery
Massachusetts General Hospital
Boston, Massachusetts
Approach to the Patient with a Painful Prosthetic Hip or Knee

John Kwon, MD
Orthopedic Surgery
Massachusetts General Hospital
Boston, Massachusetts
Approach to the Patient with Foot & Ankle Pain

Grant H. Louie, MD, MHS
Assistant Professor of Medicine
Division of Rheumatology
Johns Hopkins University School of Medicine
Baltimore, Maryland
Reactive Arthritis; Psoriatic Arthritis

C. Benjamin Ma, MD
Associate Professor
Chief, Sports Medicine and Shoulder Surgery
University of California
San Francisco, California
Approach to the Patient with Knee Pain

C. Ronald MacKenzie, MD
Hospital for Special Surgery
New York Presbyterian Hospital
New York Weill Cornell Medical Center
New York, New York
Perioperative Management of the Patient with
    Rheumatic Disease

Andrew L. Mammen, MD, PhD
Associate Professor of Neurology and Medicine
Co-Director of Johns Hopkins Myositis Center
Johns Hopkins University School of Medicine
Baltimore, Maryland
Dermatomyositis, Polymyositis, & Immune-Mediated
    Necrotizing Myopathy

Anthony Marchie, MD
The Oregon Clinic
Medical Director, The Providence Center
  for Partkinson's Disease
Affiliate Professor of Neurology
Oregon Health and Sciences University
Portland, Oregon
Approach to the Patient with a Painful Prosthetic Hip or Knee

Simon C. Mears, MD, PhD
Chairman
Department of Orthopeadic Surgery
Johns Hopkins University/Johns Hopkins
  Bayview Medical Center
Baltimore, Maryland
Approach to the Patient with Hip Pain

Lester D. Miller, MD
Associate Clinical Professor of Medicine
Rheumatology Division
University of California San Francisco Medical Center
San Francisco, California
Rheumatoid Arthritis

John A. Mills, MD
Associate Professor Emeritus
Harvard Medical School
Courtesy Staff, Massachusetts General Hospital
Boston, Massachusetts
Physical Examination of the Musculoskeletal System

David R. Moller, MD
Professor of Medicine
Johns Hopkins University School of Medicine
Baltimore, Maryland
Sarcoidosis

Paul S. Mueller, MD, MPH
Professor of Medicine,
College of Medicine
Mayo Clinic
Rochester, Minnesota
Amyloidosis

Mary C. Nakamura, MD
Associate Professor in Residence
Department of Medicine
University of California, San Francisco
San Francisco VA Medical Center
San Francisco, California
Laboratory Diagnosis

Anne Louise Oaklander, MD, PhD
Associate Professor of Neurology
Harvard Medical School
Assistant in Pathology (Neuropathology)
Massachusetts General Hospital
Boston, Massachusetts
Complex Regional Pain Syndromes (Reflex Sympathetic Dystrophy) & Posttraumatic Neuralgia

James R. O'Dell, MD
Bruce Professor and Chief
Division of Rheumatology & Immunology
Vice-Chairman, Department of Internal Medicine
University of Nebraska Medical Center
Omaha, Nebraska
Rheumatoid Arthritis

Stephen A. Paget, MD
Hospital for Special Surgery
Weill Medical College of Cornell University
New York, New York
Perioperative Management of the Patient with Rheumatic Disease

Shanique R. Palmer, MD
Instructor in Medicine and Oncology
Fellow, Hematology/Medical Oncology
Mayo Clinic
Rochester, Minnesota
Amyloidosis

Dimitrios A. Pappas, MD
Assistant Professor of Medicine
Columbia University College of Physicians and Surgeons
New York, New York
Musculoskeletal Ultrasound

Marzouq Awni Qubti, MD
Department of Medicine
Division of Rheumatology
CVPH Medical Center
Plattsburg, New York
Ankylosing Spondylitis & the Arthritis of Inflammatory Bowel Disease

Manuel Ramos-Casals, MD, PhD
Consultant
Department of Systemic Autoimmune Diseases
Hospital Clinic
Barcelona, Spain
Primary Sjögren Syndrome

James T. Rosenbaum, MD
Professor of Ophthalmology
Medicine & Cell Biology
Edward E. Rosenbaum Professor of Inflammation Research
Chief
Division of Arthritis & Rheumatic Diseases
Director, Uveitis
The Oregon Clinic
Oregon Health and Sciences University
Portland, Oregon
Ocular Inflammatory Diseases for Rheumatologists

Richard Rosenbaum, MD
Medical Director
The Providence Center for Parkinson's Disease
Affiliate Professor of Neurology
Oregon Health and Sciences University
Portland, Oregon
Selected Topics in Neurology for the Rheumatologist

Peggy Schlesinger, MD
Clinical Professor of Medicine and Pediatrics
University of Washington School of Medicine
Seattle, Washington
*Approach to the Adolescent with Arthritis;
   Juvenile Idiopathic Arthritis*

Philip Seo, MD, MHS
Associate Professor of Medicine
Johns Hopkins University School of Medicine
Director, Johns Hopkins Vasculitis Center
Director,
Johns Hopkins Rheumatology Fellowship
Baltimore, Maryland
*Eosinophilic Granulomatosis with Polyangiitis (Churg-Strauss
   Syndrome); Miscellaneous Forms of Vasculitis*

Margaret Seton, MD
Assistant Professor of Medicine
Harvard Medical School
MGH Rheumatology, Allergy and Immunology
Massachusetts General Hospital
Boston, Massachusetts
Paget Disease of Bone

Dolores Shoback, MD
Professor of Medicine
University of California, San Francisco
Staff Physician
San Francisco Department of Veterans
   Affairs Medical Center
San Francisco, California
Osteoporosis & Glucocorticoid-Induced Osteoporosis

Stanford T. Shulman, MD
Virginia H. Rogers Professor of Pediatric Infectious
   Diseases
Northwestern University Feinberg School of Medicine
Chief, Division of Infectious Diseases
Lurie Children's Hospital
Chicago, Illinois
Rheumatic Fever

Bernadette C. Siaton, MD
Assistant Professor
Division of Rheumatology & Clinical Immunology
University of Maryland School of Medicine
Baltimore, Maryland
Pregnancy & Rheumatic Diseases

Antoni Sisó-Almirall, MD, PhD
Hospital Clinic of Barcelona
Barcelona, Spain
Primary Sjögren Syndrome

Umasuthan Srikumaran, MD
Assistant Professor of Orthopaedic Surgery
Johns Hopkins Shoulder & Sports Medicine
Johns Hopkins Community Physicians
Columbia, Maryland
Approach to the Patient with Shoulder Pain

John H. Stone, MD, MPH
Professor of Medicine
Harvard Medical School
Director, Clinical Rheumatology
Massachusetts General Hospital
Boston, Massachusetts
*Relapsing Polychondritis; Granulomatosis
   with Polyangiitis (Wegener Granulomatosis);
   Microscopic Polyangiitis; Eosinophilic Granulomatosis
   with Polyangiitis (Churg-Strauss Syndrome);
   Polyarteritis Nodosa; Mixed Cryoglobulinemia;
   Hypersensitivity Vasculitis; Henoch-Schönlein Purpura;
   Buerger Disease; Miscellaneous Forms of Vasculitis;
   Common Rheumatologic Problems Encountered
   by the Hospitalist: Pearls & Myths; Sensorineural
   Hearing Loss (Immune-mediated Inner Ear Disease);
   IgG4-Related Disease*

Sangeeta D. Sule, MD
Assistant Professor
Pediatric Rheumatology
Johns Hopkins University
Baltimore, Maryland
Raynaud Phenomenon

Alex Truong, MD
Assistant Professor of Medicine
Emory University Hospital
Atlanta, Georgia
Dermatomyositis, Polymyositis, & Immune-Mediated Necrotizing Myopathy

Jennifer K. Turner, MD
Assistant Professor Seattle Children's Hospital
University of Washington
Seattle, Washington
Approach to the Adolescent with Arthritis; Juvenile Idiopathic Arthritis

Dimitrios Vassilopoulos, MD
Associate Professor of Medicine and Rheumatology
Athens University School of Medicine
Athens, Greece
Rheumatic Manifestations of Acute & Chronic Viral Arthritis; Evaluation of Rheumatic Complaints in Patients with HIV

Fredrick M. Wigley, MD
Professor of Medicine
Associate Director, Division of Rheumatology
Johns Hopkins University School of Medicine
Baltimore, Maryland
Raynaud Phenomenon; Scleroderma

John H. Wilckens, MD
Associate Professor of Orthopedics
Johns Hopkins School of Medicine
Baltimore, Maryland
Approach to the Patient with Shoulder Pain

David Wofsy, MD
Professor of Medicine and Microbiology/Immunology
University of California
San Francisco, California
Treatment of Systemic Lupus Erythematosus

Robert L. Wortmann, MD
Professor Emeritus, Rheumatology Section
Geisel School of Medicine at Dartmouth
Lebanon, New Hampshire
Gout; Pseudogout: Calcium Pyrophosphate Dihydrate Crystal Deposition Disease

Preface

Progress in the rheumatic diseases since the year 2000—the dawn of biologic therapies for immune-mediated conditions—has been astonishing. As *Current Diagnosis and Treatment: Rheumatology* now enters its third edition, we are both invigorated and delighted by the necessity of updating and often changing radically nearly every chapter. In addition, we have been compelled to add new chapters that capture emerging currents in the field.

Among the new chapters in the third edition are those addressing IgG4-related disease, Whipple disease, and Paget disease. In acknowledgment of the growing attention to the lung in rheumatic diseases, we have added chapters on interstitial lung disease and pulmonary hypertension. As a nod to the increasing utility of imaging in the practice of rheumatology, we have added thorough chapters on both musculoskeletal magnetic resonance imaging (MRI) and ultrasound.

We have supplemented existing chapters with new sections when appropriate. To the chapter previously entitled Polymyositis & Dermatomyositis has been added "Immune-Mediated Necrotizing Myopathy," in recognition of new clinical entities in this area (particularly statin-induced myopathy). Similarly, "Scleroderma Mimickers" has been added to the chapter on scleroderma.

A hallmark of previous editions of *Current Diagnosis & Treatment: Rheumatology* has been the collaboration with authors from other specialties and subspecialties whose expertise is essential to practicing rheumatology well. In the past, we have engaged experts from otolaryngology, ophthalmology, orthopedics, and endocrinology to write critical chapters. These are reprised in the third edition, sometimes under different titles (and/or new authors), eg, Immune-Mediated Inner Ear Disease, Inflammatory Diseases of the Eye for Rheumatologists, Osteonecrosis, and Glucocorticoid-Induced Osteoporosis. In this edition, we continue this tradition with Neurology for the Rheumatologist. In further acknowledgment of the need to collaborate effectively with other specialties, we commissioned a chapter on Perioperative Management of the Patient with Rheumatic Disease.

This third edition is illustrated much more thoroughly than its predecessors with a substantial full-color insert as well as outstanding, integrated clinical and radiologic images. As an example, the extensive images shown and described in the chapter on Musculoskeletal MRI serve as an excellent complement to the clinical chapters on rheumatoid arthritis, psoriatic and reactive arthritis, ankylosing spondylitis, osteonecrosis, and gout. This edition has 60 color figures that demonstrate major teaching points.

We have made these changes while bearing in mind the principal target of this book: the practicing clinician. The book is a guide to the diagnosis and management of the complete range of rheumatologic problems encountered in clinical medicine, from common musculoskeletal complaints to complex, multiorgan system inflammatory diseases. Practical chapters on the evaluation of common musculoskeletal symptoms are accompanied by concise, authoritative reviews of multiorgan system disorders, supplemented by unique chapters on clinical topics of special interest.

We anticipate that the third edition of *Current Diagnosis & Treatment: Rheumatology* will have a broad readership among clinicians:

- Rheumatologists will find the book to be a quick, reliable, and up-to-date reference.
- The book will prove to be invaluable for those studying for board certification or recertification in rheumatology.
- Primary care physicians will appreciate the book's problem-oriented approach to musculoskeletal symptoms and its emphasis on the clinical features, laboratory findings, differential diagnosis, and treatment of specific rheumatic diseases.
- Fellows, house officers, and medical students will appreciate this engaging introduction to clinical rheumatology.

We hope that this book will engage and guide you in the study of the rheumatic diseases.

John B. Imboden, MD
David B. Hellmann, MD, MACP
John H. Stone, MD, MPH

Acknowledgments

Dr. Imboden wishes to acknowledge the ongoing support of the Rosalind Russell Medical Research Center for Arthritis.

Dr. Hellmann wishes to acknowledge the support of Mrs. Aliki Perroti and the Aliki Perroti Professorship in the Johns Hopkins Center for Innovative Medicine.

Dr. Stone wishes to acknowledge his support as Hugh and Renna Cosner Scholar in the Center for Innovative Medicine at the Johns Hopkins Bayview Medical Center.

Physical Examination of the Musculoskeletal System

1

John A. Mills, MD

A thorough knowledge of musculoskeletal anatomy is essential to the performance of an accurate and meaningful examination. As a quick reference, an atlas should be near at hand (or only a few computer strokes away). Manifestations that are elicited objectively, eg, swelling, warmth, effusions, or clearly limited range of motion, must be distinguished from more subjective findings such as tenderness and pain on motion.

The musculoskeletal system constitutes a demanding part of the physical examination in terms of both knowledge and time. The skillful examiner focuses this critical task through information obtained in a careful history.

OBTAINING A HISTORY

The clinician may begin the patient interview by asking the following two questions: (1) Are the patient's symptoms articular in nature? and (2) Do they derive from a musculotendinous location? If the answer to either of these questions is yes, then the examiner can begin to focus his or her efforts on the specific anatomic parts referred to by the patient in the history, bearing in mind two points:

- Referred pain and an incomplete understanding of the anatomy may affect the patient's localization of the complaint. For example, "hip pain" perceived over the lateral side while rolling over in bed at night is more likely to be trochanteric bursitis than pathology of the true hip joint.
- Musculoskeletal complaints are sometimes part of overarching, systemic disorders that affect the joints, muscles, bones, and tendons.

Pain present at rest usually indicates an acute inflammatory, neurologic, or neoplastic process. In addition to determining which musculoskeletal structures are the source of the patient's symptoms, the overall objectives of the examination, which are outlined in Table 1–1, should be kept in mind.

SPECIFIC EXAMINATION TECHNIQUES

▶ Observation

The examiner should take the opportunity to observe the patient's posture and mobility when he or she first enters the examination room. Alternatively, if the patient is already in the examining room or on the examination table when first encountered, the examiner should request at some point during the assessment that the patient stand, walk a few yards, and sit again. Gait analysis (for limp) can help separate primary from antalgic or extra-articular manifestations of musculoskeletal disease, such as weakness. This exercise also facilitates the identification of certain deformities. Genu varum or pes planus, for example, become more evident with weight bearing.

▶ Palpation

A bilateral comparison may be helpful in evaluating a swollen area. The anatomic extent of swelling should be verified by palpation, keeping in mind the anatomy of the part. The presence of free fluid is determined by ballottement alternatively at two positions over the swollen area. Joint effusions are most easily detected over their extensor surfaces, where they are not covered by a flexor retinaculum, nerves, and blood vessels. The bony margins of the normal joint can usually be felt on the extensor surface. The inability to feel the joint margins is evidence of synovial swelling or joint effusion. Comparing metacarpophalangeal (MCP) or metatarsophalangeal (MTP) joints in this way is a sensitive test for rheumatoid arthritis.

The presence of local warmth or erythema as signs of inflammation should be noted. The knee, ankle, and wrist joints should all be cooler than the skin over their adjoining long bones. This is gauged most effectively by placing the dorsum of the examiner's hand over the portion of the limb adjacent to the joint in question and then placing the dorsum

Table 1-1. Overall objectives of the physical examination.

A. Define the anatomic distribution of the problem. Is the process: • Monoarticular?   • Polyarticular? If so, it is symmetric or asymmetric?   • Does it involve only one extremity?   • Is it axial?   • Is it complex?
B. Ascertain whether or not there are local signs of an inflammatory process.
C. Determine if anatomic disruption is present; ie, joint instability, tendon rupture, bone fracture, or deformity.
D. Distinguish between true muscle weakness as opposed to fatigue or disuse atrophy.
E. Establish if constitutional symptoms, such as fever or weight loss, implicate a systemic process, or other symptoms are present that direct attention to other organs.

of the hand over the joint itself. A warmer temperature over these joints strongly suggests the presence of inflammation.

Pain on Motion

Almost all causes of joint pain, including rheumatoid arthritis, permit some relatively painless passive range of motion. Pain elicited by the slightest movement suggests a septic joint, gout, rheumatic fever, intra-articular hemorrhage, tumor, or joint fracture. Both passive and active range of motion should be tested. Pain caused by active but not passive motion often implicates an extra-articular source of the problem, such as a tenosynovitis.

Range of Motion

Measuring the range of motion in joints is useful for documenting the course of arthritis and the degree of disability. Several measurements systems are in use. A simple one is to use a positive sign before the measurement in degrees for flexion, abduction, internal rotation, or pronation, and a negative sign for the opposite motion, all measured from the "anatomic position." For example: Shoulder flexion −45 + 160, abduction −30 + 90. A prepared form or template saves time.

THE PHYSICAL EXAMINATION

Hands

Observe for full finger joint extension. The volar surfaces of the palms and fingers should make full contact when placed together. In making a fist, each fingertip should touch the MCP crease.

Synovial swelling of the proximal interphalangeal (PIP) and MCP joints can be detected readily by the presence of soft tissue swelling on either side of the dorsal aspects. The examiner supports the palm in individual fingers with both hands and palpates the joint margins using the thumbs. When synovial fluid swelling is present, the joint margins will be less distinct compared to the same joint on the opposite hand. Inflammation of the distal interphalangeal (DIP) joints has a limited differential diagnosis that includes osteoarthritis (typically characterized by Heberden nodes), gout (with tophi often occurring at sites of Heberden nodes), and psoriatic arthritis. Septic arthritis, trauma, sarcoidosis, and syphilis are also in the differential diagnosis. Classic rheumatoid arthritis rarely involves the PIP joint alone. Psoriatic arthritis of the PIP joints commonly stimulates the juxta-articular periosteum, giving them a fusiform, erythematous appearance called a sausage digit. Pain caused by lateral compression of the MCP joints as a group is a good screening test for small joint polyarthritis.

Secondary contracture of the intrinsic muscles of the hand in patient with rheumatoid arthritis leads to the swan-neck deformity characterized by fixed hyperextension of the PIP and flexion of the DIP joints. Ulnar deviation and inability to extend the MCP joints of the fingers are the result of the rheumatoid disruption of the soft tissue tethers that allowed the long extensor tendons to slip off the metacarpal heads. Inability to fully extend the PIP joints is a result of separation of the two slips of the long extensor tendon and their subluxation to either side of the joint. This leads to what is known as the boutonniere deformity. Extensive inflammation of finger joint capsules and ligaments in patients with systemic lupus erythematosus can result in joint laxity and diverse deformities in the absence of bone erosion.

Bony enlargements of the DIP joints (Heberden nodes) are a feature of hereditary osteoarthrosis and are often accompanied by similar changes in the PIP joints (Bouchard nodes). That process commonly affects the thumb carpometacarpal joint also, producing a squared appearance to the base of the joint and inability to extend it fully. The MCP joints are rarely, if ever, affected by osteoarthritis but a similar appearance of the second and third MCP joints may be seen in patients with hemochromatosis. Localized swelling of the tendon that restricts its motion within the sheath can be felt if the examiner palpates over the tendon at the distal palmar crease as the finger is flexed or extended.

Wrists

Arthritis of the wrists is usually caused by an inflammatory process. The exceptions are wrist pain related to carpal subluxation or fracture that can be reliably detected only by radiography. Synovitis of either the true radiocarpal or intercarpal joints is common among patients with rheumatic disorders. The absence of pain at the wrist on pronation or supination of the forearm suggests that the process is restricted to the carpus. When swelling is prominent on the dorsal or volar aspects of the joint, tenosynovitis of the extensor or flexor tendons respectively should be suspected and can be confirmed by observing the axial movement of the swelling when the fingers are moved. Swelling and tenderness over the ulnar styloid is common in rheumatoid arthritis and may be followed by dorsal subluxation of the ulnar head.

Pain and tenderness at the radial styloid is often caused by irritation of the extensor pollicis longus tendon where it crosses the radial head. This disorder, known as de Quervain tenosynovitis, is caused by repeated lifting with the palm oriented vertically. The diagnosis of de Quervain tenosynovitis can be confirmed by Finkelstein test.

▶ Elbow

The causes of inflammation of the elbow joint include rheumatoid arthritis, seronegative arthritides, septic arthritis, and gout. Swelling and effusions in the joints present at the radial head on the lateral aspect of the radiohumeral joint. Pronation and supination of the forearm is often painful and restricted. Synovial swelling in the olecranon fossa prevents full extension of the joint by limiting entry of the olecranon process. Acute inflammation of the olecranon bursa over the tip of the elbow is usually caused by gout or infection, but more chronic benign swelling can also be caused merely by direct trauma. The extensor surface of the ulna just below the olecranon is a common site for a rheumatoid nodule.

Epicondylitis is an enthesopathy of the common wrist flexor origin at the medial epicondyle (golfer's elbow) or that of the extensors at the lateral epicondyles (tennis elbow). Tenderness is present over or immediately below the epicondyle and pain is elicited by resisted wrist flexion or extension, respectively.

▶ Shoulder

The motion of the shoulder is the most complex of any joint. Consequently, it is often difficult to determine the exact cause of shoulder pain. With most activities, the glenohumeral joint moves in several planes simultaneously and scapulothoracic translocation can increase its apparent range misleadingly. The joint should be examined while scapular motion is observed or restricted by placing a hand over the shoulder on the trapezius ridge. The range of motion of the glenohumeral joint precludes ligamentous stabilization, which is replaced by dynamic control provided by the concerted action of the four rotator cuff muscles. Painful contractions of the shoulder tend to induce rotator cuff muscle dyssynergia, which is itself painful and can obscure the primary cause of the problem. Passive or active motions that minimize rotator cuff function include rotation of the humerus while the arm is hanging vertically oriented for flexion and extension in the sagittal plane. If those movements produce pain, true glenohumeral joint disease is present.

Shoulder joint pain is felt in the area of the deltoid muscle. Pain proximal to the olecranon is more often of cervical or thoracic apex origin. The capsule of the glenohumeral joint extends medially to the coracoid process. Tenderness at that site is the only place where it can be confidently assigned to the glenohumeral joint because the rest of the area is covered by the rotator cuff apparatus. Swelling of the glenohumeral joint is best appreciated at the anterior margin of the deltoid muscle just below the acromion, where an effusion, if present, can be balloted.

The shoulder drop sign is a good test for rotator cuff pathology. The shoulder should be passively flexed in the sagittal plane to 90 degrees, preferably with the elbow also flexed to reduce leverage. The humerus is supported while being rotated to the coronal plane and the forearm is extended and pronated. Support of the arm is then gently withdrawn while the patient is instructed to maintain the arm in this abducted position. The onset of pain and dropping of the arm is a positive sign. Tenderness over the lateral tip of the shoulder just below the acromion is often attributed to subacromial bursitis but is almost always attributable to supraspinatous tendon pathology. Inflammation of the long head of the biceps tendon at the groove where it crosses the humerus may cause widespread shoulder pain. In addition to tenderness immediately over the bicipital groove, the diagnosis can be confirmed by Yergason sign. The patient should sit with the elbow flexed and the forearm pronated, resting on the thigh. The examiner grasps the wrist and asks the patient to supinate the forearm against resistance, which will cause pain in the bicipital groove.

Restricted and painful active or passive motion of the shoulder in all directions is diagnostic of a frozen shoulder caused by generalized capsular inflammation and constriction. This is frequently idiopathic but may also result from traumatic injury. The patient may be able to move the arm only by scapulothoracic motion. Inflammation of the acromioclavicular or sternoclavicular joints can occur in rheumatoid arthritis or septic arthritis, the latter being especially common in injection drug users. Tenderness and swelling is easily appreciated at the site. Shrugging of the shoulder while lying on the affected side is painful.

▶ Hip

Gait analysis can help define the nature of hip disease. Dwell time on the affected hip is limited compared to its opposite. Forward lurching as the leg is extended with each step indicates either fixed hip flexion or pain caused by tensing a swollen or inflamed hip capsule. Movement of the upper trunk over the weight-bearing hip suggests either adductor (gluteus maximus) weakness or its inhibition. Joint loading, by increasing intra-articular pressure, aggravates many different causes of hip pain. A positive Trendelenburg sign will be detected. This sign is demonstrated by having the examiner place his or her hands on both iliac crests and asking the patient to raise one leg or the other. Weight bearing on the painful side cause the opposite iliac crest to drop.

Restricted hip motion can be masked by compensatory movement of the pelvis. Children with very mobile lumbar spines, for example, can nearly completely conceal a fused hip. In order to restrict pelvic motion during examination, the patient should hold the opposite hip fully flexed. Any pelvic motion will be revealed by movement of the flexed knee. Loss of motion caused by hip disease first restricts full extension followed by inversion, eversion, and then abduction. Inability to keep the extended leg on the table while fully flexing the opposite indicates some loss of full extension as a result of either hip disease or a periarticular problem, such as iliopsoas tendinitis. Passive log rolling of the extended leg while the patient is supine can detect early guarding and restricted motion. Performing the FABER maneuver (flexion, abduction, and external rotation) is a test for painful—as well as limited—motion. Because the hip joint is supplied by the femoral nerve, pain emanating from the true hip joint is perceived in the groin, anteromedial thigh, and often in the knee. In some cases, hip pain is felt only in the knee. Pain in the buttock is more often caused by a sciatic nerve problem.

Groin or anterior thigh pain when the hip is actively flexed against resistance or passively extended may be caused by iliopsoas tendinitis or bursitis. Local tenderness is usually present. Iliopsoas lesions must be distinguished from femoral hernias and enthesopathy of the thigh adductors. In the latter case, the tenderness is located at the pubic tubercle more medially. Pain located in the buttock, on passive internal rotation and adduction of the hip (as an initiating a golf swing) is symptomatic of piriformis tendinitis or bursitis. When felt deep inside the pelvis it may be a symptom of obturator bursitis, which can be confirmed by palpating the margin of the lesser sciatic foramen per rectum.

Apparent and true leg length discrepancy may reflect either fixed hip abduction, abduction, or lumbar spine scoliosis. It can be distinguished from true leg shortening by measuring each side from the anterior/superior iliac spine to the medial tibial plateau or medial malleolus. True leg length shortening occurs in superior subluxation of the hip or severe destructive disease of the joint.

Pain over the greater trochanter points to trochanteric bursitis or, equally commonly, gluteus enthesopathy (usually of the gluteus medius) or a tear of the gluteus muscle. Because the gluteus tendons insert into the trochanter, it can be difficult to differentiate these problems by palpation. Pain felt while rolling over in bed is most likely due to bursitis. In contrast, trochanteric pain aggravated by prolonged standing or stair climbing typically indicates gluteus medius tendinitis.

▶ Knee

The knee is the most commonly painful joint because it is subject to almost all causes of articular pathology. The alignment of the knee should be observed while the patient is standing. Varus or valgus malalignment may be congenital or acquired. Erosion of articular cartilage from either the medial or lateral tibiofemoral compartment is a common cause. Valgus alignment results in abnormal compression of the lateral opposing surfaces of the patellofemoral articulation. In individuals who are symptomatic, manual displacement of the patella on an extended knee produces discomfort. This is known as the **apprehension sign**. The lateral angle at the extended knee, the acute angle, is measured along the axis of the femur and through the midpoint of the patella to the tibial tubercle. The valgus angles in young women of less than 20 degrees can be ignored and corrects as the skeleton matures. Activities that involve excessive weight bearing on partially flexed knees cause chondromalacia of the undersurface of the patella. This condition is associated with a feeling of crepitus when the hand is placed over the patella as the knees are extended against gravity. When severe, it can be a cause of the pain. Crepitus can also indicate the presence of loose bodies within the joint.

Most knee disorders are accompanied by a synovial effusion that is best detected by eliciting the bulge sign. The knee must be as fully extended as possible. The effusion is demonstrated by first directing the fluid entered into the suprapatellar synovial recess by stroking upward over the medial patellofemoral articulation. Fingers are then immediately drawn downward from above the lateral patellofemoral groove while carefully observing the hollow between the patella and a medial condyle for a bulge. Chronic and relatively painless effusions may also protrude posteriorly into the popliteal space to produce a Baker cyst. Although such cysts can be sizable and track down beneath the gastrocnemius muscle, they are more often felt as a firm lump in the popliteal space. The knee must be fully extended since even slight flexion increases the capacity of the joint and a small effusion will diminish. Chronic synovial swelling, as in patients with rheumatoid arthritis, will produce a collar-like thickening immediately above the patella where the suprapatellar recess creates a double layer of the joint lining. It is frequently tender to palpation.

Because the tibial plateau is almost flat, translocation of the femoral condyles (rolling across the examination table) during flexion and extension is prevented by the menisci, which form a shallow cup, and the cruciate ligaments. A tendency within knee to give way while bearing weight or to lock suggests the presence of damage to the structures or a loose soft tissue fragment in the joint. Displaced menisci may be palpated along the margin of the tibial plateau but can be more reliably detected by the McMurray test. The McMurray test is performed by flexing the knee as far as possible, grasping the foot holding the thigh with the other hand and either internally or externally rotating the tibia while exerting either a varus or valgus strain. During knee extension, a torn meniscal fragment may become caught in the joint, producing pain and arrested motion.

Classically, the torn meniscus is opposite to the direction of tibial rotation, although that is not invariable. An injured infrapatellar synovial fold (plica), which is attached to the intracondylar notch, can result in symptoms that are similar to those of a torn meniscus, especially in young athletes.

Traumatic elongation or rupture of the cruciate ligaments allows abnormal anteroposterior translocation of the femoral condyles onto the tibial plateau. The anterior cruciate ligament limits posterior condylar translocation (ie, it prevents the tibia from sliding anteriorly) and the posterior cruciate ligament limits anterior displacement of the femur. The drawer test demonstrates increased anteroposterior instability of the joint by attempting to move the proximal tibia back and forth over the femoral condyles. Because the anterior cruciate ligament is normally relaxed by flexion of the knee, any abnormal laxity of that structure should be tested within knee and no more than 20–30 degrees of flexion. When the posterior cruciate ligament has been damaged, hamstring spasm may draw the tibia posteriorly. This must be minimized by flexing the knee to 90 degrees when testing for the integrity of the posterior cruciate ligament.

Pain caused by medial or collateral ligament injury or insufficiency is listed by supporting the knee in a fully extended position and abruptly applying a valgus or varus strain to the tibia. Some slight laxity is usually observed, especially in young or loose-jointed individuals. Comparison of the two sides is necessary.

There are several bursae around the knee. Inflammation in these bursae can cause pain upon weight bearing. The prepatellar bursa can be injured by prolonged kneeling. Another bursa under the patellar tendon is subject to both direct pressure and excessive quadriceps tension. The anserine bursa, which is located below the medial tibial plateau between the tibia and the biceps femoris tendon, becomes painful and swollen in individuals who are overweight and have valgus knee alignment.

Ankle

Careful examination is required to distinguish between true talotibial and subtalar joint pathology as well as injury to the complex ligamentous support of those joints. In addition, the tendons to the foot may be injured where they turn sharply behind the malleolae. Examination by sequential active, passive, and resisted isometric maneuvers can usually distinguish between those possible sources of pain. Synovial swelling and effusions of the talotibial joint are appreciated best over the anterior joint line, on either side of the tibialis anterior tendon and over the synovial fold below the flexor retinaculum over the neck of the talus. Swelling in relation to the malleolae is usually present also but is difficult to distinguish from that caused by injury to a ligament or tendon in the area.

Pain and limitation of motion related to the subtalar joint is detected by grasping the heel and applying a varus or valgus strain while holding the tibia. A normal range of motion is variable. The ankle and foot should also be examined while the patient is standing in order to detect eversion of the hindfoot, manifested as valgus deviation of the calcaneus and Achilles tendon. This may reflect either deltoid ligament insufficiency or weakness of the tibialis posterior muscle. Pes planus is also best seen on standing.

Inflammation of the joints or tendon sheaths in the compartment below the medial malleolus can compress the posterior tibial nerve and cause chronic pain in the foot and ankle.

Foot

Pain around the heel has several possible causes. It is a common manifestation of reactive arthritis. Tenderness near the insertion of the Achilles tendon reflects either enthesopathy or inflammation of the bursa that lies immediately above the upper corner of the calcaneus and the tendon insertion. Plantar surface heel pain and tenderness is usually caused by so-called plantar fasciitis, which includes enthesopathy of the plantar ligament or the origin of the flexor digitorum brevis at its attachment to the calcaneus just anterior to the heel pad. The heel pad itself may become painful by prolonged standing on hard surface without adequate heel cushioning. Pain elicited by lateral compression of the heel distinguishes talalgia from plantar enthesopathy.

Inflammation of the intertarsal and tarsometatarsal joints is often difficult to localize. There is variable intraconnectivity of the synovial cavities in the midfoot, and this region may become diffusely swollen. In patients with rheumatoid arthritis or its seronegative variants, the MTP and PIP joints are affected as much as the hands, and they should be examined in the same way. Chronic inflammation that results from damage to the transverse metatarsal ligaments leads to cockup deformities of the toes and prolapse of the metatarsal heads. The metatarsal arch is flattened and the metatarsal heads can be felt as tender, pebble-like structures on the plantar service at the base of the toes. Transverse compression of the metatarsals is a good sign for arthritis of any of the MTP joints. This maneuver can also identify pain from a Morton neuroma in one of the intraosseous nerves.

Stiffness of the first MTP joint (hallux rigidus) or valgus toe deviation that may be associated with varus positioning of the metacarpal can cause chronic foot pain.

Spine

For the detection of scoliotic or kyphotic deformities, the patient should be observed standing, preferably barefoot. The range of normal lumbar lordosis is considerable but a curve of more than 30 degrees or none at all is usually abnormal. Have the patient bend forward as far as possible. A rotational deformity will be revealed by twisting of the thorax. The Schober index, a measure of a loss of flexibility of the lumbar spine, is useful in the longitudinal evaluation of patients with ankylosing spondylitis. The Schober index is measured by marking the lumbosacral junction (the first "valley" detected while probing up toward the midline over the sacrum), measuring up a distance of 10–15 cm, and making a second mark. The patient is then asked to flex forward as far as possible. The line should separate by a distance about 50% greater than that originally measured. The index is more useful for following disease progression than for initial diagnosis. Measuring the distance between the fingertips and the floor when fully flexed is also useful; however, it can be limited by reduced hip flexion.

Observe neck rotation, flexion, and extension. Patients with normal neck flexion and extension can touch the tip of the jaw to the sternum and to extend the neck to form a straight line from the surface of the sternum to the horizontal ramus of the mandible. The ability to bend the neck in the coronal plane (ie, tilt the head) is variable but is often the most painful motion with intravertebral disk disease or the presence of nerve root compression. Measuring the distance between the occiput and the wall while the patient is standing with his heels against it is a good way to document flexion deformity of the upper trunk and neck.

Lateral bending of the thoracolumbar spine is assessed with the patient standing. The spine should form a smooth curve from the lower lumbar to midthoracic levels. A straight segment indicates either an abnormality of that level or paraspinous muscle spasm. This can be an early manifestation of ankylosing spondylitis.

The spondyloarthropathies often affect the costovertebral joints, thus limiting chest expansion. Measuring chest expansion helps identify and follow those disorders. Inflammation of the sacroiliac joints is a common early manifestation of the spondyloarthropathies. It is often asymmetric in psoriatic or reactive arthritis. Local tenderness may be detected over the joints at the "dimples of Venus." A sensitive test for sacroiliac inflammation is the McCunnell maneuver. This is performed by having the patient lie on the side of the less painful joint and grasp and hold the dependent leg fully flexed while the examiner supports and extends the other leg with one hand. The examiner restricts pelvic motion during leg extension by placing the other hand on the iliac crest. The McCunnell maneuver, which causes a twisting strain through the joints, should be performed gently because it can be quite painful in the presence of sacroiliitis.

Joint Aspiration & Injection

2

Kenneth H. Fye, MD*
John B. Imboden, MD

ESSENTIAL FEATURES

▶ The major components of synovial fluid analysis are assessing fluid clarity and color, determining the cell count, examining for crystals, and obtaining culture.

▶ Joint aspiration should be performed promptly whenever septic arthritis is suspected because synovial fluid cell count, Gram stain, and culture are necessary to establish or exclude joint space infection.

▶ Synovial fluid analysis can be diagnostic in cases of crystalline arthritis.

▶ The synovial fluid white cell count is the most reliable means of distinguishing noninflammatory (<2000 cells/mcL) from inflammatory (>2000 cells/mcL) forms of arthritis.

▶ Joint injections with glucocorticoid are often the swiftest means of providing relief to patients with inflamed joints.

▶ Indications for Joint Aspiration

Joint aspiration with subsequent synovial fluid analysis, Gram stain, and culture should be performed promptly whenever there is clinical suspicion of septic arthritis (eg, unexplained, acute monoarticular arthritis). The presence of crystals in synovial fluid can be diagnostic of gout as well as pseudogout and calcium pyrophosphate dehydrate deposition disease (CPPD). The synovial fluid white cell count is the most reliable means of distinguishing noninflammatory from inflammatory forms of arthritis. As a general guide, synovial fluid should be examined when the underlying cause of arthritis is uncertain and arthrocentesis is feasible.

---

*Deceased.

▶ Synovial Fluid Analysis

The major components of synovial fluid analysis are (1) assessing fluid clarity and color, (2) determining the cell count, (3) examining for crystals, and (4) obtaining cultures. When septic arthritis is suspected, a Gram stain should also be performed. Determinations of synovial fluid glucose and protein have little diagnostic value and should not be ordered. Although the viscosity of synovial fluid decreases with inflammation, evaluations of viscosity are not standardized and add little to the diagnostic value of synovial fluid analysis.

A. Clarity and Color

Examination of the synovial fluid begins with a visual determination of clarity and color. Although crystals, lipids, and even cellular debris may affect clarity, the major determinant of synovial fluid clarity and color is the cell count. Noninflammatory fluid, such as that associated with osteoarthritis, has a low cell count and is clear. Synovial fluid from moderately inflammatory forms of arthritis, such as systemic lupus erythematosus or mild rheumatoid arthritis, has higher cell counts and is translucent and yellow. Fluid from intensely inflammatory processes, such as septic joints or crystal-induced arthropathies, has very high cell counts and is opaque and white to yellow. Bleeding into a joint leads to a hemarthrosis with characteristic opaque, red synovial fluid.

B. Cell Count

Normal synovial fluid has <200 white cells/mcL, most of which are mononuclear. In pathologic effusions, the synovial fluid white cell count discriminates between noninflammatory forms of arthritis (<2000 white cells/mcL) and inflammatory arthritis (>2000 white cells/mcL with a neutrophil predominance). The synovial fluid white cell count can be an approximate guide to the cause of the underlying inflammatory arthritis (see below, "Classes of Synovial Fluid").

C. Crystals

Crystal analysis is best performed on a fresh wet preparation with a clean slide and cover slip. Synovial fluid analysis for crystals is performed under polarized light. The strength of birefringence and shape of the crystals are helpful in distinguishing among the different forms of microcrystalline disease.

- Monosodium urate crystals are needle-shaped and negatively birefringent (ie, the crystal is yellow when the long axis of the crystal is parallel to the slow axis of vibration of the red compensator used with polarized lenses to identify crystals under the microscope). Because of their strong birefringence, monosodium urate crystals are easily seen with a polarized light microscope. The sensitivity of an examination for urate crystals in acute gout is >90%.
- Calcium pyrophosphate dihydrate crystals are rhomboid-shaped and positively birefringent (ie, the crystal is blue when the long axis of the crystal is parallel to the slow axis of vibration of the red compensator used with polarized lenses to identify crystals under the microscope). Because they are weakly birefringent, calcium pyrophosphate dihydrate crystals are dim and difficult to detect even with a polarized light microscope.
- Calcium oxalate crystals can be seen in patients with primary oxalosis or in renal failure. These crystals are rod- or tetrahedron-shaped and positively birefringent.
- Cholesterol crystals are rectangular and tend to have notched corners. Lipids form spherules with birefringence in the shape of a Maltese cross. Because the arms of the cross that parallel the slow axis of vibration of the red compensator are blue, these spherules are positively birefringent.
- Hydroxyapatite crystals are not birefringent and form amorphous clumps that stain red with alizarin red S.
- Glucocorticoids from previous joint injections, talc from gloves, and even debris can form birefringent crystals and lead to mistaken diagnoses of microcrystalline disease.

The presence of intracellular crystals in synovial fluid inflammatory cells is diagnostic of a crystal-induced arthropathy. However, this diagnosis does not rule out infection, so it is always wise to culture the fluid from an acute monoarticular arthritis even when crystals are identified. In addition, a patient may have more than one crystal-induced arthropathy. Fifteen percent of patients with gout also have CPPD.

When aspirating a small joint, such as the first metatarsophalangeal joint, it is important to remember that monosodium urate crystals can be identified in interstitial fluid. Even when synovial fluid cannot be drawn into the syringe, enough interstitial fluid for crystal analysis can be pulled into the needle by maintaining negative pressure as the needle is withdrawn. The needle is then removed, the syringe is filled with air, the needle is replaced, and the air is used to express the contents of the needle onto a slide. The small amount of material obtained is often enough to allow detection of monosodium urate crystals.

D. Culture and Gram Stain

Gram stain and culture should be performed on synovial fluid from any patient in whom infection is suspected. The sensitivity of synovial fluid cultures for nongonococcal septic arthritis is approximately 90%. Gram stain of synovial fluid has lower sensitivity (in the range of 50–75%) but high specificity. Microbiologic analysis usually is performed on fluid collected in a sterile tube. However, if the aspiration is difficult, material in the needle may be expressed onto a swab and sent for culture and sensitivity studies. Some significant pathogens are difficult to culture. Synovial fluid cultures are usually negative in the early phases of gonococcal arthritis; in cases of mycobacterial infection, cultures may require several weeks of incubation to isolate the causative agent.

E. Classes of Synovial Fluid

Four classes of synovial fluid have been defined and can serve as a guide to differential diagnosis.

Class I (noninflammatory) synovial fluid is defined by a synovial fluid white cell count of **<2000/mcL.** Class I fluid is transparent with a color ranging from clear to yellow. Osteoarthritis is the most common cause of class I synovial fluid. Other causes include post-trauma, chondromalacia patella, osteonecrosis, hypothyroidism (often with especially viscous fluid), Charcot arthropathy, amyloidosis, and sarcoidosis (which also can cause inflammatory synovial fluid).

Class II (inflammatory) synovial fluid has white cell counts from **2000/mcL to 75,000/mcL**, occasionally up to 100,000/mcL. Polymorphonuclear leukocytes predominate. The appearance of class II synovial fluid ranges from translucent to opaque and is yellow or white; it is characteristic of noninfected, inflammatory forms of arthritis. In systemic lupus erythematosus, white cell counts are usually between 2000 cells/mcL and 30,000 cells/mcL. The cell counts in rheumatoid arthritis and the spondyloarthropathies are typically 5000–50,000 cells/mcL; however, the pseudoseptic presentations of these disorders can generate higher counts (but rarely ≥100,000 cells/mcL). In crystal-induced arthropathies, cell counts of 30,000–50,000 cells/mcL are typical, but ≥100,000 cells/mcL are sometimes observed. Other causes of class II fluid include systemic rheumatic diseases, such as dermatomyositis and mixed connective tissue disease; Still disease; relapsing polychondritis; postinfectious arthritis; and the systemic vasculitides.

Class III (septic) synovial fluid has white cell counts that are often **>100,000/mcL**, and the appearance is opaque and yellow (sometimes white). Class III synovial fluid is typical of septic arthritis caused by infection with *Staphylococcus aureus*, streptococci, and gram-negative organisms.

Although these infections classically cause very inflammatory fluid (≥100,000 cells/mcL), synovial fluid cell counts can be considerably lower early in the course of the infection, in partially treated infection, or in cases of overwhelming sepsis. Counts <50,000 cells/mcL are common in gonococcal arthritis and in chronic infections, such as those caused by mycobacteria or fungi.

Class IV (hemorrhagic) fluid is red and opaque. In contrast to bloody returns due to a traumatic aspiration, class IV fluid is "defibrinated" and does not clot ex vivo. Class IV synovial fluid is typical of trauma, tuberculosis, pigmented villonodular synovitis, neoplasia, coagulopathies, and Charcot arthropathy.

▶ Therapeutic Aspiration or Injection

A. Aspiration

The removal of synovial fluid from an acutely inflamed joint may provide significant benefit. This is particularly true in infected joints, from which removal of synovial fluid will decrease intra-articular synovial pressure, the number of activated inflammatory cells, and the concentration of destructive enzymes and cytokines that can damage articular and periarticular structures. Although septic joints can be aspirated daily to prevent reaccumulation of inflammatory synovial fluid, current practice has moved to arthroscopic lavage, debridement, and drain insertion rather than repeated arthrocenteses. Removing blood from a hemarthrosis may also be beneficial. A significant collection of blood may increase intra-articular pressure, thereby stretching periarticular supporting structures and resulting in subsequent joint laxity. Intra-articular blood can also lead to the development of adhesions, eventually resulting in decreased range of motion.

B. Injection

A number of locally injected pharmacologic agents have been used in the treatment of rheumatic disorders. Local glucocorticoids in conjunction with lidocaine are valuable in the treatment of the arthritic conditions. Joints, tenosynovium, bursae, soft tissue tender points (such as the medial and lateral epicondyles in tennis or golfer elbow or the lateral thigh in meralgia paresthetica), and even the epidural space can be injected with a reasonable expectation of benefit. Although most target tissues can be injected without radiographic help, it is always wise to inject the hip or the epidural space under computed tomographic guidance to ensure that the medication is delivered to the proper tissue space.

The response to joint injection can have diagnostic implications. For example, in a patient with prominent knee pain and osteoarthritis of both the hip and knee, relief of pain following injection of lidocaine into the hip points to hip arthritis with referred pain as the primary source of symptoms.

▶ Technique

A. Equipment

The specific procedure and size of the joint determine the size of the syringe needed for aspiration. Syringes 3 mL and smaller are usually adequate for injecting lidocaine and glucocorticoids into a peripheral target. Three- to 10-mL syringes are preferred for aspiration of small joints, and 10- to 20-mL syringes are best for intermediate joints, such as the elbow or ankle. For larger joints, such as the knee or glenohumeral joint, or when copious amounts of synovial fluid must be aspirated, a 60-mL syringe may be more appropriate. When using a large syringe, it is important to break the vacuum in the syringe before introducing it into the joint. Aspiration should be performed slowly to avoid generating significant negative pressure that can draw synovial tissue into the opening of the needle and actually prevent adequate withdrawal of fluid. To aspirate ≥100 mL from an arthritic joint, several large syringes or a stopcock on the end of a syringe may be used. If using several syringes, a Kelly clamp can stabilize the needle (which can be left in place) while the syringes are changed.

The size of the needle also depends on the procedure. Needles as small as 25 or 30 gauge are most appropriate for injecting lidocaine into articular or periarticular structures before aspiration or for injecting glucocorticoids into small joints. A 25-gauge needle also can be used to aspirate synovial fluid or periarticular interstitial fluid from small, acutely inflamed joints, such as the first metatarsophalangeal joint in acute gout. A 1.5-inch, 22-gauge needle is useful for injecting large joints, such as the knee, or deep structures, such as the trochanteric bursa. These 22-gauge needles also can be used to aspirate small joints, but 19- or 20-gauge needles are indicated for the aspiration of large joints, joints with large amounts of synovial fluid, or joints or cysts with inspissated synovial fluid.

Joint infection after aspiration or injection is extremely rare, but the possibility of complications must always be minimized. Povidone-iodine should be applied to the arthrocentesis site and allowed to dry. An alcohol swab then should be used to wipe off the excess to prevent skin irritation in those patients sensitive to iodine or iodine derivatives. Sterile gloves are indicated, particularly if the anatomy is equivocal and the clinician must reexamine the procedure site after preparing the area with povidone-iodine. Very experienced clinicians can use a "no touch" technique: the clinician simply marks the injection target with a ballpoint pen, applies appropriate antisepsis, and then proceeds using nonsterile gloves. Gloves are important in protecting the clinician from the patient's body fluids.

B. Medications

Some clinicians use ethyl chloride to numb the skin before the procedure. However, this technique is somewhat cumbersome and of equivocal benefit.

Lidocaine (1–2%, without epinephrine) is a safe and effective local anesthetic that can be injected into the capsule and periarticular supporting structures before aspiration is attempted. Aspiration without benefit of anesthesia can be quite painful. To provide anesthesia as glucocorticoids are being injected into the target tissue, lidocaine should be drawn up with the glucocorticoids to be given. Single-dose vials of lidocaine, although more costly, are less likely to be contaminated.

Local injections are an efficient way to administer high concentrations of glucocorticoids directly into target tissues, maximizing the desired anti-inflammatory effects of the medication and minimizing the many unpleasant side effects associated with systemic glucocorticoids. Glucocorticoids can be injected with reasonable expectation of clinical benefit into joints, synovial cysts, peritendinous structures, bursal sacs, ligamentous attachments, tender points, and periarticular tissues. Patients should be aware that injection of local glucocorticoids, although frequently helpful, is not always curative. The long-term efficacy of the procedure depends in large part on the nature of the underlying problem.

Several preparations of glucocorticoids are available. Dexamethasone can be obtained in a crystalloid solution, dissolved in lidocaine. It is short acting and less likely to lead to atrophy, even when injected into soft tissues. Both dexamethasone and triamcinolone diacetate are available as colloidal suspensions. These suspensions remain in target tissues longer and may be more effective in the treatment of chronic inflammatory processes. However, they are more likely to lead to atrophy or cutaneous pigment changes when injected into superficial structures, such as the lateral epicondyle in the treatment of lateral epicondylitis. Some very stable (and therefore extremely long-acting) agents, such as triamcinolone hexacetonide, should be used only for the injection of large joints or deep structures because of the possibility of atrophy of superficial tissues. Repeat glucocorticoid injections should be administered judiciously. Too many injections sometimes lead to laxity of the periarticular

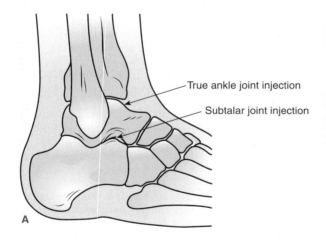

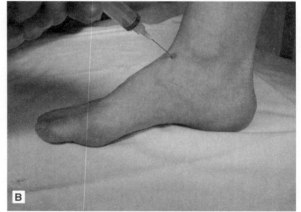

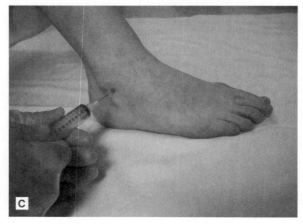

▲ **Figure 2–1. A:** Lateral view of the ankle. **B:** Injection of the true ankle joint, just medial to the extensor hallucis longus. **C:** Injection of the subtalar joint, just inferior and anterior to the tip of the lateral malleolus.

supporting structures, soft tissue atrophy, or bone dissolution. No solid data provide guidance on which to base definitive recommendations. However, a single joint or soft tissue target probably should not be injected more than three times a year.

Several preparations of injectable hyaluronic acid are available. Evidence suggests that a series of three injections of hyaluronic acid into an affected joint (particularly the knee) in a patient with degenerative arthritis can give short-term relief of pain equal to the response observed in patients receiving glucocorticoid injections into the joint. However, 6 months after injection, no significant difference in pain or function was noted among groups of patients receiving hyaluronic acid, glucocorticoids, or placebo. Although no difference has been reported in the long-term clinical benefits of

hyaluronic acid and glucocorticoid injections, the cost difference is significant. The prohibitive expense of a series of hyaluronic acid injections makes glucocorticoid injection the preferred therapy.

C. Approach

The optimal approaches to the ankle, shoulder, wrist, knee, elbow, and metacarpophalangeal joints are shown in Figures 2–1 through 2–6. The optimal approach to the trochanteric bursa is shown in Figure 2–7.

Aspiration of a joint should be performed with the joint positioned to maximize intra-articular pressure, allowing easier withdrawal of synovial fluid. Intra-articular pressure is usually highest at maximum extension or flexion. For

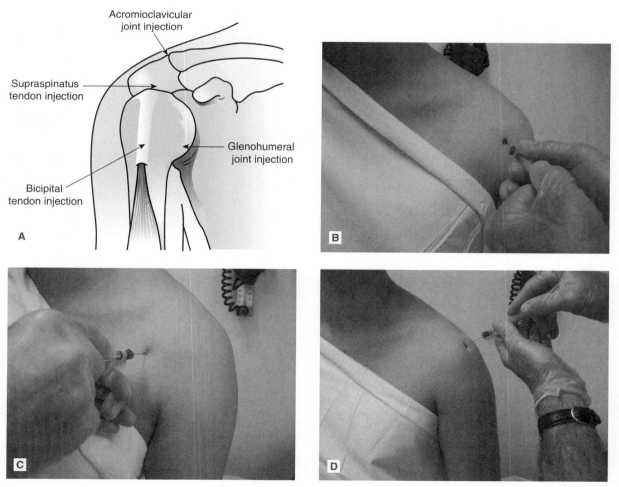

▲ **Figure 2–2. A:** Anterior view of the shoulder. **B:** Technique for infiltration of the bicipital groove of the humerus with a glucocorticoid preparation (treatment for biceps tendinitis). **C:** Injection of the glenohumeral joint from the anterior position. **D:** Injection of the shoulder just inferior to the acromion (the preferred approach to shoulder injection).

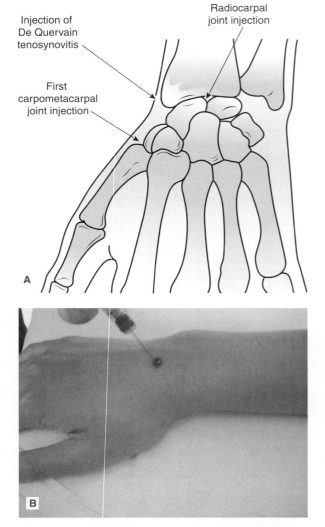

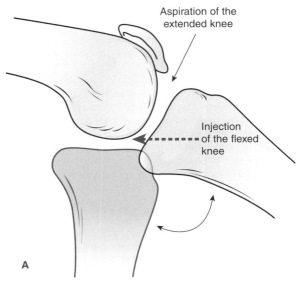

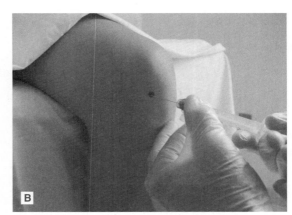

▲ **Figure 2–3.** **A:** Dorsum of the left wrist. **B:** Injection of the radiocarpal joint.

example, in the knee, the intra-articular pressure is highest when the knee is in full extension (see Figure 2–4). Conversely, joint injection (without aspiration) is performed most easily with the joint semiflexed to minimize intra-articular pressure (see Figure 2–4). The simplest approach for a knee injection is to seat the patient on an examining table, with the leg dangling down and the knee flexed at a 90-degree angle. This flexed position minimizes intra-articular pressure. Gravity pulls the lower leg down, thus opening the joint and facilitating introduction of the needle. The best position for aspiration alone or with injection depends on the anatomy of the specific target joint.

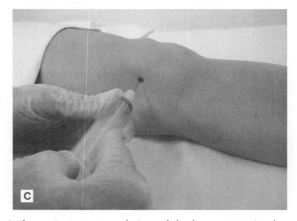

▲ **Figure 2–4.** **A:** Lateral view of the knee. **B:** Optimal positioning of the knee for joint injection. **C:** Optimal positioning of the knee for joint aspiration.

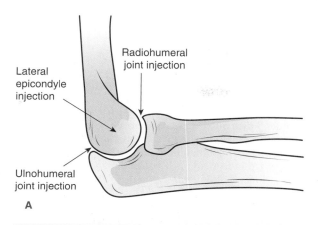

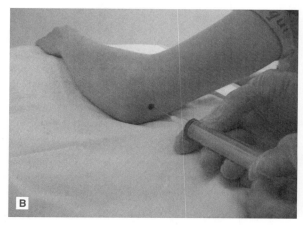

Lateral epicondyle injection

Radiohumeral joint injection

Ulnohumeral joint injection

A

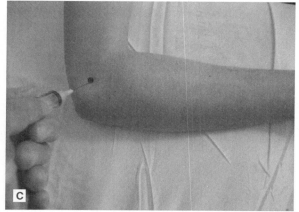

C

▲ **Figure 2–5.** **A:** Lateral view of the elbow flexed to 90 degrees. **B:** Injection of the ulnohumeral joint, into the olecranon fossa. **C:** Injection of the lateral epicondyle, just proximal to the radial head.

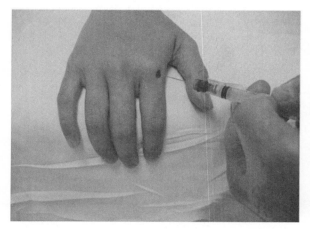

▲ **Figure 2–6.** Injection of the metacarpophalangeal joint.

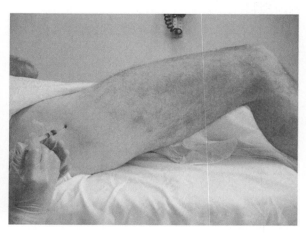

▲ **Figure 2–7.** Injection of the trochanteric bursa.

The best approach for aspiration or injection of soft tissues also depends on the anatomy of the target. Aspiration or injection of the olecranon or prepatellar bursae is performed most effectively with the elbow or knee in full flexion, thereby maximizing intrabursal pressure. Positioning is less important when injecting ligaments or tendinous attachments, such as the lateral epicondyle in tennis elbow (see Figure 2–5), because the target is a tissue plane or area of swelling, nodularity, tenderness, or pain, rather than a distinct structure. When treating tendinitis, the target tissue is the tendon sheath, not the tendon itself.

Care must be taken *not* to inject against resistance, because an unusual degree of resistance may indicate that the tip of the needle is in the tendon. Injection directly into an inflamed tendon may increase the likelihood of tendon rupture.

D. Difficulty in Obtaining Adequate Samples

On occasion, initial efforts at aspiration may fail to produce an adequate sample of synovial fluid. This may occur because the needle is not in the joint space, and simple repositioning of the needle may result in a successful aspiration. If the needle is properly positioned but the synovial fluid is too viscous to be withdrawn easily, a larger gauge needle must be used.

Sometimes chronic inflammatory arthritis results in the formation of loculations that make adequate joint drainage difficult. In such cases, arthroscopic surgery should be considered.

In some attempts at aspiration, synovial fluid flows easily at first and then stops. This may be the result of too much negative pressure and can be resolved either by slowing the rate of fluid withdrawal or using a smaller syringe.

Synovial fluid debris can easily clog the needle. The needle can be cleared by reinjecting a small amount of synovial fluid from the syringe; aspiration is then resumed.

When enough synovial fluid has been removed to significantly lower intra-articular pressure, aspiration becomes increasingly difficult. In aspiration from the knee, an assistant can apply external pressure to the joint, thereby increasing intra-articular pressure and facilitating the aspiration.

E. Contraindications to Joint Injection and Aspiration

Cellulitis overlying the joint is a contraindication to arthrocentesis. The aspirating/injecting needle should never be passed through infected tissue because of the risk of introducing infection into the joint space. Similarly, the aspirating/injecting needle should never be passed through psoriatic plaques, which often are heavily contaminated with bacteria and are difficult to sterilize. Therapeutic anticoagulation with warfarin is not a contraindication, provided the international normalized ratio (INR) is less than 3.0 and a small (eg, 22 gauge) bore needle is used.

▶ Synovial Biopsy

Sometimes an arthritic condition cannot be diagnosed by synovial fluid analysis. Diagnoses of indolent infections or noninfectious forms of granulomatous arthritis (such as sarcoidosis) usually require synovial biopsy. Although synovial fluid cytologic studies can sometimes reveal the presence of malignant cells, neoplastic arthritic conditions are usually diagnosed by histologic analysis of synovial biopsy material. Finally, several infiltrative, metabolic, or presumably infectious disorders (such as amyloidosis, ochronosis, hemochromatosis, Wilson disease, and Whipple disease) that can affect the joints are difficult to detect by synovial fluid analysis but are easily recognized by synovial biopsy.

American College of Rheumatology Ad Hoc Committee on Clinical Guidelines. Guidelines for the initial evaluation of the adult patient with acute musculoskeletal symptoms. *Arthritis Rheum.* 1996;39:1. [PMID: 8546717]

Margaretten ME, Kohlwes J, Moore D, Bent S. Does this adult patient have septic arthritis? *JAMA.* 2007;297:1478. [PMID: 17405973]

Shmerling RH. Synovial fluid analysis: a critical reappraisal. *Rheum Dis Clin North Am.* 1994;20:503. [PMID: 8016423]

Laboratory Diagnosis

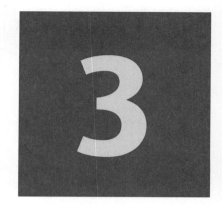

Mary C. Nakamura, MD
John B. Imboden, MD

In general, laboratory tests are useful adjuncts in establishing a rheumatologic diagnosis but are not absolutely diagnostic of any specific disease. Two features of rheumatologic diseases contribute to the difficulties of interpreting laboratory tests. First, many rheumatic diseases are chronic systemic inflammatory diseases and, therefore, share many laboratory abnormalities with other such diseases, particularly chronic infections and malignancies. Second, the prevalence of certain rheumatologic diseases is low in most patient populations. Therefore, even if sensitivity and specificity of a test are high for a specific disease, the positive predictive value of the test may be low. Considering these statistical characteristics of laboratory tests can help the clinician interpret the data within the context of the clinical case.

▶ Statistical Characteristics of Laboratory Tests

Appropriate use of laboratory tests requires awareness of the rates and causes of false-positive and false-negative test results (see box, Defining Statistical Characteristics of Laboratory Tests). The **sensitivity** of a test demonstrates the ability of the test to detect a patient with disease and is measured by the proportion of people with disease who have a positive test result. The **specificity** of a test demonstrates the ability of the test to avoid detecting patients without disease and is measured by the proportion of people without disease who have a negative test result. The usefulness of a laboratory test is best reflected in the **positive predictive value**, which determines the proportion of patients with a positive test result who truly have the disease. The **positive predictive value** of a test depends on the **prevalence** of the disease in the population being examined (or the pretest probability of disease); thus, even if the sensitivity and specificity of a test are 99%, the positive predictive value of the test can be low if the prevalence of the disease in the population is extremely low. The **negative predictive value** of a test determines how many patients with a negative test result truly do not have the disease. The negative predictive value also depends on the prevalence of the disease. The generally low prevalence of rheumatologic disease in the overall population means that many rheumatologic laboratory tests will only have a high positive predictive value when the tests are selected on the basis of clinical presentations that are highly suggestive of a rheumatologic disorder, which increases the pretest probability of disease.

The American College of Rheumatology (ACR) has published guidelines on some immunologic tests following review of the literature. Studies were evaluated for quality, and likelihood ratios were calculated through summary of the "best quality" studies.

The **likelihood ratio** (LR) is the likelihood that a given test result would be expected in a patient with the target disorder compared to the likelihood that that same result would be expected in a patient without the target disorder. The LR is used to assess the usefulness of a diagnostic test and to help the provider select appropriate tests for a given patient. The LR has the advantage of being independent of disease prevalence and indicates how much a given test result will raise or lower the odds of having disease relative to the pretest probability of the disease. An LR of 1 means that the posttest probability is exactly the same as the pretest probability.

Thus, an LR greater than 1 produces a posttest probability that is higher than the pretest probability. If the pretest probability lies between 30% and 70%, then positive test results with a very high LR (over 10) would rule in the disease.

An LR less than 1 produces a posttest probability that is lower than the pretest probability. A negative test result with a very low LR (below 0.1) virtually rules out the chance that the patient has the disease. A test is considered to be very useful if weighted average positive LR >5 or negative LR <0.2. A test is considered not useful if weighted average positive LR <2 or negative LR >0.5.

AUTOANTIBODIES

▶ Methods for Detecting Autoantibodies

A variety of basic assays are used to detect autoantibodies. More than one type of assay may be available for any given autoantibody, and the particular test used may vary from institution to institution. In general, there has been a trend away from labor-intensive tests, such as agglutination assays and countercurrent immunoelectrophoresis, and toward assays amenable to automation, such as nephelometry, enzyme-linked immunoabsorbent assay (ELISA), and high throughput multiplex bead assays.

Indirect immunofluorescence assays identify autoantibodies reactive with antigens, in particular tissues or subcellular compartments (eg, nuclear antigens). Fixed tissue samples or cells are overlayed with patient sera and then washed. The presence of autoantibodies bound to the tissue sample is revealed by staining with a fluorescein-labeled antiserum against human immunoglobulin and observed by immunofluorescent microscopy. The antinuclear antibody (ANA) test has traditionally been done by this method.

Agglutination assays identify autoantibodies through the aggregation of particles, such as latex beads, coated with a defined autoantigen.

Immunodiffusion assays detect the formation of immune complexes in a semisolid support, such as an agar gel. Patient sera and antigen, placed in separate wells in the gel, diffuse toward one another and form a line of precipitation when insoluble immune complexes form. Placing

the gel in an electrical field (**countercurrent immunoelectrophoresis**) increases the rate of diffusion and facilitates complex formation.

Nephelometry measures the interaction of antibodies and antigens in solution, detecting immune complex formation by monitoring changes in the scattering of an incident light.

ELISA uses an enzymatic readout to detect reactive antibodies. Sera to be tested for an autoantibody is incubated with the relevant autoantigen immobilized on a surface. After extensive washing, a detecting antibody (eg, an antiserum to human immunoglobulin) that has been conjugated to an enzyme is added. In the final step, substrate is added, and the product of the enzymatic reaction is measured. The amount of product reflects the quantity of detecting antibody bound to the autoantibody. There are several modifications of the basic ELISA, but all take advantage of the remarkable sensitivity imparted by the enzymatic readout.

High throughput multiplex bead assays use antigen-coated beads that are prelabeled with fluorescent label and mixed with serum and fluorescent-labeled secondary antibody. Multiplex bead assays can identify multiple autoantibodies and their specificities in single, high throughput assay. There is increasing use of this technology for ANA testing because (1) a small amount of serum is required, (2) the test is fully automated and more cost effective than measuring ANA by indirect immunofluorescence, and (3) the test provides simultaneous detection of ANA and identification of specific autoantibodies. However, a disadvantage is that only a limited group of antigens—*not* all nuclear antigens—are used, potentially lowering sensitivity. The test detects only autoantibodies to the selected set of nuclear antigens and does not detect all antibodies reactive with all nuclear proteins. Consequently, a negative multiplex test for ANA does not have the same negative predictive value for systemic lupus erythematosus (SLE) as does a negative indirect immunofluorescence test for ANA. Recent ACR guidelines state that the indirect immunofluorescence test for ANA remains the gold standard, and laboratories should inform providers of the method used to assess for ANA.

RHEUMATOID FACTOR

Rheumatoid factor is an autoantibody directed against the Fc region of IgG. The most commonly used methods of detecting rheumatoid factor are latex fixation (using latex beads coated with human IgG) and nephelometry (using human IgG as the target antigen). Both assays primarily detect IgM rheumatoid factors. The results of latex fixation assays are reported as the greatest dilution that retains agglutination activity; in most laboratories, sera with titers of >1:40 are considered abnormal. Rheumatoid factor measured by nephelometry is quantified in international units, with ≥20 international units reported as abnormal in most laboratories. ELISAs for rheumatoid factor are also available but are not in wide use. ELISAs can measure IgG, IgA, and IgM rheumatoid factors.

Table 3–1. Disorders associated with a positive test for rheumatoid factor.

Autoimmune disorders[a]
Rheumatoid arthritis[a]
Primary Sjögren syndrome[a]
Mixed connective tissue disease[a]
Polymyositis/dermatomyositis
Scleroderma
ANCA-associated vasculitis[a]
Polyarteritis nodosa
Primary biliary cirrhosis[a]
Chronic infections
Subacute bacterial endocarditis[a]
Tuberculosis
Leprosy
Syphilis
Hepatitis C[a] (with or without mixed cryoglobulinemia)
Hepatitis B[a]
Other viral infections
Parasitic infections
Miscellaneous conditions
Sarcoidosis
Idiopathic pulmonary fibrosis
Silicosis
Asbestosis
Malignancy
Age ≥65

[a]Prevalence of rheumatoid factor >50% in most series.
ANCA, antineutrophil cytoplasmic antibodies.

A. Associated Conditions

Rheumatoid factor is present in 70–90% of patients with rheumatoid arthritis. Despite its name, rheumatoid factor is not specific for rheumatoid arthritis. Positive tests for rheumatoid factor occur in a wide range of autoimmune disorders, inflammatory diseases, and chronic infections (Table 3–1). Also, the prevalence of positive rheumatoid factor tests increases with age; as many as 25% of persons over the age of 65 may have a positive test result. In the absence of disease, the titer for rheumatoid factor is usually low (≤1:160). High titer for rheumatoid factor (≥1:640) almost always reflects an underlying disease.

B. Indication

Rheumatoid factor should be ordered when there is clinical suspicion of rheumatoid arthritis.

C. Interpretation of Results

Because of the large number of disorders associated with rheumatoid factor (see Table 3–1), the value of a positive test for rheumatoid factor depends on the pretest probability of the disease. In the proper clinical setting, a positive test provides strong support for the diagnosis of rheumatoid

arthritis. However, it should be kept in mind that the combination of arthritis and a positive test for rheumatoid factor is not specific for rheumatoid arthritis and can be seen in patients with SLE; mixed connective tissue disease; systemic vasculitis; polymyositis; dermatomyositis; sarcoidosis; subacute bacterial endocarditis; and viral infections, particularly hepatitis C.

A negative test for rheumatoid factor should not be the only reason to rule out the possibility of rheumatoid arthritis. Between 10% and 30% of patients with long-standing disease are "seronegative." At the time of presentation, however, the prevalence of a positive rheumatoid factor test is substantially lower (in the range of 50%). Therefore, the sensitivity of the test is lowest when the diagnosis is most likely to be in doubt. Although a positive rheumatoid factor test in a patient with clinical rheumatoid arthritis is associated with more severe, erosive disease and increased extra-articular manifestations of rheumatoid arthritis, there is no role for serial measurement of rheumatoid factor during the course of the disease for evaluation of disease activity.

ANTIBODIES TO CYCLIC CITRULLINATED PEPTIDES

Proteins that contain citrulline are the target of an autoantibody response that is highly specific for rheumatoid arthritis. Citrulline, a neutral amino acid, is not genetically encoded. Citrullinated proteins arise through a posttranslational modification in which arginine residues are converted enzymatically to citrulline. Currently, autoantibodies to citrullinated proteins are detected using ELISA with synthetic cyclic citrullinated peptides (CCP).

A. Associated Conditions

The presence of anti-CCP antibodies appears to be quite specific for rheumatoid arthritis. The second-generation ELISA tests for anti-CCP antibodies (anti-CCP2) have a specificity for rheumatoid arthritis as high as 97%. The sensitivities of anti-CCP tests are in the range of 70–80% for established rheumatoid arthritis and of 50% for early-onset rheumatoid arthritis. Thus, compared with rheumatoid factor, the currently available anti-CCP ELISA tests have superior sensitivity and comparable sensitivity for the diagnosis of rheumatoid arthritis. Recent studies suggest that a rheumatoid factor test does not add to the ability of an anti-CCP2 test to predict joint damage in patients with rheumatoid arthritis and does not add to ability of anti-CCP2 to predict progression from undifferentiated arthritis to rheumatoid arthritis.

The likelihood of rheumatoid arthritis developing in individuals with positive test results for both rheumatoid factor and CCP2 is nearly 100%. Most patients with rheumatoid arthritis are positive for both anti-CCP antibodies and rheumatoid factor, but some have only one of these autoantibodies, and others have neither. A meta-analysis of studies of anti-CCP in rheumatoid arthritis demonstrated a pooled sensitivity of 67%, specificity of 95%, a positive LR of 12.46, and a negative LR of 0.36. The risk of radiographic progression was shown to be greater with positive anti-CCP than positive rheumatoid factor in patients with rheumatoid arthritis.

B. Indication

Anti-CCP antibodies should be ordered when there is clinical suspicion of rheumatoid arthritis.

C. Interpretation of Results

The presence of anti-CCP antibodies provides strong support for the diagnosis of rheumatoid arthritis. Moreover, in patients with early onset, undifferentiated, inflammatory arthritis, the presence of anti-CCP antibodies is a strong predictor of progression to rheumatoid arthritis and for the development of joint erosions. A positive anti-CCP antibody test or a positive rheumatoid factor test is part of the 2010 ACR diagnostic criteria for rheumatoid arthritis. A negative test for anti-CCP antibodies does not exclude the possibility of rheumatoid arthritis, particularly at the time of initial presentation when approximately 50% of patients lack detectable anti-CCP antibodies.

The specificity of the anti-CCP ELISA tests suggests that this test will prove useful when determinations of rheumatoid factor are not. For example, initial studies indicate that anti-CCP antibodies are not associated with chronic hepatitis C infection. In contrast to rheumatoid factor, therefore, testing for anti-CCP antibodies may help distinguish concomitant rheumatoid arthritis from viral arthritis in patients infected with hepatitis C.

Levasque MC, Zhou Z, Moreland LW. Anti-cyclic citrullinated peptide testing for the diagnosis of rheumatoid arthritis and the quest for improved sensitivity and predictive value. *Arthritis Rheum.* 2009;60:2211. [PMID: 19644881]

Nijenhuis S, Zendman AJ, Vossenaar ER, Pruijn GJ, vanVenrooij WJ. Autoantibodies to citrullinated proteins in rheumatoid arthritis: clinical performance and biochemical aspects of an RA-specific marker. *Clin Chim Acta.* 2004;350:17. [PMID: 15530456]

Nishimura K, Sugiyama D, Kogata Y, et al. Meta-analysis: diagnostic accuracy of anti–cyclic citrullinated peptide antibody and rheumatoid factor for rheumatoid arthritis. *Ann Intern Med.* 2007;146:797. [PMID: 17548411]

Wener MH, Hutchinson K, Morishima C, Gretch DR. Absence of antibodies to cyclic citrullinated peptide in sera of patients with hepatitis C virus infection and cryoglobulinemia. *Arthritis Rheum.* 2004;50:2305. [PMID: 15248231]

ANTINUCLEAR ANTIBODIES

Antinuclear antibodies (ANAs) are autoantibodies directed against histones, double-stranded and single-stranded DNA, ribonucleoprotein (RNP) complexes, and other nuclear components. ANAs are measured using either indirect immunofluorescence assays, ELISA, or high throughput multiplex bead assays.

Current indirect immunofluorescence assays for ANA use HEp-2 cells, a human epithelial cell line, as the source of nuclei and are more sensitive than older tests that used rodent liver and kidney. These assays for ANA report the titer of the ANA and the pattern of nuclear staining and are considered the gold standard for ANA testing. In most laboratories, ANA with titers ≥1:40 are considered positive. The staining patterns are diffuse or homogeneous (due to antibodies to histone), rim (an uncommon pattern due to antibodies to nuclear envelope proteins and to double-stranded [ds] DNA), speckled (due to antibodies to Sm, RNP, Ro/SS-A, La/SS-B, and other antigens), nucleolar (see the section, Antibodies to Nucleolar Antigens, below), and centromeric. In general, there is a poor correlation between the pattern of the ANA and the identity of the underlying disease. An exception is the centromeric pattern, which has considerable specificity for limited scleroderma (see the section, Anticentromere Antibodies, below). Patients often have antibodies to multiple nuclear components, and the staining pattern of certain autoantibodies (eg, antihistone antibodies) can prevent detection of others. The pattern of the ANA should not preclude, or substitute for, the ordering of more specific tests that are otherwise indicated.

A. Associated Conditions

Positive tests for ANA occur in a wide range of conditions, including SLE and other rheumatic diseases, organ-specific autoimmune diseases, lymphoproliferative diseases, and chronic infections (Table 3–2). A number of drugs induce ANA and, less commonly, a lupus-like syndrome (Table 3–2). Low-titer ANA are relatively common among healthy adults; in one analysis, an ANA titer of ≥1:40 was seen in 32% of healthy adults and ≥1:160 was seen in 5%.

B. Indications

Testing for ANA by indirect immunofluorescence is a very useful initial laboratory investigation when there is clinical suspicion of SLE, drug-induced lupus, mixed connective tissue disease, or scleroderma. The ANA may provide useful prognostic information for patients with isolated Raynaud phenomenon, identifying those at greater risk for systemic rheumatic disease.

C. Interpretation of Results

The sensitivity of an ANA test determined by an indirect immunofluorescence assay for SLE is very high (>95%). A negative result, therefore, is very strong evidence against this diagnosis and usually precludes the need to pursue tests for antibodies to specific nuclear antigens (eg, dsDNA, Sm, RNP). In contrast, a false-negative ANA test determined by

Table 3–2. Conditions associated with ANA by indirect immunofluorescence assays.

Rheumatic diseases
  Systemic lupus erythematosus
  Mixed connective tissue disease
  Scleroderma
  Sjögren syndrome
  Rheumatoid arthritis
  Polymyositis
  Dermatomyositis
  Discoid lupus
Organ-specific autoimmune diseases
  Autoimmune thyroid disease
  Autoimmune hepatitis
  Primary biliary cirrhosis
  Autoimmune cholangitis
Other
  Drug-induced lupus[a]
  Asymptomatic drug-induced ANA[a]
  Chronic infections
  Idiopathic pulmonary fibrosis
  Primary pulmonary hypertension
  Lymphoproliferative disorders

[a]Drugs that can induce lupus and/or positive tests for ANA include procainamide, hydralazine, minocycline, antitumor necrosis factor agents, interferon-α, isoniazid, quinidine, methyldopa, chlorpromazine, penicillamine, and anticonvulsants.
ANA, antinuclear antibodies.

ELISA or multiplex bead testing can occur in SLE. Thus, a negative ELISA or other high throughput test for ANA should not be the sole grounds for excluding the diagnosis of SLE; when clinical suspicion warrants, ANA should be determined by indirect immunofluorescence.

A positive ANA test is one of the diagnostic criteria for drug-induced lupus and mixed connective tissue disease. The sensitivity of the ANA for scleroderma is >85%.

In general, the probability of an underlying autoimmune disease increases with the titer of the ANA. Nonetheless, because the specificity of the ANA is limited, the value of a positive test depends on the pretest probability of disease. In the proper clinical context, a positive ANA by immunofluorescence provides supportive evidence of disease and should prompt tests for antibodies to specific nuclear antigens (Table 3–3).

Serial determinations of ANA are not useful for monitoring disease activity.

Meroni PL, Schur PH. ANA screening: an old test with new recommendations. *Ann Rheum Dis.* 2010;69:1420. [PMID: 20511607]
Solomon DH, Kavanaugh AJ, Schur PH, and the American College of Rheumatology Ad Hoc Committee on Immunologic Testing Guidelines. Evidence-based guidelines for the use of immunologic tests: antinuclear antibody testing. *Arthritis Rheum.* 2002;47:434. [PMID: 12209492]

ANTIBODIES TO DEFINED NUCLEAR ANTIGENS

1. Antibodies to Double-Stranded DNA

Antibodies to dsDNA recognize its base pairs, its ribose-phosphate backbone, and the structure of its double helix. ELISA is the most commonly used method to detect antibodies to dsDNA and has largely supplanted the Farr radioimmunoassay and the crithidia immunofluorescence assay, which measures binding to the dsDNA of the protozoan *Crithidia luciliae.*

Table 3–3. Selected antinuclear antibodies with high sensitivity or specificity for rheumatic diseases.

Condition	High Sensitivity[a]	High Specificity[b]
SLE	ANA[c]	Anti-dsDNA, anti-Sm
Drug-induced lupus	ANA, anti-histone[d]	—
Neonatal cutaneous lupus	Maternal anti-Ro/SS-A (90%)	—
Congenital complete heart block	Maternal anti-Ro/SS-A	—
Mixed connective tissue disease	ANA, anti-RNP[e]	—
Sjögren syndrome	Anti-Ro/SS-A (75%)	—
Limited and diffuse scleroderma	ANA (>85%)	Anti-centromere anti-Scl-70 and other anti-nucleolar antibodies

[a]Sensitivity (probability of a positive test result in a patient with the disease) >95% except where noted.
[b]Specificity (probability of a negative test result in a patient without the disease) >95%.
[c]ANA determined by immunofluorescence using HEp-2 cells.
[d]Anti-histone antibodies occur in only a minority of cases of minocycline-induced lupus.
[e]The presence of antibodies to RNP is required for diagnosis.
ANA, antinuclear antibodies; SLE, systemic lupus erythematosus.

A. Associated Conditions

Antibodies to dsDNA occur in SLE and are rare in other diseases and in healthy persons. When detected outside the context of SLE, antibodies to dsDNA are almost always of low titer. Antibodies to dsDNA do not occur in most forms of drug-induced lupus but have been observed during treatment with penicillamine, minocycline, and antitumor necrosis factor agents.

B. Indications

Antibodies to dsDNA should be measured when there is clinical suspicion of SLE and the ANA test is positive. The yield of testing for anti-dsDNA antibodies is low when ANAs are not detected by indirect immunofluorescence on HEp-2 cells. Longitudinal determinations of the levels of antibodies to dsDNA may aid in the analysis of disease activity for patients with known SLE.

C. Interpretation of Results

The specificity of anti-dsDNA antibodies for SLE is 97% overall and approaches 100% when the antibody titer is high. A positive test, therefore, is a very strong argument for the diagnosis of SLE.

Antibodies to dsDNA occur in 60–80% of patients with SLE. Because titers can fluctuate in and out of the normal range over time, the sensitivity of an isolated test for anti-dsDNA antibodies is probably in the range of 50% for SLE. A negative test, therefore, does not argue strongly against the diagnosis of SLE.

Studies of patient populations indicate that the level of anti-dsDNA antibodies correlates with certain manifestations of SLE activity, such as lupus nephritis, but not others. The strength of this relationship, however, varies from patient to patient. For most patients, a rise in antibody titer often precedes—or occurs concomitantly with—a disease flare. However, there are subsets of patients who manifest disease flares in the absence of anti-dsDNA antibodies and others whose disease is quiescent despite elevated levels of this autoantibody.

Kavanaugh AF, Solomon DH, and the American College of Rheumatology Ad Hoc Committee on Immunologic Testing Guidelines. Guidelines for immunologic laboratory testing in the rheumatic diseases: anti-DNA antibody tests. *Arthritis Rheum.* 2002;47:546. [PMID: 12382306]

2. Antibodies to Sm & RNP

Smith (Sm) and RNP were initially identified as extractable nuclear antigens. Antibodies to Sm recognize nuclear proteins that bind to small nuclear RNAs, forming complexes involved in the processing of messenger RNA. Antibodies to RNP recognize a complex of protein and the small nuclear RNA designated U1. ELISA has largely replaced immunodiffusion assays for the measurement of antibodies to Sm and RNP. Antibodies to Sm or to RNP produce a speckled pattern on indirect immunofluorescence assays for ANA.

A. Associated Conditions

Antibodies to Sm are specific for SLE. Antibodies to RNP occur in SLE and mixed connective tissue disease. The prevalence of these autoantibodies in other conditions is very low.

B. Indications

Antibodies to Sm and RNP should be determined when there is clinical suspicion of SLE or mixed connective tissue disease and the ANA test determined by indirect immunofluorescence is positive.

C. Interpretation of Results

Antibodies to Sm are highly specific for SLE but occur in only 10–40% of patients. The prevalence of anti-Sm antibodies appears to be lower in white patients than in black and Asian patients.

Antibodies to RNP occur in 30–40% of patients with SLE. The diagnosis of mixed connective tissue disease requires the presence of antibodies to RNP; by definition, therefore, 100% of patients with this disease have anti-RNP antibodies.

Serial determinations of antibodies to Sm and RNP are not useful for monitoring disease activity.

3. Antibodies to Ro (SS-A) & La (SS-B)

The Ro (also known as Sjögren syndrome A or SS-A) and La (SS-B or Sjögren syndrome B) antigens are distinct RNP particles. ELISA and immunoblot assays are supplanting the older immunodiffusion assays for detection of anti-Ro and anti-La antibodies. Antibodies to Ro and La produce a speckled pattern on immunofluorescence assays for ANA. When rodent tissues were used for this assay, antibodies to Ro often went undetected and were a cause of "ANA-negative" lupus if these were the dominant autoantibody system. The use of HEp-2 cells enhances detection of anti-Ro antibodies and has led to a decline in the prevalence of ANA-negative lupus.

A. Associated Conditions

Antibodies to Ro are uncommon in the normal population and in patients with rheumatic diseases other than Sjögren syndrome and SLE. Antibodies to Ro are present in 75% of patients with primary Sjögren syndrome but only in 10–15% of patients with secondary Sjögren syndrome associated with rheumatoid arthritis. In SLE, anti-Ro antibodies are present in up to 50% of patients and are associated with photosensitivity, subacute cutaneous lupus, and interstitial lung disease. Transfer of maternal anti-Ro antibodies across the placenta appears to be important in the pathogenesis of neonatal cutaneous lupus and congenital complete heart block (see Table 3–3). Mothers of babies with neonatal cutaneous lupus or congenital complete heart block secondary to maternal anti-Ro antibodies may or may not have clinical signs of a systemic rheumatologic disease.

Antibodies to La occur, almost always in association with anti-Ro antibodies, in primary Sjögren syndrome (40–50%), SLE (10–15%), congenital complete heart block (90%), and neonatal cutaneous lupus (70%).

B. Indications

Antibodies to Ro and La should be measured when there is clinical suspicion of primary Sjögren syndrome or SLE. Even when ANA are not detected by indirect immunofluorescence, testing for anti-Ro antibodies is still indicated for patients with suspected subacute cutaneous lupus or with recurrent photosensitive rashes. Mothers of children with neonatal cutaneous lupus and congenital complete heart block should be tested for antibodies to Ro and La; many of these women are asymptomatic. Testing is also indicated for patients with SLE who become pregnant or who are planning to become pregnant.

C. Interpretation of Results

The presence of antibodies to Ro, or to Ro and La, is a strong argument for the diagnosis of Sjögren syndrome in a patient with sicca symptoms. Although not a sensitive test for SLE, a positive test for anti-Ro antibodies can facilitate a diagnosis of subacute cutaneous lupus. Chapter 69 reviews the monitoring of pregnancy in the setting of maternal antibodies to Ro and the evaluation of asymptomatic mothers found to have anti-Ro antibodies.

4. Anticentromere Antibodies

Antibodies to centromere proteins produce a characteristic pattern of staining in indirect immunofluorescence assays using HEp-2 cells. Anticentromere antibodies can be measured by ELISA, but indirect immunofluorescence is the most commonly used method of detection.

A. Associated Conditions

Anticentromere antibodies occur in limited scleroderma and scleroderma. They are rare in other rheumatic conditions and in healthy persons.

B. Indications

Anticentromere antibodies should be determined when there is clinical suspicion of scleroderma or its CREST variant (calcinosis, Raynaud phenomenon, esophageal dysmotility, sclerodactyly, telangiectasias).

C. Interpretation of Results

Anticentromere antibodies occur in approximately 60% of patients with CREST and in 15% of those with scleroderma. The specificity of this test is remarkable (>98%). A positive test for anticentromere antibodies, therefore, is a very strong argument for the presence of CREST or scleroderma. The presence of anticentromere antibodies early in the course of disease predicts limited cutaneous involvement and a decreased likelihood of interstitial lung disease. Anticentromere antibodies and antibodies to Scl-70 rarely coexist. Serial determinations of anticentromere antibodies are not useful for monitoring disease activity.

ANTIBODIES TO NUCLEOLAR ANTIGENS

1. Antibodies to Scl-70 (Topoisomerase-I)

Antibodies to Scl-70 (or topoisomerase I) produce nucleolar staining on indirect immunofluorescence and are measured by immunodiffusion assays, immunoblotting, and ELISA.

A. Associated Conditions

Antibodies to Scl-70 occur in scleroderma and are rare in patients with other systemic rheumatic diseases and in healthy persons.

B. Indications

Antibodies to Scl-70 should be measured when there is clinical suspicion of scleroderma.

C. Interpretation of Results

Immunodiffusion assays identify antibodies to Scl-70 in 20–30% of patients with scleroderma; approximately 40% of patients have antibodies to Scl-70 detectable by immunoblotting or ELISA. The specificity of anti-Scl-70 antibodies approaches 100% for the immunoblotting and immunodiffusion assays. A positive test by these assays, therefore, is a very strong argument for the diagnosis of scleroderma. The specificity of ELISA is not certain but may be lower. The presence of antibodies to Scl-70 has prognostic value in scleroderma and carries an increased likelihood of diffuse skin involvement and of interstitial lung disease. Serial determinations of anti-Scl-70 antibodies are not useful for monitoring the disease.

2. Antibodies to Other Nucleolar Antigens

Antibodies to nucleolar antigens other than Scl-70 occur in scleroderma. Antibodies with high specificity for scleroderma include anti-RNA polymerase I, anti-RNA polymerase III, anti-U3 small nucleolar RNP (or anti-fibrillarin), and anti-Th small nucleolar RNP. The low sensitivity of these antibodies limits their usefulness in the diagnosis of scleroderma. Antibodies to RNA polymerase II are present in scleroderma, SLE, and overlap syndromes. Antibodies to PM-Scl occur in scleroderma and in an overlap syndrome of myositis and scleroderma.

Reveille JD, Solomon DH, and the American College of Rheumatology Ad Hoc Committee of Immunologic Testing Guidelines. Evidence-based guidelines for the use of immunologic tests: anticentromere, Scl-70, and nucleolar antibodies. *Arthritis Rheum.* 2003;49:399. [PMID: 12794797]

ANTIBODIES TO HISTONES

Antibodies to histones usually produce a homogeneous staining on indirect immunofluorescence assays for ANA. Antihistone antibodies are almost always present in lupus induced by drugs such as procainamide, hydralazine, and isoniazid (sensitivity >95%). An important exception is minocycline-induced lupus; antihistone antibodies are present in only a minority of patients with this disorder. Antibodies to histones are common in SLE (prevalence 50–70%) and occur at low frequency in a range of rheumatic and nonrheumatic disorders. The clinical usefulness of testing for antibodies to histones is limited. Antihistone antibodies are nonspecific and do not distinguish drug-induced lupus from SLE. Although the absence of antihistone antibodies is strong evidence against most forms of drug-induced lupus, the clinical diagnosis of drug-induced lupus is based on the clinical manifestations, a positive test for ANA by indirect immunofluorescence, and resolution of symptoms following withdrawal of the implicated drug.

MYOSITIS-ASSOCIATED ANTIBODIES (SEE CHAPTER 27)

1. Anti-Jo-1 & Other Antisynthetase Antibodies

Autoantibodies against amino acyl-tRNA synthetases occur almost exclusively in inflammatory myosis and can cause cytoplasmic staining when sera are analyzed for ANA by indirect immunofluorescence. The most common of these autoantibodies (anti-Jo-1) is directed against histidyl-tRNA synthetase and is present in 20–30% of the patients with polymyositis. Patients with antisynthetase antibodies tend to have interstitial lung disease, arthritis, mechanic's hands, and Raynaud phenomenon as well as myositis.

2. Antibodies to Signal Recognition Particle

These antibodies recognize a cytoplasmic RNP, occur in 4% of myositis patients, and are associated with acute onset and severe disease.

3. Anti-Mi-2 Antibodies

These antibodies are directed against helicase activities and produce homogeneous nuclear staining on indirect immunofluorescence assays for ANA. Anti-Mi-2 antibodies have high specificity for dermatomyositis and occur in 15–20% of patients with that disorder.

ANTINEUTROPHIL CYTOPLASMIC ANTIBODIES

Antineutrophil cytoplasmic antibodies (ANCA) are reviewed in Chapter 32.

MEASUREMENT OF THE ACUTE PHASE RESPONSE

The acute phase response develops in the setting of a wide range of acute and chronic inflammatory conditions: severe bacterial, viral, or fungal infections; rheumatic and other inflammatory diseases; malignancy; and tissue injury or necrosis. These conditions elicit a response in which interleukin-6 and other cytokines trigger the synthesis by the liver of a variety of plasma proteins, including C-reactive protein (CRP) and fibrinogen. The detection and monitoring of this response can be clinically useful and is accomplished by measuring the level of CRP or by determining the erythrocyte sedimentation rate (ESR), which is influenced by the binding of protein, particularly fibrinogen, to erythrocytes. As a general rule, CRP is a more sensitive and dynamic reflection of the acute phase response than the ESR.

C-REACTIVE PROTEIN

CRP likely has a physiologic role in the innate immune response to infection and may participate in the clearance of necrotic and apoptotic cells. The availability of highly sensitive assays of CRP has allowed accurate determination of baseline CRP levels and has revealed a correlation between baseline CRP and cardiovascular disease. The median baseline level for young adults is 0.8 mg/L, and the 90th percentile is 3.0 mg/L. The baseline levels of CRP increase with age and with body mass index. Obesity alone can raise CRP levels up to 10 mg/L. Laboratories sometimes offer a choice between a routine CRP assay (suitable for the detection and monitoring of inflammatory disease) and a highly sensitive CRP assay for the determination of cardiac risk.

During the acute phase response, levels of CRP rapidly increase up to 1000-fold, reaching a peak at 48 hours. With resolution of the acute phase response, CRP declines with a relatively short half-life of 18 hours. Because there are a large number of disparate conditions that can induce CRP production, an elevated CRP level does not have diagnostic specificity. An elevated CRP level, however, can provide support for the presence of a clinically suspected inflammatory disease, such as polymyalgia rheumatica or giant cell arteritis, when other objective findings are absent. Values >10 mg/L indicate clinically significant inflammation. Monitoring CRP levels can provide useful information on the activity of diseases such as rheumatoid arthritis and giant cell arteritis.

Despite their apparent inflammatory nature, scleroderma, polymyositis, and dermatomyositis often elicit little or no

CRP response. CRP levels also tend not to be elevated in SLE unless serositis or synovitis is present.

Elevations of CRP in the absence of clinically important inflammation can occur in renal failure.

ERYTHROCYTE SEDIMENTATION RATE

The ESR is determined by allowing anticoagulated blood to sediment for 1 hour in a glass tube (200 mm in length for the commonly used Westergren method; 100 mm for the Wintrobe method). Normal ranges for the ESR are 0–10 mm/hour and 0–15 mm/hour for men and women, respectively, but the upper limit of normal increases with age and with obesity.

Because fibrinogen and certain other acute phase proteins (not including CRP) bind to erythrocytes and increase their sedimentation rate, the ESR is a measure of the acute phase response. The ESR responds slower (over days) to the onset and resolution of an acute phase response than does the level of CRP, and the dynamic range of the ESR is less than that of CRP. More so than CRP, the ESR can be influenced by factors other than the acute phase response.

The ESR is a useful diagnostic test when there is clinical suspicion of polymyalgia rheumatica or giant cell arteritis. While ESR is commonly used to monitor the disease activity in both polymyalgia rheumatica and giant cell arteritis, several studies have demonstrated that extremely high ESR levels are not necessarily correlated with the severe outcome of cranial ischemia in giant cell arteritis or temporal arteritis. Extremely strong inflammatory responses with systemic symptoms of fever, weight loss, anemia, and ESR over 100 mm/hour were associated with a lower risk of visual loss in giant cell arteritis. ESR is also commonly used to monitor the activity of rheumatoid arthritis. Due to the wide range of disorders associated with an acute phase response, elevations of the ESR have little diagnostic specificity. Transient mild to moderate elevations, moreover, can occur in the absence of clinical disease. Marked elevations of the ESR (>100 mm/hour by the Westergren method), however, are almost always due to a clinically significant condition, usually infection, malignancy, or rheumatic disease.

The ESR is of very limited value in patients with the nephrotic syndrome or end-stage renal disease because virtually all have an elevated ESR (some >100 mm/hour), probably due to high levels of fibrinogen. Elevations of the ESR in the absence of clinically important inflammation also occur in pregnancy, anemia, erythrocyte macrocytosis, and hypercholesterolemia. Conversely, hypofibrinogenemia, polycythemia, microcytosis, sickle cell disease, and congestive heart failure lower the ESR.

Pepys MB, Hirschfield GM. C-reactive protein: a critical update. *J Clin Invest.* 2003;111:1805. [PMID: 12813013]

Salvarani C, Cimino L, Macchioni P, et al. Risk factors for visual loss in an Italian population-based cohort of patients with giant cell arteritis. *Arthritis Rheum.* 2005;53:293. [PMID: 15818722]

MEASUREMENT OF COMPLEMENT

Complement is a complex system of at least 30 proteins that play key roles in the innate and adaptive immune responses. Effector functions of complement include opsonization, chemotaxis and activation of leukocytes, lysis of bacteria and cells, promotion of antibody responses, and clearance of immune complexes and apoptotic cells. Three enzymatic complement cascades (the classic pathway, the alternative pathway, and the mannose-binding lectin pathway) lead to the generation of a convertase that cleaves C3, releasing C3a (an anaphylatoxin) and producing C3b, which binds to the target surface. C3b, a potent opsonin, forms a complex that cleaves C5 to C5a (another anaphylatoxin) and C5b, which sequentially binds C6, C7, C8, and C9 to form the membrane attack complex, a channel that can induce osmotic lysis of the target cell.

▶ Indications for Measurement of Complement

Complement should be measured when there is clinical suspicion of a disease that is associated with hypocomplementemia (Table 3–4) or an inherited or acquired abnormality of the complement system (Table 3–5). Complement levels also can be used to monitor the activity of diseases such as SLE. Some components of the complement system, including C3 and C4, are acute phase proteins, and their synthesis increases during the acute phase response. Because the liver synthesizes many complement components, severe hepatic failure can produce hypocomplementemia.

There are three commonly used measurements of complement in clinical practice: the CH50 and determination of the levels of C4 and C3.

A. CH50

The CH50 is a functional assay for the classical pathway (components C1 through C9) of complement activation (Figure 3–1). The test measures the complement-dependent lysis of sheep red blood cells, using patient sera as a source of

Table 3–4. Immune complex diseases associated with hypocomplementemia.

Systemic lupus erythematosus
Vasculitis
Hypocomplementemic urticarial vasculitis
Polyarteritis nodosa (especially hepatitis B-associated)
Glomerulonephritis
Poststreptococcal
Membranoproliferative
Cryoglobulinemia (types II and III)
Subacute bacterial endocarditis
Serum sickness

Table 3–5. Clinical syndromes associated with deficiencies of components of the classical pathway of complement activation.

Component	Syndrome
Pathway components	
C1q, C4, C2	Lupus-like syndromes
C3	Recurrent pyogenic infections; immune complex glomerulonephritis
C5, C6, C7, C8	Recurrent Neisserial infections
Regulatory proteins	
C1 inhibitor	Angioedema

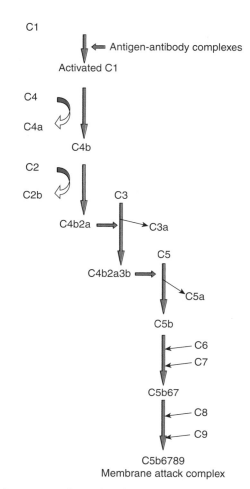

▲ **Figure 3–1.** Classical pathway of complement activation. Antigen-antibody complexes activate C1 esterase, which acts on C4 and then C2, forming the C3 convertase (C4b2a) that cleaves C3. C4b2a3b acts on C5, releasing C5a and generating C5b, which interacts with C6, C7, C8, and C9 to form the membrane attack complex. (Adapted, with permission, from Parslow T, Stites D, Terr A, Imboden J, eds. *Medical Immunology*. McGraw-Hill, 2001.)

complement and rabbit antibodies to sheep red blood cells. Units are standardized with a known source of complement and may vary from laboratory to laboratory if the standard reagents differ. Immune complex diseases (see Table 3–4) can lead to the activation of the classical pathway, the depletion of complement components, and a depressed CH50. In general, a reduction in the CH50 requires at least a 50% reduction of one or more components. Because each component of the classical pathway has an essential role in this assay, the CH50 is an excellent screen for deficiencies of the classical pathway (Table 3–5). The CH50 is undetectable when there is complete deficiency of any individual component, and a persistently undetectable CH50 should raise the possibility of such a deficiency. Conversely, a detectable CH50 rules out complete deficiency of components of the classical pathway.

B. C4 Levels

The concentration of C4 is determined by immunoassay, usually by rate nephelometry. Low levels of C4, or of both C4 and C3, usually reflect activation of the classical pathway by immune complex disease. Deficiency in C1 inhibitor leads to unregulated C1 esterase activity and to depression of C4 levels. Thus, C4 is an excellent screen for C1 inhibitor deficiency and should be performed before more specific (and costly) determinations of C1 inhibitor protein levels and enzymatic activity. Two tandem genes on chromosome 6 encode C4. Although null alleles for these genes are relatively common, complete deficiency of C4 is rare because four genes encode C4 protein. Partial deficiencies (due to the presence of one, two, or three null alleles) can produce persistently low levels of C4 and predispose to SLE.

C. C3 Levels

The concentration of C3 is determined by immunoassay, usually by rate nephelometry. The classical and alternative pathways converge on C3. Depression of both C4 and C3 indicates activation of the classical pathway. A depressed C3 with normal C4 suggests activation of the alternative pathway.

Complete deficiency of C3 is rare and usually manifests in childhood as severe, recurrent infections with pyogenic organisms. C3 nephritic factor, an autoantibody associated with membranoproliferative glomerulonephritis and partial lipodystrophy, stabilizes the alternative pathway C3 convertase, leading to dysregulated cleavage of C3 and low levels of C3 with normal levels of C4.

Walport MJ. Complement. *N Engl J Med*. 2001;344:1140,1058. [PMID: 11297706, 11287977]

CRYOGLOBULINS

▶ Classification

Cryoglobulins are cold-insoluble immunoglobulins that precipitate with cold and dissolve on rewarming. The Brouet classification describes three categories.

Type I is a monoclonal immunoglobulin that precipitates in the cold. Type I cryoglobulins are often associated with underlying lymphoproliferative disorders and may cause cold-induced hyperviscosity symptoms if the monoclonal immunoglobulin precipitates at physiologically relevant temperatures.

Type II cryoglobulins are immune complexes composed of a monoclonal immunoglobulin (usually IgMκ) with rheumatoid factor activity and polyclonal IgG. Most cases of type II cryoglobulinemia are associated with chronic hepatitis C infection and manifest clinically as an immune complex–mediated vasculitis with palpable purpura (see Chapter 36). The levels of C4 are usually low. Tests for serum rheumatoid factor are positive unless handling of the sample at temperatures lower than 37°C produces a false-negative test.

Type III cryoglobulins are immune complexes composed of polyclonal rheumatoid factor and polyclonal IgG. Type III cryoglobulinemia occurs in hepatitis C; other chronic infections, including subacute bacterial endocarditis; and autoimmune diseases, such as SLE and rheumatoid arthritis.

▶ Measurement

Blood to be tested for cryoglobulins is drawn in prewarmed tubes, is allowed to clot at 37°C, and then is centrifuged at 37°C; exposure to temperatures lower than 37°C during these steps can result in a false-negative test due to premature precipitation of the cryoglobulin. The resulting serum is placed at 4°C for 2–7 days (usually 2–3) and then is examined for a precipitate. A "cryocrit" provides a crude estimate of quantity of cryoglobulin. The highest levels are usually seen in type I cryoglobulinemia, but in general, the cryocrit correlates poorly with clinical severity. Analysis of resolubilized cryoglobulins by immunofixation electrophoresis permits classification as type I, II, or III.

Approach to the Patient with Arthritis

John B. Imboden, MD

Many diseases can cause arthritis. Obtaining a history and performing a physical examination are the first steps in allowing the clinician to accurately characterize the arthritis and approach the differential diagnosis in a focused, logical fashion based on the duration of symptoms, the presence or absence of joint inflammation, the number of joints affected, and the pattern of joint involvement (Table 4–1).

When evaluating a patient with joint symptoms, it is important to determine whether the symptoms are due to an articular process and not to bursitis, tendinitis, or other soft tissue conditions. The physical examination should also establish whether there are objective findings of arthritis, such as swelling, in the symptomatic joints. Arthralgias in the absence of objective arthritis commonly occur in systemic lupus erythematosus (SLE) and acute viral illnesses but have less diagnostic significance than true arthritis.

Laboratory tests cannot substitute for clinical evaluation and should never be used as a "screen" for disease. Musculoskeletal complaints are common in the general population, but the prevalence of inflammatory rheumatic diseases is relatively low. Hence, the positive predictive value of many rheumatologic tests is low when tests these are ordered indiscriminately. In general, radiographs add little to the evaluation of acute presentations of arthritis (except in cases of suspected trauma) but often are critical for the assessment of chronic arthritis.

▶ Inflammatory versus Noninflammatory Arthritis

The distinction between inflammatory arthritis and noninflammatory arthritis is a critical bifurcation point in the differential diagnosis of arthritis. The most reliable means for making this distinction is analysis of the white blood cell (WBC) count in the synovial fluid. The synovial fluid WBC count is >2000/mcL in inflammatory arthritis and is <2000/mcL in noninflammatory arthritis (see Chapter 2). Arthrocentesis should be performed whenever feasible because although clinical features and other laboratory investigations also help distinguish inflammatory and noninflammatory arthritis, no single finding is definitive.

Patients with an inflammatory arthritis usually complain of pain and stiffness in involved joints; typically these symptoms are worse in the morning or after periods of inactivity (the so-called "gel phenomenon") and improve with mild to moderate activity. On examination, the larger joints can be warm and, when severely inflamed as in acute gout or septic arthritis, can have erythema of the overlying skin. Laboratory investigations often reveal an elevated erythrocyte sedimentation rate (ESR) and a high C-reactive protein (CRP) level. In contrast, patients with noninflammatory arthritis have pain that worsens with activity and improves with rest. Stiffness is generally mild, lasts <30 minutes in the morning, and is not a prominent symptom. The ESR and CRP are usually normal.

▶ Constitutional Symptoms

The presence of fever raises the possibility of infection. Most patients with septic arthritis or disseminated gonococcal infection are febrile. Fever can also accompany arthritis that is not due to active infection (Table 4–2). Indeed, intermittent high-grade fever ≥39°C is characteristic of Still disease. SLE can also cause fever ≥39°C. However, fever more often occurs when serositis, rather than polyarthritis, is the major manifestation of SLE. On the other hand, fever ≥38.3°C is unusual in rheumatoid arthritis, occurring in <1% of patients.

Significant weight loss is common at the initial presentation of reactive arthritis, systemic vasculitis, enteropathic arthritis, and paraneoplastic arthritis but is unusual in rheumatoid arthritis of recent onset. Constitutional symptoms rarely accompany noninflammatory forms of arthritis.

Table 4–1. Initial clinical characterization of arthritis.

- Duration: acute (presenting within hours to days) or chronic (persisting for weeks or longer)
- Number of joints involved: monoarticular, oligoarticular (2–4 joints), or polyarticular (5 joints or more)
- If more than one joint is involved: symmetric or asymmetric; additive or migratory
- Accurate delineation of the involved joints
- Inflammatory or noninflammatory

▶ Extra-articular Manifestations

Extra-articular manifestations, such as glomerulonephritis, pulmonary abnormalities, oral ulcerations, ocular inflammation, and peripheral neuropathy, may signal that arthritis is a manifestation of a systemic rheumatic disease or vasculitis. The presence of rash can be a very helpful clue to the diagnosis (Table 4–3).

▶ Comorbid Conditions

Certain chronic conditions predispose to the development of particular musculoskeletal problems. For example, patients with long-standing, poorly controlled diabetes mellitus are at greatly increased risk for Charcot arthropathy in the feet and limited joint mobility in the hands. Certain medications can trigger drug-induced lupus, which can present as a polyarthritis, often with serositis. The resurgence in the use of hydralazine for the treatment of hypertension has led to

Table 4–2. Fever and arthritis.

Active infection
   Septic arthritis
   Disseminated gonococcal infection
   Endocarditis
   Acute viral infections
   Mycobacterial
   Fungal
Post infection
   Reactive arthritis (particularly in its early phases)
   Acute rheumatic fever and poststreptococcal arthritis
Not due to infection
   Systemic lupus erythematosus
   Drug-induced lupus
   Still disease
   Gout
   Pseudogout
   Inflammatory bowel disease
   Paraneoplastic arthritis
   Acute sarcoidosis
   Systemic vasculitis
   Familial Mediterranean fever and other inherited periodic fever syndromes

Table 4–3. Rash and arthritis.

Skin Manifestation	Associated Conditions
Erythematous maculopapular rash	Superimposed drug reaction Still disease Viral syndromes Kawasaki disease Secondary syphilis Chronic meningococcemia
Urticaria	SLE Hypocomplementemic urticarial vasculitis Serum sickness Acute hepatitis B Still disease Schnitzler syndrome
Palpable purpura	ANCA-associated vasculitis SLE Hypersensitivity vasculitis Cryoglobulinemia Henoch-Schonlein purpura Subacute bacterial endocarditis
Papulosquamous lesions	Psoriatic arthritis Reactive arthritis Discoid lupus Subacute cutaneous lupus erythematosus Secondary syphilis
Annular lesions	Subacute cutaneous lupus erythematosus Lyme disease (erythema chronicum migrans) Acute rheumatic fever (erythema marginatum)
Pustular lesions	Disseminated gonococcal infection Pustular psoriasis Reactive arthritis (keratoderma blenorrhagicum) Behçet disease Acne-associated rheumatic syndromes Sweet syndrome (also painful papule/nodules)

Subcutaneous nodular lesions	Erythema nodosum
	  Sarcoidosis
	  Inflammatory bowel disease
	  Behçet disease
	SLE (lupus profundus)
	Polyarteritis nodosa
	Weber-Christian disease

ANCA, antineutrophil cytoplasmic antibodies; SLE, systemic lupus erythematosus.

an increase in the incidence of hydralazine-induced lupus as well as the more serious hydralazine-induced, antineutrophil cytoplasmic antibody (ANCA)-associated vasculitis. Prior glucocorticoid therapy and alcohol abuse are the leading risk factors for osteonecrosis, which commonly presents as hip pain. Osteonecrosis and bone pain are common manifestations of Gaucher disease. Injection drug use carries the risk of septic arthritis; endocarditis; and infection with hepatitis B, hepatitis C, and HIV—each of which is associated with rheumatic conditions.

Family History

A positive family history, particularly among first-degree relatives, increases the likelihood of certain forms of arthritis. Most notably, the risk of ankylosing spondylitis for children or siblings of a patient with ankylosing spondylitis is as much as 75-fold that of the general population. The relative risk for SLE among first-degree relatives ranges from 20 to 30. A positive family history of rheumatoid arthritis is less helpful. The relative risk for siblings may be as low as 3, and family histories of rheumatoid arthritis can be inaccurate due to confusion with osteoarthritis.

ACUTE ARTHRITIS

Except in cases of trauma, arthritis that is acute in onset is usually inflammatory. Septic arthritis and crystal-induced arthritis typically have an acute onset, and patients often seek medical attention within hours to days after the onset of symptoms. These disease processes, therefore, always warrant serious consideration in cases of acute arthritis. Nonetheless, the differential diagnosis of acute arthritis is broad and includes such entities as rheumatoid arthritis and the spondyloarthropathies; however, these entities more commonly present as chronic conditions.

1. Acute Monoarthritis

ESSENTIAL FEATURES

▶ Septic arthritis is the major diagnostic concern.
▶ Arthrocentesis is the most important diagnostic test.

Initial Clinical Evaluation

The history and physical examination should determine whether the process is acute (onset over hours to days), involves the joint rather than surrounding tissues or bone, and is truly monoarticular. The most common causes of acute monoarthritis are infection, crystal-induced arthritis, and trauma (Table 4–4). In cases of suspected trauma, it is important to ascertain whether the reported trauma was sufficiently severe to account for the joint findings. (Patients with new-onset joint effusions often attribute the joint abnormality to incidental bumps, turns, or other minor trauma.) Joint space infection is the foremost concern in patients with acute pain and swelling in a single joint not clearly due to trauma.

Table 4–4. Common causes of acute monoarthritis.

Cause	Example
Bacterial infection of the joint space	Nongonococcal: especially, *Staphylococcus aureus*, β-hemolytic streptococci, *Streptococcus pneumoniae*, gram-negative organisms Gonococcal: often preceded by a migratory tenosynovitis or oligoarthritis associated with characteristic skin lesions
Crystal-induced arthritis	Gout (monosodium urate crystals) Pseudogout (calcium pyrophosphate dihydrate crystals)
Trauma	Hemarthrosis

A. Laboratory Evaluation

Arthrocentesis is indicated for all cases of unexplained acute monoarthritis. Synovial fluid should be sent for culture (for bacteria, mycobacteria, and fungus), cell count, Gram stain, and examination for crystals by polarized light microscopy. Routine laboratory determinations (eg, complete blood cell count, serum electrolytes and creatinine, and urinalysis) can provide helpful ancillary information. Blood cultures should be obtained if septic arthritis is suspected.

The characteristics of the synovial fluid guide the initial differential diagnosis. Nongonococcal septic arthritis usually causes synovial fluid WBC counts >50,000/mcL and often generates very high counts (>100,000/mcL). The synovial fluid WBC count in gonococcal arthritis is generally lower than in nongonococcal septic arthritis (mean synovial fluid WBC as low as 34,000/mcL in some series). Crystal-induced arthritis is also very inflammatory, with synovial fluid WBC counts often >50,000/mcL; WBC counts >100,000/mcL, however, are uncommon.

Gram staining for bacteria in synovial fluid is relatively insensitive (false-negative rates range from 25% to 50% for nongonococcal septic arthritis and are substantially higher for gonococcal infections). On the other hand, examination of synovial fluid by polarized light microscopy is a sensitive test for urate crystals. Calcium pyrophosphate dihydrate crystals are somewhat more difficult to visualize due to their weaker birefringence, but their detection should not present difficulties for the experienced observer. Thus, the absence of crystals is a strong argument against microcrystalline disease, but a negative Gram stain does not exclude infection. Occasionally, infection and microcrystalline disease coexist; therefore, the finding of crystals in the synovial fluid does not exclude the possibility of infection.

Properly performed cultures of synovial fluid are a sensitive test for nongonococcal septic arthritis (positive in up to 90% of cases). In contrast, synovial fluid cultures are positive in only 20–50% of cases of gonococcal arthritis, and the diagnosis often depends on identification of *Neisseria gonorrhoeae* at other sites by culture or nucleic acid amplification tests. In some cases, however, the diagnosis of disseminated gonococcal infection rests on the response to appropriate antibiotic therapy.

B. Imaging Studies

Radiographs can demonstrate fractures in cases of trauma but usually contribute little to the diagnosis of nontraumatic monoarthritis if the process is truly acute. Radiographic evidence of chondrocalcinosis can be seen in cases of pseudogout and, when there have been recurrent attacks of gout, radiographs may reveal erosions characteristic of gout. Occasionally, imaging studies can be misleading. For example, radiographs may demonstrate osteoarthritis or other chronic conditions that predispose to the development of septic arthritis but are not the proximal cause of the acute joint inflammation.

▶ Differential Diagnosis

A. Inflammatory Monoarthritis

The leading causes of acute inflammatory monoarthritis— infection and crystal-induced arthritis—are difficult to differentiate in the absence of synovial fluid analysis and culture. Patients with septic arthritis may be afebrile and may not manifest a peripheral leukocytosis. Conversely, patients with crystal-induced arthritis can have fever and an elevated peripheral blood WBC count. An elevated serum uric acid level does not establish a diagnosis of gout, and patients with gout can have a normal serum uric acid level at the time of an acute attack.

Septic arthritis indicates the presence of a potentially life-threatening infection and requires prompt treatment with appropriate antibiotics. Delay in the treatment of nongonococcal septic arthritis also causes substantial morbidity due to the rapid destruction of articular cartilage. Acute inflammatory monoarthritis should be considered septic arthritis until there is compelling evidence either against bacterial infection or in favor of an alternative diagnosis.

The differential diagnosis of acute inflammatory monoarthritis not due to septic arthritis, gout, or pseudogout is broad. Many of these entities more commonly present as subacute or chronic processes (see below). Diseases that are typically oligoarticular or polyarticular, such as the spondyloarthropathies and rheumatoid arthritis occasionally begin as an inflammatory monoarthritis ("pseudoseptic" presentation).

B. Noninflammatory Monoarthritis

Noninflammatory synovial fluid can be seen with internal derangements (ie, torn meniscus of the knee). Osteoarthritis of a single joint usually presents with chronic complaints but, on occasion, can cause the acute onset of pain. Similarly, neuropathic arthropathy, amyloidosis, and osteonecrosis usually cause chronic noninflammatory arthritis of one or several joints but occasionally present with acute symptoms.

C. Hemarthrosis

Frank blood on arthrocentesis can be indicative of a fracture or other joint trauma. Hemarthrosis also occurs in patients who are receiving anticoagulant therapy or have a clotting factor deficiency, such as hemophilia. Bloody synovial fluid can be seen in pigmented villonodular synovitis, a rare proliferative disorder of the synovium that presents as a chronic monoarthritis, typically of the knee, in young adulthood.

2. Acute Oligoarthritis

ESSENTIAL FEATURES

▶ Disseminated gonococcal infection, nongonococcal septic arthritis, and the spondyloarthropathies are leading causes of acute inflammatory oligoarthritis.
▶ Arthrocentesis and appropriate cultures are important diagnostic tests.

▶ Initial Clinical Evaluation

Acute oligoarthritis is usually due to an inflammatory process (Table 4–5). Infectious causes of the arthritis need to be excluded. Disseminated gonococcal infection is the most common cause of acute oligoarthritis in sexually active young people. Nongonococcal septic arthritis is usually monoarticular but involves more than one joint in up to 20% of cases.

Spondyloarthropathies typically cause an asymmetric oligoarthritis. Of these, reactive arthritis is most likely to present with acute onset of arthritis and, early in its course, can be difficult to distinguish from disseminated gonococcal infection.

Gout is a common cause of acute oligoarthritis. Oligoarticular gout usually develops after years of antecedent attacks of acute monoarthritis, but it occasionally can be the initial manifestation.

The use of four joints as a dividing line between oligoarthritis and polyarthritis is somewhat arbitrary, and there is overlap between disorders that cause oligoarthritis and polyarthritis. For example, rheumatoid arthritis can be oligoarticular in its early stages. Erythrovirus (parvovirus B19) infection usually causes a true polyarthritis but on occasion produces an oligoarthritis. Conversely, many of the entities listed in Table 4–4 sometimes involve more than four joints.

A. Laboratory Evaluation

Complete blood cell count, serum electrolytes and creatinine, and urinalysis should be obtained. Synovial fluid should

Table 4–5. Differential diagnosis of acute inflammatory oligoarthritis.

- Infection
    - Disseminated gonococcal infection[a]
    - Nongonococcal septic arthritis
    - Bacterial endocarditis[b]
    - Viral[c]
- Post infection
    - Reactive arthritis[b]
    - Rheumatic fever (poststreptococcal arthritis)[d]
- Spondyloarthropathy
    - Reactive arthritis[b]
    - Ankylosing spondylitis[b]
    - Psoriatic arthritis[b]
    - Inflammatory bowel disease[b]
- Oligoarticular presentation of rheumatoid arthritis, systemic lupus erythematosus,[a] adult-onset Still disease, relapsing polychondritis,[a] or other polyarthritis
    - Gout and pseudogout

[a]Often migratory.
[b]Can be associated with back pain.
[c]Usually causes polyarthritis but occasionally oligoarticular and sometimes noninflammatory.
[d]Migratory in children but usually not in adults.

be sent for culture, cell count, Gram stain, and examination for crystals. When disseminated gonococcal infection is suspected, samples from pharynx, urethra, cervix, and rectum—even when asymptomatic—should be tested for *N gonorrhoeae*. Cultures of pharynx, urethra, cervix, and rectum are, in aggregate, positive in 80–90% of cases of disseminated gonococcal infection. Nucleic acid amplification tests of samples from these sites and from urine have greater sensitivity than culture for detection of *N gonorrhoeae*. Urethral and cervical swabs also should be tested for Chlamydiae. If bacterial endocarditis is a possibility, at least 3 blood cultures should be obtained, and a transesophageal echocardiogram may be indicated. Antibodies to streptococcal antigens (eg, streptolysin O) should be determined in cases of suspected acute rheumatic fever or poststreptococcal arthritis. The presence of antibodies to cyclic citrullinated peptides (CCP) is a strong predictor of evolution to rheumatoid arthritis.

B. Imaging Studies

Radiographs usually are of little help if the onset of the oligoarthritis is truly acute.

▶ Differential Diagnosis

Disseminated gonococcal infection usually presents as a migratory tenosynovitis, often with characteristic skin lesions; meningococcemia can cause a similar syndrome but is much less common. Bacterial endocarditis can cause

an oligoarthritis with either septic joints (due to hematogenous spread) or sterile inflammatory synovial fluid (likely due to immune complex disease); back pain is common, particularly in acute bacterial endocarditis (Table 4–5). Reactive arthritis classically follows within 1 to 4 weeks of enteric or genitourinary tract infections, but the triggering infection is sometimes subclinical. In its presenting phase, reactive arthritis has a predilection for the lower extremities and can be associated with significant constitutional signs and symptoms including prominent weight loss and fever. Most patients with the new onset of psoriatic arthritis either have or have had psoriasis, but, in a minority (15%), the arthritis precedes the skin disease. Acute rheumatic fever produces a migratory arthritis in children; in adults, however, poststreptococcal arthritis is usually not migratory and is rarely associated with the other distinctive manifestations of rheumatic fever (eg, rash, subcutaneous nodules, carditis, and chorea). Early disseminated Lyme disease can cause an acute oligoarthritis or monoarthritis (especially of the knee) but more commonly presents as migratory arthralgias.

3. Acute Polyarthritis

 ESSENTIAL FEATURES

▶ Viral infections and rheumatoid arthritis are the leading causes of acute polyarthritis.

▶ Observation to distinguish persistent from self-limited polyarthritis is critical.

▶ Initial Clinical Evaluation

Viral polyarthritis typically resolves over days to a few weeks. Thus, the longer polyarthritis persists, the less likely viral polyarthritis becomes. Rheumatoid arthritis usually has an insidious onset, and patients seek medical care after weeks or months of symptoms. Nonetheless, it begins abruptly in enough patients to warrant consideration as a cause of acute polyarthritis. Acute polyarthritis can also be the initial manifestation of SLE and drug-induced lupus as well as a variety of uncommon entities, including systemic vasculitis (Table 4–6).

A. Laboratory Evaluation

The clinical setting should guide the decision to send tests for specific viral infections (eg, erythrovirus [parvovirus B19] or hepatitis B). If viral polyarthritis is thought unlikely, then routine laboratory studies (including complete blood cell count, serum electrolytes and creatinine, liver function tests, and urinalysis), determinations of the ESR or CRP, and tests for serum rheumatoid factor, antibodies to CCP, and antinuclear antibodies (ANAs) are indicated.

Table 4–6. Differential diagnosis of acute polyarthritis.

- Common
    - Acute viral infections
    - Early disseminated Lyme disease
    - Rheumatoid arthritis
    - Systemic lupus erythematosus
- Uncommon or rare
    - Paraneoplastic polyarthritis
    - Remitting seronegative symmetric polyarthritis with pitting edema
    - Acute sarcoidosis, usually with erythema nodosum and hilar adenopathy
    - Adult-onset Still disease
    - Secondary syphilis
    - Systemic autoimmune diseases and vasculitides
    - Whipple disease

B. Imaging Studies

Joint radiographs are rarely of value in acute polyarthritis and may be deferred until it is clear that the polyarthritis is persistent.

▶ Differential Diagnosis

Many acute viral infections cause joint symptoms, with polyarthralgias being considerably more common than true polyarthritis. The prevalence of polyarthritis is high, however, in adults with acute erythrovirus (parvovirus B19) infection. The pattern of viral polyarthritis often mimics that of rheumatoid arthritis. Adults with acute erythrovirus (parvovirus B19) infection, the cause of "slapped cheek fever" in children, usually have only a faint rash on the trunk or no rash at all. IgM antibodies to erythrovirus (parvovirus B19) are generally present at the onset of joint symptoms and persist for approximately 2 months. Acute hepatitis B causes an immune complex–mediated arthritis, often with urticaria or maculopapular rash, during the preicteric phase of infection; tests for hepatitis B surface antigen are positive. Effective vaccination programs in the United States have substantially reduced the incidence of acute hepatitis B and have eliminated acute rubella infection, which is also associated with acute polyarthritis.

Acute-onset rheumatoid arthritis can be difficult to distinguish from virally induced acute polyarthritis, and many rheumatologists are hesitant to make a diagnosis of rheumatoid arthritis in the acute setting. The joint American College of Rheumatology (ACR) and European League Against Rheumatism (EULAR) 2010 Rheumatoid Arthritis Classification Criteria are weighted toward polyarthritis, the involvement of "small joints" (metacarpophalangeal [MCP] joints, proximal interphalangeal [PIP] joints, second through fifth metatarsophalangeal [MTP] joints, thumb interphalangeal joints, and wrists), the presence of either anti-CCP antibodies or rheumatoid factor, particularly in high titer.

Testing for ANA has sensitivity for SLE but low specificity. When ANAs are detected by indirect immunofluorescence assays using human cell lines (eg, HEp-2 cells), the sensitivity for SLE approaches 100%. False-negative results, however, can occur when ANAs are measured by enzyme-linked immunoabsorbent assays (ELISA) or by high throughput assays using multiplex beads. In a patient with polyarthritis or polyarthralgias, a positive assay for ANA should prompt a careful evaluation for other manifestations of SLE and additional serologic tests (see Chapter 3).

Aletaha D, Neogi T, Silman AJ, et al. 2010 Rheumatoid Arthritis Classification Criteria: an American College of Rheumatology/European League Against Rheumatism Collaborative Initiative. *Arthritis Rheum.* 2010;62:2569. [PMID: 20872595]

CHRONIC ARTHRITIS

1. Chronic Monoarthritis

ESSENTIAL FEATURES

- ▶ Distinguishing between inflammatory and noninflammatory arthritis is a key step toward establishing a diagnosis.
- ▶ Arthrocentesis and imaging studies are important diagnostic tests.

▶ Initial Clinical Evaluation

It is important to determine whether the symptoms and signs point to an inflammatory or noninflammatory process. Indolent infections are a concern with inflammatory monoarthritis of weeks to even months in duration. The particular joint involved influences the differential diagnosis.

A. Laboratory Evaluation

A critical step is to determine whether the monoarthritis is inflammatory or noninflammatory, preferably by analysis of synovial fluid. Synovial fluid should be sent for culture (for bacteria, mycobacteria, and fungus), cell count, and Gram stain and should be examined for crystals by polarized light microscopy.

Routine laboratory studies (eg, complete blood cell count, serum electrolytes and creatinine, and urinalysis) and determinations of the ESR or CRP can provide helpful ancillary information. Patients with inflammatory monoarthritis and negative bacterial cultures should be tested for Lyme disease and for reactivity to purified protein derivative (PPD).

B. Imaging Studies

In contrast to acute monoarthritis, radiographs can be helpful in the evaluation of processes present for weeks or more and

Table 4–7. Differential diagnosis of chronic inflammatory monoarthritis.

- Infection
    - Nongonococcal septic arthritis
    - Gonococcal
    - Lyme disease and other spirochetal infections
    - Mycobacterial
    - Fungal
    - Viral[a]
- Crystal-induced arthritis
    - Gout
    - Pseudogout
    - Calcium apatite crystals[b]
- Monoarticular presentation of an oligoarthritis or polyarthritis
    - Spondyloarthropathy
    - Rheumatoid arthritis
    - Lupus and other systemic autoimmune diseases
- Sarcoidosis[a]
- Familial Mediterranean fever and other inherited periodic fever syndromes[c]
- Amyloidosis[a,c]
- Foreign-body synovitis due to plant thorns, sea urchin spikes, wood fragments, etc.[c]
- Pigmented villonodular synovitis[c,d]

[a]Also can cause noninflammatory synovial fluid.
[b]Not detected by polarized light microscopy.
[c]Uncommon or rare.
[d]Commonly associated with bloody, or blood-tinged brown, synovial fluid.

Table 4–8. Differential diagnosis of chronic noninflammatory monoarthritis.

Osteoarthritis
Internal derangements (eg, torn meniscus)[a]
Chondromalacia patellae[a]
Osteonecrosis[a]
Neuropathic (Charcot) arthropathy[c]
Sarcoidosis[a-c]
Amyloidosis[a-c]

[a]Radiograph of the affected joint often normal at presentation.
[b]Can also cause inflammatory synovial fluid.
[c]Uncommon or rare.

can point to the correct diagnosis in cases of infection, osteoarthritis, osteonecrosis, neuropathic joints, and other entities.

▶ Differential Diagnosis

A. Inflammatory

A wide range of disease processes can cause inflammatory arthritis in a single joint for several weeks or longer (Table 4–7). Most patients with septic arthritis and gonococcal arthritis experience significant pain in the infected joint and seek medical attention within hours to days of the onset of symptoms. However, patients occasionally seek medical care after a delay of several weeks, particularly if symptoms have been partially masked by the use of nonsteroidal anti-inflammatory drugs, antibiotics, or glucocorticoids (systemic or intra-articular).

Untreated indolent infections, on the other hand, commonly present after weeks or more of symptoms. These are associated with negative synovial fluid cultures for bacteria and require additional diagnostic tests and cultures to establish the correct diagnosis. Chronic Lyme disease can cause an inflammatory monoarthritis, often of the knee, with synovial fluid WBC typically in the 10,000–25,000/mcL range. Tuberculous infection of a joint can present after days, weeks, or months of symptoms. Smears for acid-fast bacilli are positive in only 20% of cases; cultures for mycobacteria are positive in 80% but take weeks. Synovial biopsy can greatly expedite the diagnosis of tuberculous arthritis and is also indicated in suspected cases of fungal arthritis.

B. Noninflammatory

Osteoarthritis is the leading cause of chronic noninflammatory monoarthritis, particularly when the hip, knee, first carpometacarpal joint, or acromioclavicular joint is involved (Table 4–8). Internal derangements, such as a torn meniscus in the knee, often produce mechanical symptoms and characteristic findings on physical examination. Pain is frequently a prominent feature of osteonecrosis, which can produce large knee effusions when the distal femur is involved. Radiographs are often normal early in the course of osteonecrosis, and diagnosis may require MRI. Hip pain with a normal radiograph should raise the possibility of early osteonecrosis, particularly if the patient is relatively young and has a risk factor for osteonecrosis. Diabetes mellitus is the most common underlying cause of neuropathic arthropathy, which should be considered in a diabetic patient with foot, ankle, or knee arthritis. The involved joint may be warm and painful, but the joint fluid is typically noninflammatory. Radiographs usually show characteristic neuropathic changes.

2. Chronic Oligoarthritis

 ESSENTIAL FEATURES

▶ Careful delineation of the arthritis and detection of extra-articular disease facilitate accurate diagnosis.

▶ Radiographs are often of diagnostic value.

Table 4–9. Differential diagnosis of chronic oligoarthritis.

Inflammatory Causes	Noninflammatory Causes
Common	
Spondyloarthropathy	Osteoarthritis
Reactive arthritis[a]	
Ankylosing spondylitis[a]	
Psoriatic arthritis[a]	
Inflammatory bowel disease[a]	
Atypical presentation of rheumatoid arthritis	
Gout	
Uncommon or rare	
Subacute bacterial endocarditis	Hypothyroidism
Sarcoidosis[b]	Amyloidosis
Behçet disease	
Relapsing polychondritis	
Celiac disease[a]	

[a]Can be associated with involvement of the axial skeleton.
[b]Can be a migratory arthritis and have either inflammatory or noninflammatory synovial fluid.

▶ Initial Clinical Evaluation

Spondyloarthropathies are the most common cause of chronic inflammatory oligoarthritis (Table 4–9). For months or longer, however, it may be difficult to distinguish spondyloarthropathies from early-onset rheumatoid arthritis. Osteoarthritis commonly presents as a noninflammatory oligoarthritis of the hips or knees and usually does not present diagnostic difficulties.

A. Laboratory Evaluation

Synovial fluid should be analyzed for crystals and cultured. The distinction between inflammatory and noninflammatory chronic oligoarthritis often can be made on clinical grounds but is confirmed by the synovial fluid WBC count.

Antibodies to CCP and rheumatoid factor have similar sensitivity in identifying rheumatoid arthritis, but the antibodies to CCP have greater specificity and can help establish the diagnosis in the proper clinical context. Testing for HLA-B27 has usefulness in certain circumstances.

B. Imaging Studies

Radiographs can be of considerable value. An experienced radiologist or rheumatologist often can distinguish among the erosions of the spondyloarthropathies, rheumatoid arthritis, and gout. Radiographic demonstration of sacroiliitis points to a spondyloarthropathy and narrows the differential diagnosis considerably.

▶ Differential Diagnosis

Although spondyloarthropathies typically cause an asymmetric oligoarthritis and rheumatoid arthritis is usually a symmetric polyarthritis, it can be difficult to differentiate these entities in patients with early disease. Several features are helpful in making this distinction. Ankylosing spondylitis always, and the other spondyloarthropathies often, produce inflammatory axial skeleton disease with sacroiliitis that causes pain and stiffness in the low back, particularly in the morning. Sacroiliitis is not a feature of rheumatoid arthritis, which involves the cervical spine but no other part of the axial skeleton. The prominent tenosynovitis of the spondyloarthropathies can produce dactylitis ("sausage digits") of the toes or fingers. Dactylitis is not seen in rheumatoid arthritis. (Dactylitis is not specific for the spondyloarthropathies; it also occurs in sarcoidosis and gout). Reactive arthritis and the arthritis of inflammatory bowel disease have a predilection for the lower extremities. Rheumatoid arthritis invariably involves the hands, and >90% of cases eventually have wrist arthritis.

Many of the entities that cause chronic oligoarthritis have extra-articular manifestations that point to the correct diagnosis but that are easily overlooked. For example, psoriasis may be subtle, and the patient may be unaware of psoriatic lesions, particularly in the umbilicus, the external auditory canal, the scalp, and the anal cleft. The oral ulcers of reactive arthritis are painless and usually not detected unless specifically sought by the examining physician. Patients with inflammatory bowel disease may not volunteer that they have chronic diarrhea, particularly if bowel symptoms are intermittent. Antecedent anterior uveitis can be an important clue to the presence of a spondyloarthropathy, but patients generally do not associate ocular inflammation with arthritis and may not mention a past episode of anterior uveitis unless asked directly.

3. Chronic Polyarthritis

 ESSENTIAL FEATURES

▶ Rheumatoid arthritis and osteoarthritis are the leading causes of chronic polyarthritis.
▶ Careful delineation of the joints involved, particularly in the hands, can help point to the correct diagnosis.

▶ Initial Clinical Evaluation

Rheumatoid arthritis is the leading cause of chronic inflammatory polyarthritis, and osteoarthritis is the most common cause of chronic noninflammatory polyarthritis. Nonetheless, polyarthritis that persists for weeks or more has many possible etiologies and warrants careful diagnostic

Table 4–10. Differential diagnosis of chronic polyarthritis.

Inflammatory Polyarthritis	Noninflammatory Polyarthritis
Common	
Rheumatoid arthritis	Primary generalized osteoarthritis
Systemic lupus erythematosus	Hemochromatosis[a]
Spondyloarthropathies (especially psoriatic arthritis) Chronic hepatitis C infection Gout Drug-induced lupus syndrome	Calcium pyrophosphate deposition disease[a]
Uncommon or rare	
Paraneoplastic polyarthritis Remitting seronegative symmetric polyarthritis with pitting edema Adult-onset Still disease Systemic autoimmune diseases and vasculitides Sjögren syndrome Viral infections other than hepatitis C Whipple disease	

[a]Degenerative changes are seen on radiographs; can cause flares with inflammatory synovial fluid.

evaluation (Table 4–10). As is the case with other forms of arthritis, the distinction between inflammatory and noninflammatory processes is critical.

A. Laboratory Evaluation

If arthrocentesis is feasible, synovial fluid should be obtained and sent for cell count and analysis for crystals. Routine laboratory investigations (complete blood cell count, serum electrolytes and creatinine, and urinalysis) should be done. If the process appears inflammatory, studies also should include determinations of the ESR or CRP and tests for serum rheumatoid factor, anti-CCP antibodies, ANA, and hepatitis B and C infection.

B. Imaging Studies

Radiographs are indicated in most cases of chronic polyarthritis of the hand. Radiographs of the hand usually show characteristic changes at the time of presentation of primary generalized osteoarthritis, hemochromatosis, calcium pyrophosphate deposition disease, and chronic tophaceous gout. In cases of rheumatoid arthritis and the spondyloarthropathies, however, the likelihood of radiographic joint erosions and other characteristic findings increases with the duration of the polyarthritis; hand radiographs may be normal or demonstrate nonspecific changes only, for months or longer. Radiographs of the feet can reveal rheumatoid erosions even when hand films are unrevealing. The polyarthritis of

SLE, drug-induced lupus, and chronic hepatitis C is usually nonerosive and does not produce characteristic radiographic findings.

► Differential Diagnosis

Osteoarthritis and rheumatoid arthritis have different patterns of joint involvement in the hand. Osteoarthritis involves the distal interphalangeal (DIP) and PIP joints and the first carpometacarpal joint. Rheumatoid arthritis, in contrast, involves the PIP and MCP joints and the wrists.

Osteoarthritis and rheumatoid arthritis typically spare certain joints. Osteoarthritis usually does not involve the MCP joints, wrists, elbows, glenohumeral joints, and ankles; degenerative arthritis of these joints raises the possibility of antecedent trauma, calcium pyrophosphate deposition disease, underlying osteonecrosis, or neuropathic arthropathy. Rheumatoid arthritis usually spares DIP joints, the thoracic and lumbosacral spine, and sacroiliac joints.

In generalized osteoarthritis, interphalangeal joints, particularly the DIPs, may appear to be inflamed ("inflammatory osteoarthritis") and thus cause some diagnostic uncertainty. Radiographs, however, usually show typical degenerative changes (irregular joint-space narrowing, sclerosis, and osteophytes). Psoriatic arthritis also commonly involves the DIP joints, usually with radiographic changes distinct from those of osteoarthritis. Psoriatic changes of the fingernail on the same digit often occur concomitantly with psoriatic involvement of a DIP joint.

Table 4–11. Clinical findings and their associated diagnoses that can mimic chronic rheumatoid arthritis.

Clinical Finding	Examples of Associated Diagnoses
Arthritis with radiographic erosions	Spondyloarthropathies, especially psoriatic arthritis Gout
Arthritis with positive rheumatoid factor	Chronic hepatitis C infection Systemic lupus erythematosus Sarcoidosis Systemic vasculitides Polymyositis/dermatomyositis Subacute bacterial endocarditis
Arthritis with nodules	Chronic tophaceous gout Granulomatosis with polyangiitis (formerly Wegener granulomatosis) Eosinophilic granulomatosis with polyangiitis (Churg-Strauss syndrome) Hyperlipoproteinemia (rare) Multicentric reticulohistiocytosis (rare)
Arthritis of metacarpophalangeal joints and/or wrists	Hemochromatosis Calcium pyrophosphate deposition disease

Many diseases can mimic rheumatoid arthritis, but several warrant particular emphasis (Table 4–11). Features that distinguish rheumatoid arthritis and the spondyloarthropathies are discussed above. Chronic infection with hepatitis C can produce a symmetric polyarthritis and a positive test for rheumatoid factor (but not for anti-CCP antibodies). The polyarthritis of SLE is nonerosive but can lead to reducible "swan neck" deformities of the fingers. On occasion, chronic tophaceous gout is a remarkable mimic of rheumatoid arthritis, with tophi mistaken for rheumatoid nodules. Gout is not associated with rheumatoid factor (virtually all cases of nodular rheumatoid arthritis are seropositive), and the erosions of gout and rheumatoid arthritis have different radiographic characteristics. Analysis of synovial fluid for urate crystals is the definitive diagnostic test. Hemochromatosis and other causes of calcium pyrophosphate deposition disease lead to arthritis of the MCPs (especially the second and third) and wrists; radiographs often reveal "hook-like" osteophytes of the MCPs and degenerative changes, usually with chondrocalcinosis, of the wrist.

Although rheumatoid arthritis is the leading cause of chronic inflammatory polyarthritis, physicians must be certain that rheumatoid arthritis accounts for the full clinical picture. Rheumatoid arthritis is not a plausible explanation for the following: fever >38.3°C, substantial weight loss, significant adenopathy, rashes (apart from subcutaneous nodules), hematuria, and proteinuria. Failure to account for these additional clinical findings can lead to a failure to diagnose SLE, Still disease, subacute bacterial endocarditis, paraneoplastic syndromes, vasculitides, and the like.

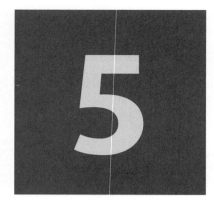

Approach to the Adolescent with Arthritis

Jennifer K. Turner, MD
Peggy Schlesinger, MD

ESSENTIAL FEATURES

▶ Inflammatory and noninflammatory conditions can cause joint pain in adolescents.
▶ Appropriate therapy for adolescents with arthritis requires not only treatment of the disease, but also attention to developmental needs and discussion of school and vocational issues.

▶ General Considerations

There are many causes of joint pain occurring in childhood and adolescence (Table 5–1). Diagnostic accuracy is very important to ensure that the patient receives appropriate treatment.

The first step in evaluating a young patient who complains of musculoskeletal discomfort is to distinguish **arthritis** (true synovitis and joint swelling) from **arthralgia** (pain in and around joints). Pain in and around the joints without synovitis or swelling is usually caused by trauma, mechanical factors, or soft tissue syndromes. Excruciating joint pain and swelling, often with erythema, may indicate malignancy. A careful history of recent infections and exposures, as well as immunizations, can highlight possible infection-related causes of joint swelling and pain in the adolescent age group. Chronic childhood arthritis is one of the five most common chronic diseases of childhood, occurring with a frequency greater than diabetes or cystic fibrosis. Juvenile idiopathic arthritis (JIA), including psoriatic arthritis and the spondyloarthropathies of childhood, is the most common cause of chronic arthritis in childhood and adolescence.

▶ Evaluation

The initial evaluation of an adolescent with a possible rheumatic disease includes a complete history and physical examination. In this age group, special attention should be paid to the following issues:

- Age at menarche.
- Is the patient skeletally mature? (A rough guide: is shoe size changing with every new pair?)
- Is the patient sexually active?
- Have there been prolonged or recurrent school absences?
- Are there barriers at school that make participation or attendance difficult?
- Has there been uninterrupted participation in physical education?
- Is there a history of participation in athletics?
- In what way does the patient make accommodations to compensate for arthritis symptoms (eg, wearing elastic waist sweat pants instead of jeans with buttons and zippers, avoiding going to the bathroom at school because of difficulty getting on and off the toilet).
- Does the patient have a best friend with whom she or he can discuss arthritis issues?
- Is there a receptive teacher or school counselor to contact if a Section 504 or Individualized Education Plan (IEP) is needed?
- Have vocational and career goals been identified?
- Has a disability application been filed?

INFECTIONS

Rubella, mononucleosis, hepatitis B and C, and varicella infections have all been associated with transient joint swelling (<6 weeks) and should be considered in the differential diagnosis of arthritis in this age group (Table 5–1). Immunization for varicella and the vaccine for MMR (measles, mumps, rubella) may be given to teenagers who did not receive their full complement of vaccinations as children.

Table 5–1. Differential diagnosis of arthritis in adolescents.

Infection-related	Metabolic/genetic
Lyme disease	Cystic fibrosis
Septic arthritis	Diabetes
Gonococcal arthritis	Sickle cell disease
Erythrovirus (parvovirus B19)	**Connective tissue diseases**
Mononucleosis	Systemic lupus
Cytomegalovirus	erythematosus
HIV	Dermatomyositis
Varicella	Mixed connective
Endocarditis	tissue disease
Streptococcal-associated arthritis	Sarcoidosis
Acute rheumatic fever	Vasculitis
Hepatitis B and C	**Noninflammatory**
Toxic synovitis	**conditions**
Malignancy	Chondromalacia patellae
Bone tumors	Hypermobility syndrome
Leukemia	Avascular necrosis
Lymphoma	Skeletal dysplasias
Neuroblastoma	Slipped capital
Juvenile idiopathic arthritis (JIA)	femoral epiphysis
Polyarticular JIA	Osgood-Schlatter disease
Systemic-onset JIA	Sever disease
Oligoarticular JIA (recurrent)	Scheuermann disease
Psoriatic arthritis	Osteochondritis dessicans
Enthesitis-related arthritis (ERA)	Synovial chondromatosis
Arthritis of inflammatory bowel	Synovial hemangioma
disease	Pigmented villonodular
Reactive arthritis	synovitis
Juvenile-onset spondylitis	

Vaccination with these attenuated viruses has also been associated with transient arthritis symptoms.

Erythrovirus (parvovirus B19) infection in the older child can cause fever and large and small joint polyarthritis with a morbilliform rash. Lyme disease, caused by *Borrelia burgdorferi*, can initially present with a rash followed by migratory, large joint arthritis, particularly the knee. A significant number of patients do not recall a tick bite or rash, so it is important to test patients who reside in or who have visited a Lyme endemic area. It is important to distinguish Lyme disease from JIA so that proper antibiotic therapy can be given. Rheumatic fever is now rare, but the syndrome of poststreptococcal arthritis is not uncommon. True synovitis can develop within 7–10 days in adolescents with antecedent streptococcal infection as a result of the molecular mimicry involved in the immune response to the streptococcal infection. In streptococcal-associated arthritis, the chorea and carditis of rheumatic fever are absent, and joint symptoms resolve completely but can recur with subsequent streptococcal infections (see Chapter 52).

Bloody diarrheal illnesses caused by *Campylobacter, Salmonella, Shigella, Yersinia*, and toxigenic *Escherichia coli* can be associated with postinfectious reactive arthritis in teenagers, particularly those who are HLA-B27 positive.

Sexually active teenagers may contract chlamydia, which is associated with reactive arthritis, or gonococcal infection, which can disseminate and produce a characteristic dermatitis-arthritis syndrome (see Chapter 46).

MECHANICAL MIMICS

Noninflammatory conditions can cause joint pain and swelling in the adolescent patient, which can mimic arthritis and be confusing diagnostically. The hallmark of this group of disorders is pain that worsens with activity in the absence of signs and symptoms of inflammation. Chondromalacia patellae, osteochondritis dessicans, Osgood-Schlatter, Sever syndrome, hypermobility syndromes, slipped capital femoral epiphysis, Legg-Calvé-Perthes disease, and Scheuermann disease, represent the most common causes of noninflammatory joint pain in this age group.

Chondromalacia patellae, or **patellofemoral syndrome,** is commonly seen in teenage girls and presents as unilateral or bilateral knee pain that worsens with activity. Any activity that involves weight bearing on a bent knee can aggravate the pain of this condition. Climbing stairs, using the clutch in a car, standing up after prolonged sitting, participation in gym class, and competitive athletic activities can be particularly troublesome. A minority of girls with chondromalacia patellae (approximately 10%) have knee swelling in addition to knee pain, and even fewer of these patients have persistent knee effusion lasting more than 6 weeks. When this does occur, chondromalacia patellae is easily confused with JIA.

The diagnosis of chondromalacia patellae is confirmed by crepitus and a positive patellar inhibition test on examination, together with a history of knee pain that worsens with activity, the absence of morning stiffness, and the absence of other affected joints, even in patients with prolonged knee swelling. Isometric quadriceps strengthening exercises (Figure 5–1)

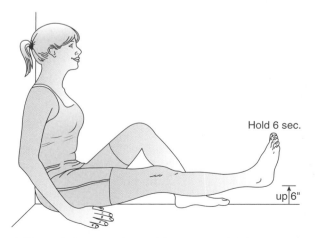

Hold 6 sec.

up 6"

▲ **Figure 5–1.** Isometric quadriceps-strengthening exercise.

with the leg held externally rotated at the hip to provide particular focus on the vastus medialis muscle reduces pain and swelling and allows for a return to normal activity, including competitive athletics. Nonsteroidal anti-inflammatory drugs (NSAIDs) (Table 5–2), ice, and occasionally joint injection with 20 mg triamcinolone hexacetonide mixed with 2 mL of a long-acting local anesthetic reduces pain and swelling, allowing continued progress in an exercise program. Failure to comply with the program of regular isometric quadriceps strengthening exercises often leads to recurrence of the knee pain, with or without swelling. The pain can be a good reminder to teenagers to make daily quadriceps exercises a part of their routine. Symptoms of chondromalacia patellae can last for several years. Despite several years of knee pain as teenagers, degenerative patello-femoral joint disease does not develop in most of these patients as they reach adulthood.

Osteochondritis dessicans and **Osgood-Schlatter disease** are common causes of knee or ankle pain in adolescent boys. In osteochondritis dessicans, a piece of cartilage fractures, producing pain and swelling in the affected joint. Knees (femoral condyles) and ankles (dome of the talus) are the most commonly affected joints. There is often a history of trauma to the affected joint, typically in the form of repeated minor trauma or overuse, and the recommended course of action is orthopedic consultation. Osgood-Schlatter disease

is caused by apophysitis (injury or inflammation at the site of growth cartilage where tendons insert) at the insertion of the patellar tendon onto the tibial tubercle, with localized pain in this area just below the knee. True synovitis is rare; however, the presence of painful swelling in close proximity to the knee joint can easily be confused with true arthritis.

Sever disease is a syndrome of similar etiology, with calcaneal apophysitis occurring at the growth plate of the heel. This disorder is commonly seen in soccer players, and treatment may include the use of a heel cup, NSAIDs, and ice. Sever disease is self-limited and unrelated to any of the HLA-B27 related spondyloarthropathies, although the occurrence of heel pain in the adolescent male may be misleading to practitioners.

Joint hypermobility syndrome is familial and can be troublesome in the adolescent. Some teenagers are "double jointed," with ligamentous laxity and freely subluxing shoulders, patellae, and hips. The increased joint range of motion often leads to pain that is aggravated by continued use or repetitive activity, especially when they participate in competitive athletics. Weight lifting and strength training can help offset the tendency to subluxation in these patients by producing tight, bulky muscles to help provide internal stability to the joint. This is particularly helpful for shoulder and knee joints, where increasing muscle bulk and tone in the rotator cuff mechanism and the quadriceps can reduce pain and bring useful joint excursion back to normal levels.

Isolated hip pain in adolescence is uncommon and should prompt investigation for a mechanical etiology, beginning with plain radiographs. **Slipped capital femoral epiphysis** is a common cause of hip pain in teenage boys. Typically, the adolescent complains of groin pain or referred pain in the knee that worsens with activity. There is often insidious onset of a limp. Obesity is a predisposing factor in the development of this idiopathic disorder. Once the primary care clinician confirms the diagnosis with a radiograph, an orthopedic consultation should be obtained. Although slipped capital femoral epiphysis is usually unilateral at onset, bilateral involvement eventually develops in 30–45% of patients.

Legg-Calvé-Perthes disease typically occurs in a somewhat younger age group, most commonly in boys 5–10 years of age, but extends into the adolescent age group. It is caused by an idiopathic avascular necrosis of the femoral head and presents with limp and hip pain. Early in the disease course, plain radiographs may appear normal, and MRI has greater sensitivity for early detection of disease. Orthopedic consultation is recommended, but it is unclear whether surgical intervention results in a better outcome than splinting.

Scheuermann disease, or vertebral apophysitis, can cause back pain in adolescents. It typically involves three contiguous vertebrae with involvement of the end plates at each level; lower thoracic vertebrae are most commonly affected and thoracic kyphosis can develop in later life. This condition is easily confused with juvenile onset spondylitis because both cause back pain in teenagers. Imaging with plain radiographs

Table 5–2. Nonsteroidal anti-inflammatory drugs (NSAIDs) used in pediatric patients.[a]

Drug	Dose	Formulation
Naproxen	20 mg/kg/d 10 mg/kg/dose twice daily up to 1000 mg/d	Liquid: 125 mg/5 mL Tablet: 220 mg, available over the counter Twice-daily dosing is convenient
Ibuprofen	40 mg/kg/d 10 mg/kg/dose four times daily up to 2400 mg/d	Liquid: 100 mg/5 mL Tablet: 200 mg, available over the counter
Tolmetin	30 mg/kg/d 10 mg/kg/dose four times daily up to 1800 mg/d	Tablets: 200, 400, and 600 mg
Indomethacin	1–3 mg/kg/d three or four times daily up to 200 mg/d	Liquid: 25 mg/5 mL Approved for patients younger than 14 years Used in younger patients with systemic-onset JIA or spondylitis
Meloxicam	0.125 mg/kg/d up to 7.5 mg/d	Liquid: 7.5 mg/mL Tablet: 7.5 and 15 mg Once-a-day dosing is convenient

[a]As of this writing, other NSAIDs have not been approved by the Food and Drug Administration for use in the pediatric age group. JIA, juvenile idiopathic arthritis.

can be helpful in establishing the diagnosis, and a lateral view shows anterior vertebral wedging and irregularity of the vertebral end plates (Schmorl nodes).

JUVENILE IDIOPATHIC ARTHRITIS

JIA is a heterogeneous group of several different disorders, all of which can cause persistent synovitis lasting 6 weeks or longer in patients younger than 17 years. The subtypes of JIA are systemic onset (Still disease), enthesitis-related arthritis (ERA), psoriatic arthritis, oligoarticular, polyarticular seronegative, polyarticular seropositive, and undifferentiated arthritis. The systemic onset, ERA, and polyarticular seropositive subgroups are more commonly seen in the adolescent age group. The diagnosis of JIA is based on the following clinical criteria: (1) the age of disease onset; (2) the number and type of joints involved; and (3) the presence of associated symptoms, such as rash, fever, or iritis. The subgroup of JIA is determined by the pattern of the illness during the first 6 months of symptoms. There is no definitive test or radiographic finding that can confirm the diagnosis of JIA, but laboratory tests and radiographs can help exclude alternative causes of arthritis in children. JIA is reviewed in Chapter 20.

RHEUMATIC DISEASES & SYNDROMES

Other rheumatic syndromes that are well known in adults, such as Raynaud phenomenon and fibromyalgia, can present initially in adolescence. The majority of teenagers who have Raynaud phenomenon have no associated rheumatic disease, and reassurance regarding the prognosis can be given liberally. Although a positive antinuclear antibody test may be present in these patients, it is not as useful as nailfold capillaroscopy in predicting in which patients systemic rheumatic disease will develop. In young adults with Raynaud phenomenon, abnormal nailfold capillaroscopy showing the typical pattern of dilation and dropout of capillary loops strongly correlates with the development of systemic disease, either progressive systemic sclerosis or juvenile dermatomyositis. Normal nailfold capillaries are seen in adolescents with isolated Raynaud phenomenon. In adolescents with Raynaud phenomenon in association with other rheumatic diseases, such as systemic lupus erythematosus (SLE), the nailfold capillary pattern is normal.

Treatment of Raynaud phenomenon is directed at reducing the frequency of vasospastic episodes by keeping the hands and feet warm. Unfortunately, asking teenagers to wear socks and gloves to keep their extremities warm can be as effective as asking them to turn in homework early. Fortunately, treatment with biofeedback, solid fuel hand warmers, and medications (such as extended-release niacin, diltiazem, and transdermal nitroglycerin) can be used when needed, giving the patient better control over their symptoms.

Sleep issues loom large in adolescence. Teenagers seem to require much more sleep than adults—and also more than younger children. The growth spurt and pubertal changes at this age are fueled by hormones, such as growth hormone, that are secreted in a circadian rhythm with the highest output during the night. Sleep disorders can present in early adolescence with fibromyalgia-like arthralgias and myalgias. The good news is that these symptoms are amenable to therapeutic intervention. Proper sleep hygiene is essential, including the removal of televisions, video games, and telephone and text-messaging systems from the bedroom. If the patient regularly snores, a sleep study should be done to evaluate for obstructive sleep apnea. Treatment with low-dose amitriptyline (10–30 mg each night at bedtime) or cyclobenzaprine (10–30 mg each night at bedtime) can correct a nonrestorative sleep pattern, relieving the pain that keeps them from falling asleep as well as the pain that wakens them throughout the night. Once the sleep cycle has been reset, a gradually increasing exercise program helps build specific muscle strength and improve endurance, thus allowing the patient to return to normal activity. As in adults, the disability from this fibromyalgia-like syndrome can be extreme; however, with proper treatment the outlook for a return to normal activity is excellent.

Regional pain syndromes and soft tissue rheumatism present special challenges when they occur in the adolescent age group. Treatment is focused on returning the patient to normal activity as quickly as possible and addressing the accompanying psychosocial issues that can complicate recovery. Intensive physical therapy combined with psychological support for the patient and family is the usual treatment of choice.

SLE can present in adolescence and cause arthritis in this age group. The female to male ratio of SLE is approximately 2:1 before puberty and 8:1 after puberty. The changing hormonal milieu of teenage girls can be incendiary, causing flares of this disease during these difficult years. Neuropsychiatric involvement with SLE can be particularly challenging to diagnose and treat in adolescent girls with frequent mood swings.

Vasculitides, including granulomatosis with polyangiitis (formerly Wegener granulomatosis), microscopic polyangiitis, polyarteritis nodosa, Henoch-Schönlein purpura, leukocytoclastic vasculitis, among others, are also seen in the adolescent age group with signs and symptoms at presentation very similar to the adult form of the disease.

SCHOOL ISSUES

The goal of treatment should be to help the teenager return to normal function, which in most cases involves regular school attendance as well as participation in after school activities. Public Law 94-142 guarantees students with disabling conditions access to an education in the public schools and requires modifications in order to accomplish this. Adjustment of the school program may be needed to accomplish the goal of regular attendance. Examples of common modifications that can be done in public school include scheduling core classes later in the day or allowing a late start to accommodate morning stiffness, arranging classes all on one level of the building or providing access to an elevator to avoid stairs, offering an adaptive physical education program, and providing an extra set of textbooks to keep at home. Providing additional time for in class writing assignments and allowing stretch breaks during the day can also be helpful. The necessary changes can be made on an individual basis or by utilizing the Section 504 or IEP process. Parent advocacy programs are in place in many states to help educate parents on the rights of disabled students, and how to work within the public school system to ensure quality education for their children.

DEVELOPMENTAL STAGES OF ADOLESCENCE

During the teenage years, the adolescent begins to establish relationships outside the family, with the ultimate goal of achieving independence from the nuclear family. In the process, teenagers deconstruct and reconstruct their self-image, finding an identity that encompasses their new experiences. During this period, the parents' roles change from primary caregivers to advocates, allowing and encouraging more independence in their offspring.

It is important that these changes be incorporated into the medical setting as well. Adolescents want to be taken seriously in the physician-patient encounter. The adolescent may be more comfortable transitioning to an internal medicine physician for their primary care rather than their previous pediatric caregiver. They may prefer to see the practitioner by themselves, without a parent present. The physician can use this time alone with the young person to talk over feelings about many sensitive subjects such as body image concerns, sexuality, worries about the future, and the impact of disability on everyday activities. Alcohol and drug use should be discussed, as these substances can interact with medications used to treat rheumatic diseases, and may affect decisions about which therapies are most appropriate for a particular patient. Some useful tasks that older teenagers can do to help them prepare for their own self care include filling out their own health history forms and, when they reach age 18 years, calling to schedule their own appointments and medication refills.

Parents must be heard as well, often in a separate session, so that the physician has an accurate picture of the situation as a whole. Parental concerns can overwhelm both the patient and the physician; parents tend to be overprotective toward teenagers with a chronic illness. Opportunities will arise when the physician can point out to parents how appropriately their teenager is responding to his or her illness. This will help parents begin to see their teenagers as capable managers of their illness. Camps for children with arthritis of all ages are another good place to encourage independence and appropriate self-care, while also building self-esteem. Parents can help facilitate independence in the older teenager by finding out the age limits of their health care policy as the teenager approaches adulthood, as well as working together with the teenager to fill out a prior health history form (examples available at several online sites) including immunizations, major illnesses, and previous medications, which the patient can take to appointments with future health care providers.

The task of adolescents is to put together a healthy self-concept as they near adulthood, ideally one that incorporates their illness but is not solely defined by it. They must also take on the responsibility of caring for themselves and their disease. The physician's role is to encourage this development in the adolescent patient, while helping parents evolve comfortably into a secondary role by pointing out examples when the patient is responding appropriately and by modeling encouragement for such behaviors. For a time, it may feel as if there are two patients in the family—the adolescent and the parents—until such time as the adolescent can feel comfortable taking primary responsibility for his or her health. This transition is absolutely necessary if patients are to become effective advocates for themselves and responsible members of the healing partnership.

VOCATIONAL ISSUES

In addition to the transition from adolescence to adulthood, the teenager must navigate the road from high school to post-secondary education and the world of employment. There are approximately 200 transition-planning programs in the United States that address the vocational needs of teenagers with chronic and potentially disabling conditions, but they cannot reach everyone who needs assistance. Vocational rehabilitation services can begin career counseling and the employment identification process with teenagers during the senior year of high school. Case management services may continue depending on whether or not the patient qualifies for Social Security disability benefits. Working with patients to identify specific career goals and individual abilities can help adolescents focus their studies and make appropriate plans for their future. The assistance of the clinician in this area is essential to making this transition to adulthood a success.

[Adolescent Health Transition Project]
    http://depts.washington.edu/healthtr/

[Arthritis Foundation]
    http://www.arthritis.org/AFAStore/StartRead.
        asp?idProduct=3370
    http://www.arthritis.org/ja-kgat.php

Cassidy JT. *Textbook of Pediatric Rheumatology.* 4th ed. Philadelphia, Pa: WB Saunders Co; 2001.

Isenberg DA, Miller JJ, eds. *Adolescent Rheumatology.* London: Martin Dunitz; 1999.

[Kidhealth]
    http://kidshealth.org/teen/diseases_conditions/bones/juv_
        rheumatoid_arthritis.html

McDonagh JE, Southwood TR, Ryder CAJ. Bridging the gap in rheumatology. *Ann Rheum Dis.* 2000;59:86.

Tucker LB, Cabral DA. Transition of the adolescent patient with rheumatic disease: Issues to consider. *Pediatr Clin North Am.* 2005;52:641. [PMID: 15820382]

White PH. Transition: a future promise for children and adolescents with special health care needs and disabilities. *Rheum Dis Clin North Am.* 2002;28:687. [PMID: 12380376]

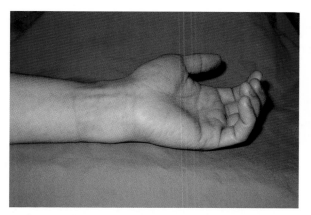

▲ **Plate 1.** The normal repose cascade. When the hand is at rest, the fingers should be held with the small finger flexed slightly more than the ring finger. The ring finger is slightly more flexed than the long finger, and the long finger is slightly flexed more than the index finger.

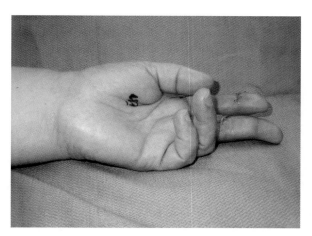

▲ **Plate 2.** This patient has flexor tendon lacerations of the left index and long fingers. Note the disturbance in the repose cascade, as the index and long fingers are extended.

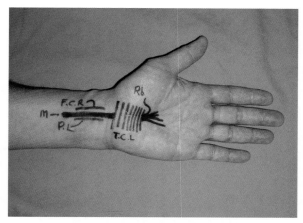

▲ **Plate 3.** The left hand drawn with the relevant structures at the proximal hand and distal forearm. The median nerve (M) becomes more superficial as it approaches the distal one third of the forearm, but still deep to both the palmaris longus tendon (P.L.) and the flexor carpi radialis (F.C.R.). As the median nerve continues distally into the hand, it enters the carpal tunnel. The roof of the carpal tunnel is formed by the transverse carpal retinaculum (T.C.L). The recurrent branch (Rb) generally emerges at the distal edge of the transverse carpal ligament. Occasionally, it will emerge through the fibers of the ligament. The median nerve continues through the proximal hand and then divides into its digital sensory branches.

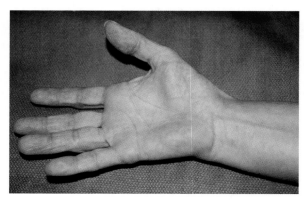

▲ **Plate 4.** A patient with long-standing carpal tunnel syndrome with extreme hand weakness. Note the thenar atrophy. There is a hollowness at the proximal radial side of the palm. This is the classic appearance of thenar muscle atrophy due to severe and chronic median nerve compression at the wrist causing the carpal tunnel syndrome.

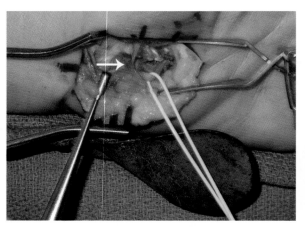

▲ **Plate 5.** Picture of the ganglion cyst (arrow). It is located under the ulnar motor (deep branch).

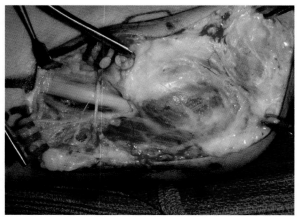

▲ **Plate 7.** Picture of the ulnar nerve at the elbow being compressed by a very muscular anconeous epitrochlearis prior to division.

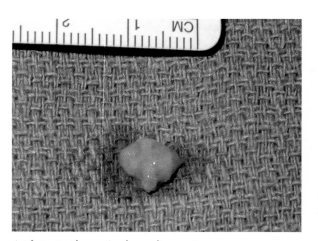

▲ **Plate 6.** The excised ganglion cyst measures approximately 1 cm in diameter.

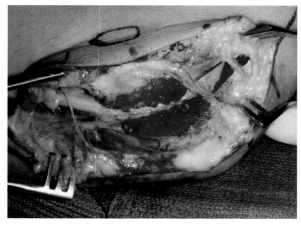

▲ **Plate 8.** The ulnar nerve released after the anconeous epitrochlearis has been divided.

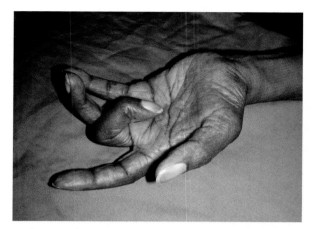

▲ **Plate 9.** This patient has locking of the left long finger due to stenosing flexor tenosynovitis, known commonly as trigger finger. She is unable to extend her affected finger without having to take the other hand and passively extend the long finger.

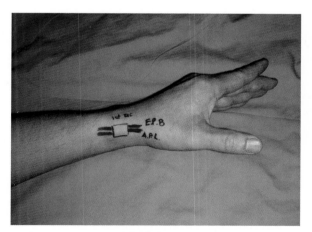

▲ **Plate 10.** Picture of the left extensor pollicis brevis (EPB) and the abductor pollicis longus (APL) tendons at the first dorsal extensor compartment.

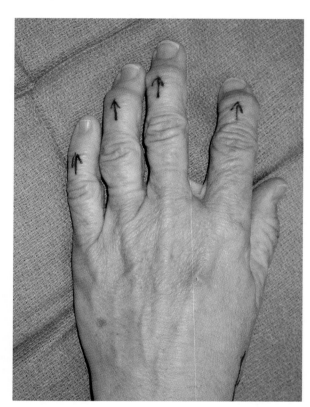

▲ **Plate 11.** Clinical picture of the same hand prior to surgery for DIP joint arthrodesis (fusion).

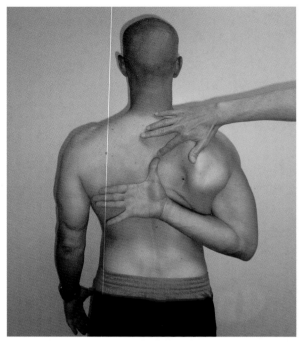

▲ **Plate 12.** Measure internal rotation by documenting the vertebral level reached by both the **right** and left hands.

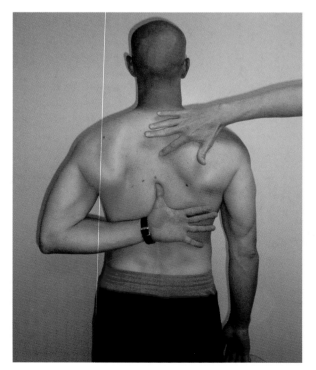

▲ **Plate 13.** Measure internal rotation by documenting the vertebral level reached by both the right and **left** hands.

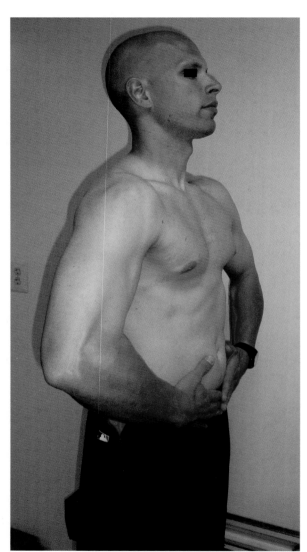

▲ **Plate 14.** The belly-press test is used to evaluate the subscapularis.

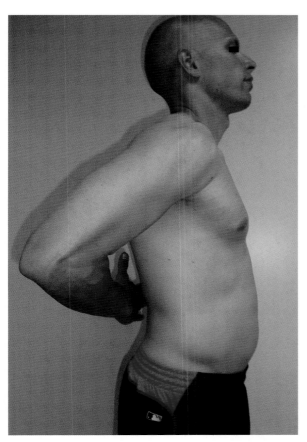

▲ **Plate 15.** The lift-off test is used to evaluate the subscapularis.

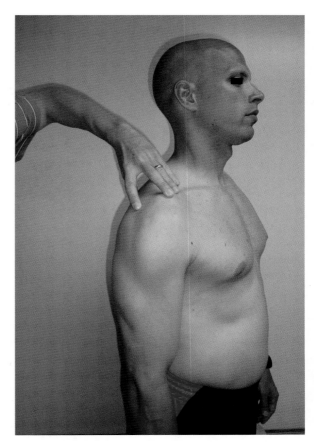

▲ **Plate 16.** The sulcus sign test evaluates inferior shoulder laxity.

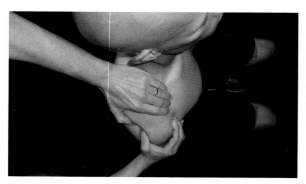

▲ **Plate 17.** The load and shift test evaluates the degree of anterior instability.

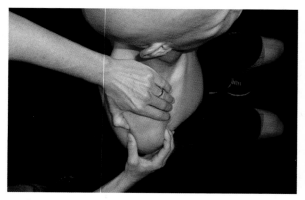

▲ **Plate 18.** The load and shift test evaluates the degree of posterior instability.

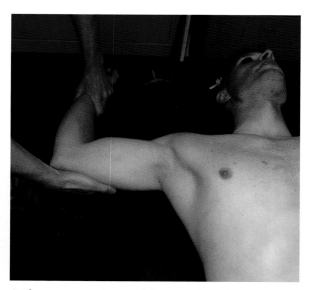

▲ **Plate 19.** Anterior instability is evaluated by the apprehension test.

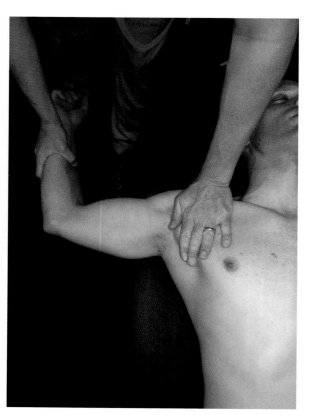

▲ **Plate 20.** Anterior instability is evaluated by the Jobe relocation maneuver.

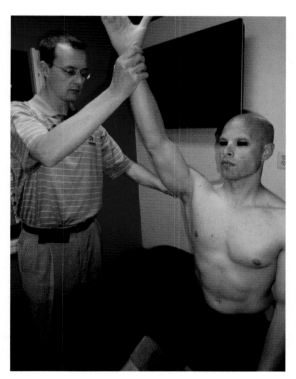

▲ **Plate 21.** The Neer test evaluates rotator cuff impingement.

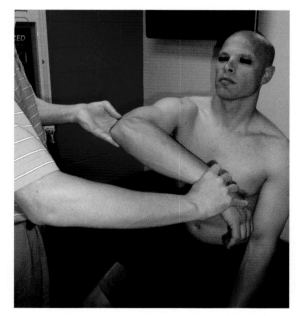

▲ **Plate 22.** The Hawkins test evaluates rotator cuff impingement.

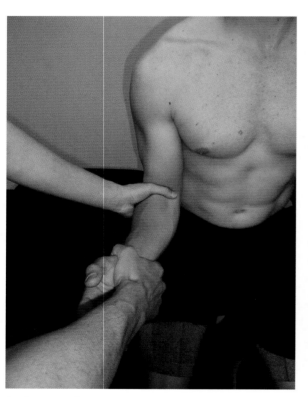

▲ **Plate 23.** The Yergason test evaluates biceps tendinitis.

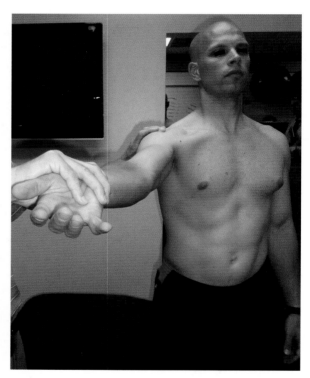

▲ **Plate 24.** The Speed test evaluates biceps tendinitis.

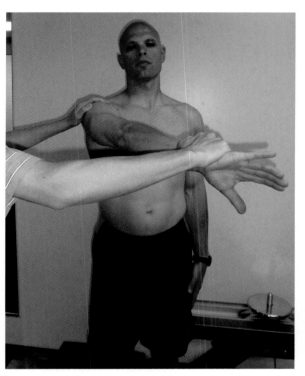

▲ **Plate 25.** The O'Brien test evaluates superior labrum anterior and posterior (SLAP) lesions.

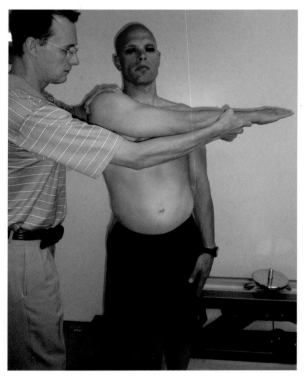

▲ **Plate 26.** The cross-arm adduction test evaluates for AC joint abnormality.

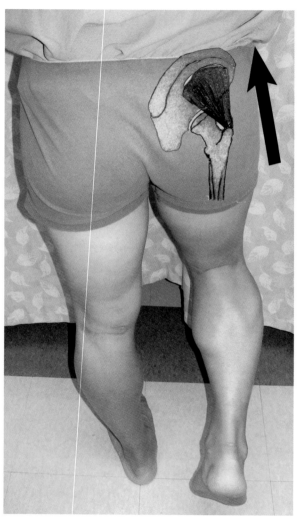

▲ **Plate 27.** A Trendelenburg gait results from a weakened gluteus medius muscle (a hip abductor). An intact gluteus medius keeps the pelvis level during a normal single-leg stance.

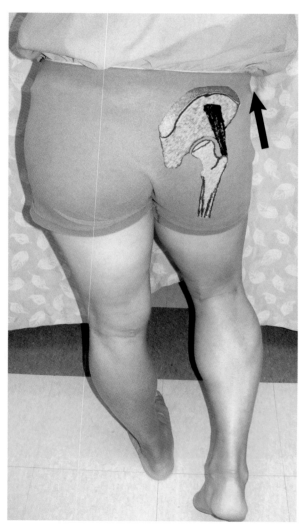

▲ **Plate 28.** A Trendelenburg gait results from a weakened gluteus medius muscle (a hip abductor). With a weak gluteus medius, the pelvis droops, and the body then swings laterally over the affected side.

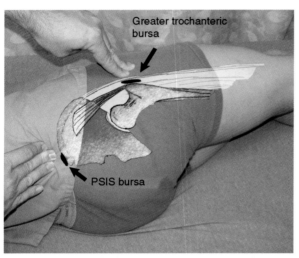

Greater trochanteric bursa

PSIS bursa

▲ **Plate 29.** The bursae around the hip are examined with the patient lying in a lateral position on the unaffected side. The two most common areas of tenderness are over the greater trochanter and over the insertion of the iliacus onto the posterosuperior iliac spine (PSIS). Many patients have tenderness at both of these sites. The ischiogluteal bursa may also be tender over the top of the ischium.

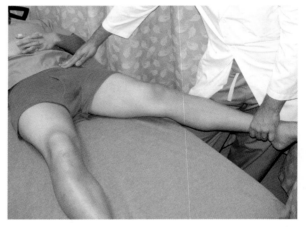

▲ **Plate 30.** The limit of hip abduction is determined by stabilizing the pelvis with one hand pressing down on the opposite anterosuperior iliac spine and with the other hand grasping the ankle and abducting the extended leg. The normal abduction of the hip is 45–50 degrees. Limited hip abduction is common in patients with hip arthritis.

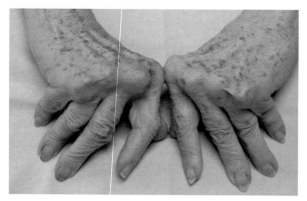

▲ **Plate 31.** Prominent rheumatoid nodules over the metacarpophalangeal joints.

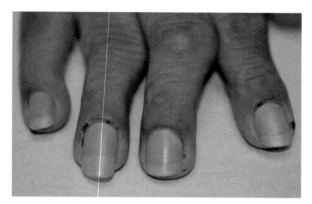

▲ **Plate 32.** Rheumatoid vasculitis: periungual and dermal infarcts.

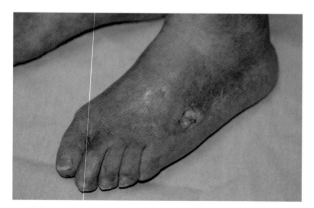

▲ **Plate 33.** Rheumatoid vasculitic leg ulcer.

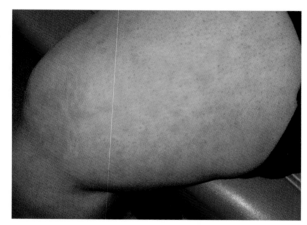

▲ **Plate 34.** The rash of adult-onset Still disease. The rash is an evanescent salmon-colored, maculopapular eruption, usually on the trunk and extremities. Occasionally, as in this case, the rash also has an urticarial quality.

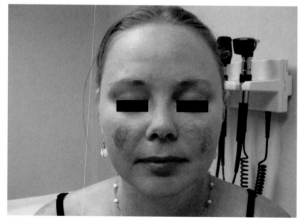

▲ **Plate 35.** Malar rash of systemic lupus erythematosus.

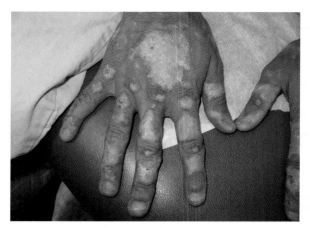

▲ **Plate 36.** Discoid lupus with erythematous plaques and scale.

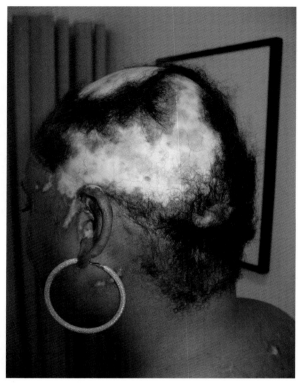

▲ **Plate 38.** Discoid lupus with prominent scarring and atrophy and alopecia.

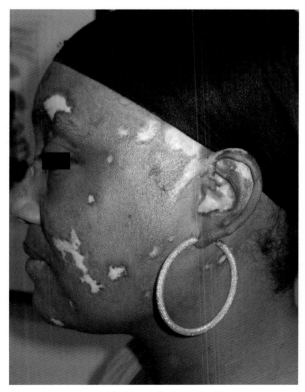

▲ **Plate 37.** Discoid lupus with prominent scarring and atrophy.

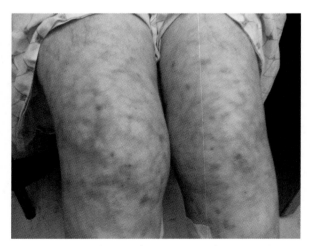

▲ **Plate 39.** Livedo reticularis as a manifestation of antiphospholipid antibody syndrome.

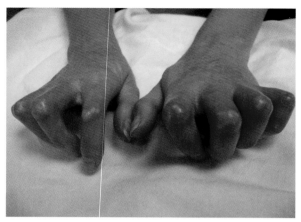

▲ **Plate 40.** Finger joint contractures in diffuse systemic sclerosis. Sclerosis of the skin of the fingers has led to contractures of the joints. The skin is shiny and there are areas of potential skin breakdown over the knuckles. Both active and passive range of motion of the joints is limited and painful.

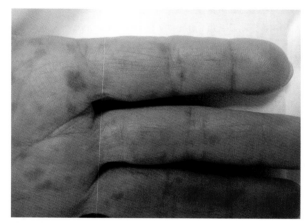

▲ **Plate 42.** Extensive telangiectasias over the fingers of a patient with limited systemic sclerosis. Although the lesions in this case have an ischemic appearance, in fact they are highly vascular and blanch intensely upon pressure, requiring several seconds to resume the morphology seen here.

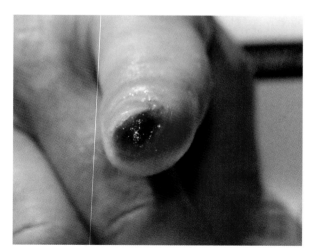

▲ **Plate 41.** Digital ulcer over the fingertip of a patient with limited systemic sclerosis.

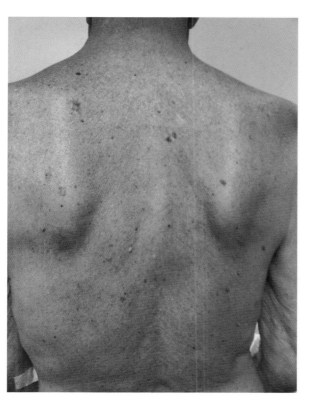

▲ **Plate 43.** Evaluation of scapular winging (see Plate 44).

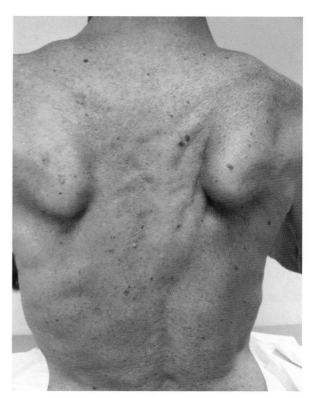

▲ **Plate 44.** Scapular winging on attempted forward arm flexion.

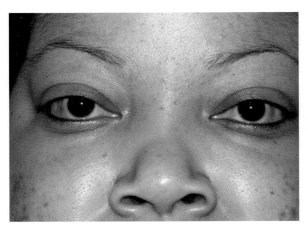

▲ **Plate 45.** Scleral thinning is a patient with relapsing polychondritis and a history of scleritis. Note also the depressed nasal ridge caused by a saddle-nose deformity.

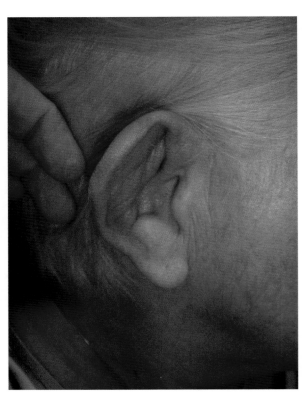

▲ **Plate 46.** Cauliflower ear in a patient with poorly-controlled inflammation of the auricle.

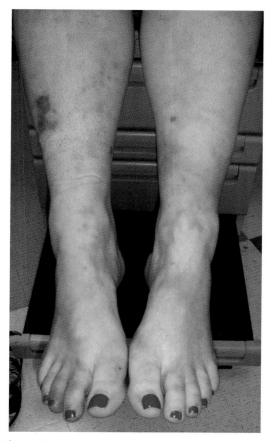

▲ **Plate 47.** Livedo reticularis as a manifestation of microscopic polyangiitis. Livedo reticularis and ulcers occurring on the lower extremities of a patient with microscopic polyangiitis. This patient's presenting manifestation was neuropathic pains from a sensorimotor vasculitic neuropathy. The cutaneous manifestations developed later.

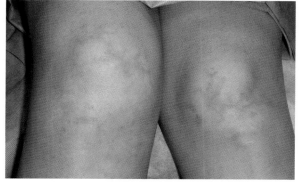

▲ **Plate 48.** Livedo racemosa as a manifestation of polyarteritis nodosa.

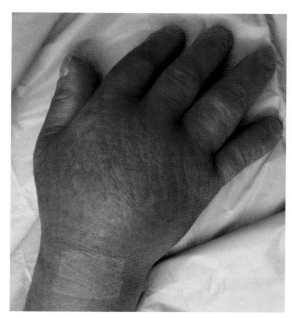

▲ **Plate 49.** Tenosynovitis of the hand due to infection with *Mycobacterium marinum.* The patient, a middle-aged man employed as a fishmonger, sought medical attention after having diffuse hand swelling for 6 months. Culture of synovial fluid obtained by aspiration of a metacarpophalangeal joint grew *M marinum,* an organism associated with fresh-water fish and aquaria. Control of the infection required extensive surgical debridement and prolonged antimicrobial therapy with clarithromycin.

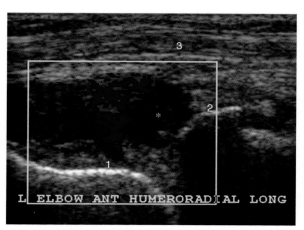

▲ **Plate 50.** Elbow synovitis with Doppler signal. A Doppler signal indicative of inflammation related hyperemia is demonstrated in the center of the hypoechoic collection. **Key:** 1, humeral capitellum; 2, radial head; 3, biceps tendon; *, the center of a hypoechoic collection corresponding to synovitis.

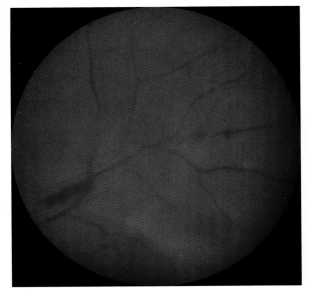

▲ **Plate 51.** Fundus photograph of the retina illustrating one form of retinal vasculitis manifesting as an intraretinal hemorrhage and vessels showing narrowing, occlusion, and dilation.

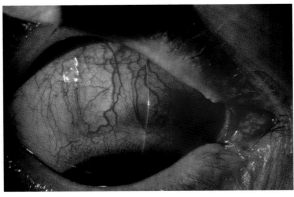

▲ **Plate 53.** Scleritis and scleral thinning that exposes bluish sclera in a patient with severe rheumatoid arthritis.

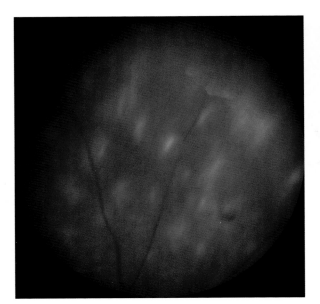

▲ **Plate 52.** Multiple yellowish chorioretinal lesions in the retina. These lesions are typical of birdshot chorioretinopathy.

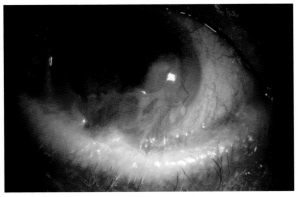

▲ **Plate 54.** Advanced ocular cicatricial pemphigoid with symblepharon (adherence between the palpebral conjunctiva and the bulbar conjunctiva) and opacification and neovascularization of the inferior cornea.

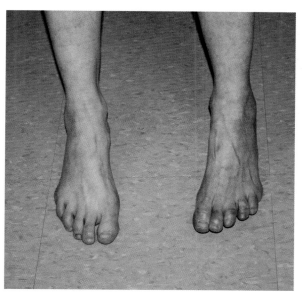

▲ **Plate 55.** This 51-year-old woman has had severe left foot complex regional pain syndrome after orthopedic surgery and 12 weeks of casting complicated by wound infection. Discoloration and foot edema fluctuate but are gradually improving. She reports excess left foot sweating and loss of hair on her left lower leg. She has a Tinel sign at her left but not right fibular head; palpation here causes burning on the dorsum of her left foot consistent with an underlying peroneal nerve injury.

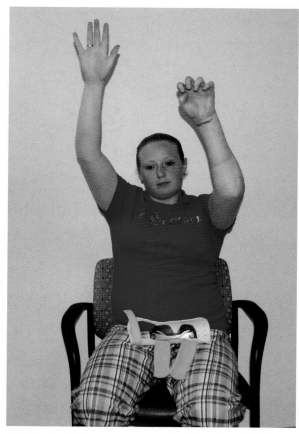

▲ **Plate 56.** This young woman had developed left hand complex regional pain syndrome spontaneously 3 months earlier without known trauma or injury; forearm burning and then edema developed over 2 days. Range of motion later became limited at her left shoulder. Left wrist extension is limited to horizontal, her hand is carried closed and she is not able to fully extend or flex her fingers. She had allodynia to touch over the back of her left hand and profound loss to pin on all fingertips believed caused by ischemia.

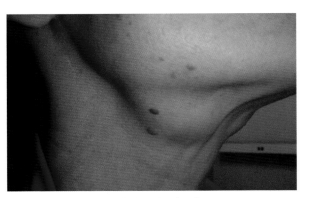

▲ **Plate 57.** Submandibular gland enlargement in a patient with IgG4-related disease.

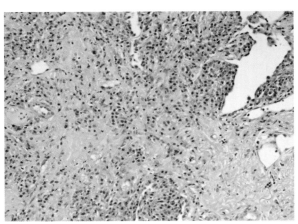

▲ **Plate 59.** Histopathologic and immunostaining features of tissues affected by IgG4-related disease. This lung biopsy shows a lymphoplasmacytic infiltrate with storiform fibrosis (the pink strands of tissue running through the sample).

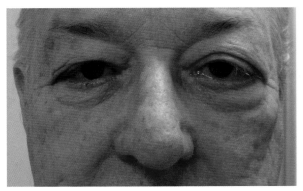

▲ **Plate 58.** Lacrimal gland involvement by IgG4-related disease. This patient had bilateral lacrimal gland biopsies that were positive, but proptosis of the left eye is particularly evident.

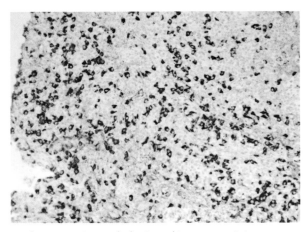

▲ **Plate 60.** Histopathologic and immunostaining features of tissues affected by IgG4-related disease. This lung biopsy shows diffuse IgG4-staining of plasma cells within the tissue. All of the brown-staining cells are plasma cells that are positive for IgG4.

Approach to the Patient with Hand, Wrist, or Elbow Pain

6

James C. Johnston, MD

E. Gene Deune, MD

The causes of upper extremity pain can be categorized as neurologic, musculoskeletal, joint-related, and vascular. A thorough history is critical to characterize the pain. Clinicians should ask specific questions about the quality of the pain (eg, aching, stabbing, throbbing, tingling, pins and needles, numbness). Radiologic and diagnostic testing can help the clinician differentiate between the sources of pain, thereby limiting the differential diagnosis. However, because pain is subjective, the objective physical, radiologic, and electrophysiologic findings sometimes correlate poorly with the intensity of the patient's perceived pain.

▶ Anatomy & Common Terminology

Describing anatomic locations in the hand and the finger can be difficult because of their complex, three-dimensional structures. To avoid confusion and potential errors, standardized terminology should be used. While the surface of the palm can be referred to as either the palmar or the volar surface, palmar is the preferred term to avoid confusion. The back of the hand is referred to as the dorsal surface. The terms "ulnar" and "radial" are used instead of "medial" and "lateral" to describe the sides of the hand because lateral and medial sides can change based on the rotational position of the arm at the time of the examination. The side of the hand toward the small finger is referred to as the "ulnar" side, and the side toward the thumb is referred to as the "radial" side. The fingers should be referred to by name, such as the thumb, the index finger, the middle (or long) finger, the ring finger, and the small finger rather than as the first, second, third, fourth, or fifth fingers. It not infrequent that the index finger is called the first finger and the small finger is called the fourth finger. In truth, however, the thumb is the first finger and the small finger is the fifth finger.

There are 27 bones within the hand: 8 carpal bones, 5 metacarpal bones, and 14 phalangeal bones. The 8 carpal bones are arranged in two rows (a proximal and a distal) that contain 4 bones each. The scaphoid, lunate, triquetral, and pisiform form the proximal row. The distal row is formed by the trapezium (under the thumb metacarpal), the trapezoid, the capitate (which is directly under the middle finger metacarpal), and the hamate (on the ulnar side). The carpal bones are connected to each other by strong ligamentous connections. There are 5 metacarpal bones, and they should be referred to by name rather than by numbers based on the fingers to which they are attached: thumb, index, long, ring, or small metacarpal bones. The phalanges are the bones in the fingers. The thumb has 2 phalanges: the distal and the proximal phalanges. The four other fingers have 3 phalanges: the distal, middle, and the proximal phalanges. To avoid confusion, the phalanges should also be referred to by name (distal, middle, or proximal) rather than by numbers, such as P1, P2, or P3.

The vascular supply of the hand comes from the brachial artery, which separates into the radial and the ulnar arteries at the proximal forearm. These two arteries course along the ulnar and radial borders of the forearm before entering the hand. The ulnar artery feeds the superficial vascular arch of the hand, supplying blood flow to the small, ring, and long fingers. The radial artery at the distal forearm gives rise to the dorsal metacarpal artery, which supplies the dorsal hand. After this, the radial artery continues into the hand and becomes the deep palmar vascular arch, which supplies most of the arterial flow to the thumb and the index finger. In most people, the superficial and the deep vascular arches have arterial connections. The crucial consequence of this is that the hand can be perfused by either the radial or the ulnar artery in most people.

The median, ulnar, and the radial nerves are the three major nerves that provide motor and sensory function to the hand. The ulnar nerve provides the sensation to the small finger and the ulnar half of the ring finger and the dorsal ulnar surface of the hand, the dorsal small finger, and the ulnar dorsal side of the ring finger. The median nerve provides the sensation to the radial palm, the palmar surface of the thumb, index, long, and the radial half of the ring fingers.

The median nerve also innervates the dorsal tips of these fingers. The dorsal radial sensory nerve, as the name suggests, provides sensation to the dorsal radial side of the hand, the dorsal surface of the thumb, index, long, and the radial dorsal side of the ring finger.

The ulnar motor fibers provide most of the innervation to the intrinsic hand muscles. The thenar muscles are primarily innervated by the recurrent branch of the median nerve. The median and ulnar nerves innervate the extrinsic long flexor muscles outside the hand in the forearm to provide finger and wrist flexion. The radial nerve innervates the extrinsic extensor muscles that extend the thumb, the fingers, and the wrist.

▶ Assessment of the Patient

A. History

When evaluating the patient with hand pain, the history is critical to the diagnosis. The examiner should determine the patient's age, handedness, and vocation. The pain should be characterized with such details as the initial onset, the duration, its specific location, if the pain radiates, and if the pain is changing and if it is, whether it is improving or worsening. The patient should be asked if there are any motor functional changes noted in the hand or the finger when the pain occurs, such as finger trigger or locking. The examiner should inquire about any aggravating and relieving factors, including specific activities at work or at home and if there is any diurnal or nocturnal variation. If there is a history of recent trauma, a precise description of the mechanism of any injuries to the area should be noted. A fracture or ligamentous injury at a joint can cause pain. A history of remote trauma is also important because it might indicate that the pain is due to degenerative changes from an untreated fracture or soft tissue injuries. Treatments including nonsteroidal anti-inflammatory drugs (NSAIDs), splinting, hand therapy, prior injections or surgeries should be noted. The patient's medical and surgical histories including prior fractures, history of autoimmune disorders, and infections can also lead to a diagnosis.

The patient should also be asked for other symptoms that are associated with nerve compression, tendinopathies, vascular abnormalities, and arthritis. Unremitting aching and radiating pain with paresthesias that occurs at night and improves with motion or shaking the hand is likely neurogenic. Focal tenderness and swelling with repetitive activity, relieved with rest, is more likely tendinopathy. Joint pain from osteoarthritis or osteochondral injuries is often deep aching pain associated with loss of joint motion, instability, and swelling. Vascular pain is often unremitting with severe throbbing pain that is worsened with cold temperatures that can then lead to ischemic ulcerations and wound healing issues. Other causes of pain include trauma and infection. Complete physical and neurologic examinations of both upper extremities are therefore important.

B. Observation

Much information can be gathered just by observing the patient's hands while taking the history. Observe both of the hands for symmetry and posture. It is helpful to have a diagram of the hand present, so that the examiner can easily mark on the diagram the fingers that have pain or are affected (Figure 6–1). Look for calluses, scarring (traumatic or surgical), and swelling. With the hand is at rest, the fingers should be held in a normal cascade (Plate 1). This means that the small finger is flexed slightly more than the ring finger, the ring finger slightly more flexed than the long finger, and the long finger slightly flexed more than the index finger. Should the hand not have this posture, there may be a tendon rupture, laceration (Plate 2), inflammation of the tendons such as in trigger finger (see Plate 9), or fascial cords (Dupuytren contractures) that alter this repose cascade. Tenderness to palpation and stability should be assessed in each joint. Although it is tempting to touch the part of the hand that is in pain first, it is sometimes more helpful to examine the entire hand first as a unit.

C. Physical Examination

The physical examination begins at the neck, assessing for pain, crepitus, and decreased range of motion. Spurling test can reproduce cervical radiculopathy pain by hyperextending the neck while turning the chin toward the affected side in order to compress the neural foramina around exiting nerve root. Reflexes at the biceps, triceps, and brachioradialis should be measured with the simple goal of determining whether the patient is hyperreflexic or hyporeflexic. The Hoffmann sign, the so-called Babinski test of the upper extremity, involves flicking the distal phalanx of the middle finger and monitoring for reflexive flexion of the thumb interphalangeal joint. Any hyperreflexia, especially when combined with an unsteady gate or difficulty with fine motor activities, should raise concern for neurologic compression and may require further evaluation by a neurologist or a spine surgeon.

The shoulder should be taken through a range of motion and all bony prominences should be palpated. Pain with passive internal rotation of the shoulder due to bony impingement can be mistaken for distal arm pain. Pain in the "shoulder patch" distribution over the deltoid can indicate rotator cuff pathology. Sensation over the shoulder, upper arm, and forearm should be tested and compared to the contralateral side to evaluate for cervical based dermatomal paresthesias. Muscle strength in the biceps (musculocutaneous nerve) and triceps (radial nerve) should be evaluated, along with the strength of forearm pronation and supination. The range of motion at the elbow as well as stability should be tested.

The sensory examination should assess the radial, ulnar, and median nerve distributions in the hand with comparisons made for both hands. Two-point discrimination testing and Semmes-Weinstein monofilament testing are sensitive

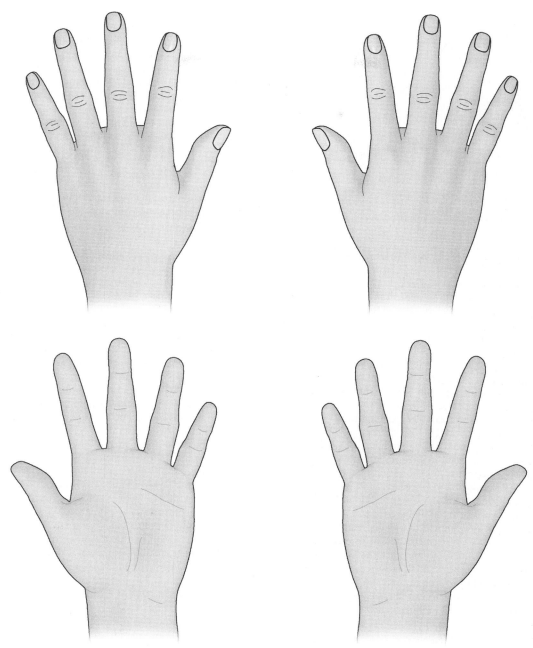

▲ **Figure 6–1.** Diagram of the hands, palmar, and dorsal views. These are helpful to have during the examination to document any findings.

early indicators of nerve dysfunction. A positive Tinel sign test over the common compression sites of the median, ulnar, and radial nerves can indicate nerve irritation due to an injury or compression.

The motor examination should assess strength. The most commonly used method is based on a numerical gradation from zero (0) to five (5) (Table 6–1). The motor and sensory function of the major nerves to the hand (radial,

Table 6–1. Medical Research Council method for assessing motor strength.

Numerical Gradation	Clinical Finding
0	No muscle movement
1	Flicker
2	Muscle moves the joint when gravity is eliminated
3	Muscle cannot hold the joint against resistance but moves the joint fully against gravity
4	Muscle holds the joint against a combination of gravity and moderate resistance
5	Full strength

median, and ulnar nerves) should be assessed. Thumb opposition to the small finger indicates a functional recurrent branch of the median nerve. Ability to flex the index finger interphalangeal joint and thumb interphalangeal joint indicates that the anterior interosseous nerve branch of the median nerve is intact. The ability to adduct the fingers indicates that the ulnar motor nerve is functional. The ability to extend the fingers, the thumb, and the wrist indicates that the radial motor nerve is functional. Weakness, lack of function, or sensory changes should prompt the clinician to order a nerve conduction velocity/electromyography (NCV/EMG) study.

The upper extremity vascular examination begins with a thorough inspection of the skin for discoloration, scars, rashes, hair pattern, and ulceration. Touching the hand gives the examiner a qualitative assessment of the hand vascularity based on the temperature, moisture, and quality of the skin. The fingertips should be warm and well-perfused with capillary refill less than 2 seconds. Also noted should be any temperature differences between digits; the presence of vascular masses; thrills; or the strength of brachial, radial, and ulnar arterial pulsation. As noted, the hand usually has dual blood supply through the radial and ulnar arteries, which interconnect through the superficial and deep vascular palmar arches. An Allen test should be done to ascertain perfusion to the hand via either the ulnar artery or the radial artery. The Allen test is performed by applying simultaneous pressure to the patient's radial and ulnar arteries with the examiner's thumb and fingers at the wrist. The patient is asked to flex the fingers three times fully before keeping the fingers fully extended. At this point, the fingers and the hand should be pale. The examiner then releases the pressure on the radial artery while maintaining pressure on the ulnar artery. If the communication between the deep arch (radial artery) and the superficial arch is patent, the fingers and the hand will reperfuse and the hand will turn pink within 2 seconds. The patient is asked again to squeeze three times and then to keep the fingers

extended. This time the pressure is released from the ulnar artery while pressure is maintained on the radial artery. If the connection between the superficial arch (ulnar artery) and the deep arch is patent, the fingers and hand will reperfuse. The results of the Allen test are best stated as "the Allen test was performed, and perfusion was present through both the radial and the ulnar arteries." If an abnormality is noted, the results are best stated as "the Allen test was performed and there is poor (or delayed) perfusion by the ulnar (or radial) artery." When stated in this fashion, there is no confusion what a "positive" or a "negative" Allen test means.

D. Imaging

Plain radiographs, computed tomography scans, and magnetic resonance imaging studies all have roles to play in selected musculoskeletal conditions and should be used as required to elucidate the diagnosis.

NEUROLOGIC CAUSES OF PAIN

Pain due to peripheral nerve dysfunction can present with varying symptoms, ranging from pure sensory dysfunction to pure motor paralysis or a combination of both. Most commonly, the dysfunction is due to external compression or trauma. This is in contrast to intrinsic neurologic dysfunction from metabolic causes, such as diabetes mellitus, or from demyelinating conditions, such as the Charcot-Marie-Tooth or Guillain-Barré syndromes. These symptoms tend to manifest in multiple limbs and are more global within each limb. Patients who present with these symptoms should undergo a thorough medical evaluation. Generally mild symptoms are transient and spontaneously resolve. If the pain persists and there are other symptoms, such as paresthesias and weakness, further evaluation and treatment by a hand surgeon should be recommended. The initiation of the evaluation by the primary care physician with radiographs and NCV/EMG studies can shorten the time between presentation, diagnosis, and the institution of treatment.

Compression neuropathies affect up to 10% of the population. As the peripheral nerves travel from the vertebral foramina to their end organs, they pass through several anatomic sites of potential compression. The pathophysiology of compression and neurologic pain can be explained by the localized nerve ischemia and the interference of the axonal transport of metabolic products. The level of compression determines the clinical symptoms. Proximal compression of the nerves as they exit the vertebral bodies produces symptoms in a dermatomal distribution, whereas distal nerve compression produces symptoms in the defined region of the specific nerve(s) that cross multiple dermatomes. Symptoms of intrinsic neurologic dysfunction, eg, metabolic or demyelinating neuropathies, tend to manifest in multiple limbs and are more global within each limb. After the physical examination, the next step in the patient's work-up should be an electrodiagnostic evaluation. The level and severity of compression can be elucidated by NCVs. Motor dysfunction and muscle denervation due to nerve compression can be elucidated with an EMG. Multiple levels of compression can occur simultaneously at the various sites. This is referred to as a "double crush" phenomenon.

Intrinsic nerve dysfunction may be symptoms of an underlying systemic disease, such as hypothyroidism, rheumatologic disease, diabetes mellitus, and pregnancy. The patient therefore should undergo a thorough medical evaluation. If the hand symptoms are mild and of recent onset secondary to an underlying medical condition, they will often resolve when the underlying cause is treated. However, severe pain, weakness, or paresthesias warrant evaluation and treatment by a hand surgeon, because permanent damage can occur in the absence of timely intervention.

1. Median Nerve Compression at the Wrist (Carpal Tunnel Syndrome)

ESSENTIALS OF DIAGNOSIS

▶ Paresthesias of the palmar aspect of the thumb, index, and long fingers, and radial aspect of the ring finger.

▶ Positive Phalen maneuver and Tinel sign at the wrist.

▶ Thenar atrophy and weakened pinch with long-standing compression.

▶ General Considerations

A. Anatomy

The carpal tunnel is an anatomic structure located in the proximal part of the hand distal to the junction with the forearm. The carpal tunnel is the space defined by the carpal bones on the radial, ulnar, and dorsal sides with a tough ligamentous structure called the transverse carpal ligament on its palmar roof. The transverse carpal ligament attaches on the radial side to the tuberosity of the trapezium distally and proximally to the tuberosity of the scaphoid and the styloid process of the radius. On the ulnar side, the ligament attaches to the hook of the hamate distally and to the pisiform proximally. The transverse carpal ligament maintains the carpal arch and serves as a pulley for the flexor tendons. Within this space, there are nine flexor tendons (four flexor digitorum superficialis tendons, four flexor digitorum profundus tendons, and the flexor pollicis longus), and the median nerve.

After the median nerve passes through the carpal tunnel, it divides into the digital sensory branches to the thumb, index and long fingers, and to the radial side of the ring finger. The only motor nerve that branches from the median nerve at this level of the wrist is the recurrent motor branch, which provides the motor innervation to the majority of the thenar musculature. This recurrent branch has variable branching patterns, with the most frequent being the branch curling over the distal edge of the ligament (Plate 3).

B. Risk Factors and Common Causes

Carpal tunnel syndrome is the most common nerve entrapment syndrome; up to 1% of all people will develop symptoms during their lifetime. It is more common after the fourth decade of life and occurs three times more often in women than in men. Medical risk factors include diabetes mellitus, pregnancy, hypothyroidism, and renal disease. It may also be associated with any activity that produces repetitive motion and vibration. Controversy exists about whether carpal tunnel syndrome is a work-related entity.

The most common cause of idiopathic carpal tunnel syndrome is the inflammation of the tenosynovium of the nine tendons within the carpal tunnel, resulting in the compression of the median nerve within the carpal tunnel. Other causes include space-occupying lesions (ganglion cyst, lipoma, giant cell tumors [Figure 6–2]), trauma, hematoma, and proliferative wrist arthritis. Traumatic causes are often acute and may require urgent surgical decompression.

▶ Clinical Findings

A. Symptoms and Signs

The classic symptoms of carpal tunnel syndrome include numbness and tingling in the median sensory nerve distribution (thumb, index and long fingers, and the radial side of the ring finger). These symptoms may be worse at night due to the wrist flexion that occurs with the fetal position during sleep. Patients often describe alleviation of the pain when they shake the affected hand or placing the hand in a dependent position, perceiving vascular insufficiency as the cause of the hand feeling cold and numb. Symptoms may be exacerbated during the day when the wrist is hyperflexed or hyperextended, such as with driving or using a computer. With long-standing compression, there can be profound grip and pinch weakness and complete loss of sensation in the affected fingers.

B. Physical Examination

Both hands are visually examined. The thenar muscles in a normal hand should be well developed and full. In mild carpal tunnel syndrome, there should be no change in the appearance of the thenar musculature. With advanced carpal tunnel syndrome, the thenar muscles can atrophy due to decreased innervation of the abductor pollicis brevis muscle by the recurrent motor branch, resulting in a depressed or hollowed appearance (Plate 4). This results in hand weakness and difficulty in thumb opposition to the small finger. Spontaneous fibrillation in the thenar muscles can sometimes be seen.

Sensation in the fingers should be assessed. Light touch perception is done by touching the fingers lightly with either

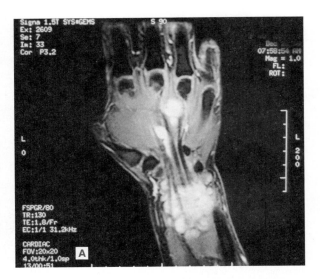

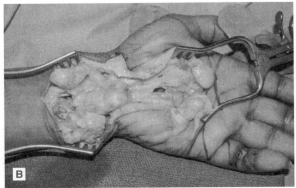

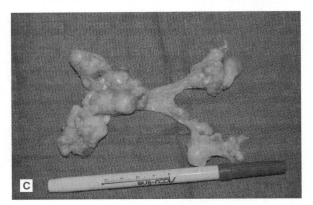

▲ **Figure 6–2. A:** Magnetic resonance image of a giant cell tumor spanning the carpal tunnel. The patient was having carpal tunnel syndrome symptoms with paresthesia of the fingers in the median nerve distribution. **B:** Intraoperative view of the giant cell tumor in the carpal tunnel. **C:** The giant cell tumor excised.

a gauze or a cotton swab. Perception of noxious stimuli is done with either a paper clip or the relatively sharp end of a toothpick. For more sophisticated testing, sensation can be measure by a two-point discrimination test or the Semmes-Weinstein monofilament testing. Grip and pinch strength should be done for baseline measurements. Provocative testing can be done to look for the Tinel sign, Phalen sign, or Durkan sign. A positive Tinel sign is when the patient perceives electrical shooting pains into the distal distribution of the nerve when the nerve is percussed. In the case of the median nerve, the percussion is done over the median nerve at the wrist. If the patient perceives the electrical shocks at the site of the percussion and it radiates into the thumb, index, and long fingers, then this is a positive Tinel sign of the median nerve.

A Phalen test is performed with the patient passively flexing both wrists by touching the dorsal surfaces of one hand to the other dorsal surface. The wrist is held in flexion for 60 seconds. If the patient's symptoms are reproduced, this is a positive Phalen test. In Durkan carpal tunnel compression test, the examiner's thumbs are placed over the carpal tunnel over the median nerve just above the carpal tunnel. If the patient has symptoms of carpal tunnel within 1 minute of compression, the test is considered positive. The Durkan test is not widely used.

C. Imaging Studies and Special Tests

Despite a classic history, the clinical hand examination may be normal in early stages of carpal tunnel syndrome. The nerve conduction study though should show prolonged motor latencies with slowing of nerve conduction velocities if there is compression. With prolonged median nerve compression, there may be muscle denervations that can be detected with the EMG.

If the cause of the nerve compression is due to a tumor or suspected to be a tumor, an MRI should be ordered (see Figure 6–2). A diagnostic biopsy of the mass is done if required and followed by surgical resection.

▶ Treatment

A. Conservative Therapy

Conservative management for idiopathic carpal tunnel syndrome should aim at reducing the tenosynovial inflammation and swelling within the carpal tunnel. Splinting and the use of over-the-counter NSAIDs, such as ibuprofen, should be the first-line therapy. The patients are fitted with prefabricated wrist splints that maintain the wrist at 5–10 degrees of extension. These wrist splints are available in the hand surgeon's office or over-the-counter as "carpal tunnel splints." Splints can also be custom fabricated by the hand therapists. The patients are instructed to wear the splints during the most symptomatic times, which often is during the night when the patients flex their wrist during the fetal sleeping position or during the day when the patient is more active. The patients are instructed on proper ergonomics during the awake and sleeping hours to avoid any positions that cause compression of the median nerve. Approximately one-third of patients managed nonoperatively in this fashion respond favorably.

B. Injection Therapy

Glucocorticoid injections into the carpal tunnel can alleviate the symptoms, although they can be associated with median nerve injury if done incorrectly. The relief of symptoms by the glucocorticoid injection is often only temporary, as patients who require such injections generally have pathology severe enough to warrant surgical decompression. The injections are done by identifying the palmaris longus tendon at the distal forearm at the wrist. Triamcinolone or decadron is mixed with 1% lidocaine without epinephrine, and the injection is given through a 30-gauge needle by inserting it into the forearm from the ulnar side of the palmaris longus tendon. Once inserted, the needle is gently advanced through the forearm fascia so the tip is just above the median nerve but below the level of the fascia. It is important the patient is awake during the injection so the patient can inform you of any electrical discharges, which indicates that the needle has encountered the median nerve. If there is no paresthesia, slowly administer the volume. If the needle is too superficial and is above the forearm fascia, there will be a skin wheal and no noticeable paresthesia in the median nerve. This is not optimal as the superficial location of the glucocorticoid may cause significant skin atrophy and depigmentation. If the glucocorticoid is injected into the right plane, the patient will have paresthesia in the median nerve distribution. Some experts prefer to avoid glucocorticoid injections unless the patient is a poor candidate for surgery and the injection is the only viable treatment option.

C. Surgical Therapy

If symptoms persist after a 2- to 3-month period of diligent splinting, NSAID use, and glucocorticoid injections, surgical intervention is indicated to avoid permanent damage to the median nerve and its innervated muscles. Surgical release can be done by either the classic open carpal tunnel release (or its multiple variations) or through the endoscopic approach. As with any surgical procedure, there are advantages and disadvantages of each technique. Most patients have decreased discomfort and pain with the endoscopic approach in the early postoperative period and tend to return to work earlier than those patients who undergo the open release procedure. Multiple studies suggest that patients' satisfaction and long-term results are equivalent. The most common cause of incomplete resolution of symptoms is incomplete release of the carpal tunnel.

2. Proximal Median Nerve Compression: Pronator Syndrome & Anterior Interosseous Nerve Syndromes

ESSENTIALS OF DIAGNOSIS

▶ Can mimic carpal tunnel syndrome.

▶ Deep aching pain in the forearm is a typical symptom.

▶ General Considerations

Proximal median nerve compression syndromes are far less common than carpal tunnel syndrome, but their symptoms can mimic closely those of carpal tunnel syndrome. The proximal median nerve compression syndromes include the pronator syndrome and the anterior interosseus nerve (AIN) syndromes.

▶ Clinical Findings

In the **pronator syndrome**, the median nerve is compressed just below the elbow by the fibrous bands of the pronator teres, flexor digitorum superficialis, or lacertus fibrosis. These patients suffer from deep aching pain in their forearm, which can be made worse with forceful gripping and pronation of the proximal forearm. Because the median palmar cutaneous nerve branches proximal to the carpal tunnel, patients with pronator syndrome have decreased sensation at the thenar eminence. Three provocative tests that reproduce the compression can reproduce the symptoms of pain and paresthesias. First, the patient's hand is held as if in a handshake posture and the patient is asked to pronate against resistance. This will cause the pronator teres to contract. Second, with the palm up, the fingers are passively extended by the examiner and the patient is asked to flex the middle finger against resistance, resulting in contraction of the flexor digitorum superficialis and increased pressure on the median nerve. In the third test, the patient's hand is gripped as if to arm wrestle. The arm is pronated and simultaneously extended against resistance. This will isolate the lacertus fibrosus. In addition, the medial elbow should be palpated during resisted wrist flexion to look for medial epicondylitis, which can occur with pronator syndrome. All three of these maneuvers lead to exacerbations of the patient's symptoms if the pronator syndrome is present.

The AIN innervates the index finger flexor digitorum profundus (FPD) and the flexor pollicis longus (FPL) tendon to the thumb, allowing for active flexion of the index distal interphalangeal (DIP) joint and the interphalangeal joint of the thumb. In an **AIN syndrome**, the patient has an aching forearm pain along with inability to flex the thumb interphalangeal joint or the index finger DIP joint. This results in the inability to form an "O" shape when pinching the index finger with the thumb. Because there is no sensory component to the AIN, there is no sensory disturbance noted in the hand. Differential diagnosis includes Parsonage-Turner syndrome (brachial plexus neuritis) and flexor tendon rupture.

▶ Treatment

Pronator syndrome improves with activity modification, NSAIDs, splinting, and treatment of concomitant medial epicondylitis, if present. Surgical decompression is not often necessary. The AIN syndrome, from which patients usually recover within 3 months, is treated with observation while maintaining range of motion. If the AIN function does not return, tendon transfers or nerve neurotization may be needed.

3. Compression of the Ulnar Nerve at the Wrist (Guyon Canal Syndrome)

ESSENTIALS OF DIAGNOSIS

▶ Paresthesias of the palmar aspect of the ring and small fingers.

▶ Absence of paresthesias on the dorsal ulnar aspect of the hand.

▶ General Considerations

If a patient's numbness is described as being in the palmar aspect of the small and ring fingers and not the dorsal ulnar hand, with or without weakness in the hypothenar muscles, it is likely due to ulnar nerve compression at Guyon canal. Guyon canal is a small triangular space located at the proximal hypothenar eminence and bound by the hook of the hamate on the radial side, the pisiform on the ulnar side, and the volar transverse carpal ligament as its floor. The roof is defined by the palmar fascia. The ulnar nerve and the ulnar artery pass through this canal as they travel from the forearm to the hand. The lack of numbness on the dorsal ulnar aspect of the hand isolates the ulnar nerve compression to the wrist rather than to the elbow. This is because the dorsal ulnar sensory nerve separates from the main trunk of the ulnar nerve 5 cm proximal to Guyon canal. The remainder of the ulnar nerve continues distally as the palmar ulnar sensory and the ulnar motor branch. As the ulnar nerve crosses into the palm within Guyon canal, the motor branch, which is ulnar to the palmar sensory branch, dives deep, and crosses dorsally under the ulnar sensory nerve from the ulnar to the radial side and enters into the muscular compartment of the hand under the confluent fascial origins of the hypothenar muscles to innervate most of the intrinsic muscles of the hand.

▶ Clinical Findings

A. Symptoms and Signs

Compression of the ulnar nerve within Guyon canal can result in a sensory deficit, an isolated ulnar motor deficit, or both. The key differential between ulnar nerve compression at Guyon canal versus ulnar nerve compression at the cubital tunnel in the elbow is that with ulnar nerve compression at Guyon canal only the ulnar palmar surface of the hand and the small and ring fingers are numb. With ulnar nerve compression at the cubital tunnel, there is both palmar and dorsal ulnar hand numbness.

Motor hand weakness may be subtle or not present and usually is not the overriding presenting symptom. In contrast to carpal tunnel syndrome, which is thought to be primarily caused by inflammation, Guyon canal syndrome is caused by compression from a soft tissue mass. The most common cause is a ganglion cyst (Figure 6–3 and Plates 5 and 6), followed by a lipoma. Trauma resulting in hook of the hamate fracture, or ulnar artery thrombosis (that occurs with hypothenar hammer syndrome) may cause similar symptoms. Hypothenar hammer syndrome is a constellation of symptoms, occurring mostly in manual laborers who use their hand as a "hammer" during their work activities. This repetitive trauma can result in scar adhesions to the ulnar nerve or the presence of an ulnar artery pseudoaneurysm causing ulnar nerve compression and ischemia due to intraluminal thrombosis or embolism should be suspected.

B. Imaging Studies and Special Tests

Electrodiagnostic studies can show slowing of the ulnar nerve across the canal but often may be normal. Plain films with a

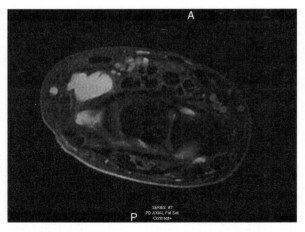

▲ **Figure 6–3.** Magnetic resonance image of a ganglion cyst within Guyon canal. The cyst was dorsal to the ulnar motor branch and caused a purely motor dysfunction without sensory changes in the ulnar sensory distribution.

carpal tunnel view can aid in the diagnosis of a hook of the hamate fracture, and an MRI may be useful to delineate a mass impinging on the canal. The diagnosis is often made based on strong clinical suspicion, subjective positive findings, and abnormal ulnar nerve conduction across the wrist with a normal ulnar NCVs through the cubital tunnel at the elbow.

▶ Treatment

The tortuosity of Guyon canal precludes glucocorticoid injections, and splinting is often ineffective. Surgical decompression is recommended. With mild ulnar nerve compression at the wrist in the presence of carpal tunnel syndrome, division of the transverse carpal ligament during the carpal tunnel surgery is often effective in decompressing Guyon canal. If it is more severe, a formal decompression of Guyon canal is recommended. It is important during a formal decompression of Guyon canal, that both the sensory and the motor nerves are decompressed along with the excision of the space occupying mass. If hypothenar hammer syndrome is suspected, an upper extremity vascular Doppler examination, a magnetic resonance arteriogram, or a formal arteriogram should be ordered. Vascular reconstruction of the ulnar artery may also be required.

4. Compression of the Ulnar Nerve at the Elbow (Cubital Tunnel Syndrome)

ESSENTIALS OF DIAGNOSIS

- ▶ Pain in the proximal forearm.
- ▶ Paresthesias of the palmar and dorsal aspects of the small finger and of the ulnar side of the ring finger.
- ▶ Positive Tinel sign with percussion of the ulnar nerve at the elbow.
- ▶ Weakness and atrophy of the intrinsic muscles of the hand with long-standing compression.

▶ General Considerations

The cubital tunnel syndrome is the second most common nerve entrapment syndrome and often coexists with the most common, carpal tunnel syndrome. Proximal to the elbow, the ulnar nerve is located next to the medial head of the triceps and on the posterior surface of the medial intermuscular septum. As it approaches the elbow, it lies between the olecranon and the medial humeral epicondyle and enters the cubital tunnel. In the strictest definition, the cubital tunnel is defined by the elbow joint laterally, the flexor carpi ulnaris origin medially, and the medial epicondyle anteriorly. However, often the term "cubital tunnel" is used to include the region spanned by proximal fascial covering of the ulnar

nerve proximal to the medial epicondyle and distal fascia between the two heads of the flexor carpi ulnaris. When this distal fascia is thickened, it is referred to as Osborne ligament. Another potential cause of compression is the anconeus epitrochlearis muscle located at the proximal elbow (Plates 7 and 8). This anomalous muscle is believed to be present in about 10% of the population. The muscle arises from the medial border of the olecranon and the adjacent triceps and inserts into the medial epicondyle. It runs superficial to the ulnar nerve and maintains the ulnar nerve in place. The Arcade of Struthers was thought in the past to be another site of ulnar nerve compression. This arcade was described as stretching from the medial head of triceps to the medial intermuscular septum and was found in patients undergoing secondary surgeries for persistent ulnar nerve compression. Most surgeons now believe that the Arcade of Struthers is not a distinct anatomic structure but rather the fibrosis of the proximal fascial bands that were not released with the prior surgery.

▶ Clinical Findings

A. Symptoms and Signs

Clinically with ulnar nerve compression, there is an extreme aching or lancinating pain in the proximal forearm and elbow, and paresthesias radiating distally to the ulnar side of the ring finger, the small finger, and the dorsal ulnar hand. These symptoms are exacerbated by elbow flexion due to traction and compression of the tethered ulnar nerve as it traverses the cubital tunnel. This is because the cubital tunnel is below the pivot point of the elbow flexion, so elbow flexion causes stretching of the nerve. Weakness and intrinsic muscular atrophy, or "clawing," are usually late symptoms. Two classic late physical findings are Wartenberg sign and Froment sign. In Wartenberg sign, patients have an annoying difficulty putting their hand in their pocket because the small finger gets stuck outside the pocket. This occurs because from an unopposed abductor digiti quinti muscle, innervated by the PIN (radial nerve) by the weakened ulnar nerve. In Froment sign, a patient is asked to hold a piece of paper between the thumb and the palm of the hand while the examiner pulls the paper away from them. Inability to hold the paper indicates weakness of the ulnar nerve innervated adductor pollicis. Patients will often flex their median innervated flexor pollicis longus to compensate. Percussion of the ulnar nerve at the elbow will produce discomfort and paresthesia, a positive Tinel sign.

B. Imaging Studies and Special Tests

Patients with primarily ulnar nerve symptoms who are smokers and report concomitant shoulder pain should have a chest radiograph to evaluate for Pancoast tumor. EMG and NCVs are extremely helpful to establish the diagnosis as well as the severity of the compression. Fibrillations noted on electromyography indicate neurologic compromise to the muscles.

▶ Differential Diagnosis

Other common diagnoses to consider include thoracic outlet syndrome and C8-T1 radiculopathy. Less common disorders that can mimic cubital tunnel syndrome include Charcot-Marie-Tooth, amyotrophic lateral sclerosis, and Guillain-Barré syndrome.

▶ Treatment

Conservative therapy is indicated in patients with minimal compression. Patients are advised against maintaining postures that involve severe elbow flexion, such as arm crossing during awake hours and the fetal position during sleep. To prevent elbow flexion during sleep, patients wear custom-made long arm splints to maintain the elbow at about 45 degrees of flexion. For those with coexisting carpal tunnel syndrome, the splint is extended beyond the wrist to keep the wrist at neutral. If both sides are affected, bilateral splints are made and the patients are instructed to alternate the splints nightly, so that one arm is free to function in its normal capacity such as removing eyeglasses, turning the light off at night, and reaching for the clock. The patients are referred to occupational therapists for ergonomic exercises and posture modifications. The use of NSAIDs is recommended.

If symptoms do not improve over 2 to 3 months or there is worsening symptoms, surgical decompression may be indicated to relieve the symptoms. Several surgical techniques have been proposed, each with its own proponents. Several recent randomized controlled trials indicate that in situ decompression of the nerve has equivalent outcomes to transposition. Some experts prefer an in situ decompression of the ulnar nerve without submuscular anterior transposition.

5. Radial Nerve Compression (Radial Tunnel & Posterior Interosseous Nerve Syndrome)

ESSENTIALS OF DIAGNOSIS

▶ Idiopathic entrapment is uncommon.
▶ Aching pain in the extensor and supinator muscle masses in the proximal forearm.
▶ Difficult to distinguish from lateral epicondylitis.

▶ General Considerations

Compression of the radial nerve like other nerves can occur in predictable regions of the upper extremity along its course. The radial tunnel starts 10 cm above the lateral epicondyle where the radial nerve enters the anterior compartment and extends to the dorsal compartment of the forearm where the posterior interosseous nerve (PIN) pierces through the supinator muscle.

▶ Clinical Findings

A. Symptoms and Signs

Symptoms vary based on if the compression is above or below the bifurcation of the sensory and motor branches of the radial nerve at the proximal forearm. Radial tunnel syndrome, the most common entrapment of the radial nerve, results from compression of the PIN in the region from the radial head to the supinator. Patients describe aching pain in the extensor and supinator muscle mass in the proximal forearm without any sensory or motor deficit.

Physical findings include tenderness of the radial nerve upon palpation along its path. Although not entirely reliable, radial tunnel syndrome should be strongly suspected if the symptoms are reproduced over the radial tunnel by resisted supination with the elbow in extension, or resisted extension of the long finger. The diagnosis is made more difficult by lateral epicondylitis, which has similar symptoms, is extremely common, and coexists in 5% of cases. One common clinical scenario with radial tunnel syndrome is that lateral epicondylitis has been diagnosed and the patient is treated with a compressive strap at the elbow but has worsening of the symptoms because of the compression.

B. Special Tests

Neurodiagnostic studies are usually not helpful unless there is evidence of muscle denervation, which is usually a late symptom of chronic compression. Often, therapeutic and diagnostic injections with lidocaine at the lateral epicondyle or within the radial tunnel are the best means of determining the etiology of proximal forearm pain.

▶ Treatment

A 2- to 3-month course of NSAIDs, splinting, and muscle stretching exercises are often helpful. For refractory cases, an MRI can evaluate for a space occupying lesion, and the patient should be referred for surgical exploration and decompression.

6. Compression of the Superficial Radial Nerve at the Distal Forearm (Wartenberg Syndrome)

ESSENTIALS OF DIAGNOSIS

▶ Paresthesias of the dorsal aspects of the thumb, index, and long fingers.
▶ Nerve often compressed by a wristwatch or other constrictive band.

General Considerations

The superficial branch of the radial nerve provides sensation to the dorsal thumb, index and long fingers, and the radial dorsum of the hand and wrist. Its proximity to the bony prominence of the radius makes it vulnerable to extrinsic compression, such as from a tight wrist watch, splint, handcuffs, or a slingshot as reported in a literature case report.

Clinical Findings

Presenting symptoms may include numbness and paresthesias in the radial sensory distribution with dull aching pain in the wrist. There is no associated weakness. A positive Tinel sign over the radial sensory nerve can aid in the diagnosis. Radiographs will evaluate for arthritis, and injection of a short-acting local anesthetic into the area of most severe pain can be both diagnostic and therapeutic.

Differential Diagnosis

The differential diagnosis includes de Quervain tenosynovitis and basilar joint arthritis of the thumb. Occasionally, radial sensory neuritis can be caused by de Quervain tenosynovitis due to the adjacent inflammation.

Treatment

The treatment is to remove the offending causes. If the symptoms persist after several weeks, referral to a hand surgeon should be made, for potential exploration and neurolysis of the radial nerve.

MUSCULOSKELETAL UPPER EXTREMITY PAIN

1. Trigger Finger (Stenosing Tenosynovitis)

ESSENTIALS OF DIAGNOSIS

▶ Racheting motion during flexion of the affected finger.
▶ Locking of the finger.

Clinical Findings

Triggering of the finger is caused by entrapment of the smooth hand flexor tendon in the retinacular A1 annular pulley, resulting in the classic trigger position (finger in the position of pulling a gun's trigger) or ratcheting motion during finger flexion. This is thought to be caused by irritation and subsequent swelling of the flexor tendon tenosynovium at the proximal edge of the A1 pulley. The constant motion of the inflamed tenosynovium causes intense pain. Further swelling results in locking of the finger in extension or more commonly in flexion, as the swollen tendon can no longer glide through the A1 pulley. Once, the finger is locked, the patient needs to passively extend the finger to "unlock" it (Plate 9). Acquired trigger fingers can be associated with rheumatoid arthritis and diabetes mellitus and are more common in females. Most cases are idiopathic and thought to be due to minor injuries such as that from repetitive motion or blunt trauma.

Treatment

Conservative therapy is initially indicated in acquired adult trigger finger. The patients are educated about possible etiology, such as the preferential use of the finger during typing or forceful grasping of objects that causes minor direct blunt trauma to the proximal edge of the A1 pulley. Finger splints and NSAIDs are recommended as initial treatment for a trial of several weeks.

If the patient has already tried this or the triggering is severe, glucocorticoid injections are given into the potential space between the A1 pulley and the flexor tendon. Glucocorticoid injections may be repeated several times but usually should not exceed three injections, unless there are medical contraindications to surgery. If triggering recurs, surgical release of the A1 pulley is indicated. This can be accomplished quite easily under local anesthetic, with low morbidity, although digital nerve laceration, stiffness, and infection with delayed wound healing have been reported.

2. de Quervain Tenosynovitis

ESSENTIALS OF DIAGNOSIS

▶ Radial wrist pain.
▶ Pain with extension and abduction of the thumb.
▶ Positive Finkelstein sign.

General Considerations

A common cause of radial-sided wrist pain is tendinitis of the first dorsal extensor compartment. The dorsal compartments act as pulleys for the wrist and finger extensors. Within the first dorsal compartment are the extensor pollicis brevis and the abductor pollicis longus (Plate 10).

Clinical Findings

When the first dorsal compartment and the tenosynovium around these two tendons are inflamed, there can be severe pain with thumb extension and abduction. There is usually pain on direct palpation of the compartment when the patient extends the thumb against resistance. Finkelstein test assesses pain over the first dorsal compartment with the thumb clasped by the other fingers. Occasionally, palpable crepitance is present in the compartment when the patient ranges the thumb, and a radial osteophyte may also be visible on radiographs.

▶ Differential Diagnosis

Differential diagnoses include thumb basilar joint arthritis and compression of the dorsal radial sensory nerve.

▶ Treatment

Conservative treatment is the first-line therapy, consisting of NSAIDs, a thumb spica splint, and glucocorticoid injections into the first dorsal compartment. Care must be taken to infiltrate over both the abductor pollicis longus and extensor pollicis brevis tendons, which are often separated by a septum within the first dorsal extensor compartment. Failure of conservative treatment will necessitate surgical first compartment release, which can be performed as an outpatient procedure, under local anesthesia and intravenous sedation, with a low rate of morbidity and a high rate of success.

3. Ganglion Cysts

ESSENTIALS OF DIAGNOSIS

▶ Firm cystic masses adjacent to joints.
▶ Usually painless.

▶ General Considerations

A ganglion cyst is the most common benign tumor in the hand or wrist. Despite the name, a ganglion cyst is not related to a nerve. It is thought that its etiology is due to leakage of joint fluid along with its synovial lining through a weakness in the joint capsule. The inciting factor may be a tear or localized degenerative change in the tenosynovium.

▶ Clinical Findings

A localized check-valve effect occurs at the base of the stalk, allowing ingress but not egress of synovial fluid from the joint into the protrusion. As fluid accumulates, a cyst forms. With partial resorption of the fluid by the cyst lining, the fluid inside becomes more concentrated, making aspiration of the fluid difficult. The most common location is at the dorsal wrist with the origin at the scapholunate joint. The second most common location is on the palmar aspect of the wrist on the radial side. Cysts can also occur in the fingers, elbow,

and shoulder. Ganglion cysts are generally painless but can cause pain due to compression of the overlying nerve or the joint space. On examination, the mass is mobile and should transilluminate with a light source.

▶ Treatment

The fluid within the ganglion cyst has a gel-like consistency and must be aspirated with a wide-gauge needle, such as an 18 or 20 gauge. Aspiration is sometimes successful but high recurrence is reported (up to 95%). Surgical exploration is the most effective means of long-term control in which the entire cyst, check-valve, and underlying cause of the localized synovial degeneration (such as an osteophyte) are resected.

4. Medial & Lateral Humeral Epicondylitis

ESSENTIALS OF DIAGNOSIS

▶ Pain and tenderness over the involved epicondyle.
▶ Wrist flexion exacerbates the pain of medial epicondylitis.
▶ Wrist extension exacerbates the pain of lateral epicondylitis.

▶ General Considerations

The forearm flexors originate from the medial humeral epicondyle, and the extensors originate from the lateral humeral epicondyle. Inflammation at the insertions of these muscles is referred to as epicondylitis. The term "tennis elbow" for lateral epicondylitis was initially used in the nineteenth century because of the lateral elbow pain exacerbated with forceful wrist extension and supination to achieve topspin during the backhand stroke. Tennis is certainly not the only cause of this overexertion syndrome.

▶ Clinical Findings

Clinically, there is pain at the epicondyle, which is worsened with contraction of the involved muscles. In lateral epicondylitis, the pain is worse with wrist extension and in medial epicondylitis with wrist flexion. Patients may complain of difficulty with simple tasks, such as holding a coffee cup. Histologic preparations from surgical debridements show evidence of microtrauma at the origin of the extensor carpi radialis brevis and longus with evidence of neovascularization and healing without any evidence of acute inflammation. There is also weakness of the associated muscles secondary to pain. Epicondylitis is seen more commonly in the fourth and fifth decades of life. Younger patients should be examined for other causes of pain, such as elbow instability, tumors, or osteochondritis dissecans. Pain over the medial elbow with valgus stress can indicate ulnar collateral ligament injury, especially in a throwing athlete.

Treatment

The large majority (85–95%) of patients respond to conservative therapy, with a 2–3 week course of rest, splinting, and NSAIDs, followed by a course of gentle strengthening exercises and the use of a commercially available forearm support band. Glucocorticoid injections may be helpful to alleviate severe discomfort, with care taken to avoid more than three injections or superficial injections, since there can be severe skin atrophy. Surgical options include (1) debridement of the flexor or extensor tendon origins at the epicondyle; (2) lengthening or fasciotomy of the tendon origin if there is tension; (3) decompression of the radial sensory branches around the elbow; or (4) elbow joint arthroplasty with ligament division, synovectomy, or epicondylectomy. Results of surgery can be excellent, although not always predictable.

5. Dupuytren Contractures

ESSENTIALS OF DIAGNOSIS

▶ Thickened cords of the palmar fascia that lead to flexion contractures.
▶ Strong familial tendency and a predilection for males.

General Considerations & Clinical Findings

Dupuytren contractures are thickened cords of the palmar fascia that cause flexion contractures of the metacarpophalangeal and proximal interphalangeal (PIP) joints. The cords progress slowly and become tender ad limit hand function. The ring finger and little finger are most commonly affected. The index finger and the thumb are generally not involved. The etiology is poorly understood, but there is a strong genetic predisposition and is more common in people of Scandinavian or Northern European ancestry. This condition is ten times more likely to develop in men than in women.

Treatment

Traditionally, surgical release and debridement of the cords has been the mainstay of treatment for symptomatic patients, but there is considerable morbidity and risk of recurrence. Needle aponeurotomy is a less invasive technique in which the fascial cords are punctured with a needle and released by extending the finger; however, high rates of recurrence have

been reported. Collagenase injections into the fascial cords are a promising new treatment with lower morbidity than surgery yet with similar low recurrence rates.

JOINT RELATED CAUSES OF PAIN

Hand, elbow, and wrist pain are often due to either an inflammatory or degenerative arthritis.

1. Nodal Osteoarthritis

ESSENTIALS OF DIAGNOSIS

▶ Heberden and Bouchard nodes.
▶ Radiographic evidence of osteoarthritis at the DIP and PIP joints.

Clinical Findings

Nodal osteoarthritis, a common condition in patients over 45 years of age, represents proliferative changes in joints in response to chronic loss of joint cartilage. Some patients have acute flares, with redness and joint swelling that can be confused with an acute attack of microcrystalline or rheumatoid arthritis. As the inflammatory process subsides, permanent bony changes at the affected joints develop, known as Heberden nodes when they are at the DIP joints and Bouchard nodes when they are at the PIP joints (Figure 6–4 and Plate 11). A common associated finding is a ganglion cyst (sometimes referred to as a mucous cyst in this location) on the dorsal surface of the finger, distal to the DIP joint and proximal to the nailfold.

It is important to note that osteoarthritis can coexist with the various crystalline and rheumatoid arthritides, making the diagnosis more challenging. Unlike the hip and the knee, the hand is relatively non-weight bearing, so patients can present with radiographs with advanced arthritis including joint-space narrowing, subchondral cysts and osteophytes, and will be asymptomatic. The arthritis can be of rapid onset and can be quite destructive.

Treatment

DIP and PIP joint arthritis is generally treated with oral anti-inflammatory medications, hand therapy for range of motion, and splinting for relief of pain. Symptomatic ganglion cysts can be aspirated and injected with glucocorticoids. Patients should be informed of the chronic, progressive nature of the condition, which can be indolent in some, while in others can be crippling. Arthrodesis can be done for severe pain in the DIP joint. For the PIP joint arthritis, surgical options include either joint arthrodesis (fusion) or joint arthroplasty (replacement). In the PIP

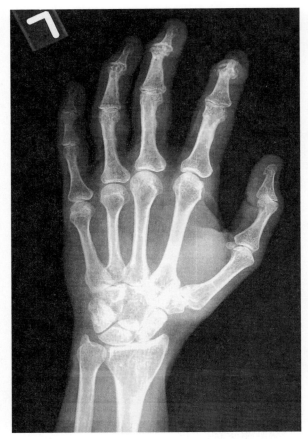

▲ **Figure 6–4.** Radiograph of a left hand with significant arthritis in the distal interphalangeal (DIP) and proximal interphalangeal joints.

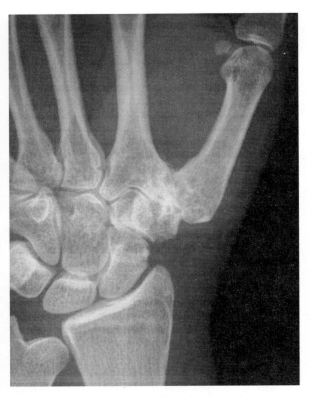

▲ **Figure 6–5.** Radiograph of the left thumb shows loss of the joint space between the proximal thumb metacarpal and the trapezium bone. There is also bony sclerosis and bony cysts noted in both bones and faint osteophytes. Both are characteristic of carpometacarpal (CMC) joint arthritis. There is also proximal and radial subluxation of the thumb metacarpal, indicative of CMC joint ligament laxity, caused by the progressive arthritis.

joint, it is preferable to preserve motion when possible, as arthrodesis can be quite limiting for hand function.

2. Basilar Thumb Osteoarthritis (Thumb Carpometacarpal Joint Osteoarthritis)

ESSENTIALS OF DIAGNOSIS

▶ Pain at the base of the thumb made worse by pinching activity.
▶ Pain and crepitance with passive rotation and compression of the thumb carpometacarpal (CMC) joint.
▶ Degenerative changes of the thumb CMC joint on radiographs.

▶ General Considerations

The base of the thumb is the area in the hand most commonly affected by osteoarthritis (Figure 6–5). It is more common in women 50 years and older. Thumb motion is ubiquitous in daily activities and acts as a lever arm with the fulcrum at the CMC joint causing large physiologic loads in people who perform repeated pinching activities. Pinch power at the tip of the thumb is amplified 25 times at the base of the thumb, because of the long lever arm. Patients report pain with turning a key, turning the door knob, and opening a jar. The Eaton classification defines the initial stage of the disease as rupture of the palmar "beak" ligament, which destabilizes the joint and converts compressive forces to shear forces. The next two stages show slight then severe narrowing with osteophytes of the CMC joint. The final stage, stage IV, involves pan-trapezial arthritis.

Clinical Findings

Physical examination findings include pain and crepitus on passive rotation and compression of the joint. This is referred to as a positive "CMC grind test." de Quervain tendinitis should be ruled out as the two have similar symptoms. With advanced CMC joint arthritis, there will be a palpable and visible protrusion of the thumb base on the radial dorsal side with the thumb held in a slightly flexed and clasped position into the hand. This is due to the erosion of the surrounding ligaments of the thumb CMC joint and loss of joint stability causing collapse of the thumb base. The pull of the long extensor and the flexor tendons cause the flexed or the "clasp" position of the thumb. Physical examination is usually sufficient to make this diagnosis, but radiographs can also be confirmatory (see Figure 6–4).

Treatment

Osteoarthritis of the thumb CMC joint is treated initially with oral anti-inflammatory medicines and a wrist-based thumb splint to immobilize the CMC joint. Should this not work, glucocorticoids can be injected into the joint to relieve the pain and the inflammation temporarily. The patients are told that the injections can relieve the pain although they do not reverse the degenerative process. Unless there are overriding reasons, patients should not receive more than three glucocorticoid injections into the joint. As the cartilage and joint destruction progresses, pain and stiffness may eventually necessitate surgical intervention.

One surgical option includes tendon interpositional arthroplasty, with removal of the trapezium followed by ligamentous tendon reconstruction of the joint. Silicone interposition arthroplasties have been performed in the past but are no longer advised because of prosthetic failure and silicone synovitis. Arthrodesis between the thumb metacarpal and the trapezium is another option in treating CMC joint arthritis. This limits the range of motion in the thumb and is contraindicated in patients who have progressed to stage III or IV disease involving the scaphoid-trapezium-trapezoid joints.

3. Scapholunate Advanced Collapse

ESSENTIALS OF DIAGNOSIS

▶ Deep, aching pain in the wrist associated with activity.
▶ A long-term consequence of rupture of the scapholunate ligament following untreated wrist trauma.

General Considerations & Clinical Findings

Scapholunate advanced collapse, also known as a SLAC wrist, is the most common pattern of wrist arthritis. This condition, due to the rupture of the scapholunate ligament, is often associated with a scaphoid fracture. Patients often present years after an untreated wrist injury with deep aching pain associated with activity. A common clinical scenario is the patient with an unrecognized or an untreated scaphoid fracture in the distant past, which has de-stabilized the wrist, causing the degenerative changes. Stage I is radial sided joint narrowing with a radial styloid osteophyte. Stage II involves radio-scaphoid arthritis, and stage III involves proximal migration or "collapse" of the capitate bone through the scapholunate joint with capitolunate arthrosis.

Treatment

Treatment depends on the stage of presentation. It is important to recognize scaphoid fractures so that they can be treated at the time of the injury. For stage I disease, the scapholunate joint is re-approximated and the radial styloid removed. For stage II disease, a larger stabilization procedure is necessary. The options include a proximal row carpectomy, four corner fusion, or wrist fusion. For stage III disease, the wrist is generally fused.

4. Triangular Fibrocartilage Complex & Distal Radial Ulnar Joint Injuries

ESSENTIALS OF DIAGNOSIS

▶ Common injury following fall onto an outstretched wrist.

General Considerations & Clinical Findings

An increasingly recognized source of chronic ulnar sided wrist pain is a triangular fibrocartilage complex (TFCC) injury. Patients present with activity-related aching pain without sensory or motor deficits. They often have a history of a fall onto the outstretched wrist. The TFCC is a fibrous hammock that stretches from the ulnar styloid to the radial articular surface and supports the carpal bones. When the TFCC is injured, the ulnar side of the wrist is destabilized allowing ulnar impaction. In severe cases, the TFCC injury can destabilize the distal radial ulnar joint (DRUJ), resulting in severe pain that can be disabling. On physical examination, the patients have ulnar sided wrist pain with ulnar deviation of the wrist and axial compression. Pain may be reproduced when using their hands to help them rise from a seated position. Radiographs may show an old ulnar styloid fracture. An MRI arthrogram is the most sensitive imaging modality.

Treatment

A course of nonsurgical management with splinting and NSAIDs is indicated for a stable DRUJ as assessed by physical examination. Arthroscopic debridement or repair of the TFCC may be of benefit. If ulnocarpal impaction is causing the pain, an ulnar shortening osteotomy may be necessary. Ulnar styloid fractures may need to be repaired to tension the TFCC.

VASCULAR CAUSES OF PAIN

Ischemic symptoms range from mild (such as cold intolerance, decreased digital temperature, or intermittent color changes) to severe (such as excruciating ischemic pain, fingertip ulceration, or necrosis). The patient may also point out the presence of a mass that could represent an aneurysm or an arteriovenous malformation. Once vascular insufficiency is established, the cause of the insufficiency has to be determined. This may be due to an underlying medical condition, such as hypercoagulable disorder, atherosclerosis, embolic disorder, connective tissue diseases, malignancy, or diabetes mellitus. The patient should also be asked about occupational and recreational exposure to vibration or other repetitive hand trauma that could cause hypothenar hammer syndrome. It is important to ask about exposure to tobacco and toxic chemicals that might cause distal capillary spasms. Symptoms that increase with arm position or exercise may tip off the examiner to thoracic outlet syndrome or proximal occlusive disease.

Hand perfusion should be assessed with the Allen test, testing for perfusion through either the ulnar or the radial artery. Although there may some false-positive and false-negative results, the Allen test is easy and useful. To increase the sensitivity of circulation, the Doppler should be used to evaluate the radial and ulnar arteries, as well as the digital arteries on both the ulnar and radial sides of the finger. The use of advanced noninvasive imaging, such as the magnetic resonance or computed tomographic angiography, can image a vessel as small as 1 mm with good resolution. However, the gold standard in evaluating the vascular anatomy in the hand is still an arteriogram, which visualizes the entire vascular tree from the aortic root to the distal finger.

A comprehensive survey of the many vascular disorders of the upper extremity is beyond the scope of this chapter. If a circulatory urgency or emergency is found on history and physical examination, it is incumbent on the physician to make a speedy referral to a qualified hand surgeon.

Badalamente MA, Hurst LC. Efficacy and safety of injectable mixed collagenase subtypes in the treatment of Dupuytren's contracture. *J Hand Surg Am.* 2007;32:767. [PMID: 17606053]

Calfee RP, Patel A, DaSilva MF, Akelman E. Management of lateral epicondylitis: current concepts. *J Am Acad Orthop Surg.* 2008;16:19. [PMID: 18180389]

Cranford CS, Ho JY, Kalainov DM, Hartigan BJ. Carpal tunnel syndrome. *J Am Acad Orthop Surg.* 2007;15:537. [PMID: 17761610]

Deune EG, Mackinnon SE. Endoscopic carpal tunnel release. The voice of polite dissent. *Clin Plast Surg.* 1996;23:487. [PMID: 8826685]

Drucker WR, Hubay CA, Holden WD, Bukovnic JA. Pathogenesis of post-traumatic sympathetic dystrophy. *Am J Surg.* 1959;97:454. [PMID: 13627386]

Ferdinand RD, MacLean JG. Endoscopic versus open carpal tunnel release in bilateral carpal tunnel syndrome. A prospective, randomized, blinded assessment. *J Bone Joint Surg Br.* 2002;84:375. [PMID: 12002496]

Gervasio O, Gambardella G, Zacone C, Branca D. Simple decompression versus anterior submuscular transposition of the ulnar nerve in severe cubital tunnel syndrome: a prospective randomized study. *Neurosurgery.* 2005;56:108. [PMID: 15617592]

Goergen T, Dalinka MK, Alazraki N, et al. Chronic elbow pain. American College of Radiology. ACR Appropriateness Criteria. *Radiology.* 2000;215: 339. [PMID: 11037446]

Green DP, Hotchkiss, RN, Pederson WC: *Green's Operative Hand Surgery,* 4th ed. New York: Churchill Livingstone, 1999.

Hui AC, Wong S, Leung CH, et al. A randomized controlled trial of surgery vs steroid injection for carpal tunnel syndrome. *Neurology.* 2005;64:2074. [PMID: 15985575]

Kerr CD, Gittins ME, Sybert DR. Endoscopic versus open carpal tunnel release: clinical results. *Arthroscopy.* 1994;10:266. [PMID: 8086018]

Li Z, Smith TL, Koman LA. Diagnosis and management of complex regional pain syndrome complicating upper extremity recovery. *J Hand Ther.* 2005;18:270. [PMID: 15891984]

Mackinnon SE, Dellon AL. Ulnar nerve entrapment at the wrist. In Mackinnon SE, Dellon AL (eds). *Surgery of the Peripheral Nerve.* New York: Thieme; 1988;97–216.

Medical Research Council of the United Kingdom. Aids to Examination of the Peripheral Nervous System: Memorandum No 45. Palo Alto, Calif: Pedragon House. 1978.

Nagle DJ. Endoscopic carpal tunnel release. In favor. *Clin Plast Surg.* 1996;23:477. [PMID: 8826684]

Nagle DJ. Endoscopic carpal tunnel release. *Hand Clin.* 2002;18:307. [PMID: 12371033]

Nagle DJ. Evaluation of chronic wrist pain. *J Am Acad Orthop Surg.* 2000;8:45. [PMID: 10666652]

O'Connor D, Marshall S, Massy-Westropp N. Non-surgical treatment (other than steroid injection) for carpal tunnel syndrome. *Cochrane Database Syst Rev.* 2003;(1):CD003219. [PMID: 12535461]

Trumble TE, Budoff JE. *Hand Surgery Update IV,* Rosemont IL, American Society for Surgery of the Hand 2007.

Approach to the Patient with Foot & Ankle Pain

Richard J. de Asla, MD

John Kwon, MD

The foot and ankle are marvelous biomechanical creations. Tasked with forward propulsion, shock absorption, and providing balance for more than one hundred and twenty million steps in the average lifetime, it is a wonder that more people do not have more problems than they already have with their feet.

It is useful to divide the foot into the following three anatomic regions for evaluation: forefoot, midfoot, and hindfoot. Each region has its own unique pathology. Similarly, when evaluating the ankle it is helpful to consider whether the complaint is generated from an intra-articular or extra-articular source. In either case, a working knowledge of the anatomy is essential.

The forefoot includes the phalanges and the metatarsals. The midfoot boundaries include the tarsometatarsal joint (or Lisfranc joint complex) and the midtarsal joints (talonavicular and calcaneal-cuboid joints). The hindfoot consists of the talus and calcaneus (Figure 7–1).

The ankle (tibiotalar) joint is largely responsible for dorsiflexion and plantarflexion of the foot. The joint itself is composed of the distal tibia, the distal fibula, and the talus. Inversion and eversion motion of the foot occurs cooperatively through the subtalar (talocalcaneal), talonavicular, and calcaneal- cuboid joints. The joints in the midfoot region contribute very little to foot motion.

There are five major peripheral nerves that innervate the foot. Three of these run superficial to the fascia (sural nerve, superficial peroneal nerve, and saphenous nerve) and two are deep to the fascia (the posterior tibial nerve and the deep peroneal nerve) (Figure 7–2).

▼ FOREFOOT PAIN

METATARSALGIA

Metatarsalgia is plantar pain under the metatarsal heads or under the "ball" of the foot from abnormal loading. This term is often used incorrectly to describe any plantar forefoot pain

and should be reserved for pain localized under the metatarsal heads with loading from standing or gait. Although multiple etiologies of forefoot pain exist, symptoms from metatarsalgia are typically under the second or third metatarsal heads. Careful physical examination reveals tenderness directly under the metatarsal head with less or no tenderness dorsally, with toe motion, or with palpation in the web spaces. The differential diagnosis is extensive but includes stress fracture, metatarsophalangeal joint (MTP) synovitis, Freiberg disease, Morton neuroma, bursitis/neuritis, and either degenerative or inflammatory arthritides of the MTP joints. Metatarsalgia is commonly seen with hammertoe deformities due to plantar displacement of the metatarsal head secondary to tendon imbalance. It is also commonly associated with bunion deformity as increased angulation leads to decreased load bearing by the first ray during gait and transfer of the weight-bearing load to the relatively longer second metatarsal.

METATARSAL STRESS FRACTURE

 ESSENTIALS OF DIAGNOSIS

► Insidious development of dorsal forefoot pain after increased physical activity or change in shoe wear.
► Pain to direct palpation of the metatarsal.

► Clinical Findings

A. Symptoms and Signs

Metatarsal stress fractures are incomplete metadiaphyseal or diaphyseal breaks that typically involve the metatarsal neck or shaft. Although any metatarsal can be involved, classically these are seen in the second or third metatarsals. Fatigue stress fractures occur with repeated overload of normal bone past its remodeling capabilities or with normal loading in

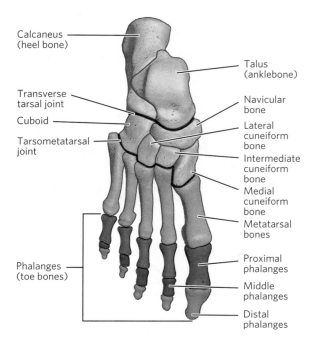

Calcaneus (heel bone)

Talus (anklebone)

Transverse tarsal joint

Navicular bone

Cuboid

Lateral cuneiform bone

Tarsometatarsal joint

Intermediate cuneiform bone

Medial cuneiform bone

Metatarsal bones

Phalanges (toe bones)

Proximal phalanges

Middle phalanges

Distal phalanges

▲ **Figure 7–1.** Anatomy of the foot.

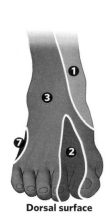
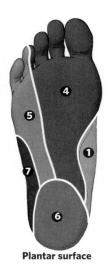

Dorsal surface **Plantar surface**

▲ **Figure 7–2.** Cutaneous innervation of the foot. Key: (1) Saphenous nerve. (2) Deep peroneal nerve. (3) Superficial peroneal nerve. (4) Medial plantar nerve. (5) Lateral plantar nerve. (6) Calcaneal branch (tibial nerve). (7) Sural nerve.

osteoporotic bone. Although most patients with fatigue stress fractures have a history of increased physical activity or loading, this is not always the case.

Metatarsal stress fracture typically presents subacutely; patients often do not have a history of significant trauma. Forefoot pain with ambulation and dorsal forefoot swelling is common. Pain is localized directly over the stress fracture.

B. Imaging Studies and Special Tests

Plain weight-bearing radiographs should be obtained. Because early radiographs are often normal, repeat examination in 10 days is warranted if high clinical suspicion persists. MRI can reveal bone marrow edema or occult cortical breaks earlier than radiographs, but repeat examination with a radiograph is the more cost effective strategy.

▶ Treatment

Treatment consists of immobilization in either a postoperative shoe or fracture boot for up to 4–6 weeks. Weight bearing should be allowed as tolerated but rest is recommended as long as the patient has pain. Patients should take calcium/ vitamin D supplementation when appropriate and should limit high-dose glucocorticoids they may delay bone healing in the early stages. Tobacco use increases the rate of delayed or nonunion of the fracture, and smoking cessation is therefore recommended. Close follow-up should be considered because there is a small risk for displacement.

METATARSOPHALANGEAL JOINT STRESS SYNDROME

ESSENTIALS OF DIAGNOSIS

▶ Increased incidence of central metatarsalgia involving the second and third MTP joints.

▶ Point tenderness over the metatarsal heads with palpation.

▶ Clinical Findings

A. Symptoms and Signs

The MTP joint stress syndrome occurs when increased stress from load bearing is transferred abnormally to these joints. Since the second and third tarsometatarsal joints are relatively fixed, these MTP joints are affected most commonly. The first, fourth, and fifth tarsometatarsal joints are in comparison more mobile and are less affected as a result, but sesamoiditis can manifest as metatarsalgia of the first ray. Predisposing factors include synovitis, spondyloarthropathies, and multiple biomechanical alterations of the foot that may predispose to abnormal forefoot loading. Examples of such biomechanical alterations include the cavo varus deformity, Achilles/gastrocnemius contracture, fat pad atrophy, arthritis, posttraumatic deformities. Bunion deformities often lead to second MTP metatarsalgia due to an increased angulation between the first and second metatarsals and decreased relative loading of the first ray with ambulation. Although initially presenting as plantar forefoot pain secondary to inflammation, long-standing metatarsalgia can lead to MTP joint dislocation, stress fracture, and digital deformities (hammer toe, claw toe, cross-over toe).

Pain is described as a dull ache under the plantar forefoot ("ball of the foot") with symptoms exacerbated by increased activity or the use of high heels that increase forefoot loading. Lesser toe deformities may exist. Morton neuroma must be considered if the patients complain of pain radiating into the toes. Patients typically have point tenderness under the metatarsal heads or at the MTP joint with increased pain with toe motion. If there is no tenderness in the plantar region and the patient reports pain with toe motion, isolated MTP synovitis should be considered. Patients with long-standing symptoms of MTP pain may have joint instability. In such cases, an evaluation for MTP joint subluxation should be performed. The Lachman or vertical load test assesses the stability and integrity of the ligaments and capsular structures. To perform this test, the examiner stabilizes the metatarsal with one hand while lifting the digit at the proximal phalanx dorsally with the other, assessing the patient for joint stability and symptom exacerbation.

B. Imaging Studies and Special Tests

Plain radiographs of the foot are usually unremarkable but are essential to exclude other conditions. Weight-bearing radiographs are required.

▶ Treatment

Treatment consists of shoe wear modification, nonsteroidal anti-inflammatory drugs (NSAIDs), and activity modification. Stiff sole shoes and the avoidance of high heels is recommended. Often times a shoe with a rocker bottom may help alleviate symptoms. An orthosis with a metatarsal bar and recess under the metatarsal heads is usually beneficial. Toe strapping may be helpful to limit motion. Glucocorticoid injections should be used sparingly as ligament and capsular weakening and rupture can occur.

MORTON NEUROMA

ESSENTIALS OF DIAGNOSIS

▶ *Plantar* forefoot pain with possible radiation into the toes.

▶ Tenderness on compression of the involved web space.

▶ Presence of a "Mulder click" is highly suggestive of the condition.

▶ Clinical Findings

A. Symptoms and Signs

Morton neuroma is an entrapment neuropathy of the small interdigital nerves. This is associated with perineural fibrosis and soft tissue swelling. The third MTP interspace is the most common location, although the second is often involved. Rarely are the first or fourth interspaces involved. The hallmark of Morton neuroma is a burning pain radiating into the toes. Patients often complain of plantar foot pain as well and often describe the sensation of "walking on a pebble" or as if their socks were bunched in the forefoot area. Symptoms are often exacerbated with tight shoe wear and high heels and alleviated when barefoot. Compression of the webspace often elicits symptoms. Often the nerve can be subluxed with forefoot compression and dorsal pressure in the interspace (Mulder click) although the sensitivity and specificity of this test is questionable. The clinician should consider other diagnoses if the patient denies any radiating pain into the toes.

B. Imaging Studies and Special Tests

Plain radiographs are often normal although are useful to rule out other causes of pain. MRI and ultrasound have limited usefulness, since normal or abnormal radiographic findings do not correlate well with clinical presentation.

▶ Treatment

Initial treatment consists of shoe wear modification, NSAIDs, and activity modification. If these measure fail, glucocorticoid injection may be considered but there exists a risk of ligament and capsular weakening from repeated use. Recalcitrant cases should be referred for neurectomy.

DEEP PERONEAL NERVE ENTRAPMENT

ESSENTIALS OF DIAGNOSIS

▶ Pain, paresthesias, and dysesthesias in the first web space.

▶ Positive Tinel sign with percussion.

▶ Pain relief after nerve block.

▶ Clinical Findings

A. Symptoms and Signs

Deep peroneal nerve entrapment is a compression neuropathy of the deep peroneal nerve. This often occurs more proximally at the anterior tarsal tunnel or distally as the nerve passes over the midfoot. Proximal entrapment occurs when the nerve is affected as it passes under the anterior ankle extensor retinaculum. The anterior ankle extensor retinaculum is a fibrous band of tissue that encases the neurovascular bundle as well as the extensor tendons of the ankle and foot. More distal entrapment can occur as the nerve passes intimately over the midfoot and is often secondary to trauma, scarring, and arthritis or bone spurs.

Patients with deep peroneal nerve entrapment present with pain, paresthesias or dysesthesias isolated to the dorsal first web space (dermatome of the deep peroneal nerve). Ankle and foot plantar flexion, compression or percussion exacerbate symptoms over the site of entrapment (Tinel sign). Increased physical activity, particularly while wearing shoes that increase dorsal pressure on the nerve, also exacerbates symptoms. Most patients have a component of rest pain as well. Late in the disease, weakness of the extensor hallucis brevis may occur. This is heralded by weakness to hallux extension with resistance placed against the proximal phalanx.

B. Imaging Studies and Special Tests

Weight-bearing radiographs are important to assess for bone spurring or arthritis, which can lead to nerve compression, and to exclude other etiologies of pain. MRI may be a useful adjuvant to assess for ganglion cysts or other masses that may be causing compression.

▶ Treatment

Symptomatic treatment includes the use of NSAIDs, rest, and stiff shoes with the avoidance of dorsal pressure. Topical analgesics and medications for neuropathic pain may help. Immobilization and injections should be considered for recalcitrant cases. If all conservative measures fail, referral for decompression and neurolysis is warranted.

HALLUX RIGIDUS

ESSENTIALS OF DIAGNOSIS

▶ Limited or absent motion of the first MTP joint.
▶ Radiographic evidence of osteoarthritis.

▶ Clinical Findings

A. Symptoms and Signs

Hallux rigidus is secondary to degenerative arthritis of the first MTP joint. Patients may have a history of trauma, although this may seem benign. Patients complain of pain with attempted weight bearing and with activities that require increased motion at the MTP joint. Pain is centered over the hallux MTP joint and is worse with walking barefoot, on the beach or with high heels. Patients may notice decreased symptoms when wearing stiff soled shoes. Patients may report tenderness with pressure due to bone spurring and often complain of nerve symptoms into the hallux secondary to mild compressive neuropathy of the digital nerves from swelling or spurs. Patients often confuse their condition with a bunion deformity due to the appearance of a "bump" on the great toe. Hallux rigidus can coexist with hallux valgus deformity. A personal and family history of gout or other crystalline arthropathy should be elicited. The swelling associated with hallux rigidus is often less severe, less acute, and with less redness than that seen in podagra.

Hallux dorsiflexion should equal lesser toe dorsiflexion and limited dorsiflexion with elicitation of pain is the hallmark sign of hallux rigidus. Plantar flexion is often limited and can cause pain due to the stretching of soft tissues over the prominent dorsal spur. With advanced arthritis, the grind test (axial loading of the joint) is positive. Patients often have tenderness with palpation of the spurs.

B. Imaging Studies and Special Tests

Weight-bearing plain radiographs reveal joint-space narrowing, sclerosis, subchondral cysts, spurring, and sometimes malalignment. Periarticular erosions are classic for a gouty arthropathy.

▶ Treatment

Initial treatment consists of rest, NSAIDs, activity modification, and shoe wear modification. Stiff sole shoes, rocker bottom shoes, and the avoidance of high heels are recommended. A rigid orthosis, such as a Morton extension, can help alleviate symptoms. Surgery is indicated if conservative measures fail.

HALLUX VALGUS

ESSENTIALS OF DIAGNOSIS

▶ Lateral deviation of the hallux with medial bunion causing pain.

▶ Clinical Findings

A. Symptoms and Signs

Hallux valgus (bunion) consists of lateral deviation of the hallux with medial MTP joint irritation and is associated with shoe wear, female gender, and hyperlaxity conditions. Hallux valgus results from angular deformity at multiple joints in the foot and is not a result of simple medial bone growth. Patients typically complain of pain directly over the bunion that is often exacerbated by shoe wear and hallux motion. With more advanced conditions, patients may complain of forefoot pain due to metatarsalgia or commonly associated lesser toe deformities such as hammer and cross-toe deformities. Patients may also complain of toe numbness due to the stretching of the medial digital nerves. Patients have tenderness most often over the bunion itself but can have pain with MTP motion and metatarsalgia.

B. Imaging Studies and Special Tests

Weight-bearing plain radiographs are essential for diagnosis.

▶ Treatment

Initial conservative treatment should consist of shoe wear modification (open toe shoes or those with a wide, tall toe box), NSAIDs, and activity modification. Toe straps and spacers may be helpful although they do not permanently correct or limit the progression of hallux valgus. Night bunion splints have no utility and may be harmful, particularly in the neuropathic patient or those with vascular compromise. Orthotics may help with symptoms secondary to metatarsalgia but have a limited role in the treatment of hallux valgus. When conservative measures fail and the patient has continued pain and disability, surgery may be indicated. Surgery is not indicated for cosmetics in the absence of pain.

▼ SUBTALAR JOINT & MIDFOOT DISORDERS

Subtalar motion is responsible for inversion and eversion of the hindfoot and helps assist ambulation on uneven ground. Midfoot motion, although relatively small compared to ankle or subtalar motion, is a complex coupling of abduction, adduction, rotation and translation of smaller joints and helps translate hindfoot motion to the forefoot during gait.

Multiple conditions can interfere with hindfoot and midfoot motion including trauma, posttraumatic arthritis, coalitions, and rheumatologic conditions such as osteoarthritis and inflammatory arthropathy. Congenital or acquired malalignment conditions such as pes planus (flat foot) and cavo varus foot deformities (high arches) inherently create limitations in subtalar and midfoot motion by altering normal foot kinematics.

A pes planus or flat foot deformity exists if the hindfoot is in valgus/eversion, the midfoot is collapsed plantar medially and abducted with the foot in a pronated position. This malpositioning results in unlocking of the transverse tarsal joints, which manifest as midfoot instability with gait and attempted heel rising and a general sense of weakness with plantar flexion. As increased motion in the sagittal plane occurs through the midfoot with gait, the Achilles tendon or gastrocnemius often becomes contracted over time. Pes planus can be either congenital such as in the case of coalitions or accessory navicular or secondary to various rheumatologic conditions, posterior tibial tendon insufficiency, trauma or acute rupture (or both) of the posterior tibialis tendon, hypermobility conditions, or neuropathic arthropathy. The asymptomatic flatfoot is not necessarily pathologic as arch height has a relatively wide spectrum of normal.

A cavo varus or high arch deformity exists if the hindfoot is in varus/inversion, the midfoot has an abnormally high medial arch and the foot is in a supinated position. Although this deformity can simply fall within the spectrum of normal arch height, one must consider other etiologies as neuromuscular disorders such as Charcot-Marie-Tooth present with this classic foot deformity.

Symptoms often depend on the underlying etiology although patients with symptomatic pes planus deformity typically complain of medial ankle or foot pain initially. With progress deformity, patients complain of medial plantar foot pain secondary to increased loading of the plantar medially displaced talar head with ambulation and lateral ankle pain secondary to subfibular impingement. Patients with symptomatic caro varus typically complain of lateral ankle pain, ankle instability, and lateral foot pain secondary to overload.

Along with other conservative modalities, initial treatment should consist of orthosis. With flexible deformities a semi-rigid posted orthotic to correct the deformity is often effective. With long-standing symptomatic rigid deformities, these modalities become less effective and ankle bracing or surgery may be required.

▼ HINDFOOT PAIN

HEEL PAIN

A range of disorders manifest as heel pain (Table 7–1). Accurate diagnosis starts with identifying the location of the pain source. Most heel pain occurs under the plantar, weight-bearing surface or over the posterior aspect.

PLANTAR FASCIITIS

ESSENTIALS OF DIAGNOSIS

▶ Pain with the first steps of the morning or with rising from a seated position.
▶ Pain elicited by deep palpation of the plantar fascia origin.

Table 7–1. Causes of heel pain.

Infracalcaneal pain
 Plantar fasciitis
 Infracalcaneal nerve entrapment
 Fat pad atrophy
 Infracalcaneal bursitis
 Calcaneal stress fracture
 Tarsal tunnel syndrome
 Radiculopathy
 Spondyloarthropathy
 Infection
 Tumor
 Fractured heel spur
Retrocalcaneal heel pain
 Achilles tendinitis
 Haglund deformity
 Pre-Achilles bursitis
 Retrocalcaneal bursitis
 Posterior lateral calcaneal exostosis
 Lateral calcaneal adventitious bursitis
Tenderness with lateral compression of the heel
 Stress fracture of the calcaneus
 Osteomyelitis (especially in children)
 Calcaneal apophysitis (ie, Sever disease, especially in boys
  ages 8–15 years)

► Clinical Findings

A. Symptoms and Signs

The most common cause of plantar heel pain is plantar fasciitis and much misinformation surrounds this topic. Plantar fasciitis is a benign, self-limited enthesopathy that occurs at the origin of the plantar fascia on the plantar medial tubercle of the calcaneus (Figure 7–3). Plantar fasciitis is often mistakenly attributed to "heel spurs," most of which are asymptomatic and unrelated to the pain. The exact etiology of plantar fasciitis is unknown but may be more common in runners, patients with pes planus, and associated with a tight Achilles tendon. A nearly universal complaint is pain in the plantar heel with the first steps after rising out of bed. Pain initially diminishes with activity only to recur after a period of prolonged activity. Less commonly, pain may occur in the plantar aspect of the medial arch along plantar fascia's medial cord.

B. Imaging Studies and Special Tests

The diagnosis of plantar fasciitis is based on the history and physical examination findings. Radiographs are of little value in the diagnosis of plantar fasciitis but may be needed to rule out other disorders such as calcaneal stress fractures or a fractured infracalcaneal heel spur. The presence of infracalcaneal heel spurs on radiographs correlates poorly with symptoms.

► Treatment

It is important to reiterate that plantar fasciitis is a *self-limited condition*. Therefore, every attempt should be made to avoid invasive procedures. Initial treatment focuses on plantar fascia and Achilles tendon stretching, NSAIDs, and use of a heel cushion to provide symptomatic relief. Night splints may reduce morning symptoms. There is little evidence to suggest that orthotics provide relief. Custom molded orthotics have no proven benefit over prefabricated commercially available inserts. Taping techniques can provide temporary relief but frequent re-taping is required for prolonged relief. High-energy ultrasound and use of magnetic insoles have failed to demonstrate efficacy in randomized, controlled studies. Judicious use of glucocorticoid injections may provide symptomatic relief but multiple injections are associated with fat pad atrophy and plantar fascia rupture. Walking casts and boots are also considered.

Extracorporeal shock wave therapy (ESWT) is considered in refractory cases. Patients who respond best have point tenderness over the heel and no associated pathology (eg, nerve entrapment). The modality is safe with limited side effects. About two-thirds of patients experience pain relief. ESWT is generally not covered by insurance plans.

Surgical release of the plantar fascia is considered only in the most refractory of cases when symptoms persist for over a year and have not responded to more conservative measures.

BAXTER NERVE SYNDROME (ENTRAPMENT OF THE FIRST BRANCH OF THE LATERAL PLANTAR NERVE)

 ESSENTIALS OF DIAGNOSIS

► Burning pain that persists in the plantar heel even after weight bearing (so-called "after burn").
► Pain to direct palpation over the region of the Baxter nerve.

► Clinical Findings

Entrapment of first branch of the *lateral plantar nerve* (ie, *Baxter nerve*) between the deep fascia layers of the abductor hallucis muscle and the quadratus plantae results in signs and symptoms very similar to those experienced with plantar fasciitis. The condition commonly coexists with plantar fasciitis. The classic patient is a male runner in his mid to late thirties. Pain may radiate from the inferomedial aspect of the heel to the medial ankle or across the plantar aspect to the lateral foot. Symptoms are

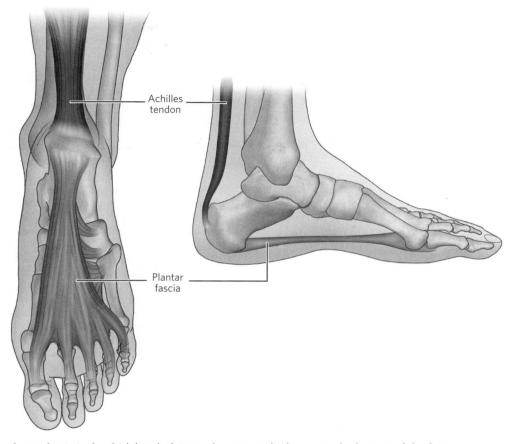

Achilles tendon

Plantar fascia

▲ **Figure 7–3.** Plantar fascia is the thick band of tissue that covers the bones on the bottom of the foot.

exacerbated by impact loading. Pain typically lingers even when weight-bearing activities have ceased. This so-called "after burn" can help differentiate Baxter nerve syndrome from plantar fasciitis.

Knowledge of the local anatomy is required for accurate diagnosis. The pathognomonic finding in these patients is reproduction of tenderness and radiating pain with direct pressure over Baxter nerve deep to the abductor hallucis muscle.

▶ Treatment

The condition can be quite frustrating for patients as symptoms often persist for nearly 2 years. Modalities used to alleviate pain associated with plantar fasciitis are often ineffective. Orthotics may exacerbate symptoms due to direct pressure on the nerve branch. Orthotics with a soft or viscous material built into the arch have been recommended. Neuropathic pain medications can also be tried. Surgical release of Baxter nerve is considered when symptoms persist.

FAT PAD ATROPHY

 ESSENTIALS OF DIAGNOSIS

▶ Diffuse, central heel pain aggravated by impact loading activity.
▶ Palpable atrophy of the heel pad.

▶ Clinical Findings

The fat pad of the heel consists of irreplaceable, specialized, separate hydraulic fat chambers designed to absorb shock and transmit mechanical forces to the calcaneus. The fat pad atrophies with age, certain rheumatologic diseases, vascular disease, multiple glucocorticoid injections, and trauma. The heel pain is central and diffuse. In severe cases, the underlying bone is palpable.

Treatment

Treatment consists of shoe modification and flexible heel cups that cushion and absorb shock. There is no surgical solution.

NONINSERTIONAL & INSERTIONAL ACHILLES TENDINOSIS

ESSENTIALS OF DIAGNOSIS

▶ Pain with direct palpation of Achilles tendon.

▶ Thickening (fusiform enlargement) of the tendon.

Clinical Findings

A. Symptoms and Signs

The gastrocnemius and soleus tendon form a twisting convergence to become the Achilles tendon, the largest and strongest tendon in the body. The tendon inserts onto the plantar-posterior aspect of the calcaneus. Just proximal to its insertion, the Achilles passes a posterior prominence on the dorsal calcaneus known as Haglund deformity. In the potential space between the Achilles tendon and posterior aspect of the calcaneus exists the retrocalcaneal bursa (Figure 7–4A–B).

Achilles tendinopathy is a form of enthesopathy that afflicts the Achilles tendon in one of two locations: at the insertion of the tendon on the calcaneus or 2–6 cm proximal to the insertion. Hence, the terms **insertional** and **non-insertional tendinosis.** The condition is degenerative, not inflammatory, and is characterized histologically by the presence of altered collagen synthesis, fibroblast proliferation, and neovascularization. In contrast, **Achilles tendinitis** refers to inflammation of the paratenon associated with

Table 7–2. Differential diagnosis of Achilles tendinopathy.

Rheumatoid arthritis
Gout
Seronegative arthropathies
Diffuse idiopathic skeletal hyperostosis (DISH)
Fluoroquinolone antibiotic treatment
Systemic glucocorticoids

paratenon thickening, swelling and, sometimes, crepitus. Differentiating between Achilles tendinitis and tendinosis can be difficult.

Achilles tendinosis occurs in both active and sedentary persons. Younger patients with the condition tend to be runners, and there is a correlation between injuries and the intensity level of a training program. Tendon rupture can occur but this is not at all common.

Pain is typically directed over the tendon and is worst when initiating activity. Symptoms tend to improve with activity. For runners, pain occurs at the start and after the end of a run. Women gravitate toward high-heeled shoes to help alleviate symptoms. Pain is aggravated by stair climbing and in the case of insertional tendinosis, by shoes with a stiff heel counter.

The diagnosis is usually made quite easily based on history and physical examination findings alone. Pain is reproduced by direct palpation over the diseased portion of the tendon. Retrocalcaneal bursitis is often concomitant with insertional tendinosis and characterized by painful medial and lateral swelling in the posterior heel. Noninsertional tendinosis is characterized by the presence of a painful nodule in the tendon or by fusiform enlargement of the tendon. The differential diagnosis of Achilles tendinopathy is shown in Table 7–2.

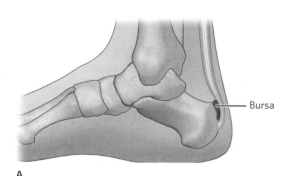

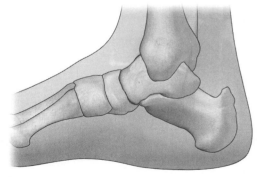

Bursa

A

B

▲ **Figure 7–4. A:** Normal. **B:** Haglund deformity.

B. Imaging Studies and Special Tests

Imaging is generally not required for diagnosis but a weight-bearing lateral radiograph is usually obtained. The presence of a large Haglund deformity is thought to contribute to the development of insertional Achilles tendinosis. A thickened soft tissue shadow depicting the Achilles tendon is usually noted. Insertional tendinosis is very commonly associated with a posterior calcaneal spur. MRI is generally obtained prior to surgery to assess the extent of disease but is almost never necessary for diagnostic purposes.

▶ Treatment

Physical therapy consisting of eccentric exercises and deep tissue manipulation is the conservative treatment modality of choice because it is well studied and shown to be effective in reducing symptoms. Noninsertional tendinosis responds better to conservative measures than insertional tendinosis. Physical therapy is more effective in the early stages of the condition. Heel lifts and activity modification are often recommended. NSAIDs may be no more effective than placebo but may be helpful in cases of retrocalcaneal bursitis or concomitant Achilles paratenosynovitis. Topical treatment with glyceryl trinitrate is described but not well studied. Glucocorticoid injections are discouraged. ESWT has been shown to be effective in relieving symptoms. Currently, there is little evidence that platelet rich plasma injections are effective.

When conservative measures fail to provide acceptable relief, surgery is considered. Surgical intervention involves debridement of diseased tendon and, in the case of insertional tendinosis, excision of Haglund deformity. In more severe forms of the disease, tendon debridement followed by tendon reconstruction may be required.

▼ ANKLE PAIN

INTRA-ARTICULAR CAUSES OF ANKLE PAIN

ESSENTIALS OF DIAGNOSIS

▶ Ankle joint effusion.
▶ Pain or crepitus (or both) with passive ankle joint motion.

▶ Clinical Findings

A. Symptoms and Signs

Intra-articular pathology is often associated with joint effusion. Ankle joint effusion is best observed over the anterolateral aspect where the soft tissue is thinnest. Severe soft tissue edema and patient body habitus can obscure the physical examination and needs to be differentiated from a true effusion. Pain or crepitus (or both) with passive dorsiflexion and plantarflexion of the ankle are also indicative of an intra-articular process. Occasionally, determining whether the tibiotalar joint or the subtalar joint is the source of the discomfort is difficult. In these cases, a diagnostic injection of a local anesthetic into the ankle joint helps determine the source of pain. Direct palpation of the ankle joint line anteriorly also provokes pain. However, the overlying structures make this method less reliable.

B. Imaging Studies and Special Tests

The choice of imaging modality depends on the differential diagnosis. Radiographs of the ankle are obtained to evaluate for osteochondral lesions, fractures, loose bodies, and arthritic changes. A standard three-view study includes anteroposterior, lateral, and internal oblique (mortise) views and is preferred. When possible, *weight-bearing* radiographs should be obtained. MRI is useful for evaluating intra-articular soft tissues such as the synovial lining and joint cartilage and screening for osteochondral defects. When bony detail is required, CT scan is the study of choice.

▶ Differential Diagnosis

Obtaining a careful patient history is essential when formulating a meaningful differential diagnosis for ankle joint pain. Key aspects of the patient history to be ascertained include previous trauma (posttraumatic arthritis, osteochondral lesion of the talus, soft tissue impingement, septic arthritis), diabetes or neuropathy (Charcot arthropathy), recent ankle joint injection (septic arthritis, drug allergy), endocarditis (septic arthritis, synovitis), locking or catching of the joint in dorsiflexion or plantarflexion (loose body) and known inflammatory disorders (gout; pseudogout; and reactive, psoriatic, or rheumatoid arthritis). A timely diagnosis of septic arthritis is imperative if the joint is to be preserved. Sometimes infection is difficult to differentiate from an acute, aseptic, inflammatory condition or Charcot. In such cases, joint aspiration is performed to verify the presence of crystals or bacteria, and determine a white blood cell count. Unlike the hip and knee, primary osteoarthritis of the ankle joint is quite uncommon. Most cases result from previous trauma. Charcot arthropathy may present with spontaneous painful or painless swelling and deformity. Pigmented villonodular synovitis is also known to involve the ankle joint.

▶ Treatment

Ankle arthritis can be quite debilitating for patients. Conservative measures for reducing pain include NSAIDs, avoidance of impact loading activities, and intermittent periods of cast or walking boot immobilization. Glucocorticoid and hyaluronic acid injections can also be considered. A variety of commercially available and custom made braces are available and commonly used for long-term management. Tibiotalar joint arthrodesis remains the "gold standard" surgical treatment option. This procedure is durable and can provide good pain relief but results in an altered gait pattern limiting activity. Total ankle replacement is becoming more popular with the newest generation of prostheses. Indications for the procedure remain narrow and patient selection is critical for success.

Septic arthritis mandates some form of joint irrigation that includes open or arthroscopic approaches or serial joint aspirations in patients considered poor surgical candidates.

Charcot arthropathy of the ankle poses a therapeutic challenge because of the inherent instability associated with the condition. Attempted bracing often leads to ulcer formation over the malleoli creating further treatment difficulties. Therefore, surgical stabilization is an early consideration.

OSTEOCHONDRAL LESIONS OF THE TALUS (OSTEOCHONDRITIS DISSECANS)

 ESSENTIALS OF DIAGNOSIS

► Ankle joint pain exacerbated by weight-bearing activity.

► No pathognomonic clinical examination findings.

► Advanced imaging (MRI or CT scan) often necessary to make diagnosis.

► Clinical Findings

A. Symptoms and Signs

An osteochondral lesion can be described as a local condition that results in the detachment of a segment of cartilage and its corresponding subchondral bone from an articular surface. They occur most commonly in the knee and third most commonly in the ankle. The term "osteochondritis dissecans" is pervasive in the medical literature and is suggestive of an inflammatory process. However, investigators have not demonstrated the presence of inflammatory cells by histologic sections. Therefore, the term should probably be abandoned. Multiple etiologies have been proposed for osteochondral lesions of the talus (OLTs) including direct trauma, repetitive microtrauma, ischemia, ossification defects, and genetic predisposition.

Most experts agree that trauma is the principle predisposing factor for the development of OLTs, particularly for lateral lesions.

Clinically, OLTs are generally located anterolaterally or posteromedially on the talar dome weight-bearing surface. Central lesions have also been reported. Anterolateral lesions tend to be broad but superficial and wafer-like while posteromedial lesions tend to be deep but involve less articular surface area. A history of trauma is reported in approximately 98% of lateral dome lesions whereas trauma was noted in approximately 70% of medial lesions. The mechanism of their occurrence is often similar to a typical ankle sprain. As a result, acute cases are often misdiagnosed or not detectable at the time of injury on plain radiographs. High-energy injuries resulting from a fall from a height or motor vehicle accident may also create an OLT.

In acute cases, the signs and symptoms are similar to those found in ankle sprains: ecchymosis, ligament pain, ankle swelling, and limited range of motion. Mechanical locking can occur but is not a common complaint. In chronic cases, stiffness, activity-related pain, and intermittent swelling are typical complaints. There are essentially no pathognomonic clinical signs of OLT.

B. Imaging Studies and Special Tests

A minimum work-up includes anteroposterior, lateral, and internal oblique (mortise view) radiographs of the ankle. The mortise view is usually most helpful. Up to 30–40% of OLT are not visualized on plain radiographs. Either MRI or CT scan is indicated for further work-up. The former is a better screening tool and the latter is often chosen to better characterize a lesion detected on plain radiographs.

► Treatment

Occasionally OLT are discovered as incidental findings on imaging studies. Asymptomatic lesions require no treatment. For symptomatic lesions, treatment depends on the age, size, and stage of the defect. For low-stage lesions, whether acute or chronic, a period of immobilization in a cast or walking boot is recommended along with avoidance of impact loading activities. Acute lesions in younger patients tend to do better with this treatment. For chronic unstable lesions, surgery is usually required to alleviate symptoms. Displaced lesions that result in an ankle joint loose body or lesions that cause mechanical locking to motion of the ankle joint are an absolute indication for surgery.

With the advent of distraction and small joint arthroscopes, the arthroscopic approach to OLT has become the preferred method of treatment. The goals of surgical management of OLT include the debridement of the necrotic sequestrum, addressing cystic lesions, and the reestablishment of a joint surface by fibrocartilage ingrowth, hyaline cartilage replacement, or fixation of a loose fragment. All loose bodies in the joint must be removed. Surgical treatment of OLT should be performed by foot and ankle subspecialty surgeons or surgeons facile with arthroscopic techniques and familiar with OLT treatment algorithms.

EXTRA-ARTICULAR CAUSES OF ANKLE PAIN

Extra-articular causes of ankle pain tend to localize to the posterior medial, the posterior lateral, or the anterolateral aspects of the ankle and produce characteristic findings depending on which structures are involved (Table 7–3).

1. Posterior Tibial Tendinosis

ESSENTIALS OF DIAGNOSIS

▶ Pain over posterior tibial tendon in early stages.
▶ Progressive planovalgus deformity characterized by a valgus heel, collapsed medial arch, and abducted forefoot.

▶ Clinical Findings

A. Symptoms and Signs

The posterior tibial tendon courses directly posterior to the medial malleolus of the ankle before finding its primary insertion on the medial aspect of the navicular. Its purpose is to secure (or "lock") the midfoot thereby converting the foot from an accommodating platform for balance and shock absorption to a rigid lever arm for efficient forward propulsion. Having the patient perform a toe rise on one foot and observing the heel shift from a valgus posture to a varus posture can test posterior tibial tendon function.

Degenerative changes to the posterior tibial tendon may occur without prior injury. Typically, this occurs in a region between the medial malleolus and the insertion on the navicular. Stage 1 tendinosis is characterized by pain and swelling localized to the posterior tibial tendon but the patient notes no deformity developing in the foot. Furthermore, the tendon still functions normally as seen on

Table 7–3. Extra-articular causes of ankle pain.

Posterior medial ankle pain
Flexor hallucis longus dysfunction
Tibialis posterior tendon dysfunction
Tarsal tunnel syndrome
Posterior lateral ankle pain
Posterior talar impingement syndrome
Peroneal tendinopathy
Tarsal coalition of the subtalar joint posterior facet
Sural nerve neuropathy
Anterior lateral ankle pain
Sinus tarsi syndrome
Superficial peroneal nerve neuropathy
Lateral ankle ligament pathology
Coalition of the talocalcaneal or calcaneal-navicular joints

a single heel rise test. In stage 2, the tendon becomes elongated reducing its ability to stabilize the midfoot. The result is progressive deformity of the foot that consists of a sagging arch, a more valgus hindfoot posture and an abducted forefoot (so-called planovagus deformity). In addition to pain over the posterior tibial tendon, some patients develop *lateral*-sided hindfoot pain directed just distal to the tip of the lateral malleolus. This so-called "impingement" pain results from deformity as the calcaneus drifts into the lateral malleolus. In very chronic cases of posterior tibial tendinosis, the medial pain resolves as the tendon eventually fails completely. Single toe rise becomes difficult if not impossible to perform in stage 2 but the deformity remains "flexible." In other words, the heel may be passively returned to varus and the forefoot may be easily rotated. A tight gastrocnemius is common. In stage 3, the deformity becomes rigid or fixed. This makes bracing and surgical corrections more difficult. In stage 4, the talus has rotated into a valgus position within the ankle mortise.

B. Imaging Studies and Special Tests

Weightbearing anteroposterior and lateral radiographs of the foot are mandatory. The deformity can be well characterized by plain radiographs aiding surgical correction, and arthritic changes can be identified. A weight-bearing anteroposterior ankle radiograph is needed to identify stage 4 deformity.

▶ Treatment

Orthotics can be effective in early stages. As deformity progresses bracing may become necessary if surgery is to be avoided. Glucocorticoid injections are ill advised. Surgery is indicated if symptoms cannot be adequately alleviated with nonoperative treatment. A relative indication for surgical intervention is stage 4 deformity. Surgical corrective procedures for flexible deformities are quite varied depending on severity and include debridement or resection of the diseased posterior tibial tendon, flexor digitorum longus tendon transfer to the navicular, medializing calcaneal osteotomy, and selected midfoot fusions, and osteotomies. For stage 3 deformity, a triple arthrodesis is typically necessary (fusion of the subtalar, talonavicular, and calcaneal cuboid joints). Surgery should be performed by a foot and ankle specialist.

2. Posterior Ankle Impingement (Os Trigonum Syndrome)

ESSENTIALS OF DIAGNOSIS

▶ Posterolateral or direct posterior ankle pain.
▶ Pain is reproducible with forced plantar flexion of the ankle.

▶ Clinical Findings

A. Symptoms and Signs

Posterior ankle impingement most commonly manifests as pain over the posterolateral aspect of the ankle or, less often, over the posterior aspect of the ankle deep to the Achilles tendon. The condition may arise from repetitive activity in the plantar flexed position or from a violent plantar flexion injury of the ankle. It occurs as the dorsal aspect of the calcaneal body approaches the posterior aspect of the tibial plafond essentially "pinching" the bony or soft tissues in between. The presence of an os trigonum or large Stieda process predisposes one to the condition. However, the presence of an os trigonum is *not* required. Fractures of the posterior process of the talus (Shepherd fracture) can mimic posterior impingement.

Patients complain of a dull aching pain with activity particular when the foot is plantar flexed. Descending stairs seems particularly problematic. Some patients convey a sense of popping or clicking in the ankle with activity. In the patient with a history of trauma who reports severe pain, fracture of the posterior talus needs to be ruled out.

On examination, posterolateral swelling may be present. Reproduction of pain with forced plantar flexion of the foot is nearly pathognomonic for the condition. Pain can also be elicited with palpation directed over the posterior aspect of the subtalar joint (just anterior to the lateral edge of the Achilles tendon). In equinus athletes, posterior ankle impingement and flexor hallucis longus (FHL) tenosynovitis often coexist and should be considered during the examination.

B. Imaging Studies and Special Tests

A lateral radiograph is often adequate for identifying the presence of an os trigonum or large Stieda process. If a fracture needs to be ruled out and plain radiographs prove to be inadequate, then CT scan is warranted. MRI is helpful if the FHL tendon is also to be evaluated.

▶ Treatment

It should be noted that treatment for posterior impingement differs from fracture treatment. In acute cases of impingement, a rigid walking boot is favored along with avoidance of offending activities. NSAIDs are also considered. Glucocorticoid injections into the anatomic space posterior to the subtalar joint are offered in more refractory cases. The needle is introduced just posterior to the peroneal tendons approximately 1 cm proximal to the distal-most aspect of the lateral and aimed 15 to 20 degrees posterior. When nonsurgical measures fail, operative intervention is considered. Surgery involves excision of the os trigonum (if present) or excision of inflamed soft tissue.

3. Flexor Hallucis Longus Tendinopathy

ESSENTIALS OF DIAGNOSIS

▶ Pain with palpation of the flexor hallucis longus tendon.
▶ Pain with active plantarflexion of the hallux against resistance.

▶ Clinical Findings

A. Symptoms and Signs

The FHL is the strongest flexor of the great toe. Repetitive use may result in a spectrum of tenosynovitis resulting in nodule formation and degenerative tears. FHL tendinopathy is relatively uncommon but more prevalent in ballet dancers. Posteromedial ankle pain is most typical and is reproducible with active plantar flexion of the hallux against resistance. Active flexion may be absent or weak depending on the degree of stenosis or the presence of a partial rupture. Development of a tendon nodule may result in "triggering" of the hallux as the nodule is forced to pass through the fibroosseous tunnel. Entrapment or scarring of the FHL following distal tibial, ankle, or calcaneus fractures present differently and is important to recognize. Distinguishing between posterior ankle impingement and FHL tendinitis can be a diagnostic challenge and therefore attention to diagnostic nuances is important.

FHL tenosynovitis may also occur in the medial arch at the "knot of Henry," an anatomic region where the FHL intertwines with the flexor digitorum longus tendon. Repetitive use is the usual culprit but ill-fitting orthotics with excessively high arch supports may also produce symptoms. This condition may be mistaken for plantar fasciitis as the two anatomic structures are in close proximity.

B. Imaging Studies and Special Tests

In cases where the diagnosis is in question MRI may be helpful.

▶ Treatment

Conservative measures may include NSAIDS, activity modification, immobilization in a walking boot, and physical therapy. Glucocorticoid injections into the tendon sheath are used judiciously. Intratendinous injections are avoided to reduce risk of rupture.

When conservative measures fail, surgery can be considered and includes tenosynovectomy, debridement or repair of the tendon, and decompression of the tendon sheath.

4. Sinus Tarsi Syndrome

ESSENTIALS OF DIAGNOSIS

▶ History of inversion sprain.

▶ Pain over the sinus tarsi.

▶ Diagnosis of exclusion. Relief of symptoms after injection into the sinus tarsi.

▶ Clinical Findings

A. Symptoms and Signs

The sinus tarsi (a sulcus between the neck of the talus and distal calcaneus) is an area containing fat and other soft tissues located just distal to the anterior talo-fibular ligament. Sinus tarsi syndrome is often a result of damage to the tarsal canal ligaments but can be due to chronic inflammation of the fatty soft tissues, synovitis secondary to impingement from underlying foot deformities, or the development of a ganglion cyst. Patients often have a history of inversion sprains and sinus tarsi syndrome is often misdiagnosed as such.

Patients complain of pain in the area of the sinus tarsi, often exacerbated by activity and somewhat alleviated by rest. Patients may complain of sensations of hindfoot instability, but this is less common and should point to other etiologies of lateral ankle and foot pain. Patients have point tenderness in the sinus tarsi, which may be exacerbated with inversion and plantar flexion of the foot or with subtalar motion. Injection of anesthetic directly into the sinus tarsi is a useful diagnostic tool. Sinus tarsi syndrome is a diagnosis of exclusion and differential diagnosis to be considered include ankle sprains, superficial nerve entrapment syndromes, anterior calcaneal process fractures, peroneal tendon pathology, tumor or ganglion cysts, coalitions, and arthritis.

B. Imaging Studies and Special Tests

Plain radiographs are often normal but are useful to rule out other possible diagnosis. MRI is a useful adjuvant especially when there is a higher suspicion for other etiologies or if the diagnosis cannot be made on clinical grounds. Inflammatory changes are often seen in the sinus tarsi area.

▶ Treatment

Most cases respond to conservative measures including glucocorticoid injection, rest, ice, NSAID use, physical therapy as well as a brief period of immobilization. Correction of foot biomechanics through the use of orthosis may be a useful adjuvant for patients with foot deformities such as pes planus. If conservative measures fail, surgery may be indicated.

5. Tarsal Tunnel Syndrome

ESSENTIALS OF DIAGNOSIS

▶ Entrapment of the posterior tibial nerve in the tarsal tunnel typically produces unilateral pain, paresthesias or dysesthesias along the plantar aspect of the foot and toes.

▶ Percussion (Tinel sign) or compression of the posterior tibial nerve along the posteromedial heel elicits symptoms.

▶ Clinical Findings

A. Symptoms and Signs

The tarsal tunnel is a compartment in the posteromedial heel created by a retinacular ligament overlying tendinous and neurovascular structures against the medial calcaneus. Although each tendinous structure may have a separate fascial overlying band, the tarsal tunnel typically encompasses the posterior tibial tendon; flexor digitorum longus; posterior tibial artery, vein, and nerve; and the FHL. The posterior tibial nerve branches distally into the medial and lateral plantar nerve, which gives sensory branches to the plantar foot and toes although this branching often occurs within the tarsal tunnel or proximal. Anomolous branching can create nerve symptoms from tarsal tunnel syndrome in either the medial, lateral, or entire plantar foot.

Compression of the posterior tibial nerve within the tarsal tunnel can be a result of multiple etiologies, including space occupying lesions such as ganglion, vascular malformations, tenosynovitis, hindfoot malalignment or as a result of bony malformation from trauma. Compression typically elicits pain, paresthesias, or dysesthesias in the plantar foot and toes. This is often worse with prolonged weight bearing and activity although rest pain is common. Typically, this is unilateral but can be bilateral. Conditions such as neuropathy, lumbosacral spine pathology and rheumatologic conditions should be considered when bilateral symptoms are present.

Compression of the tibial nerve or percussion often elicits symptoms. Dorsiflexion at the ankle and holding the hindfoot in an exaggerated inverted or everted position can also reproduce symptoms.

B. Imaging Studies and Special Tests

Plain radiographs should always be obtained initially to rule out osseous abnormalities that may be causing increased pressure within the tarsal tunnel. MRI is valuable to rule out space occupying lesions and inflammatory processes. Electromyography and nerve conduction studies are important as diagnostic and confirmatory studies. However, a negative study does not necessarily rule out tarsal tunnel syndrome.

Careful injection of an anesthetic into the tarsal tunnel can be used for diagnostic purposes although care must be taken due to the close proximity of the vascular structures to the posterior tibial nerve.

▶ Treatment

Initial conservative treatment includes rest, ice, NSAIDs, immobilization, and physical therapy. Orthosis, such as orthotics and ankle bracing, may decrease symptoms caused by hindfoot alignment problems. Injections can be initiated for patients refractory to the above treatments. Medications for neuropathic pain as well as topical anesthetics may be effective.

If conservative treatment fails, surgical release of the tarsal tunnel should be considered. Surgical treatment is most successful when a space occupying lesion is present and when nerve conduction studies are positive.

Approach to the Patient with Shoulder Pain

John H. Wilckens, MD
Michael T. Freehill, MD
Umasuthan Srikumaran, MD
Johnathan A. Bernard, MD

8

The shoulder complex consists of four joints—the glenohumeral, acromioclavicular (AC), sternoclavicular (SC), and scapulothoracic joints—with encapsulating ligaments and muscles (Figure 8–1). It is the most mobile joint of the body, with the primary role of positioning the hand in space to function. A detailed history and physical examination with appropriate imaging can help narrow the extensive differential diagnosis and guide treatment. Most conditions can be treated initially with medication and physical therapy. Resistant shoulder pain should be referred for orthopedic consultation.

▶ History

Much like pain elsewhere, shoulder pain can be initially categorized by onset of symptoms, character of pain, and what activities relieve and aggravate the pain.

The onset of pain may follow a recent injury (≤4 weeks) or remote injury (>4 weeks). Recent injury usually has an acute onset of pain, whereas a remote injury may be episodic or insidious. Because the shoulder is involved in many repetitive functions, pain can result from overuse.

Character, location, timing, and radiation of pain can also be helpful. Sharp or stabbing pain usually suggests a structural cause. Dull and aching pain, especially related to early mornings and weather changes, suggests arthritis. Burning and radiating pain suggests a neurologic cause. Lateral upper arm pain is typical of rotator cuff pain. Pain radiating below the elbow or to the medial border of the scapula suggests a cervical spine or neurologic source of the pain. Pain at night is also typical of rotator cuff disease, but it can be noted in metastatic bone disease. Pain with overhead activity is a very common symptom and can be generally categorized as "impingement" pain. It is most commonly caused by rotator cuff dysfunction or disease. Constitutional symptoms, such as fever and weight loss, should alert the clinician that the cause of pain is infectious, metabolic, or neoplastic.

Other symptoms associated with shoulder pain include stiffness, weakness, and instability. A helpful way to frame the magnitude of shoulder pain is to identify the activities that are limited by the pain, such as overhead use, lifting, dressing, combing or shampooing hair, washing, and hygiene. Recreational and occupational limitations should also be sought.

▶ Physical Examination

For an accurate examination, the shoulder needs to be visible; for female patients, privacy can be respected by using special examination gowns or by having the patient wear a sports bra, swimsuit top, or strapless blouse.

Both shoulders should be examined not only from the front but also from the back and side. Particular attention should be paid to shoulder symmetry to allow the clinician to appreciate subtle muscle atrophy. Atrophy suggests neurologic injury or chronicity of the underlying problem.

Palpating the shoulder and assessing its range of motion are the next steps in the physical examination.

A. Palpation

Palpation begins at the SC joint and moves lateral over the clavicle to the AC joint and should be sensitive to deformity, pain, and crepitance. The presence of SC and AC joint pain or deformity can suggest injury or arthritis or both. A painful acromion may indicate an os acromiale. Next, the greater and lesser tuberosities (insertions of the supraspinatus and subscapularis, respectively) should be palpated; if pain is present, a rotator cuff abnormality should be suspected. Between the tubercles, the intertubercular groove (the course of the long head of the biceps) can be palpated. Pain at this location suggests biceps tendinitis, which can occur on its own or with rotator cuff abnormality and superior labral tears.

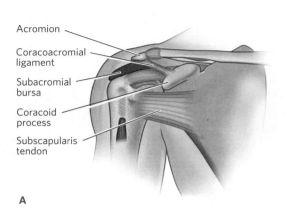

Acromion

Coracoacromial ligament

Subacromial bursa

Coracoid process

Subscapularis tendon

A

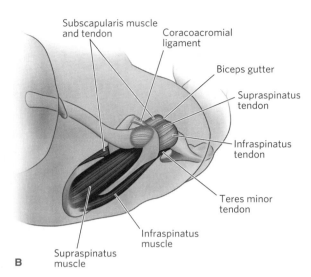

Subscapularis muscle and tendon

Coracoacromial ligament

Biceps gutter

Supraspinatus tendon

Infraspinatus tendon

Teres minor tendon

Infraspinatus muscle

Supraspinatus muscle

B

▲ **Figure 8–1.** Shoulder and rotator cuff muscle anatomy, frontal (**A**) and superior (**B**) views.

B. Range of Motion (ROM)

Because of the shoulder's mobility, its ROM should be checked in several planes, in overhead elevation, and in internal and external rotation. In addition, ROM should be assessed actively and passively. Overhead motion should be observed from the front and back of the patient. From the back, asymmetry of excursion of the scapulae should be assessed. Winging can be observed with serratus anterior, trapezius, and infraspinatus weakness. More subtle medial border elevation is commonly seen with the painful shoulder from weak or misfiring scapular stabilizers, which contribute to the closing of the coracoacromial arch and shoulder impingement.

Internal rotation can be measured by having patients place their thumbs midline on their spines as high as they can; the level of the vertebrae touched should be recorded (Plates 12 and 13). In addition, internal and external rotation can be measured with the arm abducted 90 degrees and the elbow flexed 90 degrees.

ROM of the affected shoulder should be compared with that of the opposite side. Active ROM that is more painful and restricted than passive ROM suggests a rotator cuff component to the pain. Painful restricted passive ROM is seen in adhesive capsulitis, or "frozen shoulder." The painful arc of motion should also be noted.

Finally, ROM of the cervical spine should also be examined, including flexion, extension, lateral bending, and rotation, because restricted or painful neck motion can refer pain to the shoulder.

▶ Neurologic Examination

Muscle testing should be performed next, with special attention to assessment of rotator cuff strength. Abduction against resistance tests the supraspinatus. External rotation versus resistance tests the posterior rotator cuff muscles, infraspinatus, and teres minor. The "belly-press" test and "lift-off" tests assess the anterior rotator cuff muscle, the subscapularis (Plates 14 and 15).

If cervical neck abnormality is considered, a more formal neurologic examination, including sensory, distal motor function, and reflexes, should be conducted.

▶ Special Tests

In addition to the basic examination of the shoulder, numerous abnormality-specific tests or maneuvers can be used to help determine the cause of shoulder pain or dysfunction. Examination of adjacent anatomy (arm, elbow, forearm, hand, and cervical spine) should be performed before these tests. However, many of these tests can elicit pain and apprehension and should therefore be performed after less painful aspects of the examination; results of the affected shoulder should be compared with those of the normal side. Special tests, including the sulcus sign test, load and shift test, apprehension and relocation test, the Neer test, the Hawkins test, the Yergason test, the Speed test, and the O'Brien test, can be used to assess for abnormalities ranging from instability and rotator cuff impingement, to labral and biceps tendon disease, to disorders of the AC joint.

A. Instability

The shoulder joint is inherently lax, affording it a great degree of mobility. Abnormal laxity represents a spectrum of disease, ranging from painful subluxation to traumatic dislocation. Because there is a wide range of normal laxity, a determination of abnormal laxity should be made only with consideration of the individual history, baseline examination, or contralateral "normal" examination. Conditions resulting in generalized laxity of several joints should also be considered. The following are specific tests to evaluate and characterize shoulder instability.

1. Sulcus sign test—The goal of this test is to evaluate for inferior shoulder laxity. With the patient seated, the degree of translation between the lateral border of the acromion and the humeral head is noted as downward force is applied to the distal arm in neutral rotation (Plate 16). A "sulcus," or depression in the skin between the acromion and humeral head, is seen. Some practitioners suggest this result should be graded (grade 0, no translation; grade I (≤1 cm), mild translation; grade II (1–2 cm), moderate translation; grade III (>2 cm), severe translation), whereas others suggest the result should simply be reported as positive or negative. A positive or high-grade sulcus sign in both shoulders may suggest multidirectional instability, whereas a unilateral sulcus sign may suggest inferior instability, particularly if associated with pain or symptoms of instability.

2. Load and shift test—The load and shift test measures humeral translation on the glenoid in the anterior and posterior directions. With the patient seated, the examiner places one hand over the top of the shoulder from the posterior position. The other hand grasps the upper arm, gaining control of the humeral head and controlling rotation (neutral). The first part of this maneuver involves "loading" the joint by applying axial pressure through the arm, centering the humeral head in the glenoid. From this position, anterior or posterior force can be applied (Plates 17 and 18). The examiner should then note and grade the degree of translation or subluxation that is felt as the humeral head slides over the glenoid surface. The modified Hawkins classifications assigns three translation grades: I, the humeral head does not move over the glenoid rim; II, the humeral head moves over the rim but returns to a central position; and III, the humeral head moves beyond the rim and requires a reduction maneuver to return to anatomic position. The load and shift test is highly specific: a negative result indicates a high likelihood that anterior or posterior instability is not present.

3. Apprehension and relocation tests—The apprehension test evaluates anterior instability by attempting to reproduce symptoms with the arm in a position of abduction and external rotation. The test can be performed with the patient seated or supine. The examiner positions the patient's arm in increasing amounts of abduction and external rotation while determining whether the patient becomes apprehensive about impending subluxation or dislocation (Plates 19 and 20). A positive test, indicated by the patient's feeling of apprehension, not simply pain, is suggestive of anterior instability. The positive predictive value of this test approaches 98%.

The relocation test is performed in the supine position after the patient's arm is in a position that produces apprehension. The examiner then places one hand anteriorly on the shoulder and applies a posterior force, reducing any humeral head translation. The test is considered positive if this maneuver relieves the sense of apprehension. This test is also very specific and has a 100% positive predictive value for anterior instability.

B. Rotator Cuff Impingement

Patients with rotator cuff pain often note positional pain at night and with overhead activity; however, the pain is usually poorly localized around the anterior or lateral aspect of the shoulder. The Neer and Hawkins tests are frequently used to reproduce this pain and assess for "impingement," which is believed to be a major cause of rotator cuff tendinitis.

1. Neer test—The Neer test is performed by first stabilizing the scapula and then passively raising the patient's arm in forward elevation (Plate 21). The patient's report of pain constitutes a positive result and usually occurs at approximately 80 degrees to 120 degrees of elevation (the point at which the anterior rotator cuff impinges on the undersurface of the acromion). This test is nonspecific for rotator cuff abnormality and may yield a positive result for other conditions, such as adhesive capsulitis, subacromial bursitis, instability, and arthritis.

2. Hawkins test—The Hawkins test is a variation of the Neer test and involves the examiner internally rotating the patient's 90-degree forward-elevated arm with the elbow in flexion (Plate 22). The exact anatomic mechanism for pain generation with this maneuver is unclear, but rotator cuff abnormality is suggested with a high sensitivity and low specificity.

C. Biceps and Labral Abnormality

Abnormality of the biceps tendon is difficult to diagnose because tenderness of the anterior aspect of the shoulder is difficult to isolate anatomically. Likewise, lesions of the labrum (such as superior labrum anterior and posterior [SLAP] lesions) can also be difficult to isolate with the physical examination. Nevertheless, the following tests can help suggest abnormality of these structures.

1. Yergason test—The Yergason test attempts to evaluate for biceps tendon synovitis. With the patient's elbow held at 90 degrees of flexion and the forearm fully pronated, the examiner holds the wrist and resists active supination by the patient (Plate 23). Reproduction of pain isolated to the region of the bicipital groove indicates a positive test and likely biceps tendon inflammation. Patients with a rotator cuff tear who also experience anterior shoulder pain should have a negative Yergason test. This test has been found to have moderate accuracy with a specificity of 79%.

2. Speed test—The Speed test also attempts to assess for biceps tendon synovitis. The test is performed by having the patient forward-flex the shoulder with the elbow in extension and the forearm in supination against resistance from the examiner at 60 degrees to 90 degrees (Plate 24). A positive test causes pain at the bicipital groove. This test has been found to have a specificity of 75% and a sensitivity of 32% in some studies, whereas in others, it has had a sensitivity of 72% and a specificity of 28% for detecting type II SLAP lesions.

3. O'Brien test (active compression sign)—The O'Brien test attempts to discern SLAP lesions. The test is performed by having the patient stand and forward-flex the shoulder to 90 degrees at 10 degrees of adduction, with the elbow extended, the forearm in pronation, and the thumb pointing down. The examiner then applies a downward-directed force on the patient's arm. The test is then repeated with the forearm in supination (Plate 25). The patient's description of a "click" or pain deep within the shoulder when the arm is pronated, combined with relief or minimal pain with the arm in supination, is considered a positive result and suggestive of a SLAP tear.

D. AC Joint Abnormality

Osteoarthritis, AC separations, and osteolysis are common conditions causing pain around the AC joint. Pain in this anterior region of the shoulder can also be caused by rotator cuff or labral abnormality. In addition to information garnered from the history and physical examination (inspection, palpation), the cross-arm adduction test can help localize pain to the AC joint.

This test is performed by compressing the AC joint by passively adducting the arm at 90 degrees of forward elevation (Plate 26). Pain localized to the AC joint is considered a positive test. Sensitivity and specificity are moderately high at 77% and 79%, respectively.

▶ Imaging

A. Radiographs

Radiographs are often used as the initial imaging modality approach to the patient with shoulder pain and can help evaluate the integrity of osseous structures and their anatomic relationship in the shoulder girdle. Radiographs may reveal additional findings that suggest a diagnosis such as the so-called "vacuum phenomenon" seen with an intact rotator cuff. In addition, radiographs can document the lack of normal anatomic findings, which may indicate inflammatory conditions. For example, the absence of the peribursal fat plane may indicate rheumatoid arthritis or calcific tendinitis. Signs of rotator cuff impingement, including acromial and supraspinatus outlet morphology, can also be noted on radiographs.

Because there is an association among cuff tears and greater tuberosity sclerosis and hyperostosis, osteophytes, subchondral cysts, and osteolysis in the shoulder, radiography is a reasonable first-line imaging modality for identifying such findings. There are four variations of acromial morphology: flat, curved, convex, and hooked. The hooked type has the highest prevalence for subacromial spurs. Similarly, acromial angle and ossification of the coracoacromial ligament, best seen on outlet view, are also associated with clinical impingement and rotator cuff tears.

There are many radiographic views, all of which yield varying degrees of diagnostic value. A Grashey or true anteroposterior (AP) view with internal or external rotation can be used to assess acute problems. This view is particularly useful in the setting of trauma to identify fractures or dislocations. It can also be useful in chronic conditions, such as the identification of any narrowing of the glenohumeral space consistent with osteoarthritic changes. However, the true AP view is not useful for the detection of an anterior or posterior dislocation, nor does it help evaluate the lateral shoulder. On the other hand, dislocations can be evaluated on the scapular Y view because this view allows the assessment of the humeral head within the glenoid fossa. The axillary view also allows evaluation of the humeral head and glenoid, making it another study useful for evaluating anterior or posterior subluxation or dislocation. It can also be used to evaluate bony Bankart lesion of the glenoid rim. The West Point view is another option for evaluating the glenoid rim and can be used to identify a bony Bankart lesion. Conversely, the Stryker notch view allows for evaluation of the posterolateral aspect of the humeral head and can document any condition that alters its integrity (eg, a Hill-Sachs or Bennett lesion).

B. Arthrography

Shoulder arthrography is used to evaluate full-thickness rotator cuff tears, rupture of the long head of the biceps, and diagnosis and treatment of adhesive capsulitis. This imaging modality, which can be performed as a single-contrast or double-contrast study, involves the fluoroscopic injection of a radiopaque contrast agent into the glenohumeral joint space, which aids in defining the shoulder anatomy and the detection of rotator cuff tears. With arthrography, detection of full-thickness rotator cuff tears approaches 98%–99%. Leakage of contrast from the glenohumeral joint into the subacromial bursa or the subdeltoid bursa, which represents the rupture of the joint capsule, is indicative of a rotator cuff tear. Limitations of shoulder arthrography include false-negative results, which can occur when the glenohumeral joint capsule is not ruptured but a rotator cuff tear has occurred. Shoulder arthrography has some drawbacks: it is not helpful in identifying partial-thickness tears, its use for soft-tissue assessment is limited, its value for rotator cuff assessment is inferior to that of MRI, and its ability to identify labral injuries is limited. Increasingly, shoulder arthrography is combined with CT and MRI to assess shoulder abnormalities.

Shoulder arthrography can be helpful in diagnosing and treating adhesive capsulitis. Increased resistance on injection of a small amount of the radiopaque contrast agent into the glenohumeral joint and documentation of a small axillary pouch and subscapular recess are diagnostic for adhesive capsulitis. This imaging modality can confirm the placement of intra-articular injection of therapy.

C. Ultrasound

Ultrasound is a dynamic examination that is able to evaluate tendons and bursa of the rotator cuff. It can also be useful in the evaluation of the patient with shoulder instability, and in the postoperative patient with hardware where MRI findings may be obscured by metal artifact. However, it requires the use of an experienced technician and appropriate ultrasound equipment, notably a high-resolution transducer, to generate the most accurate and reliable information.

Ultrasound is useful for rotator cuff disease, including partial-thickness and full-thickness tears. Full-thickness tears have been more completely characterized than partial-thickness tears. Findings of full-thickness tears on ultrasound include nonvisualization, focal thinning, and discontinuity of the rotator cuff. Partial-thickness tears assessed by ultrasound often have increased echogenicity secondary to granulation tissue or hypertrophied synovium and focal thinning around the rotator cuff. The sensitivity of ultrasound drops from 100% for full-thickness tears to 47% for partial-thickness tears, whereas the specificity for both is 98%.

Ultrasound can provide information about the appearance of the biceps tendon and supraspinatus tendon. It can also help evaluate bursal surfaces, including the subacromial bursa and subdeltoid bursa, Hill-Sachs lesions, glenoid rim fractures, and glenohumeral ligaments. In addition, ultrasound can be used to evaluate the labrum under dynamic conditions to assess for degeneration, tears, and inflammatory joint disease.

D. CT and Computed Arthrotomography

CT is most useful in evaluating the integrity of bony morphology of the shoulder. Through the delivery of ionizing radiation in the axial plane, multidetector CT can reconstruct sagittal and coronal projections, giving great insight to the complicated three-dimensional anatomy of the shoulder girdle. Although it does not detect soft-tissue abnormalities well, CT is of great use in evaluating shoulder pain in the trauma patient, where assessment of complicated osseous structures, such as the body of the scapula, glenohumeral articular surfaces, and humeral head fractures, is essential.

The combination of CT and arthrography allows for extensive evaluation of the glenoid labrum and may be important for patients with recurrent glenohumeral instability. CT imaging can detect osseous lesions associated with instability, such as Hill-Sachs defects, periosteal reaction, and loose fragments.

E. MRI

MRI is an extremely useful imaging modality in the evaluation of the patient with a painful shoulder. MRI is used to assess the rotator cuff, glenoid labrum, articular surfaces, bony anatomy, and surrounding soft tissues. The AC joint can be evaluated for osteoarthritis, capsular hypertrophy, or spurs. Similarly, the morphology of the acromion, whether it is downsloping, lateral, or anterior overhang, can be assessed as the cause of shoulder pain. The subacromial space can be evaluated for bursitis or to find evidence for a clinical diagnosis of subacromial impingement. MRI also provides a detailed look at all of the muscles that comprise the rotator cuff. Information generated from MRI about the rotator cuff muscles includes degree of tendinopathy, partial- or full-thickness tear, atrophy of the muscle, and calcific tendinitis.

In addition to the rotator cuff tendons, the biceps tendon can also be evaluated. Like the rotator cuff, the biceps tendon can be evaluated for a partial- or full-thickness tear and for tendinopathy. The biceps tendon insertion is also evaluated, yielding information about the integrity of the superior labrum of the glenoid. MRI can effectively provide information about the glenohumeral joint and structures, including Hill-Sachs lesions of the humeral head, nondisplaced fractures of the humeral head, and osteonecrosis of the proximal humerus. It can also identify osseous Bankart lesions of the glenoid rim and a glenohumeral joint effusion. Furthermore, it can yield information about the superior, middle, and inferior glenohumeral ligaments, information about the capsule, and the cause of the related abnormality (degeneration or inflammation). MRI also provides information about the rotator interval (disruption of which can be the source of anterior shoulder pain) and about osseous and soft tissue tumors of the shoulder. Such tumors are relatively infrequent, but when they do occur, they can be assessed for various characteristics, such as size, aggressiveness, and metastases.

▶ Diagnosis & Treatment

With a detailed history, physical examination, and indicated imaging, the differential diagnosis for shoulder pain can be narrowed. The differential diagnosis includes the following conditions: rotator cuff disease, instability, adhesive capsulitis, arthritis, cervical abnormality, neurologic disorders, congenital anomalies, and tumors.

A. Rotator Cuff Disease

Rotator cuff abnormality can be secondary to a spectrum of disease processes, including inflammation, partial- or full-thickness tears, and cuff tear arthropathy. Factors underlying rotator cuff disease include intrinsic degeneration because of senescence and tearing because of avascular regions of the tendon, trauma, or mechanical impingement.

Physical examination with observation and maneuvers can lead the physician to a high suspicion for rotator cuff tears. Atrophy in the supraspinatus or infraspinatus fossa compared with the contralateral side, weakness, or pain with the examination can all help narrow the diagnosis of rotator cuff abnormality. Weakness or pain against resistance in internal or external rotation with the elbow at the side and bent to 90 degrees is often present with a rotator cuff insult. Likewise, the empty can test against resistance at 45 degrees from the midline and forward flexion to 90 degrees is also a good indication of supraspinatus abnormality. Palpation of the greater tuberosity should be firm, but not hard enough to elicit a painful response from pressing on the periosteum of the bone. The affected shoulder should always be compared to the contralateral one.

Impingement syndrome is one of the most common causes of shoulder pain. A decreased space between the humeral head and the acromion suggests subacromial impingement. A distance of <5 mm between these structures as shown on an AP radiograph usually confirms the diagnosis of rotator cuff abnormality. An outlet view can show the presence of subacromial bone spurring and abnormal acromial morphology. A subacromial injection of lidocaine is useful in diagnosing impingement and as an initial treatment modality. Physical therapy for rotator cuff strengthening, stretching, ROM, and modalities for pain relief are other first-line treatments options. If nonoperative management fails, the treatment is acromioplasty. If rotator cuff strength is compromised with the pain secondary to the impingement, suspicion should be high for an associated rotator cuff tear. Along with weakness, rotator cuff tears are often associated with recalcitrant pain and night pain.

Imaging modalities are extremely useful for the diagnosis of rotator cuff tears. Conventional MRIs have been found to have a sensitivity of 100% and specificity of 95% for diagnosing full-thickness rotator cuff tears, and a sensitivity of 82% and specificity of 85% for partial-thickness rotator cuff tears. Partial-thickness tears are best visualized with an MRI arthrogram. Although ultrasound has been found to be a valuable tool for diagnosing full-thickness rotator cuff tears, it is extremely operator-dependent and therefore less practical in many settings.

The treatment of rotator cuff tears varies depending on tear size and should be individualized to each patient. Most partial-thickness tears are initially treated nonsurgically. Arthroscopic evaluation, acromioplasty, rotator cuff debridement, and possible repair are recommended in cases of recurrent symptoms. A full-thickness rotator cuff is not an absolute indication for surgery. Indications for repair of the torn rotator cuff include severity of pain, functional limitations, patient demands or occupation, and an unsuccessful

trial of nonoperative treatment. Early surgical intervention is usually recommended for acute traumatic tears or when weakness is prominent or progressive. There is a high rate of cuff tears in the asymptomatic population, and 51% of patients more than 80 years old have rotator cuff tears. It is important to understand that patients with rotator cuff tears can exhibit relatively normal shoulder function. A longitudinal analysis of asymptomatic rotator cuff tears detected by ultrasound found that of 58 patients with a symptomatic rotator cuff tear and contralateral asymptomatic rotator cuff tear, 51% of the asymptomatic cuff tears became symptomatic over a mean of 2.8 years. The natural disease progression of rotator cuff tears remains largely unknown.

B. Instability

Instability includes the spectrum from acute traumatic dislocation to multidirectional instability secondary to generalized ligamentous laxity. The most common sequela of traumatic anterior shoulder dislocation is recurrence. The recurrence rate is documented in the literature as ≥90% in patients less than 20 years old.

After a fracture or dislocation, pain and guarding of the arm will be present. ROM is limited and the contour of the shoulder compared with the contralateral side is altered. A thorough neurovascular examination is essential because an associated axillary neuropraxia occurs in 5% to 35% of first-time dislocators. Comparing the light touch sensation over the lateral deltoid is the best method of evaluating the competency of the axillary nerve.

After a traumatic dislocation, associated rotator cuff tears need to be ruled out. As a general rule, young patients suffer ligamentous injuries after dislocation, whereas patients more than 50 years old have a higher incidence of rotator cuff tears. Axillary neuropraxia can be differentiated from rotator cuff tears by testing the sensation over the lateral deltoid.

Imaging modalities include AP, Grashey (true AP in the plane of the glenoid), and axillary radiographic views for the assessment of the glenohumeral articulation. An axillary view is critical in this setting; an inability to obtain this view makes a CT scan mandatory. The axillary radiographic view and CT are good for the examination of bony abnormality or fracture of the inferior glenoid. MRI is used to diagnose a rotator cuff tear or ligamentous injury.

Closed reduction of the dislocated shoulder can be obtained via one of several reduction maneuvers, usually with conscious sedation. Postreduction attempts should always be evaluated with conventional radiographic imaging, including an axillary view. Immobilization in a sling is warranted after reduction; however, in instances of a glenoid fracture or gross instability, an abduction brace in internal rotation can aid in immobilization.

Treatment is aimed at physical therapy with strengthening of the rotator cuff and scapular stabilizers. In the active population, acute surgical stabilization should be considered. Recurrent episodes of instability with failed nonoperative management may require surgical intervention. Depending on the injury (soft-tissue versus bony involvement), an arthroscopic or open procedure may be used. Repair of the capsulolabral tissue, with possible stabilization of a bony Bankart lesion, of the glenoid is the goal of the procedure.

Overhead athletes, including gymnasts, swimmers, and weight-lifters, are predisposed to multidirectional instability, i.e., symptomatic subluxation or dislocation in more than one plane (anterior, posterior, or inferior). The cause of the instability in this setting is a loose shoulder capsule. Physical examination maneuvers show gross ligamentous laxity in both shoulders. Prolonged physical therapy emphasizing strengthening and conditioning of the large and small muscles of the shoulder is instituted. Differentiation from voluntary dislocators must be established because, historically, such patients are poor surgical candidates. If nonoperative management fails after ≥6 months, surgical stabilization aimed at tightening and decreasing the shoulder capsular volume is recommended.

C. Adhesive Capsulitis

Adhesive capsulitis, or "frozen shoulder," is a common cause of shoulder pain. With this condition, pain is constant, deep, poorly localized, and made worse with any motion. Patients typically have night pain. Onset can be insidious or acute after incidental trauma. It is seen with endocrine disorders, most commonly diabetes. Many times, the cause is unknown. The hallmark of this condition is a restricted passive ROM, especially interior and external rotation, making activities of daily living difficult. Imaging, particularly MRI, is not helpful with this diagnosis but is used to rule out other causes of shoulder pain.

Although a benign and self-limiting condition (1–2 years), most patients seek treatment because the pain and restricted motion affect their daily activities. Most patients respond to supervised physical therapy that stretches and mobilizes the shoulder joint. Severe and recalcitrant cases can undergo manipulation under anesthesia to restore motion. Arthroscopic capsular release can be conducted to restore motion in the most resistant cases. Because pain occurs at the limits of ROM, pain becomes less problematic as the patient regains ROM.

D. Arthritis

Arthritis can involve the glenohumeral, AC, or SC joints. The cause of the arthritis can be degenerative, infectious, or inflammatory. Physical examination and radiographic appearances are the mainstays of diagnosing the anatomic site and type of arthritis. A long history of repetitive motion (from manual labor or overhead sporting activities) with chronic pain is more suggestive of degenerative arthritis. The insidious onset of pain, with a positive family history and the presence of rashes, fevers, or involvement of multiple joints, may indicate an inflammatory arthritis.

An acute onset of fevers, erythema, warmth, or pain with movement predisposes to a higher diagnosis of infectious arthritis. Limited, painful passive ROM with fevers and elevated inflammatory markers is more predictive of an infectious process. Aspiration of the joint and synovial fluid can confirm the diagnosis; white cell counts >100,000 cells/mL strongly suggest infection.

AC arthritis can be diagnosed by local tenderness at the AC joint. This finding is considered the sine qua non of diagnosing AC joint abnormality. The "one-finger" test is useful for determining the precise location of the pain. Generally, the patient will point directly to the AC joint at the top of the shoulder. Local tenderness at the AC joint when compressed by forcible adduction of the arm across the chest is also diagnostic of AC joint arthritis. Although sepsis of the AC joint produces pain and swelling, other symptoms such as fever, redness, and warmth will likely be present. A higher index of suspicion should be present in immunosuppressed individuals.

SC arthritis is the most common diagnosis at the SC joint when there is pain without associated trauma or swelling. Tenderness to palpation is usually present over the joint in the region of the proximal clavicle sternal attachment. In an infectious process of the SC joint, pain, swelling, warmth, and erythema are present. The SC joint can be readily evaluated by comparing both sides of the disrobed patient.

Conventional radiographs of patients with degenerative arthritis usually show sclerosis, asymmetric joint space narrowing, and osteophytes. Infectious arthritis can have normal radiographs in the early stages, and joint destruction and a mixed pattern of sclerosis and osteopenia in later stages. Arthritis secondary to an inflammatory process usually is associated with symmetric joint space narrowing, a lack of osteophytes, and osteopenia.

The initial treatment of degenerative and inflammatory arthritis is composed of nonoperative interventions such as physical therapy, including ROM, strengthening, and local modalities. Intra-articular injection of cortisone can be administered to the glenohumeral or AC joint to relieve symptoms of pain. After nonoperative treatment fails, degenerative arthritis can be treated with total shoulder arthroplasty or hemiarthroplasty, and AC and SC joint arthritis can be treated with distal clavicle excision or medial clavicle excision, respectively. A diagnosis of septic arthritis requires immediate surgical irrigation and debridement of the involved joint with appropriate antibiotics sensitive to the aggravating organism.

E. Cervical Abnormality

Cervical disc disease and spondylosis can refer pain to the shoulder. Typically, such patients have restricted cervical ROM and, in the presence of a radicular component, distal neurologic findings. Radiographs, CT scans, and MRI scans are all helpful in making this diagnosis and localizing the level(s) of abnormalities. Early nonoperative treatment includes medication, physical therapy, and a soft cervical collar. More severe and resistant cases should be referred to pain management specialists for more sophisticated treatment modalities and/or a spine surgeon, if a surgical indication exists.

F. Neurologic Disorders

Several neurologic disorders about the shoulder can create pain. Brachial plexopathy can involve a stretch or compression injury, typically from trauma, such as a tackle in football or a fall. Patients complain of "burning" or "stinging" pain. Usually such injuries are self-limiting. Persistent symptoms necessitate a work-up, including MRI, to rule out cervical root injury. Less common causes of brachial plexopathy include tumor, viral illness, and vaccinations.

Stretch or compression to the long thoracic nerve (that innervates the serratus anterior) or the accessory nerve (that innervates the trapezius) can cause shoulder pain. Because these muscles are scapular stabilizers, these neurologic conditions cause scapular winging. Most of the palsies are self-limiting, with recovery over a 12- to 18-month period. Electromyography or a nerve conduction study can assist in making this diagnosis, and serial studies can monitor recovery. Physical therapy during this period can be helpful in improving function.

The suprascapular nerve innervates the supraspinatus and infraspinatus, and compression of this nerve can cause posterior shoulder pain and muscles weakness and/or atrophy. In addition to compression at the suprascapular notch or spinoglenoid notch, the nerve can be compressed by a perilabral ganglion cyst. Electromyography or a nerve conduction study and MRI can help locate the area of compression. If symptoms persist for >6 months, decompression at the site of compression is indicated. Ganglion cyst decompression can be achieved with image-guided aspiration, arthroscopic decompression, or open excision.

G. Congenital Anomalies

Congenital anomalies represent a rare cause of shoulder pain. Such conditions include disorders of the bones, muscles, and neurovascular system. Work-up and treatment of these conditions requires the appropriate subspecialist.

H. Tumor

Tumors represent an uncommon cause of shoulder pain. Primary soft-tissue and bony tumors are identified by radiography and MRI. Once suspected, a systematic work-up to include biopsy is best conducted by an oncologist. In addition, metastatic disease should be considered for a patient with shoulder pain who has a history of cancer. Referral to an oncologist for work-up is recommended.

▶ Injection Techniques

Injections for the painful shoulder can be diagnostic and therapeutic. Informed consent for an injection should include risks of infection, subcutaneous fat atrophy, hypopigmentation (especially in darker-skinned patients), and allergic reaction. The injection solution usually includes a short-acting anesthetic, a longer-acting anesthetic, and a corticosteroid. The injection site can be infiltrated with a local anesthetic or sprayed with ethyl chloride to reduce the discomfort of the injection. Injection is delivered observing sterile technique.

A. Subacromial Injection

Typically, 10–12 mL of fluid is injected into the subacromial space. The injection can be delivered from a posterior, lateral, or anterior direction, just under the edge of the acromion. This injection relieves pain associated with rotator cuff disease and shoulder impingement.

B. Glenohumeral Injection

This injection is used for glenohumeral arthritis and may include corticosteroid or investigational use of a hyaluronic acid. A volume injection of the glenohumeral space may also help in the management of pain with adhesive capsulitis. More commonly, the glenohumeral joint is aspirated to rule out infection. The technique commonly used is a spinal needle inserted one fingerbreadth below and medial to the posterolateral corner of the acromion, directed toward the coracoid process anteriorly. Fluoroscopy can assist and document needle placement.

C. AC Injection

The AC joint can be injected for patients with a painful AC joint, which includes AC joint separation, clavicle osteolysis, and AC arthritis. This small joint can accommodate only a 3-mL injection. Entry point is just lateral to the distal clavicle, angled approximately 15 degrees.

Holtby R, Razmjou H. Accuracy of the Speed's and Yergason's tests in detecting biceps pathology and SLAP lesions: comparison with arthroscopic findings. *Arthroscopy.* 2004;20:231. [PMID: 15007311]

McFarland EG. *Examination of the Shoulder: The Complete Guide.* New York: Thieme; 2006.

Sanders TG, Jersey SL. Conventional radiography of the shoulder. *Semin Roentgenol.* 2005;40:207. [PMID: 16060114]

Tzannes A, Murrell GAC. Clinical examination of the unstable shoulder. *Sports Med.* 2002;32:447. [PMID: 12015806]

Yamaguchi K, Tetro AM, Blam O, Evanoff BA, Teefey SA, Middleton WD. Natural history of asymptomatic rotator cuff tears: a longitudinal analysis of asymptomatic tears detected sonographically. *J Shoulder Elbow Surg.* 2001;10:199. [PMID: 11408898]

Approach to the Patient with Neck Pain

9

David Borenstein, MD

Neck pain is a common musculoskeletal symptom and accounts for a sizeable portion of the 9.3 million physician visits annually in the United States for soft tissue disorders. Of those individuals with neck pain, 81% were between the ages of 18 and 64 years as reported by the United States Bone and Joint Decade in 2008. Mechanical disorders cause 90% of neck pain episodes. Mechanical neck pain may be defined as pain secondary to overuse of a normal anatomic structure or pain secondary to trauma or deformity of an anatomic structure (Figure 9–1). Mechanical disorders are characterized by exacerbation and alleviation of pain in direct correlation with particular physical activities. Neck pain due to mechanical disorders decreases within 2–4 weeks in over 50% of patients; symptoms usually resolve within 2–3 months.

INITIAL EVALUATION

The goal of the initial evaluation is to differentiate patients with probable mechanical disorders from those with neck pain that requires more thorough immediate evaluation (Figure 9–2). A history should be taken and an examination should be performed in all patients with new-onset neck pain. The neurologic examination should determine whether there are any signs of cervical nerve root or cervical cord involvement (ie, spastic weakness, hyperreflexia, clonus, and positive Babinski signs).

Diagnostic radiographic or laboratory tests are not necessary during the initial evaluation of patients with probable mechanical neck pain. These tests, however, are indicated for patients whose history and physical findings suggest persistent compression of the spinal cord or nerve roots or raise the possibility of neck pain as a component of an underlying systemic disease.

▶ History

The history should establish the character, onset, location, radiation, aggravating and alleviating factors, intensity, and chronologic development of neck pain. Mechanical disorders cause pain that increases with activity. The end of the day is associated with more severe distress, and recumbency and rest are associated with improvement. Tingling pain that radiates down an arm is suggestive of nerve impingement. Aching pain of slow onset that localizes to the base of the cervical spine suggests muscle or joint involvement. The history should determine whether the neck pain has unusual qualities that suggest a focal destructive process (due to tumor or infection) or pain referred from the heart or other viscera, whether there is an underlying systemic disease that could predispose to a serious neck problem (Table 9–1).

The duration of mechanical neck pain is typically a few days to weeks. Disk herniations may require 8–12 weeks to resolve. Medical conditions tend to cause persistent chronic pain.

▶ Physical Examination

Abnormalities of the cervical spine may be observed while the spine is in motion or static. Observation of the spine from 360 degrees identifies any misalignments of the neck or shoulders. Pain in the neck may cause deviation that can be toward or away from the painful side.

Palpation can detect painful structures as well as increased paraspinous muscle tension. Posterior elements of the cervical spine are more easily identified than those located anteriorly. In general, midline tenderness is related to an intrinsic spinal disorder, while sensitivity to pressure in structures off the midline suggests soft tissue pathology.

Active range of motion in all planes is helpful in documenting the extent but not the cause of cervical spine problems. Active and passive movement of the shoulders can help discriminate abnormalities of the appendicular skeleton from those of the cervical spine.

Neurologic evaluation, including reflex, sensory, and motor function both in the upper and lower extremities

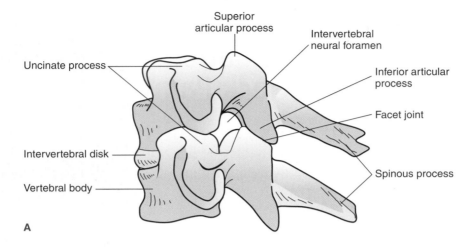

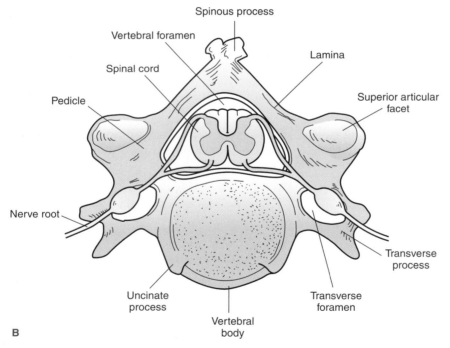

▲ **Figure 9–1.** Schematic representation of a lateral view of the mid-cervical spine (**A**) and the superior aspect of C5 (**B**). The inferior articular processes from synovial-lined **facet joints** (also called **apophyseal joints**) with the superior articular processes of the vertebra below. The uncinate processes or posterolateral lips located on the superior aspect of the vertebral bodies interact with the inferolateral aspects of the vertebral body above, forming the small, non-synovial-lined **uncovertebral joints** (also referred to as the joints of Luschka). The spinal cord lies within the vertebral foramen formed by the vertebral body anteriorly, the pedicles laterally, and the laminae posteriorly. The cervical nerve roots course along "gutters" formed by the pedicles and exit through an intervertebral foramen. The vertebral artery passes through the transverse foramen. (Reproduced, with permission, from Polley HF, Hunder GS. *Rheumatologic Interviewing and Physical Examination of the Joints,* 2nd ed. WB Saunders; 1978.)

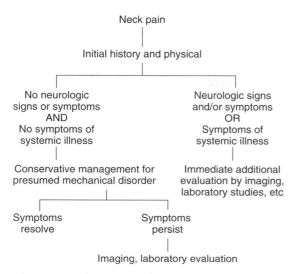

▲ Figure 9–2. The initial evaluation of the patient with neck pain.

is essential to determine the extent of compromise of the central and peripheral nervous systems. The presence of long-tract signs is indicative of more severe spinal cord compression.

The Spurling maneuver is performed by extending and rotating the head to one side and then the other. A positive result is the reproduction of radicular pain. This test is useful in confirming the presence of a cervical radiculopathy.

The Adson test for thoracic outlet obstruction is performed by palpating the pulse at the wrist while abducting, extending, and externally rotating the arm. The patient takes a deep breath and rotates the head to the affected side. If there is compression of the subclavian artery, a marked diminution of the radial pulse is observed and is a positive test.

Table 9–1. Symptoms that point to the need for urgent evaluation in a patient with neck pain.

- Constitutional symptoms such as fever, night sweats, weight loss
- Unusual quality of the neck pain
  - Greatest at night; exacerbated by recumbency
  - Well-localized within the neck
  - Occurring in a regular pattern and extending to structures outside the neck
- Neurologic symptoms
  - Lower extremity weakness; difficulty walking
  - Combination of upper and lower extremity symptoms
  - Rectal or urinary incontinence (or both)
- Associated medical conditions
  - Cancer, diabetes mellitus, AIDS, and injection drug use, for example

Laboratory Tests

Laboratory tests are not necessary for the diagnosis of mechanical neck pain. Erythrocyte sedimentation rate and C-reactive protein tests are useful in the minority of patients with a systemic disorder causing neck pain.

Imaging Studies

Radiographic studies are needed for the small minority of patients who do not respond to a 6–8 week course of medical therapy, who demonstrate severe neurologic compromise, or who have signs or symptoms of a systemic illness.

Plain radiographs are easily obtained but offer few specific findings that identify the cause of neck pain. Many anatomic abnormalities are asymptomatic.

MRI is a useful technique for individuals with clinical symptoms and signs of nerve compression who do not respond to medical therapy. MRI is a sensitive means of identifying disk herniations, narrowing of the spinal canal, and increased inflammation in osseous and soft tissue structures. CT is a better technique at delineating bony structures. A disadvantage of CT is the exposure to ionizing radiation needed to obtain images of the spine.

Special Tests

Electrodiagnostic tests, electromyography, and nerve conduction tests are useful in the differentiation of central versus peripheral nerve compression (a more difficult distinction with cervical spine disorders compared with lumbar spine problems). For example, electromyography and nerve conduction tests can help distinguish between the individual who has median nerve compression at the wrist and the patient with a C6 or C7 spinal nerve compression from a herniated cervical disk.

DISORDERS REQUIRING URGENT EVALUATION

Suspected cervical myelopathy and neck pain in the setting of systemic disease require urgent evaluation in the form of imaging studies, laboratory investigation, and often, referral to the appropriate specialist.

1. Cervical Myelopathy

 ESSENTIAL FEATURES

- ▶ Symptoms of weakness in upper and lower extremities; urinary or rectal incontinence.
- ▶ Upper motor neuron signs on examination of the lower extremities.

General Considerations

Cervical myelopathy occurs secondary to compression of the neural elements (spinal cord or nerve roots) in the cervical spinal canal. Cervical spondylitic myelopathy is the most common cause of spinal cord dysfunction in persons older than 55 years. The cause of the compression is usually a combination of osteophytes and degenerative disk disease that leads to a decrease in the volume of the spinal canal. The distribution and severity of symptoms depend on the location, duration, and size of the lesion.

Clinical Findings

A. Symptoms and Signs

The most frequent presentation of myelopathy is a combination of arm and leg dysfunction. Patients with cervical myelopathy may have symptoms in four limbs, difficulty walking, and urinary or rectal incontinence. Only one-third of patients with cervical myelopathy mention neck pain. Older patients may describe leg stiffness, foot shuffling, and a fear of falling. Physical examination reveals weakness of the appendages in association with spasticity; hyperreflexia, clonus, and a positive Babinski sign are findings in the lower extremities.

B. Imaging Studies

MRI detects the extent of spinal cord compression and is the imaging test of choice for most cases. CT myelogram helps distinguish between osteophytes and protruding disks. Plain radiographs reveal advanced degenerative disease with narrowed disk spaces, facet joint sclerosis, and osteophytes but do not image neural compression.

Treatment

The natural history of cervical spondylitic myelopathy is gradual progression. Although some patients improve with conservative therapy, progressive myelopathy requires surgery to prevent further cord compression, vascular compromise, and myelomalacia. Outcomes are best when surgery is performed before severe neurologic deficits appear.

2. Neck Pain Associated with Systemic Medical Illness

ESSENTIAL FEATURES

► The history and physical examination help identify patients whose neck pain is not due to a mechanical disorder.

► The differential diagnosis and clinical context of each case determine the urgency and nature of the evaluation.

Clinical Findings

Patients with neck pain require urgent evaluation if they have constitutional symptoms, symptoms that suggest either a focal process or referred pain, a history of cancer, or a condition that predisposes to infection (see Table 9–1). If present, signs or symptoms of radiculopathy or spinal cord compression add to the urgency of the situation. The differential diagnosis, clinical setting, and findings of the individual case dictate the use of imaging, laboratory investigations, and need for consultations.

Differential Diagnosis

Neck pain in the presence of fever, night sweats, weight loss, or a predisposing condition (such as injection drug use, AIDS, or diabetes) raises the possibility of **infection.** MRI and CT are indicated in cases of suspected vertebral osteomyelitis, diskitis, and epidural abscess. In these conditions, radiographs of the cervical spine may demonstrate alterations of bone integrity but are often unrevealing, especially early in the disease course.

Spinal cord infiltrative processes and vertebral column **tumors** tend to produce pain that is greatest at night or with recumbency. Patients with these symptoms and neurologic signs should undergo MRI of the central nervous system. Patients with nocturnal pain and with normal neurologic examinations may have a bone tumor. Benign bone tumors affect the posterior elements of vertebral bodies, while malignant lesions affect the vertebral bodies. If plain radiographs are unable to detect alterations in bone architecture, bone scan is a sensitive means to detect lesions over the entire axial skeleton. CT scan clarifies the nature of abnormalities seen on bone scan.

Pain localized directly over the bony structures of the cervical spine is usually associated with either **fracture** or **expansion of bone.** Any condition that replaces bone with abnormal cells or increases mineral loss from trabeculae causes fractures that occur spontaneously or with minimal trauma. Fractures cause pain in the area of the lesion. Physical examination identifies the maximum point of tenderness. A bone scan may identify the area of fracture if the radiograph is normal. MRI can identify the presence of malignancies, such as **myeloma**, that do not stimulate osteoblast activity and thus are not detected by bone scan.

The **spondyloarthropathies** and **rheumatoid arthritis** can cause early morning stiffness of the cervical spine lasting for hours. Patients with neck symptoms due to these diseases usually have extensive disease of other joints, but women with ankylosing spondylitis may have neck disease without low back pain. Flexion-extension views of the cervical spine can reveal the presence of C1–C2 subluxation in either the spondyloarthropathies or rheumatoid arthritis. MRI is an important technique to identify synovitis affecting the C1–C2 articulation in rheumatoid arthritis. MRI can also visualize the presence of bone marrow inflammation and edema in vertebral structures affected by ankylosing spondylitis.

Patients with **viscerogenic pain** (ie, neck pain secondary to cardiovascular, gastrointestinal, or neurologic disorders) have symptoms that recur in a regular pattern in structures that extend beyond the cervical spine. Pain with exertion raises the possibility of myocardial ischemia. Carotidynia is pain and tenderness over the carotid arteries. Esophageal disorders should be considered if neck pain occurs in association with eating. Posterior esophageal lesions, in particular, may affect the prevertebral space, causing neck pain. Disorders of the cranial nerves can cause cervical spine and facial pain.

Patients with **polymyalgia rheumatica** are over 50 years of age and have severe early morning muscle stiffness. Pain is localized to the proximal muscles of the shoulders and thighs. The erythrocyte sedimentation rate is elevated in most cases.

ACUTE NECK PAIN DUE TO A PROBABLE MECHANICAL DISORDER

ESSENTIAL FEATURES

▶ There are no signs or symptoms of systemic disease, and the neurologic examination is normal.

▶ A trial of nonsurgical therapy is indicated.

▶ General Considerations

Patients with neck pain but without symptoms or signs of myelopathy or an associated systemic disorder should receive nonsurgical therapy for 3–6 weeks. In general, imaging studies and laboratory investigations are not necessary unless the neck pain persists.

▶ Treatment

Nonselective nonsteroidal anti-inflammatory drugs (NSAIDs) help decrease pain and localized inflammation that is associated with acute neck pain. Nonsurgical management also includes muscle relaxants, nonopioid analgesics, temperature modalities, local injections, and range of motion and strengthening exercises.

Medications that have rapid onset of action and are effective analgesics are preferred. In addition, drugs with sustained relief properties may offer more constant pain relief with fewer tablets each day. Muscle relaxants do not produce peripheral muscle relaxation but do offer additional pain relief for persons with increased paracervical muscle contractions. Patients must be informed of the potential sedative effects of these medications. Patients may use ice massage on painful areas for 10 minutes for additional analgesia. Some patients may find the application of heat to the neck improves range of motion by decreasing muscle tightness.

A local injection with 10 mg of triamcinolone and 2–4 mL of lidocaine into the area of maximum tenderness in the paravertebral musculature or trapezii may decrease pain.

Because of the pain, patients often have difficulty complying with the recommendation of returning to normal motion of the cervical spine. Patients will limit motion and prefer to wear a cervical collar. Short-term immobilization is useful, particularly at night when motion during sleep increases neck pain. A soft collar that does not extend the neck is appropriate in most cases. Patients should understand that the eventual goal of therapy is a return to normal neck motion. Therefore, the collar should be used less frequently as neck pain improves.

PERSISTENT NECK PAIN

Most patients, including those with cervical radiculopathy, improve within 2 months. If initial nonsurgical treatment fails after 6 weeks, symptomatic patients are separated into two groups: patients with neck pain alone and patients with arm pain as the predominant complaint.

1. Neck Pain Predominant

ESSENTIAL FEATURES

▶ Osteoarthritis is a frequent cause of local neck pain.

▶ Muscle tightness is a common exacerbating factor.

▶ Differential Diagnosis & Treatment

Cervical strain causes pain in the middle or lower portion of the posterior aspect of the neck. The pain may cover a diffuse area or both sides of the spine. Physical examination reveals local tenderness in the paracervical muscles, decreased range of motion, and loss of cervical lordosis. No abnormalities are found on neurologic or shoulder examination. Laboratory tests are normal. Cervical spine radiographs of patients with cervical strain may be normal or demonstrate a loss of cervical lordosis. Management of chronic cervical strain includes pharmacotherapy with NSAID, muscle relaxant, and local injections as well as nonpharmacotherapy with neck exercises, including strengthening and range of motion.

Cervical spondylosis is associated with disk degeneration and the approximation of articular structures. This instability results in osteoarthritis with osteophyte formation in the uncovertebral and apophyseal joints. Neck pain is diffuse and may radiate to the shoulders, occipital area, or the interscapular muscles. Physical examination may reveal midline tenderness and pain at the limit of motion with extension and lateral flexion. Factors that exacerbate and alleviate neck pain help differentiate among the various causes of mechanical neck pain. Plain radiographs of the cervical spine demonstrate intervertebral narrowing and facet joint sclerosis. MRI of the neck reveals degenerative disk disease in over 50% of persons 40 years of age or older, many of whom are asymptomatic. The radiographic findings are significant only if they correlate with the clinical symptoms of the patient. Therapy for osteoarthritis of the cervical spine requires a balance between stability and maintenance of motion. Patient education is essential to maximize neck flexibility with range of motion exercises while decreasing pain by restricting neck movement with a cervical collar. NSAIDs and local injections may also diminish neck and referred pain. Most patients with cervical spondylosis have a relapsing course with recurrent exacerbations of acute neck pain.

Cervical hyperextension injuries (whiplash) of the neck are most often associated with rear-impact motor vehicle accidents, but diving, falls, and other sports injuries also cause whiplash. Whiplash is an acceleration-deceleration injury to the soft tissue structures in the neck. Paracervical muscles are stretched or torn, and with severe injury, cervical intervertebral disk injuries occur. Severe whiplash also can damage the sympathetic ganglia, resulting in Horner syndrome, nausea, hoarseness, or dizziness. Symptoms of stiffness and pain on motion generally develop 12–24 hours after the accident. Patients may have difficulty swallowing or chewing. Physical examination reveals soreness of the neck with palpation, paracervical muscle contraction, and decreased range of motion. Neurologic examination is unrevealing, and radiographs demonstrate loss of cervical lordosis. Structural damage identified on radiographs occurs in patients with severe injuries that require immediate stabilizing therapy. Treatment of most whiplash injuries includes the use of a cervical collar for a minimal period of time. Longer use of collars may result in greater pain and decreased motion. Nonopioid analgesics, NSAIDs, and muscle relaxants decrease pain and facilitate motion of the neck. Patients with persistent symptoms have pain secondary to apophyseal joint injury. Patients with persistent symptoms for greater than 6 months rarely experience significant improvement.

If a patient with persistent neck pain does not have muscle tenderness and if the neurologic examination and imaging studies are unrevealing, the patient should have a complete psychosocial evaluation. Patients with neck pain who have psychiatric conditions may have conversion reactions or substance dependence as the cause of their symptoms.

2. Arm Pain Predominant

ESSENTIAL FEATURES

► Herniated intervertebral disks are a frequent cause of radicular pain.

► Cervical spinal stenosis is a cause of radicular pain in older persons.

► Differential Diagnosis & Treatment

Patients with arm pain refractory to nonsurgical management frequently have symptoms and signs owing to mechanical pressure from a herniated disk or hypertrophic bone and secondary inflammation of the involved nerve roots. Cervical disk herniation occurs with the sudden exertion of heavy lifting. A **herniated cervical disk** causes radicular pain that radiates from the shoulder to the forearm and hand. The pain may be so severe that the use of the arm is limited. Neck pain is minimal or absent. Physical examination reveals increased radicular pain with any maneuver that narrows the intervertebral foramen and places tension on the affected nerve. Compression, extension, and lateral flexion of the cervical spine (Spurling sign) cause radicular pain. Neurologic examination reveals sensory abnormalities, reflex asymmetry, or motor weakness corresponding to the damaged spinal nerve root and degree of impingement (Table 9–2). MRI is the best technique to identify the location of disk herniation and nerve root impingement. Electromyography and nerve conduction tests document nerve dysfunction and are able to differentiate nerve root impingement from peripheral entrapment syndromes (eg, carpal tunnel syndrome).

If arm pain occurs during exertion, vascular evaluation is indicated. Patients who complain of neck and arm pain that occurs with exertion should be evaluated for coronary artery disease, particularly if chest pain occurs in conjunction with arm pain. If the exertional pain is limited to the arm alone, an evaluation for thoracic outlet syndrome, using the Adson test, is also appropriate. Patients with thoracic outlet syndrome should be evaluated by appropriate imaging to rule out a Pancoast tumor (apical lung tumor). Patients with idiopathic thoracic outlet obstruction may benefit from isometric shoulder girdle exercises, improved posture, and limiting movements of the arm above the head. Surgery is helpful in a minority of patients.

Nonsurgical treatment for radiculopathy secondary to an acute herniated cervical disk is successful in 80% of

Table 9–2. Characteristics of radicular pain caused by cervical nerve root compression.

Nerve Root	Area of Pain	Sensory Loss	Motor Loss	Reflex Loss
C5	Neck to outer shoulder, arm	Shoulder	Deltoid	Biceps, supinator
C6	Outer arm to thumb, index finger	Index finger, thumb	Biceps	Biceps, supinator
C7	Outer arm to middle finger	Index, middle fingers	Triceps	Triceps
C8	Inner arm to ring and little fingers	Ring, little fingers	Hand muscles	None

patients. Nonsurgical therapy includes patient education of natural history of improvement, limited use of cervical collars, therapeutic exercises, cervical traction, and NSAIDs. Low-dose glucocorticoids, administered orally or epidurally, may have additional benefit in relieving radicular pain. However, the benefit compared to placebo has not been demonstrated consistently in clinical trials. For patients in whom nonsurgical therapy fails, anterior diskectomy with fusion relieves arm pain in over 90% of patients. Cervical disk arthroplasty has been offered as an alternate surgical approach as a means of maintaining spinal motion while relieving nerve root compression. Selecting appropriate patients is essential for a good outcome with disk replacement. Contraindications to cervical disk replacement include facet joint arthritis, vertebral body deformity, spinal instability, predominant neck pain, poor bone quality or severe spondylosis.

[American Academy of Orthopaedic Surgeons]
http://www.aaos.org

Bogduk N. The anatomy and pathophysiology of neck pain. *Phys Med Rehabil Clin N Am.* 2003;14:455. [PMID: 12948338]

Borenstein DG. Chronic neck pain: How to approach treatment. *Curr Pain Headache Rep.* 2007;11:436. [PMID: 18173978]

Carette S, Fehlings MG. Cervical radiculopathy. *N Engl J Med.* 2005;353:392. [PMID: 16049211]

[Dr. David Borenstein America's Back Doctor]
http://www.drborenstein.com

Mink JH, Gordon RE, Deutsch AL. The cervical spine: radiologist's perspective. *Phys Med Rehabil Clin N Am.* 2003;14:493. [PMID: 12948340]

[NYU Langone Medical Center's Hospital for Joint Diseases]
http://www.hjd.med.nyu.edu

Rao R. Neck pain, cervical radiculopathy, and cervical myelopathy: pathophysiology, natural history, and clinical evaluation. *Instr Course Lect.* 2003;52A:479. [PMID: 12690874]

Riew KD, Buchowski JM, Sasso R, Zdeblick T, Metcalf NH, Anderson PA. Cervical disc arthroplasty compared with arthrodesis for the treatment of myelopathy. *J Bone Joint Surg Am.* 2008;90:2354. [PMID: 18978404]

[The American College of Rheumatology]
http://www.rheumatology.org

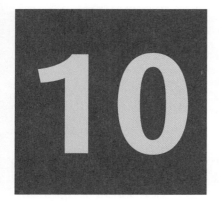

Approach to the Patient with Low Back Pain

Rajiv K. Dixit, MD

ESSENTIAL FEATURES

▶ Most patients with acute low back pain improve spontaneously within 4 weeks.

▶ Degenerative change in the lumbar spine is the most commonly identified cause of low back pain.

▶ Diagnostic testing is rarely indicated in the absence of significant neurologic involvement or suspicion of systemic disease unless symptoms persist beyond 4 weeks.

▶ Imaging abnormalities must be interpreted carefully because they are frequently seen in asymptomatic persons.

▶ Patients with neurologic involvement or an underlying systemic disease (eg, infections, malignancies, and spondyloarthropathies) may need urgent or specific treatment, including surgery.

▶ Surgery is rarely needed for patients who respond to analgesia, education, aerobic conditioning, and physical therapy.

▶ General Considerations

Low back pain (LBP) is the most common musculoskeletal complaint and a leading cause of work disability. An estimated 80% of the population experiences it during their lifetime.

LBP affects the area between the lower rib cage and gluteal folds and frequently radiates into the thighs. Most LBP is benign and self-limited. Ninety percent of patients with acute LBP improve spontaneously within 4 weeks, although low-grade symptoms may persist in some. Approximately half of the patients with acute LBP experience one or more episodes of LBP over the next few years, but these, too, are generally self-limited. Less than 1% of the patients with acute LBP have true sciatica, which is defined as pain in the distribution of a lumbar nerve root, often accompanied by sensory and motor deficits (Table 10–1 and Figure 10–1).

Risk factors that have been associated with LBP include heavy lifting, driving motor vehicles, jogging, weaker trunk strength, obesity, pregnancy, psychosocial factors, and cigarette smoking.

▶ Clinical Findings

A. History

An important aspect of history-taking in a patient with LBP is the identification of "red flags" to ensure that conditions that require early diagnostic testing are not missed (Table 10–2).

Mechanical LBP is due to an anatomic or functional abnormality that is not associated with inflammatory or neoplastic disease. Mechanical LBP increases with physical activity and upright posture and is relieved by rest and recumbency. Degenerative change in the lumbar spine is the most common cause of mechanical LBP. Severe and acute mechanical LBP in a slender and elderly woman is suspicious for a vertebral compression fracture secondary to osteoporosis. **Nonmechanical LBP**, especially when accompanied by nocturnal pain, suggests the possibility of underlying infection or neoplasm.

Inflammatory LBP, as seen in the spondyloarthropathies, typically worsens with rest, improves with activity, and is accompanied by morning stiffness that lasts half an hour or longer. Some patients complain of alternating buttock pain. Sciatica and pseudoclaudication suggest neurologic involvement. **Sciatica** results from nerve root compression, generally from a herniated disk, and produces lancinating pain in a radicular distribution. Sciatica should be differentiated from nonneurogenic **sclerotomal** pain, which arises from pathology within the disk, facet joint, or lumbar paraspinal muscles and ligaments. Like sciatica, sclerotomal pain is often referred into the lower extremities, but unlike sciatica, sclerotomal pain is nondermatomal in distribution, is dull in quality, and

Table 10–1. Neurologic features of lumbosacral radiculopathy.

Disk Herniation	Nerve Root	Motor	Sensory (Light Touch)	Reflex
L3–4	L4	Dorsiflexion of foot	Medial foot	Knee
L4–5	L5	Dorsiflexion of great toe	Dorsal foot	None
L5–S1	S1	Plantar flexion of foot	Lateral foot	Ankle

Table 10–2. "Red flags" that indicate need for early diagnostic testing.

Spinal fracture
 Significant trauma
 Prolonged glucocorticoid use
 Age >50 years
Infection or cancer
 History of cancer
 Unexplained weight loss
 Immunosuppression
 Injection drug use
 Nocturnal pain
 Age >50 years
Cauda equina syndrome
 Urinary retention
 Overflow incontinence
 Fecal incontinence
 Bilateral or progressive motor deficit
 Saddle anesthesia
Spondyloarthritis
 Marked morning stiffness in the back that lasts >30 min
 Low back pain that improves with activity but not rest
 Alternating buttock pain
 Age <40 years

pain usually does not radiate below the knee or have associated paresthesias.

Persistence of LBP may be associated with depression, job dissatisfaction, and pursuit of disability compensation or litigation.

B. Physical Examination

Examination of the back usually does not lead to a specific diagnosis. A general physical examination, including a

neurologic examination, may help identify those few patients who have a systemic disease or neurologic involvement.

Inspection may reveal the presence of **scoliosis**. Scoliosis can be either **structural** or **functional**. A structural scoliosis is associated with structural changes of the vertebral column and sometimes the rib cage as well. In adults, structural scoliosis is usually secondary to degenerative changes, although some individuals have a history of adolescent idiopathic scoliosis. As the patient bends forward (flexing the spine), structural scoliosis persists whereas functional scoliosis usually disappears. Paravertebral muscle spasm and leg length discrepancy are leading causes of functional scoliosis.

Palpation can detect paravertebral muscle spasm that often leads to loss of the normal lumbar lordosis. Point tenderness over the spine has sensitivity but not specificity for vertebral osteomyelitis. A palpable step-off between adjacent spinous processes indicates spondylolisthesis.

Limited spinal motion (flexion, extension, lateral bending, and rotation) is not associated with any specific diagnosis, since LBP due to any cause may limit motion. Range-of-motion measurements, however, can help in monitoring treatment.

The hip joints should be examined for any decrease in range of motion because hip arthritis, which normally causes groin pain, may occasionally present as LBP. Tenderness over the greater trochanter of the hip is seen in trochanteric bursitis, which can be confused with LBP. The presence of more

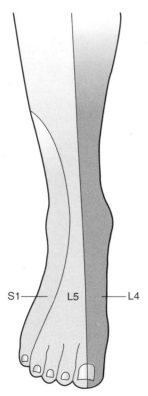

▲ **Figure 10–1.** Lower extremity dermatomes.

widespread tender points suggests the possibility that LBP may be secondary to fibromyalgia.

A **straight-leg raising test** should be performed on all patients with sciatica or pseudoclaudication. Straight leg raising places tension on the sciatic nerve and thereby stretches the sciatic nerve roots (L4, L5, S1, S2, and S3). If any of these nerve roots is already irritated, such as by impingement from a herniated disk, further tension on the nerve root by straight-leg raising will result in radicular pain that extends below the knee. The test is done by the examiner cupping the patient's heel in his or her hand and flexing the hip while keeping the knee extended. The test is positive if radicular pain (not merely back or hamstring pain) is produced when the leg is raised less than 60 degrees. The straight-leg raising test is very sensitive (95%) but not specific (40%) for clinically significant disk herniation at the L4–5 or L5–S1 level, which are the sites of 95% of clinically meaningful disk herniations. False-negative tests are seen more frequently with herniation above the L4–5 level. The straight-leg raising test is usually negative in patients with spinal stenosis. The crossed straight-leg raising test (with sciatica reproduced when the opposite leg is raised) is insensitive (25%) but highly specific (90%) for disk herniation.

The neurologic examination (see Table 10–1) should always include motor testing with focus on dorsiflexion of the ankle (L4), great toe dorsiflexion (L5), and foot plantar flexion (S1); determination of knee (L4) and ankle (S1) deep tendon reflexes; and tests for dermatomal sensory loss (see Figure 10–1). The inability to toe walk (mostly S1) and heel walk (mostly L5) may indicate muscle weakness. Muscle atrophy can be detected by circumferential measurements of the calf and thigh at the same level bilaterally.

C. Laboratory Findings

Laboratory studies play a minor role in the investigation of LBP. They are used mostly in identifying patients with systemic causes of LBP. A patient with normal blood cell counts, erythrocyte sedimentation rate, and radiographs of the lumbar spine is unlikely to have an underlying systemic disease as the cause of LBP.

D. Imaging Studies

Diagnostic tests should be done early for patients who have evidence of a major or progressive neurologic deficit and those in whom an underlying systemic disease is suspected (see Table 10–2). Otherwise, diagnostic tests are not required unless symptoms persist for more than 4 weeks. Because 90% of patients with LBP recover spontaneously within 4 weeks, this approach avoids unnecessary early testing.

A major problem with imaging studies is that many of the anatomic abnormalities seen are common in asymptomatic persons. These abnormalities are often the result of age-related degenerative changes and are frequently present after the age of 30. Making causal inferences based on imaging abnormalities can be hazardous in the absence of corresponding clinical findings and can lead to unnecessary and costly interventions with a potential for iatrogenic complications.

Plain radiographs of the spine do not usually help in determining the cause of LBP. Abnormalities such as single disk degeneration, facet joint degeneration, Schmorl nodes (intraspongy disk herniation), spondylolysis, mild spondylolisthesis, transitional vertebrae (lumbarization of S1 or sacralization of L5), spina bifida occulta, and mild scoliosis are equally prevalent in persons with and without LBP. Plain radiography should be limited to patients with clinical findings suggestive of infection, cancer, spondyloarthritis, or trauma, or those who continue to have LBP after 4–6 weeks of conservative care. It is noteworthy that radiation exposure to the female gonads from standard views of the lumbar spine is equivalent to that of a daily chest radiograph for several years.

Computed tomography (CT) and magnetic resonance imaging (MRI) should be reserved for patients in whom there is a strong clinical indication of underlying infection or cancer, or for the evaluation of patients with significant or progressive neurologic deficits. MRI is the preferred modality for the detection of spinal infection and cancers, herniated disks, and spinal stenosis. When interpreting the results of MRI and CT, it is important to remember that most asymptomatic adults above age 30 have evidence of either disk bulges (symmetric, circumferential extension of the disk material beyond the interspace) or disk herniation (focal or asymmetric extension of the disk bulge). Herniations are classified according to whether they are protrusions or extrusions. Protrusions are broad-based but extrusions have a neck, so that the base of an extrusion is narrower than the extruded material. Bulges and protrusions are common in asymptomatic adults. Thus, when these findings are seen in a patient, they are not necessarily the cause of LBP. Extrusions are less common but are also not invariably symptomatic. MRI with the intravenous contrast agent gadolinium is useful for the evaluation of patients with prior lumbar spine surgery (with no hardware present) to help in the differentiation of scar tissue from recurrent disk herniation.

The significance of a focal high signal (high-intensity zone) in the posterior annulus on a T2-weighted image is controversial. It is thought to represent annular tears and to correlate with positive findings on provocative diskography (which itself is a controversial procedure). **Discogenic LBP** has been diagnosed in patients with these high-intensity zones, and spinal fusion surgery is often recommended. The high prevalence of high-intensity zones in asymptomatic individuals, however, calls this approach into question.

Bone scanning is used primarily to detect infection, bony metastases, and occult fractures. Bone scans have limited specificity due to poor spatial resolution, and thus abnormal findings often require confirmatory imaging, such as MRI.

E. Special Tests

Electrodiagnostic studies can confirm nerve root compression and define the distribution and severity of involvement. Nerve conduction studies and electromyography are unnecessary when a patient has an obvious radiculopathy or isolated LBP. Electrodiagnosis, however, may be helpful in differentiating the limb pain of peroneal nerve palsy from that of L5 radiculopathy or in evaluating possible factitious weakness. Electromyographic changes depend on the development of muscle denervation following nerve injury and may not be detected until a few weeks after the injury.

▶ Differential Diagnosis

LBP usually originates from the lumbar spine or associated muscles and ligaments (Table 10–3). Rarely, pain is referred to the back from visceral disease. More than 95% of LBP is mechanical (Table 10–4). Degenerative change, also called lumbar spondylosis or lumbar osteoarthritis, is by far the most common disorder seen within the spine and the most important cause of mechanical LBP. However, even when one is certain that the cause of LBP is lumbar spondylosis, identification of the "pain generator" is challenging. The precise disk(s) or facet joint(s) responsible for the patient's pain is difficult to localize.

The focus of the initial diagnostic evaluation is to identify the small proportion of patients with systemic disease (infection, neoplasm, and spondyloarthropathy together account for only 1% of patients with LBP) or with neurologic involvement that requires urgent or specific intervention.

A. Lumbar Spondylosis

Lumbar spondylosis, or osteoarthritis of the lumbar spine, is the most commonly identified cause of LBP. Degenerative changes occur in both the intervertebral disk and facet joints (Figure 10–2), predisposing patients to disk herniation, spondylisthesis, and spinal stenosis.

Symptomatic patients complain of mechanical LBP. Recurrent attacks of acute LBP may occur in some patients while chronic LBP may develop in others. In patients with facet joint osteoarthritis, the pain may radiate into the posterior thigh and be exacerbated by bending ipsilateral to the involved joint (**facet syndrome**).

Imaging evidence of degenerative changes increases with age and is common (Figure 10–3). However, the relationship between these changes and back pain is complex. Patients with severe LBP may have minimal radiographic changes, and conversely, patients with advanced changes may be asymptomatic.

Spinal instability (in the absence of fractures or spondylolisthesis) remains a controversial diagnosis. Spinal instability is identified by demonstrating abnormal vertebral motion (anteroposterior displacement or excessive angular change of adjacent vertebrae) on flexion-extension radiography.

Table 10–4. Mechanical causes of low back pain.

Lumbar spondylosis[a]
Disc herniation[a]
Spondylolisthesis[a]
Spinal stenosis[a]
Diffuse idiopathic skeletal hyperostosis
Fractures (mostly osteoporotic)
Idiopathic (sprain and strain, lumbago)

[a]Related to degenerative changes.

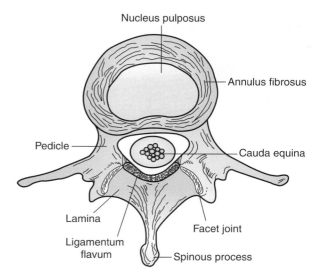

▲ **Figure 10–2.** Schematic drawing showing a cross-sectional view through a normal lumbar vertebra. The facet joints are formed by the articulation between the superior facet of the vertebra below and the inferior facet of the vertebra above.

Table 10–3. Causes of low back pain.

Originating from spine
Mechanical
Neoplastic
Infectious
Inflammatory
Metabolic
Originating from viscera

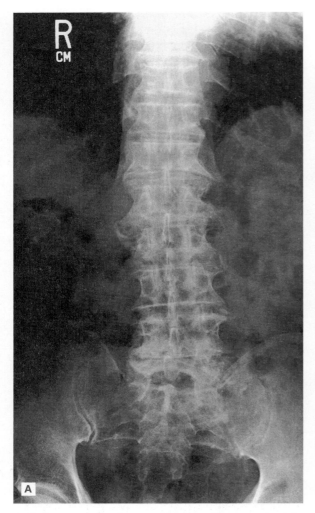
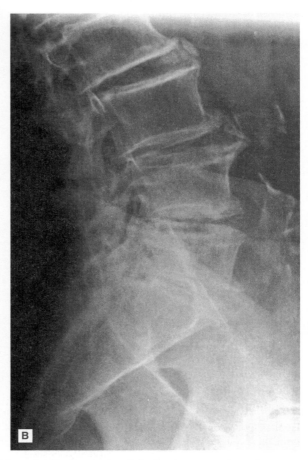

▲ **Figure 10–3.** Lumbar spondylosis. Anteroposterior (**A**) and lateral (**B**) radiographs of the lumbar spine show the cardinal features of disk-space narrowing, marginal osteophytes, and endplate sclerosis. (Used with permission from John Crues, MD, University of California, San Diego.)

However, such spinal motion may be seen in asymptomatic persons, and its relationship to the causation of pain is unclear.

B. Disk Herniation

The nucleus pulposus in a degenerated disk may prolapse and push out the weakened annulus, usually posterolaterally. Imaging evidence of disk herniation is commonly seen, even in asymptomatic adults. Occasionally, however, disk herniation results in a nerve root impingement syndrome (Figure 10–4 and 10–5). This accounts for less than 1% of patients with LBP but is nevertheless important to identify.

Such disk herniation may be precipitated by a wide range of activities from heavy lifting to trivial movement.

Ninety-five percent of clinically significant lumbar disk herniations involve either the L4–5 or L5–S1 disk. In general, the more caudal nerve root is impinged, that is, the L5 nerve root with L4–5 herniation and the S1 nerve root with L5–S1 herniation. Nerve root impingement results in sciatica. Indeed, sciatica has such a high sensitivity (95%) that its absence makes clinically significant lumbar disk herniation unlikely.

The natural history of disk herniation is favorable. Studies using sequential MRI testing reveal that the herniated portion

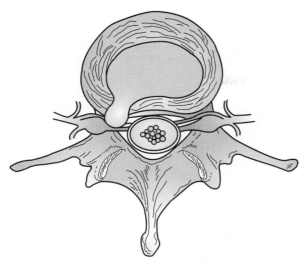

▲ **Figure 10–4.** Schematic drawing showing posterolateral disk herniation resulting in nerve root impingement.

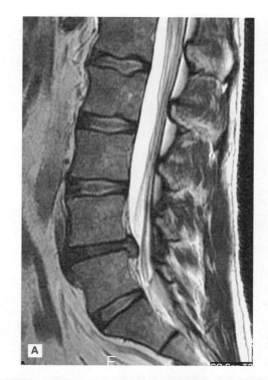

of the disk tends to regress with time. In most patients, the radicular pain resolves over a period of weeks, and less than 10% of patients with nerve root impingement require surgical decompression.

Rarely, a massive midline disk herniation, usually L4–5 (Figure 10–6), compresses the cauda equina causing **cauda equina syndrome**. This is a surgical emergency since neurologic results are affected by the time to decompression. Patients usually complain of bilateral sciatica and motor deficits. Sensory loss in the perineum (saddle anesthesia) is common, and urinary retention with overflow incontinence is usually present. Fecal incontinence may also occur.

Internal disk disruption is a controversial disorder diagnosed by provocative diskography. Following contrast injection into the disk, the radiographic appearance and induced pain are assessed. Diskographic anatomic abnormalities and induced pain are detected frequently in asymptomatic persons, however. More importantly, the discogenic pain attributed to disk disruption frequently improves spontaneously.

C. Spondylolisthesis

Spondylolisthesis is the anterior displacement of a vertebra on the one beneath it. This displacement is usually the result of degenerative changes in the disk and facet joints (**degenerative spondylolisthesis**) but also can be due to a developmental defect in the pars interarticularis of the vertebral arch that produces **isthmic spondylolisthesis** (Figure 10–7).

Degenerative spondylolisthesis is approximately four times more common in women and occurs most often at the L4–5 level. The spondylolisthesis may be missed if standing

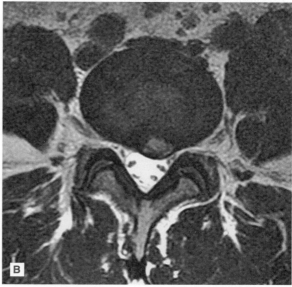

▲ **Figure 10–5.** Lumbar disk extrusion. **A:** The sagittal T2-weighted MRI shows an extruded disk at the L4–5 level. **B:** The axial image through the L4–5 level shows disk extrusion extending to the left side of the neural canal and compressing the exiting L5 nerve root against the left lamina. (Used with permission from John Crues, MD, University of California, San Diego.)

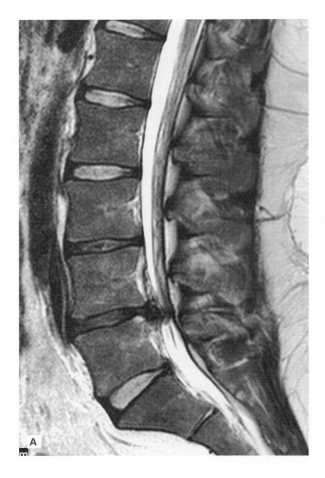

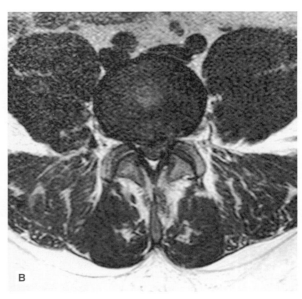

▲ **Figure 10–6.** Cauda equina syndrome. **A:** The sagittal T2-weighted MR image shows an extruded disk at the L4–5 level. **B:** The axial image through this level reveals a large central disk extrusion causing severe loss of cross-sectional area of the thecal sac. (Used with permission from John Crues, MD, University of California, San Diego.)

lumbar radiographs are not obtained because of its potential dynamic nature. Most patients with a minor degree of spondylolisthesis are asymptomatic, although some patients may have mechanical LBP. Greater degrees of spondylolisthesis may result in nerve root impingement (usually L5) or spinal stenosis (Figure 10–8). Rarely, extreme slippage results in cauda equina syndrome.

D. Spinal Stenosis

Lumbar spinal stenosis is defined as a narrowing of the spinal canal, its lateral recesses, and neural foramina that may result in a compression of lumbosacral nerve roots. Lumbar stenosis can be asymptomatic; up to 20% of asymptomatic adults older than age 60 have evidence of spinal stenosis on imaging. Spinal stenosis can occur at one or more levels and the narrowing can be asymmetric.

Degenerative changes are the cause of spinal stenosis in an overwhelming majority of cases (Table 10–5). The intervertebral disk loses vertical height as it degenerates; this results in a bulging of the now redundant and often hypertrophied

ligamentum flavum into the posterior part of the canal. Any herniation of the degenerated disk narrows the anterior part of the canal. Hypertrophied facets and osteophytes may compress nerve roots in the lateral recess or intervertebral foramen (Figures 10–9 and 10–10).

The hallmark of spinal stenosis is **pseudoclaudication** (neurogenic claudication). The symptoms of pseudoclaudication are usually bilateral. The patient complains of pain and discomfort together with weakness or paresthesias in the buttocks, thighs, and legs. Unsteadiness of gait is a frequent complaint. The lumbar component of pain is frequently mild. Pseudoclaudication is induced by standing or walking and relieved by sitting or flexing forward. In fact, the most important finding may be a history of no pain when the patient is seated with the spine flexed. This forward flexion increases the canal diameter and may lead to the patient adopting a simian stance. It has been hypothesized that spinal flexion relieves venous congestion along the spinal nerves. Other evidence, however, suggests that direct pressure on the nerve roots is the major mechanism. Factors that favor a diagnosis of pseudoclaudication over vascular claudication include

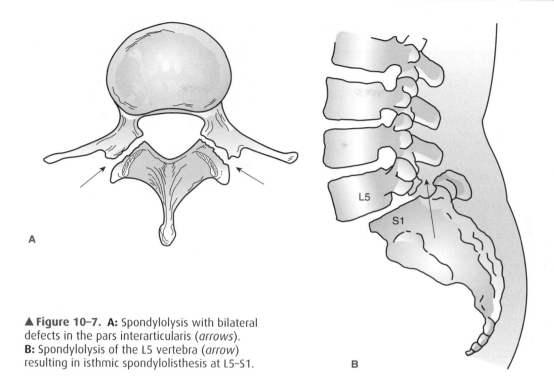

▲ **Figure 10–7. A:** Spondylolysis with bilateral defects in the pars interarticularis (*arrows*). **B:** Spondylolysis of the L5 vertebra (*arrow*) resulting in isthmic spondylolisthesis at L5–S1.

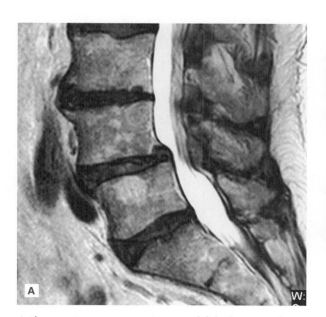

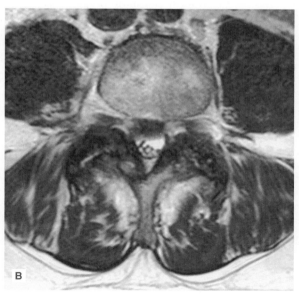

▲ **Figure 10–8.** Degenerative spondylolisthesis. **A:** The sagittal T2-weighted MRI shows an anterior slippage of the L4 vertebral body with respect to the L5 vertebral body compromising the thecal sac at this level. **B:** The axial image through the L4–5 disk space confirms the loss of cross-sectional area of the thecal sac. (Used with permission from John Crues, MD, University of California, San Diego.)

Table 10–5. Causes of lumbar spinal stenosis.

Congenital
Idiopathic
Achondroplastic
Acquired
Degenerative
Hypertrophy of facet joints
Hypertrophy of ligamentum flavum
Disc herniation
Spondylolisthesis
Scoliosis
Iatrogenic
Postlaminectomy
Postsurgical fusion
Miscellaneous
Paget disease
Fluorosis
Diffuse idiopathic skeletal hyperostosis

the preservation of pedal pulses, provocation of symptoms by standing just as readily as by walking, and location of the maximal discomfort to the thighs rather than the calves.

The physical examination of a patient with lumbar spinal stenosis is often unimpressive. Severe neurologic deficits are rarely seen. Lumbar range of motion may be normal or reduced and the result of straight-leg raising is usually negative. Deep tendon reflexes and vibration sense may be reduced. Mild weakness is seen in some. The significance of these findings is often difficult to determine in elderly

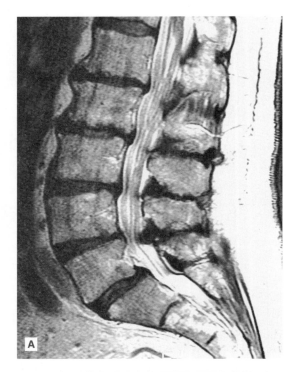

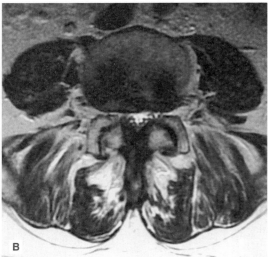

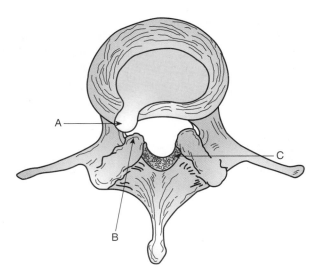

▲ **Figure 10–9.** Spinal stenosis secondary to a combination of disk herniation (**A**), facet joint hypertrophy (**B**), and hypertrophy of the ligamentum flavum (**C**).

▲ **Figure 10–10. A:** Degenerative spinal stenosis. The sagittal T2-weighted MR image shows decreased anteroposterior diameter of the neural canal at the L4–5 level due to redundancy of the ligamentum flavum. **B:** The axial image through the L4–5 disk shows decreased cross-sectional area of the thecal sac from hypertrophic changes of the facet joints posterolateral to the thecal sac. (Used with permission from John Crues, MD, University of California, San Diego.)

patients. The diagnosis of spinal stenosis is most often suspected when a history of pseudoclaudication is elicited and is best confirmed by MRI.

Spinal stenosis is generally an indolent condition, and the symptoms evolve gradually. Most patients remain stable, although some gradually worsen over a period of years.

E. Diffuse Idiopathic Skeletal Hyperostosis

Diffuse idiopathic skeletal hyperostosis is characterized by florid hyperostosis of the spine. Marginal bony proliferation leads to the formation of anterior osseous ridges that fuse and give the appearance of flowing wax on the anterior bodies of the vertebrae on radiography. Ossification of paraspinous ligaments, such as the anterior and posterior longitudinal ligaments, may be seen. The thoracic spine is most commonly involved, although the cervical and lumbar regions may also be affected. Lesions are most prominent anteriorly and along the right lateral aspect of the spine. Involvement of the left lateral aspect in patients with situs inversus has led to speculation that the descending thoracic aorta plays a role in the location of calcification. Intervertebral disk spaces are preserved, unless there is coexisting lumbar spondylosis, and sacroiliac and facet joints appear normal. This helps differentiate diffuse idiopathic skeletal hyperostosis from spondylosis and the spondyloarthritis. Extraspinal manifestations include irregular new bone formation ("whiskering") and large bone spurs that are often seen at the olecranon process and calcaneus. Severe ligamentous calcification may be seen in the patellar, sacrotuberous, and iliolumbar ligaments.

Diffuse idiopathic skeletal hyperostosis is usually seen in the middle-aged and the elderly. In spite of the extensive radiologic abnormalities, pain is often minimal or absent with only moderate limitation of spinal motion. Stiffness, which may be generalized, is a common complaint. Rarely, dysphagia or cervical myelopathy can occur secondary to extensive ossification of the anterior or posterior longitudinal ligaments, respectively. An association with diabetes mellitus has been noted.

F. Idiopathic Lower Back Pain

A definitive pathoanatomic diagnosis cannot be made in 80% of patients with LBP, largely because of the weak association between symptoms and the results of imaging. Thus, nonspecific terms such as lumbago, strain, and sprain have come into use. Strain and sprain have never been anatomically or histologically characterized. Therefore, idiopathic LBP is a more accurate label for these patients who have a mostly self-limited syndrome of back pain.

G. Neoplasm

Cancer is an unusual cause of LBP. Most cases result from involvement of the spine by metastatic carcinoma (especially prostate, lung, breast, thyroid, or kidney) or multiple myeloma.

Patients are usually older than 50 years and may give a history of weight loss or cancer in the past. Recumbency often does not improve the LBP and nocturnal pain is common. Missing the diagnosis can lead to irreversible neurologic compromise, ranging from cord compression to cauda equina syndrome.

Radiographs can reveal a compression fracture or lytic or blastic lesions that may be present in one or several vertebral bodies with sparing of the disk space. MRI is the test of choice to confirm bony metastases.

Patients with neurologic involvement may need urgent radiation therapy or surgical decompression.

H. Infection

Vertebral osteomyelitis, epidural abscess, and septic diskitis are infrequent but important causes of LBP. Osteomyelitis usually results from hematogenous seeding, direct inoculation at the time of spinal surgery, or contiguous spread from an infection in the adjacent soft tissue. It can lead to the formation of an epidural abscess. The most common organism is *Staphylococcus aureus,* followed by *Escherichia coli.* Coagulase-negative staphylococci and *Propionibacterium acnes* are the microorganisms that are almost always the cause of exogenous osteomyelitis after spinal surgery. Risk factors for osteomyelitis and epidural abscess include immunosuppression, diabetes, injection drug use, alcoholism, and renal failure. The primary focus of infection is often the urinary tract, skin, soft tissue, a site of vascular access, or endocarditis. Tuberculosis and nontubercular granulomatous infections (blastomycosis, cryptococcosis, actinomycosis, coccidioidomycosis, and brucellosis) of the spine are rare but should be considered in the appropriate clinical setting.

Back pain that is not relieved by rest or recumbency, spine tenderness over the involved segment, and an elevated erythrocyte sedimentation rate are the most common findings. Fever may only be seen with abscess formation, and the white blood cell count is often normal. An untreated epidural abscess can result in spinal cord compression or cauda equina syndrome. Radiographs may show a narrowed disk space with erosion of adjacent vertebrae, but these changes often take weeks to appear. MRI is the most sensitive and specific imaging technique to detect spinal infections. A biopsy for culture is recommended, especially if blood cultures are negative. Treatment consists of intravenous antibiotics initially, with a total duration of at least 6 weeks of antimicrobial treatment. The presence of an epidural abscess generally requires surgical decompression.

I. Inflammation

The spondyloarthritides (see Chapters 17–19) cause inflammatory LBP (Table 10–2).

J. Metabolic Disease

The major consideration is the occurrence of acute LBP secondary to a vertebral compression fracture in a patient with osteoporosis (see Chapter 58). Most patients are postmenopausal women.

Paget disease of bone is often detected in an asymptomatic patient by the incidental finding of either an elevated alkaline phosphatase or characteristic radiographic abnormality. Back pain secondary to involvement of the spine is most common in the lumbar area. The pain may be due to the pagetic process itself, to secondary osteoarthritis in the facet joints, or rarely to a pathologic fracture of a vertebra. Spinal cord and cauda equina compression secondary to Paget disease have been seen on rare occasions.

K. Visceral Pathology

Disease in organs that share segmental innervation with the spine can cause pain to be referred to the spine. In general, pelvic diseases refer pain to the sacral area, lower abdominal diseases to the lumbar area, and upper abdominal diseases to the lower thoracic spine area. Local signs of disease, such as tenderness to palpation, paravertebral muscle spasm, and increased pain on spinal motion, are absent.

A partial list of causes includes a contained rupture of an abdominal aortic aneurysm, pyelonephritis, ureteral obstruction due to renal stones, chronic prostatitis, endometriosis, ovarian cysts, inflammatory bowel disorders, colonic neoplasms, and retroperitoneal hemorrhage (usually in a patient taking anticoagulants).

▶ Treatment

Specific treatment is available only for the small fraction of patients with LBP who either have major neural compression or have an underlying systemic disease (infection, malignancy, or spondyloarthritis). In the vast majority of patients with LBP, either the precise cause cannot be determined, or when the cause is determined, no specific treatment is available. These patients are treated with a conservative program centered on analgesia, education, and physical therapy. Less than 1% of patients with LBP need surgery.

One should be wary of the proliferation of unproven medical, surgical, and alternative therapies. Most have not been rigorously tested in randomized controlled trials; uncontrolled studies can produce a misleading impression of efficacy due to fluctuating symptoms and the favorable natural history of LBP.

For management purposes, patients with LBP are considered to have either **acute LBP** (duration less than 3 months), **chronic LBP** (duration greater than 3 months), or a **nerve root compression syndrome.**

A. Acute Lower Back Pain

Patients often seek medical attention for sudden onset of severe mechanical LBP. Examination usually reveals paravertebral muscle spasm, often resulting in loss of the normally present lumbar lordosis, and severe decrease in range of motion secondary to pain.

Patients with acute LBP are advised to stay active and continue ordinary daily activities within the limits permitted by pain. Bed rest of more than 1 or 2 days is discouraged.

Medications are used for symptomatic relief. Aspirin, acetaminophen, and nonsteroidal anti-inflammatory drugs are effective analgesics. Some patients, however, may need short-term opioid analgesia. Muscle relaxants, used for a few days, may help some patients. Oral glucocorticoids are of no benefit in patients with acute LBP, including those with sciatica.

Back exercises are not helpful in the acute phase, and a physical therapy referral is usually unnecessary in the first month. Later, a program of regular back exercises including stretching exercises, aerobic conditioning, and loss of excess weight are used to prevent recurrences. The purpose of back exercises is to stabilize the spine by strengthening the trunk muscles. Flexion exercises strengthen the abdominal muscles and extension exercises strengthen the paraspinal muscles. Various exercise programs have been developed and appear to be equally effective. Educational booklets that include back exercises and safe lifting techniques are helpful. Back school may be effective for worksite-specific patient education but has not been shown to be effective in nonoccupational settings.

There is no evidence that spinal manipulative therapy is superior to other standard treatments for patients with acute or chronic LBP.

There is limited evidence to support the use of epidural glucocorticoid injections for short-term relief of radicular pain but these offer no significant functional benefit and do not reduce the need for surgery. Epidural injections are not recommended for LBP without radiculopathy. Injections of trigger points, ligaments, sacroiliac joints, and facet joints with anesthetic agents or glucocorticoid are of unproven efficacy and are not recommended in the management of LBP. Nerve root blocks are also not recommended for therapeutic or diagnostic purposes.

Self-application of heat or cold is an easy and inexpensive option. Shoe lifts are considered only when the leg length inequality is more than 1 inch.

Modalities such as ultrasound, cutaneous laser treatment, shortwave diathermy, electrical stimulation, and transcutaneous electrical nerve stimulation are not effective in the treatment of LBP. Other treatments such as lumbar braces, traction, acupuncture, dry-needling, biofeedback, and massage are also largely ineffective and not recommended.

LBP is common in pregnancy and although it frequently starts before the twelfth week it is rarely progressive. Back pain can be reduced in most pregnant patients by the use of an inelastic low sacroiliac belt that does not compress the abdomen.

Kyphoplasty (Figure 10–11) and vertebroplasty (percutaneous injection of bone cement into a fractured vertebral body through bone biopsy needles) are two increasingly popular, technically demanding, and expensive procedures that are used for treating the pain associated with osteoporotic compression fractures. However, two recent randomized

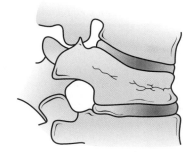

Fractured vertebra

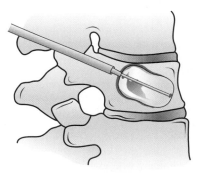

Balloon inflation

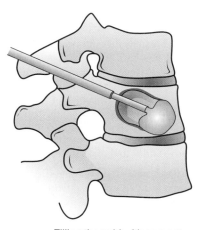

Filling the void with cement

▲ **Figure 10–11.** Balloon kyphoplasty. The first illustration is of a fractured osteoporotic vertebra. In the next illustration an orthopedic balloon has been percutaneously guided into the fractured vertebral body and inflated, reducing the fracture and elevating the superior endplate. The balloon is then deflated and removed, thereby creating a void. The final illustration shows filling of the void with cement. (Reproduced with permission from Kyphon Pictures.)

controlled trials of vertebroplasty for painful osteoporotic spinal fractures found no beneficial effect of vertebroplasty compared with a sham procedure. Therefore, based on current evidence, the routine use of vertebroplasty or kyphoplasty for relief of pain from osteoporotic compression fractures cannot be justified.

B. Chronic Lower Back Pain

In most patients, the specific pathoanatomic diagnosis of the pain generator is unclear. The clinical spectrum in these patients with chronic pain is wide. Some patients complain of severe unremitting pain, but most have a nagging mechanical LBP that may radiate into the buttocks. Patients with chronic LBP may experience periods of acute exacerbation. Treatment is centered on relief of pain and restoration of function. Results are often unsatisfactory, and complete relief of pain is unrealistic for most. However, the large majority of patients with chronic back pain continue working.

Acetaminophen and nonsteroidal anti-inflammatory drugs may provide some degree of analgesia, but the evidence for their efficacy is not compelling. Long-term use of opioid analgesics should be avoided, but this is not always possible. Antidepressants are useful in the one-third of patients who have associated depression. Low-dose tricyclic antidepressants (eg, amitriptyline 10–75 mg at bedtime) may help some patients without depression, but anticholinergic side effects are common.

Back exercises (see section on Acute Lower Back Pain, above), aerobic conditioning, loss of excess weight, and patient education are effective in managing chronic LBP. Multidisciplinary pain centers offer a combination of drug therapy, behavioral therapy, physical therapy, and patient education. These therapies may be helpful in selected patients as long as the center is not procedure oriented and avoids the use of unproven and expensive therapies, including invasive procedures.

Massage, when combined with exercise and education, may be beneficial for patients with chronic LBP. As with patients with acute LBP, there is no evidence to support the use of injection therapies and modalities for chronic LBP.

Prolotherapy is an injection-based treatment that has been used for chronic LBP. Proponents of prolotherapy hypothesize that back pain in some patients stems from weakened ligaments. Repeatedly injecting the ligaments with an irritant sclerosing agent is believed to strengthen the ligaments and reduce pain. However, there is no evidence that prolotherapy injections are more effective than control injections.

Radiofrequency denervation of the small nerves to the facet joints is sometimes recommended for patients with the facet syndrome. There is no evidence of benefit beyond a few weeks following this procedure.

Spinal cord stimulation is yet another modality used for the relief of chronic LBP. An electrical generator delivers pulses to a targeted spinal cord area through leads implanted via laminectomy or percutaneously. The mechanism of action is poorly understood, and there are insufficient data to support its use. The use of intraspinal drug infusion systems for intrathecal delivery of analgesics (usually morphine) is also not supported by adequate data.

The exact pathophysiology of pain in degenerative disease of the lumbar spine remains elusive. It is therefore not surprising that as a general principle, the results of back surgery are disappointing when the goal is relief of back pain rather than relief of radicular symptoms resulting from neurologic compression. The role of surgical treatment of chronic disabling LBP without neurologic involvement remains controversial. The most common surgical treatment in these patients with degenerative changes is spinal fusion. The rationale for fusion is based on its successful use at painful peripheral joints. A growing body of clinical evidence now suggests that functional restoration through a cognitive behavioral therapy–based intensive rehabilitation program can generate improvements similar to spinal fusion.

Intradiskal electrothermal annuloplasty is another unproven procedure for the relief of chronic LBP in patients with positive diskography. A wire-containing catheter is inserted into the disk, positioned against the posterior annulus, and then heated. This presumably shrinks collagen fibrils and cauterizes granulation and nerve tissue.

The use of lumbar artificial disks for spinal arthroplasty, in patients with degenerative disk disease at one level from L4–S1 and no spondylolisthesis, is approved in the United States. Approval was based on data showing efficacy equal to that of spinal fusion. This may be faint praise given the controversy regarding the efficacy of spinal fusion for isolated LBP. Few data support the hypothetical advantage that, unlike spinal fusion, artificial disks will protect adjacent levels from further degeneration by preserving motion.

C. Nerve Root Compression Syndromes

1. Disk herniation—Patients with radicular pain in whom a disk herniation with nerve root compression is suspected should be treated nonsurgically, as described in the section on Acute Lower Back Pain, for the first 6 weeks unless they have a severe or progressive neurologic deficit. Most patients (approximately 90%) respond. Elective surgery may be considered in the few patients who have a significant persistent neurologic deficit or severe sciatica after 6 weeks of conservative care (Table 10–6).

Laminotomy with limited diskectomy is generally the procedure of choice. A microdiskectomy is the same procedure but with the use of a microscope. Percutaneous techniques are less effective.

2. Spinal stenosis—The symptoms of spinal stenosis remain stable for years in most patients and may actually improve in a few. Even when symptoms progress, there is little likelihood of irreversible neurologic impairment. Therefore, nonoperative treatment is a rational choice for most patients. Analgesics, nonsteroidal anti-inflammatory drugs, loss of excess weight, physical conditioning and exercises (including

Table 10–6. Indications for surgical referral.

Disk herniation
Cauda equina syndrome (emergency)
Clinically significant neurologic deficit
Progressive neurologic deficit
Greater than 6 weeks of sciatica (elective)
Persistence of significant neurologic deficit
beyond 6 weeks (elective)
Spinal stenosis
Clinically significant neurologic deficit
Progressive neurologic deficit
Persistent and disabling pseudoclaudication (elective)
Spondylolisthesis
Significant or progressive neurologic deficit

those that reduce lumbar lordosis) may provide symptomatic relief. Limited data suggest that epidural glucocorticoid injections may temporarily relieve leg pain. They do not, however, influence functional status or subsequent need for surgery.

Patients with a progressive or severe neurologic deficit are surgical candidates (see Table 10–6). Elective surgery may be considered in patients with severe and disabling pseudoclaudication. Surgical treatment is aimed at decompression of the neural elements. This is accomplished by laminectomy or laminotomy with excision of the ligamentum flavum and medial aspect of the hypertrophied facet joints and removal of any protruding disk material. If spinal instability is present (as with spondylolisthesis) or results from surgical decompression, fusion of vertebral segments may be required. Unfortunately, the routine use of complex fusion techniques in the absence of evidence of greater efficacy is rapidly increasing. The techniques include instrumentation (use of hardware including screws and plates), bone graft augmentation (with bone cement and human bone morphogenetic proteins), and combined anterior and posterior fusion (often at multiple levels). These techniques are associated with increased perioperative mortality, major complications, rehospitalization, and cost.

3. Spondylolisthesis—The vast majority of patients are treated conservatively. Rarely, a patient may need decompression surgery with fusion if a significant or progressive neurologic deficit develops from nerve root impingement or if disabling pseudoclaudication develops secondary to spinal stenosis. Surgical fusion for spondylolisthesis with severe chronic disabling pain but no neurologic deficit may yield better results than nonsurgical treatment. Unfortunately, long-term follow-up shows that this benefit is not sustained.

Carragee EJ. Clinical practice. Persistent low back pain. *N Engl J Med.* 2005;352:1891. [PMID: 15872204]

Carragee EJ. The increasing morbidity of elective spinal stenosis surgery: is it necessary? *JAMA.* 2010;303:1309. [PMID: 20371793]

Chou R, Atlas SJ, Stanos SP, Rosenquist RW. Nonsurgical interventional therapies for low back pain: a review of the evidence for an American Pain Society Clinical Practice Guideline. *Spine.* 2009;34:1078. [PMID: 19363456]

Chou R, Baisden J, Carragee EJ, Resnick DK, Shaffer WO, Loeser JD. Surgery for low back pain: a review of the evidence for an American Pain Society Clinical Practice Guideline. *Spine.* 2009;34:1094. [PMID: 19363455]

Chou R, Fu R, Carrino JA, Deyo RA. Imaging strategies for low-back pain: systematic review and meta-analysis. *Lancet.* 2009;373:463. [PMID: 19200918]

Chou R, Loeser JD, Owens DK, et al. American Pain Society Low Back Pain Guideline Panel. Interventional therapies, surgery, and interdisciplinary rehabilitation for low back pain: an evidence-based clinical practice guideline from the American Pain Society. *Spine.* 2009;34:1066. [PMID: 19363457]

Chou R, Qaseem A, Snow V, et al. Clinical Efficacy Assessment Subcommittee of the American College of Physicians; American College of Physicians; American Pain Society Low Back Pain Guidelines Panel. Diagnosis and treatment of low back pain: a joint clinical practice guideline from the American College of Physicians and the American Pain Society. *Ann Intern Med.* 2007;147:478. [PMID: 17909209]

Cochrane Review
http://www.cochrane.org/cochrane-reviews

Deyo RA, Weinstein JN. Low back pain. *N Engl J Med.* 2001;344:363. [PMID: 11172169]

Dixit RK, Schwab JH. Low back and neck pain. In: Stone JH, editor. *A Clinician's Pearls and Myths in Rheumatology.* Springer; 2009.

Institute for Clinical Systems Improvement
http://www.icsi.org

Katz JN, Harris MB. Clinical practice. Lumbar spinal stenosis. *N Engl J Med.* 2008;358:818. [PMID: 18287604]

National Guideline Clearinghouse
http://www.guideline.gov

Weinstein JN. Balancing science and informed choice in decisions about vertebroplasty. *N Engl J Med.* 2009;361:619. [PMID: 19657127]

11 Approach to the Patient with Hip Pain

Simon C. Mears, MD, PhD

Hip pain is a common complaint which patients may describe in the thigh, back, or groin areas. Pain in these areas may be due to pathology in or about the hip joint or may be referred, which commonly occurs with spinal stenosis. The hip joint and its periarticular structures are relatively inaccessible to evaluation by palpation for possible tenderness. Therefore, accurate evaluation of patients with "hip" pain depends on the identification of specific historical features of the symptoms, the determination of the exact cause of the pain (through careful medical history and appropriate physical examination), a basic understanding of common radiographic findings, and a thorough understanding of the potential differential diagnosis. The particular cause of hip pain often correlates with the age of the patient.

▶ Clinical Findings

A. History

The history should (1) determine the location of the pain within the hip area, (2) distinguish between acute and chronic pain, (3) establish whether the onset of pain was abrupt or gradual, (4) delineate the circumstances associated with the onset of pain, and (5) identify activities that exacerbate or ameliorate the pain.

Pain located primarily in the groin and associated with weight bearing or range of motion is most typical of intra-articular hip abnormalities. Pain beginning in the low back and radiating down the buttock and back of the leg to the side of the calf and lateral side of the foot is more likely to be due to a lumbar radiculopathy than to an intra-articular hip abnormality. Pain localized to the side of the hip and exacerbated by lying on the affected side is most likely greater trochanteric bursitis. Hip pain due to infections or malignancy is severe, generalized, constant, and often worse at night.

A traumatic event associated with the acute onset of pain strongly suggests fracture or injury to the soft tissues about the hip. In cases of acute onset pain, the history also should include questions regarding changes in activity, such as new exercise programs or injuries. For example, abnormal mechanics during running, such as the feet crossing the midline (increased adduction), wide pelvis and genu valgum, or running on oval tracks that lack banks can predispose to trochanteric bursitis. Repetitive loading activities can result in a femoral stress fracture.

Pain that has been slow and progressive over time is common in arthritic conditions. A person with osteoarthritis of the hip experiences a gradual onset of slowly worsening hip pain and decreasing range of motion. It becomes progressively harder to walk normally, especially going up and down stairs.

The age of the patient influences the differential diagnosis of hip pain. Children are susceptible to particular hip problems, such as slipped capital femoral epiphysis and Legg-Calvé-Perthes disease. Adolescents and young adults commonly have avascular necrosis, hip dysplasia, labral tears, or femoroacetabular impingement. Middle-aged and older patients often have hip arthritis, low back pain, or trochanteric bursitis.

Snapping in and around the hip, suggests one of the "snapping hip syndromes," which are divided into internal and external causes. Internal snapping can be caused by the iliopsoas tendon slipping over the osseous ridge of the lesser trochanter or the anterior acetabulum or by the iliofemoral ligament riding over the femoral head. Acetabular labral tears or loose bodies can cause intra-articular snapping associated with sharp pain in the groin and anterior thigh. External snapping results from a tight iliotibial band or gluteus maximus tendon riding over the greater tuberosity of the femur. These types of snapping occur during hip flexion and extension, especially during internal rotation.

In rare instances, an intrapelvic, intra-abdominal, or retroperitoneal abnormality (ranging from uterine fibroids to a sports hernia to a retroperitoneal hematoma or infection) may be the cause of hip symptoms.

Another presentation of hip pathology is pain felt in the in the knee alone. Branches of the obturator nerve innervate the knee and the hip joint and may cause hip pathology to refer pain to the knee. All patients with knee pain should have an examination of the hip.

B. Physical Examination

A basic understanding of the hip anatomy and biomechanics is the cornerstone of an accurate physical examination of the patient with hip pain. The hip is formed by the proximal femur and the articulation with the pelvis. The bony anatomy of the proximal femur includes the femoral head, the femoral neck, and the greater and lesser trochanters. The acetabulum, the mating socket for the femoral head, is coated with articular cartilage, and a rim of fibrocartilage (the labrum) adds to the stability of the hip and circumscribes the outer edge of the acetabulum. The iliotibial band originates along the brim of the iliac wing (along the anterior and posterior margins), consolidates over the greater trochanter, travels laterally along the thigh, and inserts in the proximal leg. These tendinous insertions have an associated bursa that decreases friction where the tendon crosses a bony protuberance. The trochanteric bursa is located between gluteus maximus and the greater trochanter, the gluteofemoral bursa is between the gluteus maximus and the vastus lateralis origin, and the ischial bursa lies between the ischial tuberosity and gluteus maximus. The muscles around the hip can be summarized into four main groups (Figure 11–1).

1. Inspection of gait—Examination of the hip begins with the careful observation of the patient's gait. Two phases of gait need to be observed: stance phase (when the foot is on the ground and bears weight) and swing phase (when the foot moves forward and does not bear weight). Most of the problems appear during the weight-bearing stance phase.

The width of the gait, the shift of pelvis, and flexion of the knee should be observed as well as the lumbar portion of the spine. With the patient in the supine position, the lumbar spine reflects a slight lordosis. Loss of lordosis may reflect vertebral spasm, and excess lordosis may suggest a flexion deformity of the hip. Therefore, this observation should always be followed with the assessment of leg-length symmetry. Leg shortening and external rotation with pain suggest hip fracture. The anterior and posterior surfaces of the hip should be inspected for areas of muscle atrophy or bruising related to a traumatic event or neuromuscular disease.

Pain is a common cause of limp. The characteristic of an **antalgic limp** is shortened standing time on the affected side. When pain arises in the hip joint, the trunk also shifts toward the painful side. Moving the body's center of gravity toward the painful hip decreases the moment arm of bodyweight to hip joint, reducing total force on the hip. This maneuver should not be confused with a **Trendelenburg gait**, which is secondary to a weakened gluteus medius muscle. In the Trendelenburg gait pattern, the opposite side of the pelvis tilts downward during the stance phase on the weakened side and, in an effort to compensate for the weakness, the trunk lurches toward the weakened side during the same walking cycle phase (Plates 27 and 28). This action moves the center of gravity nearer the fulcrum on the weak side and shortens the moment arm from the center of gravity to the hip joint to produce the characteristic waddle.

A limp is common in patients with substantial hip arthritis or disease in other joints of the lower extremity. The limp may be caused by pain, shortening of the leg, flexion contracture, or weakness in the pelvic girdle muscles or in other parts of the lower limb (such as in a paralyzed quadriceps gait pattern, triceps surae gait pattern, and dorsiflexor gait pattern). Therefore, a thorough evaluation of the lower extremity muscle strength is essential for diagnosing the cause of the limp. Manual muscle testing is useful for evaluating flexors (iliopsoas and rectus femoris), extensors (gluteus maximus and hamstrings), abductors (gluteus medius and minimus), and adductors (adductor longus, magnus and brevis, pectineus and gracilis). Muscle testing should be performed on the lower leg muscles (ankle and toe dorsiflexors and plantarflexors) to evaluate for weakness as a result of a radiculopathy.

2. Palpation—With the patient supine, the clinician should ask the patient to place the heel of the leg being examined on the opposite knee. This position facilitates palpation along the inguinal ligament. Bulges along the ligament can be inguinal hernias or aneurysms, which can be secondary causes of hip pain outside the hip joint (eg, ischemia secondary to vascular disease or compression of an aneurysm). From lateral to medial, a sequence of nerve, artery, vein, and lymph nodes can be palpated. Enlarged nodes suggest infection. Tenderness over the femoral greater trochanter indicates local bursitis rather than arthritis. With the patient lying on the unaffected side and the hip flexed and internally rotated, the trochanteric bursa over the greater trochanter and the bursa over the posterosuperior iliac spine can be palpated (Plate 29). The ischiogluteal bursa cannot be palpated unless it is inflamed. When it is inflamed, this bursitis can mimic sciatica. Bursitis is one of the major causes of tenderness around hip joint, but other causes of such tenderness include synovitis of the hip joint or psoas abscess. Tenderness without swelling on the posterolateral surface of the greater trochanter suggests localized tendinitis or muscle spasm from referred hip pain. Crepitus, or a grating sensation in the joint, felt by the patient or determined by the examiner, is a late manifestation of arthritic condition and is not a sensitive or specific indicator. Sensory examination of the skin around the hip may reveal a condition called meralgia paresthetica, or compression of the lateral femoral cutaneous nerve. This nerve innervates the lateral aspect of the thigh and may be compressed at the waist by tight belts or clothing leading to numbness or pain.

3. Range of motion—Motions of the hip include flexion, extension, abduction, adduction, and rotation (Table 11–1). The hip can flex further when the knee is also flexed. In the

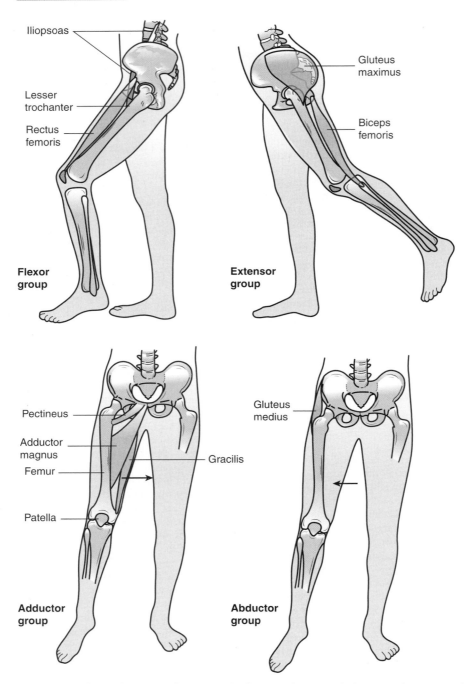

▲ **Figure 11–1.** Four powerful muscle groups that move the hip are shown with their attachments to the femur and pelvis. The primary hip flexor is the iliopsoas tendon, which inserts on the lesser trochanter. The main hip extensor muscle is the gluteus maximus. The hip adductors include the pectineus, adductor brevis, magnus, and longus, and the gracilis. The main abductors of the hip are the gluteus medius and minimus. Abductor function is critical to the hip and weakness leads to a Trendelenburg gait. (Reproduced, with permission, from Bickley LS, Szilagyi PG. The musculoskeletal system. In: *Bates' Guide to Physical Examination and History Taking,* 8th ed. Philadelphia: Lippincott Williams & Wilkins; 2003.)

Table 11–1. Normal range of motion of the adult hip.

Motion	Normal Range (degrees)
Flexion	0 to 135
Extension	0 to 15
Abduction	0 to 45
Adduction	0 to 25
Internal rotation	0 to 35
External rotation	0 to 45

case of a hip with a flexion deformity, flexion of the unaffected hip prevents full leg extension of the affected hip, which appears flexed (Figure 11–2). With the patient supine, the examiner places one hand on the patient's iliac crest. As the patient attempts to extend the hip to neutral, the clinician can detect pelvic movement that might be mistaken for hip movement. Flexion deformity may be masked by an increase in lumbar lordosis and an anterior pelvic tilt. Assessment of the extension can be aided by positioning the patient face down and extending the thigh toward the clinician in a posterior direction.

Stabilizing the pelvis by pressing down on the opposite anterosuperior iliac spine with one hand, grasping the ankle with the other, and abducting the extended leg marks the limit of hip abduction (normal range, 45–50 degrees; Plate 30). Restricted abduction is common in hip osteoarthritis. In the same manner, moving the leg medially across the body and over the opposite extremity marks

the adduction limit. Flexing the leg to 90 degrees at hip and knee, stabilizing the thigh with one hand, grasping the ankle with the other, and rotating the lower extremity externally (normal, 45 degrees) and internally (normal, 35 degrees) identifies the hip's rotation limits (Figure 11–3). Loss of internal rotation is an especially sensitive indicator of hip disease and is often the earliest change in range of motion. As the disease progresses, prolonged joint stiffness and other limitations of movements become more evident. Limitation of joint movement may be secondary to flexion contractures or mechanical obstructions.

There are two tests for evaluating elicited hip pain. The Stinchfield resisted-hip-flexion test evaluates the pain response caused by an increase in hip joint reactive force and is a valuable tool for distinguishing intra-articular and extra-articular hip abnormalities causing groin, thigh, buttock, and even pretibial leg pain. While the patient is in a supine position, he or she is asked to elevate the leg while the examiner applies gentle manual resistance to the ankle with the knee extended. Reproduction of pain in a typical pattern related to the sensory innervation of the hip (groin, thigh, buttock, or knee) makes the test positive for a hip abnormality. In Patrick test, the patient lies supine, and the clinician holds the affected leg and rotates it externally. Pain elicited suggests sacroiliitis, hip abnormality, or an L4 nerve root lesion.

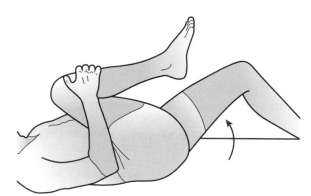

▲ **Figure 11–2.** In flexion deformity of the hip (in this case, the left), the affected hip does not allow full leg extension when the opposite hip is flexed. Therefore, the affected hip appears flexed. (Reproduced, with permission from Bickley LS, Szilagyi PG. The musculoskeletal system. In: *Bates' Guide to Physical Examination and History Taking*, 8th ed. Philadelphia: Lippincott Williams & Wilkins; 2003.)

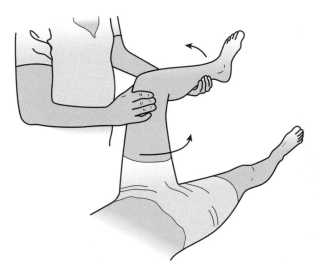

▲ **Figure 11–3.** Establishing the rotation limits of the hip is done by flexing the leg to 90 degrees at the hip and knee, stabilizing the thigh with one hand, and with the other hand grasping the ankle and rotating the lower extremity externally (normal, 45 degrees) and internally (normal, 35 degrees). (Reproduced, with permission, from Bickley LS, Szilagyi PG. The musculoskeletal system. In: *Bates' Guide to Physical Examination and History Taking*, 8th ed. Philadelphia: Lippincott Williams & Wilkins; 2003.)

C. Laboratory Findings

Examination and culture of synovial fluid (see Chapter 2) is essential whenever infection of the hip is suspected. Intensely inflammatory effusions suggest pyogenic infection, requiring immediate antibiotic therapy and aspiration or other drainage to establish the diagnosis and prevent joint destruction. Hemorrhagic joint fluid suggests fracture, bleeding diathesis, or malignancy.

Usually, imaging modalities are preferred as the first-line diagnostic tools once involvement of the hip joint is established, and laboratory investigations have a limited role. The erythrocyte sedimentation rate and serum C-reactive protein are typically elevated in inflammatory conditions. Isolated involvement of the hip (pseudoseptic presentation) is an uncommon presenting manifestation of rheumatoid arthritis; specific serologic tests (ie, antibodies to cyclic citrullinated peptides, rheumatoid factor) can be helpful in these unusual cases.

D. Imaging Studies

1. Conventional radiography—Conventional radiographs of the hip and pelvis should be ordered as the first diagnostic tests for patients with hip pain. Conventional radiographs can delineate the alignment, bone mineralization, articular cartilage, and soft tissue. Alignment abnormality may indicate a fracture, a dislocation, or secondary causes of osteoarthritis such as congenital dislocation of the hip or slipped capital femoral epiphysis. Bone mineralization indicates osteoporosis or osteopenia as the underlying cause of pain. An anteroposterior pelvic radiograph and a "frog-leg" lateral hip radiograph may reveal fractures, provide a better view of the anterolateral femoral head, and help evaluate for osteonecrosis. For patients in the later stages of osteonecrosis, radiographs show a break in the cortex and a rim sign (a subcortical black lucent line) characteristic of femoral head collapse. A 40-degree cephalad anteroposterior view is useful for elucidating subtle femoral neck and pubic fractures. Radiographs may reveal evidence of hip dysplasia shown by the lack of femoral head coverage. Femoroacetabular impingement may be indicated by a deformity of the femur (such as an osteophyte on the femoral neck causing cam impingement), or by a deformity on the acetabulum (such as coxa profunda, protrusio, or acetabular retroversion leading to pincer impingement). On conventional radiographs, joint-space narrowing is indicative of articular cartilage loss, spurs or osteophytes are indicative of arthritic change, segmental radiolucency or sclerotic changes of the femoral head are indicative of avascular necrosis, calcifications are indicative of synovial chondromatosis, and soft-tissue calcification is indicative of calcific tendinitis (Figure 11–4).

2. Arthrography—Arthrography is a useful tool for showing labral abnormalities, especially when it is performed in conjunction with MRI. Magnetic resonance arthrography is the most sensitive and specific test for labral tear of the hip. Injection with local anesthetic agents during the arthrogram can be a powerful tool for the diagnosis of hip abnormalities. If the injection does not help the pain, other diagnoses should be ruled out. Arthrography continues to have a role in the diagnosis of infection and loosening of the prosthesis in the patient with a painful total joint arthroplasty.

3. CT scanning—CT of the hip and pelvis is most useful in the assessment of fractures, particularly complex fractures. Pelvic and acetabular fractures, osseous sequelae of hip dislocation, and intra-articular osseous fragments are better visualized by CT than by conventional radiographs. CT is also useful in characterizing calcifications secondary to tumor matrix within bone or soft tissue or to ossification, and CT is the best modality for imaging cortical bone.

4. MRI—MRI provides excellent visualization of medullary bone and soft tissues. The diagnosis of osteonecrosis of the femoral head is made earlier by MRI than by any other technique, including bone scintigraphy, CT, and conventional radiographs. MRI is also the method of choice for the diagnosis of occult hip fracture in the elderly and, despite its expense, can be cost-effective for this purpose. MRI is the most accurate method for the diagnosis of stress fractures around the hip and pelvis, and it is the best test for the diagnosis of transient osteoporosis of the hip. It is also the most valuable test for the staging of bony and soft tissue tumors around the hip. MRI is frequently helpful in documenting synovitis of the hip joint by revealing effusion (eg, in pigmented villonodular synovitis). Magnetic resonance arthrography is useful in defining labral abnormalities and in examining for evidence of impingement, such as a high angle or herniation pits in the lateral femur.

5. Bone scans—Bone scans are useful for detecting metastatic disease (when suspected), osteonecrosis, arthritis, and Paget disease of bone. Scintigraphy delineates the regions of increased metabolic activity ("hot spots") by increased uptake of a radioactive tracer.

E. Special Tests

1. Electromyography and nerve conduction velocity studies—Electromyography and nerve conduction velocity studies are used in the differential diagnosis of hip pain to evaluate referred lumbosacral plexopathies and to assess local nerve entrapment or nerve damage from trauma such as meralgia paresthetica, surgery, or other disease states.

2. Injections—Differential block of the hip joint can be a valuable adjunct in differentiating the source of intra-articular hip joint pain. This procedure is best undertaken in the fluoroscopy suite, with arthrography used to confirm the location of the injection. The technique may be particularly useful in distinguishing intra-articular hip abnormalities from referred lumbosacral radiculopathy and possible soft-tissue conditions. Dye injection along the iliopsoas tendon

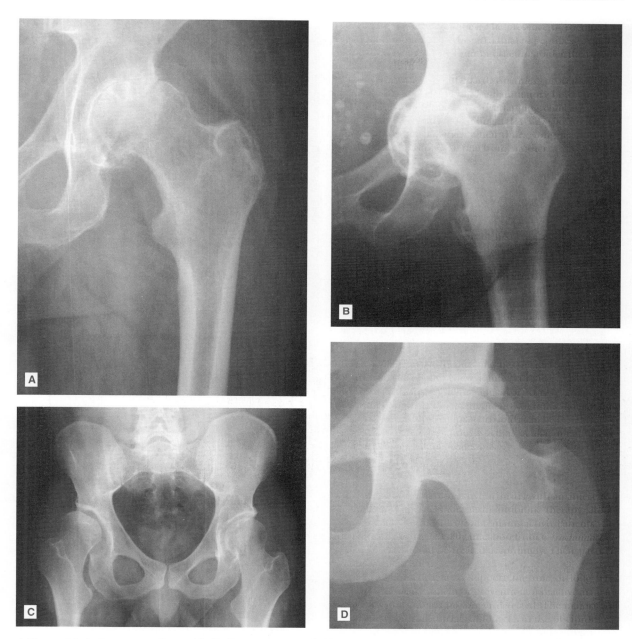

▲ **Figure 11–4.** Common radiographic findings. **A:** Osteoarthritis: asymmetric joint space narrowing, joint sclerosis, osteophytes, subchondral cysts. **B:** Rheumatoid arthritis: symmetric joint space narrowing, protrusio acetabuli. **C:** Dysplasia: acetabular uncovering, increased acetabular slope. **D:** Femoroacetabular impingement: peripheral osteophytes.

sheath under fluoroscopy sometimes reveals the snapping of the iliopsoas tendon over the pelvic brim and, when accompanied by lidocaine or glucocorticoid injection, may help prove that the tendon condition is the pain generator.

▶ Differential Diagnosis & Treatment

The age of the patient is critical in diagnosing the cause of hip pain (Figure 11–5).

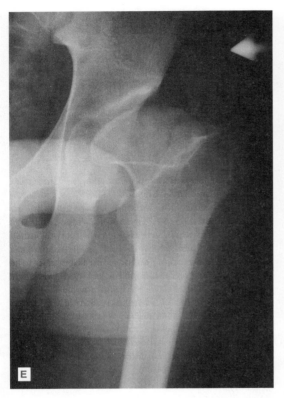

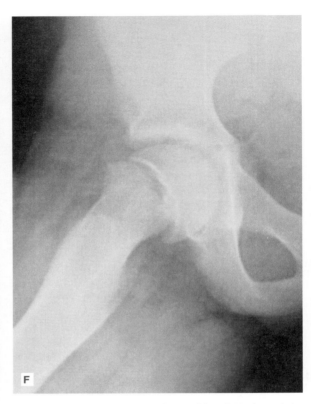

▲ **Figure 11–4.** (*Continued*) **E:** Legg-Calvé-Perthes disease: incongruent joint, misshapen femoral head. **F:** Slipped capital femoral epiphysis: fracture through epiphyseal growth plate.

A. Children

Neonates are susceptible to hematogenous infection and can present with an acute septic joint. Children 3- to 10-years-old who have hip pain most commonly have an infection, acute transient synovitis, or Legg-Calvé-Perthes disease. A normal radiograph and hip is most commonly associated with a self-limiting condition termed "acute transient synovitis of the hip." If the child has a fever or sign of infection, hip aspiration should be performed to rule out an acute septic joint. Legg-Calvé-Perthes disease is a condition that causes a portion of the femoral head to develop ischemic necrosis and collapse. Radiographs reveal evidence of Legg-Calvé-Perthes disease (Figure 11–4E). The hip then gradually remodels; however, later in life, early hip arthritis develops in up to 50% of patients. Children are treated symptomatically and may require realignment surgery if substantial collapse occurs.

The most common diagnosis in children 11- to 16-years-old who have hip pain is slipped capital femoral epiphysis. This condition represents a fracture through the growth plate or epiphysis of the femoral neck (Figure 11–4F). In 50% of

the cases, slipped capital femoral epiphysis occurs bilaterally and is treated surgically to prevent additional slippage, osteonecrosis, and chondrolysis. Fractures occur in different patterns in adolescent patients than in adults. Sudden muscular exertion can cause avulsion injuries and injury at the bony insertion of the tendons around the hip.

In addition, oncologic problems are different in children compared with adults. In children, primary osteosarcoma and Ewing sarcoma are typical, whereas in adult and elderly patients, metastatic disease is most common. Tumors seen on radiographs should be further evaluated with MRI scanning.

B. Adults

Stress fractures of the femoral neck may develop in young adults in response to an increase in exercise. Hip pain from several patterns of disease may develop in adults aged 40 years or older, gradually leading to early hip arthritis. The first pattern of disease is hip dysplasia, which occurs when the acetabulum does not develop correctly over the femoral head (Figure 11–4C). The severity of this process ranges from mild changes to full dislocation. In mild forms, hip

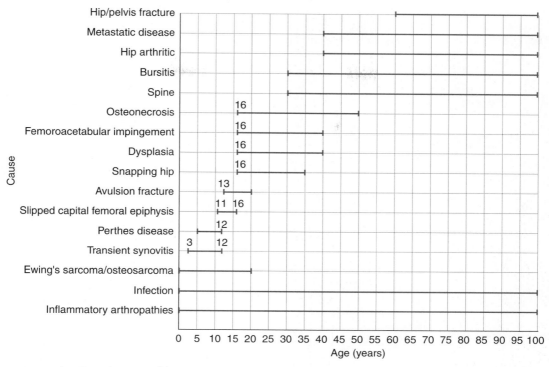

▲ Figure 11–5. Timeline of causes of hip pain.

dysplasia causes excessive anteversion of the acetabular cup, which leads to gradual wear on the labrum with labral tearing. Wear then begins to occur at the edge of the joint, causing early arthritis. It is possible to reorient the acetabulum surgically with a periacetabular osteotomy to prevent later hip arthritis.

The second condition that can lead to early arthritis and hip pain in the young adult is femoroacetabular impingement. There are two types of femoroacetabular impingement: cam impingement and pincer impingement. These types can occur concurrently. In **cam impingement,** the deformity is on the femoral side of the joint. The upper lateral portion of the femoral neck gradually impinges on the acetabulum, leading to labral tearing, osteophyte formation around the hip (Figure 11–4D), and ultimately, hip stiffness and arthritis. In **pincer impingement,** the deformity is on the acetabular side of the joint. The acetabulum is deeper than normal because of coxa profunda, protrusio acetabuli, or retroversion of the acetabulum, and the normal femur hits against the enlarged anterior rim of the acetabulum, which also leads to labral damage and subsequent arthritis. It is possible to treat impingement surgically by removing the impinging osteophytes and "reshaping" the femoral head or by removing the acetabular osteophytes and reattaching the torn labrum (see Table 11–3). In the case of acetabular

retroversion, a periacetabular osteotomy may be used to realign the acetabulum. Impingement surgery may be done open, and the use of arthroscopy and limited incision surgery is being explored. There are currently no long-term outcomes to indicate whether these procedures ultimately prevent total hip arthroplasty.

Osteonecrosis of the femoral head may develop in young adults. This condition can be associated with prednisone use, heavy alcohol use, deep sea diving, or coagulopathies. Osteonecrosis, which can develop in multiple joints (but especially the hips and knees), can cause subchondral bone in the femoral head to die. The cartilage above the necrotic bone collapses, and arthritis ensues (Figure 11–6). MRI scans are the most sensitive test for osteonecrosis and are abnormal before radiographic changes appear. In mild cases, bone grafting procedures may be successful, but in advanced cases, hip replacement surgery is required.

Transient osteoporosis of the hip is a rare condition most often seen in young women during pregnancy. Acute hip pain develops and the diagnosis is confirmed by MRI scan. Treatment involves restricted weight bearing and repeated MRI scans to make sure the bone density improves; otherwise, the patient may be at risk for fracture.

Middle-aged patients commonly have hip pain from osteoarthritis of the hip, trochanteric bursitis, or spinal

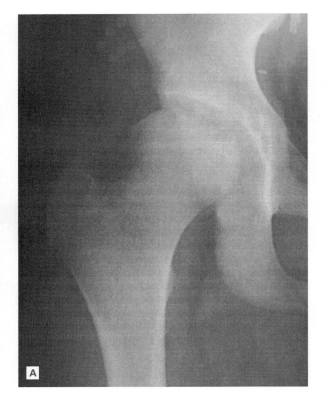

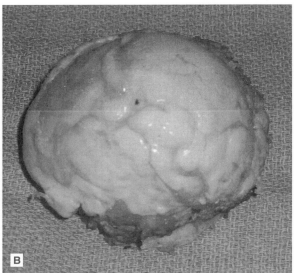

▲ **Figure 11–6.** Osteonecrosis. **A:** Radiographs reveal subchondral lucency and collapse of a segment of femoral head. **B:** At the time of hip arthroplasty, the collapsed bone has delaminated from the cartilage.

Table 11–2. Symptoms of common soft tissue pains around the hip.

Diagnosis	Symptoms
Iliopsoas bursitis	Deep anterior hip, groin pain with active flexion of the hip, possible audible or palpable snapping of the tendon
Ischial bursitis	Deep pain posteriorly over the ischial tuberosity; pain with sitting
Piriformis syndrome	Deep pain in the buttock region posteriorly
Posterosuperior iliac spine bursitis	Pain in the lateral lower back over the lateral aspect of the pelvic brim, often combined with trochanteric bursitis
Trochanteric bursitis	Lateral pain over the greater trochanter, often with sitting or laying on the side

causes. Osteoarthritis of the hip is generally unilateral, and the pain is worse with weight bearing and twisting motions of the hip (Figure 11–4A). Typically, the pain is in the groin and leads to gradual hip stiffness and limp. Trochanteric bursitis presents with lateral pain that is often worse at night when the patient lies on the affected side. Several other areas around the hip may develop soft-tissue pain (Table 11–2). Spinal problems present with radiculopathy or pain that starts in the lower back and radiates down the leg to the foot. Weakness or numbness may occur with nerve compression in the back.

Hip pain in elderly patients (>60 years old) typically comes from osteoarthritis, metastatic disease, trochanteric bursitis, spinal stenosis, or fracture. Radiographs that reveal lytic lesions of the femoral neck or hip in these patients typically are the result of metastatic disease, which requires a thorough work-up. Often, surgery is needed to strengthen or replace the bone. Elderly patients with osteoporosis are also at high risk for fracture of the femoral neck or the pelvis. Fracture should be ruled out in all elderly patients with acute hip pain because fractures in this population may occur with mild trauma, such as a fall, or with no precipitating event and an insidious onset (insufficiency fractures). Fractures causing hip pain are located in the proximal femur, the acetabulum, or the pelvis. If radiographs are normal, an MRI scan should be obtained.

C. All Ages

Infections in the hip joint may develop in patients of all ages. Immunosuppressed patients and those who use injection drugs are particularly vulnerable and often do not show systemic signs of infection. Joint infections cause unrelenting pain and fevers and should be diagnosed by hip aspiration.

Table 11–3. Interventions for common hip conditions.

Condition	Intervention
Avulsion fracture	Ice, NSAIDs, activity modification, surgery (rarely)
Dysplasia	NSAIDs, activity modification, surgery for realignment or hip arthroplasty
Femoroacetabular impingement	NSAIDs, activity modification, hip arthroscopy, surgery for hip reshaping or hip arthroplasty, activity modification
Hip fracture	Surgical fixation
Infection	Surgical drainage, intravenous antibiotic
Labral tear	NSAIDs, activity modification, intra-articular steroid injection, hip arthroscopy
Meralgia paresthetica	Relieve pressure on the lateral femoral cutaneous nerve, NSAIDs, surgical decompression
Pelvic fracture	Pain medications, ambulatory aid
Legg-Calvé-Perthes disease	Activity modification, possible surgery
Piriformis syndrome	NSAIDs, activity modification, muscle stretching
Slipped capital femoral epiphysis	Surgical fixation
Snapping syndromes	Muscle stretching, ice, NSAIDs, physiotherapy
Soft tissue injuries (eg, iliopsoas bursitis)	Muscle stretching, glucocorticoid injection, physiotherapy
Stress fracture	Activity modification, careful observation for the need for surgical stabilization
Transient osteoporosis of the hip	Activity modification, careful observation for the need for surgical stabilization
Trochanteric bursitis	Ice, NSAIDs, muscle stretching, glucocorticoid injection, physiotherapy

NSAIDs, nonsteroidal anti-inflammatory drugs.

Treatment should be intravenous antibiotics and surgical debridement of the hip (Table 11–3). Patients of all ages also are susceptible to a range of inflammatory arthritides, from juvenile rheumatoid arthritis in the young patient to rheumatoid arthritis, ankylosing spondylitis, or psoriatic arthritis in the adult patient. Inflammatory arthritis often is bilateral and generally affects both hips as well as other joints throughout the body (see Figure 11–4B).

Sierra RJ, Trousdale RT, Ganz R, Leunig M. Hip disease in the young, active patient: evaluation and nonarthroplasty surgical options. *J Am Acad Orthop Surg.* 2008;16:689. [PMID: 19056918]

Tibor LM, Sekiya JK. Differential diagnosis of pain around the hip joint. *Arthroscopy.* 2008;24:1407. [PMID: 19038713]

Williams BS, Cohen SP. Greater trochanteric pain syndrome: a review of anatomy, diagnosis and treatment. *Anesth Analg.* 2009;108:1662. [PMID: 19372352]

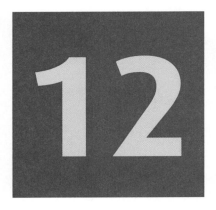

Approach to the Patient with Knee Pain

Andrew Gross, MD

C. Benjamin Ma, MD

Knee pain is a common problem, accounting for 1.9 million visits to primary care practitioners and 1 million visits to emergency departments annually. By following a systematic approach in evaluating knee pain (which includes obtaining a thorough and directed history), focusing on specific questions, using the physical examination (sometimes with the assistance of diagnostic studies), and understanding knee anatomy (Figure 12–1), physicians are able to make the correct diagnosis and formulate an appropriate therapeutic strategy.

OVERVIEW OF THE CLINICAL ASSESSMENT

The first step in the evaluation of knee pain is a thorough history that includes the core elements outlined in Table 12–1. While obtaining a history, the following key questions should be addressed:

- Has there been an acute injury?
- Is a joint effusion present?
- Is there evidence of osteoarthritis?
- Are there mechanical symptoms?
- Is there evidence of systemic disease?

The answers to these questions help the clinician narrow the differential diagnosis and formulate a strategy for a directed work-up of the knee pain.

The history should also determine whether the pain is localized to a specific region of the knee, which also can be a helpful guide to the cause of symptoms. The examiner should take into account the age and sex of the patient, both of which can influence the differential diagnosis. Finally, the clinician should bear in mind that pain can be referred to the knee from other sites, most notably the ipsilateral hip. Every patient with knee pain should have a careful examination of the hip.

► General Approach to the Physical Examination

The general physical examination has 5 major components: observation of stance and gait, range of motion, palpation, examination for a knee effusion, and stability tests. After completing these general examinations and considering the patient's history, the clinician can generate a differential diagnosis and focus the work-up accordingly (see specific injuries and conditions below).

A. Observation of Stance and Gait

Physical examination should start with observation of stance and gait. Can the patient bear weight on the affected leg? Is there a limp? Attention should be paid to medial or lateral translation of the knee upon heel strike. Angular (varus or valgus) deformities can identify bone and cartilage erosion with secondary stretching of the opposite collateral ligament. Varus alignment predisposes medial compartment arthritis. Following gait analysis, patients should be asked to perform a deep squat. Limitations in squatting may be related to patellofemoral or meniscal pathology.

B. Range of Motion

Active and passive range of motion of the knee should be recorded. Normal knee extension is 0 degrees; normal knee flexion ranges from 115 to 160 degrees. It is helpful to compare with the contralateral side.

C. Palpation

The skin overlying the anterior surface of the knee is typically cooler than the skin proximal and distal to the joint. The examiner can best detect a "warm" knee by using the dorsum of his or her hand to compare the temperature of the skin overlying the patella to the temperature of the skin "above and below" the knee (rather than comparing one knee to the other).

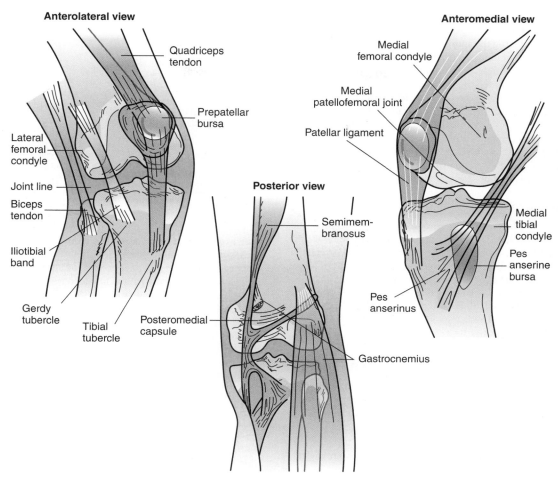

Anterolateral view
- Quadriceps tendon
- Prepatellar bursa
- Lateral femoral condyle
- Joint line
- Biceps tendon
- Iliotibial band
- Gerdy tubercle
- Tibial tubercle

Anteromedial view
- Medial femoral condyle
- Medial patellofemoral joint
- Patellar ligament
- Medial tibial condyle
- Pes anserine bursa
- Pes anserinus

Posterior view
- Semimembranosus
- Posteromedial capsule
- Gastrocnemius

▲ **Figure 12–1.** Functional anatomy of the knee.

Table 12–1. Knee pain: Core elements of the history.

Age and sex of the patient
Circumstances of the onset of pain
Exacerbating and alleviating factors
Presence of swelling and warmth
Loss of range of motion
Loss of function – inability to bear weight
Presence of mechanical symptoms (locking/catching, instability)
Duration of stiffness when arising in the morning or after inactivity
Localization of symptoms to specific regions of the knee (ie, anterior, posterior, medial, or lateral)
Involvement of other joints
Presence of systemic symptoms

Palpation should be gentle but thorough to help localize the knee pain. Palpation around the patella can identify facet tenderness or insertional tenderness of the patella tendon and quadriceps tendon. Palpable defects along the quadriceps or patella tendon can indicate tendon ruptures. Injury along the collateral ligaments can best be identified with pain elicited along their course and at their attachments. Palpation of the joint line is done both medially and laterally to elicit pain that can be caused by meniscal injury. Tenderness at the tibial tubercle can indicate Osgood-Schlatter disease or patella tendon tears. Osteochondritis dessicans of the knee can also be diagnosed with a positive Wilson sign (pain with internal rotation and extension of the knee that is relieved with external rotation).

D. Examination for a Knee Effusion

With the patient supine, an effusion is often visible as fullness in the suprapatella bursa and loss of the concavity that is usually present on the medial aspect of the knee. The effusion is confirmed by balloting the patella onto the femoral groove while compressing the suprapatellar and infrapatellar bursae. In the absence of fluid, the patella moves directly into the femoral condyles. With large effusions the patella will float above the condyles, so when the examiner quickly pushes down on the patella (balloting), a tap will be felt as the patella bumps into the condyles. Smaller effusions can be detected by compressing fluid from the medial compartment of the knee by applying a sweeping compression motion to the medial and superior aspects of the knee. If a small effusion is present, compression of the lateral aspect of the knee will generate a fluid wave that can be seen as a small bulge on the medial side.

E. Stability Tests

Stability or provocative tests should be performed when the patient is relaxed. These tests can reproduce symptoms and thus can be uncomfortable. The examiner should determine the direction of instability of the knee: anterior cruciate ligament (ACL)/posterior cruciate ligament (PCL) tears produce anterior/posterior instability; collateral ligament injuries lead to varus/valgus instability as well as internal/external rotational instability. These tests are described in detail under specific disease entities.

KNEE PAIN THAT FOLLOWS ACUTE INJURY

 ESSENTIAL FEATURES

▶ Mechanism of injury often points to the diagnosis.
▶ "Popping sound" at the time of injury suggests an ACL injury.
▶ Plain radiographs may be indicated to rule out fracture.
▶ Instability suggests ligament injuries.
▶ Locking or catching suggests a meniscal tear.

▶ General Considerations

Acute injuries can lead to fractures, patella dislocation, and internal derangements of the knee, including tears of the ligaments and meniscal cartilage (Table 12–2). Injuries also can cause acute traumatic bursitis as well as tendon strains and tears.

▶ Clinical Findings

A. History

The mechanism of injury is extremely important in the diagnosis of knee injuries (Table 12–3). The injury can be acute or chronic. Most patients can recall the specific knee position during injury and the stresses incurred. Knee injuries can

Table 12–2. Essential features of acute knee injuries.

	Injury Mechanism	Joint Swelling	Characteristics
ACL/PCL tears	Acute injury/ trauma	Immediate	Instability
Meniscus	Deep squat or twisting	Delay (first 24 hour)	Pain with twisting
Patella dislocation	Trauma or twisting	Immediate	Pain with palpation of medial facet, lateral femoral condyle
Fractures	Trauma	Immediate	Unable to bear weight

ACL, anterior cruciate ligament; PCL, posterior cruciate ligament.

occur from contact forces as well as from falls and twisting injuries not involving contact. An audible 'pop' at the time of injury is characteristic of injury to the ACL. It is important to know whether the patient is able to walk following the injury, and whether the injury affects the range of motion of the knee. This information enables the clinician to determine the severity of the injury and the likelihood of intra-articular fractures. Injuries that prevent weight-bearing typically signify a fracture or other severe knee injury.

B. Physical Examination

The patient should be in the supine position on a comfortable examination table. Since the injured knee may be

Table 12–3. Mechanisms of injuries.

Scenario	Concern
Fall from a height	Fracture
Twisting injury with foot planted	ACL with or without meniscal tear
Acute pain with deep flexion or twisting	meniscal tear
Lateral (valgus) blow to the knee	MCL injury
Medial blow (varus) blow	LCL injury
Anterior blow to the knee (dashboard injury)	PCL tear
Misstep with inability to straighten knee	Patella or quadriceps tendon rupture
Acute anterior pain and swelling with twisting motion	Patella dislocation
Gradual onset of discomfort and startup pain	Osteoarthritis or degenerative condition

ACL, anterior cruciate ligament; LCL, lateral collateral ligament; MCL, medial collateral ligament; PCL, posterior cruciate ligament.

swollen or locked and cannot be fully extended, a pillow can be placed behind the knee to relax it; another pillow can be placed behind the uninjured knee so that both knees can be inspected at the same angle. The uninjured limb should be examined first. Because there is little variation between right and left knees, the uninjured knee can serve as a good indicator for joint motion and laxity prior to injury.

After examining the uninjured knee, the injured knee should first be inspected for its skin integrity and any areas of ecchymosis. Loss of both active and passive range of motion can signify a chronic problem with contractures or a mechanical block, whereas loss of only active motion can signify pain or weakness. Location of pain should be noted during range of motion. For example, displaced meniscus tears can be painful during range of motion and can clue clinicians to the presence of medial or lateral injuries.

The presence and location of swelling is helpful in the evaluation of the acutely injured knee. The majority of acute knee swelling is secondary to hemarthrosis following intra-articular ligament tears, such as ACL tear and patella dislocation. An osteochondral fracture or peripheral tear of the meniscus can also produce a hemarthrosis. The swelling may take longer to occur if ice is applied to the knee immediately following injury. Immediate, brisk swelling should make the examiner suspicious of osteochondral fractures or ACL tears. When the effusion is drained, the presence of fat droplets signifies osteochondral fractures or nondisplaced intra-articular fractures. Swelling that occurs over the next 24 hours may represent meniscus tears or unstable cartilage injuries.

C. Imaging Studies

Patients who have difficulty with immediate weight-bearing should have orthogonal (anteroposterior and lateral) radiographs to rule out fractures. The Ottawa Knee Rules outline indications for obtaining radiographs to rule out fracture (Table 12–4). The Ottawa Knee Rules consist of 5 criteria; the absence of all 5 criteria rules out fracture with a sensitivity that approaches 100%.

Table 12–4. Ottawa Knee Rules: Indications for obtaining radiographs.

Patient is 55 years or older
Isolated tenderness of the patella (no bone tenderness of the knee other than at the patella
Tenderness of the head of fibula
Inability to flex the knee to 90 degrees
Unable to weight bear for 4 steps both immediately and at the emergency department
Patients with at least 1 positive criteria are considered to be at risk for knee fracture and should have a radiograph. Studies indicate the sensitivity of plain radiographs for fractures is 85-100%. Patients with normal radiographs but persistent symptoms should undergo follow-up imaging 1-2 weeks later.

MRI can be helpful in the evaluation of soft tissue injuries, such as ligament or meniscus injuries. MRI is 75–85% sensitive for detecting meniscal, ligamentous, or cartilage damage. The specificity, however, is lower because of frequent false-positives, particularly in older individuals. Abnormal MRI findings are common, even in asymptomatic knees. Therefore, MRI should be used to confirm a diagnosis rather than as the sole basis for a diagnosis.

▶ Treatment

Protected weight-bearing and brace for stabilization can be helpful following acute knee injuries and prior to definitive diagnosis and treatment. Fractures or severe ligament injuries should be referred to the specialists.

Bachmann LM, Haberzeth S, Steurer J, ter Riet G. The accuracy of the Ottawa knee rule to rule out knee fractures: a systematic review. *Ann Intern Med*. 2004;140:121. [PMID: 14734335]
Behairy NH, Dorgham MA, Khaled SA. Accuracy of routine magnetic resonance imaging in meniscal and ligamentous injuries of the knee: comparison with arthroscopy. *Int Orthop*. 2009;33:961. [PMID: 18506445]

1. Injuries to Collateral Ligaments

▶ Clinical Findings

A. History

Most patients with injuries to collateral ligaments describe injuries on the side of the knee. A lateral blow to the knee leads to injury of the medial collateral ligament (MCL), whereas a medial blow leads to injury of the lateral collateral ligament (LCL).

B. Physical Examination

When testing the MCL, the patient is asked to lie in a supine position with the hip abducted and the knee gently hanging off the edge of the examination table and flexed at 30 degrees. A valgus stress is applied through the examiner's left hand, which supports the ankle. The examination is repeated at full extension. When examining the LCL, an adduction or varus stress is applied. The test is performed similar to the valgus stress test, only with a varus directed force and medial placement of the hand to counteract the stress. The test is performed at full extension and at 30 degrees of flexion.

C. Imaging Studies

MRI is rarely indicated for isolated MCL tears. It is uncommon to have meniscus injuries with MCL tears. However, the ACL can be injured with MCL tears, and these complex injuries should be evaluated by MRI. LCL injuries should necessitate MRI evaluation to determine the significance of injuries. MRI has 80% sensitivity and 90% specificity in the evaluation of acute collateral ligament injuries.

▶ Treatment

MCL injuries are commonly treated with immobilization and bracing. The majority of these injuries heal without the need for surgical stabilization. Grade III (more than 1 cm opening) injuries are treated with protected weight-bearing. LCL or lateral ligament complex injuries do not respond well to nonsurgical treatment and, when recognized, should be urgently referred to an orthopedic surgeon.

LaPrade RF, Gilbert TJ, Bollom TS, Wentorf F, Chaljub G. The magnetic resonance imaging appearance of individual structures of the posterolateral knee. A prospective study of normal knees and knees with surgically verified grade III injuries. *Am J Sports Med.* 2000;28:191. [PMID: 10750995]

2. Injuries to the Anterior Cruciate Ligament

▶ Clinical Findings

A. History

Typically, the history reveals a twisting injury while the foot is planted. A tear of the ACL can occur with either contact or non-contact mechanisms of injury. Patients commonly describe a 'pop' sound.

B. Physical Examination

The **Lachman** or **Ritchey test** is a highly sensitive and specific method for assessing an ACL sprain or tear in the acute setting (Figure 12–2). It consists of an anteriorly directed

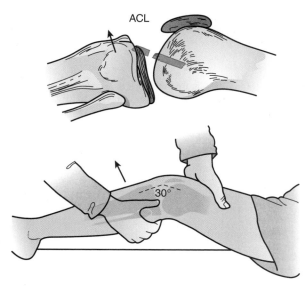

▲ **Figure 12–2.** The Lachman test for tear of the anterior cruciate ligament (ACL). The test is performed at 30 degrees of flexion; the extremity does not have to be lifted or the foot stabilized.

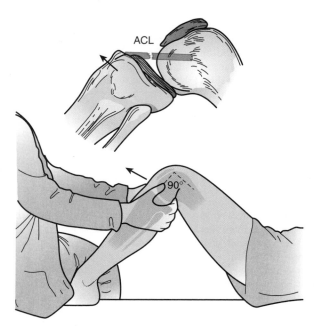

▲ **Figure 12–3.** The anterior drawer test for instability of anterior cruciate ligament (ACL). Flex the knee to 90 degrees and stabilize the foot. Note the forward shift of the tibia.

force with the knee at 30 degrees of flexion; an increase in anterior translation of the tibia compared with the contralateral side constitutes a positive test and signifies injury to the ACL. The anterior drawer test is performed with the knee flexed at 90 degrees and the hip at 45 degrees (Figure 12–3). Difficulty with having the patient relax during the anteriorly directed force can limit the usefulness of this test. The pivot shift test is the most specific test for ACL tear but has low sensitivity for the awake patient. The sensitivity of the test is highly dependent on the examiner's skill and the patient's relaxation.

C. Imaging Studies

MRI is commonly needed to confirm the diagnosis. MRI of the ACL is 93% sensitive and nearly 100% specific. MRI also can identify associated injuries, such as meniscus tear and cartilage injuries, which can affect management.

▶ Treatment

The treatment of ACL tears varies on the basis of the needs and activity level of the patient. These injuries are best managed by consultation of an orthopedic surgeon or sports medicine clinician. The patient should be evaluated within 2–3 weeks following the acute injury.

Benjaminse A, Gokeler A, van der Schans CP. Clinical diagnosis of an anterior cruciate ligament rupture: a meta-analysis. *J Orthop Sports Phys Ther.* 2006;36:267. [PMID: 16715828]

3. Injuries to the Posterior Cruciate Ligament

▶ Clinical Findings

A. History

Injuries to the PCL usually signify significant knee trauma; typically, a significant blow to the anterior portion of the tibia pushes the tibia posteriorly, thereby rupturing the large ligament. A dashboard injury or an injury that occurs when the knee is flexed and the foot is plantarflexed are typical. Associated neurovascular injuries are common and must be ruled out. PCL injuries often occur in combination with other injuries to the knee, such as ACL tears or posterolateral corner injuries.

B. Physical Examination

The most accurate test to identify a PCL injury is the posterior drawer test. This is done in the exact opposite manner as the anterior drawer test: the examiner determines the amount of excess posterior translation when a force is applied to the tibia in a posterior direction with the knee at 90 degrees of flexion. Sometimes the posterior drawer test is difficult to perform in the acute setting because the patient is unable to flex the swollen knee to 90 degrees.

C. Imaging Studies

Plain radiographs should be obtained to rule out any fractures that may occur with this significant injury. The sensitivity and specificity for MRI for the diagnosis of acute PCL tears approach 90%; MRI also is needed to evaluate possible associated injuries.

▶ Treatment

An urgent referral to an orthopaedic surgeon is needed to rule out other associated injuries. A significant percentage of patients with PCL injuries have injuries to vascular structures, peripheral nerves, other ligaments, and soft tissues.

Fanelli GC, Orcutt DR, Edson CJ. The multiple-ligament injured knee: evaluation, treatment and results. *Arthroscopy.* 2005;21:471. [PMID: 15800529]

4. Meniscal Injuries

▶ Clinical Findings

A. History

Traumatic lesions of the menisci occur most commonly when there is rotation on the flexed knee as it is moving toward a more extended position. Tears in the medial meniscus usually occur in its posterior horn, possibly because the posterior horn is less mobile and is directly loaded when the knee is flexed. In contrast, tears in the lateral meniscus, which is more mobile and is C-shaped, are usually radial. Meniscal injuries are commonly associated with ACL injures. In an acute ACL injury, the lateral meniscus is most commonly torn because the lateral tibial plateau subluxes anteriorly on the lateral femoral condyle.

Patients with meniscal tears often complain of a locking and clicking sensation. With larger tears, the knee may lock during range of motion, requiring the patient to stop and twist the knee in order to unlock the displaced meniscus and regain full motion. Small tears of the meniscus produce clicking or catching sensation but not true locking. Meniscal injuries are usually associated with pain and swelling of the knee. Swelling develops over the course of the first day of the injury in contrast to the first 1–2 hours following an ACL tear. Patients may complain of recurrent or chronic swelling in the knee following a twisting injury.

B. Physical Examination

The most important physical finding in patients is localized tenderness along the joint line, with sensitivity and specificity for meniscal tear of 63% and 77%, respectively. The McMurray and the squat tests for meniscal injuries are provocative maneuvers that 'trap' the meniscus and generate symptoms. The **McMurray test** is performed with the patient lying supine with the hip and knee flexed to about 90 degrees. With one hand on the knee to apply compression, the examiner uses the other hand to hold the foot and then to maneuver it from external rotation to internal rotation. If positive, this maneuver entraps the torn meniscus, producing a 'pop' or 'click' that can be felt by the fingers. The McMurray test is 70% sensitive and 71% specific for meniscal tear. In the **squat test,** the examiner asks the patient to perform a series of full squats, first with legs neutral, then with legs internally rotated, and finally with legs externally rotated. Pain with deep squat indicates the presence of a meniscal tear. If there is more pain with the leg externally rotated, the medial meniscus is most likely injured; conversely an injured lateral meniscus produces more discomfort when the leg is internally rotated.

C. Imaging Studies

MRI is a very sensitive tool to diagnose meniscal tears. Its specificity is limited due to the occurrence of meniscal tears in asymptomatic individuals. The prevalence of meniscus tears ranges from 19% among women age 50–59 years to 56% among men aged 70–90 years. Practitioners should use MRI to confirm, not to establish, the diagnosis of meniscal tear.

▶ Treatment

Acute symptomatic meniscal injuries are commonly treated surgically to repair or remove the torn meniscus. Chronic or degenerative conditions are usually managed with activity modification and nonsurgical treatment. Surgical debridement can be performed for chronic symptomatic meniscus injuries that did not respond well to nonsurgical treatments.

Englund M, Guermazi A, Gale D, et al. Incidental meniscal findings on knee MRI in middle-aged and elderly persons. *N Engl J Med.* 2008;359:1108. [PMID: 18784100]

Hegedus EJ, Cook C, Hasselblad V, Goode A, McCrory DC. Physical examination tests for assessing a torn meniscus in the knee: a systematic review with meta-analysis. *J Orthop Sports Phys Ther.* 2007;37:541. [PMID: 17939613]

5. Injuries to the Quadriceps Tendon

▶ Clinical Findings

A. History

Ruptures of the quadriceps tendon are more common at the latter part of life, with a peak incidence from the fifth to seventh decades of life. In addition to age, predisposing factors include systemic conditions, such as diabetes and systemic lupus erythematosus. The rupture typically occurs during eccentric contraction of the knee during a fall, missed step, or twisting injury. The patient usually experiences intense pain over the anterior part of the knee and often is unable to walk. Even when able to ambulate, the patient tends to hold the affected leg straight and to widely circumduct the leg during the swing phase of gait. There is a sensation of instability due to the lack of quadriceps pull.

B. Physical Examination

Common findings are a palpable defect above the patella and a hemarthrosis of the knee. With a complete rupture, the patient is usually unable to extend the knee from a supine position. With varying degrees of rupture, the patients may be able to extend their knee while lying supine but have difficulty when their knee is held in flexion. Quadriceps tendon rupture in the elderly can be subtle; one series reported that up to 30% of the cases were missed initially.

C. Imaging Studies

Radiographs (bilateral flexion weight-bearing standing views and lateral view of the knee) can help evaluate the location of the patella. Quadriceps tendon tear usually leads to patella baja (patella sitting abnormally low). MRI is rarely needed to establish the diagnosis but can be helpful to evaluate partial quadriceps ruptures.

▶ Treatment

Almost all complete quadriceps tendon rupture necessitate surgical repair. Nonsurgical management of quadriceps tendon injuries is reserved only for partial injuries or sedentary individuals.

6. Ruptures of the Patella Tendon

▶ Clinical Findings

A. History

Ruptures of the patella tendon usually occur during violent jumping activities or eccentric contraction. They are less common than ruptures of the quadriceps tendon and usually occur in patients under the age of 40, most often in the setting of preexisting patella tendinitis. Local glucocorticoid injections for patella tendonitis, systemic glucocorticoid use, endocrine abnormalities, and systemic lupus erythematosus predispose to rupture of the patella tendon. Patients usually complain of severe pain and are unable to ambulate.

B. Physical Examination

There is a palpable defect inferior to the patella, which usually has migrated superiorly. Virtually all patients are unable to extend the affected knee.

C. Imaging Studies

Radiographs reveal patella alta (patella sitting abnormally high). MRI is rarely needed to establish the diagnosis but can be helpful to evaluate partial quadriceps ruptures.

▶ Treatment

Ruptures of the patella tendon require urgent repair.

KNEE EFFUSION

ESSENTIAL FEATURES

- ▶ Restricted range of motion and pain with ambulation.
- ▶ An acutely swollen knee with a history of acute injury suggests mechanical derangement, particularly ACL tear.
- ▶ An acutely swollen knee in the absence of acute injury raises the concern of septic arthritis and demands immediate evaluation.
- ▶ Joint aspiration with synovial fluid analysis is the most helpful test.

▶ General Considerations

Small, asymptomatic effusions commonly occur in healthy individuals. Larger joint effusions, however, signal the presence of intra-articular pathology, the most serious of which is septic arthritis. A variety of pathologic processes cause knee effusions (Table 12–5), and these are typically grouped by fluid characteristics (see Chapter 2).

Table 12–5. Differential diagnosis for an acutely swollen knee.

Infection
Bacterial
Mycobacterial
Spirochete (Lyme, syphilis)
Viral
Crystal (gout and pseudogout)
Spondyloarthritis
Reactive arthritis
Inflammatory bowel disease
Hemarthrosis
Acute injury
Osteoarthritis
Osteonecrosis

► Clinical Findings

A. History

Patients with joint effusions often complain of swelling and stiffness, as well as loss of knee range of motion. Particularly large effusions can manifest as a Baker cyst in the popliteal fossa and cause posterior knee pain. Occasionally, very large effusions rupture the synovial capsule, resulting in dependant collection of fluid in the lower leg. Knee involvement is common in rheumatoid arthritis and other systemic diseases, usually in association with inflammation in multiple joints. Isolated knee involvement can be a manifestation of spondyloarthritis (especially reactive arthritis), late Lyme disease, osteoarthritis and, uncommonly, rheumatoid arthritis. Pseudogout, as well as gout, can cause repeated episodes of acute knee swelling. Septic arthritis of the knee usually results from hematogenous spread and rarely is caused by local penetrating injury. Patients with septic arthritis of the knee are often, but not always, febrile. Reactive arthritis and crystal-induced arthritis also can cause high fever and inflammatory knee effusions.

B. Analysis of Synovial Fluid

Arthrocentesis and subsequent synovial fluid analysis are indicated for all cases of unexplained knee effusion. The aspirated fluid should be sent for cell counts, Gram stain, cultures, and crystal analysis. Hemarthrosis is commonly caused by joint trauma, as described above; fat droplets (detected by polarized microscopy) also indicate articular fracture. Hemophilia and other clotting disorders can cause hemarthrosis in the absence of trauma. The most common cause of noninflammatory effusions of the knee (synovial fluid white blood cell count <2000 cells/mcL) is osteoarthritis; other causes include osteonecrosis, Charcot arthropathy, sarcoidosis, amyloidosis, hypothyroidism, and acromegaly. Inflammatory arthritis (synovial fluid white blood cell

>2000 cells/mcL) can be caused by infection, autoimmune disease, and crystal-induced arthritis. Aspiration of dark brown serosanguinous fluid should raise the possibility of pigmented villonodular synovitis.

C. Imaging Studies

Moderate to large knee effusions are apparent on radiographs. Acute nontraumatic arthritis rarely causes additional radiographic abnormalities. In chronic conditions, radiographs can provide valuable information regarding the etiology and severity of the arthritis. Persistent inflammatory arthritis leads to symmetric joint space narrowing as well as marginal erosions and periarticular osteopenia, whereas osteoarthritis (discussed below) causes asymmetric joint space narrowing, typically of the medial compartment. Patients with pseudogout of the knee frequently have radiographic evidence of chondrocalcinosis. Osteonecrosis causes a radiolucent lesion and flattening of the femoral condyle.

Margaretten ME, Kohlwes J, Moore D, Bent S. Does this adult patient have septic arthritis? *JAMA.* 2007;297:1478. [PMID: 17405973]

Thomsen TW, Shen S, Shaffer RW, Setnik GS. Videos in Clinical Medicine. Arthrocentesis of the knee. *N Engl J Med.* 2006;354:e19. [PMID: 16687707]

OSTEOARTHRITIS OF THE KNEE

 ESSENTIAL FEATURES

- ► Pain that increases with activity and is relieved with rest.
- ► Functional limitation.
- ► Morning stiffness lasting less than 30 minutes.
- ► Identification of osteophytes on plain radiographs is specific for the diagnosis but insensitive, especially in early disease.

► General Considerations

Osteoarthritis should be considered as a cause of knee pain in all patients over the age of 40. Osteoarthritis typically presents as long-standing discomfort, but patients can have "flares" of acute pain, often precipitated by minor injury or overuse. Clinical history alone is sensitive for detecting osteoarthritis, but the sensitivity increases to 95% when paired with the physical examination. A differential diagnosis for osteoarthritis is listed in Table 12–6.

Table 12–6. Differential diagnosis of osteoarthritis of the knee.

Inflammatory arthritis
Internal derangement, meniscal tear
Osteonecrosis
Pigmented villonodular synovitis

▶ Clinical Findings

A. History

Typical symptoms of osteoarthritis are pain with use that limits certain activities. Patients frequently describe transient stiffness in the morning or with periods of inactivity such as sitting at a desk; the stiffness almost always resolves in less than 30 minutes and typically after just a few minutes. The discomfort usually worsens toward the end of the day and is relieved with rest. As osteoarthritis advances, pain may become more persistent and problematic, causing more significant functional limitations, persistent pain at rest, and disturbances in sleep. Risk factors for knee osteoarthritis include female gender, higher body mass index, previous knee injury, malalignment, joint laxity, and family history.

B. Physical Examination

The knee is typically cool, but osteoarthritis occasionally causes mild warmth and a small or moderate effusion. Range of motion typically is limited and often provokes pain. Crepitus—a grating sensation with motion—is common. The presence of bony enlargement is highly suggestive of osteoarthritis. Joint line tenderness, particularly over the medial aspect of the knee, is a nonspecific but common finding in osteoarthritis. In some individuals, fixed flexion or varus (rarely valgus) deformity develops.

Clinical criteria for the diagnosis of osteoarthritis, established by the American College of Rheumatology, include age > 50 years, stiffness < 30 minutes, crepitus, bony tenderness, bony enlargement, and the lack of warmth. The presence of 3 of these 6 criteria in the patient with chronic knee pain is 95% sensitive and 69% specific for the diagnosis of osteoarthritis.

C. Imaging Studies

The plain radiograph is an adjunct to the diagnosis. Early manifestations of osteoarthritis occur in the absence of radiographic abnormalities, and radiographic abnormalities are only weakly related to symptoms. Classic features of osteoarthritis include osteophytes, subchondral bony sclerosis, and joint space narrowing and subchondral cysts (Figure 12–4). Osteophytes are often seen in early disease, but joint space narrowing generally is restricted to advanced disease and thus is insensitive for the detection of early osteoarthritis. Because

clinical features of osteoarthritis are highly sensitive for the diagnosis, and because early osteoarthritis is frequently not associated with any radiographic findings, plain radiographs are not necessary for routine confirmation of the clinical diagnosis of osteoarthritis.

Felson DT. Clinical practice. Osteoarthritis of the knee. *N Engl J Med.* 2006;354:841. [PMID: 16495396]

Mont MA, Baumgarten KM, Rifai A, et al. Atraumatic osteonecrosis of the knee. *J Bone Joint Surg Am.* 2000;82:1279. [PMID: 11005519]

Ofluoglu O. Pigmented villonodular synovitis. *Orthop Clin North Am.* 2006;37:23. [PMID: 16311109]

Zhang W, Doherty M, Peat G, et al. EULAR evidence-based recommendations for the diagnosis of knee osteoarthritis. *Ann Rheum Dis.* 2010;69:483. [PMID: 19762361]

MECHANICAL KNEE SYMPTOMS & NO HISTORY OF ACUTE INJURY

 ESSENTIAL FEATURES

▶ Locking or catching symptoms suggest meniscal tear.

▶ Instability symptoms suggest ligamentous laxity or tear.

▶ Knee buckling is a nonspecific symptom that is associated with knee pain and quadriceps weakness.

▶ Asymptomatic meniscal tears are common findings on MRI in middle-aged and elderly patients.

▶ Meniscal tears are associated with knee osteoarthritis.

▶ General Considerations

The middle-aged patient with chronic knee pain in the absence of any recalled trauma is a common and vexing problem. The challenge for the practitioner is to determine whether the source of the pain is from internal derangement (particularly a large meniscal tear that is best managed surgically) or whether the problem is more degenerative in nature and better managed with conservative therapy.

▶ Clinical Findings

A. History

"Mechanical" symptoms can signify the presence of meniscal tears or ligamentous sprain. A locking or catching sensation with knee extension and flexion raises the possibility of a meniscal tear but is a somewhat nonspecific symptom because it can also be caused by loose bodies in the knee. Instability is usually episodic and unpredictable. When given the history of instability, the practitioner should note the severity of these episodes and the presence

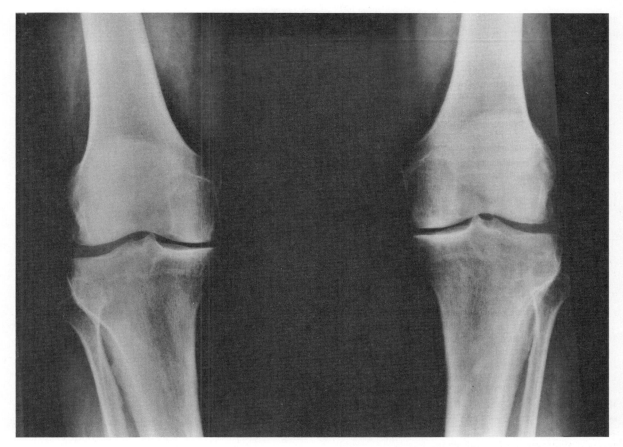

▲ **Figure 12–4.** Osteoarthritis of the knees. This weight-bearing radiograph reveals joint-space narrowing and sclerosis of both medial compartments and osteophytes of the tibial spines.

of swelling after an episode, which can point to the presence of a ligamentous tear. A third mechanical symptom is that of buckling or "giving way." This is a less specific but extremely common complaint that typically occurs during weight bearing, especially when weight loading is increased such as climbing stairs. The "giving way" is likely to occur as a reflex to pain (from osteoarthritis or meniscus injuries) or from insufficient quadriceps muscle strength to support the knee. Buckling can also be caused by ligamentous tears, but this is relatively uncommon in the absence of trauma. Complaints of buckling should be addressed by the practitioner, since buckling is associated with falls, potentially causing fracture.

B. Physical Examination

The practitioner should perform a complete knee examination, but special attention should be focused to specific structures based on the nature of the patient's complaint. When

meniscal tear is suspected, patients can be asked to perform deep knee bends to elicit pain. Tenderness elicited by joint line palpation can also suggest meniscal pathology, but both of these tests are nonspecific in the chronic setting (see acute injuries section). The McMurray test and eliciting pain with passive hyperextension have reasonable specificity for meniscal tears but limited sensitivity. Tests for ligamentous instability should be carefully performed for patients with episodes of instability (see acute injuries section). Finally, patients should be assessed for signs of osteoarthritis, including crepitus and bony enlargement, because degenerative disease increases the likelihood of meniscal tears as well as buckling symptoms secondary to pain.

C. Imaging Studies

The plain radiograph can be useful to confirm the presence osteoarthritis but is less helpful to identify the cause of locking symptoms or instability. Patients with abnormal physical examination findings, or complaints highly suggestive of meniscal or ligamentous pathology in the absence of arthritis, can be referred for MRI evaluation of the knee structures.

Treatment

In the middle age patient, knee pain is very common, but the management is far less straight-forward than in the young athlete who sustains an acute injury. Meniscal tears are common findings on knee MRI in patients with knee pain, and the incidence of tears increases with the age of the population studied. The incidence of meniscal tears is even higher in patients who have radiographic evidence of osteoarthritis. However, many meniscal tears detected by MRI are asymptomatic. This emphasizes 2 important concepts: (1) There is a complex but strong relationship between degenerative arthritis and meniscal damage, with evidence suggesting that the presence of each drives the development of the other and (2) the presence of meniscal tears detected on MRI are weakly associated with knee pain in middle age and elderly patients. Consequently, management issues are complex. In the young athlete with good healing potential, large tears can be successfully repaired surgically. In the middle-aged patient, total meniscectomy was once used, but this has fallen out of favor because it has been shown to accelerate the development of osteoarthritis. Even arthroscopy with partial meniscectomy has been shown to be no better than exercise for the treatment of knee pain in patients with meniscal tear and minimal or no evidence of knee osteoarthritis on radiographs. Consequently, in the absence of trauma, expert opinion recommends monitoring middle-aged patients with knee pain. In general, practitioners should direct patients toward exercise to treat symptoms. However, those patients with distinct symptoms of an unstable meniscal tear—particularly locking or recurrent effusion—should be referred to an orthopedic surgeon for consideration of surgical intervention.

Englund M, Guermazi A, Gale D, et al. Incidental meniscal findings on knee MRI in middle-aged and elderly persons. *N Engl J Med.* 2008;359:1108. [PMID: 18784100]

Englund M, Guermazi A, Lohmander LS. The meniscus in knee osteoarthritis. *Rheum Dis Clin North Am.* 2009;35:579. [PMID: 19931804]

Felson DT, Niu J, McClennan C, et al. Knee buckling: prevalence, risk factors, and associated limitations in function. *Ann Intern Med.* 2007;147:534. [PMID: 17938391]

Herrlin S, Hållander M, Wange P, Weidenhielm L, Werner S. Arthroscopic or conservative treatment of degenerative medial meniscal tears: a prospective randomised trial. *Knee Surg Sports Traumatol Arthrosc.* 2007;15:393. [PMID: 17216272]

Lowery DJ, Farley TD, Wing DW, Sterett WI, Steadman JR. A clinical composite score accurately detects meniscal pathology. *Arthroscopy.* 2006;22:1174. [PMID: 17084293]

KNEE PAIN WITH EVIDENCE OF SYSTEMIC DISEASE

Knee pain can be a manifestation of systemic diseases, such as rheumatoid arthritis and psoriatic arthritis. In general, these are polyarticular diseases with obvious clinical signs of involvement of multiple joints. Occasionally, however, monoarticular knee involvement is the initial manifestation of a spondyloarthritis or rheumatoid arthritis, as well as of chronic infections such as Lyme disease, Whipple disease, mycobacteria infection, and brucellosis.

Prolonged morning stiffness (typically > 30 minutes), elevated serum inflammatory markers (erythrocyte sedimentation rate and C-reactive protein), and inflammatory synovial fluid point to the presence of an underlying autoimmune disease or chronic infection as the cause of knee pain. Radiographic findings of marginal erosions or narrowing of both the medial and lateral tibial-femoral compartments can point to the presence of inflammatory arthritis but require months or years to develop. In addition, a complete review of systems should be carefully evaluated to determine if extra-articular manifestations of disease are present. Particular attention should be given to ophthalmologic, dermatologic, gastrointestinal, and genitourinary complaints because each of these can herald the presence of systemic disease.

PROBLEMS BY LOCATION OF PAIN WITHIN THE KNEE

Patients often describe pain localized to specific regions of the knee. While this is not always helpful to identify the etiology of the pain, practitioners should be aware of regional knee pain problems.

1. Anterior Knee Pain

 ESSENTIAL FEATURES

▶ Pain underneath the patella.
▶ Pain across the patella tendon or quadriceps insertion.
▶ Swelling in the anterior aspect of the knee.
▶ Patella feels unstable.

General Considerations

Anterior knee pain is a common complaint with a variety of causes (Table 12–7). Several factors are responsible for normal patellofemoral mechanics. The quadriceps tendon guides tracking of the patella. Of the four muscles, the vastus medialis obliquus is the primary stabilizer of the patella against the lateral pull of the vastus lateralis. Other factors that can affect normal patellofemoral mechanics include the shape of the patella, the shape of the trochlea groove, the shape of the

Table 12–7. Causes of anterior knee pain.

Problem	Location
Patellofemoral pain syndrome (runner's knee)	Pain underneath patella and along extensor mechanism Usually related to change in activity level
Patella instability	Pain over the medial facet of patella Apprehension on examination
Quadriceps tendinitis	Pain at the proximal pole of the patella
Patella tendinitis	Pain at the distal pole of the patella
Osgood-Schlatter disease	Seen in adolescents Pain and swelling over tibial tubercle
Anterior horn meniscus tear	Uncommon injury Can be present in runners or gymnasts Pain along the anterior joint line
Patellofemoral osteoarthritis	Pain underneath patella Difficulty with stairs, more with descents Patellofemoral crepitus

Table 12–8. Prevalent causes of anterior knee pain by age.

Age	Diagnosis	Clinical Characteristics
Skeletal immature	Osgood-Schlatter disease	Pain over tibial tubercle
16–40	Patellofemoral syndrome	Pain underneath patella
20–40	Patella tendinitis/ruptures	Pain over distal pole For rupture, difficulty with active leg extension, palpable defect between patella and tibial tubercle
50–70	Quadriceps tendinitis and ruptures	Pain over proximal pole For ruptures, difficulty with active leg extension, palpable defect between patella and quadriceps tendon
50–80	Osteoarthritis	Start up pain Pain under patella

femoral condyles, the length of the patella tendon, the patellofemoral articulating cartilage as well as tension of the extensor mechanism. Disruption or abnormality in any facet of this complex joint can lead to dysfunction and subsequent pain.

▶ Clinical Findings

A. History

When eliciting a history from a patient with anterior knee pain, it is important to attempt to distinguish whether the pain is derived from the anterior structures of the knee, or whether it is referred from the tibial-femoral compartments. Acute onset of anterior knee pain, with or without trauma, can signify quadriceps tendon rupture (see acute injury section) and prepatellar bursitis. Mild trauma may also result in patellar dislocation in individuals with anatomic malalignment causing excess lateral traction on the patella. It is important to distinguish a true dislocation that required reduction by trained personnel from a sensation of "dislocation" experienced by the patient, because this represents a difference in instability and severity. The cause of subacute or chronic anterior knee pain can often be narrowed based on the age of the patient (Table 12–8). Patellofemoral pain syndrome is one of the most common causes of anterior knee pain in the younger patient, especially in women, whereas osteoarthritis of the patellofemoral compartment is the most common cause in the older patient. In either case, pain is typically worsened by activity that puts increase load and pressure on the patella, such as ascending and descending stairs, squatting, or even rising from a sitting position. With knee extension, patients sometimes describe a grinding sensation.

Pain typically localizes around or under the patella. Patients may note a sensation of knee buckling or giving way, but as stated earlier, this is a nonspecific finding that seems to be largely related to pain rather than pathologic process.

B. Physical Examination

The examination starts with the evaluation of gait and the evaluation of limb alignment. Any valgus or varus deformity of the limb, internal or external rotation of the leg should be noted. Patients, especially young females, with valgus alignment of their lower limb, commonly complain of anterior knee pain due to a weak quadriceps muscle, lateral pull of the patella, and lateral facet tenderness. The presence or absence of flexion contractures, recurvatum or abnormal position of the feet should also be noted. Significant recurvatum can reflect generalized ligament laxity that is prone to patella instability. Pronated feet also can lead to valgus alignment, which can lead to lateral subluxation of the patella and anterior knee pain. The examiner should note the position of the patella, whether it is in alta (patella sits high in the patellar grove relative to the femur) or baja (sits low). Patella alta usually leads to increased patella instability as the patella engages into the trochlea groove at a higher knee flexion angle. Patella baja usually presents after tendon injury or knee surgery and can present with increased anterior knee pain due to increased stress of the patellofemoral joint.

The examination should also include slow active unassisted range of motion of the knee to assess patella tracking.

The 'J' sign can be appreciated when the patella slides laterally at terminal extension of the knee. This indicates an excessive pull of the vastus lateralis muscle, an increase Q angle, patella alta, shallow trochlea groove, a deficient vastus medialis obliquus, or all of the above.

Through careful palpation, the examiner can identify the source of anterior knee pain (Table 12–7). Focal tenderness at the superior or inferior pole of the patella represents quadriceps and patella tendinitis. Patients who have acute patella dislocation have tenderness over the medial facet with associated bruising. The patella should then be compressed against the femoral groove to elicit patellar pain. Crepitus during range of motion or pain with 'grinding' of the patella on the trochlea groove indicates patellofemoral arthritis. Patellar mobility or glide should also be evaluated. Medial and lateral glide of the patella is performed at full extension and at 30 degrees of flexion. The amount of glide is being quantified using a quadrant system with respect to the widest portion of the patella. The first quadrant means that the patella can be subluxed over the femoral condyle by less than 25% of the widest width of the patella, second quadrant is when the patella can be subluxed between 25% and 50% of the patella width and so forth. It is important to repeat the test at 30 degrees of flexion because most patella dislocations do not occur at full extension. They usually occur at gentle flexion, around 20–30 degrees. The lateral displacement of the patella is also known as the 'apprehension test.' An increase in pain or apprehension on the part of the patient for fear of the patella dislocating is a positive finding. The apprehension test is the most specific test for patella dislocation or instability. A normal patella should not be displaced beyond the second quadrant in either direction.

The quadriceps, or Q, angle is also an important physical examination. The Q angle is formed by the line of pull of the quadriceps and the patella tendon as they intersect at the patella. Clinically, the angle is measured between a line drawn from the anterior-superior iliac spine to the patella and a line drawn from the patella and the tibial tubercle. Normal Q angle should be 8 to 10 degrees for males and less than 15 degrees for females. The Q angle should be measured at full extension and at 90 degrees of flexion. Any value greater than 10 degrees for males is considered abnormal. Increased Q angle is one of the risk factors for patellofemoral syndrome.

▶ Treatment

Most patellofemoral injuries are treated nonsurgically. Rarely, patients undergo patellofemoral realignment for chronic problems that are nonresponsive to nonsurgical measures. Most of these ailments can be treated with physical therapy focusing on quadriceps strengthening, core stability, and hip strengthening exercises.

Dixit S, DiFiori JP, Burton M, Mines B. Management of patellofemoral pain syndrome. *Am Fam Physician.* 2007;75:194. [PMID: 17263214]

Table 12–9. Causes of medial knee pain.

Problem	Location
Medial meniscus	Medial joint line, often posterior
MCL	Pain along the course of the ligament from medial epicondyle to pes anserine
Medial compartment osteoarthritis	Medial joint line, but more specifically along the bony edges Varus alignment of the patient's limb
Pes anserine	Pain along the anteromedial tibia where the hamstring and sartorius muscles insert

MCL, medial collateral ligament.

2. Medial Knee Pain

ESSENTIAL FEATURES

▶ Pain over medial joint line.
▶ Difficulty squatting or twisting.
▶ Pain over anteromedial portion of the proximal tibia.

Several structures on the medial aspect of the knee can cause pain. Careful palpation allows the examiner to localize the source of the discomfort (Table 12–9). Medial meniscus tears have characteristic joint line pain. MCL tears have pain along the MCL ligament, which extends from the medial epicondyle and the pes anserine area. Pes anserine bursitis causes pain over the pes insertion, which is distal to the joint line over the anteromedial tibia. Bursitis of the pes anserine bursa is very common, particularly in patients with knee osteoarthritis. Localized tenderness of the bursa can be located between the anteromedial tibial metaphysis and the insertion of the sartorius, gracilis and semitendinosus tendons at the pes anserine. MCL ligament sprain, as discussed above, is common following trauma to the lateral aspect of the knee and is associated with valgus laxity. Medial compartment osteoarthritis, as well as tears in the medial horn of the meniscus can also cause medial knee pain.

3. Lateral Knee Pain

ESSENTIAL FEATURES

▶ Pain over the lateral joint line.
▶ Difficulty squatting or twisting.
▶ Pain over fibula head.

Lateral knee pain, a somewhat uncommon complaint, can be caused by damage to several local structures (Table 12–10). In athletes, particularly runners and cyclists, tendinitis of the iliotibial band can develop from friction to the tendon as it passes over the lateral femoral condyle. Compression of the tendon typically causes pain. Lateral compartment osteoarthritis is unusual but can cause lateral joint line tenderness, particularly in patients with valus deformity. Lateral meniscus tears, which are less common than tears medial meniscus, cause pain along the lateral joint line.

4. Posterior Knee Pain

 ESSENTIAL FEATURES

▶ Fullness over the back of the knee.
▶ Difficulty achieving full flexion.

While there are few weight-bearing structures in the posterior knee, there are a few causes of posterior knee pain (Table 12–11). The neurovascular bundle of the leg travels through the popliteal fossa, so vascular events can be manifested by posterior knee pain, including acute arterial thrombosis as well as deep venous thrombosis. Large synovial effusions can cause a Baker cyst to develop in the popliteal fossa. Patients typically complain of symptoms of a synovial effusion, including pain with range of motion and on ambulation, but they may also complain of posterior knee pain or fullness. Occasionally, Baker cysts rupture, resulting in extravasation of synovial fluid into the calf and mimicking a deep venous thrombosis. Finally, tendonitis of the hamstrings or referred pain from lumbar spine osteoarthritis can cause posterior knee pain.

Table 12–10. Causes of lateral knee pain.

Problem	Location
Lateral meniscus	Lateral joint line, often posterior
LCL ligament sprain	Pain along the course of the ligament from lateral epicondyle to fibular head
Lateral compartment arthritis	Lateral joint line, but more specifically along the bony edges Valus alignment of the patient's limb
Iliotibial band syndrome	Pain along the Gerdy tubercle or along the iliotibial band near the lateral epicondyle Common with runners or patients who have recent changes in activity level
Biceps femoris tendinitis	Tenderness along the posterior portion of the fibular head and the insertion of the biceps femoris tendon
Peroneal nerve entrapment	Tinel sign along the fibular neck, usually 2 cm distal to the proximal tip of the fibular head

LCL, lateral collateral ligament.

Table 12–11. Causes of posterior knee pain.

Problem	Location
Popliteal cyst	Posterior joint level, can sometime feel a mass
Gastronemius tightness	Tenderness along the heads of the gastronemius muscle insertion the distal portion of the femur, above the joint line
Generalized osteoarthritis	Diffuse pain
Thrombosis	Common with pain and positive Homan sign (50% of the cases). Distal limb swelling. Occasional with palpable cords

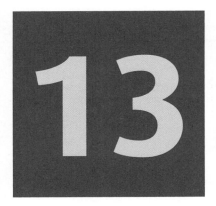

Approach to the Patient with a Painful Prosthetic Hip or Knee

Anthony Marchie, MD

Andrew A. Freiberg, MD

Young-Min Kwon, MD, PhD

ESSENTIAL FEATURES

▶ A thorough clinical history and a detailed physical examination are essential to delineate various intrinsic and extrinsic causes of pain in patients with hip and knee total joint replacements.

▶ Radiographs with orthogonal and weight-bearing views should be ordered to assess signs of implant-related complications.

▶ Laboratory investigations should include both erythrocyte sedimentation rate (ESR) and C-reactive protein (CRP) as screening serologic markers for joint infection.

▶ A high index of suspicion for infection must always be maintained, especially in patients with comorbidities such as diabetes, inflammatory arthritis, and compromised immunity.

▶ Awareness of adverse soft-tissue reaction to metal wear debris in patients with painful metal-on-metal total hip replacements is important in light of its increasing use in young and active patients.

▶ General Considerations

Total hip and knee joint replacement surgery is one of the most successful operations in medicine in terms of patient satisfaction, reduction in pain, and improvement in function. Despite the overwhelming success of total joint arthroplasty, the painful hip and knee prosthetic joint remains a challenge for the physician to evaluate and manage. Because a painful prosthetic hip and knee joint has various intrinsic and extrinsic causes (Table 13–1), a thorough clinical history, a detailed physical examination, as well as radiographic and laboratory tests are essential to delineate the potential causes of the pain (Figure 13–1).

▶ Clinical Findings

A. History

A complete history is critical in the evaluation of patients with painful hip and knee replacements. The temporal onset, duration, severity, location, and character of the pain help narrow the differential diagnosis. The presence of pain since surgery suggests either infection, failure to obtain initial implant stability, a periprosthetic fracture, or a misdiagnosis of the initial reason the arthroplasty was performed. If the pain comes after a pain-free interval following surgery, the likely causes include aseptic loosening or late infection.

Activity-related pain that is relieved with rest suggests implant loosening, fracture, or either neurogenic or vascular claudication. The presence of persistent pain, pain at rest, or night pain may indicate sepsis or malignancy.

Precipitating causes of the pain should be elucidated. Onset of pain after trauma may be caused by fracture or loosening. A history of delayed wound healing, chronic drainage, postoperative hematoma formation, pain after dental or gastrointestinal procedures, and distant sites of infection are all clues to potential joint sepsis. Risk factors that increase likelihood for infection include immunosuppression, obesity, diabetes mellitus, and inflammatory arthritis.

B. Physical Examination

After a general examination, evaluation of a painful prosthetic joint should focus on the joints above and below the prosthesis, and the spine. A comprehensive neurovascular examination is necessary to rule out neurogenic and vascular causes of pain. When examining the lower extremity, gait should be observed for antalgia, limb-length discrepancy, and Trendelenburg lurch. Because lumbar spine disease and fixed pelvic obliquity may be present, true and apparent leg lengths should also be assessed.

Table 13–1. Differential diagnosis for the painful prosthetic joint.

INTRINSIC CAUSES
Prosthesis-related
Infection
Mechanical loosening
Dislocation
Osteolysis
Extensor mechanism problems in knee replacement:
Maltracking, tendon disruption, patellar fracture,
unresurfaced patella
Periprosthetic fracture
Soft-tissue-related
Inflammatory bursitis, tendinitis
Arthrofibrosis
EXTRINSIC CAUSES
Spine disease: Stenosis; disk herniation; spondylolysis or
spondylolisthesis
Peripheral vascular disease
Complex regional pain syndrome
Psychological disorder
Hernia (femoral, inguinal)
Peripheral nerve injury (eg, sciatic, femoral,
meralgia paresthetica)
Malignancy or metastases
Metabolic bone disease (eg, Paget disease, osteomalacia)

Inspection of the skin should note previous scars and signs of infection, including warmth, erythema, fluctuance, drainage, and sinus tracts. Range of motion (ROM) should be examined to determine the positions that elicit the patient's pain. Pain with active ROM or with extremes of motion often indicate loosening, while pain with passive ROM suggests infection.

C. Laboratory Findings

In addition to radiographic studies, laboratory tests such as the complete blood count and differential, ESR, and CRP can provide additional information in evaluating the painful prosthetic joint.

The ESR can help distinguish septic from aseptic loosening after joint replacement surgery. However, the ESR typically increases to a peak at 5–7 days postoperatively and then declines gradually to its preoperative baseline level over a 3-month period. In some patients, the ESR remains elevated for up to 1 year after surgery.

The CRP has been reported to be a better marker for infection than ESR. When ESR and CRP levels are measured together as a screening battery, the sensitivity is 95%, and the negative predictive value is 97%. When both the ESR and CRP are elevated, specificity for infection has been reported to be as high as 93%. Conversely, if both ESR and CRP are within normal limits, the diagnosis of infection can be excluded.

D. Imaging Studies

After a complete history is obtained and a physical examination is performed, serial plain radiographs should be obtained to look for signs of implant-related complications, such as loosening, migration, or osteolysis. Signs of implant loosening include a progressive increase in the radiolucent line, change in component position and subsidence, fracture of the cement mantle, or bony reaction around the tip of the component. There are also certain radiographic findings suggestive of infection. These signs include periosteal new bone formation (Figure 13–2), endosteal scalloping, soft-tissue swelling, osteopenia, and premature loosening of the component.

Technetium bone scanning has been reported to have a lower sensitivity and specificity than serial plain radiographs for diagnosing component loosening. Thus, bone scans should be obtained only when plain radiography is equivocal with regard to the questions of loosening or infection. Furthermore, increased uptake of radioisotope with bone scintigraphy may occur up to 2 years after uncomplicated cemented and cementless total hip and knee arthroplasty.

E. Prosthetic Joint Aspiration

Aspiration of the prosthetic joint is indicated when clinical suspicion for infection is high, such as when the ESR or CRP or both are elevated. During synovial fluid analysis of prosthetic joints, a white blood cell count (WBC) as low as >3000/mcL has a high sensitivity and specificity for infection, and the possibility of infection must be considered seriously in this setting.

▶ Differential Diagnosis & Treatment

A. Infection

Infection is always considered foremost in the differential diagnosis of the painful prosthetic joint. Signs and symptoms include fever, chills, night sweats, and pain at rest. A history of previous infection at the incision site, distant infections in the body, and recent invasive procedures (including dental, gastrointestinal, or urologic procedures) are all risk factors for infection of the prosthetic joint.

On physical examination, the wound and surrounding joint areas should be examined carefully for evidence of swelling, erythema, and drainage. Laboratory tests may show a leukocytosis, with an elevated ESR and CRP. When aspiration is indicated, Gram stain and cultures for aerobic and anaerobic organisms as well as acid-fast bacilli and fungal organisms are essential.

Radiographic findings suggestive of infection include periosteal new bone formation (Figure 13–2), endosteal

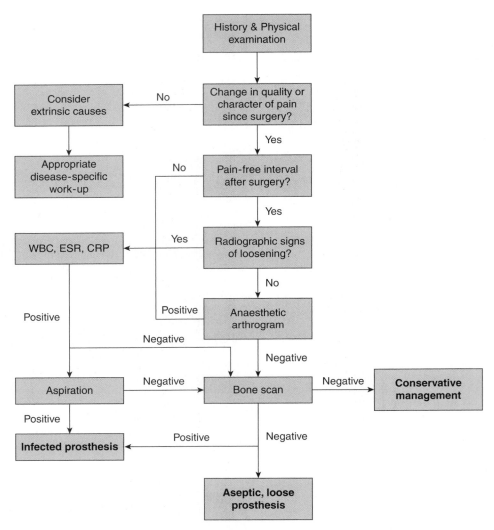

▲ **Figure 13–1.** Clinical evaluation of a patient with painful total hip and knee arthroplasty. CRP, C-reactive protein; ESR, erythrocyte sedimentation rate; WBC, white blood count.

scalloping, soft-tissue swelling, osteopenia, and premature loosening of the component. Infections are considered to be acute if diagnosed within 6 weeks of symptom onset. Acute infections can be treated with surgical irrigation, debridement, and exchange of the modular components. For infections that have persisted longer than 6 weeks, a two-stage reimplantation is currently the standard of care. The first stage surgery involves removal of all foreign material, including the prosthetic implant, methylmethacrylate, metal cables, plates, and screws. A 6-week course of intravenous antibiotics follows the first stage. After this initial treatment, joint aspiration is recommended following an antibiotic "holiday";

ie, the antibiotic is discontinued for a minimum of 2 weeks before joint aspiration is performed. Once there is no clinical evidence of infection, the ESR and CRP values have returned to their baseline levels, and the joint aspiration is negative for infection, the definitive second stage reimplantation surgery is performed. Reimplantation surgery is not undertaken until the infection has been eradicated.

B. Prosthetic Loosening

On average, a well-implanted prosthesis remains viable for 10–25 years or more, depending on multiple factors, such

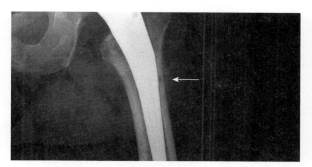

▲ **Figure 13–2.** The periosteal reaction (*arrow*) in the setting of infection is seen in the lateral aspect of the proximal femur.

as implant design, material, patient age, and activity level. Longevity of implant survival is improved with modern bearing surfaces, such as highly cross-linked polyethylene, because these have significantly lower wear rates compared with materials used in the past. The most common cause of prosthetic failure, however, is aseptic loosening.

The pain associated with aseptic prosthetic loosening is usually aggravated by weight-bearing activities, such as lifting objects or simply rising from a seated position. This pain can also be present immediately after surgery if there has been inadequate fixation of the prosthesis to the bone.

Patients with prosthetic loosening in the lower extremity are likely to have an antalgic gait or limp, and pain may be elicited with range of motion. There may also be more pain in the area of loosening with an active straight leg raise (raising the leg off the examination table with the knee fully extended), than with a passive straight leg raise.

The radiographic signs of prosthetic joint loosening include subsidence of the implant, cement or prosthetic fracture, debonding between the cement mantle and implant, and pedestal formation with a cementless femoral stem (Figure 13–3).

C. Osteolysis

Periprosthetic osteolysis (or bone resorption) is initiated by osteoclasts, which are stimulated by inflammatory mediators produced through the macrophage response to wear debris. Wear debris stimulates a foreign body inflammatory response, which leads to the bone resorption. Osteolysis manifests itself as a lucent area around the prosthesis on plain radiographs and is the most common cause for implant loosening. In the absence of loosening, osteolysis can still account for pain. Radiographs normally do not demonstrate osteolysis until the bone mass in the area of lucency has decreased by at least 30% (Figure 13–4).

Treatment of osteolysis may be expectant if the patient is asymptomatic or only mildly symptomatic. Revision arthroplasty is indicated if there is significant pain, dysfunction, or impending fracture.

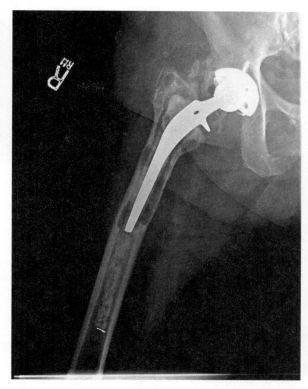

▲ **Figure 13–3.** Aseptic loosening of the femoral implant with periprosthetic osteolysis, areas of debonding between cement mantle and implant.

D. Periprosthetic Fracture

Fracture around the implant is uncommon and is typically related to osteolysis, implant loosening, or trauma. There may be antecedent minor trauma, especially in patients with significant osteolysis. Standard radiographs almost always reveal the fracture (Figure 13–5).

Fracture of the bone around a prosthesis typically requires surgery, and surgical considerations include the quality of the bone, stability of the implant, and location of the fracture.

E. Prosthetic Dislocation

Prosthetic dislocation is most common at the hip and rare in the knee. Joint dislocation leads to pain, deformity, and loss of function. Standard radiographs are necessary to help confirm dislocation (Figure 13–6). Radiographic evaluation should always include two orthogonal views (eg, anteroposterior and lateral), since the diagnosis can be missed if only one view is obtained.

Prosthetic dislocation is treated with closed reduction under sedation, although open reduction may be required for patients in whom closed reduction is unsuccessful. Once

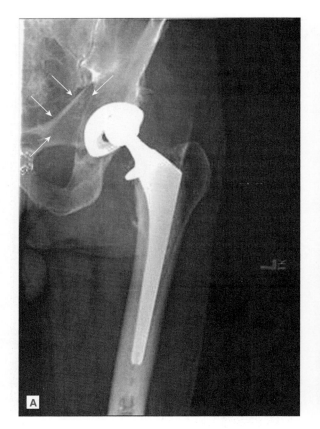

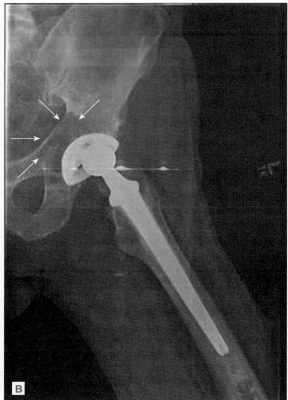

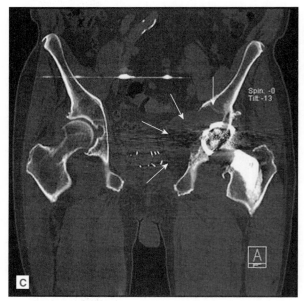

▲ **Figure 13–4.** Osteolysis (*arrows*) in the acetabulum seen on radiographic (**A** and **B**) and CT assessment (**C**).

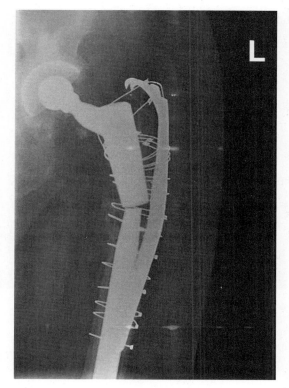

▲ **Figure 13–5.** Fracture of prosthesis.

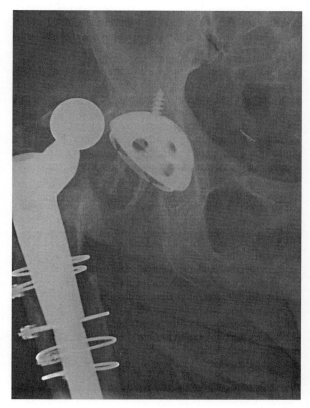

▲ **Figure 13–6.** Prosthetic dislocation.

the joint has been reduced, patients are counseled on activity modification to prevent further dislocation or subluxation. Revision surgery is indicated in cases of recurrent dislocation.

F. Referred Pain

A common cause of referred pain to the lower limb is a spinal disorder. Nerve impingement in the cervical or lumbar spine can cause pain similar to that of a loose prosthesis. Indeed, tumors in the neck, shoulder, abdomen, or pelvis can also cause referred pain. Signs and symptoms of nerve root impingement include atrophy, weakness, paresthesia, and neuropathic pain. This pain is not normally aggravated by weight-bearing.

Pain caused by spinal stenosis is typically relieved by forward flexion or the assumption of a stooped, forward-leaning posture. CT and MRI of the spine are useful in arriving at the diagnosis. Treatment of spinal disorders includes both conservative and surgical measures. Depending on the diagnosis, there may be a role for activity modification, physiotherapy, core body strengthening activity, and pain management modalities. Patients whose symptoms are refractory to these conservative measures may require spinal decompression or fusion.

G. Bursitis

Bursae around prosthetic joints remain potential sites of inflammation and sources of pain after total joint arthroplasty. Patients with trochanteric, pes, patellar or anserine bursitis describe pain in the bursal region and localized tenderness to palpation.

The treatment approach to bursitis following joint arthroplasty is different to that of bursitis in a native joint. Following surgery, patients are less likely to have a capsular boundary between the bursa and the joint space. Thus, bursal injections are discouraged as contamination of the bursa is associated with an increased risk of joint infection. Use of a nonsteroidal anti-inflammatory medication and other multimodal therapy may help with resolution of the pain. Surgical intervention for bursitis refractory to conservative management has a variable outcome.

H. Neuroma or Chronic Regional Pain Syndrome

Any nerve transected at surgery may cause pain postoperatively. The infrapatellar branch of the saphenous nerve, normally cut with a midline incision during knee arthroplasty, can be a potential source of complaint. Symptomatic neuromas generally cause pain disproportionate to the physical examination and can lead to cutaneous hypersensitivity with dysesthesia, allodynia, and hyperalgesia.

Patients with chronic regional pain syndrome generally have pain that is diffuse. There may be associated joint stiffness, hyperhidrosis, and skin discoloration, along with motor disturbances such as weakness, spasm, and tremor. Local osteopenia can often be seen in the affected extremity on radiographs.

In the absence of another diagnosis, resection of the neuroma may be useful in patients with symptoms of at least 6 months duration and refractory to conservative treatment. In addition to the use of tricyclic antidepressant and anticonvulsant agents, physiotherapy modalities and sympathetic nerve block may offer relief to patients with chronic regional pain syndrome. Nevertheless, these conditions remain difficult to treat and usually require multimodal treatments.

I. Adverse Soft-Tissue Reaction to Metal-on-Metal Hip Resurfacing

Metal-on-metal hip resurfacing arthroplasty has undergone a resurgence as an alternative treatment option for young and active patients with significant hip osteoarthritis. The proposed potential advantages of metal-on-metal hip resurfacing arthroplasty over conventional total hip arthroplasty include bone conservation, greater implant stability, and easier revision surgery. Despite the satisfactory short-term implant survival, there is concern regarding the long-term biologic consequences of exposure to cobalt (Co) and chromium (Cr), the principal elements in the CoCr alloy used in the modern metal-on-metal bearings. One of the local adverse biologic responses is the occurrence of abnormal periprosthetic soft-tissue reactions, which have become popularly described as pseudotumors (Figure 13–7).

Pseudotumors can cause a wide spectrum of clinical presentations, including hip pain, lump/mass, and joint dislocation. These lesions are characterized histologically by the presence of T-lymphocytes and macrophages with extensive necrosis, often difficult to distinguish morphologically from a necrotic tumor, hence the term "pseudotumor." However, these periprosthetic soft-tissue lesions have also been described by other names, such as bursae, cysts, inflammatory masses, or adverse reactions to metal debris. The association between the increased serum and hip aspirate metal ion levels suggests that pseudotumors are likely to represent a biologic response to the large amount of metal wear debris generated from excessive wear in vivo. Although the exact prevalence is unknown, it has been reported to be approximately 2%.

Clinicians need to be aware of the potential for pseudotumor development when evaluating patients with painful metal-on-metal hip resurfacing arthroplasty. Because patients with pseudotumors may have normal radiographs, further radiographic investigation using soft-tissue imaging modalities, such as ultrasound or MRI with metal artifact reduction sequence, is recommended to confirm the diagnosis. In the

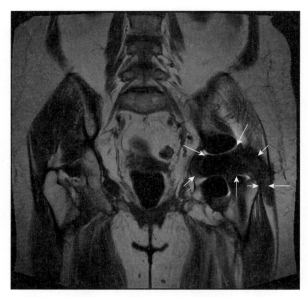

▲ **Figure 13–7.** MRI scan with metal artifact reduction sequence showing a pseudotumor with both cystic and solid components in a patient with painful metal-on-metal hip replacement.

majority of patients with pseudotumors, the treatment is revision surgery to non-metal-on-metal total hip replacements.

Della Valle CJ, Sporer SM, Jacobs JJ, Berger RA, Rosenberg AG, Paprosky WG. Preoperative testing for sepsis before revision total knee arthroplasty. *J Arthroplasty.* 2007;22(6 Suppl 2):90. [PMID: 17823024]

Glyn-Jones S, Pandit H, Kwon YM, Doll H, Gill HS, Murray DW. Risk factors for inflammatory pseudotumour formation following hip resurfacing. *J Bone Joint Surg Br.* 2009;91:1566. [PMID: 19949118]

Kwon YM, Glyn-Jones S, Simpson DJ, et al. Analysis of wear of retrieved metal-on-metal hip resurfacing implants revised due to pseudotumours. *J Bone Joint Surg Br.* 2010;92:356. [PMID: 20190305]

Kwon YM, Thomas P, Summer B, et al. Lymphocyte proliferation responses in patients with pseudotumours following metal-on-metal hip resurfacing arthroplasty. *J Orthop Res.* 2010;28:444. [PMID: 19834954]

Kwon YM, Xia Z, Glyn-Jones S, Beard D, Gill HS, Murray DW. Dose-dependent cytotoxicity of clinically relevant cobalt nanoparticles and ions on macrophages in vitro. *Biomed Mater.* 2009;4:025018. [PMID: 19349653]

Mabilleau G, Kwon YM, Pandit H, Murray DW, Sabokbar A. Metal-on-metal hip resurfacing arthroplasty: a review of periprosthetic biological reactions. *Acta Orthop.* 2008;79:734. [PMID: 19085489]

Toms AD, Mandalia V, Haigh R, Hopwood B. The management of patients with painful total knee replacement. *J Bone Joint Surg Br.* 2009;91:143. [PMID: 19190044]

The Patient with Diffuse Pain

14

Ernest H. S. Choy, MD, FRCP

Musculoskeletal pain is the one of the most common reasons for medical consultations in the community. Nonarticular rheumatic pain syndromes (eg, tendinitis, bursitis, enthesitis, or muscular tear) constitute a major proportion of these consultations. In most cases, these conditions are self-limited and respond to treatment.

Diffuse pain may be caused by inflammatory and noninflammatory conditions. Polymyalgia rheumatica (see Chapter 30), rheumatoid arthritis (see Chapter 15), and systemic lupus erythematosus (see Chapter 21) are common causes of diffuse inflammatory pain, while fibromyalgia and primary generalized osteoarthritis (see Chapter 43) are common causes of noninflammatory diffuse pain. Both inflammatory and noninflammatory diffuse pain conditions sometimes occur in the same patient, causing confusion in diagnosis and treatment. Because inflammatory conditions are covered elsewhere in this book, fibromyalgia is the main focus of this chapter.

Although some experts argue that fibromyalgia is not a distinct disease entity and that labeling patients with the diagnosis encourages chronic illness behavior and increases healthcare consumption, data from the General Practice Research Database has shown this premise to be false. The General Practice Research Database has collected information from over 750 practices, with more than 3 million patients and 35 million patient years of data. Based on this data, a 2006 study showed that healthcare utilization among fibromyalgia patients was already very high in the 8 years preceding the diagnosis. Furthermore, healthcare utilization decreased after diagnosis, indicating that the diagnosis could be used constructively to reassure and educate patients.

ESSENTIALS OF DIAGNOSIS

▶ Diffuse pain for longer than 3 months. Pain is defined as above and below the waist bilaterally; axial skeletal pain must also be present.

▶ Increased tenderness to light pressure (allodynia).

▶ Fatigue and nonrestorative sleep.

▶ Depression and anxiety disorders are common, but mood disorder is not universal and response to antidepressants is independent of any change in mood.

General Considerations

Fibromyalgia is one of the most common causes of chronic diffuse pain. It is associated with increased tenderness to light pressure (allodynia). Although the term **fibromyalgia** has only been used in the last 2 decades, it is not a new disease. In 1850, Froriep described hard places in the muscles of patients with "rheumatism" that were painful to light touch. Gowers used the term **fibrositis** to describe patients who complained of tenderness with light pressure in the absence of any signs of local or systemic inflammation. Subsequently, fibrositis was found to be a common cause of muscular pain, although many clinicians considered it as "psychogenic rheumatism."

Pathophysiology

Patients with fibromyalgia have altered pain processing compared to normal individuals. This includes greater subjective pain, decreased pain threshold, increased pain ratings, and a steeper rise of response to repeated stimulation. These abnormalities have been attributed to an underlying central sensitization. **Central sensitization** is a term denoting a state of enhanced, or amplified, neural processing within the central nervous system. The normal physiologic role of central sensitization is thought to protect an injured area from further damage and maximize healing by immobilization. Central sensitization may involve the abnormal ascending and descending pain pathways in the spinal cord. Consistent with this hypothesis is the finding that in patients with fibromyalgia, increased levels of substance P are found in the cerebrospinal fluid. Neuroimaging studies have shown different neuronal activation pattern in patients with fibromyalgia compared with controls, supporting the notion that pain processing is abnormal.

▶ Clinical Findings

A. Symptoms and Signs

1. Pain—Pain is the dominant symptom and principal complaint in fibromyalgia. Most patients have suffered from pain for many years before seeking medical advice. In some cases, pain may start in childhood. The reason for seeking medical advice is often because pain has become widespread or more severe, and patients may find it difficult to cope. Typically, patients complain of "pain all over their body," although often it starts in one or two areas and then spread to other parts of the body. The severity of pain may vary in difficult parts of the body and from day to day. Most often, patients complain of a chronic ache with occasional severe sharp spasms or electric shocks. Others describe their muscles as tense and liken it to being "tied in knots."

Pain is often worsened by exertion or physical activities, although many patients also complain of spontaneous pain without any obvious precipitating factor. Simple analgesics, such as acetaminophen or nonsteroidal anti-inflammatory drugs, are rarely effective. Some patients notice pain is worsened by stress. Indeed, some patients associate the onset of the illness with a physical or emotional stressful event, such as an illness or road traffic accident.

For a patient to meet the 1990 or 2011 American College of Rheumatology (ACR) classification criteria for fibromyalgia (see Diagnostic Criteria below), he or she must have a history of diffuse pain lasting more than 3 months, defined as pain on both sides of the body and pain above and below the waist. In addition, axial skeletal pain (cervical spine, anterior chest, thoracic spine, or low back) must be present. Low back pain is considered lower segment pain.

Tenderness, an increased sensitivity to light touch or pressure (allodynia and hyperalgesia), is one of the characteristic features of fibromyalgia. **Hyperalgesia** is defined as excessively severe pain induced by a noxious stimulus, while **allodynia** is pain induced by an innocuous stimulus. In some patients, the slightest touch can make them recoil in pain. They have to avoid physical contact, including gentle patting by their partners. As pain is aggravated by physical activity, most patients find it disabling and limits their ability to perform routine household chores, especially shopping and cleaning. Those patients who are employed often find it difficult to cope at work.

Concomitant chronic painful conditions, such as migraine, noncardiac chest pain, heartburn, dysmenorrhea, and irritable bowel syndrome, are common in patients with fibromyalgia and may pre-date the diagnosis.

2. Fatigue—Fatigue is common in fibromyalgia, affecting 80–90% of patients. Typically, patients describe fatigue as an "overwhelming tiredness" and feeling "completely washed out." In some patients, severe episodic attacks may come on suddenly. Some patients find it more difficult to cope with the fatigue than with the pain, since rest and sleep rarely improve fatigue. Although many patients complain that fatigue is a disabling symptom, it is less severe and disabling than in chronic fatigue syndrome. When fatigue is overwhelming and the muscular pain is less prominent, chronic fatigue syndrome should be considered as an alternative diagnosis.

3. Nonrestorative sleep—Nonrefreshing sleep is a feature of fibromyalgia in over 90% of patients. In most patients, it is not insomnia; they can fall asleep, but they do not feel refreshed in the morning, which is due to poor sleep quality. Often, poor sleep quality is associated with feeling tired and difficulty in performing physical activity and poor cognitive performance. In addition, some fibromyalgia patients complain of sleepiness during the day. Other patients complain of waking up frequently during the night. Some patients also suffer from restless leg syndrome. Impaired sleep quality was found to be predictive of pain, fatigue, and social functioning in one study. Polysomnographic studies have found correlation between sleep disturbance in patients with fibromyalgia with specific patterns of alpha intrusion and decrease slow wave sleep, suggesting "wakefulness" or lack of quality deep restful sleep may be an important part of the pathophysiology. Indeed, inducing sleep disturbance in healthy individuals can cause myalgia and increase tenderness. However, loud snoring and disturbances of breathing during the night are uncommon in fibromyalgia; the presence of these symptoms should alert clinicians to possible primary sleep disorders, such as obstructive sleep apnea. These patients may need referral to sleep clinics for further evaluation.

4. Depression and anxiety—History of depression and anxiety disorders is common in patients with fibromyalgia. The prevalence of concomitant depression and anxiety is higher among patients in secondary care than those in the community. This contributes significantly to the view among specialists that mood disorders are the cause of fibromyalgia. However, epidemiologic studies showed that mood disorder is not universal and response to antidepressants in patients with fibromyalgia is independent of any change in mood. These studies suggest that mood disturbance is not the sole pathogenic factor in most patients with fibromyalgia. In patients with fibromyalgia, depression is often associated with more severe fatigue as well as poor sleep quality and pain control. Patients with anxiety often experience palpitation and dizziness, sweating, and paresthesia. In severe cases, some patients may experience panic attacks. Occasionally, some patients may have severe depression, so it is important to assess mood and suicidal risk. Patients with severe depression and those with suicidal thoughts need urgent referral to a psychiatrist.

5. Impaired cognition—Cognition problems are common in patients with fibromyalgia. Poor short-term memory as well as difficulty in learning a new task, processing information, and problem solving are common complaints. Many patients describe suffering from "brain fog." In many cases, impaired cognition occur as episodic attacks and last for a few hours or days, although in some cases, they may be more prolonged. Impaired cognition is a major contributor of frustration and psychosocial stress, especially in patients whose employment is mentally demanding.

6. Morning stiffness—Traditional prolonged early morning stiffness is regarded as a symptom of inflammatory disorders, such as rheumatoid arthritis. However, patients with fibromyalgia also suffer from prolonged early morning stiffness, resulting in diagnostic confusion with inflammatory arthritis, especially if they also complain of swollen hands or feet. One of the distinguishing features of early morning stiffness in fibromyalgia is that it is not relieved by exercise. Furthermore, although patients may complain of swelling in the hands and feet, objective evidence of synovitis is lacking, and the patient points to more diffuse swelling rather than discrete swelling around the joints.

7. Other symptoms—Patients with fibromyalgia may complain of symptoms affecting other systems, including gastrointestinal (nausea, vomiting, bloating, abdominal pain, diarrhea, and constipation), urogynecologic (urgency, frequency, incontinence, pelvic pain, and dysmenorrhea), and neurologic (dizziness, vertigo, paresthesia, and tinnitus).

However, fever, weight loss and swollen lymph glands are rare. The presence of these suggest an alternative diagnosis.

B. Physical Examination

The goal of the physical examination is to confirm diagnosis and rule out other differential diagnoses, which are listed in Table 14–1.

Given the differential diagnoses, a full medical examination is important to assess joint swelling, deformities, skin rashes, muscle bulk, and strength and tendon reflexes. In patients with fibromyalgia, clinical findings are usually unremarkable except for the presence of increase tenderness and "tender points."

Table 14–1. Differential diagnosis of fibromyalgia.

Osteomalacia
Hypermobility syndrome
Primary generalized osteoarthritis
Polymyalgia rheumatica
Rheumatoid arthritis
Connective tissue diseases: Systemic lupus erythematosus and Sjögren syndrome
Inflammatory muscle diseases
Myopathies
Hypothyroidism
Malignancies

The presence of multiple allodynic tender point is a typical finding in fibromyalgia and is part of the ACR 1990 classification criteria (see below). It is normal to experience pain when sufficient pressure is applied over any part of our body. However, patients with fibromyalgia have a lower pressure pain threshold and experience pain at pressure that is normally innocuous (ie, allodynia). The tender points stipulated by the 1990 ACR classification criteria for fibromyalgia are the occipital, low cervical, trapezius, supraspinatus, second rib, lateral epicondyle, gluteus, greater trochanter, and at the medial fat pad of the knee bilaterally. Each point is palpated with the thumb of the examiner, using gradually increasing pressure until the patient reports the pressure to be painful. A point is considered "positive" if the patient reports pain when less than 4 kg of pressure (the color under the nail blanches) is applied. At least 11 of 18 tender point sites were required to meet the 1990 ACR classification criteria, but this provision was revised by the 2011 guidelines (see below).

C. Laboratory Findings

The sole purpose of laboratory tests in fibromyalgia is to exclude alternative diagnoses, since there are no specific diagnostic tests for fibromyalgia. Many patients with fibromyalgia undergo a large number of blood tests and imaging studies. Aside from being expensive, false-positive or weakly positive results, such as rheumatoid factor and antinuclear antibodies, are not uncommon. In the absence of relevant clinical symptoms or signs, these tests are unwarranted. In general, complete blood count, biochemistry, erythrocyte sedimentation rate (ESR) or C-reactive protein (CRP), and thyroid function tests are all that is necessary. Another potential pitfall of excessive investigation is that patients often associate investigations with serious illnesses. They often feel confused when told the results are normal. It is, therefore, important to anticipate this problem by forewarning patients that the results of the investigations are expected to be normal.

D. Imaging Studies

Single photon emission computer tomography (SPECT) and functional magnetic resonance imaging (fMRI) have demonstrated reduced thalamic blood flow under resting conditions in patients with fibromyalgia. When pressure stimuli are applied to the thumbnail, fibromyalgia patients demonstrated activity in the pain-processing regions of the brain at much lower stimulus intensities than in healthy controls.

▶ Subtypes of Fibromyalgia

Several studies have suggested that fibromyalgia is a heterogenous condition. While chronic widespread pain and increased tenderness are universally present, other associated symptoms are not present in all patients. One study using cluster analysis of community recruited fibromyalgia suggested that there may be three different subtypes:

Group 1: Moderate anxiety, depression, catastrophizing; poor control over pain; the highest pain thresholds and low tenderness.

Group 2: High levels of anxiety, depression, and catastrophizing; low pain control and considerable tenderness.

Group 3: Low levels of anxiety, depression, and catastrophizing; good control over pain but very low pain threshold and the most tenderness.

In this study, the first subtype was the most common, with over half the patients falling within this group. Therefore, patients in group 1 were considered to represent "typical fibromyalgia." It is important to note, however, that in these studies patients were recruited from the community. The proportion of patients in each subtype may change if patients in secondary care were studied, since the latter tends to include a higher prevalence of mood disturbance and psychosocial stress.

Another study conducted a cluster analysis based on musculoskeletal, nonmusculoskeletal, and cognitive and psychological symptoms gathered from 2182 female patients who completed an internet survey. The analysis revealed four groups:

Group 1: High on all three symptom domains.

Group 2: Moderate on the musculoskeletal and nonmusculoskeletal domains and high on cognitive/psychological symptoms.

Group 3: Moderate on the musculoskeletal and nonmusculoskeletal domains and low on cognitive/psychological symptoms.

Group 4: Low on all symptom domains.

Group 1 patients reported the greatest amount of health care utilization and difficulty in coping with symptoms.

Recently, an analysis of data from clinical trials of duloxetine again suggested there are patient subgroups. In this study, these subgroups also predicted response to treatment.

▶ Diagnostic Criteria

In 1977, the seminal work of Smythe and Moldofsky laid the foundation for the current classification and diagnostic criteria for fibromyalgia. They noted that at certain anatomic locations, patients with fibromyalgia have more tenderness than patients without fibromyalgia. Subsequent studies confirmed the diagnostic utility of these tender points, leading to several proposed diagnostic criteria based on presence of pain and tender points, with or without supplementary symptoms, after excluding other rheumatic or systemic diseases.

In 1990, the ACR criteria for the classification of fibromyalgia were published. These criteria include the presence of chronic widespread pain (defined as bilateral, above and below the waist, and axial) for at least 3 months and the presence of at least 11 out 18 tender points. Over the last 2 decades, the ACR classification criteria have enhanced research by ensuring homogenous populations of patients could be studied. Although this was the primary aim of the ACR classification criteria, it is commonly used in routine practice for diagnosing fibromyalgia.

In 2011, the ACR published new diagnostic criteria for fibromyalgia and a further modified version was published later in the same year. The new criteria do not require the presence of tender points, but patient must have widespread pain for at least 3 months and does not have a disorder that would otherwise explain the pain. In addition, patients must have a Widespread Pain Index (WPI) >7 and Symptom Severity Scale (SSS) score >5 or WPI 3–6 and SSS score >9. The WPI is assessed by asking patients to indicate the regions (maximum 19) of the body where they have experienced pain over the past week with each positive region scoring 1 point.

SSS is the sum of the severity of the following symptoms: fatigue, unrefreshed upon waking, and cognitive symptoms plus the extent of somatic symptoms. For fatigue, unrefreshed upon waking and cognitive symptom, severity is scored using a numeric rating scale between 0 to 3. The rating of 0 = no problem; 1 = slight or mild problems, generally mild or intermittent; 2 = moderate, considerable problems, often present or at a moderate level; 3 = severe, pervasive, continuous, life-disturbing problems over the last week.

For assessing the extent of somatic symptoms, the following are acceptable: muscle pain, irritable bowel syndrome, fatigue/tiredness, thinking or remembering problem, muscle weakness, headache, pain/cramps in the abdomen, numbness/tingling, dizziness, insomnia, depression, constipation, pain in the upper abdomen, nausea, nervousness, chest pain, blurred vision, fever, diarrhea, dry mouth, itching, wheezing, Raynaud phenomenon, hives/welts, ringing in ears, vomiting, heartburn, oral ulcers, loss of/change in taste, seizures, dry eyes, shortness of breath, loss of appetite, rash, sun sensitivity, hearing difficulties, easy bruising, hair loss, frequent urination, painful urination, and bladder spasms. This is scored between 0 and 3. The rating of 0 = no symptoms; 1 = few symptoms; 2 = a moderate number of symptoms; and 3 = a great deal of symptoms. Therefore, the range of SSS is 0–12.

Removing the reliance on tender point count is the major advantage of the new criteria for fibromyalgia. In addition, the SSS includes characteristic features of fibromyalgia and may be used to monitor disease activity. These criteria are not intended to replace the ACR 1990 classification criteria, but to represent an alternative method of diagnosis.

▶ Treatment

Because fibromyalgia is a heterogenous condition associated with a wide range of symptoms, there is no single universal panacea, since it is unlikely that a single treatment will target all the symptoms involved. As indicated above, different subgroups of patients are likely to respond differently to treatment strategies, highlighting the fact that patients should be treated according to their individual needs, rather than following a uniform approach. Treatment needs to be tailored to the individual. For many patients, a multidisciplinary approach to treatment is needed, using both nonpharmacologic and pharmacologic interventions as required.

A. Nonpharmacologic Management

A wide range of nonpharmacologic approaches have been tested with varying success in fibromyalgia. These interventions are generally safe, and some (such as exercise) have general health benefit. Their importance and potential benefits in the management of fibromyalgia should not be overlooked by practitioners when treating fibromyalgia patients. They can be implemented in isolation or combined with other nonpharmacologic or pharmacologic agents, depending on the patients' needs.

1. Patient education—Like all chronic medical conditions, patient education is an important aspect of management. Patients need information on the nature of fibromyalgia as well as its prognosis and treatment. Patients need to understand that the chance of spontaneous remission is unlikely, but positive management can help them cope and live with the condition. Providing more realistic health beliefs is a key part of management. Patients with fibromyalgia often feel frustrated because their spouses, relatives, friends, and employer cannot understand why they are unwell. Educating the relatives and colleagues can help the patient reestablish their social life.

2. Graded exercise—A number of studies have shown that aerobic exercise and strength training are beneficial in fibromyalgia. Fibromyalgia patients are equally able to carry out exercise as healthy people. When performing strength training they can experience the same strength gains, which lead to functional performance and improve quality of life. Patients should be warned that exercise may not improve pain, indeed it can be worsened at first. However, there is good evidence that it can lead to improvement in physical function, tender point count, aerobic performance, and global well-being if patient can persevere. Adherence to exercise program is important, so educating patients on the benefits and risks of exercise is vital. First, patients should be reassured that exercise is not harmful. It does not cause any muscle damage or worsening of fibromyalgia. Regular exercise in fibromyalgia is safe and has other health gains. However, exercise program should be tailored and graded according to the functional ability of the patient. Education can improve adherence to exercise program. Patients should be advised before and during their exercise program so that they do not have unrealistic treatment goals or worries. Muscle deconditioning and wasting can result from inactivity and worsen fibromyalgia in the long-term. Patients should be warned against inactivity.

Many patients find heated pool-based exercise particularly beneficial. Buoyancy reduces pressure load from the muscles, and the heated water provides relaxation. Warm water hydrotherapy can relieve pain even without exercise. Pain relief is often transient, treatment is safe. Although the availability of a hydrotherapy pool may be a limiting factor, many patients find taking a warm water bath at night can relieve pain and improve sleep.

3. Cognitive behavioral therapy—In clinical trials, cognitive behavioral therapy (CBT), is often combined with patient education as a multidisciplinary treatment package. It has been shown to improve pain and function in fibromyalgia either as sole therapy or in combination with exercise. CBT may be of particularly beneficial to patients with fibromyalgia soon after the diagnosis to help the patient understand fibromyalgia, thereby avoiding chronic illness behavior and learning how to develop more effective coping strategies.

4. Other nonpharmacologic therapies—A range of dietary interventions and complementary therapies, including acupuncture, have been studied in fibromyalgia; however, the evidence supporting their efficacy is very limited.

B. Pharmacologic Treatments

In general, medications should be added to nonpharmacologic interventions in the management of fibromyalgia. Currently, in the United States, three medications are licensed by the Food and Drug Administration (FDA) for the treatment of fibromyalgia: pregabalin, milnacipran, and duloxetine.

1. Analgesics—Tramadol improves pain but not function in fibromyalgia. Tramadol, which is a mu opioid receptor agonist, is classified as a moderate strength opioid analgesic; however, it also inhibits norepinephrine and serotonin reuptake. Since clinical trials of strong opioid analgesics produced disappointing benefit in fibromyalgia, the therapeutic effect of tramadol may be attributed to its norepinephrine and serotonin reuptake. The most commonly reported adverse events of tramadol include nausea, somnolence, constipation, and dizziness.

Most studies of nonsteroid anti-inflammatory drugs produced negative results in fibromyalgia. They may be considered if patients have other concomitant diseases (such as osteoarthritis), but they should not be considered as an option for long-term management of fibromyalgia due to their gastrointestinal effects and low benefit to risk profile.

2. Antidepressants—There is strong evidence to support the use of antidepressants in patients with fibromyalgia. Tricyclic antidepressants (TCAs), such as amitriptyline, are the most widely used antidepressants in the management of fibromyalgia. They inhibit serotonin and norepinephrine reuptake. In addition, TCAs also affect glutaminergic neurotransmission by acting on histamine, acetylcholine, and glutamate channels. A meta-analysis of clinical trials in fibromyalgia confirmed that TCAs improve pain, sleep, and fatigue. The best result for amitriptyline was demonstrated at 25 mg rather than 50 mg, indicating that the benefit in fibromyalgia is independent to its antidepressant effect. The limitation of amitriptyline is its poor tolerability. Adverse effects are mainly anticholinergic and include dry mouth, nausea, neuropsychiatric disturbances, and excessive daytime drowsiness.

Two serotonin norepinephrine reuptake inhibitors (SNRIs), milnacipran and duloxetine, have been approved by the FDA for the treatment of fibromyalgia. They have similar efficacy to TCAs without the anticholinergic side effects, resulting in better tolerability. Their most common side effects are headaches and nausea.

Duloxetine was the first SNRI approved by the FDA for the treatment of fibromyalgia. In clinical trials, duloxetine, 30 and 60 mg/d reduced pain and improved function. The recommended starting dose is duloxetine 30 mg once a day for 1 week, the dose may be increased to duloxetine 60 mg/d. It is effective in patients irrespective of the presence or absence of depression. Common side effects of duloxetine include nausea, dry mouth, constipation, decreased appetite, somnolence, increased sweating, and agitation. It is contraindicated in patients taking monoamine oxidase inhibitors or thioridazine and in patients who suffer from uncontrolled narrow-angle glaucoma.

Milnacipran was the second SNRI approved by the FDA. The normal starting dose is 25 mg/d for 2 days, increasing gradually to 50 mg twice daily. In clinical trials of milnacipran, all patients with significant depression were excluded. In these studies, milnacipran reduced pain and improved function. Nausea is the most common side effect. Noradrenergic side effects (such as dry mouth, hyperhidrosis, headache, hot flush, and constipation) are also common. Increases in blood pressure and heart rate are uncommon but monitoring is recommended. It is also contraindicated in patients taking monoamine oxidase inhibitors.

Selective serotonin reuptake inhibitors (SSRIs), such as fluoxetine, have been examined in clinical trials in fibromyalgia. They have the advantage of less anticholinergic side effects than TCAs. However, randomized controlled trials of SSRIs in fibromyalgia produced mixed results.

3. Antiepileptic drugs—

Pregabalin and gabapentin are agonists of the $\alpha_2\delta$ subunit of the voltage-dependent calcium channel in neurons. They reduce calcium influx into the nerve terminals and decrease the release of neurotransmitters, such as glutamate, norepinephrine, and substance P. Initially, they were developed as antiepileptic agents.

Pregabalin was the first drug that received approval from the FDA for treatment of fibromyalgia in the United States. The recommended target dose is 300–450 mg/d. In clinical trials, pregabalin 300 mg/d and 450 mg/d reduced pain and fatigue as well as improved physical function and sleep quality. Common side effects include dizziness, drowsiness, dry mouth, edema, weight gain, constipation, and increased appetite.

Gabapentin has also been studied in a randomized controlled trial. It improves pain, physical function, and quality of

life. Taken together, these results suggest that the α_2-calcium channel is a good therapeutic target in fibromyalgia.

4. Other pharmacologic interventions—

Dopamine agonist such as pramipexole is used in the treatment of Parkinson disease. However, there is evidence to suggest that it also affects the mesolimbic system, particularly sleep control. In a randomized controlled trial, pramipexole demonstrated efficacy for improvements in pain, fatigue, function, and global well-being with good tolerance; however, this is based on one study in which patients were allowed to continue with current medications if at a stable dose. Large randomized controlled trials are needed to confirm the benefits and risks of pramipexole in the treatment of fibromyalgia.

Arnold LM, Crofford LJ, Martin SA, Young JP, Sharma U. The effect of anxiety and depression on improvements in pain in a randomized, controlled trial of pregabalin for treatment of fibromyalgia. *Pain Med.* 2007;8:633. [PMID: 18028041]

Bradley LA, Choy EH, Van Wambeke P, Lipkovich IA, Deberdt W. Typology of Patients with Fibromyalgia: Cluster Analysis of Duloxetine Study Patients. *Arthritis Rheum.* 2009;60(supp l):S212.

Bradley LA, Sotolongo A, Alberts KR, et al. Abnormal regional cerebral blood flow in the caudate nucleus among fibromyalgia patients and non-patients is associated with insidious symptom onset. *J Musculoskel Pain.* 1999;7:285.

Carville SF, Arendt-Nielsen S, Bliddal H, et al. EULAR. EULAR evidence-based recommendations for the management of fibromyalgia syndrome. *Ann Rheum Dis.* 2008;67:536. [PMID: 17644548]

Curran MP. Duloxetine: in patients with fibromyalgia. *Drugs.* 2009;69:1217. [PMID: 19537838]

Froriep R. On the Therapeutic Application of Electro-Magnetism in the Treatment of Rheumatic and Paralytic Affections. Translated by RM Lawrance. London, Henry Renshaw, 1850.

Giesecke T, Williams DA, Harris RE, et al. Subgrouping of fibromyalgia patients on the basis of pressure-pain thresholds and psychological factors. *Arthritis Rheum.* 2003;48:2916. [PMID: 14558098]

Gowers WR. A Lecture on Lumbago: Its Lessons and Analogues: Delivered at the National Hospital for the Paralysed and Epileptic. *Br Med J.* 1904;1:117. [PMID: 20761312]

Gracely RH, Petzke F, Wolf JM, Clauw DJ. Functional magnetic resonance imaging evidence of augmented pain processing in fibromyalgia. *Arthritis Rheum.* 2002;46:1333. [PMID: 12115241]

Hadler NM, Ehrlich GE. Fibromyalgia and the conundrum of disability determination. *J Occup Environ Med.* 2003;45:1030. [PMID : 14534442]

Hughes G, Martinez C, Myon E, Taïeb C, Wessely S. The impact of a diagnosis of fibromyalgia on health care resource use by primary care patients in the UK: an observational study based on clinical practice. *Arthritis Rheum.* 2006;54:177. [PMID: 16385513]

Moldofsky H, Scarisbrick P. Induction of neurasthenic musculoskeletal pain syndrome by selective sleep stage deprivation. *Psychosom Med.* 1976;38:35. [PMID: 176677]

Nishishinya B, Urrútia G, Walitt B, et al. Amitriptyline in the treatment of fibromyalgia: a systematic review of its efficacy. *Rheumatology.* 2008;47:1741. [PMID: 18697829]

Owen RT. Milnacipran hydrochloride: its efficacy, safety and tolerability profile in fibromyalgia syndrome. *Drugs Today.* 2008;44:653. [PMID: 19137120]

Russell IJ, Orr B. Littman, Vipraio GA, et al. Elevated cerebrospinal fluid levels of substance P in patients with the fibromyalgia syndrome. *Arthritis Rheum.* 1994;37:1593. [PMID: 7526868]

Smythe HA, Moldofsky H. Two contributions to understanding of the "fibrositis" syndrome. Bull Rheum Dis. 1977;28:928. [PMID: 199304]

Staud R. Abnormal pain modulation in patients with spatially distributed chronic pain: fibromyalgia. *Rheum Dis Clin North Am.* 2009;35:263. [PMID: 19647141]

Wilson HD, Robinson JP, Turk DC. Toward the identification of symptom patterns in people with fibromyalgia. *Arthritis Rheum.* 2009;61:527. [PMID: 19333980]

Wolfe F, Clauw DJ, Fitzcharles MA, et al. Fibromyalgia criteria and severity scales for clinical and epidemiological studies: a modification of the ACR Preliminary Diagnostic Criteria for Fibromyalgia. *J Rheumatol.* 2011;38:1113. [PMID: 21285161]

Wolfe F, Clauw DJ, Fitzcharles MA, et al. The American College of Rheumatology preliminary diagnostic criteria for fibromyalgia and measurement of symptom severity. *Arthritis Care Res.* 2010;62:600. [PMID: 20461783]

Wolfe F, Smythe HA, Yunus MB, et al. The American College of Rheumatology 1990 Criteria for the Classification of Fibromyalgia. Report of the Multicenter Criteria Committee. *Arthritis Rheum.* 1990;33:160. [PMID: 2306288]

Rheumatoid Arthritis

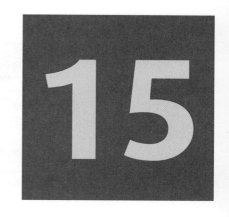

James R. O'Dell, MD

John B. Imboden, MD

Lester D. Miller, MD

Rheumatoid arthritis (RA) is a chronic, systemic disease that primarily targets the synovium, leading to synovial inflammation and proliferation, loss of articular cartilage, and erosion of juxtarticular bone. The natural history of the disease is one of progressive joint damage and deformity and, in a sizeable minority, the development of extra-articular manifestations. Fortunately, current therapeutic strategies, particularly if the disease is diagnosed and treated early, result in substantial clinical benefit for most patients.

RA affects approximately 1% of the adult population worldwide and is more common in women (female:male, 3:1) (Table 15–1). Although RA may present at any age, the typical age of onset in women is the late childbearing years; in men, RA develops more often in the sixth to eighth decade.

The causes of RA remain elusive. The **genetic contribution** to RA is substantial, and more than 30 loci conferring risk for RA have been identified thus far. Most genes linked to RA influence immune responses (eg, T cell activation, cytokine signaling). The strongest known association is with alleles of *HLADRB1*, which encodes the β chain of HLA-DR, a major histocompatiblity class II molecule directly involved in the presentation of antigen to T cells. Allelic variants of *HLADRB1* associated with risk for RA encode a similar sequence (amino acids 70–74) known as the "shared epitope."

Studies of genetic risk reinforce the concept that clinical RA is not a single entity. Most notably, shared-epitope-encoding *HLADRB1* alleles confer risk only for RA associated with **antibodies to citrullinated protein epitopes** (present in approximately 70% of all patients with RA). Citrullination—a post-translational modification of proteins in which arginine residues are converted to citrulline—occurs at sites of inflammation. How patients with RA lose tolerance to citrullinated protein epitopes is uncertain. Interestingly, **epidemiologic data** links smoking (which induces inflammation and citrullinated proteins in the lung) and periodontitis (which is associated with the citrullination of proteins in periodontal tissues) to risk of developing anti-CCP-positive RA.

ARTICULAR MANIFESTATIONS & TREATMENT

James R. O'Dell, MD & John B. Imboden, MD

ARTICULAR MANIFESTATIONS OF RA

ESSENTIALS OF DIAGNOSIS

▶ Chronic symmetric polyarthritis.

▶ Symptoms often start in proximal interphalangeal (PIP), metacarpophalangeal (MCP), and metatarsophalangeal (MTP) joints.

▶ Serum rheumatoid factor, antibodies to cyclic citrullinated peptides (anti-CCP), or both in 70%.

▶ Radiographic changes include juxtarticular erosions and joint-space narrowing.

▶ Clinical Findings

A. Symptoms and Signs

1. Onset—In most patients, RA presents with the insidious onset of pain, stiffness, and swelling in multiple joints over the course of weeks to months. Others, however, may have a fulminant presentation or an onset so insidious that the patient hardly notices. Alternatively, patients may have persistent monoarthritis or oligoarthritis for prolonged periods before manifesting the more typical pattern of polyarticular involvement. Palindromic rheumatism (episodic, self-limited attacks of polyarthritis) may evolve into RA. Rarely, extra-articular features of RA (eg, scleritis) may present before the joint problems occur.

2. Systemic symptoms—Most patients have fatigue and many have low-grade fevers (≤38°C). Significant weight loss can occur but is uncommon in early onset disease.

Table 15–1. Classic manifestations.

- Gender: Female (3:1 ratio)
- Age: Late childbearing years in women (sixth to eighth decade in men)
- Onset: Insidious (builds up over several weeks to months)
- Distribution: Symmetric small joints—MCP, PIP, and MTP (spares DIP) joints
- Systemic: Fatigue, possible weight loss, occasional low-grade fevers
- Symptoms: Joint stiffness (worse in morning), pain, swelling
- Laboratory: Anemia, elevated ESR or CRP or both, thrombocytosis, positive rheumatoid factor in 60–80%

CRP, C-reactive protein; DIP, distal interphalangeal; ESR, erythrocyte sedimentation rate; MCP, metacarpophalangeal; MTP, metatarsophalangeal; PIP, proximal interphalangeal.

Although genetics play a large role in determining risk of RA, most patients have no significant family history.

3. Distribution of involved joints—Figure 15–1 illustrates the different joint distribution in RA and osteoarthritis (OA). Most patients with RA report involvement of small joints first, classically the PIP, MCP, and MTP joints, with involvement of large joints occurring later. Symptoms include pain, swelling, and stiffness, with stiffness often dominating. Patients with early disease often complain that rings no longer fit and that they have pain on the balls of the feet while walking to the bathroom in the morning.

4. Morning stiffness—Morning stiffness is a hallmark of inflammatory arthritis and is a prominent feature of RA. Patients with RA are characteristically at their worst upon arising in the morning or after prolonged periods of rest. This stiffness in and around joints often lasts for hours and improves with activity. Routine activities like brushing teeth and combing hair may be very difficult early in the morning, and patients sometimes report running warm water over their hands to "get them working."

5. Articular manifestations—RA can affect any of the synovial joints (Figure 15–1). Most commonly, the disease starts in the MCP, PIP, and MTP joints followed by the wrists, knees, elbows, ankles, hips, and shoulders in roughly that order. Early treatment helps limit the number of joints involved. Of particular importance, RA almost always spares the distal interphalangeal (DIP) joints (in contrast, these joints are often involved in OA and psoriatic arthritis). Less commonly, and usually only in more advanced cases, RA may involve the temporomandibular, cricoarytenoid and

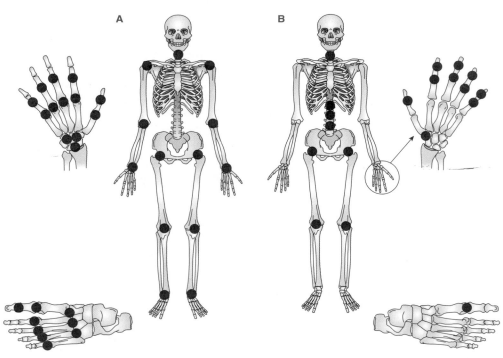

▲ **Figure 15–1.** The joint distribution of the two most common types of arthritis are compared: rheumatoid arthritis **(A)** and osteoarthritis **(B)**. Rheumatoid arthritis involves almost all synovial joints in the body. Osteoarthritis has a much more limited distribution. Importantly, rheumatoid arthritis rarely, if ever, involves the distal interphalangeal joints, but osteoarthritis commonly does.

sternoclavicular joints. RA may involve the upper part of the cervical spine, particularly the C1–C2 articulation, but, unlike the spondyloarthropathies, rarely, if ever, involves the rest of the spine.

The hands are involved in almost all patients with RA; hand involvement is responsible for a significant portion of the disabilities caused by RA. Typical early disease is shown in Figure 15–2A with the swelling of the PIP joints easily seen. The DIP joints are almost always spared unless the patient also has OA; both diseases are common and can coexist, particularly in elderly patients. Radiographs can detect evidence of articular damage early in the course of RA and long before the appearance of joint deformities (Figure 15–3). Late, established disease all too commonly causes **ulnar deviation** of the fingers at the MCPs, **swan neck deformities** (hyperextension of the PIP joints and flexion at the DIP joints; Figure 15–2B), and **boutonnière (or buttonhole) deformities** (flexion of the PIP joints and hyperextension of the DIP joints). If the clinical disease remains active, hand function slowly deteriorates.

Wrists are involved in most patients with RA. Early in the course of the disease, synovial proliferation in and around the wrists can compress the median nerve, causing carpal tunnel syndrome. Chronic synovitis can lead to radial deviation of the wrist and, in severe cases, to volar subluxation. Synovial proliferation of the wrist can invade extensor tendons, lead to rupture and abrupt loss of function of individual fingers.

The feet, particularly the MTP joints, are involved early in almost all cases of RA and are second only to hand involvement in terms of the problems they cause. Radiographic erosions occur at least as early in the feet as in the hands. Subluxation of the toes at the MTP joints is common and leads to the dual problem of skin ulceration on the top of the toes and painful ambulation because of loss of the cushioning pads that protect the heads of the metatarsals. Symptoms from MTP subluxation can respond to orthotics but may require surgery.

Involvement of **large joints** (knees, ankles, elbows, hips, and shoulders) is common but generally occurs somewhat later than small joint involvement. Characteristically, the entire joint surface is involved in a symmetric fashion. Therefore, RA is not only symmetric from one side of the body to the other but is also symmetric within the individual joint. In the case of the knee (Figure 15–4A), the medial and lateral compartments are both severely narrowed in RA, whereas OA usually involves only one compartment (Figure 15–4B). Total joint replacements of hips and knees can dramatically improve function and quality of life and should be considered in patients with severe mechanical damage.

Synovial cysts present as fluctuant masses around involved joints (large or small). Synovial cysts from the knee are perhaps the best examples of this phenomenon. The inflamed knee produces excess synovial fluid that can accumulate posteriorly because of a one-way valve effect between the knee joint and the popliteal space (popliteal or **Baker cyst**). Baker cysts cause problems by compressing the

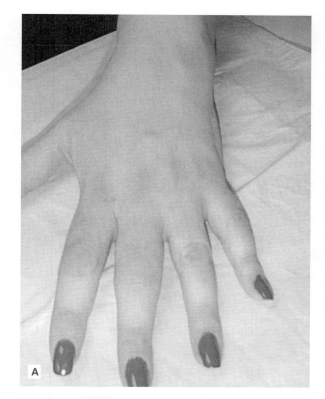

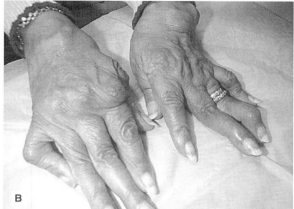

▲ **Figure 15–2. A:** A patient with early rheumatoid arthritis. There are no joint deformities, but the soft tissue synovial swelling around the third and fifth proximal inter-phalangeal (PIP) joints is easily seen. **B:** A patient with advanced rheumatoid arthritis with severe joint deformities including subluxation at the metacarpophalangeal joints and swan-neck deformities (hyperextension at the PIP joints).

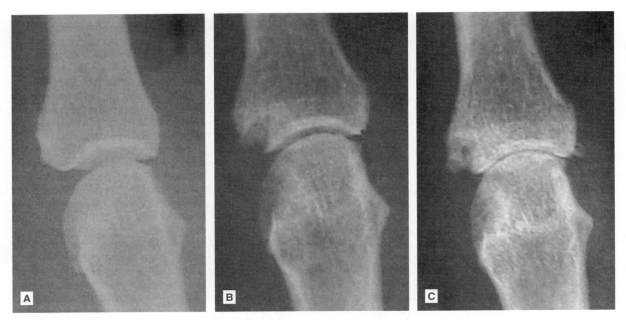

▲ **Figure 15–3.** Progressive destruction of a metacarpophalangeal joint by rheumatoid arthritis. Shown are sequential radiographs of the same second metacarpophalangeal joint. **A:** The joint is normal 1 year prior to the development of rheumatoid arthritis. **B:** Six months following the onset of rheumatoid arthritis, there is a bony erosion adjacent to the joint and joint-space narrowing. **C:** After 3 years of disease, diffuse loss of articular cartilage has led to marked joint-space narrowing.

popliteal nerve, artery, or veins; by dissecting into the tissues of the calf (usually posteriorly); and by rupturing into calf. Dissection usually produces only minor symptoms such as a feeling of fullness. Rupture of a Baker cyst, however, leads to extravasation of the inflammatory contents into the calf, producing significant pain and swelling that may be confused with thrombophlebitis (pseudothrombophlebitis syndrome). Ultrasonography of the popliteal fossa and calf is useful to confirm the diagnosis and to rule out thrombophlebitis, which may be precipitated by popliteal cysts. Short-term treatment of popliteal cysts usually involves injecting the knee anteriorly with glucocorticoids to interrupt the inflammatory process.

RA commonly affects **the cervical spine** (especially the C1–C2 articulation) but spares the thoracic, lumbar and sacral components of the spine. As with RA elsewhere, bony erosions and ligament damage can occur in this area and can lead to subluxation. Most often, subluxation is minor, and patients and caregivers need only be cautious and avoid forcing the neck into positions of flexion. Occasionally, C1–C2 subluxation is severe and requires complex surgical intervention in an attempt to prevent compromise of the cervical cord and, in some cases, death.

Wherever synovial tissue exists, RA can cause problems; the temporomandibular, cricoarytenoid, and sternoclavicular joints are examples. The cricoarytenoid joint is responsible for abduction and adduction of the vocal cords. Involvement of this joint may lead to a feeling of fullness in the throat, to hoarseness, or rarely to a syndrome of acute respiratory distress with or without stridor when the cords are essentially frozen in a closed position. In this latter situation, emergent tracheotomy may be lifesaving.

B. Laboratory Findings

Anemia of chronic disease is seen in most patients with RA, and the degree of anemia is proportional to the activity of the disease. Therapy that controls the disease results in normalization of the hemoglobin. White blood cell counts may be elevated, normal or, in the case of Felty syndrome, profoundly depressed. **Thrombocytosis** is common when RA is active, with platelet counts returning to normal as the inflammation is controlled.

An acute phase response, reflected in elevated **erythrocyte sedimentation rates** (ESR) and serum levels of **C-reactive protein** (CRP), often parallels the activity of the disease. Persistent elevation of ESR and CRP portends a poor prognosis, both in terms of joint destruction and mortality.

Autoantibodies occur in most patients. The autoantibodies most specific for RA are directed against citrullinated

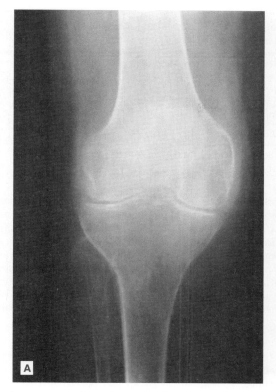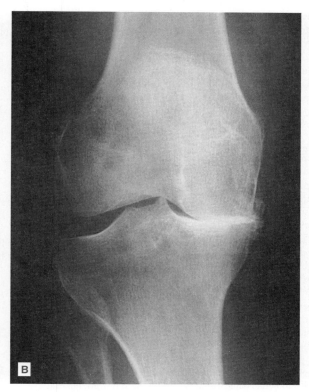

A

B

▲ **Figure 15-4.** The radiographic features of rheumatoid arthritis and osteoarthritis are compared with regard to large joint involvement. **A:** Symmetric loss of cartilage space that is typical of inflammatory arthritis such as rheumatoid arthritis. Note that both the medial and lateral compartments are severely narrowed. Despite this severe narrowing, there is very little in the way of subchondral sclerosis or osteophyte formation since these repair mechanisms are generally shut off in active rheumatoid arthritis. **B:** Complete loss of the cartilage in the medial joint compartment with significant subchondral sclerosis and osteophyte formation. The lateral compartment in this patient is not involved. These features are typical of osteoarthritis.

protein epitopes and are detected by use of synthetic cyclic citrullinated peptides. These **anti-CCP antibodies** are present in 60–70% of patients with RA at diagnosis, are 90–98% specific for RA, are often present in the serum years before RA is diagnosed, and correlate strongly with erosive disease. The first autoantibody to be associated with RA was **rheumatoid factor,** an autoantibody directed against the constant (Fc) region of IgG. Rheumatoid factor is positive in about 50% of cases at presentation and an additional 20–35% of cases become positive in the first 6 months after diagnosis. Rheumatoid factor has an unfortunate name because it is not unique to RA and occurs in many other diseases, particularly those characterized by chronic stimulation of the immune system (Table 15–2). In RA, the presence of rheumatoid factor is associated with more severe articular disease, and essentially all patients with the extra-articular features are seropositive for rheumatoid factor. RA is associated with multiple other autoantibodies, including **antinuclear**

Table 15-2. Differential of a positive rheumatoid factor.

Rheumatic diseases
Rheumatoid arthritis
Sjögren syndrome
Systemic lupus erythematosus
Others
Infections
Viral: Hepatitis C, EBV, erythrovirus (parvovirus), influenza, others
Bacterial: Endocarditis, osteomyelitis, others
Chronic inflammatory conditions
Liver disease, inflammatory bowel disease, others
Aging

EBV, Epstein-Barr virus.

antibodies (ANA; ~30% of patients) and antineutrophil cytoplasmic antibodies (ANCA), particularly of the perinuclear type (~30% of patients).

Synovial fluid in RA is inflammatory; white blood cell counts typically range from 5000/mcL to 50,000/mcL with approximately two-thirds of the cells being neutrophils. No synovial fluid findings are pathognomonic of RA.

C. Imaging Studies

Radiographs of rheumatoid joints may demonstrate **juxta-articular demineralization** and **bony erosions**. Early erosions typically occur at the margins of the joint ("marginal erosions") where synovium directly contacts bone and there is no articular cartilage (Figure 15–3). Cartilage loss leads to **joint-space narrowing** which, in RA, is uniform (in contrast to OA, which cause irregular narrowing) (Figures 15–3 and 15–4). Radiographs of the hands and feet are an important component of the evaluation of the patient with RA and should be obtained at the outset and then assessed thereafter at intervals of a year or more. Radiographs are often normal early in the course of RA; the presence of erosions at presentation is associated with a more aggressive course. Erosions of MTPs may be detected prior to radiographic changes in the hands. Progression of erosions and joint-space narrowing is an indication of ongoing joint damage. Radiographs are not sensitive for early changes in hips, knees, elbows and other large joints but can be very helpful in the assessment of damage in these joints in chronic disease. Radiographs of the cervical spine in flexion and extension can demonstrate C1–C2 subluxation; MRI is the preferred imaging technique to evaluate possible impingement on the spinal cord.

▶ Making the Diagnosis

Unfortunately, there is no one single finding on physical examination or laboratory testing that is diagnostic of RA. Instead, the diagnosis of RA is a clinical one, requiring a collection of historical and physical features, as well as an alert and informed clinician. While a history of arthralgias is important, the diagnosis of RA requires the objective evidence of joint inflammation (swelling or warmth or both) on examination.

In 1987 the American College of Rheumatology provided classification criteria that, although not designed specifically for the purpose, were widely used as an aid to diagnosis of RA (Table 15–3). The first five criteria are clinical; only the last two criteria require laboratory tests or radiographs. Of note the first four criteria need to be present for at least 6 weeks before a diagnosis of RA can be made. This time requirement was imposed because a number of conditions, most notably viral-related syndromes, can cause self-limited polyarthritis (generally of 2–4 week duration) indistinguishable from RA (Table 15–4). The 1987 classification criteria perform well for the diagnosis of

Table 15–3. 1987 American College of Rheumatology classification criteria for rheumatoid arthritis.

- Morning stiffness[a]
- Arthritis of three joint areas[a]
- Arthritis of the hands[a]
- Symmetric arthritis[a]
- Rheumatoid nodules
- Serum rheumatoid factor
- Radiographic changes

[a]These criteria must be present for more than 6 weeks.

established RA but are of limited usefulness for the diagnosis of early disease and do not incorporate testing for anti-CCP antibodies, which are highly specific for RA. In 2010 the American College of Rheumatology and the European League Against Rheumatism collaborated to develop new classification criteria with the explicit goal of improved sensitivity and specificity for early RA. The 2010 classification criteria, which require synovitis in at least one joint and the absence of a more plausible alternative diagnosis, use

Table 15–4. 2010 classification criteria for rheumatoid arthritis.

Criteria[a,b]	Score
A. Joint involvement	
1 large joint	0
2–10 large joints	1
1–3 small joints	3
>10 joints (at least 1 small joint)	4
B. Serology	
Negative RF and anti-CCP	0
Low-positive RF or anti-CCP	2
High-positive RF or anti-CCP	3
C. Acute-phase reactants	
Normal CRP and ESR	0
Abnormal CRP or ESR	1
D. Duration of symptoms	
<6 weeks	0
≥6 weeks	1

[a]Criteria apply only to patients who have objective signs of synovitis in at least 1 joint and who do not have a better alternative explanation for synovitis.

[b]A patient is classified as having rheumatoid arthritis if the sum of A–D is >6.

CRP, C-reactive protein; ESR, erythrocyte sedimentation rate; CCP, citrullinated peptides; RF, rheumatoid factor.

Adapted from Aletaha D, Neogi T, Silman AJ, et al. 2010 Rheumatoid arthritis classification criteria: an American College of Rheumatology/European League Against Rheumatism collaborative initiative. *Arthritis Rheum.* 2010;62:2569.

a composite scoring system based on four domains: (1) the number and site of affected joints; (2) the presence and level of anti-CCP antibodies and rheumatoid factor; (3) acute phase reactants (ESR and CRP); (4) duration of symptoms for more than 6 weeks (Table 15–4).

▶ Differential Diagnosis

Many diseases can mimic RA (Table 15–5). Accurate diagnosis of early RA can be particularly challenging. Acute viral syndromes, especially acute hepatitis B, erythrovirus (parvovirus B19), rubella (infection or vaccination), and Epstein-Barr virus can produce a polyarthritis that mimics early RA but is self-limited, usually resolving over 2–4 weeks. Atypical early presentations of RA can be difficult to distinguish from the initial stages of undifferentiated spondyloarthropathy, psoriatic arthritis, and reactive arthritis; a targeted history and examination may elucidate associated clinical features of these diseases, such as rash, oral ulcers, nail changes, dactylitis, and urethritis. There can be considerable clinical and serologic overlap between RA and systemic lupus erythematosus. Anti-Jo-1-positive polymyositis can present with an erosive polyarthritis, a positive test for serum rheumatoid factor, and minimal muscle symptoms. Chronic infection with hepatitis C commonly causes polyarthralgias (less often, polyarthritis) in a joint distribution similar to that of RA as well as serum rheumatoid factor (but not anti-CCP antibodies or radiographic erosions); RA and hepatitis C can coexist, causing diagnostic uncertainty. In the elderly with abrupt onset of polyarthritis, remitting seronegative symmetric synovitis with pitting edema (RS3PE), paraneoplastic syndromes, and drug-induced lupus should be considered. The diagnosis of chronic, deforming RA is usually obvious. However, chronic tophaceous gout can mimic severe nodular RA, and chondrocalcinosis can cause a destructive "pseudorheumatoid" arthropathy of the wrists and MCPs. Finally, OA with severe deformities of the hands from bony proliferation of the DIP and PIP joints (Heberden and Bouchard nodes) may confuse inexperienced clinicians; the keys here are DIP joint involvement and the bony, instead of soft tissue, joint abnormalities.

Table 15–5. Differential diagnosis.

Viral syndromes, especially hepatitis B and C, Epstein-Barr virus, erythrovirus (parvovirus), rubella
Psoriatic arthritis, reactive arthritis
Tophaceous gout
Systemic lupus erythematosus
Calcium pyrophosphate disease
Polymyalgia rheumatica
Paraneoplastic syndromes
Osteoarthritis, especially hereditary osteoarthritis of the hand
Sarcoidosis, Lyme disease, rheumatic fever, etc

▶ Complications

RA is a lifelong, progressive disease that can produce significant morbidity and premature mortality. Long-term studies have found that 50% of RA patients have had to stop working after 10 years (approximately 10 times the average rate). Patients who have anti-CCP antibodies, who are rheumatoid factor positive, or who have *HLADRB1* alleles expressing the shared epitope have a worse prognosis with more erosions and more extra-articular disease. Once deformities are found on examination or erosions on radiography, the damage is largely irreversible. Erosions develop in the majority of patients in the first 1 or 2 years of disease; early effective therapy clearly slows the rate of radiographic damage.

TREATMENT

For most patients, RA is a chronic disease requiring lifelong treatment. Fortunately, available therapies can be very effective, particularly if treatment is started early in the course of the disease.

Early RA appears to be a "window of opportunity" in which aggressive treatment with disease-modifying antirheumatic drugs (DMARDs) leads to better long-term outcomes. Therapy should be escalated to ensure maximal suppression of disease while making efforts to minimize toxicity and expense.

Therapeutic approaches should be more aggressive for patients with early RA and features of poor prognosis (eg, functional limitation, seropositivity for rheumatoid factor or anti-CCP antibodies, erosive disease on radiographs, extra-articular disease). In such cases, aggressive therapy is important because once deformities are present the mechanical component is refractory to medical therapy.

Because RA is a dynamic disease and because its therapeutic regimens are complex, it is essential that rheumatologists monitor patients.

▶ Pharmacotherapy

There are three broad categories of medications that are effective in managing RA: synthetic DMARDs (Table 15–6), biologic DMARDs (Table 15–7), and low-dose glucocorticoids. Almost all patients require more than one type of medication and, with rare exceptions, all patients should receive DMARD therapy. Optimal control of disease activity often requires combinations of different synthetic DMARDs or combinations of synthetic DMARDs and a biologic DMARD. Prior to starting DMARD therapy, patients should receive vaccinations (see recommendations of the American College of Rheumatology); live attenuated vaccines are contraindicated once individuals have started biologic DMARDs.

A. Synthetic DMARDs

Synthetic DMARDs are a group of medications that have the ability to modify or change the course of RA. Drugs

Table 15–6. Synthetic disease modifying antirheumatic drugs.

Methotrexate
Hydroxychloroquine
Sulfasalazine
Leflunomide
Minocycline

included in this class have, in most cases, met the "gold standard" of halting or slowing the radiographic progression of RA. The synthetic DMARDs in current use are methotrexate, sulfasalazine, hydroxychloroquine, leflunomide, and minocycline. These medications take 2–6 months to reach maximal effect. Therefore, other measures, such as low-dose glucocorticoid therapy, may be needed to control the disease while these medications are starting to work. The choice of synthetic DMARD depends on the activity of the disease, comorbid conditions, concerns about toxicity, and monitoring issues. Synthetic DMARDs are often used in combination with one another (most often, various combinations of methotrexate, sulfasalazine, and hydroxychloroquine) or with a biologic DMARD.

Methotrexate is the preferred synthetic DMARD of most rheumatologists. Many patients with RA have a durable, clinically meaningful response to methotrexate, which also slows radiographic progression of the disease. While effective as monotherapy, methotrexate also is the anchor drug in most successful combinations of synthetic DMARDs, and biologic agents are more effective when used concomitantly with methotrexate.

Methotrexate is administered as a **single dose once a week**, never on a daily basis (toxicity is substantially greater when the same amount of drug is administered on a daily basis rather than as a weekly pulse). The typical starting dose is 7.5 mg orally once a week; the dose then is increased by 2.5 mg to 7.5 mg increments as needed to a maximum of 20–25 mg. Oral absorption of methotrexate is variable; therefore, subcutaneous methotrexate may be effective if the response to oral methotrexate is suboptimal. Oral folate (1–4 mg daily) reduces side effects and should be administered concomitantly. Monitoring of blood cell counts, liver transaminase levels, and serum creatinine should be done every 12 weeks (every 2–4 weeks during initiation or after dose adjustments) for the duration of methotrexate therapy. Serious toxicities are rare with careful monitoring.

Contraindications to methotrexate include preexisting liver disease, infection with hepatitis B or C, ongoing alcohol use, and renal impairment (creatinine clearance <30 mL/minute). Oral ulcers, nausea, hepatotoxicity, bone marrow suppression, and pneumonitis are the most commonly encountered toxicities. With the exception of pneumonitis (which is a hypersensitivity reaction), these toxicities respond to dose adjustments and are reduced by the concomitant use of folic acid. Renal function is critical for clearance of methotrexate and its active metabolites; previously stable patients may experience severe toxicities when renal function deteriorates. Pneumonitis, while rare, is unpredictable and may be fatal, particularly if the methotrexate is not stopped or is restarted.

Hydroxychloroquine is frequently used for the treatment of RA, usually in combination with other synthetic DMARDs, particularly methotrexate. It has the least toxicity of any of the DMARDs but also is the least effective as monotherapy. Hydroxychloroquine is given orally at a dose of 200–400 mg daily. An uncommon but serious complication is retinal toxicity, which correlates with cumulative dose and can be prevented by regular screening. The risk of retinal

Table 15–7. Biologic disease-modifying antirheumatic drugs.

Agent	Structure	Target	Route of Administration
Infliximab	Chimeric mouse/human IgG1 mAb	TNF-α	Intravenous infusion
Etanercept	Fusion of human p75 TNF receptor and human IgG1 Fc	TNF-α Lymphotoxin	Subcutaneous injection
Adalimumab	Human IgG1 mAb	TNF-α	Subcutaneous injection
Golimumab	Human IgG1 mAb	TNF-α	Subcutaneous injection
Certolizumab pegol	Humanized Fab' linked to PEG	TNF-α	Subcutaneous injection
Abatacept	Fusion protein of human CTLA4 and Fc of human IgG1	CD80, CD86	Intravenous infusion or subcutaneous injection
Rituximab	Chimeric mouse/human IgG1 mAb	CD20	Intravenous infusion
Tocilizumab	Chimeric mouse/human IgG1 mAb	Interleukin-6 receptor	Intravenous infusion

PEG, polyethylene glycol.

toxicity increases substantially after 5–7 years of use or a cumulative dose of 1000 g. At a minimum, patients should have a baseline ophthalmologic examination within 1 year of initiation of hydroxychloroquine and annual screening examinations after 5 years of therapy. Earlier, more frequent screenings are indicated for patients with risk factors (daily dose >400 mg or >6.5 mg/kg ideal body weight for patients of short stature, kidney or liver dysfunction, other retinal disease, age >60 years).

Sulfasalazine is an effective treatment when given in doses of 1–3 g daily, often in combination with methotrexate, hydroxychloroquine, or both. Recommendations for laboratory monitoring are the same as for methotrexate.

Leflunomide, a pyrimidine antagonist, appears comparable in effectiveness to methotrexate. It is given daily in an oral dose of 10–20 mg and has a very long half-life. The most common toxicity is diarrhea, which may respond to dose reduction. Like methotrexate, leflunomide has hepatotoxicity, and recommendations for laboratory monitoring are the same as for methotrexate. Because leflunomide is teratogenic and has an exceptionally long half-life, women who have previously received leflunomide (even if therapy was years ago) should have blood levels drawn if they wish to become pregnant. Oral cholestyramine can rapidly eliminate leflunomide if toxicity occurs or if pregnancy is being considered.

Minocycline, 100 mg twice daily, is an effective treatment for RA, particularly when used in early seropositive disease. The mechanism of action in RA is uncertain but probably is independent of its antibacterial effects. Long-term therapy (more than 2 years) may lead to cutaneous hyperpigmentation.

B. Biologic DMARDs

Biologic DMARDs are bioengineered protein drugs (antibodies or receptor-antibody chimeras) and must be administered by subcutaneous injection or intravenous infusion (Table 15–7). Biologic DMARDs inhibit tumor necrosis factor-α (anti-TNF agents), deplete CD20+ B cells (rituximab), inhibit T-cell costimulation (abatacept), and block the receptor for interleukin-6 (tocilizumab). The efficacy of biologic DMARDs is well established. All reduce the signs and symptoms of synovitis—even in patients who have active disease despite treatment with methotrexate—and substantially diminish radiographic progression of RA. The onset of action of biologic DMARDs is rapid: days to weeks. All have greater efficacy when used in combination with methotrexate. The major disadvantages are cost and concerns about long-term toxicities.

An increased risk of infection is a concern with all biologic agents. All patients should be screened for latent tuberculosis with either a tuberculin skin test or an interferon-γ-release assay. Active tuberculosis or untreated latent tuberculosis is an absolute contraindication to the use of biologic DMARDs. Reactivation of latent tuberculosis has occurred within weeks of starting anti-TNF agents (particularly infliximab), which

also confer greatly increased risk of infection with other intracellular pathogens (eg, *Histoplasma capsulatum, Coccidioides immitis,* and *Listeria monocytogenes*). Biologic DMARDs should not be administered to patients with untreated hepatitis B infection.

There is a paucity of data regarding the use of biologic DMARDs in patients with a history of malignancy. Currently, biologic agents (except rituximab) are not recommended for patients with a solid malignancy or nonmelanoma skin cancer treated within 5 years, a history of treated skin melanoma, or a history of treated lymphoproliferative malignancy.

Anti-TNF agents should not be administered to patients with New York Heart Association class III or IV congestive heart failure or with ejection fractions less than 50%.

C. Glucocorticoids

Glucocorticoids in low doses (eg, prednisone 5–10 mg daily) can provide rapid, symptomatic improvement of articular disease and significantly slow the radiographic progression of RA. Glucocorticoids should be used rarely, if ever, as monotherapy for RA but can help control synovial inflammation while initiating therapy with the slow-acting synthetic DMARDs or when the response to DMARDs is suboptimal. The toxicities of long-term glucocorticoid therapy are considerable and are dose-dependent. Therefore, prednisone, the most commonly used glucocorticoid, generally should not be used in doses higher than 10 mg daily to treat articular disease and, after initiation of DMARD therapy, should be slowly tapered off or to the lowest effective dose. Long-term therapy with prednisone in doses of ≥7.5 mg/d orally is associated with an increased risk of both vertebral and hip fractures (see Chapter 58).

Nonsteroidal anti-inflammatory drugs (NSAIDs) play only a minor role, if any, in slowing progression of RA and, therefore, **should not be used as the sole therapy for RA**. The role of NSAIDs in RA is limited to symptomatic relief. The gastrointestinal toxicity of NSAIDs is a major issue for RA patients, who often have multiple risk factors for gastrointestinal toxicity. The use of protein pump inhibitors reduces the incidence of clinically significant gastrointestinal side effects.

Intra-articular injections of glucocorticoids (see Chapter 2) can suppress joint inflammation for several months and can be a useful addition to DMARD therapy, especially when there is residual activity in large joints (eg, wrists, knees). In many cases, patients benefit from consultation with physical and occupational therapists regarding range of motion exercises, joint protection, and assistive devices.

▶ Assessment of Disease Activity

Accurate assessment of disease activity by objective measures is essential to judge the effectiveness of treatment but

Table 15–8. Standardized assessments disease activity for rheumatoid arthritis.

Assessment	Components	Disease Activity by Numerical Score			
		Remission	Low	Moderate	High
PAS	Questionnaire Pain scale Patient global	≤0.25	0.26-3.7	3.71-<8.0	≥8.0
RAPID3	Questionnaire Pain scale Patient global	≤1.0	>1.0-2.0	>2.0-4.0	>4.0
CDAI	Patient global Physician global Swollen joints Tender joints	≤2.8	>2.8-10.0	>10.0-22.0	>22.0
SDAI	Patient global Physician global Swollen joints Tender joints CRP	≤3.3	>3.3-<11	11.0-≤26.0	>26.0
DAS28	Patient global Swollen joints Tender joints ESR or CRP	<2.6	>2.6-<3.2	≥3.2-≤5.1	>5.1

Joints examined: proximal phalangeal joints, interphalangeal joints of thumbs, metacarpophalangeal joints, wrists, elbows, shoulders, knees.
CRP, C-reactive protein; CDAI, clinical disease activity index; DAS28, disease activity score 28 joints; ESR, erythrocyte sedimentation rate; PAS, patient activity scale; RAPID, routine assessment of patient index data; SDAI, simplified disease activity index.

is a difficult task for a complex, systemic disorder such as RA. In practice, rheumatologists often gauge activity by their "clinical gestalt" which, in most cases, is heavily influenced by the results of the joint examination. However, the American College of Rheumatology recommends the use of standardized clinical assessments of disease activity to judge the effectiveness of treatment (Table 15–8). Several of these assessments are based solely on self-report (the Patient Activity Scale [PAS], and Routine Assessment of Patient Index [RAPID]) or on joint counts and visual analogue scales (the Clinical Disease Activity Index [CDAI]). Assessments such as the Disease Activity Scale 28 joints (DAS28) and the Simplified Disease Activity Index (SDAI) use joint counts and visual analogue scales but also incorporate a marker of inflammation (the ESR or CRP). Each assessment yields a numeric score and has cut points corresponding to remission and to low, moderate, and high disease activity (Table 15–8).

▶ Managing Comorbidities

Optimal care of patients with RA requires recognition of the comorbid conditions that are associated with RA. These include increased risk of cardiovascular death, osteoporosis, infections, and certain cancers.

The well-documented excess mortality (median life years lost: 8 years for males and 10 years for females) associated with RA is due largely to **cardiovascular disease** that is not explained by the traditional risk factors of family history, smoking history, hypertension, diabetes mellitus, and serum cholesterol levels. RA is a systemic inflammatory disease, and chronic systemic inflammation has complex, deleterious effects on lipoproteins and the vascular system. Effective treatment of RA appears to have a beneficial effect on the excess cardiovascular risk. Observational studies suggest that methotrexate and use of anti-TNF agents reduce cardiovascular events and mortality. In addition to RA-directed therapies, clinicians should aggressively address other cardiovascular risk factors (eg, hypertension, serum cholesterol) in these patients.

Osteoporosis is ubiquitous in patients with RA, and early therapy directed at this problem will result in long-term benefits. Patients with RA are at an increased risk for infections, including **septic arthritis** (almost always due to *Staphylococcus aureus*). The risk of infection is further increased by some therapies. Patients should be cautioned to seek medical attention early for even minor symptoms suggestive of infection, especially if receiving anti-TNF therapy. All patients with RA should receive pneumococcal and yearly influenza vaccinations (live attenuated viruses should not be administered to patients receiving biologic therapies). Finally, patients with RA have an increased risk of **lymphomas**. Occasionally, B-cell lymphomas may be associated with immunosuppression and regress after immunosuppression is discontinued. Interestingly, RA patients have significantly decreased risk (odds ratio = 0.2) of developing colon cancer. This is thought to be secondary to chronic inhibition of cyclooxygenase by the NSAIDs commonly used in this group of patients.

Aletaha D, Neogi T, Silman AJ, et al. 2010 Rheumatoid arthritis classification criteria: an American College of Rheumatology/European League Against Rheumatism collaborative initiative. *Arthritis Rheum.* 2010;62:2569. [PMID: 20872595]

[American College of Rheumatology] http://www.rheumatology.org

Saag KG, Teng GG, Patkar NM, et al. American College of Rheumatology. American College of Rheumatology 2008 recommendations for the use of nonbiologic and biologic disease-modifying antirheumatic drugs in rheumatoid arthritis. *Arthritis Rheum.* 2008;59:762. [PMID: 18512708]

Singh JA, Furst DE, Bharat A, et al. 2012 update of the 2008 American College of Rheumatology recommendations for the use of disease-modifying antirheumatic drugs and biologic agents in the treatment of rheumatoid arthritis. *Arthritis Care Res* (Hoboken). 2012;64:625. [PMID:22473917]

van der Linden MP, Knevel R, Huizinga TW, van der Helm-van Mil AH. Classification of rheumatoid arthritis: comparison of the 1987 American College of Rheumatology criteria and the 2010 American College of Rheumatology/European League Against Rheumatism criteria. *Arthritis Rheum.* 2011;63:37. [PMID: 20967854]

▼ EXTRA-ARTICULAR MANIFESTATIONS

Lester D. Miller, MD

Extra-articular disease develops in approximately one- third of patients with RA at some point in the course of their illness. The extra-articular manifestations of RA are diverse (Table 15–9) and range in clinical impact from the minor nuisance of a few isolated subcutaneous nodules to the life-threatening consequences of progressive interstitial pulmonary fibrosis and rheumatoid vasculitis. Extra-articular manifestations occur almost exclusively in patients who are seropositive for rheumatoid factor, and they often cluster together (eg, the co-occurrence of subcutaneous nodules and interstitial fibrosis). The incidence of extra-articular disease appears to be decreasing, probably as a result of the widespread use of aggressive therapy (eg, methotrexate in combination with anti-TNF agents) for early RA (see above). Nonetheless, extra-articular rheumatoid disease remains clinically important, and familiarity with its broad spectrum is critical for the appropriate management of the patient with RA.

Table 15–9. Extra-articular manifestations.

Dermatologic	Rheumatoid nodules with and without ulceration Periungual vasculitic infarcts Vasculitic leg ulcers Pyoderma gangrenosum (rare)
Mucosal	Sicca symptoms Ocular, oral, vaginal mucosa Sjögren syndrome
Ocular	Keratoconjunctivitis sicca Episcleritis Scleritis Scleromalacia perforans Peripheral ulcerative keratitis
Pulmonary	Nonspecific interstitial pneumonitis Usual interstitial pneumonitis Cryptogenic organizing pneumonitis Bronchiectasis Bronchiolitis obliterans Pleuritis and pleural effusion Rheumatoid nodulosis in the lungs Caplan syndrome
Cardiac	Pericarditis and pericardial effusion Constrictive pericarditis Valvular thickening and nodulosis Conduction abnormalities Coronary vasculitis Myocarditis
Hematologic and Lymphatic System	Anemia of chronic disease Felty syndrome Large granular lymphocyte leukemia Extremity lymphedema—unilateral or bilateral
Neurologic	Compression neuropathies Atlantoaxial subluxation Peripheral neuropathy Mononeuritis multiplex Rheumatoid pachymeningitis
Renal	AA amyloidosis Necrotizing crescentic glomerulonephritis (rare)

RHEUMATOID NODULES

ESSENTIALS OF DIAGNOSIS

► Usually manifest as subcutaneous nodules over pressure points.

► Strongly associated with rheumatoid factor.

Clinical Findings & Treatment

Subcutaneous nodules occur in 20–35% of patients with RA and are usually nontender, firm, and 1 cm or less in diameter. Subcutaneous nodules can be fixed or mobile and occur most frequently over pressure point areas such as the extensor aspect of the elbows, within the olecranon bursa, and over the Achilles tendon but also can overlie joints (Figure 15–5 and Plate 31). Nodulosis over the sacrum, ischial tuberosities, occipital region of the scalp, or borders of the scapulae may develop in bedridden patients. Rarely, nodules develop within organ systems including the scleral layer of the eye, heart valves, lung, on the dural surface of the brain, or in the larynx.

Rheumatoid nodules are strongly associated with rheumatoid factor (positive in >95% of cases). Recent epidemiologic studies demonstrate that patients with RA who smoke have a higher risk of developing nodules. Strongly seropositive individuals with nodulosis tend to carry a worse prognosis, with a higher propensity toward erosive and destructive rheumatoid disease.

The mimics of subcutaneous rheumatoid nodules include tophi, xanthomas, Garrod knuckle pads (fibrous nodules on the dorsal surfaces of the PIP joints of patients with Dupuytren contractures), the nodules of multicentric reticulohistiocytosis and, in children, the nodules of acute rheumatic fever. On clinical grounds alone, even experienced rheumatologists may be unable to distinguish RA with olecranon nodulosis from polyarticular gout with olecranon tophi. Excisional biopsy is sometimes necessary to establish the correct diagnosis. Rheumatoid nodules have characteristic—but not specific—histologic findings of central fibrinoid necrosis with a rim of palisading fibroblasts. Histologically, rheumatoid nodules are indistinguishable from granuloma annulare (dermal or subcutaneous nodules not associated with arthritis) or from "benign nodules" which occur exclusively in children

<18 years of age and are not associated with arthritis or with rheumatoid factor.

Subcutaneous rheumatoid nodules may resolve with effective therapy of the associated articular disease. A subset of rheumatoid patients, however, experience paradoxical **accelerated nodulosis with methotrexate therapy**. Nodules in these patients are often found over the extensor aspect of the MCP and PIP joints of the fingers. Methotrexate should be discontinued when there is extensive proliferation of nodules, particularly with ulceration of overlying skin. Unfortunately, there is no effective therapy for this situation. Most alternative DMARDs have been tried in these cases but with only occasional success.

Symptomatic subcutaneous nodules located over pressure points can be surgically removed. The effectiveness of this surgical approach, however, is limited by high rates of recurrence of nodules, poor wound healing, and secondary infection at the operative site, often with *S aureus*.

Rheumatoid nodules in the lung may be solitary or multiple, and some are necrotic. Isolated reports suggest a possible link between leflunomide therapy and necrotic pulmonary nodules. Distinguishing **rheumatoid pulmonary nodules** from carcinoma can be a particularly difficult problem, even after extensive imaging evaluation with computed tomography (CT) and positron emission tomographic scans. CT-guided biopsy is usually the only certain means of differentiating between these possibilities.

A variant of rheumatoid pulmonary nodulosis is **Caplan syndrome**. In 1953, Caplan described multiple rheumatoid nodules, some with cavitation, in the lungs of Welsh coal miners with RA. This pattern has also been reported in RA patients exposed to silica dust and asbestos, raising the question of whether Caplan syndrome is a combined "pneumoconiosis—RA" entity.

SJÖGREN SYNDROME

 ESSENTIALS OF DIAGNOSIS

▶ Dryness of eyes and mouth.

▶ The most common ocular manifestation of RA.

Clinical Findings

Approximately 30% of patients with RA have sicca symptoms due to secondary Sjögren syndrome. Mucosal dryness most commonly affects the mouth, the conjunctival surfaces of the eyes, and vagina. Dental caries, gingivitis, and accelerated tooth loss may occur due to the lack of adequate salivary lubrication. Patients frequently experience chronic "foreign body" sensations in their eyes, and women often develop recurrent monilial infections of the vaginal mucosa.

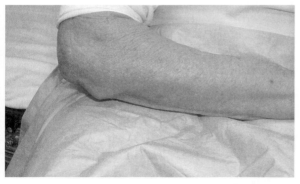

▲ **Figure 15–5.** A rheumatoid nodule in a typical location on the extensor surface of the forearm is apparent in this patient with seropositive, erosive rheumatoid arthritis.

Care must be exercised in distinguishing typical Sjögren symptoms from xerostomia due to medications, particularly antidepressants. Chronic hepatitis C infection, which can cause polyarthritis, sicca symptoms, and rheumatoid factor, also can mimic RA with secondary Sjögren syndrome. Occasionally, it is difficult to distinguish RA with secondary Sjögren syndrome from primary Sjögren syndrome with polyarthritis.

The diagnostic evaluations to establish xerophthalmia and xerostomia are those used for primary Sjögren syndrome (see Chapter 26). In contrast to primary Sjögren syndrome, antibodies to SS-A/Ro and to SS-B/La are not prevalent in the secondary Sjögren syndrome associated with RA.

Compared to patients with primary Sjögren syndrome, hypergammaglobulinemia, interstitial nephritis, and distal renal tubular acidosis uncommonly develop in patients with RA and secondary Sjögren syndrome. Additional rare complications include the development of non-Hodgkin large B cell lymphomas or mucosal associated lymphoid tumors (MALT).

▶ Treatment

Treatment of secondary Sjögren syndrome is symptomatic. Artificial tears or cyclosporine 0.05% emulsion drops twice daily can ease ocular symptoms. Pilocarpine hydrochloride 5 mg orally three to four times daily or cevimeline 30 mg three times daily may be effective in promoting increased salivary production but can cause hyperhidrosis.

OCULAR INFLAMMATION

ESSENTIALS OF DIAGNOSIS

- ▶ RA can cause episcleritis, scleritis, and peripheral ulcerative keratitis.
- ▶ Nodular scleritis and peripheral ulcerative keratitis threaten vision and require aggressive immunosuppressive therapy.

▶ Clinical Findings & Treatment

Keratoconjunctivitis sicca due to secondary Sjögren syndrome is the most common ocular manifestation of RA. However, RA also can cause ocular inflammation, leading to episcleritis, scleritis, and peripheral ulcerative keratitis.

Episcleritis, or inflammation of the episclera, manifests as a red eye due to hyperemia of this superficial ocular layer. Episcleritis produces irritation more than pain; it is not a vision-threatening condition. Episcleritis may be self-limited but is often treated with topical corticosteroid drops.

Of greater concern is inflammation of the sclera, the deeper, poorly vascularized layer of the eye. **Scleritis** is most commonly seen in patients who have had RA for 10 years or longer. Patients who are both rheumatoid factor and anti-CCP positive tend to have more intense ocular disease. Scleritis is a painful, persistent condition. The eye typically is deep red. With time, thinning of the sclera can occur, imparting a bluish hue from the underlying choroid. Scleritis can be complicated by rheumatoid nodules forming and enlarging within the scleral layer. Unchecked, scleritis can produce scleromalacia perforans and can threaten the structural integrity of the globe. Inadequate or unsuccessful treatment can lead to irreversible blindness. Nodular scleritis is an urgent ophthalmologic problem that requires initiation of immunosuppressive therapy, most often with cyclophosphamide in combination with high-dose oral prednisone (eg, 1 mg/kg/d).

An additional serious ocular complication of RA is **peripheral ulcerative keratitis** with "melting" of the corneal epithelial layers. Again, this is seen in long-standing RA, often accompanied by rheumatoid vasculitis or other serious extra-articular manifestations. Peripheral ulcerative keratitis must be aggressively treated with immunosuppression using high-dose glucocorticoids and often cyclophosphamide. If the inflammation is successfully ameliorated, a corneal transplant can be performed to salvage vision.

PULMONARY INTERSTITIAL FIBROSIS

ESSENTIALS OF DIAGNOSIS

- ▶ Risk factors include rheumatoid factor, male sex, and smoking.
- ▶ High-resolution CT is the imaging modality of choice.
- ▶ Nonspecific interstitial pneumonitis is glucocorticoid-responsive but usual interstitial pneumonitis is often refractory to therapy.

▶ General Considerations

Interstitial fibrosis of the lungs is one of the most dreaded complications of RA and often carries a guarded prognosis. The prevalence of clinically evident pulmonary fibrosis among RA patients is approximately 2–3%, and the prevalence of asymptomatic pulmonary fibrosis detected by high-resolution CT (HRCT) is substantially higher. The cumulative incidence of clinical pulmonary fibrosis approaches 10%.

▶ Clinical Findings & Treatment

Virtually all patients with interstitial fibrosis are seropositive for rheumatoid factor and have anti-CCP antibodies. Risk factors include male sex and smoking; patients often have subcutaneous nodules.

Dyspnea on exertion and nonproductive cough are the most common symptoms of interstitial fibrosis. On examination, there may be fine crackles at the bases. The chest radiograph may show an interstitial pattern but is inadequate for assessing the extent of pulmonary fibrosis. HRCT scanning is the current imaging gold standard. Pulmonary function tests reveal a restrictive defect and decreased diffusing capacity.

Nonspecific interstitial pneumonitis (NSIP) and usual interstitial pneumonitis (UIP) are the most common pathologic types of fibrosis encountered. NSIP has a more uniform distribution on plain radiographs and a "ground glass" appearance on HRCT. UIP has a more basilar distribution of fibrosis; HRCT scanning in UIP demonstrates honeycomb patterns and, frequently, traction bronchiectasis (Figure 15–6). If a biopsy is being considered, it is best to obtain a more robust specimen by video-assisted thoracoscopy because transbronchial biopsies through a flexible bronchoscope yield inadequate pathologic material. It is not uncommon to have equivocal or inconsistent interpretations of pulmonary biopsies as specimens may contain pathologic features of both NSIP and UIP.

NSIP is often responsive to glucocorticoids, but there are no current treatments capable of halting the progression of UIP. Nonetheless, most rheumatologists and pulmonologists will initiate a trial of oral prednisone (1 mg/ kg/d) regardless of the whether the pathology indicates UIP or NSIP. Prednisone is then tapered in accordance with the clinical picture and the results of serial pulmonary function tests, especially the diffusing capacity. There is little evidence for an ameliorative effect of anti-TNF agents on interstitial fibrosis.

Patients with preexisting interstitial lung disease may be at increased risk for methotrexate-induced pneumonitis—a hypersensitivity reaction to the drug. Because of this concern, many clinicians obtain a pretreatment chest radiograph and do not use methotrexate if there are radiographic signs of early interstitial lung disease.

OTHER PULMONARY MANIFESTATIONS OF RA

Cryptogenic organizing pneumonia produces a characteristic pattern on HRCT (multiple patches of consolidation in the subpleural areas) and is often responsive to glucocorticoids. Additional pulmonary complications of RA include **bronchiectasis**, which is present in approximately 3% of patients, and **bronchiolitis obliterans**, which is rare, is poorly responsive to therapy, and frequently leads to severe pulmonary compromise with hypoxia.

PLEURAL INVOLVEMENT

 ESSENTIALS OF DIAGNOSIS

▶ Rheumatoid pleurisy and pleural effusions can precede the articular manifestations of RA.

▶ Very low levels of pleural-fluid glucose are characteristic.

▶ Clinical Findings

Pleurisy or pleural effusion or both can be the initial manifestation of RA, preceding the onset of articular disease. This infrequent event occurs in approximately 1–3% of patients, most of whom are male. Analysis of pleural fluid is necessary to exclude malignancy, bacterial empyema, and infections with *Mycobacterium tuberculosis* and other granulomatous organisms; in some cases, a pleural biopsy is indicated as well. Rheumatoid pleural fluid is exudative and characterized by an extremely low level of pleural-fluid glucose, with the result frequently approaching zero. Some believe that a pleural-fluid glucose in this range is diagnostic of a rheumatoid effusion. The low glucose is thought to be secondary to a defect in glucose transport across the pleural membrane.

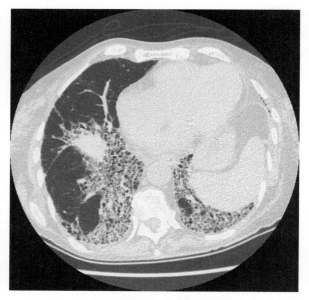

▲ **Figure 15–6.** Rheumatoid interstitial lung disease: usual interstitial pneumonitis.

Treatment

Treatment of rheumatoid pleuritis consists of moderate- to high-dose prednisone tapered in accordance with the clinical response. Pleurodesis or decortication may be required in unresponsive cases.

PERICARDIAL & CARDIAC INVOLVEMENT

Clinically evident **pericarditis** is uncommon in RA, but postmortem and echocardiographic examination reveal evidence of pericardial involvement in 30–50% of patients. Pericardial fluid shows findings similar to those of pleural fluid, notably a very low glucose. Rarely, pericardial involvement leads to **constrictive pericarditis**. This complication requires pericardiectomy with removal of the fibrotic and adherent pericardium. Additional cardiac involvement includes valvular thickening with nodules, valvular insufficiency, conduction abnormalities secondary to localized granulomatous inflammation, coronary vasculitis, and myocarditis. Advances in ultrasonography, particularly transesophageal echocardiography, have uncovered a higher prevalence of these cardiac abnormalities than previously recognized.

FELTY SYNDROME

 ESSENTIALS OF DIAGNOSIS

▶ Development of neutropenia and splenomegaly in long-standing seropositive RA.

▶ Increased risk of serious infection and of lower extremity ulcers due to rheumatoid vasculitis.

▶ Large granular lymphocytic leukemia present in 30% of patients.

General Considerations

In 1924, Augustus Felty, then a medical resident, described the co-occurrence of RA, splenomegaly, and neutropenia. Now uncommon, Felty syndrome develops in patients with long-standing (usually >10 years duration), erosive RA who are seropositive for rheumatoid factor and have anti-CCP antibodies.

Clinical Findings

The hallmarks of the syndrome are leukopenia (<4000 white blood cells/mcL), neutropenia (<1500 neutrophils/mcL), and splenomegaly. The hematologic components of the syndrome, however, can be present without frank splenomegaly. Approximately 30% of patients with Felty syndrome have large granular lymphocytic leukemia (see below). Chronic

neutropenia puts patients with Felty syndrome at risk for serious infections, but many patients remain asymptomatic.

Interestingly, patients with Felty syndrome often have synovitis that appears bland and "burnt out." However, these patients are far from inactive. About one-third have evidence of rheumatoid vasculitis with necrotic leg ulcers. Some are positive for perinuclear antineutrophil cytoplasmic antibodies (P-ANCA), anti-myeloperoxidase antibodies, and cryoglobulins.

Rarely, fibrosis develops in the hepatic portal system, which leads to portal hypertension, esophageal varices, congestive splenomegaly, and ascites. Ultrasound or CT imaging of the liver reveals "pseudotumors," which represent the pathologic lesion of nodular regenerative hyperplasia.

Treatment

Treatment of Felty syndrome is directed at the underlying RA, usually with standard oral doses of weekly methotrexate. In neutropenic patients considering surgery, such as a total joint arthroplasty, it may be necessary to enhance the neutrophil count by preoperative treatment with granulocyte colony-stimulating factor. Splenectomy can be performed in patients who have complications of neutropenia and who do not respond to DMARD therapy, but the results are not always long-lasting, with late recurrence of neutropenia.

LARGE GRANULAR LYMPHOCYTIC LEUKEMIA

A chronic, indolent form of leukemia due to clonal expansion of T lymphocytes that have the appearance of large granular lymphocytes (T-LGL leukemia) develops in approximately 1% of patients with long-standing RA. The complete blood count, which often is the initial clue to the presence of T-LGL leukemia, reveals neutropenia and a higher than expected percentage of lymphocytes relative to neutrophils (eg, a differential count showing 60% lymphocytes and 35% neutrophils). Approximately 30% of patients with Felty syndrome have T-LGL leukemia. The leukemic cells typically have the cell-surface phenotype $CD3^+CD8^+CD16^+CD57^+$; Southern blot analysis of T-cell receptor gene rearrangement confirms clonality. T-LGL leukemia patients may respond to low-dose oral methotrexate at standard doses (10–20 mg weekly) for the treatment of RA. Systemic infections remain the major potential danger to these patients.

LYMPHOMA

Non-Hodgkin lymphoma occurs 2–3 times more frequently in patients with RA than in the general population. RA itself is a risk factor for lymphoma, and the incidence of lymphoma increases in those with very active rheumatoid disease. The most frequently reported form is diffuse large B-cell lymphoma. Development of B-cell lymphomas, particularly those linked to Epstein-Barr virus, is a rare complication of methotrexate therapy for RA. The use of anti-TNF agents is associated with slightly increased risk of lymphoma, but a cause and effect relationship has not been established.

RHEUMATOID VASCULITIS

ESSENTIALS OF DIAGNOSIS

▶ A complication of long-standing seropositive RA.

▶ Most common form is a smoldering small-vessel vasculitis leading to nailbed infarctions.

▶ Less common is a medium vessel vasculitis that can cause digital ischemia and mononeuritis multiplex.

▶ Rarely, rheumatoid vasculitis can have a course similar to polyarteritis nodosa.

▶ General Considerations

Rheumatoid vasculitis, like other serious extra-articular manifestations of RA, typically develops after 10–15 years of disease and occurs almost exclusively in patients who are seropositive for rheumatoid factor and have anti-CCP antibodies. It affects approximately 1–3% of patients.

▶ Clinical Findings

The most common form of rheumatoid vasculitis is a smoldering small-vessel vasculitis that produces painless nailbed infarctions (Plate 32), usually in patients with nodular disease. This form of rheumatoid vasculitis usually does not reflect life-threatening systemic vasculitis and can be managed by more aggressive treatment with DMARDs.

Less often, RA causes a medium-vessel vasculitis whose clinical manifestations include necrotic leg ulcers (Plate 33), digital gangrene, and mononeuritis multiplex. Rarely, a systemic necrotizing arteritis develops, which is indistinguishable from polyarteritis nodosum and can lead to infarction of small or large bowel. The ESR and levels of serum CRP are almost always elevated. ANCAs, cryoglobulinemia, and hypocomplementemia are sometimes present. Initial treatment consists of high doses of glucocorticoids and, often, cyclophosphamide. There are reports of successful treatment of refractory cases with rituximab, but more data are required.

NEUROLOGIC MANIFESTATIONS

The most common neurologic complications of RA are compression neuropathies, particularly compression of the median nerve at the wrist (carpal tunnel syndrome)

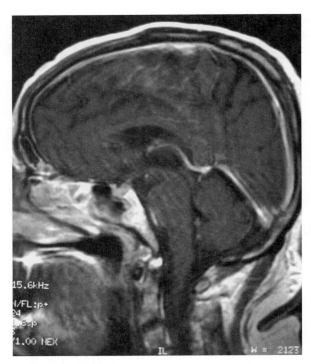

▲ **Figure 15–7.** Magnetic resonance imaging with gadolinium revealing prominent meningeal enhancement of rheumatoid pachymeningitis.

and compression of the ulnar nerve at the elbow or wrist. Rheumatoid vasculitis can cause mononeuritis multiplex and a mixed motor-sensory peripheral neuropathy. Atlantoaxial subluxation and basilar invagination can produce cervical myelopathy and brainstem compression. An unusual complication of RA is pachymeningitis—inflammation and thickening of dura mater—which presents as a clouded sensorium, cranial nerve abnormalities, and retardation of motor activity (Figure 15–7). Once an infectious etiology has been excluded, pachymeningitis is treated vigorously with glucocorticoids and appropriate DMARDs.

RENAL MANIFESTATIONS

In general, the kidney is spared in RA, and renal impairment in RA patients is most often due to drug toxicity (especially NSAIDs) or to comorbidities such as hypertension or diabetes mellitus. There are, however, rare cases of pauci-immune, necrotizing crescentic glomerulonephritis complicating RA, usually in patients who have P-ANCAs and evidence of extra-renal vasculitis. Renal amyloidosis is a rare complication of long-standing RA.

AMYLOIDOSIS

Although amyloidosis has been detected in approximately 6% of RA patients at autopsy, it is rare for amyloidosis to be a dominant clinical feature of RA. Amyloidosis in RA is type AA, which is a cleavage product of serum amyloid A (SSA). Systemic inflammation in RA leads to increased production of SSA by the liver, mediated in large part by interleukin-6. The diagnosis, clinical course, and treatment of AA amyloid are reviewed in Chapter 57.

PYODERMA GANGRENOSUM

Pyoderma gangrenosum is an ulcerative neutrophilic dermatitis of unknown cause. It occurs in less than 1% of patients with RA and usually manifests a lower-extremity, deep ulcer with purplish, overhanging borders. Initial therapy most commonly involves glucocorticoids; there are some reports of success with anti-TNF agents and with cyclosporine.

LYMPHEDEMA

On rare occasions, lymphedema of the extremities presents in patients with RA. Surprisingly, the lymphedema can be unilateral as well as bilateral. This painful condition can affect an entire upper or lower extremity. Some patients have been studied with lymphangiography, which demonstrates obstruction in the deep lymphatics. The etiology of the obstruction is unclear, but it may be the consequence of an underlying lymphangitis. Compression bandaging and massage may be helpful, together with the initiation of DMARD therapy.

Baecklund E, Iliadou A, Askling J, et al. Association of chronic inflammation, not its treatment, with increased lymphoma risk in rheumatoid arthritis. *Arthritis Rheum.* 2006;54:692. [PMID: 16508929]

Hochberg MC, Johnston SS, John AK. The incidence and prevalence of extra-articular and systemic manifestations in a cohort of newly-diagnosed patients with rheumatoid arthritis between 1999–2006. *Curr Med Res Opin.* 2008;24:469. [PMID: 18179735]

Kim DS. Interstitial lung disease in rheumatoid arthritis: recent advances. *Curr Opin Pulm Med.* 2006;12:346. [PMID: 16926650]

Yamamoto T. Cutaneous manifestations associated with rheumatoid arthritis. *Rheumatol Int.* 2009;29:979. [PMID: 19242695]

Young A, Koduri G. Extra-articular manifestations and complications of rheumatoid arthritis. *Best Pract Res Clin Rheumatol.* 2007;21:907. [PMID: 17870035]

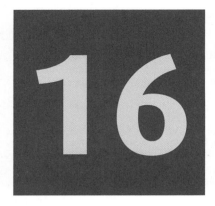

Adult-Onset Still Disease

John B. Imboden, MD

ESSENTIALS OF DIAGNOSIS

▶ Quotidian fever, frequently >39°C.

▶ Evanescent, salmon-colored macular rash on trunk and extremities, often coincident with fever spikes.

▶ Clinical manifestations include pharyngitis, polyarthralgias, lymphadenopathy, splenomegaly, and serositis.

▶ Leukocytosis and elevations of the erythrocyte sedimentation rate, serum C-reactive protein, and serum ferritin are common laboratory abnormalities.

▶ General Considerations

Adult-onset Still disease (AOSD) is a multisystem inflammatory disease of unknown cause. It affects women and men equally and is rare, with a reported incidence of 0.16 cases per 100,000 in one series. AOSD typically begins in the late teenage to early adult years, but disease onset occurs after the age of 35 in approximately 25% of patients. The onset of AOSD is systemic, with fever and rash; however, the subsequent disease course is variable. AOSD may consist of single (monocyclic) or recurrent (polycyclic) episodes of systemic disease lasting weeks to months. Alternatively, chronic articular disease, with or without recurrent systemic flares, may follow the initial systemic episode. Pediatric patients with systemic-onset juvenile idiopathic arthritis can have a recurrence of active Still disease at any age into adulthood. There are no definitive laboratory findings or diagnostic histologic abnormalities. The diagnosis is made on clinical grounds and often is one of exclusion (Table 16–1).

▶ Clinical Findings

A. Symptoms and Signs

1. Fever—Fever is a hallmark of AOSD. Typically, the fever is quotidian, with spikes to ≥39°C (often in the afternoon or

evening) followed by return to normal temperature in the absence of antipyretic medications. Shaking chills and sweating can accompany these daily temperature swings, which can be as high as 4°C. Occasionally, the fever is double quotidian (two spikes daily). In a small percentage of patients, a low-grade baseline fever persists between spikes. Untreated, the fever of AOSD is relentless, frequently lasting weeks at a time. Constitutional symptoms of profound fatigue, weight loss, and anorexia are common.

2. Rash—The rash of AOSD is a salmon-colored, macular or maculopapular eruption (Plate 34). Occasionally, it has an urticarial appearance. The rash usually affects the trunk and the extremities and spares the face, palms, and soles. It is evanescent, often appearing during febrile episodes and then clearing when the temperature returns to normal. The rash of AOSD usually is asymptomatic, but it may be mildly pruritic. Scratching uninvolved skin can elicit the rash (Koebner phenomenon). Biopsy of involved skin reveals a neutrophilic infiltration of the dermis and perivascular spaces; these histologic findings are not specific for AOSD and can be seen with urticaria of any cause, cellulitis, and other conditions.

3. Pharyngitis—A sore throat due to nonsuppurative pharyngitis is often the earliest symptom of AOSD and may precede fever, rash, and arthralgias by days to weeks.

4. Arthritis—Marked polyarthralgias are common at the onset of AOSD and usually occur without clinically detectable joint inflammation. With time, however, synovitis can develop, particularly in large joints (the hips, knees, ankles, shoulders and wrists) and less often in the small joints of the hands and feet. Articular involvement can persist after resolution of fever and leads to a chronic, destructive arthritis in approximately 20% of patients with AOSD.

5. Lymphadenopathy—Lymphadenopathy (particularly of cervical nodes) and splenomegaly are present in approximately 50% of patients at the time of initial presentation. Fine-needle aspirates and excisional biopsies of affected nodes reveal reactive hyperplasia.

Table 16–1. Yamaguchi classification criteria for adult-onset Still disease.

Major criteria	Fever ≥39°C, intermittent, lasting 1 week or more Arthralgias or arthritis lasting 2 weeks or more Characteristic rash WBC ≥10,000/mcL with neutrophils ≥80%
Minor criteria	Pharyngitis or sore throat Lymphadenopathy Hepatomegaly or splenomegaly Liver enzyme abnormalities Negative tests for rheumatoid factor and antinuclear antibodies
Exclusion criteria	Absence of infection Absence of malignant diseases Absence of inflammatory disease

Classification as adult-onset Still disease requires the presence of five or more criteria, of which at least two must be major criteria.

WBC, white blood cell count.
Data from Yamaguchi M, Ohta A, Tsunematsu T, et al. Preliminary criteria for classification of adult Still's disease. *J Rheumatol.* 1992;19:424–430.

6. Miscellaneous—Most patients have **myalgias**, but weakness is uncommon. **Serositis** leading to symptomatic pleuritis or pericarditis occurs in a sizeable minority. **Hepatomegaly** is less common than elevations of the serum hepatic transaminases.

B. Laboratory Findings

No laboratory finding, or combination of test results, is diagnostic for AOSD. However, several nonspecific laboratory abnormalities are characteristic of active AOSD. Most patients (>80%) have a leukocytosis that is neutrophil-predominant and often exceeds 15,000 cells/mcL. Virtually all patients have an elevated erythrocyte sedimentation rate and an elevated level of serum C-reactive protein. A modest normochromic normocytic anemia ("anemia of chronic disease"), low serum albumin, and mild elevations of serum hepatic transaminases are common. Only a minority of patients have thrombocytosis. Typically, the serum creatinine and urinalysis are normal. Tests for antinuclear antibodies and rheumatoid factor are negative in almost all cases. Serum complement levels are normal or elevated.

Most patients with AOSD (>90%) have elevated levels of serum ferritin, and very high levels (>10,000 mcg/L) occur in approximately 30%. The proportion of serum ferritin that is glycosylated is often lower (<20%) in AOSD than in other conditions associated with elevated levels of serum ferritin, but measurements of glycosylated ferritin are not routinely available in clinical practice.

Differential Diagnosis

The initial presentation of AOSD presents a diagnostic challenge, even for the experienced clinician. The diagnosis of AOSD is clinical, but the major manifestations of AOSD (fever, rash, polyarthralgia) also occur in a wide range of infectious, neoplastic, and immune-mediated disorders (Table 16–2). The incorporation of exclusions into the classification criteria for AOSD underscores the difficulty of diagnosis (Table 16–1).

Clinical features that are atypical for AOSD should always raise "red flags." AOSD rarely causes rash that is intensely pruritic or that affects the face. Fever patterns should be observed in the absence of antipyretic medications. The intermittent administration of antipyretic medications to a patient with a hectic fever (uncommon in AOSD) can produce a spiking fever that is more consistent with AOSD.

The patient's history and physical examination findings as well as results of laboratory studies, serologic tests, and cultures usually narrow the diagnostic possibilities considerably.

Table 16–2. Differential diagnosis of adult-onset Still disease.

Category	Examples
Malignancy	Hodgkin disease Non-Hodgkin lymphoma Renal cell carcinoma
Acute viral infections	Adenovirus Erythrovirus (parvovirus B19) Rubella Epstein-Barr virus Cytomegalovirus Hepatitis B HIV
Other infections	Acute Lyme disease Secondary syphilis Brucellosis Relapsing fever Chronic meningococcemia Subacute bacterial endocarditis Miliary tuberculosis Acute fungal infections (histoplasmosis, coccidioidomycosis, blastomycosis)
Postinfectious disorders	Acute rheumatic fever Poststreptococcal arthritis Reactive arthritis
Autoimmune diseases	Systemic lupus erythematosus Systemic vasculitides
Hereditary periodic fever syndromes	Tumor necrosis factor receptor- associated periodic syndrome
Miscellaneous	Drug hypersensitivity Reactive hemophagocytic syndromes Schnitzler syndrome

However, the exclusion of occult malignancy can be particularly difficult. There should be a low threshold for CT imaging of the chest, abdomen, and pelvis. Because Hodgkin and non-Hodgkin lymphomas can be remarkable mimics of AOSD, enlarged lymph nodes should be subjected to fine-needle aspiration and, in some cases, excisional biopsy.

▶ Treatment

Most patients with AOSD require systemic glucocorticoids (eg, oral prednisone in doses up to 1 mg/kg/day) for treatment of fever and other debilitating symptoms. During the initial diagnostic evaluation, nonsteroidal anti-inflammatory drugs (NSAIDs) can reduce fever, joint pain, and muscle aches, but few patients with AOSD have an adequate response to NSAIDs as monotherapy. NSAIDs can cause marked elevations in serum transaminases in patients with AOSD.

Oral methotrexate (7.5–20 mg once a week) is commonly used for AOSD that is refractory to glucocorticoids. Methotrexate also can facilitate tapering of glucocorticoids and is used to manage chronic articular disease. There is increasing use of biologic therapies, particularly anakinra and tocilizumab, for refractory AOSD. Inhibitors of tumor necrosis factor appear to have efficacy, but observational studies suggest that the responses are partial. Cyclosporine and intravenous immunoglobulin are sometimes used in refractory disease.

Therapy should be continued until resolution of clinical disease and laboratory parameters show no signs of inflammation. Medication can then be tapered slowly with the hope of maintaining a remission on the lowest effective dose. Methotrexate and other disease modifying agents should be continued for a 1-year disease-free interval before being discontinued altogether.

▶ Complications

Reactive hemophagocytic syndrome (macrophage activation syndrome) is a life-threatening manifestation of AOSD. The syndrome closely resembles virus-associated and familial hemophagocytic lymphohistiocytosis. Like these disorders, it is associated with the proliferation and activation of nonmalignant histiocytes, the overproduction of cytokines, and hemophagocytosis in the bone marrow and other sites.

Clinically, reactive hemophagocytic syndrome shares features with monocyclic systemic AOSD (ie, fever ≥39°C, rash, pharyngitis, lymphadenopathy, hepatosplenomegaly), but patients frequently are critically ill with hypotension, neurologic abnormalities, acute renal failure, acute liver injury, or coagulopathy (or any combination of these). Cytopenias and markedly elevated levels of serum ferritin are the laboratory hallmarks of reactive hemophagocytic syndrome. In particular, the presence of leukopenia or thrombocytopenia (or both) in the setting of systemic AOSD should raise the possibility of reactive hemophagocytic syndrome and serves to distinguish this entity from typical systemic AOSD, which is associated with leukocytosis and normal or elevated platelet counts. Diagnosis requires bone marrow aspiration and biopsy, which demonstrate hemophagocytosis by activated macrophages and histiocytes in nearly all cases. Treatment is empiric and usually consists of high doses of glucocorticoids (administered initially as pulses of intravenous methylprednisolone) in conjunction with intravenous immunoglobulin.

▶ Prognosis

The clinical course of AOSD is variable. Remission occurs in one-third of patients after one extended symptomatic period that can last up to 1 year. In another third of patients, AOSD has a polycyclic course. In these patients, relapses can occur years after the initial episode with remissions between flares. Another third of patients with AOSD have a persistent active clinical course with chronic active arthritis being the main ongoing symptom.

Chen PD, Yu SL, Chen S, Weng XH. Retrospective study of 61 patients with adult-onset Still's disease admitted with fever of unknown origin in China. *Clin Rheumatol.* 2011 Jul 20. [Epub ahead of print] [PMID: 21773715]

Hot A, Toh ML, Coppéré B, et al. Reactive hemophagocytic syndrome in adult-onset Still disease: clinical features and long-term outcome: a case-control study of 8 patients. *Medicine (Baltimore).* 2010;89:37. [PMID: 20075703]

Kim HA, Sung JM, Suh CH. Therapeutic responses and prognosis in adult-onset Still's disease. *Rheumatol Int.* 2011 Jan 29. [Epub ahead of print] [PMID: 21274538]

Kong XD, Xu D, Zhang W, Zhao Y, Zeng X, Zhang F. Clinical features and prognosis in adult-onset Still's disease: a study of 104 cases. *Clin Rheumatol.* 2010;29:1015. [PMID: 20549276]

Ankylosing Spondylitis & the Arthritis of Inflammatory Bowel Disease

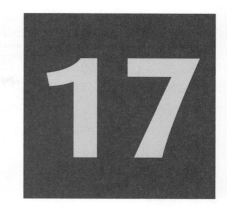

17

Marzouq Awni Qubti, MD

John A. Flynn, MD, MBA

SPONDYLOARTHRITIS

The term "spondyloarthritis" is used to describe an overlapping group of diseases that are characterized by inflammation of the sacroiliac joints (sacroiliitis); axial spine (spondylitis); tendon, fascia, and ligament insertion sites (enthesitis); and, in some patients, an oligoarthritis, rash, or inflammatory eye disease (uveitis). This group of diseases has also been referred to as seronegative spondyloarthritis based on the absence of rheumatoid factor. These diseases include ankylosing spondylitis, psoriatic arthritis, the arthritis of inflammatory bowel disease, and reactive arthritis. Although these conditions share common features, each one has distinct clinical and epidemiologic characteristics (Table 17–1). However, in some patients, especially early in the disease presentation, the diagnosis is not clear; these patients are considered to have undifferentiated spondyloarthritis. The overall prevalence of these conditions has been estimated to be between 0.5% and 1.5%.

The entheses are an important site of inflammation and subsequent pathology in spondyloarthritis. These are locations where tendons, fascia, and ligaments insert into bone. Clinical manifestations include heel pain with involvement of the Achilles tendon, foot pain at the site of insertion of the plantar aponeurosis, or swelling of an entire digit (dactylitis or sausage digit) due to inflammation of the flexor and extensor tendons of the fingers or toes.

Histologically, the synovial inflammation in spondyloarthritis is characterized by chronic inflammatory infiltrates that are nonspecific and indistinguishable from that of rheumatoid arthritis. While erosive bone disease does occur, unlike the rheumatoid process, this inflammatory process is also accompanied by new bone formation across previous articulations. This ossification of the articular and ligamentous structures of the spine leads to syndesmophyte formation and may result in eventual fusion and characteristic radiographic findings.

The dominant clinical problems that bring the patient with spondyloarthritis to a clinician and require careful management over many years are axial pain, limitation of motion, and deformity of the spine. In all forms of spondyloarthritis, the same principles of diagnosis and management of the axial problem apply with attention directed to the cutaneous, gastrointestinal, ocular, and peripheral articular manifestations of the primary disorder.

ANKYLOSING SPONDYLITIS

ESSENTIALS OF DIAGNOSIS

▶ Inflammatory back pain in young adults.
▶ Radiographic demonstration of sacroiliitis.
▶ Reductions in spinal mobility, particularly lumbar flexion.
▶ Association with anterior uveitis.
▶ Increased relative risk conferred by inheritance of HLA-B27.
▶ Positive family history.

▶ General Considerations

The pathogenesis of spinal inflammation is unknown; however, there is a strong hereditary component marked by the only known susceptibility gene, HLA-B27. This genetic marker is strongly associated with sacroiliitis and spondylitis regardless of clinical setting. More than 85% of patients with ankylosing spondylitis have HLA-B27. The prevalence of ankylosing spondylitis parallels the frequency of HLA-B27 in different populations in the United States and in other regions of the world. This gene occurs in 8–10% of white Americans, and the disease occurs in 0.1–0.2% of that population. Blacks have a much lower frequency of both disease and the HLA-B27 gene. On the other hand, there is a high frequency of spondylitis and of HLA-B27 in certain Native American and Eskimo groups. Ankylosing spondylitis is

Table 17–1. Clinical and epidemiologic features of spondyloarthritis.

	Ankylosing Spondylitis	Psoriatic Arthritis	Reactive Arthritis	Enteropathic Arthritis
Prevalence	0.1%	<1% 5–20% in psoriasis patients	0.03–0.05%	<0.1% 20% in IBD patients
Male:female ratio	3:1	1:1	Enterogenic source M:F 1:1 Urogenital source: predominantly male	1:1

Axial arthritis
  Frequency
  Radiographic features
    Sacroiliitis
    Syndesmophytes
	
	100%
	
	Symmetric
	Bilateral
	Marginal
		
		20%
		
		Asymmetric
		Unilateral
		Bulky
			
			20%
			
			Asymmetric
			Unilateral
			Bulky
				
				10–15%
				
				Symmetric
				Bilateral
				Marginal

Peripheral arthritis
  Frequency
  Distribution
 	
  Joints affected
	
	50%
	Oligoarticular,
	  monoarticular
	Hip, shoulder, knee
		
		60–90%
		Oligoarticular,
		  polyarticular
		Hands including DIP, knee
			
			90%
			Oligoarticular,
			  monoarticular
			Knee, ankle
				
				5–20%
				Oligoarticular,
				  monoarticular
				Knee, ankle

Uveitis	25–40%	15%	15–20%	5%
Dactylitis	Uncommon	20–30%	30–50%	Uncommon
Cutaneous findings	None	Psoriasis Nail pitting Onycholysis	Oral ulcers, Circinate balanitis, Keratoderma blennorrhagica	Erythema nodosum, Pyoderma gangrenosum

HLA positivity
  All patients
  With axial disease
	
	85–90%
	85–90%
		
		30%
		50%
			
			50–80%
			90%
				
				20–30%
				50–60%

DIP, distal interphalangeal; IBD, inflammatory bowel disease.

common in Europeans and most Asian groups but is found rarely in Japanese, again reflecting the relative frequency of the B27 marker. If normal persons with HLA-B27 are carefully assessed, clinical or radiographic evidence of disease can be found in only 2%.

The typical patient with ankylosing spondylitis is a young white man under the age of 40 years (Table 17–2). Occasionally, the diagnosis is made in older patients, but careful questioning often reveals that symptoms began years earlier. The impression that women are affected less often than men (ratio 1:3) may be caused by underrecognition of the disease in

women. The initial symptoms of the disorder in women may include more peripheral joint or cervical spine involvement. Therefore, one should be mindful of these differences between men and women and must consider an emerging process in young women in whom arthritis presents.

▶ **Clinical Findings**

A. Symptoms and Signs

1. Axial spine—The usual presenting symptom of ankylosing spondylitis is inflammatory back pain. The pain and stiffness are in the low back or deep within the buttocks. This discomfort begins insidiously, and the patient would typically have noticed this for several months to several years before seeking medical attention. Unlike mechanical low back syndromes, the pain and stiffness of inflammatory disease are usually worsened by rest and improved by exercise. The patient may be unable to sleep through the night or sit for prolonged periods and must arise and stretch to obtain relief, with morning stiffness lasting greater than 30 minutes. As in discogenic disease, however, symptoms of shooting pains into the buttocks and down the posterior or lateral thighs may occur and mimic sciatica. These pains are usually

Table 17–2. Clues to early ankylosing spondylitis.

A young man (less often a woman) with inflammatory back symptoms
Pain/stiffness in buttocks, low back, chest wall worst with rest and
  better with exercise
Reduced spinal mobility
Family history of ankylosing spondylitis
Oligoarticular/monoarticular large joint involvement (hips and
  shoulders)
History of eye pain, redness, blurry vision that may have been
  diagnosed as anterior uveitis

Table 17–3. Physical examination in ankylosing spondylitis.

Sacroiliac joints	Thoracic spine
Tenderness	Increased kyphosis
Pain with compression/stress	Tenderness
Lumbar spine	Pain with rib cage compression
Tenderness	Decreased chest expansion
Paravertebral muscle spasm	(<2.5 cm)
Loss of lordosis	Cervical spine
Decreased flexion: Schober	Tenderness
test (<5 cm)	Pain on motion
Decreased lateral motion and	Muscle spasm
extension	Decreased motion
Hips, shoulders	Kyphosis, decreased lordosis
Pain on motion	Occiput to wall distance
Decreased range of motion	

transient, may alternate to the opposite side and are not associated with any demonstrable neurologic deficits. There are few measurable abnormalities in patients with early disease (Table 17–3). In fact, the patient with sacroiliitis may have an entirely normal physical examination despite significant symptoms of pain and stiffness in the low back region, contributing to delays in diagnosis. At most, there may be tenderness on direct palpation of these joints in the buttocks or on compression of the pelvis.

Abnormalities that eventually appear in the patient with progressive disease relate to loss of range of motion and deformity in mobile structures. The patient with lumbar involvement has often lost the normal lordosis, and there is flattening of that segment of the back. In addition, there is loss in range of motion when the patient attempts to bend forward. It should be recalled that hip motion accounts for 90 degrees of the flexion of the trunk on the lower extremities and that the lumbar spine provides the remaining stretch by reversing its lordosis and becoming kyphotic. An objective measurement of lumbar motion is the **Schober test.** With the patient standing erect, a horizontal line is drawn at the L5–S1 region at the level of the sacral dimples and another line 10 cm above that in the midline of the back. With forward flexion, the distance between these two ends of the 10-cm line should increase from 10 cm to 15 cm in the normal lumbar spine. A modified Schober test is negative if the distance between the 5 cm mark below the sacral dimples and the 10 cm above it increases to 20 cm on forward flexion. Lateral lumbar flexion is assessed by having the patient bend laterally without flexing forward or bending the knees, with measurements scored between the middle finger and the floor. A difference of >10 cm from start to end positions is normal. These tests are best applied and interpreted in the young patient because lumbar motion normally decreases with age.

Involvement of the thoracic spine is determined subjectively by the patient's description of pain or stiffness in that region and by demonstrable tenderness along the vertebral column and paravertebral muscles. Compression of the rib cage laterally and over the sternum may also elicit discomfort. Objective determination of fusion of the costovertebral joints is obtained by measuring the chest expansion. A tape measure is placed around the patient's chest wall at the nipple line or fourth intercostal space, and the change in circumference from full expiration to full inspiration is measured. Less than 2.5 cm is considered abnormal.

The range of motion of the cervical spine should be determined; extension, right and left rotation, lateral flexion, and forward flexion should be measured. Loss of extension is usually the earliest abnormality, and as the disease progresses, fixed deformity in the forward flexed position tends to develop. Developing cervical kyphosis is assessed by the occiput-to-wall measurement. The patient places both heels against the base of the wall and attempts to extend the neck fully to touch the wall with the back of the head. If this is accomplished readily, then extension measurement is normal.

2. Peripheral arthritis—Although peripheral small joints (hands and feet) are uncommonly affected, the root joints (hips and shoulders) eventually become involved in nearly 50% of patients. Occasionally, involvement of the back may be entirely asymptomatic, and the patient seeks medical attention only when the disease reaches the hips or shoulders. Examination of the range of motion and elicitation of any pain on motion of both shoulders and hips is important. Spondyloarthritis may present as a pauciarticular juvenile form of arthritis with asymmetric lower extremity involvement and enthesitis. The usual age of presentation is close to 10 years, but cases have been reported in patients as young as 6 years.

3. Enthesitis—Chronic inflammatory enthesitis in the spine is a first step to spinal fusion and ankylosis. Enthesitis of costosternal joints leads to chest wall pain that can mimic pleuritic, pericardial, or anginal pain syndromes. Pain in the heels either at the Achilles tendon insertion or over the attachment of the plantar aponeurosis in the sole of the foot develops in approximately 10% of patients with ankylosing spondylitis. Swelling is not always apparent in these areas, but tenderness to direct palpation is found.

4. Ocular—Acute anterior uveitis occurs in approximately 30% of patients with ankylosing spondylitis and does not necessarily parallel the course of the articular disease. It may be the sentinel symptom. Its onset is usually abrupt and unilateral, with intense pain, redness, and photophobia as the cardinal symptoms. Immediate ophthalmologic attention is required to prevent serious damage to the anterior chamber of the eye. Topical corticosteroids are usually successful in treating an acute episode.

5. Cardiac—Heart abnormalities occur in less than 5% of patients with ankylosing spondylitis. The most common, first-degree atrioventricular block, can be determined only electrocardiographically. A history of palpitations or syncope and the finding of a slow or irregular pulse on examination should alert the clinician to higher degrees of atrioventricular block. A cardiac pacemaker may be required for serious arrhythmias or complete atrioventricular dissociation. Aortic regurgitation caused by inflammatory thickening of the aortic valve and root is another serious cardiac complication. Once the diastolic murmur becomes apparent, cardiac decompensation requiring valve replacement can develop within 1–2 years.

6. Neurologic—The cauda equina syndrome is a rare but serious neurologic complication of ankylosing spondylitis. It is believed to be related to entrapment of exiting lumbar and sacral nerves through the inflamed spinal column. Compressive inflammatory lesions within the spinal column may be found in some cases. Patients with ankylosing spondylitis should be asked regularly about paresthesias and pain or weakness in the legs and about symptoms of bladder or bowel sphincter dysfunction. This can be mistaken for the insidious symptoms of prostatic hypertrophy. Spontaneous atlantoaxial subluxation can occur in a small percentage of patients. A distance of greater than 3–4 mm between the anterior aspect of the odontoid and the posterior aspect of the anterior arch of the atlas in the lateral maximal flexion view is considered diagnostic for atlantoaxial subluxation. Other neurologic sequelae of the disorder include injuries to the spinal cord from fracture and dislocation of a rigid and brittle spine. The neck is especially prone to fracture with the potential for resulting paraplegia or quadriplegia.

7. Other associated conditions—Secondary renal amyloidosis is the most common cause of renal involvement in ankylosing spondylitis, usually occurring only after many decades of persistent inflammatory disease. Proteinuria and nephrotic syndrome indicate renal involvement, which is usually the most serious manifestation of amyloidosis. IgA nephropathy has been reported as another cause of proteinuria and renal insufficiency in this disease. Apical pulmonary fibrosis, sometimes with cavity formation, is rare and usually of no clinical consequence. This radiographic abnormality may mimic tuberculosis, and vice versa. Fusion of the costovertebral joints and ankylosis of the thoracic spine may lead to a restrictive disease pattern on pulmonary function testing. Osteoporosis is more common in patients and adequate vitamin D and calcium supplementation is vital in this condition.

B. Laboratory Findings

1. Routine studies—There is no diagnostic laboratory study in ankylosing spondylitis. Hematologic studies are usually normal. In patients with severe disease, there may be a mild normocytic–normochromic anemia reflective of chronic disease. The white blood cell count is usually normal, as is the platelet count, although patients with highly inflammatory

disease may demonstrate mild thrombocytosis. The erythrocyte sedimentation rate and C-reactive protein are elevated in about half of cases and tend to be more associated with peripheral disease activity. Serologic studies for rheumatoid factor and antinuclear antibodies are negative, and serum complement levels are normal.

2. Testing for HLA-B27—HLA-B27 is strongly associated with ankylosing spondylitis, occurring in over 85% of patients. This genetic marker also occurs in 8–10% of the normal white American population. It must be emphasized that indiscriminate HLA typing cannot be substituted for a thorough clinical and radiographic evaluation of the patient. Spondyloarthritis will not develop in the vast majority (>90%) of people with HLA-B27. In fact, determination of HLA-B27 is rarely needed in making the diagnosis of spondyloarthritis. There are unusual circumstances in which the patient gives a strong history suggestive of inflammatory back disease but the radiographs are not yet diagnostic of sacroiliitis. In such situations, HLA typing may be helpful, as well as in women with early or atypical disease. Even then, a positive HLA-B27 does not establish a diagnosis of sacroiliitis but only provides supporting data for the diagnosis when the most specific finding (radiographic sacroiliitis) is not present. It is in this setting that MRI is being more commonly used to determine whether there is any evidence of sacroiliac inflammation.

Patients who already know that they are HLA-B27 positive may seek genetic counseling because of the hereditary impact of disease on their family. It should be emphasized that ankylosing spondylitis is not usually a life-threatening or crippling disorder and that symptoms can be controlled medically in most patients. The likelihood that inflammatory back disease will develop in a family member is low. Because HLA antigens, including HLA-B27, are inherited in a mendelian dominant fashion, the risk of inheriting this tissue antigen type is 50% for each of a patient's children (this assumes that the patient is heterozygous and the other parent is negative for HLA-B27). Even if a child inherits this tissue antigen type, the likelihood of developing arthritis is only around 20%. Therefore, without any knowledge of HLA status, every child of a patient with HLA-B27 positive spondylitis has roughly a 10% chance of developing spondylitis. The 90% probability of never developing this form of arthritis must be emphasized to patients concerned about this hereditary factor.

C. Imaging Studies

1. Sacroiliac joints—Radiographic evaluation of the sacroiliac joints is the single most specific test for this disorder. Although a diagnosis of spondyloarthritis can be suspected based on the history and physical examination, definitive diagnosis of established ankylosing spondylitis cannot be made without radiographic findings. A single anteroposterior view of the pelvis may be adequate to define sacroiliitis; however, Ferguson or oblique views are sometimes necessary to fully evaluate the integrity of the sacroiliac joints. The earliest radiographic change is usually bony sclerosis on the iliac

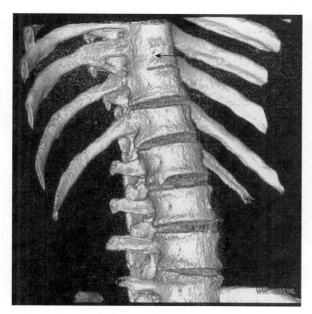

▲ **Figure 17–1.** A three-dimensional reconstruction of a thoracic spine MRI showing ankylosis across three vertebrae (*arrow*) in a patient with ankylosing spondylitis.

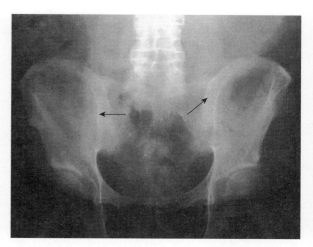

▲ **Figure 17–2.** Plain anteroposterior radiograph showing bilateral sacroiliac joint sclerosis (*arrows*) in a patient with ankylosing spondylitis.

sides of the joint margins. Thereafter, bony erosions occur. "Pseudo" widening of the joint may subsequently becomes apparent. There is eventual fusion (Figure 17–1) across the sacroiliac joint space with subsequent loss of the early sclerotic changes. These changes generally start in the lower third of the sacroiliac joint with bilateral symmetric changes typical for ankylosing spondylitis and enteropathic arthritis. This is distinct from the unilateral sacroiliac progression typical for psoriatic and reactive arthritis. MRI has proven to be more sensitive and specific in detecting changes seen early in spondyloarthritis. Using short T1 inversion recovery (STIR) imaging technique, acute sacroiliitis and spondylitis can be determined as well as enthesitis, synovitis, and bone-related inflammation. In clinical practice, this is very useful in patients, early in the course of inflammatory back symptoms, when the plain radiographs fail to show any findings consistent with sacroiliitis.

Findings suggestive of sclerosis in one or both sacroiliac joints in the absence of features of inflammatory back pain or axial spondyloarthritis will usually point to osteoarthritis of the sacroiliac joints. Sacroiliitis can be confused with the radiographic anomaly osteitis condensans ilii, in which there is symmetric sclerosis on the iliac side of each sacroiliac joint without any erosion. This finding is mostly seen in young multiparous women. Pyogenic sacroiliitis, usually related to staphylococci and mainly seen in injection drug users, is usually unilateral and is associated with other signs of infection.

Less common causes of unilateral sacroiliitis include tuberculosis, syphilis, and brucellosis. Acute gouty arthritis and calcium pyrophosphate deposition disease as causes of sacroiliitis are rare.

2. Spine—An early radiographic finding on lateral lumbar spine films is "shiny corners" or Romanus lesions, which are osseous erosions at the anterosuperior and anteroinferior corners of the vertebral bodies and are associated with bone resorption and reactive sclerosis. The process of inflammatory erosions and subsequent periosteal bone formation results in vertebral bodies appearing "square." Romanus lesions may also be seen in the thoracic and cervical regions. Calcification and ossification of the ligamentous structures between vertebral bodies result in the characteristic syndesmophytes seen on imaging (ie, the bamboo spine) (Figure 17–2). The apophyseal joints of the spine become fused with resulting immobility. Large "flowing" osteophytes, typically most prominent in the right thoracic spine but also common in the lumbar and cervical areas, are seen in diffuse idiopathic skeletal hyperostosis (DISH), which may clinically and radiographically mimic ankylosing spondylitis (Figure 17–3). Such patients can usually be discriminated by disease onset in late middle age and the absence of sacroiliitis.

3. Peripheral joints—Radiographic findings from the peripheral joints typically result from synovitis of proximal joints or from enthesitis. With synovitis, there is symmetric joint-space narrowing while enthesitis may lead to a periosteal reaction at the tendon insertion site. The pubis symphysis, a cartilaginous joint, can undergo both erosive and sclerotic change. Narrowing and irregularity at the pubic symphysis can be readily seen on pelvic films. Whiskering as a

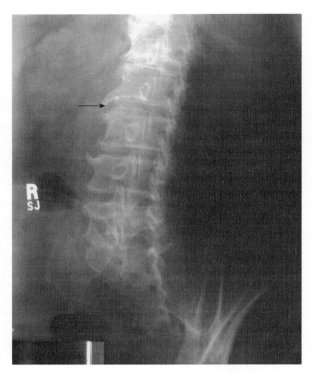

▲ **Figure 17–3.** Lumbosacral spine radiograph showing asymmetric bridging osteophytes in a patient with diffuse idiopathic skeletal hyperostosis (DISH).

manifestation of enthesitis due to erosions and reactive bone formation can be seen at the ischial tuberosities.

▶ Diagnostic Criteria

Based on the modified New York criteria (Table 17–4), radiographic evidence of sacroiliitis is considered the sine qua non for the classification of established ankylosing spondylitis. These criteria carry a sensitivity and specificity of 83% and 98%, respectively. Given that radiographic evidence may take years to develop, the Assessment of Spondyloarthritis International Society has proposed separate criteria to facilitate an earlier diagnosis for axial spondyloarthritis (see Box: Assessment of Spondyloarthritis International Society classification criteria for axial spondyloarthritis [SpA]).

The sensitivity and specificity of these criteria are 83% and 84%, respectively.

▶ Treatment

It is impossible to predict the ultimate course of any patient with ankylosing spondylitis. The inflammatory process may remain confined to the sacroiliac joints or may involve the lumbar, thoracic, and cervical spinal segments. Likewise, the

Table 17–4. Modified New York diagnostic criteria for ankylosing spondylitis.[a]

Clinical
   Low back pain and stiffness for more than 3 months that improves with exercise but is not relieved by rest.
   Limitation of motion of the lumbar spine in the sagittal and frontal planes.
   Limitation of chest expansion to 2.5 cm (1 inch) or less, measured at the level of the fourth intercostal space.
Radiographic
   Sacroiliitis: Unilateral grade 3 (sclerosis and erosions of the joint margins) or grade 4 (fusion across the joint).
   Bilateral grade 2 (sclerosis or joint margins) to 4.

[a]Definite ankylosing spondylitis: unilateral grade 3 or 4, or bilateral grade 2 to 4 sacroiliitis and any of the clinical criterion.
Reproduced, with permission, from van der Linden S, et al. Evaluation of diagnostic criteria for ankylosing spondylitis. A proposal for modification of the New York criteria. *Arthritis Rheum.* 1984;27:361.

duration of time from onset of symptoms to fusion of spinal segments is highly variable. Thus, each patient should understand the nature of this illness and the need for continued medical surveillance, as well as the principles of physical and pharmacologic management of the disorder.

A. Physical Therapy

An important function of physical therapy is the promotion of the patient's ability to prevent spinal deformity and

---

Box 17–A. Assessment of Spondyloarthritis International Society Classification Criteria for Axial Spondyloarthritis (SpA).

(In patients with back pain ≥3 months and age at onset of <45 years)

Sacroiliitis on imaging*		HLA-B27
Plus	OR	**Plus**
≥1 SpA feature**		≥2 other SpA features**

Sacroiliitis on imaging:
Active (acute) inflammation on MRI highly suggestive of sacroiliitis associated with SpA or
   Definite radiographic sacroiliitis according to modified New York criteria

****SpA Features:***
Inflammatory back pain, arthritis, uveitis, dactylitis, psoriasis, inflammatory bowel disease, good response to nonsteroidal anti-inflammatory drugs, family history of SpA, HLA-B27, or elevated C-reactive protein.

Data from Rudwaleit M, et al. The development of Assessment of SpondyloArthritis international Society classification criteria for axial spondyloarthritis (part II): Validation and final selection. *Ann Rheum Dis.* 2009;68:777.

loss of motion in the joints. Such a program is best instituted when symptoms have been brought under control. The natural history of the disease should be explained so that the patient understands the rationale for the exercise program that must be followed over many years. An erect posture when sitting or standing should be encouraged. The patient's bed should be firm and the smallest possible pillow should be used to prevent flexion of the neck. Sleeping in the prone position is best for promoting spinal extension, but the supine position is adequate if there is good support. The patient should refrain from sleeping on the side in a curled up position. An active exercise program to promote extension of the back and increase range of motion of the axial and peripheral joints, as well as breathing exercises to maintain chest expansion, should be performed two to three times a day. Referral to a physical therapist to provide specific instructions and determine that the patient is performing well is a good investment. Swimming is an excellent recreational exercise for the patient with ankylosing spondylitis.

B. Nonsteroidal Anti-inflammatory Drugs

Nonsteroidal anti-inflammatory drugs (NSAIDs) are used as first-line medical therapy to relieve the pain and stiffness of the disease and to promote the patient's ability to perform the physical exercises so important to maintaining a good posture. If the response to the initial trial is inadequate, it is appropriate to provide another class of NSAID. Occasionally, when symptoms remit, the NSAID may be tapered over several weeks and reinstituted if symptoms recur. Silent progress of the disease may occur; therefore, the clinician should closely monitor these patients even when they are not taking medication. There is some evidence that continuous use of NSAID therapy does reduce the degree of radiographic progression at 2 years.

C. Disease-Modifying Antirheumatic Drugs

Overall, this class of medications has not demonstrated efficacy in treating the spinal disease of spondyloarthritis, although it can produce some moderate improvement in the peripheral arthritis sometimes seen in these conditions. Sulfasalazine, a drug used for inflammatory bowel disease, has been found to be effective as an early therapy for ankylosing spondylitis with peripheral joint involvement. A small number of trials have used oral methotrexate in ankylosing spondylitis refractory to NSAIDs and sulfasalazine. A meta-analysis of these trials did not find a significant benefit of methotrexate.

D. Antitumor Necrosis Factor Agents

The use of the tumor necrosis factor (TNF) inhibitors has led to impressive clinical improvement. However, not all patients require TNF inhibitors. Guidelines that have been developed by international consensus to facilitate the judicious use of this therapy recommend anti-TNF agents for patients who have definitive ankylosing spondylitis with active disease, as measured by validated metrics, and who have not responded to a trial of two NSAIDs. The anti-TNF agents currently approved are etanercept, infliximab, adalimumab, and golimumab. In studies with these agents, efficacy has been demonstrated in reducing symptoms of as well as markers of inflammation, including C-reactive protein and erythrocyte sedimentation rate within several weeks of initiation of therapy.

For patients who have responded to anti-TNF agents, continued therapy is usually necessary and generally well-tolerated. Discontinuation of therapy may result in reactivation of the disease within several months time. While these agents have been a remarkable advance in the therapy of ankylosing spondylitis, their use provokes many unanswered questions regarding long-term safety issues, the proper timing of initiation of therapy, and the potential role of future biologic agents in combination when these become available.

E. Surgery

Spinal surgery is rarely performed, unless it is needed for stabilization of a fracture site. More frequently, up to 5% of patients require total hip arthroplasty. This procedure is generally well tolerated with decreased hip pain, increased mobility, and 20-year joint survival exceeding 50%. Care must be taken to perform a careful preoperative assessment for cervical spine disease in order to avoid spinal cord damage that can occur during endotracheal intubation.

▶ Prognosis

The prognosis for patients with ankylosing spondylitis is excellent. Most patients can be treated successfully by physical and pharmacologic means. Most patients continue to lead productive lives and change in vocational plans is usually not indicated. The morbidity from articular and extra-articular complications is low, and lifespan is not reduced significantly, if at all. These facts should be optimistically presented to the patient. It is also vital to ensure close follow-up of all extra-articular manifestations many years after the initial articular process as many of these organs only become involved later in the course of ankylosing spondylitis.

ENTEROPATHIC SPONDYLOARTHRITIS

▶ General Considerations

Enteropathic arthritis develops in nearly 20% of all patients with Crohn disease and ulcerative colitis. Enteropathic arthritis most commonly presents with a peripheral arthritis that can correlate with bowel activity and is usually self-limiting; it can also present with a spondylitis that may progress in the absence of active bowel disease, although this is less commonly seen than peripheral arthritis.

▶ Clinical Findings

The peripheral arthritis is often migratory and rarely erosive. Erythema nodosum and pyoderma gangrenosa may be cutaneous manifestations with the peripheral arthritis. The spondylitis is generally more benign than in ankylosing spondylitis but may be indistinguishable. The male predominance of ankylosing spondylitis is not found in enteropathic spondyloarthritis. Isolated sacroiliitis without spine involvement may also occur. No laboratory marker is specific for either condition.

It is important to rule out septic arthritis secondary to fistulization or avascular necrosis in patients with inflammatory bowel disease who have sacroiliitis or hip symptoms. Hypertrophic osteoarthropathy, which may develop in Crohn disease and ulcerative colitis, is differentiated from enteropathic arthritis due to the dominant features of periostitis and clubbing.

▶ Treatment

Frequently, treatment of the underlying bowel disease leads to remission of the peripheral arthritis. If this persists, sulfasalazine can be effective. In general, NSAIDs are avoided as first-line therapy because they may lead to exacerbations of the inflammatory bowel disease, although other studies have not demonstrated worsening flares with cyclooxygenase (COX)-2 inhibitors in patients with ulcerative colitis. This should be addressed on a case-by-case basis in conjunction with a gastroenterologist. If an adequate trial of sulfasalazine has failed to fully control symptoms, then anti-TNF agents have been demonstrated to control both Crohn disease and the associated arthritis.

Reveille JD, Arnett FC. Spondyloarthritis: update on pathogenesis and management. *Am J Med.* 2005;118:592. [PMID: 15922688]

Rudwaleit M, van der Heijde D, Landewe R, et al. The development of Assessment of SpondyloArthritis international Society classification criteria for axial spondyloarthritis (part II): Validation and final selection. *Ann Rheum Dis.* 2009;68:777. [PMID: 19297344]

Salvarani C, Fries W. Clinical features and epidemiology of spondyloarthritides associated with inflammatory bowel disease. *World J Gastroenterol.* 2009;15:2449. [PMID: 19468993]

Sandborn WJ, Stenson WF, Brynskov J, et al. Safety of celecoxib in patients with ulcerative colitis in remission: a randomized, placebo-controlled pilot study. *Clin Gastroenterol Hepatol.* 2006;4:203. [PMID: 16469681]

The American College of Rheumatology website http://www.rheumatology.org/

The European League Against Rheumatism http://www.eular.org/

The Spondylitis Association of America http://www.spondylitis.org

Wanders A, Heijde D, Landewe R, et al. Nonsteroidal anti-inflammatory drugs reduce radiographic progression in patients with ankylosing spondylitis: a randomized clinical trial. *Arthritis Rheum.* 2005;52:1756. [PMID: 15934081]

Reactive Arthritis

18

Grant H. Louie, MD, MHS
Clifton O. Bingham III, MD

ESSENTIALS OF DIAGNOSIS

▶ Inflammatory arthritis triggered by antecedent gastrointestinal or genitourinary infections.

▶ Asymmetric oligoarthritis most commonly affecting the lower extremities.

▶ Enthesitis and dactylitis.

▶ Association with extra-articular manifestations, such as conjunctivitis, anterior uveitis, urethritis, circinate balanitis, oral ulcers, and keratoderma blennorrhagicum.

▶ General Considerations

Reactive arthritis is an inflammatory arthritis that develops after certain infections of the gastrointestinal or genitourinary tracts. Symptoms can frequently be self-limited with spontaneous remission after several weeks to months, while other times the symptoms can become chronic. At onset, the arthritis is usually an acute, asymmetric oligoarthritis of peripheral joints that occurs within several weeks after the infection. While isolating the causative infectious agent aids in the diagnosis, this is neither required nor always possible. Treatment of an active infection with antibiotics is indicated but is frequently ineffective in preventing the acute arthritis from becoming chronic.

Currently, there is still no consensus on the classification and diagnostic criteria for reactive arthritis. Nonetheless, it is generally classified as one of the spondyloarthropathies, a group of diseases that also includes psoriatic arthritis, ankylosing spondylitis, and inflammatory bowel disease–associated arthritis. Arthritis of the axial skeleton (ie, the sacroiliac joints and spine), enthesitis (inflammation of the insertion sites of tendons to bone), asymmetric oligoarthritis or symmetric polyarthritis of peripheral joints, and the absence of rheumatoid factor are shared characteristics of the spondyloarthropathies. A more restrictive definition of

reactive arthritis, formerly known as Reiter syndrome, is the classic triad of peripheral arthritis, conjunctivitis, and urethritis or cervicitis.

Reactive arthritis usually occurs in young adults between 20 and 40 years of age. The post-gastrointestinal tract infection subtype of reactive arthritis equally affects men and women, while the post-genitourinary tract infection subtype overwhelmingly affects men more frequently than women (9:1 ratio). The prevalence of reactive arthritis is estimated to be 30 to 40 per 100,000, and the incidence is estimated to be 5 to 28 per 100,000 per annum.

▶ Pathogenesis

Reactive arthritis frequently develops 1–4 weeks after a bout of gastroenteritis caused by *Shigella*, *Salmonella*, *Campylobacter,* or *Yersinia*, or after acquisition of a sexually transmitted infection, most commonly *Chlamydia trachomatis* and occasionally HIV. In up to 25% of patients, however, there are no symptoms of an antecedent infection. This observation suggests that reactive arthritis ensues either after a subclinical infection or that other environmental triggers are involved.

In addition to environmental triggers, genetic factors may also play a role in disease susceptibility. Approximately 30–50% of patients with reactive arthritis are positive for HLA-B27. As such, there is a greater prevalence of the disease in whites, in contrast to other ethnic groups that have a lower frequency of HLA-B27, such as blacks. A strong family history may be elicited in patients with reactive arthritis. The exact role of HLA-B27 in the disease pathogenesis remains elusive.

The triggering microbial agents and their chromosomal DNA occasionally have been isolated from synovial fluid of affected joints. However, the causative agents and their associated components have been discovered in joints from patients without reactive arthritis. Consequently, the significance of these findings remains to be determined.

▶ Clinical Findings

A. Symptoms and Signs

1. Articular manifestations—The predominant manifestation of reactive arthritis is an acute, asymmetric oligoarthritis of peripheral joints, frequently 1–4 weeks after the onset of the inciting infection. Joints of the lower extremities (eg, knees, ankles, and feet) are preferentially affected compared with joints of the upper extremities. The sternoclavicular and temporomandibular joints are sometimes involved. Affected joints are usually stiff, swollen, and tender.

Axial skeleton disease most commonly presents as inflammatory low back pain, which occurs in up to half of patients with reactive arthritis. Radiographic evidence of sacroiliitis, which is often unilateral, develops in approximately 20–25% of patients. This is in contrast to the bilateral, symmetric sacroiliitis of ankylosing spondylitis. A minority of patients with sacroiliitis have spondylitis with extensive fusion of the spine resembling severe ankylosing spondylitis. The prevalence of axial skeleton disease is greater among those with chronic disease and those with HLA-B27 (90% of patients with radiographic evidence of sacroiliitis are HLA-B27 positive).

2. Enthesitis—A prominent feature of reactive arthritis is enthesitis, inflammation of sites where tendons attach to bone. Common sites for enthesitis are the Achilles tendon, plantar fascia, and pelvic bones. Findings of enthesitis include soft tissue swelling with overlying warmth and tenderness to palpation.

3. Dactylitis—The combination of synovitis and enthesitis in a toe or finger can cause the entire digit to become diffusely swollen, producing dactylitis or "sausage digit." Dactylitis is a feature of the spondyloarthropathies, frequently observed in reactive arthritis and psoriatic arthritis. Toes are more commonly affected than the fingers.

4. Mucocutaneous lesions—Circinate balanitis is an inflammatory lesion on the glans or shaft of the penis, and it is one of the characteristic lesions associated with reactive arthritis. In an uncircumcised man, these lesions are shallow, moist, serpiginous, painless ulcers with raised borders. In a circumcised man, these lesions can appear as dry, hyperkeratotic plaques resembling psoriasis and be painful.

Another cutaneous lesion associated with reactive arthritis is keratoderma blennorrhagicum, a papular, waxy rash that affects primarily the palms and soles. At first, the rash can be vesicular and then evolve into maculopapular nodules before turning into scaly, hyperkeratotic lesions resembling psoriasis. These lesions can coalesce to cover large areas of skin, extending proximally beyond the palms and soles.

If a genitourinary infection is the initial trigger of reactive arthritis, urethritis or cervicitis (or both) can be observed.

Aphthous ulcers, usually shallow and painless, can involve both oral and genital mucosal surfaces.

Lastly, nail changes resembling those of psoriatic arthritis can occur. However, nail pitting does not usually occur.

These so-called "Reiter nails" are nail beds that may become thickened and eventually undergo onychodystrophy. The clinical appearance can be confused with similarly appearing onychomycosis.

5. Ocular inflammation—Ocular inflammation (ie, conjunctivitis, but also iritis, scleritis, episcleritis, and keratitis) is associated with reactive arthritis in up to one-fourth of cases. The ocular inflammation is often intermittent, and presents as scleral injection, eye pain, and visual changes. Corneal clouding, due to the presence of inflammatory cells and protein exudates in the anterior chamber, can be seen on slit lamp examination. A chronic uveitis that can cause permanent visual impairment or even blindness develops in a minority of patients with relapsing uveitis.

6. Visceral involvement—Although rare, aortitis has been reported in a few patients with long-standing reactive arthritis. In addition, valvular heart disease (specifically aortic valve regurgitation) may result with thickening of the aortic root from chronic inflammation. If the conduction system involving the atrioventricular node is affected, complete heart block may result.

B. Laboratory Findings

There are no laboratory tests diagnostic for reactive arthritis. The diagnosis may be particularly challenging when patients have asymptomatic infections that trigger reactive arthritis. The various classification criteria for reactive arthritis rely principally on clinical symptoms of inflammatory arthritis that follow a gastrointestinal or genitourinary infection.

Synovial fluid is notable for a cloudy, viscous, nonhemorrhagic appearance. Cell count with differential normally shows 5000–50,000 white blood cells per microliter with a predominance of polymorphonuclear cells. Gram stain is absent of bacteria, and cultures of the synovial fluid are negative. Microscopic analysis of crystalline disease (eg, gout or pseudogout) would be unremarkable. Occasionally, "Reiter cells" may be found. These are large mononuclear cells that have phagocytized several polymorphonuclear cells, which themselves contain inclusion bodies. These inclusion bodies represent bacterial antigens, thus completing the link of reactive arthritis and infectious etiologies.

Because of the strong infectious link with reactive arthritis, great effort should be made to identify the causative microorganism if it is not already known. Hence, cultures should be taken from the blood, urine, stool, and throat as indicated. If a sexually transmitted infection is suspected, *Neisseria gonorrhoeae*, *C trachomatis*, and HIV should be assessed. Conversely, if gastroenteritis were the inciting event, then serologic tests for antibodies against *Salmonella*, *Shigella*, *Yersinia*, and *Campylobacter* should be considered. A negative serology does not definitively rule out infection (especially early in disease course), as antibody titers increase over time, and as the complete list of infections that can cause reactive arthritis is still unknown.

During an acute attack, acute phase reactants such as C-reactive protein (CRP) and erythrocyte sedimentation rate (ESR) are frequently elevated. Leukocytosis, thrombocytosis, and elevated serum immunoglobulins may also be present. In long-standing disease, a mild normocytic, normochromic anemia may be found secondary to chronic inflammation.

The presence of HLA-B27 may be useful diagnostically, since it is found in up to one-half of patients with reactive arthritis. It may be important also prognostically, as HLA-B27 positivity is associated with more chronic disease.

C. Imaging Studies

The most common radiographic abnormalities found in reactive arthritis are fluffy periostitis, which represent proliferative changes along the shaft of bones, and bony erosions, often found at the sites of joint inflammation. Osteolytic destruction and bony ankylosis may also occur, although they occur more frequently in psoriatic arthritis.

Radiographic sacroiliitis can be detected in up to 20% of patients. When present, it is frequently unilateral. There may be syndesmophytes (abnormal ossified spinal ligaments) resembling those in ankylosing spondylitis. However, they tend to be more asymmetric and less confluent than in ankylosing spondylitis.

Most radiographic findings in reactive arthritis occur months after disease onset, and the findings can be subtle.

▶ Differential Diagnosis

Other diagnoses to consider include septic arthritis, a true joint infection. Although this may be difficult to differentiate from reactive arthritis based purely on physical examination, arthrocentesis followed by synovial fluid analysis can be immensely useful. Synovial fluid from a septic joint usually demonstrates leukocyte counts between 50,000 cells/mcL and 150,000 cells/mcL (predominantly neutrophils) and frequently a positive culture, whereas reactive arthritis has lower leukocyte counts between 5000 cells/mcL and 50,000 cells/mcL and almost always a sterile culture.

Other disseminated infections, such as gonorrhea or bacterial endocarditis, can also present with acute oligoarthritis of peripheral joints. Acute viral infections, such as erythrovirus (parvovirus B19) and HIV, can present as polyarthritis.

Gout or pseudogout presents usually with an oligoarthritis of the peripheral joints. As in septic arthritis, arthrocentesis is the critical diagnostic procedure that aids to differentiate this from reactive arthritis. The presence of monosodium urate crystals and calcium pyrophosphate dihydrate crystals are pathognomonic for gout and pseudogout, respectively.

Rheumatoid arthritis is usually distinguishable from reactive arthritis by the pattern of joint involvement. Rheumatoid arthritis frequently begins with inflammatory polyarthritis of the small joints of the hands and feet and progresses in a symmetric, additive fashion, whereas reactive arthritis manifests usually as an asymmetric oligoarthritis of the peripheral joints of the lower extremities. The presence of rheumatoid factor or antibodies to cyclic citrullinated peptides (or both) will be much more likely found in rheumatoid arthritis than in reactive arthritis.

Lastly, the other spondyloarthropathies (psoriatic arthritis, ankylosing spondylitis, and inflammatory bowel disease-associated arthritis) may have overlapping clinical findings with reactive arthritis, including HLA-B27 positivity and radiographic abnormalities. Often times, long-term follow-up is needed to distinguish one from another.

▶ Treatment

A. Nonsteroidal Anti-Inflammatory Drugs (NSAIDs)

NSAIDs remain the treatment of first choice for the articular manifestations of reactive arthritis. Prescription-strength doses (eg, ibuprofen 600–800 mg orally every 6–8 hours) are needed to achieve adequate anti-inflammatory and analgesic effects. Continuous use of NSAIDs, rather than an as-needed basis, may be necessary to control the symptoms. Gastrointestinal prophylaxis should be considered.

B. Glucocorticoids

Intra-articular glucocorticoids may be considered for peripheral arthritis involving a few joints. For more widespread peripheral arthritis, systemic glucocorticoids can provide significant pain relief but are frequently of limited benefit for axial symptoms. Topical glucocorticoids can be beneficial for extra-articular manifestations, such as ocular inflammation or inflammatory cutaneous lesions.

C. Antibiotics

Given the association of reactive arthritis with an antecedent infection, appropriate short-term antibiotic therapy should be administered if the infection remains active. Patients with reactive arthritis triggered by infection from *C trachomatis* or *N gonorrhoeae* should be treated accordingly. Their partners should also be treated.

There is limited data to support the role of long-term antibiotics in the treatment or prevention of reactive arthritis when active infection is no longer detected. The majority of randomized controlled trials of long-term use of ciprofloxacin, doxycycline, and azithromycin in patients with reactive arthritis have failed to demonstrate significant efficacy of long-term outcomes compared with placebo.

Most recently, a 9-month randomized, double-blind, placebo-controlled trial of patients with at least 6 months of reactive arthritis triggered by *C trachomatis* or *Chlamydophila pneumoniae* (detected by polymerase chain reaction in synovial tissue or peripheral blood mononuclear cells) demonstrated significant clinical benefit with combination antibiotics (rifampin with doxycycline or rifampin with azithromycin) compared with placebo. Patients were treated for 6 months and followed up for 3 additional months. Adverse events were statistically similar in the three treatment arms. Limitations of the study include small sample size resulting in an underpowered study to determine which of the combination of antibiotics is more efficacious. Moreover, optimal long-term duration and dosing of antibiotics in patients with *Chlamydia*-induced reactive arthritis remain to be determined.

D. Disease-Modifying Anti-rheumatic Drugs (DMARDs)

DMARDs may be considered in patients with reactive arthritis refractory to NSAIDs and glucocorticoids. Of the ones commonly used to treat inflammatory arthritis in rheumatoid arthritis, only sulfasalazine has been tested in a randomized clinical trial. Patients with reactive arthritis treated with sulfasalazine 2000 mg daily showed a trend toward improvement of peripheral joint swelling and tenderness compared with placebo. If bowel inflammation is part of the disease process, sulfasalazine may also be beneficial. Although not tested in clinical trials, methotrexate can be considered also in reactive arthritis where peripheral arthritis predominates. Biologic therapies (eg, tumor necrosis factor inhibitors) have not been studied in randomized controlled trials and their role in reactive arthritis is unknown.

▶ Complications

Chronic arthritis of the peripheral joints or axial skeleton can lead to functional disability. Complications of visceral involvement, such as aortic regurgitation and complete heart block, may occur in long-standing disease.

▶ Prognosis

The natural history of reactive arthritis varies considerably in terms of duration of disease, frequency of relapses, and severity of relapses. The disease can be mild with a self-limited course that lasts between 3 and 5 months; alternatively, some patients progress to have chronic or recurrent symptoms. Relapses of urethritis, uveitis, and arthralgias can occur years after the initial symptoms. In a minority of patients, the condition can progress to a chronic, destructive, and disabling arthritis.

Clinical and serologic predictors of long-term outcomes are still not completely well defined, but HLA-B27 positivity, specific type of infection, strong family history of spondyloarthropathies, and chronic bowel inflammation appear to be predictors of worse prognosis.

Carter JD. Reactive arthritis: defined etiologies, emerging pathophysiology, and unresolved treatment. *Infect Dis Clin North Am.* 2006;20:827. [PMID: 17118292]

Carter JD, Espinoza LR, Inman RD, et al. Combination antibiotics as a treatment for chronic *Chlamydia*-induced reactive arthritis: a double-blind, placebo-controlled, prospective trial. *Arthritis Rheum.* 2010;62:1298. [PMID: 20155838]

Carter JD, Hudson AP. Reactive arthritis: clinical aspects and medical management. *Rheum Dis Clin North Am.* 2009;35:21. [PMID: 19480995]

Carter JD, Hudson AP. The evolving story of *Chlamydia*-induced reactive arthritis. *Curr Opin Rheumatol.* 2010;22:424. [PMID: 20445454]

Hannu T, Inman R, Granfors K, Leirisalo-Repo M. Reactive arthritis or post-infectious arthritis? *Best Pract Res Clin Rheumatol.* 2006;20:419. [PMID: 16777574]

Townes JM, Deodhar AA, Laine ES, et al. Reactive arthritis following culture-confirmed infections with bacterial enteric pathogens in Minnesota and Oregon: a population-based study. *Ann Rheum Dis.* 2008;67:1689. [PMID: 18272671]

Psoriatic Arthritis

19

Grant H. Louie, MD, MHS
Clifton O. Bingham III, MD

ESSENTIALS OF DIAGNOSIS

- ► Chronic inflammatory arthritis associated with skin and nail psoriasis.
- ► Symmetric polyarthritis or asymmetric oligoarthritis of peripheral joints (frequently with distal interphalangeal [DIP] joint involvement).
- ► Spondylitis and enthesitis may occur.
- ► Current or past history of psoriasis; family history of psoriasis.
- ► Dactylitis and characteristic nail dystrophy.
- ► Absence of rheumatoid factor.
- ► Radiographic findings of erosions, osteolytic destruction of the interphalangeal joints, and juxta-articular new bone formation.

General Considerations

Psoriatic arthritis is a chronic inflammatory arthritis associated with skin and nail psoriasis. It is one of the spondyloarthropathies, a group of inflammatory arthritides, characterized by arthritis of the axial skeleton (ie, the sacroiliac joints and spine), asymmetric oligoarthritis or symmetric polyarthritis of peripheral joints, enthesitis (inflammation at the insertion sites of tendons to bone), and the absence of rheumatoid factor. Unlike rheumatoid arthritis, psoriatic arthritis has a predilection for the DIP joints.

Psoriatic arthritis develops in approximately 20–30% (range 6–42%) of adults with psoriasis. The overall prevalence of psoriatic arthritis in the general population has been estimated to be 0.04–0.1%, but this may be an underestimate. In the United States, the incidence of psoriatic arthritis has been reported to be approximately 6–7 per 100,000 per annum. The mean age of disease onset ranges from 30 to 55 years, with men and women equally affected.

Pathogenesis

The etiology of psoriatic arthritis is unknown. Genetic susceptibility studies indicate associations with major histocompatibility alleles HLA-B27, HLA-B7, HLA-B13, HLA-B17, HLA-B57, and HLA–Cw*0602. Recent genome-wide association studies of patients with psoriasis and psoriatic arthritis have identified other susceptibility loci, including interleukin (IL)-23A, IL-23R, IL-12B, tumor necrosis factor-induced protein 3 (TNFIP3), TNFIP3 interacting protein 1 (TNIP1), IL-4, IL-13, and tumor necrosis factor receptor-associated factor 3-interacting protein 2 (TRAF3IP2). As in the pathogenesis of many other autoimmune disorders, an infectious trigger has been suspected. Group A streptococcal infections have been implicated in guttate psoriasis, and ribosomal RNA from this species has been detected in peripheral blood and synovial fluid of psoriatic arthritis patients. In addition, HIV is strongly associated with the development of psoriasis and psoriatic arthritis. Physical trauma (Koebner phenomenon) has also been implicated.

Psoriatic arthritis typically develops after or coincident with the onset of psoriasis. In 15–20% of cases, however, arthritis precedes the onset of psoriasis by as much as 2 years. An asymmetric oligoarthritis was once believed to be the usual clinical presentation of psoriatic arthritis, but recent evidence supports that symmetric polyarthritis is the most frequent presentation. Widespread destructive arthritis (arthritis mutilans) and mostly DIP joint involvement are observed less frequently but are more specific to psoriatic arthritis. The pace of joint destruction may occur over a period of months.

There may be a direct correlation between the severity of arthritis at the time of presentation and the subsequent disease course. Polyarthritis in the presence of elevated acute phase reactants, radiographic evidence of joint erosions, and inadequate response to initial pharmacotherapy predicts a more severe disease course. As seen in rheumatoid arthritis, psoriatic arthritis can significantly impact quality of life and physical function. Articular damage often develops, and destruction of single joints can occur rapidly.

► Clinical Findings

A. Symptoms and Signs

1. Articular involvement—The majority of patients with psoriatic arthritis have symmetric polyarthritis or asymmetric oligoarthritis of the hands and feet. Often the DIP joints become stiff, swollen, and tender in an asymmetric fashion. When present, involvement of the DIP joints helps distinguish psoriatic arthritis from rheumatoid arthritis, but sometimes results in confusion with osteoarthritis or gout. Other joints that are affected by psoriatic arthritis include the knees, hips, and sternoclavicular joints.

Regardless of the number of symptomatic joints at disease onset, most patients progress to additional joint involvement in the absence of effective treatment. There is ongoing destruction of joints, as evidenced clinically by the appearance of joint deformities and radiographically by the development of juxta-articular erosions, joint-space narrowing, and, in some cases, bony ankylosis. Arthritis mutilans describes the end stage of the destructive process, where loss of bony architecture allows complete subluxation and telescoping of the involved digit ("doigt en lorgnette" or opera-glass finger). This phenomenon is uncommon and is associated with long-standing, poorly controlled disease.

2. Dactylitis—Dactylitis, or "sausage digit," is the complete swelling of a single digit of the hand or foot (Figure 19–1). It is a distinctive feature of the spondyloarthropathies, and it is common in psoriatic arthritis, occurring in one-third to one-half of patients at some point during the course of the disease. Toes are more frequently involved than fingers. Dactylitis is associated with more severe radiographic joint damage.

3. Enthesitis—Enthesitis is an inflammatory process occurring at the site of insertion of tendons into bone. This is a feature common to other spondyloarthropathies and occurs in up to 40% of psoriatic arthritis patients. On physical examination, there is a soft tissue swelling usually accompanied by tenderness to palpation and sometimes by overlying erythema and warmth as well. Common sites for enthesitis are the Achilles tendon, plantar fascia, and pelvic bones. Entheseal inflammation may evolve to destruction of the adjacent bone and joints.

4. Skin and nail changes—All forms of psoriasis are associated with arthritis, although classic psoriasis vulgaris is seen most frequently. Typical psoriatic lesions are erythematous plaques that produce scaling with scratching. Interestingly, many patients with psoriatic arthritis have only mild to moderate skin disease, and there has been no consistent correlation between the degree of psoriasis and the extent of joint involvement. The psoriasis may be subtle. Therefore, careful examination of the entire skin surface must be performed when psoriatic arthritis is suspected, with particular attention to the hairline, scalp, external auditory canal, periumbilical area, and gluteal cleft.

As with uncomplicated psoriasis, nail involvement is common in psoriatic arthritis (Figure 19–2). Psoriatic nail changes include ridging, pitting, onycholysis, and hyperkeratosis, and may represent the manifestation of psoriasis before the presence of more characteristic skin lesions. Nail changes on the affected finger virtually always occur when psoriatic arthritis affects a DIP joint.

5. Spondyloarthropathy—Symptomatic involvement of the sacroiliac joints and axial skeleton is less common than peripheral joints. Inflammation of the sacroiliac joints (sacroiliitis) in psoriatic arthritis is usually unilateral and presents with pain and stiffness in the lower back or buttock. Tenderness can sometimes be elicited by direct palpation of

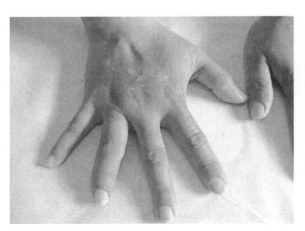

▲ **Figure 19–1.** Dactylitis of the ring finger of a patient with psoriatic arthritis. (Used with permission from Dr. J. Graf, University of California, San Francisco.)

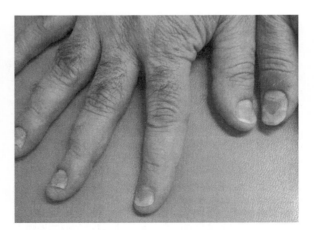

▲ **Figure 19–2.** Psoriatic nail changes with onycholysis and subungual debris. (Used with permission from Dr. J. Graf, University of California, San Francisco.)

the joints by applying firm pressure with the thumbs when the examiner places his or her palms over the patient's iliac crest—the thumbs will tend to fall directly over the joints. Another maneuver that may detect sacroiliitis is the Gaenslen test, in which the patient (in either the supine or the lateral recumbent position) flexes one leg at the hip with the knee close to the chest and hyperextends the other leg over the examination table. This applies stress to the sacroiliac joints and is considered positive if pain is elicited at the sacroiliac joint. However, the reliability of physical examination findings for detection of sacroiliitis is poor, and noninflammatory processes may elicit positive findings. Plain radiography of the pelvis and Ferguson views that focus on the sacroiliac joints may aid in the detection of inflammatory disease of this joint.

A common site of skeletal involvement in psoriatic arthritis is the cervical spine. Here, as in rheumatoid arthritis, extensive inflammation and erosion may lead to atlantoaxial (C1–C2) instability, which can produce cervical myelopathy as the odontoid process erodes. This process is often clinically silent and painless. Involvement of other levels of the spine is also seen in psoriatic arthritis with syndesmophytes, which often arise from the midpoint of a vertebral body, bridge adjacent vertebrae, and restrict motion of the spine. In contrast to the continuous ascending spinal involvement in ankylosing spondylitis, psoriatic spinal involvement is frequently discontinuous, affecting noncontiguous vertebrae or areas (Figure 19–3).

6. Extra-articular manifestations—Ocular inflammation (eg, conjunctivitis, iritis, scleritis, and episcleritis), oral ulcerations, and urethritis occur in psoriatic arthritis, but less frequently than in the other spondyloarthropathies.

B. Laboratory Findings

There are no laboratory tests diagnostic for psoriatic arthritis. Up to 20% of patients have hyperuricemia. Because of the systemic, inflammatory nature of the disease, acute phase reactants, such as the C-reactive protein and the erythrocyte sedimentation rate, may be elevated, although typically not as high as that seen in other inflammatory arthritides, such as rheumatoid arthritis. In some patients, elevations of acute phase reactants correlate with disease activity, more commonly in patients with a higher number of affected joints.

Synovial fluid analysis reveals inflammatory fluid, with white blood cell counts usually in the 5000–50,000/mcL range.

Patients with psoriatic arthritis usually do not have rheumatoid factor, but up to 10% of patients with psoriatic arthritis may test positive. A positive rheumatoid factor is not an exclusion criterion for the diagnosis of psoriatic arthritis. Antibodies to cyclic citrullinated peptides are sensitive and specific for rheumatoid arthritis. These antibodies have only rarely been reported in patients with psoriatic arthritis, and, in most cases to date have been seen in patients with polyarticular symmetric presentations that suggest

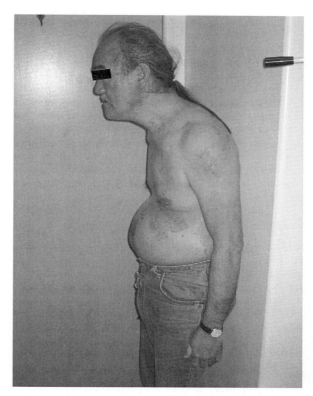

▲ **Figure 19–3.** Psoriatic spondylitis. Extensive spinal involvement has led to exaggerated thoracic kyphosis and loss of cervical extension. As a result, the patient is unable to touch the occiput to the wall when standing against the wall ("occiput-to-wall" test). There is limited chest expansion leading to a protuberant abdomen and to diaphragmatic breathing. (Used with permission from Dr. J. Graf, University of California, San Francisco.)

the co-occurrence of psoriasis with rheumatoid arthritis. Antinuclear antibodies are detected in 10–20% of patients, which is comparable to the prevalence of antinuclear antibody positivity in healthy control populations.

C. Imaging Studies

The most common radiographic findings in psoriatic arthritis are joint-space narrowing and erosions involving the DIP and proximal interphalangeal joints. Typically, these findings are asymmetric, paralleling the pattern of the clinical arthritis. The metacarpophalangeal joints and wrists are less frequently involved than in rheumatoid arthritis. In addition, periarticular osteopenia (decreased bony density adjacent to the joints) is usually absent in psoriatic arthritis, another feature that helps distinguish psoriatic arthritis from rheumatoid arthritis.

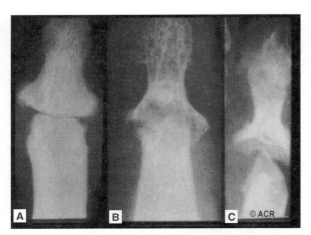

▲ **Figure 19–4.** Radiographic changes from psoriatic arthritis of the distal interphalangeal joint. **A:** Subtle periosteal erosions at the margins of the joint space are an initial appearance. **B:** Progressive erosive and proliferative changes occur over time and can be greatly destructive. **C:** Distinctive "pencil-in-cup" appearance with severe disease. (Used with permission from American College of Rheumatology Clinical Slide Collection. ©1972–1999.)

Severe destructive changes of the joints may occur with long-standing disease but may also develop rapidly in a single joint, resulting in a whittling phenomenon of the bone. When a phalanx is involved, it becomes "penciled," thus giving rise to the classic "pencil-in-cup" deformity when it abuts the base of an adjacent phalanx (Figure 19–4). Marked osteolysis results in widening of the spaces between joints and eventual complete disorganization of the joint architecture, described as arthritis mutilans. Subluxations can occur, which give the clinical manifestation of telescoping digits.

In contrast to rheumatoid arthritis, psoriatic arthritis can produce proliferative bony changes adjacent to erosive and osteolytic changes in the same bone. This new bone formation often occurs along the shaft of the metacarpal and metatarsal bones and is seen as a fluffy periostitis. Rheumatologists and radiologists may use the term "whiskering" to describe these proliferative changes.

Although not performed routinely yet in the clinical setting, joint imaging with ultrasound and MRI has gained increasing popularity among rheumatologists and can show synovitis, entheseal inflammation, and erosions on ultrasound and MRI and subchondral bone marrow changes with MRI.

▶ Differential Diagnosis

Although many classification criteria for psoriatic arthritis exist for the purposes of clinical trials, the Classification Criteria for Psoriatic Arthritis (CASPAR) criteria seem to be gaining international acceptance because of their simplicity and relatively high specificity and sensitivity, but there is not yet consensus on diagnostic criteria. The diagnosis of psoriatic arthritis may be challenging, particularly when skin manifestations are subtle or the arthritis antedates skin lesions. Clinical findings to suggest psoriatic arthritis in the absence of psoriasis include asymmetric oligoarthritis, DIP joint involvement, and characteristic nail dystrophy of psoriasis. The heterogeneity of psoriatic arthritis, the lack of defined diagnostic criteria, and the possibility of overlap syndromes with other rheumatic diseases also add to the complexity of diagnosis.

The differential diagnosis of psoriatic arthritis includes other forms of inflammatory arthritis, most notably rheumatoid arthritis and the other seronegative spondyloarthropathies (ankylosing spondylitis, reactive arthritis, and inflammatory bowel disease–associated arthritis), particularly when patients have sacroiliitis and enthesitis. When acute in onset, the monoarticular and oligoarticular forms of psoriatic arthritis can pose a diagnostic dilemma with the crystal arthropathies (gout and pseudogout) and septic arthritis, necessitating the analysis of synovial fluid to exclude these alternative diagnoses. When performing an arthrocentesis in a patient with psoriasis, it is critical to avoid passing the aspirating needle through psoriatic plaques, which are often heavily contaminated with bacteria.

▶ Treatment

A. Overview

The Group for Research and Assessment of Psoriasis and Psoriatic Arthritis (GRAPPA) has published treatment recommendations for the diverse clinical manifestations of psoriatic arthritis based on evidence from systemic reviews and consensus opinion. Treatment of psoriatic arthritis may vary, depending on the presence of peripheral arthritis, axial disease, enthesitis, skin and nail disease, or dactylitis.

B. Nonsteroidal Anti-inflammatory Drugs

Despite a lack of supporting evidence from clinical trials, nonsteroidal anti-inflammatory drugs (NSAIDs) are among the most frequently used pharmacotherapy for psoriatic arthritis. NSAIDs are particularly useful for peripheral arthritis and axial disease. Often, higher doses of nonselective NSAIDs may be required, and hence, vigilance must be maintained for gastrointestinal adverse effects. Administration of misoprostol or a proton pump inhibitor may be necessary for gastrointestinal prophylaxis.

C. Disease-Modifying Antirheumatic Drugs

Disease-modifying antirheumatic drugs (DMARDs) are considered second-line agents in psoriatic arthritis unresponsive to NSAIDs. Many DMARDs prescribed in the treatment of rheumatoid arthritis have been used in the treatment of psoriatic arthritis, including methotrexate, sulfasalazine, azathioprine, antimalarials (specifically hydroxychloroquine), and cyclosporine. The ability of DMARDs to slow and prevent joint damage and improve physical function in psoriatic arthritis remains to be demonstrated in clinical trials. Methotrexate is probably the most frequently used DMARD in the peripheral articular manifestations of psoriatic arthritis, and it is also oftentimes efficacious for the skin manifestations of psoriasis. Typical starting dose is 7.5–15 mg either orally or subcutaneously, as a single dose once weekly, with titration up to 25 mg once weekly as dictated by clinical response or by adverse events. The most common and significant side effects are nausea, hair loss, hepatotoxicity, bone marrow suppression, immunosuppression, and teratogenicity. Hence, careful follow-up, periodic laboratory monitoring with liver function tests and complete blood counts, and family planning counseling are required. Because of the hepatic metabolism of methotrexate, patients are strongly advised to limit alcohol intake to no more than one drink per week, and methotrexate use is relatively contraindicated in patients with preexisting liver disease or hepatitis B or C infection. Folic acid supplementation (1 mg/d) decreases the frequency and severity of side effects of methotrexate therapy and should be given concomitantly to all patients.

Sulfasalazine has been shown to have a good clinical effect in psoriatic arthritis. In studies conducted in patients from the Department of Veterans Affairs who were unresponsive to NSAIDs, sulfasalazine at 2 g/d decreased the joint pain and tenderness scores and swelling scores over 36 weeks. However, these findings did not reach statistical significance. Subsequent studies indicated that peripheral articular manifestations of psoriatic arthritis responded to sulfasalazine, whereas axial disease did not. Hence, axial and peripheral involvement of psoriatic arthritis may represent two distinct subgroups with regard to treatment response to sulfasalazine. While sulfasalazine was well tolerated in these studies, gastrointestinal intolerance is a commonly reported adverse event, which may be decreased with the use of enteric-coated formulations. Up to 40% of patients may discontinue this medication at higher doses secondary to gastrointestinal distress. As a result, when prescribed, it should be started at a low dose (500 mg twice daily) and slowly increased over weeks to a maximum dose of 2–3 g daily. Like methotrexate, sulfasalazine is metabolized by the liver. Hence, liver function tests should be monitored periodically. Sulfasalazine may cause allergic reactions and rash, which can be severe. It should be avoided in sulfa-allergic patients and in individuals with aspirin sensitivity. Screening for glucose-6-phosphate dehydrogenase deficiency should also be considered because patients are at increased risk for hemolysis. Because of anemia and other potential complications of sulfasalazine therapy, blood counts should also be periodically monitored.

Leflunomide (20 mg daily) has proven efficacy in treating peripheral articular manifestations of psoriatic arthritis.

Like methotrexate, it has potential hepatotoxicity and liver function tests need to be monitored periodically. It is also a teratogen with a prolonged elimination half-life, so contraception is critical.

D. Biologic Therapies

Tumor necrosis factor (TNF) is a proinflammatory cytokine that plays a central role in the pathogenesis of inflammatory arthritis and is detected in psoriatic plaques, synovium, and at entheses. Five biologic inhibitors of TNF, etanercept, infliximab, adalimumab, golimumab, and certolizumab pegol, have been approved for treating psoriasis and psoriatic arthritis. In clinical trials, all five agents had significant and early efficacy in decreasing the signs and symptoms of arthritis, as well as in the severity of psoriatic skin lesions in many patients. TNF antagonists have also been shown to slow the rate of radiographic progression of psoriatic arthritis. Four of these biologic agents (etanercept, adalimumab, golimumab, and certolizumab pegol) are given as subcutaneous injections, while infliximab is given as an intravenous infusion. The main adverse effects include injection site and infusion reactions and immunosuppression. Reactivation of latent tuberculosis has been seen with all agents as a mechanism-based side effect; thus, each patient should be screened for latent tuberculosis with a purified protein derivative skin test (or IFN release assays) and a chest radiograph prior to the initiation of a TNF inhibitor.

Another biologic agent is alefacept, a recombinant fusion protein of soluble lymphocyte function antigen with Fc fragments of IgG-1. Alefacept is approved for the treatment of moderate to severe chronic plaque psoriasis. Its mechanism of action is not completely understood, but it is thought to induce apoptosis of memory T cells, inhibit costimulation of T cells, and decrease inflammatory cell infiltration, thus leading to an anti-inflammatory effect. In an open-label extension of a randomized, double-blind, placebo-controlled study of alefacept in combination with methotrexate, alefacept-methotrexate-treated patients had a greater decrease in signs and symptoms of psoriatic arthritis than did patients in the placebo-methotrexate-treated group. There were no serious adverse reactions. Because of its effects on peripheral T cells, CD4 counts should be monitored in all patients taking alefacept.

Ustekinumab, a human monoclonal antibody against the P40 subunit of IL-12 and IL-23, has been approved for treatment of moderate to severe plaque psoriasis. In a randomized, double-blind, placebo-controlled, crossover phase II trial of ustekinumab for active psoriatic arthritis, ustekinumab significantly reduced the signs and symptoms of psoriatic arthritis compared with placebo. In one group, research participants received ustekinumab weekly for 4 weeks followed by placebo at weeks 12 and 16, and in the other group, participants received placebo weekly for 4 weeks followed by ustekinumab at weeks 12 and 16. Primary efficacy end point at week 12 was attained in 42% in the ustekinumab group compared to 14% in the placebo group ($P = 0.0002$). Serious adverse events of ustekinumab were low and not significantly different from that of placebo, but side effects included injection site reactions, infections, and reactivation of latent tuberculosis.

A phase II study demonstrated efficacy of abatacept to reduce the signs and symptoms of psoriatic arthritis. Abatacept, which has been approved for active rheumatoid arthritis, is a selective T-cell costimulation modulator that binds to the CD80/86 receptor of an antigen-presenting cell and inhibits its interaction with the CD28 receptor of the T-cell to produce the costimulatory signal necessary for T-cell activation. In a 6-month, randomized, double-blind, placebo-controlled trial comparing multiple doses of abatacept with placebo in active psoriatic arthritis, significantly higher proportions of participants receiving abatacept attained the primary efficacy end point. Abatacept was generally well tolerated but was associated with increased risk of headaches, infections (such as upper respiratory tract infections), and nasopharyngitis. Patients should be screened for latent tuberculosis before starting abatacept. Those with chronic obstructive pulmonary disease may experience worsening respiratory status and should be closely monitored.

Additional biologic agents currently being tested in psoriatic arthritis include an IL-15 inhibitor, apremilast (an oral phosphodiesterase-4 inhibitor), tocilizumab (an IL-6 antagonist), and AIN457 (an anti-IL-17 monoclonal antibody). Studies of small molecules such as Janus kinase (JAK) inhibitors are also anticipated.

E. Glucocorticoids

Intra-articular injections of glucocorticoids are an effective treatment when only one or two joints dominate a patient's symptoms. Psoriatic plaques are heavily contaminated with bacteria, and considerable care should be taken to avoid introducing an infection by passing the injecting needle through a psoriatic plaque into the joint.

Systemic glucocorticoids should be used with caution, if at all. Some rheumatologists use oral prednisone at doses of 10–20 mg daily with a gradual taper to quell an attack of psoriatic arthritis. Many dermatologists, however, avoid systemic glucocorticoids because of the risk that the glucocorticoid taper can precipitate a severe flare of pustular psoriasis. Regardless, baseline therapy in the form of NSAIDs, and in most cases, DMARDs or biologics, should be given for maintenance immunomodulatory control.

F. Surgery

Long-standing erosive and destructive disease can lead to extensive joint deformities. If severe destructive disease is present, orthopedic surgery consultation may be considered for joint replacement or stabilization.

▶ Prognosis

Because the bony destruction associated with psoriatic arthritis is irreversible, prompt diagnosis and early intervention are essential to preserve a patient's functional status and quality of life. Hence, if the appropriate diagnosis of a patient is in question, if radiographic damage is detected at presentation, or if a patient does not respond to first-line therapies with NSAIDs, referral to a rheumatologist is appropriate. More aggressive interventions, such as the initiation of DMARDs or biologics, should be overseen by a rheumatologist. If severe destructive disease is present, orthopedic surgery consultation may be considered for joint replacement or stabilization. As with all patients with psoriasis, care with a dermatologist should be coordinated.

Anandarajah AP, Ritchlin CT. The diagnosis and treatment of early psoriatic arthritis. *Nat Rev Rheumatol.* 2009;5:634. [PMID: 19806150]

Castelino M, Barton A. Genetic susceptibility factors for psoriatic arthritis. *Curr Opin Rheumatol.* 2010;22:152. [PMID: 20084005]

Fitzgerald O, Winchester R. Psoriatic arthritis: from pathogenesis to therapy. *Arthritis Res Ther.* 2009;11:214. [PMID: 19232079]

Gottlieb A, Menter A, Mendelsohn A, et al. Ustekinumab, a human interleukin 12/23 monoclonal antibody, for psoriatic arthritis: randomised, double-blind, placebo-controlled, crossover trial. *Lancet.* 2009;373:633. [PMID: 19217154]

McGonagle D, Benjamin M, Tan AL. The pathogenesis of psoriatic arthritis and associated nail disease: not autoimmune after all? *Curr Opin Rheumatol.* 2009;21:340. [PMID: 19424069]

Mease PJ. Psoriatic arthritis: update on pathophysiology, assessment and management. *Ann Rheum Dis.* 2011;70(Suppl 1):i77. [PMID: 21339225]

Mease PJ. Psoriatic arthritis assessment and treatment update. *Curr Opin Rheumatol.* 2009;21:348. [PMID: 19461518]

Ritchlin CT, Kavanaugh A, Gladman DD, et al. Treatment recommendations for psoriatic arthritis. *Ann Rheum Dis.* 2009;68:1387. [PMID: 18952643]

Soriano ER, Rosa J. Update on the treatment of peripheral arthritis in psoriatic arthritis. *Curr Rheumatol Rep.* 2009;11:270. [PMID: 19691930]

Taylor W, Gladman D, Helliwell P, Marchesoni A, Mease P, Mielants H, CASPAR Study Group. Classification criteria for psoriatic arthritis: development of new criteria from a large international study. *Arthritis Rheum.* 2006;54:2665. [PMID: 16871531]

Juvenile Idiopathic Arthritis

20

Peggy Schlesinger, MD
Jennifer K. Turner, MD
Kristen Hayward, MD, MA

Juvenile idiopathic arthritis (JIA) refers to a group of disorders that are a major cause of chronic arthritis in children. It is the most common chronic rheumatic disease of childhood and can be a significant cause of both short-term and long-term disability. In the United States, approximately 294,000 children younger than 18 years have arthritis or other rheumatic conditions.

JIA is relatively common compared to other chronic diseases of childhood. There are as many children with juvenile-onset diabetes as there are those with juvenile-onset arthritis, and there are 10 times as many children with arthritis as there are children affected with muscular dystrophy.

ESSENTIALS OF DIAGNOSIS

▶ Six weeks or more of persistent joint swelling, and the exclusion of other causes of arthritis in childhood.

▶ There is no specific laboratory test that either confirms or excludes JIA.

▶ The type of JIA is determined by the age of the child at onset of symptoms; the number and type of joints involved; the presence of extra-articular symptoms, such as rash, fever, and iritis; and the course of the illness during the first 6 months after the diagnosis is confirmed.

▶ Significant complications, including macrophage activation syndrome (MAS), contractures, growth retardation, and visual loss, can be avoided by prompt diagnosis and treatment.

SUBTYPES OF JIA

According to the International League Against Rheumatism, the types of JIA can be classified as oligoarticular, polyarticular (including seropositive and seronegative), systemic onset (SOJIA), psoriatic, enthesitis-related, and undifferentiated. The different subtypes of JIA are mainly determined by the pattern of joint involvement at the onset of the illness.

The subtypes of JIA are identified and classified based on the following factors: age at onset, number of joints involved initially, rheumatoid factor status, and associated extra-articular symptoms (Table 20–1). Identification of the correct subtype helps guide appropriate therapy and determine prognosis.

1. Oligoarticular JIA

Oligoarticular JIA occurs most commonly in very young children, ages 1–7 years.

▶ Articular Symptoms

Symptoms of joint inflammation with morning stiffness can begin at any time after the child begins to walk. An asymmetric pattern of joint involvement is common and no more than four joints are affected. Morning stiffness is a prominent finding and, although the affected joint is often swollen and quite large, the child frequently has less pain than one would expect. Knees are the most commonly involved joint; there may also be diffuse swelling of a toe or finger, and ankles, wrists, and elbows are also commonly involved. The atlanto-axial (C1–C2) joint and the temporomandibular joint (TMJ) are relatively hidden sites where joint inflammation and loss of motion can occur.

▶ Extra-articular Symptom: Iritis

Children with oligoarticular JIA, especially very young girls with a positive antinuclear antibody (ANA) test, are at increased risk for iritis. This chronic, anterior, nongranulomatous uveitis or iridocyclitis is painless and typically occurs early in the course of the illness. One of five patients

Table 20–1. Comparing the features of the subgroups of juvenile idiopathic arthritis.

Features	Subgroups of Juvenile Idiopathic Arthritis					
	Oligoarticular	Seronegative Polyarticular	Seropositive Polyarticular	Systemic Onset	Psoriatic	Enthesitis-related
Percentage of all cases	40%	20%	15%	10–20%	≤10%	≤10%
Age at onset and gender prevalence	<8 years girls >> boys	8–12 years girls = boys	Teen years girls >> boys	Any age	Any age	8–12 years boys >> girls
Number of joints involved	<5	Many	Many	Varies	Varies	Varies
Pattern	Asymmetric	Symmetric	Symmetric			Lower extremity joints
Hips involved	Rarely	No	No	Occasionally	Occasionally	Yes
Back pain	No	No	No	Myalgic	Yes	Yes
Clinical features	• Painless iridocyclitis • Requires regular slit-lamp examination at regular intervals	• Poor weight gain and growth	• Aggressive course • Poor weight gain • Can have vasculitis, nodules	• Fever • Evanescent rash • Serositis • Lymphadenopathy • Hepatosplenomegaly • MAS • Complications can be fatal	• DIP joints • Nail pitting • Psoriatic rash or positive family history for psoriasis • Dactylitis • Can resemble polyarticular or enthesitis-related arthritis	• Enthesitis • Heel pain • Sausage digits • Abnormal Shober test • Sacroiliitis • Oral ulcers
Distinguishing laboratory findings	Positive ANA	Negative rheumatoid factor	Positive rheumatoid factor	• ↑ESR • ↑WBC • ↑CRP • ↑Platelets • Anemia • Abnormal LFTs • Ferritin	Positive ANA in 30–60%	Positive HLA-B27

ANA, antinuclear antibody; CRP, C-reactive protein; DIP, distal interphalangeal; ESR, erythrocyte sedimentation rate; LFT, liver function tests; MAS, macrophase activation syndrome; WBC, white blood count.

with oligoarticular JIA has *asymptomatic* iritis identified at a screening slit lamp examination. Seventy-five percent of these children with oligoarticular JIA and iritis have a positive ANA. The iritis of oligoarticular JIA responds well to treatment when the diagnosis is made early. One or both eyes can be involved at any time in the course of the disease, not only when joints are flaring. Initial treatment with glucocorticoid eye drops and mydriatics is usually sufficient. Sub-tenon injections of long-acting glucocorticoid preparations can also be used as needed to control inflammation in the anterior chamber of the affected eye. Systemic therapy with methotrexate or biologic agents (tumor necrosis factor [TNF] inhibitors) is sometimes necessary to control ocular inflammation, even in patients whose arthritis has responded well to more conservative therapy. Serious complications, such as blindness, glaucoma, cataracts, and band keratopathy, can result from untreated eye disease. Prevention and early treatment of

both the iritis and arthritis are preferable to the disappointing results seen in cases that go unrecognized until a later stage. All children with oligoarticular JIA, regardless of ANA status, should have regular slit lamp examinations done until they reach 18 years of age, even in the absence of a red eye or ongoing joint symptoms (Table 20–2). Untreated iritis can cause serious long-term morbidity in these children, unlike the arthritis, which often resolves by the time they reach school age and typically does not lead to permanent joint damage.

► **Prognosis**

In some children, oligoarticular JIA may begin in a few joints but progress to involve more than five joints early in the course of the illness. If this progression occurs within the first 6 months of disease, the arthritis is reclassified as polyarticular JIA. If an increasing number of joints (>4) become

Table 20–2. Recommended ophthalmologic screening in juvenile idiopathic arthritis (JIA)[a].

	Schedule for Eye Examinations	
JIA Subtype	Onset Before Age 7	Onset After Age 7
Oligoarticular JIA		
Positive ANA	Every 3 months for 4 years; then every 6 months for 3 years; then yearly	Every 6 months for 4 years; then yearly
Negative ANA	Every 6 months for 7 years; then yearly	Every 6 months for 4 years; then yearly
Polyarticular JIA		
Positive ANA	Every 3 months for 4 years; then every 6 months for 3 years; then yearly	Every 6 months for 4 years; then yearly
Negative ANA	Every 6 months for 7 years; then yearly	Every 6 months for 4 years; then yearly
Systemic JIA		
Positive or negative ANA	Yearly	Yearly

ANA, antinuclear antibody.
These are surveillance recommendations for those children who do not present with iritis. If iritis develops, more frequent slit lamp exams will be indicated.
[a]Guidelines for ophthalmologic examinations in children with juvenile rheumatoid arthritis. Section on Rheumatology and Section of Ophthalmology, American Academy of Pediatrics. *Pediatrics.* 1993;92:295–296.

involved more than 6 months after diagnosis, the arthritis is referred to as **extended oligoarticular JIA.** Extended oligoarticular JIA is a more aggressive subtype, and arthritis in these children often persists into adulthood, with the possibility of joint destruction occurring over time. Patients with extended oligoarticular JIA have the same increased risk of iritis as the children with the persistent oligoarticular type and continue to require regular screening slit lamp examinations until they are 18 years old.

2. Polyarticular JIA

Polyarticular JIA presents in children of any age with persistent synovitis in five or more joints at onset. In this heterogeneous group of patients, the rheumatoid factor test is a useful prognosticator.

▶ Seropositive Polyarticular JIA

Patients who have polyarticular JIA with positive rheumatoid factor are usually teenage girls with symmetric arthritis involving the small joints of hands and feet. This is the only one of the JIA subgroups that clinically resembles the adult form of classic rheumatoid factor–positive rheumatoid arthritis, with similar HLA-DR4 associations. These girls are more likely to have aggressive, erosive joint disease. Rheumatoid nodules occur in 5–10% of patients in this subgroup, and Felty syndrome, rheumatoid vasculitis, and rheumatoid lung disease are occasionally seen. Iritis is uncommon in this subgroup, occurring in <5% of these patients.

▶ Seronegative Polyarticular Arthritis

Polyarticular JIA with negative rheumatoid factor typically affects younger children, more often girls than boys. The arthritis may or may not be symmetric but prefers large joints, knees, ankles, and wrists. There are no associated extra-articular features and iritis is rare. These children can have active arthritis for many years without erosive change seen on radiographs.

▶ Prognosis

The course is variable, and transition to the positive rheumatoid factor polyarticular subgroup can occur. In patients with psoriatic arthritis, multiple joints can be involved at presentation, but the prognosis differs from both the polyarticular rheumatoid factor–negative and rheumatoid factor–positive JIA subgroup. Both the psoriatic subgroup and the polyarticular rheumatoid factor–positive subgroup of patients may have continued active disease into adulthood.

3. Systemic Onset JIA

This disease affects children and adults at any age, with boys and girls affected equally.

▶ Articular & Extra-articular Symptoms

The hallmarks of SOJIA are the daily spiking fever in a quotidian or "rabbit ears" pattern in association with a salmon-colored, macular, evanescent rash on trunk and extremities that is present only during fever. Painful myalgias, enlarged liver, spleen, lymph nodes and pleuro-pericarditis may be present at disease onset. True arthritis may not manifest until months after the onset of fever, which can make early diagnosis difficult.

Children appear acutely ill (with significant fever, fatigue, and pain). Extensive diagnostic studies, including a bone marrow examination, may be necessary to rule out infection and malignancy. Malignancy is often suspected initially at the onset of SOJIA because the child fails to thrive due to the significant fever, fatigue, and pain.

Marked leukocytosis, very high sedimentation rates, and elevated ferritin levels are the rule in this disease. Iritis is rare in this subgroup. Recurrent episodes of active SOJIA can occur into adulthood even after an extended disease-free interval.

▶ Complications

Pericardial effusion, although common in SOJIA, usually does not become hemodynamically significant, yet children with SOJIA and pericarditis must be watched closely to ensure that cardiac function is not compromised.

Pericarditis and MAS can be life-threatening. MAS can occur at any time during the course of SOJIA and may go unrecognized until the child becomes desperately ill; thus, clinicians must always maintain a high index of suspicion for this complication. Signs and symptoms may include high unremitting fever, hepatosplenomegaly, encephalopathy, and disseminated intravascular coagulation with bruising and mucosal bleeding. Laboratory abnormalities include depression of all 3 blood cell lines (white cells, red cells, and platelets), elevated transaminases and triglycerides, low albumin, prolonged prothrombin time and partial thromboplastin time, a paradoxically normal erythrocyte sedimentation rate (secondary to dropping fibrinogen in the setting of consumptive coagulopathy), and elevated ferritin level and D-dimer. Bone marrow aspirate in children with active MAS reveals macrophages actively phagocytosing other hematopoietic cells, but bone marrow aspirate is not often needed to make this diagnosis in the appropriate clinical context. The cause of MAS is unknown, but in some patients, it seems to follow an episode of apparent viral illness. MAS can occur de novo or in association with SOJIA or other rheumatic disorders of childhood. The mortality rate for MAS is reported to be 22% in a recent case series, although older reports place it as high as 50%. This very serious complication is an important cause of morbidity and mortality in SOJIA and must be looked for assiduously. Treatment with high-dose glucocorticoids and cyclosporine should be used to control the internal cytokine storm and reduce morbidity from MAS when it complicates SOJIA.

4. Psoriatic Arthritis

▶ Articular Symptoms

The psoriatic JIA subgroup includes patients with any of the following signs and symptoms: arthritis of one or more joints, sacroiliitis, distal interphalangeal joint synovitis, dactylitis, sausage digits, nail pitting, and either a psoriatic rash or a positive family history of psoriasis (or both). A history of psoriasis in a first-degree relative can be enough to confirm this diagnosis in the child who has arthritis. In some patients, it may take years from the onset of the arthritis until the typical skin lesions appear. Radiologic findings of fluffy periostitis, dactylitis, and sacroiliac joint widening and irregularity, if present, help differentiate psoriatic JIA from polyarticular JIA.

▶ Extra-articular Symptoms

Acute anterior uveitis, with photophobia and a painful red eye, is associated with psoriatic arthritis, and patients should be advised to see an ophthalmologist if they are having these ocular symptoms. The 30–60% of patients with psoriatic arthritis who have a positive ANA are also at risk for chronic, painless, iritis indistinguishable from that seen in oligoarticular JIA. These patients in the psoriatic subgroup who have a positive ANA test should have routine slit lamp examinations on the same schedule as patients with oligoarticular JIA (Table 20–2).

▶ Prognosis

The course of psoriatic arthritis is variable, and long periods of remission with periodic exacerbations can occur.

5. Enthesitis-Related JIA

Enthesitis refers to inflammation at the site of attachment (enthesis) of tendon/ligament to the bone. The inflammation can cause point tenderness at that site. Children with enthesitis-related JIA have painful stiffness from enthesitis that can occur even in the absence of true arthritis. Inflammatory parameters, erythrocyte sedimentation rate and C-reactive protein, are frequently elevated. The HLA-B27 gene can be found in the majority of patients in this category, but it is not diagnostic. Prognosis is quite good in these children if enthesitis is recognized and treated to reduce pain and resultant disability.

The enthesitis-related JIA subgroup includes patients with juvenile-onset spondylitis, reactive arthritis, and the arthritis associated with inflammatory bowel disease. This type of JIA usually presents with synovitis in peripheral joints, mainly in lower extremities, in boys aged 8–12 years. Heel pain; rash, including pyoderma gangrenosum; oral ulcers; symptomatic sacroiliitis; and acute, painful uveitis can also occur in these patients. Pain, stiffness, and loss of flexibility in the lumbar spine may develop in older boys. Treatment of underlying inflammatory bowel disease, if present, is necessary for optimum control of arthritis and enthesitis.

6. Undifferentiated Arthritis

This category includes patients whose arthritis either does not fit into any of the other categories or whose arthritis symptoms fit into more than one of these categories.

TEMPOROMANDIBULAR JOINT ARTHRITIS

TMJ arthritis can occur in any of the JIA subtypes, although it is most commonly seen in polyarticular JIA. The TMJ may be the only joint involved in oligoarticular JIA or the first joint affected in children with one of the other subtypes. Isolated TMJ disease producing restricted jaw opening without other joint involvement can be the presenting symptom of JIA. TMJ arthritis is often difficult to recognize, and care must be taken to include evaluation of these joints in the routine joint examination. This is done by monitoring the tooth to tooth gap (normal is 3.5–4.0 cm or greater in school-aged children), assessing pain with motion and palpation of the TMJ joints, and observing the symmetry of jaw excursion. Patients should be observed for asymmetry of the mandibular arch and retrognathia, since both can be caused by undergrowth of the mandible as a direct result of unilateral or bilateral TMJ arthritis. Any abnormality should lead to imaging the joints, by Panorex or CT scan, to look for erosions at the TMJ, or by MRI of the TMJ with gadolinium contrast enhancement to look for active synovitis. Active synovitis of the TMJ can be successfully treated with intra-articular glucocorticoid injection to control symptoms and TNF inhibitors if synovitis with erosion is seen on TMJ MRI.

ETIOLOGY OF JIA

Current research suggests that the etiology of JIA is multifactorial and involves a complex interplay between environmental triggers and genetic factors. Evidence for a genetic contribution to JIA stems from family studies that indicate a 15–30 times higher prevalence of JIA among siblings of JIA patients than in the general population. However, concordance rates of 25–40% among monozygotic twins suggest that there is a complex genetic trait for JIA, and genetic predisposition alone is insufficient for disease development.

With the advent of the human genome projects and rapid advances in genotyping technology, there has been an explosion of recent research into the genetic underpinnings of JIA. In particular, multiple polymorphisms in HLA genes have been associated with JIA susceptibility. Specific HLA associations vary by JIA subtype, with certain alleles such as DRB1*04 conferring susceptibility for rheumatoid factor–positive polyarticular JIA while seeming to exert a protective effect in patients with oligoarticular or enthesitis-related disease.

Environmental triggers for JIA have been more difficult to identify. Infectious agents have long been suspected; however, no specific pathogens have been consistently identified that can trigger the onset of active disease.

CLINICAL FINDINGS

The diagnosis of JIA is made clinically when chronic synovitis is present in any one joint for 6 weeks or more in a child younger than 16 years. Synovitis is defined as inflammation of the synovial lining that manifests clinically as swelling and limited motion of a joint, often with warmth, pain, and stiffness. The chronicity of the joint involvement in JIA distinguishes this group of disorders from the many short-term causes of joint pain and swelling that can occur in childhood.

A. Laboratory Findings

There is no single laboratory test that is diagnostic of JIA. Laboratory evaluation in a child with arthritis is necessary to exclude other possible causes of arthritis, such as infection, malignancy, and other rheumatic diseases. Children in whom JIA is suspected should be evaluated with complete blood count, erythrocyte sedimentation rate, C-reactive protein quantitation, liver and renal function tests as well as an ANA and rheumatoid factor assay. The anti-cyclic citrullinated peptide antibody is currently being evaluated in this age group to identify its diagnostic potential in JIA. An HLA-B27 test can be helpful in the evaluation of patients with symptoms suggestive of enthesitis-related JIA, but it is not diagnostic. As a general screen for possible malignancy, especially in children with daily fever and joint symptoms, a uric acid level and lactate dehydrogenase should be obtained. Some children with arthritis related to leukemia can have normal blood counts at presentation, with falling counts and immature forms appearing on peripheral smears later in the course of the illness. Thyroid-stimulating hormone, albumin, and pre-albumin can help in the work-up of children with arthritis and poor weight gain and slow linear growth. In patients with suspected SOJIA, a serum ferritin level, prothrombin time, partial thromboplastin time, and D-dimer should also be done to look for evidence of MAS.

B. Imaging Studies

Plain radiographs of affected joints are helpful in the initial evaluation of joint pain and swelling in children, mainly to rule out diagnoses other than JIA. A bone scan can identify unrecognized sites of inflammation in patients in whom the diagnosis of arthritis is in question, or in patients whose symptoms are difficult to evaluate. CT scans and MRI can show joint erosions at an early stage before they are visible on plain films. An intravenous gadolinium contrast-enhanced MRI can identify active synovitis in inflamed joints. This scan is often useful in managing inflammation in patients with JIA, especially those with early erosions or TMJ disease, or both.

DIFFERENTIAL DIAGNOSIS

Most patients with JIA have swelling and synovitis in at least one joint that persists for 6 weeks or more. Pain is not the most common presenting complaint. If the provider waits for a child to complain of pain before considering the diagnosis of arthritis, then the child's stiff and swollen joint(s) plus abnormal gait pattern and morning stiffness may go undiagnosed for quite some time. Other rheumatic diseases, such as systemic lupus erythematosus (SLE) are also present in childhood and must be considered in the differential when a child presents with arthritis. There are many kinds of arthritis occurring in childhood that can cause transient swollen joints that resolve within 4–6 weeks. These disorders are beyond the scope of this chapter but should be actively investigated when children have joint swelling. See Chapter 5 for a complete discussion of the differential diagnosis of joint pain in older children.

COMPLICATIONS

Bone overgrowth secondary to increased blood flow to the inflamed joint is common in oligoarticular JIA patients, particularly at the knee joint. This can result in a leg-length discrepancy requiring the use of a shoe lift. Equalizing the leg lengths with a shoe lift can prevent or treat a flexion contracture at the affected joint and normalize the child's gait. With adequate control of inflammation, this bone overgrowth and the associated leg-length discrepancy usually resolves in time. Serious complications including mandibular asymmetry, generalized growth retardation, osteopenia or osteoporosis, gait abnormalities, muscle atrophy, difficult orthodontic problems, loss of vision, glaucoma, and cataracts can occur in the child with JIA whose arthritis is not well controlled or whose iritis goes unrecognized. In appropriately treated patients, complications of therapy, such as infection, delayed immunizations, abnormal growth, complications from glucocorticoid therapy, and medication-related dyspepsia can occur.

TREATMENT

There are several treatment options available for children with JIA that are very effective at producing remission. Early treatment should be made available to all children with JIA to minimize disability from this disease. Up to 50% of children with JIA may have continued active disease into adulthood. With early diagnosis and treatment and the use of biologic therapies, sequelae of active JIA (such as deformity and disability) as well as continued active arthritis will become less common. Consultation with a pediatric rheumatologist can ensure that every child with JIA is receiving optimal therapy, which can reduce overall morbidity from this group of diseases.

The goals of treatment are to produce remission of joint inflammation and restore the child to normal function. Once joint pain, stiffness, and swelling are reduced, then gait patterns and muscle atrophy will return to normal, making joint contracture and deformity less likely. Other sequelae, such as asymmetry of the mandible, leg length discrepancy, and generalized growth retardation, will not develop when active arthritis is well controlled. Iritis is also less likely to remain active despite treatment when arthritis is in remission.

Nonsteroidal anti-inflammatory drugs (NSAIDs) and glucocorticoids, either oral or intra-articular, are the mainstays of therapy for many children with JIA (Table 20–3).

Table 20–3. NSAIDs approved by the Food and Drug Administration for use in children with JIA.

Drug	Dose	Formulation	Comment
Etodolac	20–30 kg: 400 mg/day 31–45 kg: 600 mg/day 46–60 kg: 800 mg/day >60 kg: 1000 mg/day	Extended release tablet: 400 mg, 500 mg, 600 mg	Once daily dosing is convenient
Oxaprazocin	<31 kg: 600 mg/day, <54 kg: 900 mg/day >55 kg: 1200 mg/day	Tablet: 600 mg	Once daily dosing is convenient
Celecoxib	<25 kg: 50 mg twice daily >25 kg: 100 mg twice daily	Capsule: 50 mg, 100 mg	Twice daily dosing is convenient
Naproxen	20 mg/kg/day or 10 mg/kg/dose twice daily **Maximum dose:** 1000 mg/d	Liquid: 125 mg/5 mL Tablet: 220 mg, over the counter or 250 mg, 375 mg or 500 mg, by prescription	Twice daily dosing is convenient
Ibuprofen	40 mg/kg/day or 10 mg/kg/dose four times daily **Maximum dose:** 2400 mg/day	Liquid: 100 mg/5 mL Tablet: 200 mg, over the counter	Short half-life = four times daily dosing
Tolmetin	30 mg/kg/day or 10 mg/kg/dose three times daily **Maximum dose:** 1800 mg/day	Tablets: 200 mg, 400 mg, 600 mg	
Indomethacin	1–3 mg/kg/day three or four times daily **Maximum dose:** 200 mg/day	Liquid: 25 mg/5 mL Tablets: 25 mg, 50 mg, 75 mg (sustained release), 100 mg (extended release)	Useful in systemic onset JIA and spondylitis
Meloxicam	0.125 mg/kg/day **Maximum dose:** 15 mg/day	Liquid: 7.5 mg/5mL Tablet: 7.5 mg, 15 mg	Once daily dosing is convenient

NSAIDs, nonsteroidal anti-inflammatory drugs; JIA, juvenile idiopathic arthritis.

Table 20–4. DMARDs and TNF inhibitors used in children with JIA.

Drug	Dose	Formulation	Special Considerations
DMARDs			
Hydroxychloroquine	6 mg/kg/day once or twice daily	Tablets: 200 mg	• Yearly eye examinations recommended • Retinal toxicity is rare at these doses
Sulfasalazine	30–50 mg/kg/day2 or 3 times daily	Tablets: 500 mg	• Contraindicated in sulfa allergic or aspirin-sensitive patients • Useful in polyarticular JIA and spondylitis • Not for use in systemic onset JIA • Enteric-coated formulation is often better tolerated
Methotrexate	15 mg/m^2 or 0.5–1.0 mg/kg per dose once a week. Orally, intramuscularly, or subcutaneously **Maximum dose: 25mg/wk**	Tablets: 2.5 mg Liquid:25 mg/1 mL 2.5 mg = 0.1 mL	• Higher doses well tolerated in children • Poor oral absorption in children can lead to inadequate clinical response • Same dose subcutaneously is 100% absorbed with better clinical response • Avoid concomitant sulfa, tetracycline • Liquid can be taken orally or subcutaneously • This is the least expensive DMARD
Cyclosporine	3–5 mg/kg/day Twice daily	Capsules and Tablets: 25 mg and 100 mg Liquid: 100 mg/mL	• Modified and non-modified cyclosporine products not bioequilavent • Grapefruit juice increases absorption • Most effective in systemic onset JIA • Monitor kidney function and blood pressure • Many drug interactions
Leflunomide	100 mg/day for 1 day loading dose plus 10 mg orally every other day if <20 kg 100 mg/day for 2 days, then 10 mg orally once daily if 20–40 kg 100 mg/day for 3 days, then 20 mg/day if >40 kg	Pills: 10 mg and 20 mg	• Hair thinning occurs in 1 of 8 patients • Loose stools respond to dose adjustment and loperamide as needed • Avoid pregnancy during treatment until cholestyramine washout completed
TNF Inhibitors			
Etanercept[a]	0.8 mg/kg/dose subcutaneously weekly or 0.4 mg/kg/dose subcutaneously twice a week **Maximum dose: 50 mg/wk**	25 mg powder to reconstitute with water in prefilled syringe; or prefilled syringe 50 mg/mL Auto-injector available *Refrigerate*	• Avoid live virus immunization • Approved and indicated for polyarticular JIA • Combination with methotrexate more effective than monotherapy • Increased risk of infection
Anakinra[a]	1–2 mg/kg/day subcutaneously	Prefilled syringe 100 mg *Refrigerate*	• Very effective in systemic onset JIA • Injection is often painful • Infection risk is low
Infliximab[b]	3–10 mg/kg per infusion given intravenously at 0, 2 and 4 weeks then every 4 weeks, increase interval to 6–8 weeks as tolerated	Intravenous infusion requires premedication with diphenhydramine and acetaminophen	• Infection risk is high, especially at doses above 5 mg/kg • Chimeric molecule requires concomitant treatment with methotrexate • Avoid live virus immunization • Useful in psoriatic arthritis, inflammatory bowel disease and spondyloarthropathy
Adalimumab[a]	24 mg/m^2 subcutaneously every other week **Maximum dose: 40 mg subcutaneously every other week**	Prefilled syringe 40 mg Auto-injector available *Refrigerate*	• Early clinical response and ease of administration • Approved for JIA in patients aged 4 years and older • Increased risk of infection • Avoid live virus immunization
Abatacept[a]	10 mg/kg intravenously at 0, 2, 4 weeks and every 4 weeks ongoing **Maximum is 1000 mg/dose**	Intravenous infusion	• No increased risk of serious infection in pediatric trial • Long-term studies underway

[a]Purified protein derivative (PPD) should be done before starting therapy.
[b]Infliximab is currently under evaluation regarding usefulness in JIA.
DMARDs, disease-modifying antirheumatic drugs; JIA, juvenile idiopathic arthritis, TNF, tumor necrosis factor.

Ibuprofen and naproxen, tolmetin and indomethacin are among the nine NSAIDs that have been FDA approved for use in the pediatric age group. Meloxicam is a cyclooxygenase (COX)-2 inhibitor that has been approved for use in children with JIA, and the once-daily dosing is convenient.

Many children in the oligoarticular, seronegative polyarticular, and enthesitis-related subgroups do not need disease modifying anti-rheumatic drugs (DMARDs) to control the arthritis. They can often be treated with an NSAID or an intra-articular glucocorticoid injection of the affected joints, or both. However, if joint pain or swelling, decreased range of motion, or morning stiffness persists despite these measures, the addition of a DMARD is warranted. Because of its long record of safety and efficacy in JIA, methotrexate is typically the first DMARD of choice. Patients with seropositive polyarticular disease should be treated aggressively with DMARDs (Table 20–4) early to prevent joint erosions and deformities. Patients with SOJIA often require glucocorticoids initially to establish control of the symptoms and may need biologic therapy with an IL-1 inhibitor or methotrexate or cyclosporine to maintain remission. For patients with SOJIA patients who have evidence of MAS, high-dose intravenous glucocorticoids with cyclosporine are able to turn off the cytokine storm in most patients, though an IL-1 inhibitor (such as anakinra) is sometimes required to sustain improvement.

The FDA approval of the first biologic therapy, etanercept, for polyarticular JIA in 1999 was a very significant milestone in the treatment of JIA. Biologic therapies interrupt the immune signaling that leads to chronic inflammation in the joints. Etanercept, adalimumab, and infliximab produce remission of JIA by specific inhibition of TNF. Biologic therapies can induce remission in polyarticular disease early in the course, prior to the development of complications such as erosions, deformity, and growth abnormalities. Etanercept, adalimumab, abatacept, and anakinra are all biologic therapies that are FDA approved for the treatment of JIA. Other biologic therapies (Table 20–4) are currently in clinical trials to clarify the safety and efficacy of these agents in the pediatric age group. A tuberculin skin test (or purified protein derivative) should be performed before the initiation of any biologic therapy to rule out the possibility of reactivation of latent tuberculosis while receiving biologic treatment.

The FDA recently issued a statement regarding malignancy in the setting of TNF inhibitor use. Forty-eight malignancies were reported in pediatric patients aged 0–17 years treated with a TNF inhibitor over an 8-year period. The majority of these reported malignancies occurred in pediatric patients with inflammatory bowel disease who were receiving infliximab. Because inflammatory bowel disease itself carries an increased risk of malignancy, and because many of these patients take an additional immunosuppressive agent known to increase cancer risk (azathioprine or 6-mercaptopurine), the true risk of malignancy in children with JIA that is directly attributable to treatment with TNF inhibitors is unclear. The development of malignancies was reported in 19 patients with JIA (including 1 with psoriatic arthritis and 3 with ankylosing spondylitis) while receiving a TNF inhibitor, although the total number of children treated with these agents is not known. In all of the controlled studies of anti-TNF agents in children conducted thus far, no increased risk of malignancy has been found in this population. Based on these published studies, malignancy appears to be a rare event in treated children with JIA. At the present time, it is unlikely that treatment of children with TNF inhibitors is associated with an increased risk for malignancy. Any potential adverse event attributable to the treatment of JIA must be considered in light of the risk of allowing untreated arthritis to erode both the joints and the well being of the child involved, since untreated JIA is associated with significant morbidity and long-term disability.

The treatment team involved in the care of a child with JIA includes the primary care provider, pediatric rheumatologist, social worker, clinic nurse, and pharmacist. Others, such as a psychologist or school counselor, nutritionist, and parent advocate may also be needed. Physical and occupational therapy may be needed in some cases to suggest therapeutic exercise, provide adaptive equipment, and prevent joint contractures while working on improved joint range of motion, muscle strength, and endurance.

Recognizing the needs of the child with JIA in his or her surroundings at school as well as at home is vital to the successful management of the disease. Attention to school issues and peer acceptance, or lack thereof, is critically important. Many families benefit from the helpful involvement of a social worker for assistance with these issues. It is very important that the child with JIA be encouraged to remain active and participate fully in both school and extra-curricular activities. Participation in physical education and competitive sports can help a child with arthritis build strength and endurance as well as boost self-esteem. Participation in an arthritis camp experience can help reduce the isolation that children with JIA often feel as a result of being different from their peers. Peer, parental and school support is vital to ensuring successful treatment of this chronic illness in children.

Arthritis Foundation
  www.arthritis.org

Burgos-Vargas R. The juvenile-onset spondyloarthritides. *Rheum Dis Clin North Am.* 2002;28:531. [PMID: 12380369]

Diak P, Siegel J, La Grenade L, Choi L, Lemery S, McMahon A. Tumor necrosis factor alpha blockers and malignancy in children: forty-eight cases reported to the Food and Drug Administration. *Arthritis Rheum.* 2010;62:2517. [PMID: 20506368]

Grom AA, Glass DN. Immunopathogenesis of juvenile rheumatoid arthritis. In: UpToDate, Basow DS, editor. UpToDate. Waltham, MA; 2009.

Hayward K, Wallace CA. Recent developments in anti-rheumatic drugs in pediatrics: treatment of juvenile idiopathic arthritis. *Arthritis Res Ther.* 2009;11:216. [PMID: 19291269]

Helminck CG, Felson DT, Lawrence RC, et al. National Arthritis Data Workgroup. Estimates of the prevalence of arthritis and other rheumatic conditions in the United States. Part I. *Arthritis Rheum.* 2008;58:15. [PMID: 18163481]

Paediatric Rheumatology International Trials Organization and the Paediatric Rheumatology European Society http://www.printo.it/pediatric-rheumatology/

Petty RE, Southwood TR, Manners P, et al. International League of Associations for Rheumatology. International League of Associations for Rheumatology classification of juvenile idiopathic arthritis: second edition, Edmonton, 2001. *J Rheumatol.* 2004;31:390. [PMID: 14760812]

Prahalad S, Glass DN. A comprehensive review of the genetics of juvenile idiopathic arthritis. *Pediatr Rheumatol Online J.* 2008;6:11. [PMID: 18644131]

Ravelli A. Macrophage activation syndrome. *Curr Opin Rheumatol.* 2002;14:548. [PMID: 12192253]

Sacks JJ, Helmick CG, Luo YH, Ilowite NT, Bowyer S. Prevalence of and annual ambulatory health care visits for pediatric arthritis and other rheumatologic conditions in the United States in 2001–2004. *Arthritis Rheum.* 2007;57:1439. [PMID: 18050185]

Weiss JE, Ilowite NT. Juvenile idiopathic arthritis. *Pediatr Clin North Ama.* 2005;52:413. [PMID: 15820374]

Systemic Lupus Erythematosus

21

Maria Dall'Era, MD

ESSENTIALS OF DIAGNOSIS

- ▶ Predilection for females of childbearing age.
- ▶ Multisystem disease, often with a relapsing-remitting course.
- ▶ Photosensitive rash, polyarthritis, serositis, and fatigue are common manifestations of disease flares.
- ▶ Renal disease and central nervous system involvement are important causes of morbidity.
- ▶ Presence of antinuclear antibodies.
- ▶ Certain autoantibodies (anti-dsDNA and anti-Sm) have great specificity for the diagnosis of SLE, but lack sensitivity.
- ▶ Hypocomplementemia may occur during flares.

▶ General Considerations

Systemic lupus erythematosus (SLE) is the prototypic auto-immune disease characterized by multisystem involvement and the production of an array of autoantibodies. Clinical features in individual patients are highly variable, ranging from skin and joint involvement to organ-threatening and life-threatening disease. SLE is typically associated with a waxing and waning clinical course, but some patients have continuous disease activity.

The prevalence of SLE varies across gender, race/ethnicity, and geographic regions. SLE demonstrates a striking female predominance with a peak incidence of disease during the reproductive years. In adults, the female to male ratio is 10–15:1. In the United States, the estimated prevalence is 100 per 100,000 white women and 400 per 100,000 black women. SLE is more common in blacks in the United States but is rare among blacks in Africa. Approximately 160,000 to 320,000 people in the United States are living with SLE.

Although the etiology of SLE remains unclear, genetic, hormonal, and environmental influences play a role in disease pathogenesis. It is postulated that an environmental exposure triggers the onset of disease in a genetically susceptible person. Evidence of a genetic component to SLE is derived from studies showing strong familial risk. The disease concordance rate of 24–58% for monozygotic twins in comparison to the concordance rate of 2–5% for dizygotic twins confirms this strong genetic component. Multiple genes have been associated with SLE, including the genes within the major histocompatibility complex and genes that encode components of the complement pathway, Fcγ receptors, protein tyrosine phosphatase non-receptor type 22 (PTPN22), programmed cell death 1 gene (PDCD1), and cytotoxic T lymphocyte associated antigen 4 (CTLA4). The reasons for female sex predilection remain murky. Some observational data suggest that sex hormones might contribute to disease onset. For example, data from the Nurses Health Study suggest that early age at menarche (relative risk 2.1), oral contraceptive use (relative risk 1.5), and use of postmenopausal hormones (relative risk 1.9) increases the risk of SLE. In addition, the risk of SLE in men with Klinefelter syndrome (47, XXY) is 14-fold higher than in healthy male controls. In contrast, large controlled trials have shown that combined oral contraceptives do not increase the risk of flares in women with stable SLE, and studies examining serum sex hormone levels in patients with lupus compared with patients in a control group have been inconclusive. Thus, whether hormonal factors or non-hormonal aspects of sex are most important in influencing disease risk remains to be determined.

Various environmental factors have been examined as potential triggers for the development of SLE. Smoking is a risk factor for SLE and has been associated with anti-dsDNA production in patients with SLE. Exposure to UV light exacerbates both cutaneous and internal organ manifestations of SLE, but there is no clear evidence to suggest that UV light triggers onset of the disease.

Several viruses have been investigated as possible triggering factors for SLE, although there is no conclusive evidence linking one pathogen to development of disease. The virus that has received the most attention in this regard is Epstein-Barr virus (EBV). Studies in pediatric and adult patients have demonstrated a higher seroprevalence of antibodies to EBV antigens and a higher EBV viral load in SLE patients versus controls. Molecular mimicry between EBV and self proteins is postulated to play a role in SLE pathogenesis.

There is increasing evidence that interferon α (IFNα) plays an important role in the pathogenesis of SLE. Approximately 50% of SLE patients overexpress IFNα inducible genes, and the degree of overexpression correlates with disease activity and severity. This pattern of gene expression is referred to as the "interferon α signature." Studies have shown that plasmacytoid dendritic cells release IFNα after stimulation with immune complexes containing nucleic acid.

SLE is characterized by the production of a variety of autoantibodies to nuclear antigens (antinuclear antibodies [ANA]), cytoplasmic antigens, cell surface antigens, and soluble antigens in the circulation such as IgG and phospholipids. Subtypes of ANAs can be useful for establishing a diagnosis, detecting certain disease manifestations, and sometimes in monitoring the course of the disease. Antibodies to surface antigens on red blood cells and platelets can lead to autoimmune hemolytic anemia and immune-mediated thrombocytopenia, respectively. In the majority of SLE patients, the presence of autoantibodies predates the development of symptoms or signs of SLE, and patients accrue different autoantibodies up until the time of diagnosis. One study utilizing the Department of Defense Serum Repository demonstrated that ANA, anti-Ro/SSA antibodies, anti-La/SSB antibodies, and antiphospholipid antibodies were the first to appear and did so at a mean of 3.4 years prior to the diagnosis of SLE. Antibodies to double-stranded DNA (anti-dsDNA) appeared next at a mean of 2.2 years prior to diagnosis, and anti-Smith (anti-Sm) and anti-ribonucleoprotein (anti-RNP) were the last to appear at 1 year before diagnosis. This study also showed that the autoantibody profile at the time of SLE diagnosis remained relatively constant in the years after diagnosis.

▶ Clinical Findings

A. Symptoms and Signs

1. Constitutional—Constitutional symptoms, such as fever, fatigue, and weight changes, are common in SLE. Not infrequently, fatigue is out of proportion to other disease manifestations. In these instances, it is important to consider other factors such as deconditioning, stress, and sleep disturbance. Fever, usually low-grade, can occur in active SLE, particularly with serositis. Infection, however, is always a concern when fever develops in a lupus patient, especially in the setting of immunosuppressive therapy.

2. Mucocutaneous—Four of the 11 American College of Rheumatology (ACR) classification criteria describe mucocutaneous manifestations, and approximately 80–90% of SLE patients will have mucocutaneous involvement at some point during the course of the disease (Tables 21–1 and 21–2). Photosensitivity, defined by the ACR as "skin rash as a result of unusual reaction to sunlight, by patient history, or physician observation," occurs frequently. Patients may be sensitive to UV-A, UV-B, or visible light. Photoprovocation testing has shown that greater than 90% of lupus patients have an abnormal skin reaction to UV or visible light. SLE patients also have reported symptoms after exposure to sunlight through car glass windows and to light from fluorescent tubes and photocopiers. The majority of skin reactions occur

Table 21–1. The 1997 update of the 1982 Revised American College of Rheumatology classification criteria for SLE.[a]

Criterion	Definition
Malar rash	Fixed erythema, flat or raised, over the malar eminences, sparing the nasolabial folds
Discoid rash	Erythematous raised patches with adherent keratotic scale and follicular plugging; atrophic scarring may occur in older lesions
Photosensitivity	Skin rash as a result of unusual reaction to sunlight, by patient history or clinician observation
Oral ulcers	Oral or nasopharyngeal ulceration, usually painless, observed by a clinician
Arthritis	Nonerosive arthritis involving two or more peripheral joints, characterized by tenderness, swelling, or effusion
Serositis	a. Pleuritis b. Pericarditis
Renal disorder	a. Persistent proteinuria >0.5 g/d OR b. Cellular casts
Neurologic disorder	a. Seizures OR b. Psychosis
Hematologic disorder	a. Hemolytic anemia OR b. Leukopenia 4000/mcL OR c. Lymphopenia <1500/mcL d. Thrombocytopenia <100,000 mcL
Immunologic disorder	a. Anti-DNA OR b. Anti-Sm OR c. Antiphospholipid antibodies
Positive antinuclear antibody	An abnormal titer of antinuclear antibody by immunofluorescence or an equivalent assay in the absence of a drug

[a]The presence of four or more criteria is required for SLE classification. Exclude all other reasonable diagnoses.
SLE, systemic lupus erythematosus.

Table 21–2. Major clinical manifestations of systemic lupus erythematosus.

Organ	Manifestation
Mouth	Erythema, petechiae, or ulcers occurring most commonly on buccal mucosa, hard palate, or vermillion border
Skin	Malar rash, SCLE, discoid lupus, bullous lesions, panniculitis, palpable purpura, periungal erythema, livedo reticularis, Raynaud phenomenon, chilblain lupus
Lymph nodes	Lymphadenopathy, commonly in cervical and axillary regions
Joints	Symmetric, inflammatory polyarthritis, usually nonerosive; reducible Jaccoud-like arthropathy
Heart	Pericarditis, myocarditis, Libman-Sacks endocarditis, conduction system abnormalities, premature atherosclerosis
Lungs	Pleuritis, pneumonitis, diffuse alveolar hemorrhage, pulmonary hypertension
Gastrointestinal	Peritonitis, hepatitis, pancreatitis, mesenteric vasculitis, intestinal pseudo-obstruction
Kidney	Glomerulonephritis, interstitial nephritis, antiphospholipid nephropathy
Blood	Leukopenia, anemia, thrombocytopenia, arterial/vein thrombosis
Neuropsychiatric	Seizures, headache, acute confusional state, cognitive dysfunction, myelopathy, peripheral neuropathy

SCLE, subacute cutaneous lupus erythematosus.

more than 1 week after sun exposure and last for weeks to months. In addition to skin eruptions, some SLE patients report an exacerbation of systemic symptoms such as fatigue and arthralgias after sun exposure. Polymorphous light eruption and photosensitizing medications are additional diagnostic considerations when evaluating a SLE patient with a photosensitive rash. In contrast to SLE photosensitivity, polymorphous light eruption is characterized by an intensely pruritic papular, non-scarring rash developing hours after sun exposure and resolving after a few days. Polymorphous light eruption may occur in patients with known SLE.

Patchy or diffuse alopecia and thin, friable hair occur during active SLE flares but may also occur as a side effect of certain medications that are commonly used to treat SLE. Hair re-growth begins 6–8 weeks after disease quiescence or discontinuation of the offending drug. Permanent alopecia can occur following the development of scarring discoid lesions.

Nasal or oral ulcers, which are typically painless, commonly develop in SLE patients. This is in contrast to aphthous stomatitis which is usually painful. Lupus oral ulcers have a gradual onset and can occur anywhere on the oral mucosa.

Most lesions present as erythema, petechiae, or ulcerations. They typically occur on the hard palate, buccal mucosa, and vermillion border, and are unilateral or asymmetric. Discoid lupus erythematosus (DLE) can also occur in the oral cavity and can be very painful. Oral candidiasis and oral lichen planus can resemble the oral ulcers of SLE.

Cutaneous lupus lesions are categorized as "lupus specific" versus "lupus nonspecific" based on the presence or absence of interface dermatitis on histopathology. Acute cutaneous lupus erythematosus (ACLE), subacute cutaneous lupus erythematosus (SCLE), and chronic cutaneous lupus erythematosus (CCLE) are all considered to be lupus specific lesions. ACLE lesions can be localized or generalized. The localized form produces the classic malar or "butterfly" rash, which is characterized by sharply demarcated erythema on the cheeks and bridge of the nose, sparing the nasolabial folds (Plate 35). Induration and scaling may occur. The malar rash of SLE is sometimes confused with that of acne rosacea, seborrheic dermatitis, and flushing syndromes. Unlike SLE, rosacea is characterized by the predominance of telangiectasias and pustules that may sting and burn. Heat and alcohol intake worsen the erythema of rosacea. Seborrheic dermatitis is manifested by scaly erythematous plaques that occur on the eyebrows and the lateral sides of the nose. In contrast to the malar rash of SLE, seborrheic dermatitis is commonly found within the nasolabial folds. If the diagnosis remains unclear after clinical examination, biopsy of the rash can be helpful to distinguish SLE from these other dermatologic entities.

Generalized ACLE consists of maculopapular erythematosus lesions involving any area of the body in a photosensitive distribution. The dorsa of the hands and the extensor surfaces of the fingers are commonly involved. The erythema is typically found between the interphalangeal joints, which is in distinction to the Gottron papules of dermatomyositis, which occur over the joint. ACLE lesions heal without scarring, although post-inflammatory hyperpigmentation can be observed.

The rash of SCLE may be papulosquamous or annular and is believed to be the most photosensitive of all the lupus rashes. The scaly, erythematous papules are frequently located on the torso and limbs and spare the face. Neither scarring nor atrophy are present. Patients with such lesions often have anti-SSA/Ro antibody. Compared with other forms of cutaneous lupus, SCLE is more often induced by medications such as hydrochlorothiazide and terbinafine.

Discoid lupus is the most common subtype of CCLE. The term "discoid" refers to the disc shaped appearance of the lesions. Such lesions are raised, erythematous plaques with adherent scale occurring most commonly on the scalp, face, and neck (Plates 36–38). There is usually an erythematous ring around the lesions, which denotes the active component (Plate 36). Over time, discoid lesions can lead to scarring and skin atrophy, resulting in permanent alopecia and disfigurement (Plates 37 and 38). DLE can also occur in the oral mucosa. Squamous cell carcinoma has been reported as a late sequela of DLE; thus, surveillance of known lesions and biopsy of changing or suspicious lesions is important.

Other subtypes of CCLE include hypertrophic lupus erythematosus and lupus panniculitis. Lupus panniculitis is a lobular panniculitis that has a predilection for the scalp, face, arms, buttocks, and thighs. When a cutaneous discoid lesion overlies the panniculitis, the entity is referred to as lupus profundus. Lupus panniculitis typically presents as a deep, firm nodule that can lead to cutaneous atrophy and rarely ulceration. Biopsy is often necessary to secure the diagnosis because there are reports of T cell lymphoma mimicking panniculitis. However, biopsy should be performed carefully because the lesions have tendency to break down. Lupus panniculitis is one of the few panniculitides that can occur above the waist.

Lupus nonspecific skin findings, such as bullous lesions, periungal erythema, chilblain lupus, and livedo reticularis, can also develop in SLE patients. Bullous lupus erythematosus is a rare cutaneous manifestation that presents as blistering skin lesions. SLE may also be associated with other bullous disorders such as bullous pemphigoid and dermatitis herpetiformis. The physical examination finding of periungal erythema represents dilatation of the capillaries at the base of the nail. These capillaries can be visualized at the bedside with a dermatoscope or ophthalmoscope. Other disorders associated with periungal erythema include scleroderma and mixed connective tissue disease. Unlike scleroderma and mixed connective tissue disease, SLE is not associated with capillary drop-out. Chilblain lupus is characterized by the presence of erythematous or violaceous macules or plaques (or both) on acral surfaces that worsen after exposure to a cold, humid weather. Livedo reticularis is characterized by an erythematous to violaceous reticular or net-like pattern of the skin. It is also highly associated with the antiphospholipid antibody syndrome.

3. Lymphadenopathy—Lymphadenopathy is a common feature of SLE and can be localized or diffuse. The lymph nodes are soft and nontender, and the cervical and axillary chains are most frequently involved. Biopsy reveals reactive hyperplasia. A change in the pattern of a patient's lymphadenopathy or unusually enlarging or hard lymph nodes should prompt an evaluation for lymphoma, which has an increased incidence in SLE.

4. Musculoskeletal—Arthritis and arthralgias are noted in up to 95% of SLE patients at some time during the course of the illness and frequently involve the wrists and small joints of the hands. Swan-neck deformities and ligamental laxity are often noted. Unlike the joint findings in rheumatoid arthritis and mixed connective tissue disease, bony erosions rarely occur in SLE, and the swan-neck deformities are usually reducible (Jaccoud-like arthropathy).

5. Lupus nephritis—Renal involvement is common in SLE and is a significant cause of morbidity and mortality. It is estimated that up to 90% of SLE patients have pathologic evidence of nephritis on biopsy, but clinically significant nephritis develops in only 50% of people with SLE. Lupus nephritis

typically develops in the first 36 months of the disease, although there are exceptions. Immune complex glomerulonephritis is the most common form of SLE renal involvement, but tubulointerstitial disease and vascular disease may also be present. The clinical presentation of lupus nephritis is highly variable, ranging from asymptomatic hematuria or proteinuria (or both) to frank nephrotic syndrome to rapidly progressive glomerulonephritis with loss of renal function.

Routine screening for the presence of lupus nephritis is a critical component of the ongoing evaluation and management of SLE patients. Screening procedures include asking about new-onset polyuria, nocturia, or foamy urine and looking for the presence of hypertension or lower extremity edema. Performance of a urinalysis with microscopy is essential. Hematuria, pyuria, dysmorphic red blood cells, and red blood cell casts may all be present. Accurate measurement of proteinuria is critical because proteinuria is a very sensitive indicator of glomerular damage. Normal daily protein excretion is <150 mg. Although the gold standard tool is an accurately collected 24-hour urine protein, many clinicians are currently using the spot urine protein to creatinine ratio out of convenience. However, the use of the spot ratio is controversial because data suggest that the spot ratio often is not representative of the findings in a timed collection, especially in the range of 0.5–3.0 (the range of most lupus nephritis flares). In addition, the spot ratio is less accurate in extremely muscular or cachectic patients. Urine dipstick should not be used for the quantification of proteinuria because it reflects protein concentration and varies depending on the volume of the sample. Screening SLE patients at regular intervals for the presence of proteinuria and hematuria is recommended; in patients with active SLE, screening at 3-month intervals is prudent. Hematuria in the absence of proteinuria might also be due to urolithiasis, menstrual contamination, or bladder pathology, particularly transitional cell carcinoma in a patient with previous cyclophosphamide exposure.

Renal biopsy is a critical part of the evaluation of a patient with possible lupus nephritis. The International Society of Nephrology/Renal Pathology Society system classifies the glomerular pathology into six categories (Table 21–3) based on light microscopic, immunofluorescent, and electron-micrographic findings. An individual biopsy might exhibit just one of the pathologic classes or a combination of classes. In **class I lupus nephritis**, glomeruli appear normal on light microscopy and, on immunofluorescence, immune deposits are limited to the mesangium. **Class II disease** is characterized by mesangial proliferation on light microscopy and mesangial deposits on immunofluorescence.

Class III and IV lupus nephritis are highly inflammatory lesions with immune complex deposition in the subendothelial space. These forms of lupus nephritis are described as "proliferative" because of the presence of proliferating endocapillary cells within the glomeruli. Class III denotes that <50% of glomeruli are involved and class IV denotes

Table 21–3. International Society of Nephrology/Renal Pathology Society classification of lupus nephritis.

Class	Description
I	Minimal mesangial
II	Mesangial proliferative
III	Focal nephritis
IV	Diffuse nephritis
V	Membranous
VI	Advanced sclerosing

that ≥50% of glomeruli are involved. Class IV lesions are subcategorized according to whether the majority of glomeruli show focal (<50% of the glomerular tuft) or global (>50% of the glomerular tuft) involvement. Class IV lesions are further described as active (A), chronic (C), or a mixture of both (A/C). **Class V lupus nephritis** is characterized by immune complex deposition in the subepithelial space resulting in thickened capillary loops. This lesion commonly manifests clinically as nephrotic range proteinuria. Class V nephritis may occur in a pure histopathologic form or in combination with features of class III or class IV nephritis. **Class VI nephritis** is defined by the presence of >90% globally sclerotic glomeruli. In addition to glomerular pathology, renal histopathologic changes may include tubulointerstitial inflammation or fibrosis and a variety of vascular lesions including hyaline thrombi and thrombotic microangiopathy. Thrombotic microangiopathy is highly associated with the presence of antiphospholipid antibodies and should prompt the consideration of antiphospholipid nephropathy.

When an SLE patient has clinical or laboratory features that suggest the presence of nephritis, a renal biopsy should be performed in order to confirm the diagnosis, evaluate the degree of disease activity, and determine an appropriate course of treatment. A biopsy is especially important because urinary parameters, such as hematuria and the degree of proteinuria, imperfectly predict the underlying renal pathology. Hematuria might be absent in patients with severe class IV nephritis, and proteinuria can be modest in patients with class V nephritis. Each histopathologic class portends a different renal prognosis. Class I and class II nephritis have an excellent renal prognosis and do not require any specific therapy. In contrast, the long-term renal prognosis of class III–IV nephritis is extremely poor in the absence of immunosuppression. The long-term prognosis of class V nephritis is more favorable than class III–IV nephritis and is largely defined by the presence of associated proliferative lesions, which portend a worse prognosis. A repeat renal biopsy may be indicated in certain clinical settings, eg, if a patient is not responding appropriately to therapy or if a patient unexpectedly worsens after having achieved a good

response to therapy. Repeat renal biopsy also can detect class transformation, which occurs in 15–50% of lupus nephritis patients during the course of the disease.

6. Cardiovascular—Cardiovascular disease is a frequent complication of SLE and may involve the pericardium, valves, myocardium, and coronary arteries. Raynaud phenomenon affects approximately 30% of SLE patients and is characterized by vasospasm of the digital arteries and arterioles after exposure to cold temperature or stress.

Pericarditis may be asymptomatic; pericardial effusions are typically small and usually do not lead to hemodynamic compromise. However, on occasion lupus pericarditis can lead to life-threatening hemodynamic complications. Valvular heart disease predominantly affects the mitral and aortic valves as valve leaflet thickening, with or without nonbacterial vegetations (Libman-Sacks endocarditis). One echocardiographic study in SLE patients cited a prevalence of valvular abnormalities of 61% compared to 9% of controls. The presence of valvular disease was not associated with other clinical or serologic features of lupus disease activity. Myocarditis and conduction defects are rarer manifestations. SLE is associated with accelerated atherosclerosis and is itself a risk factor for cardiovascular disease (see below, Complications).

7. Pulmonary—SLE frequently involves the pulmonary system, with pleural involvement being the most common manifestation. Pleural effusions, which are typically small, develop in up to 50% of patients during the course of the disease. Many patients experience pleuritic chest pain, but some effusions are asymptomatic. When evaluating an SLE patient with a pleural effusion, it is important to rule out other potential etiologies such as infection, malignancy, and heart failure.

Lupus pneumonitis, characterized by an acute respiratory illness with fever, cough, and pulmonary infiltrates, is very rare and is associated with a high mortality.

Chronic interstitial lung disease, also a very rare complication of SLE, can develop in an insidious fashion or after one or more episodes of acute lupus pneumonitis.

Chest radiography may be normal early in the disease course, but high-resolution CT may show characteristic findings of lung fibrosis. Pulmonary function studies reveal a restrictive pattern.

Diffuse alveolar hemorrhage is extremely rare and frequently fatal. Presenting symptoms include dyspnea and cough; hemoptysis is not universally present at the onset of diffuse alveolar hemorrhage. Clinicians should suspect diffuse alveolar hemorrhage in the setting of acute pulmonary infiltrates, a falling hematocrit, and a hemorrhagic bronchoalveolar lavage. Lupus nephritis frequently occurs concomitantly with diffuse alveolar hemorrhage. Isolated pulmonary arterial hypertension is an uncommon manifestation of SLE but is more frequently detected in mixed connective tissue disease. Lastly, the rare manifestation of vanishing lung syndrome is characterized by progressive dyspnea and decrease in lung volume with elevated diaphragms in the absence of parenchymal or pleural abnormalities on imaging studies.

8. Gastrointestinal—SLE may involve any part of the gastrointestinal system. Abdominal pain has been reported in up to 40% of SLE patients and can be due to SLE-related causes, medication side effects, and other non–SLE-related etiologies such as infection. When evaluating an SLE patient with abdominal pain, it is critical to rule out non-SLE conditions first and to bear in mind treatment with glucocorticoids or other immunosuppressives can mask the clinical signs of an acute abdomen.

SLE-related causes of abdominal pain include peritonitis, pancreatitis, mesenteric vasculitis, and intestinal pseudo-obstruction. Pancreatitis is uncommon and is usually associated with active SLE in other organs. When considering the potential diagnosis of pancreatitis, it is important to note that elevated serum amylase may be misleading in that it has been observed in SLE patients in the absence of pancreatitis. Although glucocorticoids and azathioprine have been associated with the development of pancreatitis in patients who do not have SLE, these medications do not seem to play a major role in the development of pancreatitis in patients who do have SLE. Mesenteric vasculitis is a very rare manifestation of SLE, usually occurs in the presence of active SLE elsewhere, and typically involves the small vessels (arterioles and venules) of the small bowel submucosa. Thus, mesenteric angiography is usually nondiagnostic.

Abnormalities of liver tests occur frequently in SLE patients during the course of the illness (see below, Liver Tests). Once medications and infections have been ruled out as possible culprits, persistent liver test abnormalities should prompt an investigation with an abdominal ultrasound and possibly a liver biopsy. Lupus hepatitis is believed to be a distinct entity from autoimmune hepatitis. Lupus hepatitis is typically characterized by the presence of lobular inflammation with a paucity of lymphoid infiltrates. These findings contrast with those of autoimmune hepatitis in which periportal inflammation and dense lymphoid infiltrates usually dominate. Although ANA is frequently seen in both disorders, anti-smooth muscle antibody is more frequently noted in autoimmune hepatitis than in SLE-associated hepatitis. Lastly, vascular disorders of the liver, such as Budd-Chiari syndrome, hepatic veno-occlusive disease, and hepatic infarction, can occur in SLE, especially in the setting of antiphospholipid antibodies.

9. Neuropsychiatric—Neuropsychiatric manifestations can involve any aspect of the central or peripheral nervous system. Involvement of the nervous system is associated with a poorer prognosis.

The ACR categorized the neuropsychiatric manifestations of SLE into 19 distinct syndromes encompassing both the central and peripheral nervous system (Table 21–4). Headaches, cerebrovascular disease, seizures, mood changes,

Table 21–4. American College of Rheumatology classification of neuropsychiatric syndromes in SLE.

Central Nervous System	Peripheral Nervous System
Aseptic meningitis	Guillain-Barré syndrome
Cerebrovascular disease	Autonomic disorder
Demyelinating syndrome	Mononeuropathy, single/multiplex
Headache	Myasthenia gravis
Movement disorder	Cranial neuropathy
Myelopathy	Plexopathy
Seizure	Polyneuropathy
Acute confusional state	
Anxiety disorder	
Cognitive dysfunction	
Mood disorder	
Psychosis	

SLE, systemic lupus erythematosus.

and cognitive dysfunction are the most frequent manifestations. The pathogenic mechanisms underlying these manifestations are varied and may, in some cases, involve small vessel vasculopathy, thrombosis of arteries and veins, atherosclerotic disease, demyelination, or intrathecal production of proinflammatory cytokines.

Central nervous system events occur more frequently than peripheral nervous system events. There are several types of histopathologic changes including small vessel vasculopathy (vascular hyalinization, perivascular lymphocytosis, or endothelial proliferation), multifocal infarctions, hemorrhage, cortical atrophy, and demyelinating lesions similar to those found in multiple sclerosis. True vasculitis is rare. The most common findings on brain MRI include T2 hyperintense focal lesions in the periventricular and subcortical white matter that can appear identical to the lesions seen in multiple sclerosis. Newer imaging techniques, such as magnetic resonance spectroscopy, have demonstrated abnormalities in brains of some SLE patients that appear normal on conventional MRI. A lumbar puncture should be performed in any patient with suspected CNS involvement. Cerebrospinal fluid findings are often entirely within normal limits, but some patients may demonstrate a pleocytosis or elevated protein (or both). The primary role of lumbar puncture is to rule out central nervous system infection; cerebrospinal fluid findings are not sensitive or specific enough to confirm a diagnosis of neuropsychiatric SLE. Cognitive dysfunction, manifested primarily by deficits in thinking, memory, and concentration, is being increasingly recognized in SLE patients. Some experts have estimated a prevalence of up to 80%, although serious impairment is much less common. Cognitive dysfunction may be associated with the presence of antiphospholipid antibodies. Acute myelopathy is an uncommon but devastating neuropsychiatric manifestation characterized by the onset of bilateral lower extremity paresthesia, numbness, and weakness that can rapidly progress to involve the upper limbs and the muscles of respiration. A sensory level is usually present. MRI of the spinal cord is important to confirm the diagnosis of myelopathy; T1 and T2 signal abnormalities and widening of the cord from edema are observed. Urgent treatment is necessary to try to prevent permanent neurologic damage. SLE myelopathy should be distinguished from neuromyelitis optica (NMO), which causes myelitis and optic neuritis in the setting of a positive anti-NMO IgG antibody.

Some of the most dramatic and devastating central nervous system manifestations of SLE may reflect systemic rather than localized abnormalities. Specifically, the sudden appearance of a stroke in a patient with SLE most likely reflects thrombosis due to antiphospholipid antibodies without any inflammatory or immunologic pathology within the central nervous system.

Peripheral neuropathy has been observed in up to 20% of SLE patients and is typically characterized by a symmetric, length dependent sensory or sensorimotor polyneuropathy. Because small diameter nerve fibers are likely involved, the results of nerve conduction studies and the clinical neurologic examination may be normal. Patients typically have fluctuating numbness and tingling of the upper extremities and hands. A large fiber vasculitic neuropathy can also occur in patients with SLE. This manifestation warrants urgent treatment to prevent ongoing and irreversible nerve damage. Autonomic neuropathies and cranial neuropathies may also develop in patients with SLE.

When evaluating an SLE patient with possible neuropsychiatric manifestations, it is important to distinguish if the neurologic symptoms are due to SLE-mediated damage or to secondary factors (such as metabolic abnormalities; severe hypertension; infection; or adverse effects of medications, such as glucocorticoids). No laboratory or imaging study is sufficiently sensitive or specific to confirm the diagnosis of neuropsychiatric SLE. Instead, the diagnosis is based on a thorough clinical evaluation that is corroborated by findings (or lack thereof) on brain imaging, serologic testing, lumbar puncture, and neuropsychiatric assessment.

B. Laboratory Findings

1. Hematology

1. Hematology—All three blood cell lines can be affected in SLE. Anemia can be due to anemia of chronic disease (most common cause), autoimmune hemolytic anemia (AIHA), microangiopathic hemolytic anemia (MAHA), blood loss, renal insufficiency, pure red cell aplasia, and aplastic anemia.

AIHA should be considered in the setting of the following laboratory abnormalities: increased serum unconjugated bilirubin, increased lactate dehydrogenase, increased reticulocyte count, and reduced serum haptoglobin. The direct Coombs test is typically positive and is usually mediated by warm reacting IgG antierythrocyte antibodies. The peripheral blood smear often shows spherocytosis. There is an association between AIHA and the presence of anticardiolipin antibodies. AIHA may be the presenting manifestation of SLE but also may predate full blown SLE by many years.

MAHA, characterized by the presence of schistocytes on peripheral blood smear, should prompt the consideration of thrombotic thrombocytopenic purpura—a syndrome that consists of MAHA, thrombocytopenia, fever, neurologic symptoms, and renal involvement and that is associated with SLE. Because MAHA, thrombocytopenia, neurologic symptoms, and renal involvement can also occur in catastrophic antiphospholipid antibody syndrome, antiphospholipid antibodies should always be measured as part of the evaluation.

Leukopenia occurs in approximately 50% of SLE patients and can be secondary to lymphopenia or neutropenia or both. The presence of lymphocytoxic antibodies in some SLE patients correlates with lymphopenia. Thrombocytopenia is noted in up to 25% of SLE patients and can manifest in a severe fashion similar to immune thrombocytopenia. Chronic, low level thrombocytopenia is also a characteristic feature of the antiphospholipid antibody syndrome. Similar to AIHA, isolated immune thrombocytopenia has been shown to predate the development of complete SLE by several years. When evaluating a patient with the hematologic abnormalities described above, it is always important to consider the potential of bone marrow suppression from such medications as methotrexate, azathioprine, mycophenolate mofetil, and cyclophosphamide. In addition, glucocorticoids are a common cause of lymphopenia.

2. Chemistry

2. Chemistry—Hyperkalemia can occur as part of renal tubular acidosis in a patient with lupus nephritis. Also, hyperkalemia may be encountered in lupus nephritis patients with renal insufficiency, especially if they are being treated with an angiotensin-converting enzyme inhibitor. Serum creatinine may be elevated in lupus nephritis patients.

3. Liver tests

3. Liver tests—Liver test abnormalities have been described in up to 60% of SLE patients at some point during the course of the illness, but clinically significant liver disease is rarely a direct manifestation of SLE. For this reason, the presence of liver disease should prompt a search for other causes, including medications such as nonsteroidal anti-inflammatory drugs, methotrexate, and azathioprine, all of which can cause hepatotoxicity. Glucocorticoids can lead to hepatic steatosis. Elevated transaminases also can be seen in the setting of SLE-associated hepatitis and pancreatitis.

4. Muscle enzymes

4. Muscle enzymes—Creatine kinase can be elevated in the setting of SLE-associated myositis but is more commonly elevated in patients with mixed connective tissue disease.

5. Acute phase reactants

5. Acute phase reactants—The erythrocyte sedimentation rate (ESR) sometimes correlates with SLE disease activity, but the test is very nonspecific. The presence of anemia and renal disease (both common in SLE patients) can lead to elevations in the ESR. The majority of SLE patients have a mild elevation in the C-reactive protein (CRP) level, but very few have a marked elevation. Notable exceptions are those patients with serositis or concomitant infection in which the CRP level can be quite high (>60 mg/L). In contrast to ESR, CRP levels are not thought to correlate well with SLE disease activity.

C. Special Tests

1. Autoantibodies—The standard method for the detection of ANA is via indirect immunofluorescence using a human tumor cell line substrate (the HEp-2 cell line). When this method is used, ANA are present in virtually all SLE patients (Table 21–5). More recently, enzyme-linked immunosorbent assays (ELISA) containing a mixture of nuclear antigens are being used to detect ANA. These ELISA tests have a lower sensitivity for the detection of ANA than the HEp-2 cell immunofluorescence technique. Thus, in the appropriate clinical setting, a negative ANA by ELISA should be repeated using the immunofluorescent technique. The ANA is a nonspecific test and may be positive in a variety of other conditions including infection, malignancy, and other autoimmune diseases such as scleroderma and autoimmune thyroid disease.

Table 21–5. Autoantibodies and clinical significance in systemic lupus erythematosus (SLE).

Autoantibody	Prevalence in SLE	Clinical Significance
ANA		
Anti-dsDNA	70%	95% specificity for SLE; fluctuates with disease activity; associated with glomerulonephritis
Anti-Sm	20%	99% specificity for SLE; associated with anti-U1RNP antibodies
Anti-U1RNP	30%	Defining antibody in MCTD; associated with lower frequency of glomerulonephritis
Anti-Ro/SSA	30%	Associated with Sjögren syndrome, photosensitivity, SCLE, neonatal lupus, congenital heart block
Anti-La/SSB	20%	Associated with Sjögren syndrome, SCLE, neonatal lupus, congenital heart block, anti-Ro/SSA
Anti-histone	70%	Associated with drug-induced lupus
Antiphospholipid	30%	Associated with arterial and venous thrombosis, pregnancy morbidity

SCLE, subacute cutaneous lupus erythematosus; MCTD, mixed connective tissue disease.

Approximately 30% of healthy people have an ANA titer of 1:40 and 3% have a titer of 1:320. Thus, while a negative ANA typically excludes SLE, a positive ANA does not secure the diagnosis. Once a patient with a positive ANA and characteristic symptoms receives a diagnosis of SLE, there is usually no need to repeat the ANA test.

Anti-dsDNA antibodies are highly specific for SLE and may fluctuate with disease activity. Anti-dsDNA antibodies correlate well with the presence of lupus nephritis. Anti-Sm and anti-RNP antibodies are antibodies to small ribonucleoprotein particles that are found in some SLE patients. Anti-Sm is highly specific for the diagnosis of SLE. High titers of anti-RNP strongly suggest mixed connective tissue disease. Anti-Ro/SSA and anti-La/SSB antibodies are associated with the development of neonatal lupus and congenital heart block. In SLE patients, it is very rare to detect anti-La/SSB antibodies in the absence of anti-Ro/SSA antibodies. Anti-Ro/SSA antibodies are also associated with SCLE. Both antibodies are also commonly detected in patients with primary Sjögren syndrome.

Antiphospholipid antibodies are antibodies that are directed against phospholipids or to plasma proteins that bind to phospholipids. They are present in up to 50% of SLE patients and are associated with venous and arterial thrombosis and fetal loss. Some reports suggest an association between antiphospholipid antibodies, AIHA, and immune thrombocytopenia.

2. Complement—Hypocomplementemia may occur during SLE flares as a result of complement activation and consumption, resulting in low C4, C3, and CH50. Because other diseases that cause hypocomplementemia are uncommon, low complement levels can be a very useful clinical indicator. It is important to remember that hereditary deficiencies of the early components of the classical pathway occur with increased frequency in patients with SLE. Thus, complement deficiencies should be considered before attributing hypocomplementemia to active SLE. This distinction is most relevant when evaluating a patient with low C4. C4 is encoded by two genes: C4A and C4B. Partial deficiency of C4 is common; it is estimated that 1% of whites are homozygous for C4A null alleles and 3% of whites are homozygous for C4B deficiency. Up to 15% of whites with SLE are C4A deficient. Thus, it may be difficult to discern if low C4 in a patient with SLE is due to complement consumption or to an inherited deficiency of C4. Ongoing complement consumption due to active SLE is more likely to result in reduced levels of multiple complement components (eg, reduction in the levels of C3 as well as C4) and the levels of C4 fluctuate with disease activity. In contrast, an inherited deficiency of C4 results in a fixed low level of C4 that does not vary with disease activity. Although rare, C1q deficiency is the complement deficiency that is most highly associated with SLE. Homozygous deficiency of C2 also confers increased risk of the development of SLE.

3. Biopsy—A skin biopsy can aid in the diagnosis of cutaneous lupus in the setting of an atypical clinical presentation. Immunofluorescence should always be performed along with conventional histology. Histopathologic findings include basal layer vacuolar degeneration of keratinocytes and interface dermatitis. Dermal mucinosis is often observed. Discoid lupus lesions show follicular plugging. Immunofluorescence demonstrates deposition of IgG, IgA, IgM, and complement components along the dermoepidermal junction. IgM is the most frequent and IgA the least frequent immunoglobulin class deposited. It is important to remember that the skin biopsy of dermatomyositis can appear identical to that of SLE.

D. Imaging Studies

Chest radiography is the initial study to detect pleural effusions or alveolar infiltrates in the evaluation of pleuritic chest pain or dyspnea. However, high-resolution CT has a higher sensitivity for the diagnosis of lupus pneumonitis or diffuse alveolar hemorrhage. Echocardiography is useful for the detection of pericardial effusions, valvular lesions, and as a screening test for pulmonary hypertension. Transesophageal echocardiography provides better resolution in the evaluation of valvular abnormalities.

▶ Diagnostic Criteria

Establishing the diagnosis of lupus can be quite challenging because of the remarkable heterogeneity in clinical presentation and the lack of a definitive diagnostic test. The ACR has developed classification criteria for SLE (see Table 21–1) that are often cited to support a lupus diagnosis. A person must fulfill 4 of 11 criteria in order to be classified as having SLE, all other reasonable diagnoses having been excluded. It should be emphasized, however, that these classification criteria were developed in an effort to standardize patients being enrolled into clinical trials, and they do not always meet the diagnostic challenge in individual patients. For example, a person with unequivocal biopsy proven lupus nephritis might only meet two of the classification criteria. At the other end of the spectrum, a person might have acute erythrovirus (parvovirus B19) infection and meet 4 criteria. Although these criteria cannot always be relied upon for diagnostic purposes, they serve as useful reminders of the myriad of symptoms and signs that can be seen in SLE.

▶ Differential Diagnosis

Because of the involvement of multiple organ systems and the lack of specificity of some of the early symptoms, SLE can be readily mimicked by a variety of systemic diseases. A thorough evaluation for infectious, malignant, and other autoimmune diseases must be undertaken before SLE is diagnosed in a patient.

A number of viral infections can produce a constellation of symptoms and signs similar to SLE and, to complicate matters further, trigger the production of autoantibodies. A careful patient history and appropriate serologic testing for the potential offending virus should lead to the correct diagnosis. Erythrovirus (parvovirus B19) presents with fever, rash, anemia, and a symmetric inflammatory polyarthritis. ANA and anti-dsDNA antibodies and hypocomplementemia have been reported. Cytomegalovirus and EBV can present with constitutional symptoms; cytopenias; and gastrointestinal, hepatic, and lung abnormalities that can mimic an SLE flare. Acute HIV infection typically presents with fever, lymphadenopathy, and mucosal ulcers. Hepatitis B and C infection can also cause an inflammatory arthritis with positive autoantibodies.

Malignancy, particularly non-Hodgkin lymphoma, can present with constitutional symptoms, arthralgias, cytopenias, rash, and a positive ANA. Clinicians must be especially concerned about the possibility of malignancy in an older patient who has a new lupus-like syndrome. It is critical to ensure that the patient is up-to-date on all of their age appropriate malignancy screening tests.

Other autoimmune diseases, such as rheumatoid arthritis and dermatomyositis, can share similar features with SLE. A symmetric inflammatory arthritis with a predilection for the wrists and small joints of the hands develops in patients with rheumatoid arthritis and SLE. ANA and rheumatoid factor may be elevated in both disorders, although anti-cyclic citrullinated peptide antibody is usually absent in SLE. The photosensitive, erythematous rashes of dermatomyositis and SLE can appear clinically and histopathologically identical. A careful patient history and supporting serologic tests aid in making the correct diagnosis. Mixed connective tissue disease must also be considered when evaluating a patient for possible SLE. Mixed connective tissue disease is a syndrome characterized by a high titer anti-RNP antibody in conjunction with clinical features that are often present in SLE, scleroderma, and polymyositis. Patients frequently have puffy, swollen hands and Raynaud phenomenon. In contrast to SLE, an erosive arthritis that resembles rheumatoid arthritis can develop in patients with mixed connective tissue disease. Pulmonary arterial hypertension is a leading cause of morbidity and mortality in mixed connective tissue disease.

Drug-induced lupus usually manifests as polyarthritis, myalgia, fever, and serositis. A wide variety of drugs have been implicated in the development of drug-induced lupus; minocycline, procainamide, hydralazine, isoniazid, interferon α, and anti-tumor necrosis factor (TNF) agents are well known culprits. Hydrochlorothiazide is associated with SCLE. All these drugs cause a positive ANA and, with the exception of minocycline, anti-histone antibodies. Although characteristic of drug-induced lupus, anti-histone antibodies also are present in up to 80% of idiopathic SLE patients and cannot be used to distinguish drug-induced lupus from idiopathic SLE. Minocycline and hydralazine also can trigger production of perinuclear-staining antineutrophil cytoplasmic antibodies (pANCAs); anti-TNF agents can cause anti-dsDNA antibodies.

▶ Complications

A. Accelerated Atherosclerosis

SLE patients are at increased risk for the development of premature atherosclerotic coronary artery disease with an estimated prevalence of 6–10% of SLE patients. Myocardial infarction in women with SLE is 50-fold more common than in age-matched controls. Traditional cardiovascular risk factors do not explain this increased risk of coronary artery disease. Thus, SLE itself is thought to be an independent risk factor. Evaluation for and treatment of modifiable cardiovascular risk factors such as obesity, smoking, hypertension, and hyperlipidemia are important in mitigating the development of atherosclerotic disease.

B. End-stage Renal Disease

It is estimated that up to 10% of lupus nephritis patients progress to end-stage renal disease requiring dialysis. Some patients experience a decrease in SLE activity, while others continue to have active extrarenal manifestations and elevated serologies. SLE patients are typically good candidates for renal transplantation, although it is recommended that patients are given a 3-month dialysis period in order to allow for the possibility of recovery of renal function. The incidence of recurrent lupus nephritis in the allograft is low and does not universally result in allograft loss.

C. Infection

Infections are a major cause of illness and death in patients with SLE. Immunosuppressive medications (especially glucocorticoids and cyclophosphamide) and immunologic abnormalities of SLE itself most likely contribute to the increased risk of infection. Bacterial, viral, and opportunistic pathogens have all been described.

Progressive multifocal leukoencephalopathy (PML) is a very rare and usually fatal demyelinating disease caused by reactivation of the JC polyomavirus. Although PML has been well recognized in patients with HIV and in patients receiving heavy immunosuppression for treatment of malignancy, it has also been described in patients with rheumatic disease. The majority of reported cases of PML in the setting of rheumatic diseases have occurred in patients with SLE. Recently, PML was diagnosed in two SLE patients after they received the biologic agent rituximab. It remains to be determined whether biologic therapy poses a greater risk than conventional immunosuppressive treatments for SLE, but it should be emphasized that PML has also been reported in lupus patients whose immunosuppressive therapy was quite mild. Therefore, new, progressive neurologic deficits and white matter lesions on brain imaging should prompt

an evaluation for PML in any lupus patient. The diagnosis of PML is confirmed by the detection of JC virus by polymerase chain reaction of the cerebrospinal fluid.

Vaccination with inactivated vaccines such as the Pneumovax and the inactivated influenza vaccine is an important practice to reduce risk of certain infections. Prophylaxis against *Pneumocystis jiroveci* should be offered to selected patients, particularly those being treated with cyclophosphamide.

D. Osteoporosis and Avascular Necrosis

Glucocorticoids are a major risk factor for the development of osteoporosis and avascular necrosis in SLE patients; it is important to use the lowest possible dose to control SLE disease activity. Patients should be routinely screened for low bone mineral density, and daily calcium and vitamin D supplementation should be emphasized. The use of bisphosphonates in women of childbearing age remains highly controversial due to the prolonged half-life of those agents. Avascular necrosis often involves multiple joints in SLE patients with the femoral head being most commonly affected. SLE is an independent risk factor for avascular necrosis, even in the absence of glucocorticoid therapy. Thus, the diagnosis should be considered in any SLE patient with persistent pain in any joint that is not explained by SLE activity. Raynaud phenomenon and hyperlipidemia may be additional risk factors for avascular necrosis in patients with SLE. MRI is the most sensitive imaging modality to detect early avascular necrosis.

E. Malignancy

Patients with SLE have an increased risk of malignancy, the most common types being non-Hodgkin lymphoma, Hodgkin lymphoma, lung cancer, and cervical cancer. Interestingly, the increased cancer risk is highest in the early years after SLE diagnosis rather than after many years of disease. SLE patients should undergo age appropriate cancer screening including yearly cervical cancer screening.

▶ Prognosis

The prognosis of SLE patients has improved dramatically over the past 50 years from a 50% survival at 2 years in the 1950s to 90% survival at 10 years in developed countries in the current era. The reasons for this improvement are likely multifactorial and include earlier diagnosis, more effective treatment (glucocorticoids were introduced in the 1950s), and better medical management of such complications as infection and renal disease. However, as SLE patients live longer, complications from long-standing disease and side effects of treatments emerge. The bimodal mortality pattern in SLE was first described over 30 years ago; patient deaths early in the course of the disease are from active disease or infection, while deaths in long-standing disease are due to atherosclerotic coronary disease. Malignancy also is a cause of excess mortality in patients with long-standing disease. One study showed that the survival curve of patients with mild disease is similar to that of patients with severe disease up until 10–15 years after diagnosis at which time there is a decline in survival in the severe group. Recognition of long-term complications of disease and implementation of appropriate preventive strategies to prevent and screen for atherosclerosis and malignancy are imperative in the ongoing care of SLE patients.

Arbuckle MR, McClain MT, Rubertone MV, et al. Development of autoantibodies before the clinical onset of systemic lupus erythematosus. *N Engl J Med*. 2003;349:1526. [PMID: 14561795]

Birmingham DJ, Rovin BH, Shidham G, et al. Spot urine protein/creatinine ratios are unreliable estimates of 24 h proteinuria in most systemic lupus erythematosus nephritis flares. *Kidney Int*. 2007;72:865. [PMID: 17653137]

Helmick C, Felson DT, Lawrence R, et al. National Arthritis Data Workgroup. Estimates of the prevalence of arthritis and other rheumatic conditions in the United States. Part I. *Arthritis Rheum*. 2008;58:15. [PMID: 18163481]

Petri M, Kim MY, Kalunian KC, et al. OC-SELENA Trial. Combined oral contraceptives in women with systemic lupus erythematosus. *N Engl J Med*. 2005;353:2550. [PMID: 16354891]

Sanchez-Guerrero J, Uribe AG, Jimenez-Santana L, et al. A trial of contraceptive methods in women with systemic lupus erythematosus. *N Engl J Med*. 2005;353:2539. [PMID: 16354890]

Tsao BP. Update on human systemic lupus erythematosus genetics. *Curr Opin Rheumatol*. 2004;16:513. [PMID: 15314487]

Weening JJ, D'Agati VD, Schwartz MM, et al. International Society of Nephrology Working Group on the Classification of Lupus Nephritis; Renal Pathology Society Working Group on the Classification of Lupus Nephritis. The classification of glomerulonephritis in systemic lupus erythematosus revisited. *Kidney Int*. 2004;65:521. [PMID: 14717922]

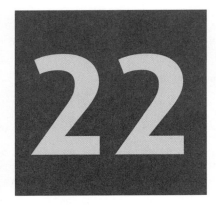

Treatment of Systemic Lupus Erythematosus

Maria Dall'Era, MD

David Wofsy, MD

Systemic lupus erythematosus (SLE) is a heterogeneous, multisystem disease. SLE manifests in a unique way in each patient, and treatment should be tailored to the type and severity of organ system involvement (Table 22–1). Unfortunately, this is more easily said than done, because there are few large studies to guide decision-making. The lack of large scale, randomized controlled trials has resulted in therapeutic strategies that are largely empiric. Despite these limitations, well-accepted community standards exist and are helpful in guiding treatment. In the end, the patient and his or her physician must weigh the potential risks and benefits of a particular therapy and agree upon a course of action.

As a foundation for any lupus treatment regimen, lifestyle modification including regular exercise, sufficient rest, a healthy diet, smoking cessation, and sun protection is critical. Lupus patients are at increased risk for accelerated atherosclerosis and, thus, aggressive risk factor modification is also required. In particular, hypertension and hyperlipidemia should be appropriately treated. Each patient should receive an inactivated influenza vaccine yearly and be up-to-date on their pneumococcal vaccine. Attention to bone health and prevention of glucocorticoid-induced osteoporosis with calcium, vitamin D, and bisphosphonates is necessary. Because of this adverse effect of glucocorticoid therapy, as well as many others, it is important to minimize the use of long-term glucocorticoids if at all possible. Studies suggest that there may be an increased risk of malignancy in patients with SLE and that these patients are less likely than the general population to undergo routine cancer screening. Thus, age appropriate cancer screening should be reinforced. Unlike the general population, women with SLE should undergo screening for cervical cancer on a yearly basis.

CONSTITUTIONAL SYMPTOMS

Fatigue is prevalent in SLE patients and can be a disabling symptom. Treatment depends on the underlying etiology of the fatigue, with reversible factors such as hypothyroidism, anemia, and diabetes needing to be being addressed first. Pain and depression are positive predictors of fatigue in SLE patients, while social support mitigates fatigue. Thus, a multidisciplinary approach with attention to these issues can be helpful. Regular aerobic exercise followed by periods of rest should also be encouraged. Not infrequently, successful treatment of other manifestations of SLE (eg, with antimalarials) has a beneficial impact on fatigue as well.

CUTANEOUS MANIFESTATIONS

▶ Sun Protection

Photosensitivity occurs in approximately 75% of SLE patients. Although sensitivity to UVB light as found in sunlight and fluorescent lights occurs most commonly, some individuals are also sensitive to UVA light or visible light. Photosensitive lesions include the malar rash, discoid lupus erythematosus (DLE), and subacute cutaneous lupus erythematosus. Prompt treatment of cutaneous lupus is necessary to prevent the development of scarring, dyspigmentation, and alopecia.

Sun protection forms the cornerstone of the management of cutaneous lupus. Patients should be educated about the use of sunscreens and the avoidance of intense sun exposure during peak daylight hours. Daily use of sunscreen with an SPF value of 30 is recommended. Patients are urged to apply the sunscreen 30–60 minutes prior to exposure and to reapply the sunscreen every 4–6 hours. Sun-protective clothing is also very important. Smoking cessation is an important goal because smokers tend to have worse skin disease than nonsmokers.

▶ Topical Therapies

Cutaneous lupus is often treated initially with topical glucocorticoids. The selection of a topical glucocorticoid is based

Table 22–1. Commonly used medications in systemic lupus erythematosus (SLE).

Agent	Typical Dose	Potential Toxicities	Follow-up	Comments
Glucocorticoids	Mild SLE: ≤10 mg/d Moderate to severe SLE: ≥10 mg/d	Hypertension, dyslipidemia, atherosclerosis, hyperglycemia, osteoporosis, avascular necrosis, infection, weight gain, adrenal insufficiency	Lipid profile yearly, urinalysis for glucose, bone densitometry, blood pressure	Regimen for organ- or life-threatening disease: prednisone, 1 mg/kg/d, or pulse intravenous methylprednisone, 1 g/d for 3 days
Hydroxychloroquine	≤400 mg/d; Not to exceed 6.5 mg/kg/d	Ocular effects including inability to focus, corneal deposits, and retinopathy; rash, hyperpigmentation, myopathy, headache, nausea	Ophthalmologic examination with fundoscopy and visual field testing yearly	Reduce dose in renal insufficiency Ophthalmologic examination every 3 months when using chloroquine
Methotrexate	7.5–15 mg/d	Myelosuppression, lymphoproliferative disorders, cirrhosis, pulmonary inflammation and fibrosis	CBC, platelets, liver function tests, albumin, creatinine every 8 weeks or more frequently during dose changes	Do not use in patients with impaired renal function; use concomitant folic acid 1 mg/d or folinic acid 2.5 mg/wk
Azathioprine	Target dose of 2 mg/kg/d	Myelosuppression, hepatotoxicity, malignancy, nausea and vomiting, infection	CBC and platelets every 2 weeks with dosage change, and every 8 weeks thereafter	Consider testing for the thiopurine methyltransferase gene prior to drug initiation; reduce dose in renal insufficiency
Mycophenolate mofetil	Target dose of 2–3 g/d	Myelosuppression, nausea, diarrhea	CBC and platelets every 2 weeks with dosage change, and every 8 weeks thereafter	Reduce dose in renal insufficiency
Cyclophosphamide	**NIH regimen:** 0.5–1.0 g/m² intravenously monthly for 3–6 months for induction; every 3 months for maintenance **Euro-lupus regimen:** 500 mg every 2 weeks for six doses, then azathioprine for maintenance **Oral dosing:** Target dose of 2 mg/kg/d	Myelosuppression, malignancy, hemorrhagic cystitis, bladder cancer, gonadal failure, infection	**Intravenous dosing:** CBC with platelets 7–14 days after dose to determine leukocyte nadir, then every 1–3 months thereafter **Oral dosing:** CBC and platelets every 1–2 weeks with dose change, every 1–3 months thereafter **Intravenous and oral:** Urinalysis and urine cytology every month while receiving treatment, every 6–12 months lifelong	Reduce dose in renal insufficiency, obesity, and advanced age; use PCP prophylaxis; ensure adequate hydration during treatment; use antiemetics and mesna with intravenous dosing; consider use of leuprolide in women receiving intravenous therapy

CBC, complete blood count; NIH, National Institutes of Health; PCP, *Pneumocystis jiroveci* pneumonia.

on the location of the lesion as well as the type of lesion. In general, a low potency glucocorticoid such as hydrocortisone is used first, with escalation to more potent, fluorinated preparations as needed. When treating facial lesions, the use of fluorinated glucocorticoids is limited to 2 weeks because of concern about side effects, such as skin atrophy, striae, depigmentation, and telangiectasias. Medium potency preparations such as triamcinolone acetonide or betamethasone valerate are often used for trunk and limb lesions, while high-potency preparations such as clobetasol are reserved for severe, hypertrophic lesions. It is thought that ointments are generally more effective than creams and

that lotions are most useful for hairy areas such as the scalp. Intralesional injections of triamcinolone acetonide are often used to treat refractory lesions, such as DLE occurring on the scalp. The injection is performed with a 30-gauge needle and is directed into the active, erythematous regions of the lesions. It is important to remember that adrenal suppression can occur as a consequence of the use of high-potency topical glucocorticoids.

Topical tacrolimus and pimecrolimus, which are approved for the treatment of atopic dermatitis, are sometimes used as second-line agents for the treatment of acute lupus lesions, subacute cutaneous lupus erythematosus, and DLE. They are often used in an attempt to minimize exposure to prolonged use of topical glucocorticoids. Enthusiasm for their use has been tempered in recent years by an FDA advisory warning clinicians about the risk of lymphoma and nonmelanoma skin cancer with topical tacrolimus. This warning was based primarily on information from animal studies and case reports from small numbers of patients. Another class of topical therapies, retinoids, might be effective in patients with DLE.

Systemic Therapies

Systemic therapies are necessary when cutaneous lupus cannot be controlled with the topical or intralesional methods described above. The antimalarial hydroxychloroquine is the initial treatment of choice. Its onset of action is approximately 1 month, and full benefit might not be seen for several months. Hydroxychloroquine is also useful in controlling mild arthritis and fatigue. In addition, there is mounting evidence that it might prevent more serious disease flares. A 24-week randomized placebo-controlled trial examining the effect of discontinuing the use of hydroxychloroquine in 47 patients with SLE determined that the risk of major and minor flares was 2.5 times greater in the patients who discontinued the hydroxychloroquine. Subsequent reports extended this observation by demonstrating that lupus patients with high serum concentrations of hydroxychloroquine had less disease activity than patients with lower serum concentrations of hydroxychloroquine. Beyond these effects on disease activity, the antithrombotic and lipid lowering effects of hydroxychloroquine are beneficial for all SLE patients, especially those who have antiphospholipid antibodies.

Hydroxychloroquine is typically given at 200 or 400 mg per day and should not exceed 6.5 mg/kg/d. At these doses, it is usually well tolerated. The most common side effects of hydroxychloroquine include gastrointestinal upset, headaches, and rashes. The most feared complication of the drug is retinal deposition leading to potentially irreversible retinopathy if it is not detected early. Thus, a baseline ophthalmologic examination followed by yearly examinations is recommended in all patients. This complication is exceedingly rare at the doses of hydroxychloroquine currently used.

The antimalarial agents chloroquine (200–500 mg/d) or quinacrine (100 mg/d) can be used in patients who do not fully respond to treatment with hydroxychloroquine. Because of the possibility of increased ocular toxicity, hydroxychloroquine should not be used in combination with chloroquine. Quinacrine does not cause retinal toxicity and, thus, can be used in combination with either hydroxychloroquine or chloroquine. In practice, quinacrine is used infrequently because it must be prepared by a compounding pharmacy and because it causes a yellow skin discoloration with long term use.

Patients with refractory cutaneous lupus may respond to treatment with a variety of other systemic agents. Dapsone (25–200 mg/d) is effective in some patients, particularly those with bullous lupus erythematosus. Open label trials have shown efficacy for thalidomide, but significant toxicities including drowsiness, dizziness, neuropathy, and teratogenicity limit its usefulness for long-term use. Azathioprine, methotrexate, mycophenolate mofetil, intravenous immunoglobulin (IVIG), and cyclophosphamide may also be beneficial for severe cutaneous disease.

MUSCULOSKELETAL MANIFESTATIONS

Arthritis and arthralgias are extremely common in patients with SLE. First-line therapy usually consists of nonsteroidal anti-inflammatory drugs (NSAIDs) or acetaminophen, or both. A proton pump inhibitor is necessary for those at risk for NSAID-induced gastropathy, especially for patients taking concomitant aspirin or glucocorticoids. Testing for and treating *Helicobacter pylori* infection is also prudent in this group of patients. Hydroxychloroquine is often added in patients who have had an incomplete response to NSAIDs. Short-term use of low doses of glucocorticoids (5–10 mg) might be necessary to obtain quick control over an inflammatory arthritis while waiting for the full effect of hydroxychloroquine. Methotrexate is frequently used as a glucocorticoid-sparing agent. Azathioprine and mycophenolate mofetil might be helpful in patients who have an incomplete response to, or are unable to tolerate, methotrexate.

SEROSITIS

Pleuritis and pericarditis often respond to treatment with NSAIDs or low-to-moderate doses of glucocorticoids, or both. Hydroxychloroquine may be helpful in patients with persistent or recurrent symptoms. Oral colchicine also may be of benefit for recurrent serositis. In patients with severe or refractory disease, moderate-to-high doses of glucocorticoids (eg, prednisone, 0.5–1 mg/kg) can be used for short periods of time. In these patients, methotrexate, azathioprine, or mycophenolate mofetil can be helpful while the prednisone is tapered.

RENAL DISEASE

Basic Principles

The treatment of lupus renal disease is divided into an induction of renal response phase and a maintenance phase. The goal of this approach is to achieve a renal response with cytotoxic agents given over several months, and then to maintain the response by using less toxic medications. In addition to addressing the inflammatory etiology of the nephritis, it is also important to treat concomitant risk factors for the progression to chronic kidney disease. Toward this end, angiotensin-converting enzyme (ACE) inhibitors and angiotensin II receptor blockers (ARBs) are used to treat proteinuria and hypertension. A combination of antihypertensive agents might be necessary to achieve the goal blood pressure of <120/80 mm Hg. Statins are often needed to lower serum low density lipoprotein cholesterol levels to the goal of <100 mg/dL.

Renal biopsy is recommended for most patients with suspected lupus nephritis. The pathologic type of nephritis, as defined by the International Society of Nephrology/Renal Pathology Society (ISN/RPS) classification system, helps guide the choice of the treatment regimen. For example, patients with proliferative disease and a high activity index usually receive cytotoxic medications and high-dose glucocorticoids. Conversely, patients with class I or class II disease can often be treated solely with ACE inhibitors or ARB medications, or both. A renal biopsy is also useful in ruling out other etiologies for the nephropathy such as diabetes, hypertension, antiphospholipid nephropathy, or focal segmental glomerulosclerosis, for which immunosuppressive medication would not be appropriate. Patients who do not respond to therapy might require a second biopsy to determine if they still have active nephritis or, alternatively, if they have developed significant renal scarring that should not be treated with further immunosuppressive drugs.

▶ Proliferative Lupus Nephritis

Several important trials conducted at the National Institutes of Health (NIH) between 1970 and 2000 established intravenous pulse cyclophosphamide as the standard of care for the treatment of proliferative lupus nephritis. Key findings from these trials area as follows: (1) treatment with pulse cyclophosphamide is superior to high-dose oral prednisone alone in preventing progression to end-stage renal disease, and (2) an extended course of cyclophosphamide (6 monthly pulses followed by quarterly pulses for 2 years) is more effective than pulse methylprednisolone and shorter courses of cyclophosphamide in preserving renal function and preventing renal relapse. Based on the regimen used in the NIH trials, cyclophosphamide is initially given at 0.5–1 g/m^2, with the lower dose range administered to elderly patients or to those with renal dysfunction or obesity. The dose is then adjusted based on the leukocyte nadir 7–10 days after the infusion.

In recent years, new treatment strategies have challenged the notion that the NIH regimen should continue to be viewed as the unequivocal standard of care. These strategies are rooted primarily in concerns about the significant toxicities associated with cyclophosphamide, which include infections (most commonly herpes zoster), cytopenias, hemorrhagic cystitis, malignancy, and premature ovarian failure. One alternative to the NIH approach involves the use of a less aggressive cyclophosphamide dosing regimen. Pioneered by investigators in Europe (and hence commonly referred to as the Euro-Lupus

regimen), this approach begins with 6 "mini-pulses" of cyclophosphamide (500 mg intravenously every 2 weeks) followed by a switch in therapy from pulse cyclophosphamide to oral azathioprine. Experience with this regimen over a period of >5 years suggests that it is comparable in efficacy to the more aggressive cyclophosphamide regimen and, in all likelihood, less toxic. Another alternative to pulse cyclophosphamide that is gaining favor involves the use of mycophenolate mofetil instead of cyclophosphamide. Recently, mycophenolate mofetil and pulse cyclophosphamide were compared directly in the largest lupus nephritis trial ever conducted. In that trial, the response rates after 6 months of therapy were the same in both treatment groups.

It remains to be determined whether standard pulse cyclophosphamide will soon be supplanted as a common therapy for lupus nephritis. For now, cyclophosphamide is still one of a small handful of options for patients with lupus nephritis. Therefore, it is important to be cognizant of measures that have been developed in an effort to minimize its toxicity. Adequate hydration and the use of mesna decrease the occurrence of bladder toxicity due to cyclophosphamide therapy. Prophylaxis against *Pneumocystis jiroveci* is recommended in patients taking cyclophosphamide. Ovarian toxicity deserves special mention because it has become a major reason why increasing numbers of patients are reluctant to receive cyclophosphamide therapy. The risk of permanent ovarian failure is related to the cumulative cyclophosphamide dose and the age of the patient. One study revealed that in patients taking the standard long course of pulse cyclophosphamide, the rate of amenorrhea was 17% for patients ≤25 years, 43% for patients between 26 and 30 years, and 100% for patients ≥31 years. Recent data suggest that administration of 3.75 mg leuprolide intramuscularly 2 weeks prior to each cyclophosphamide infusion might offer some protection against ovarian failure.

Numerous other agents are also under investigation as possible therapies for lupus nephritis. Like mycophenolate mofetil, which is widely used to facilitate organ transplantation, some of these agents have already been approved for other indications. In particular, there has been great excitement in recent years about the potential benefits of rituximab, which already is approved for the treatment of B cell lymphoma and rheumatoid arthritis. This excitement grew from several uncontrolled case series and widespread anecdotal reports, but enthusiasm was dashed recently by two large negative trials of rituximab in patients with SLE, including lupus nephritis. Further investigation is necessary to determine whether rituximab has a place in the treatment of SLE.

▶ Membranous Lupus Nephritis

The treatment of membranous nephritis is controversial. Although the renal prognosis of membranous nephropathy is better than that of proliferative nephritis, the morbid cardiovascular effects of the nephrotic syndrome are well recognized. Thus, membranous nephritis is often treated aggressively with immunosuppressive agents in hopes of retarding the extrarenal aspects of the disease. Therapeutic options include glucocorticoids, mycophenolate mofetil, cyclophosphamide, or cyclosporine. In addition, angiotensin antagonists are of paramount importance for the reduction of proteinuria.

NEUROPSYCHIATRIC SLE

Neuropsychiatric SLE encompasses a wide variety of abnormalities of the central, peripheral, and autonomic nervous systems. The specific abnormality as well as its severity dictates the appropriate treatment measures. First and foremost, it is critical to determine if a particular neuropsychiatric finding is due to active SLE or to a secondary cause such as drug side effect, infection, uremia, or a concomitant systemic disease (such as diabetes or hypertension).

If active SLE is determined to be the culprit, treatment differs widely depending on the specific manifestation. Severe neuropsychiatric manifestations include stroke syndromes, demyelinating syndromes, seizures, transverse myelopathy, and organic brain syndrome (acute confusional state). Many of these severe manifestations require high-dose glucocorticoids. Several small studies have suggested an additional benefit with pulse intravenous cyclophosphamide. However, there are exceptions to this general approach. In particular, stroke syndromes and seizures are particularly challenging. Stroke syndromes in SLE can be caused by a variety of factors including antiphospholipid antibodies, cardiac vegetations, and atherosclerosis. Long-term anticoagulation with warfarin or aspirin is the treatment of choice for strokes associated with antiphospholipid antibodies. Unless there is a concomitant SLE flare, treatment with glucocorticoids is not needed. Similarly, glucocorticoids are not the first-line of treatment for most lupus patients with seizures. Rather, seizures in SLE patients are usually treated with the same anticonvulsant medications that are used in patients who do not have SLE. However, it is sometimes difficult to determine whether seizures represent an ongoing inflammatory process or are the result of a fixed scar. If ongoing inflammation is the cause, glucocorticoids or cytotoxic drugs (or both) may be necessary. Headaches are very common in SLE patients and are treated similarly to headaches that occur in patients without SLE. Glucocorticoids are added if there are other manifestations of active SLE. Cognitive dysfunction is also present in many SLE patients. The use of glucocorticoids in these patients is controversial. If a therapeutic trial is initiated, it is important to perform serial neuropsychiatric testing to demonstrate benefit. If no benefit is seen, glucocorticoids should be discontinued. Some studies have demonstrated an association between cognitive dysfunction and the presence of antiphospholipid antibodies, but it has yet to be determined whether aspirin or any other antithrombotic therapy might be helpful in this subgroup of patients.

HEMATOLOGIC MANIFESTATIONS

Leukopenia, anemia, and thrombocytopenia are frequently noted in SLE patients, and their etiology can be multifactorial. Side effects from medication should always be considered. Because hematologic abnormalities caused by SLE are often mild, treatment is not always necessary. In patients with leukopenia in association with recurrent infections, cautious use of prednisone to raise the white blood cell count might be indicated. Granulocyte colony-stimulating factor is usually avoided because there are data to suggest that it can precipitate SLE flares.

Severe SLE-related autoimmune thrombocytopenia is generally treated according to the guidelines established for immune thrombocytopenia. The overall treatment goal is to maintain a safe platelet count while minimizing the potential toxicity of therapy. Although data suggest that life-threatening bleeding does not occur until platelet counts are <10,000/mcL, treatment is usually indicated for all patients with platelet counts of <20,000/mcL and for patients with platelet counts of <50,000/mcL with clinically important bleeding or a history of bleeding. Initial treatment consists of a course of high-dose glucocorticoids, often commencing with pulse methylprednisolone in extreme circumstances. After improvement in the platelet count (usually within 1 week), the glucocorticoids are tapered. In patients who do not respond to glucocorticoids or who relapse during tapering, IVIG is often tried. Because IVIG often produces a rapid platelet response, it should be used in conjunction with glucocorticoids from the outset in patients who are actively bleeding or in those requiring an invasive procedure. However, it is important to remember in this regard that IVIG is contraindicated in patients with IgA deficiency. Although IVIG is often initially effective, relapse is common. Splenectomy is often considered as the next therapeutic modality in refractory patients. A systematic review estimated that 66% of patients with immune thrombocytopenia achieve a complete remission after splenectomy. Laparoscopic splenectomy appears to be safer than laparotomy. The majority of patients achieve a response within 2 weeks after the procedure. Vaccinations for *Streptococcus pneumoniae, Haemophilus influenzae* b, and *Neisseria meningitidis* are recommended 2 weeks prior to the splenectomy. A variety of other agents can be tried in patients with refractory disease. Other SLE disease manifestations guide the choice of additional medications. Options include danazol, azathioprine, mycophenolate mofetil, cyclophosphamide, and rituximab.

The treatment of severe autoimmune hemolytic anemia is similar to the treatment of autoimmune thrombocytopenia. High-dose prednisone or pulse methylprednisolone is used initially, and tapering begins once the hematocrit rises. Patients with refractory disease may require additional immunosuppressive therapy. Splenectomy is occasionally necessary after all other therapeutic options have been exhausted. SLE-related microangiopathic hemolytic anemia is treated with plasmapheresis, following the standard of care for the treatment of thrombotic thrombocytopenic purpura.

UNCOMMON COMPLICATIONS

Acute pneumonitis and diffuse alveolar hemorrhage are rare pulmonary manifestations of SLE. Both syndromes carry a poor prognosis, and treatment recommendations are based on uncontrolled data and case reports. Because infection is usually part of the differential diagnosis, most patients are initially treated with broad-spectrum antibiotics. Acute pneumonitis is treated with high-dose glucocorticoids, and additional immunosuppressive agents can be added if necessary. Diffuse alveolar hemorrhage is typically treated with high-dose glucocorticoids in conjunction with pulse cyclophosphamide. In addition, plasmapheresis may be effective in some patients. Mesenteric vasculitis is another uncommon but life-threatening manifestation of SLE. Bowel perforation is the most feared complication. High-dose glucocorticoids and pulse cyclophosphamide are the most commonly used therapies.

PEDIATRIC SLE

The treatment of children and adolescents with SLE generally follows the same guidelines as the treatment of adults with SLE. However, special attention must be paid to the unique circumstances of the pediatric population. In particular, consideration of issues related to physical growth, emotional well-being, and coping with a chronic and potentially appearance changing illness are paramount to a successful treatment plan. Multidisciplinary care with education of the family is critical. In terms of pharmacologic therapies,

the negative effects of systemic glucocorticoids on bone, physical growth, and appearance are well recognized. Thus, every effort must be made to minimize the long-term use of these medications. Mild SLE is typically treated with NSAIDs and antimalarials. In patients with persistent disease, there is experience with the use of azathioprine, methotrexate, and mycophenolate mofetil as glucocorticoid-sparing agents. Organ-threatening disease is usually treated with intravenous pulse cyclophosphamide.

Appel GB, Contreras G, Dooley MA, et al. Mycophenolate mofetil versus cyclophosphamide as lupus nephritis induction treatment. *J Am Soc Nephrol.* 2009;20:1103. [PMID: 19369404]

Dall'Era M, Wofsy D. Lupus clinical trials – an interim analysis. *Nat Rev Rheumatol.* 2009;5:348. [PMID: 19491915]

Houssiau FA, Vasconcelos C, D'Cruz D, et al. The 10-year follow-up data of the Euro-Lupus Nephritis Trial comparing low-dose versus high-dose intravenous cyclophosphamide. *Ann Rheum Dis.* 2010;69:61. [PMID: 19155235]

Mittal B, Rennke H, Singh AK. The role of kidney biopsy in the management of lupus nephritis. *Curr Opin Nephrol Hypertens* 2005;14:1. [PMID: 15586009]

Ruiz-Irastorza G, Ramos-Casals M, Brito-Zeron P, et al. Clinical efficacy and side effects of antimalarials in systemic lupus erythematosus. *Ann Rheum Dis.* 2009 [Epub ahead of print]. [PMID: 19103632]

Somers EC, Marder W, Christman GM, et al. Use of a gonadotropin-releasing hormone analog for protection against premature ovarian failure during cyclophosphamide therapy in women with severe lupus. *Arthritis Rheum.* 2005;52:2761. [PMID: 16142702]

Walling HW, Sontheimer RD. Cutaneous lupus erythematosus: issues in diagnosis and treatment. *Am J Clin Dermatol.* 2009;10:365. [PMID: 19824738]

Weening JJ, D'Agati VD, Schwartz MM, et al. The classification of glomerulonephritis in systemic lupus erythematosus revisited. *Kidney Int.* 2004;65:521. [PMID: 14717922]

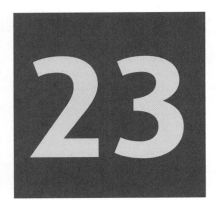

23

Antiphospholipid Antibody Syndrome

Jonathan Graf, MD

- ► Arterial or venous thrombosis.
- ► Recurrent pregnancy losses.
- ► Autoantibodies to phospholipid or β_2-glycoprotein I.
- ► Lupus anticoagulant activity.
- ► Can occur independently or in association with systemic lupus erythematosus (SLE).

► General Considerations

Antiphospholipid antibody syndrome (APS) is an acquired disorder associated with circulating autoantibodies to anionic phospholipids (eg, cardiolipin) and their protein binding complexes. The primary clinical manifestations of APS are thromboses, which can affect both the arterial and venous circulations, and pregnancy loss. APS can occur independently, in which case it is called primary APS, or it can develop in the setting of another autoimmune disease, usually SLE, in which case it is called secondary APS. The diagnosis of APS relies on recognition of its clinical presentation and detection of antiphospholipid antibodies either by enzyme immunoassays or by the presence of an anticoagulant (a "lupus anticoagulant") in a phospholipid-dependent coagulation test, such as the Russell viper venom time. Treatment usually involves anticoagulation, the level of which is still debated but depends on clinical context.

► Clinical Findings

A. Symptoms and Signs

Deep venous thrombosis (DVT) is the most common clinical manifestation of the hypercoagulability associated with primary or secondary APS. DVTs can be single or multiple and affect either large or small veins. Most common are DVTs in the lower extremities; pulmonary embolism complicates up to one third of lower extremity DVTs associated with APS. Thromboses associated with APS can involve any component of the venous circulation; APS can cause renal vein thrombosis, retinal vein occlusion, Budd-Chiari syndrome, and adrenal hemorrhage secondary to thrombosis of the adrenal veins.

APS-associated arterial disease is common and can affect the peripheral vascular, cerebrovascular, and cardiovascular circulations. The clinical sequelae of APS- associated arterial disease depend on the size and distribution of vascular beds involved (Table 23–1).

Thromboses of medium-to-large peripheral arteries can lead to cutaneous ulceration and gangrene. Involvement of dermal capillaries can produce **livedo reticularis** (Plate 39), whose dusky, mottled appearance is due to a reactive hyperemia that occurs in normal skin adjacent to the regions of relative ischemia.

Cerebrovascular involvement can result in stroke, transient ischemic attack, dural sinus thrombosis, and an encephalopathy that can be difficult to distinguish from inflammatory or infectious cerebritis or cerebral vasculitis.

The **cardiac manifestations** of APS are protean. Thrombosis of epicardial vessels can cause myocardial infarction while subendothelial microangiopathy can lead to cardiomyopathy. APS is associated with **Libman-Sacks endocarditis**, which produces verrucose lesions of the endocardium and, more commonly, of the heart valves, especially the mitral valve. The histology of the valvular lesions reveals fibrin deposits accompanied by variable extents of inflammation. The severity of the valvular disease varies. Most common is thickening of the valve leaflets, which is detected by echocardiography but is not of hemodynamic significance. At the other end of the spectrum are large vegetations leading to clinically significant valvular dysfunction (regurgitation or stenosis). Embolization from Libman-Sacks vegetations is uncommon but can occur.

Table 23–1. Arterial manifestations of antiphospholipid syndrome.

Vascular Bed	Clinical Manifestation
Skin	Ulceration, gangrene, livedo reticularis
Cerebrovascular	Stroke, transient ischemic attack, seizure, encephalopathy, chorea, myelopathy, mononeuritis
Cardiac	Myocardial infarction, cardiomyopathy, valvular vegetations and abnormalities
Renal	Renal infarction, thrombotic microangiopathy
Pulmonary	Pulmonary emboli, microvascular thromboses, pulmonary hypertension, alveolar hemorrhage
Gastrointestinal	Mesenteric ischemia, splenic infarction
Ophthalmologic	Retinal artery thrombosis and ischemia

Renal injury in APS is most often due to thrombotic microangiopathy, an increasingly recognized complication whose histopathology is similar to that of malignant hypertension or thrombotic thrombocytopenic purpura. In cases of secondary APS associated with SLE, the distinction between lupus nephritis and thrombotic microangiopathy may require renal biopsy. Other mechanisms of kidney injury due to APS include arterial thrombi and emboli as well as renal vein thrombus. There also appears to be an association between APS and renal artery stenosis.

Acute pulmonary emboli complicating proximal DVT are the most common form of **lung involvement**, but APS also causes chronic pulmonary emboli as well as in situ microvascular thromboses that can progress to pulmonary capillary obliteration, pulmonary hypertension and, in rare instances, diffuse alveolar hemorrhage.

Well-recognized but nonspecific associated hematologic abnormalities include **thrombocytopenia** and **hemolytic anemia**. Thrombocytopenia associated with APS is generally mild to moderate, although patients with APS who have thrombocytopenia are reported to have a poorer prognosis when compared with patients who have APS but do not have thrombocytopenia. Hemolytic anemia can be either antibody-mediated or a consequence of microangiopathic destruction.

Pregnancy morbidity associated with APS can vary widely in its clinical presentation. Fetal demise can occur at all gestational time points, but spontaneous abortions that occur from the second trimester onward are more specific for APS than are those that occur during the first trimester. In addition to fetal loss, APS has been linked to preeclampsia, intrauterine growth retardation, and the HELLP syndrome (*h*emolysis, *e*levated *l*iver enzymes, *l*ow *p*latelets).

Catastrophic antiphospholipid antibody syndrome (CAPS), which consists of an accelerated clinical course of thromboses and multiple organ failures (usually ≥3)

occurring over days to weeks, develops in some patients with APS. In many instances the accelerated thrombosis occurs in the microvasculature. Specific triggers can be identified in the majority of CAPS cases, including antecedent infection, surgery, withdrawal of anticoagulation, pregnancy, and use of oral contraception; up to one third of cases, however, have no identifiable cause. CAPS can mimic other forms of systemic illness, including the systemic inflammatory response syndrome, disseminated intravascular coagulation, thrombotic thrombocytopenic purpura, and HELLP. Prompt recognition of CAPS requires a high index of suspicion, and the diagnosis can be difficult to establish without adequate histopathology.

B. Laboratory Findings

According to current APS classification criteria, patients with APS must have positive test results for antiphospholipid antibodies in moderate-high titers using at least one of three general types of tests: (1) enzyme immunoassays for antibodies to cardiolipin; (2) enzyme immunoassays for antibodies to β_2-glycoprotein I; and (3) tests for lupus anticoagulant activity. All three types of tests should be used when evaluating patients with suspected APS. Anticoagulation therapy does not interfere with the enzyme immunoassays but can limit and complicate the interpretation of functional tests for lupus anticoagulants.

Occasionally, antiphospholipid antibodies may be of low titer and difficult to detect during an acute thrombosis. A more common problem is the presence of these antibodies in the absence of a clinical manifestation of APS. Antiphospholipid antibodies can be detected in 5–10% of the healthy population and in up to 50% of patients with SLE. Epidemiologic evidence suggests that the risk of thrombosis correlates strongest with lupus anticoagulant activity, followed by antibodies to β_2-glycoprotein I and then by anticardiolipin antibodies. Those patients who have positive results in all three types of assays (so called "triple positive" patients) may have the highest risk of thrombosis.

Anticardiolipin antibodies recognize one or more epitopes on cardiolipin, an anionic phospholipid that is a component of the inner membrane of mitochondria. Anticardiolipin antibodies associated with APS can cross react with the reagents used in the rapid plasma reagin (RPR) screening test for syphilis, leading to a "biological false-positive" test for syphilis. The risk of a thrombotic event may correlate with the immunoglobulin class and titer of the anticardiolipin antibody, with high titer IgG antibodies conferring greater risk than low titer IgM or IgA antibodies. Anticardiolipin antibodies have greater sensitivity, but less specificity, for APS than antibodies to β_2-glycoprotein I or lupus anticoagulants. Acute and chronic infections, particularly viral, can induce anticardiolipin antibodies that do not correlate with APS and do not confer risk of thrombosis.

Anti-β_2-glycoprotein I antibodies recognize epitopes on β_2-glycoprotein I itself or on the macromolecular complex created by the binding of β_2-glycoprotein I to cardiolipin. It is generally accepted that anti-β_2-glycoprotein I antibodies and those anticardiolipin antibodies that recognize cardiolipin in the context of β_2-glycoprotein I are more specific for APS and more closely associated with risk of thrombosis than are antibodies that recognize cardiolipin alone. Anti-β_2-glycoprotein I antibodies have greater specificity for APS than do anticardiolipin antibodies, in part because they are not as commonly seen in the setting of viral or other infections.

Lupus anticoagulant activity reflects the presence of antibodies that prolong in vitro phospholipid-dependent clotting assays, such as the Russell viper venom time. Despite its name, the lupus anticoagulant is not specific for SLE (it can be present in primary APS) and is associated with risk of thrombosis, not bleeding. Although lupus anticoagulant activity is likely due to antiphospholipid antibodies, the target antigens are not determined directly; rather, the presence of these antibodies is inferred from their ability to interfere with a functional clotting assay in vitro. Patients with APS may have lupus anticoagulant activity but lack detectable anticardiolipin and anti-β_2-glycoprotein I antibodies.

There are several different methods that can be used to test for lupus anticoagulant (Table 23–2). These are functional assays whose performance is difficult to standardize between different laboratories. Therefore, it is important for physicians who order this test to be familiar with the methods used by the laboratory and with interpretations of the results. If the index of suspicion is high in a patient whose test results are negative for lupus anticoagulant using one method, testing should be repeated using a different method. Regardless of the specific method or reagents used, a laboratory diagnosis of lupus anticoagulant requires a 3-step process (Figure 23–1). First, there must be prolongation of an in vitro coagulation test in which phospholipids are added to enhance the clotting reaction. Antiphospholipid antibodies interfere with the added phospholipid, causing prolongation of the clotting time. Second, a 1:1 mix of patient and control plasma must fail to completely correct the abnormal clotting time, indicating that an inhibitor, rather than a factor deficiency, is responsible for the abnormality. Finally, the inhibitor must be shown to be phospholipid-dependent. This

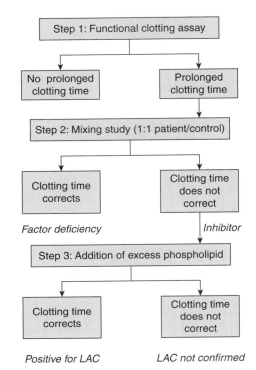

▲ **Figure 23–1.** Algorithm outlining the three steps in testing for lupus anticoagulant (LAC).

usually is accomplished by demonstrating normalization of the clotting time by the addition of molar-excess concentrations of the phospholipid reagent to the assay. Different methods and reagents exist for each of these steps and account for much variability in testing for lupus anticoagulant activity. The ability of a given assay to detect a lupus anticoagulant depends on the specific type and concentration of phospholipid reagent used in both the initial and confirmatory steps.

▶ Diagnostic Criteria

The diagnosis of APS is based on the presence of at least one clinical disease manifestation (thrombosis or pregnancy morbidity) together with laboratory evidence for the presence of antiphospholipid antibodies. Classification criteria for APS (Table 23–3) have been developed to facilitate studies of patients with this disease. While these classification criteria can be useful for the diagnosis of APS in clinical practice, the criteria sacrifice diagnostic sensitivity in favor of specificity. The actual clinical spectrum of APS is more diverse than the classification criteria would suggest. Moreover, the requirement for a second confirmatory test for antiphospholipid antibodies is not always a practical one: in many instances, clinical circumstances do not lend themselves to the luxury of waiting 12 weeks before initiating therapy.

Table 23–2. Commonly used assays to detect lupus anticoagulant.

1. Activated partial thromboplastin time (aPTT): Test of intrinsic clotting cascade requiring use of phospholipid reagents
2. Dilute aPTT: enhanced sensitivity aPTT using limiting concentrations of phospholipid reagents
3. Dilute Russell viper venom time (dRVVT): Sensitive test that uses very small amounts of phospholipid reagents
4. Hexagonal phase phospholipid (HPE) neutralization: Ratio comparing two simultaneous PTTs performed with and without HPE reagent
5. Platelet neutralization test: Similar to HPE neutralization but uses platelet extracts in the confirmatory step

Table 23–3. Classification criteria for antiphospholipid antibody syndrome.[a]

Clinical Criteria

A. Vascular thrombosis
  1. One or more clinical episodes without significant evidence of inflammation in the vessel wall.
B. Pregnancy morbidity
  1. One or more unexplained deaths of a morphologically normal fetus at or beyond the 10th week of gestation
  2. One or more premature births of a morphologically normal neonate before the 34th week of gestation because of
     a. Eclampsia or severe preeclampsia, or
     b. Recognized features of placenta insufficiency
  3. Three or more unexplained consecutive spontaneous abortions before the 10th week of gestation.

Laboratory Criteria[b]

  1. Lupus anticoagulant in plasma
  2. Anticardiolipin antibody of IgG or IgM isotype present in medium or high titer
  3. Anti-β_2-glycoprotein I antibody of IgG or IgM isotype, present in titer above the 99th percentile

[a]Patients should satisfy one or more clinical criteria and one or more laboratory criteria.
[b]Present on two or more occasions at least 12 weeks apart.
Data from Miyakis S, Lockshin MD, Atsumi T, et al. International consensus statement on an update of the classification criteria for definite antiphospholipid syndrome (APS). *J Thromb Haemost.* 2006;4:295.

▶ Treatment

The clinical manifestations of APS dictate the treatment of individual patients. The cornerstone of therapy for patients with an acute thrombotic complication of APS is anticoagulation, initially with therapeutic doses of intravenous unfractionated heparin or subcutaneous low-molecular-weight heparin and subsequently with oral warfarin. Most patients who have had an APS-associated DVT, and all patients with an APS-associated arterial thrombotic event, require lifelong anticoagulation.

Prospective studies demonstrate favorable outcomes in APS patients treated with standard-dose regimens of warfarin to obtain a target international normalized ratio (INR) of 2.0–3.0. Thus, standard-dose anticoagulation (target INR of 2.0–3.0) is recommended for APS patients with nonrecurrent venous thromboembolism. Some experts recommend a more aggressive approach (target INR >3.0) for APS patients with arterial thromboses or with recurrent venous events.

Discontinuation of warfarin therapy confers risk not only for additional thrombotic events but also for catastrophic APS. However, carefully selected patients with a single provoked DVT and a "low risk" antibody profile (eg, low titer anticardiolipin antibody and negative tests for anti-β_2-glycoprotein I antibodies and lupus anticoagulant) might be considered for warfarin therapy limited to 3–6 months.

Patients with CAPS often require immunosuppressive therapies, plasmapheresis, and intravenous immunoglobulin in addition to full therapeutic doses of intravenous unfractionated heparin or subcutaneous low-molecular-weight heparin. There are few data to guide therapies of patients with organ specific manifestations of APS, such as Libman-Sacks endocarditis.

Women who have suffered a previous pregnancy-associated complication of APS should receive prophylaxis during subsequent pregnancies with aspirin and subcutaneous unfractionated heparin or subcutaneous low-molecular-weight heparin. Warfarin should not be used because of its teratogenicity. Anticoagulation beyond the postpartum period is not recommended for women who have had a prior obstetric complication of APS but no history of thrombosis.

An area of uncertainty is the appropriate management of patients who have antiphospholipid antibodies but who do not have clinical manifestations of APS. There is general agreement that SLE patients with "asymptomatic" antiphospholipid antibodies benefit from primary prophylaxis with hydroxychloroquine. Patients who do not have SLE usually do not need prophylactic therapy. Treatment of asymptomatic individuals with antiphospholipid antibodies with low-dose aspirin does not appear to prevent future thromboses. However, some experts use prophylaxis with low-dose aspirin for selected patients with "high risk" antibody profiles, such as triple-positive patients or those with high titers of antibodies. These patients also should be considered for anticoagulation when placed in high-risk situations such as surgery or prolonged immobilization, although evidence for this approach is currently lacking. All patients with antiphospholipid antibodies should have aggressive management of hypertension, serum cholesterol, and other cardiovascular risk factors.

Asherson RA. The primary, secondary, catastrophic, and seronegative variants of the antiphospholipid syndrome: a personal history long in the making. *Semin Thromb Hemost.* 2008;34:227. [PMID: 18720302]

Asherson RA, Cervera R, Merrill JT, Erkan D. Antiphospholipid antibodies and the antiphospholipid syndrome: clinical significance and treatment. *Semin Thromb Hemost.* 2008;34:256. [PMID: 18720305]

Bertolaccini ML, Khamashta MA. Laboratory diagnosis and management challenges in the antiphospholipid syndrome. *Lupus.* 2006;15:172. [PMID: 16634372]

Branch W; Obstetric Task Force. Report of the Obstetric APS Task Force: 13th International Congress on Antiphospholipid Antibodies, 13th April 2010. *Lupus.* 2011;20:158. [PMID: 21303832]

Lim W, Crowther MA, Eikelboom JW. Management of antiphospholipid antibody syndrome: a systematic review. *JAMA.* 2006;295:1050. [PMID: 16507806]

Miyakis S, Lockshin MD, Atsumi T, et al. International consensus statement on an update of the classification criteria for definite antiphospholipid syndrome (APS). *J Thromb Haemost.* 2006;4:295. [PMID: 16420554]

Ruiz-Irastorza G, Cuadrado MJ, Ruiz-Arruza I, et al. Evidence-based recommendations for the prevention and long-term management of thrombosis in antiphospholipid antibody-positive patients: report of a task force at the 13th International Congress on antiphospholipid antibodies. *Lupus.* 2011;20:206. [PMID: 21303837]

Ruiz-Irastorza G, Hunt BJ, Khamashta MA. A systematic review of secondary thromboprophylaxis in patients with antiphospholipid antibodies. *Arthritis Rheum.* 2007;57:1487. [PMID: 18050167]

Vora SK, Asherson RA, Erkan D. Catastrophic antiphospholipid syndrome. *J Intensive Care Med.* 2006;21:144. [PMID: 16672637]

Raynaud Phenomenon

24

Sangeeta D. Sule, MD
Fredrick M. Wigley, MD

ESSENTIALS OF DIAGNOSIS

► Raynaud phenomenon (RP), a vasospastic reaction to cold temperatures or emotional stress, leads to sharply demarcated color changes of the skin.

► Classified clinically into primary or secondary forms.

► Primary RP is idiopathic and is associated with no identifiable abnormalities in blood vessel architecture.

► Secondary RP patients may have complications of digital tissue ischemia, including recurrent digital ulcerations, rapid deep tissue necrosis, and amputation.

► Avoidance of cold temperatures is critical in the management of RP. The entire body must be kept comfortably warm.

► Medications are indicated if there are signs of critical tissue ischemia (eg, digital ulcers) or if quality of life is restricted.

► General Considerations

A unique circulatory system, including both thermoregulatory and nutritional blood vessels, exists in the skin, especially in the hands, feet, and the face. In these areas of the body, local blood flow is regulated by a complex interaction of neural signals, cellular mediators, and circulating vasoactive molecules. Temperature responses are principally mediated through the sympathetic nervous system by rapidly altering blood flow through arteriovenous shunts in the skin. During hot weather, these shunts open (vasodilate), allowing heat to dissipate. In cool weather, the shunts constrict, shifting blood centrally and helping maintain a stable core body temperature.

Raynaud phenomenon (RP) is transient digital ischemia due to cold temperatures or emotional stress. This vasoconstriction of digital arteries, precapillary arterioles, and cutaneous arteriovenous shunts leads to a sharp demarcation of skin pallor or cyanosis of the digits (Figure 24–1). The ischemic phase is followed by recovery of blood flow that appears as cutaneous erythema, secondary to rapid reperfusion of the digits.

RP is classified into two categories: primary and secondary. **Primary RP** are vasospastic attacks precipitated by cold temperatures or emotional stress. Primary RP, which occurs in the absence of an identifiable disease, is most common in otherwise healthy females between 15 and 30 years of age. A family history of first-degree family members is reported in about 30% of cases. These attacks usually occur symmetrically and bilaterally in the hands. There is no underlying sign of tissue necrosis or gangrene (eg, digital pitting) and the underlying vasculature is normal. Nailfold capillary microscopy (see below) and physical examination findings are normal. If a patient meets criteria for primary RP and no new symptoms develop over 2 years of follow-up, the development of secondary disease is unlikely. The finding of abnormal nailfold capillaries on microscopy or specific autoantibodies are strong predictors of secondary RP due to an underlying rheumatologic disease.

Secondary RP is associated with an underlying pathology that alters regional blood flow by damaging blood vessels, interfering with neural control of the circulation, or changing either the physical properties of the blood or the levels of circulating mediators that regulate the digital and cutaneous circulation. Among the large number of suspected causes of secondary RP, the most likely causes are systemic sclerosis (SSc), systemic lupus erythematosus (SLE), Sjögren syndrome, or dermatomyositis. Patients with secondary RP generally have more severe, painful RP. This may be associated with evidence of digital ischemia, including fingertip ulceration and tissue loss.

► Clinical Findings

All patients with a history of RP should be asked about symptoms suggestive of an autoimmune disease, such as arthritis,

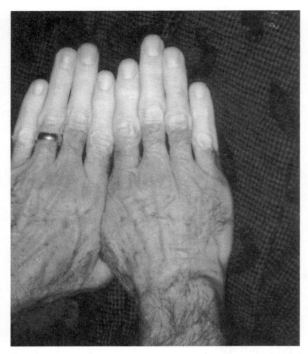

▲ **Figure 24–1.** A typical Raynaud phenomenon attack characterized by a sharp demarcation of skin pallor.

dry eyes or dry mouth, myalgias, fevers, rash, or shortness of breath. Careful physical examination for signs of immune-mediated digital ischemia should include examination of the pulses, auscultation over large arteries (eg, the subclavians), and nailfold capillary microscopy. The patient should be evaluated for specific autoantibodies if an underlying autoimmune disease is suspected (see Laboratory Findings).

A. Symptoms and Signs

RP most often affects the fingers, although attacks also occur in the toes and occasionally on areas of the face. A typical RP attack is characterized by the sudden onset of cold digits associated with a demarcation of skin pallor (white attack) or cyanosis (blue attack). After rewarming, there is vascular reperfusion, resulting in the erythema secondary to rebound of blood flow.

A diagnosis of RP may be made if a patient has a history of both cold sensitivity and associated color changes of the skin (pallor or cyanosis or both) limited to the digits. The diagnosis of RP can be made by asking the following questions: (1) Are your fingers unusually sensitive to cold? (2) Do your fingers change color when they are exposed to cold? (3) Do they turn white, blue, or both? The diagnosis of RP is confirmed if there is a positive response to all three questions but is excluded if responses to questions two and three are negative.

RP attacks typically start in a single finger and then spread to other digits of the same or both hands. The index, middle, and ring fingers are the most commonly involved digits. White attacks may lead to critical digital ischemia. In contrast, blue attacks are mainly the result of vasospasm of the thermoregulatory vessels. Low blood flow to the digits may persist for 15 minutes after rewarming. Physicians should pay careful attention to painful RP attacks because they are a symptom of ischemia.

B. Laboratory Findings

Patients with clear clinical evidence for primary RP do not need further laboratory testing. This includes patients with symmetric attacks, no evidence of peripheral vascular disease, no tissue gangrene or digital pitting, and a negative nailfold capillary examination. However, if a secondary cause of RP is suspected, specific blood work is guided by the clinical findings associated with RP and should include serum chemistries, a complete blood cell count, thyroid function tests, serum and urine protein electrophoresis, and testing for cryoglobulins or cryofibrinogens. In addition, elevated inflammatory markers, such as the erythrocyte sedimentation rate or C-reactive protein, are associated with some but not all causes of secondary RP. (SSc, for example, is seldom associated with elevated acute phase reactants [see Chapter 25].)

Antinuclear antibody (ANA) testing is useful for evaluation of autoimmune diseases. In a study of 586 patients monitored for approximately 3200 person-years, a positive ANA assay was one of the strongest predictors of progression to SSc. The pattern of ANA can provide clues to the underlying autoimmune disease. An anti-centromere pattern detected on ANA testing is associated strongly with limited scleroderma (eg, the CREST [calcinosis, Raynaud phenomenon, esophageal dysmotility, sclerodactyly, telangiectasias] syndrome. Anti-topoisomerase antibodies are found in patients with diffuse SSc. Anti-dsDNA, anti-Ro/SS-A, anti-La/SS-B, anti-Sm, and anti-RNP antibodies are most characteristic of patients with SLE (see Chapter 21), Sjögren syndrome (see Chapter 26), or mixed connective tissue disease. Anti-Jo-1 and other anti-synthetase antibodies are often associated with inflammatory myopathies (see Chapter 27).

C. Special Tests

Examination of nailfold capillaries is important for the differentiation of primary and secondary RP. To perform nailfold capillary microscopy, a drop of grade B immersion oil is placed on the patient's skin at the base of the fingernail. This area is then viewed using an ophthalmoscope set to 40 diopters or a stereoscopic microscope. Normal capillaries appear as symmetric, nondilated loops. In contrast, distorted, dilated, or absent capillaries suggest a secondary disease process. Abnormalities of the nailfold capillaries are strong independent predictors of rheumatic conditions, particularly SSc, SLE, and dermatomyositis.

Differential Diagnosis

RP is a clinical diagnosis, based on a patient's report of sudden, episodic color changes of the digits provoked by cold temperature or emotional stress. However, true RP should be distinguished from the sensitivity to cold or the nondemarcated mottling seen in a normal response to cool temperatures. True RP must also be distinguished from acrocyanosis (which has multiple potential causes, generally difficult to define precisely). Although acrocyanosis is aggravated by cold temperature, there are none of the episodic attacks or sharp demarcations of color changes observed in RP.

Mechanical stress on the nerves or vessels in the hand or fingers may also cause sensitivity to the cold temperature. Patients with complaints of color changes and numbness should be evaluated for carpal tunnel syndrome or neuropathy. Paraproteinemias and hyperviscosity syndromes should also be considered in the differential diagnosis. RP in these patients results from sluggish blood flow through cutaneous and digital vessels. Patients with cryoglobulinemia also may have RP due to the cold-sensitive proteins. The use of certain drugs (eg, sympathomimetic agents) that induce vasoconstriction can aggravate or cause RP. In addition, patients with hypothyroidism often have cold hands, acrocyanosis, or RP. Repetition injuries, such as repeated exposure to vibration, may lead to white finger or trauma that may resemble RP.

Distinguishing primary from secondary RP is critical. The connective tissue diseases are the most common secondary disorders that the internist will encounter. Thus, a thorough review of systems focusing on symptoms of a connective tissue disease is essential. Patients should be asked about dry eyes or mouth (Sjögren syndrome); painful joints or morning stiffness (arthritis); rashes, photosensitivity, or cardiopulmonary abnormalities (SLE); and skin tightening, respiratory distress, or gastrointestinal disease (SSc).

Most patients with RP report symmetric involvement of the digits. A vascular occlusion such as atherosclerosis, emboli, or arterial occlusions should be considered in patients with asymmetric RP. In particular, RP in the feet associated with lesions warrants a work-up for macrovascular disease. In such cases, vascular imaging such as a magnetic resonance arteriogram or arteriography may be appropriate.

Treatment

A. Preventive Strategies

Patient education is important in RP management. The whole body should be kept as warm as possible. This includes wearing several layers of loose fitting clothing, mittens, stockings, and headwear in cold temperatures. RP attacks are likely to be precipitated by damp windy weather or rapid shifts in ambient temperature. Even in the summer months, air-conditioning may trigger a RP attack. Emotional stress can aggravate RP and lower the threshold for temperature-induced attacks. Therefore, stress control and relaxation techniques are helpful in preventing RP attacks.

Vasoconstrictor medications such as sympathomimetic drugs (decongestants, diet pills, ephedra) and serotonin agonists (such as sumatriptan) should be avoided because they can vasoconstrict peripheral arteries and precipitate RP attacks. In addition, certain chemotherapeutic agents (bleomycin, cisplatin, carboplatin, and vinblastine) may cause vascular occlusion and RP attacks. RP patients should be counseled on smoking avoidance because nicotine reduces cutaneous and digital blood flow. Opioids can also cause cutaneous vessel vasoconstriction and should be used with caution.

B. Medications

If nonpharmacologic treatments are not successful, medications are indicated for the treatment of RP. Vasodilator therapy is the usual first-line medication therapy, particularly if digital ulcerations have developed or quality of life is affected. Calcium channel blockers are the most widely used vasodilators; however, other agents including sympatholytic agents, phosphodiesterase inhibitors, and prostaglandins are also therapeutic options. No medication has proved to be more effective or safer than the calcium channel blockers.

1. Calcium channel blockers—Calcium channel blockers are the most frequently used therapy for primary and secondary RP. They have been shown to decrease both the frequency and severity of attacks. The benefit is more robust in patients with primary RP compared to those with secondary RP. The use of calcium channel blockers appears to reduce the frequency of RP by up to five attacks per week.

Calcium channel blockers differ in their peripheral vasodilatory properties. Nifedipine, amlodipine, felodipine, nisoldipine, and isradipine have more vasodilatory effect than diltiazem and verapamil in the treatment of RP. The most significant side effects from calcium channel blockers are headache, hypotension, tachycardia, aggravation of gastroesophageal reflux, and lower extremity edema. Gum hypertrophy may also occur with long-term use of calcium channel blockers.

Slow-release preparations of calcium channel blockers are preferred because they are safer than rapid-release preparations. Oral amlodipine at doses of 5–20 mg/d is effective in RP and exerts less negative cardiac inotropy. If one calcium channel blocker is not effective, patients may be switched to another; individual responses to medications may vary. Combination therapy with calcium channel blockers and other vasodilators are often used, but this approach has not been studied rigorously.

2. Direct vasodilators—Nitroglycerin ointment is frequently used alone or in combination with other vasodilator therapy. Improvement in RP has been noted with topical nitroglycerin with 0.25–0.5 inch of 2% nitroglycerin ointment applied daily. The medication is absorbed systemically and patients often have side effects of headaches or hypotension. One can attempt to avoid the systemic effect by placing very small amounts of the ointment directly on the fingers of affected hands.

3. Autonomic nervous system blockade—The sympathetic nervous system is important in cutaneous blood vessel thermoregulation and mediates vasoconstriction, particularly α_{2c}-adrenergic receptors on the digital arteries. In severe RP, another treatment option is to block sympathetic tone with the goal of inducing vasodilatation of digital vessels. In the absence of α_{2c}-adrenergic receptor antagonist, prazosin, an α_1-adrenergic receptor blocker, is used. In two controlled trials, prazosin was more effective than placebo in primary and secondary RP. However, patients became resistant to prazosin after prolonged use. Intravascular administration of sympatholytic agents has been advocated for treatment of refractory ischemia in RP; however, there is little clinical data demonstrating benefit.

4. Prostaglandins—Prostacyclin is a potent vasodilator with inhibitory effects on platelet aggregation and antiproliferative properties on smooth muscle cells. Iloprost, a prostacyclin analogue, is beneficial in the treatment of RP secondary to scleroderma. Therapy with iloprost (0.5–2 ng/kg/min intravenous infusion for 5 days) can provide relief for several weeks with significant improvement on number and duration of vasospastic RP attacks. However, in the United States, iloprost is only available as an inhaled medication for the treatment of pulmonary hypertension. Epoprostenol and alprostadil have also been reported as helpful for severe RP and digital ulcerations secondary to scleroderma. The oral form of these agents has poor bioavailability. Thus, intravenous administration is required.

5. Phosphodiesterase inhibitors—Phosphodiesterases are enzymes that regulate intracellular cyclic nucleotide levels such as cyclic adenosine monophosphate (cAMP) and cyclic guanosine monophosphate (cGMP). In turn, these cyclic nucleotides mediate intracellular responses to prostacyclin and nitrous oxide. Selective phosphodiesterase type 5 inhibitors (eg, sildenafil, tadalafil, vardenafil) have been successfully used for the treatment of erectile dysfunction and pulmonary hypertension. Sildenafil has been reported to reduce the severity and number of RP attacks in patients with SSc. Tadalafil has also shown variable success in the treatment of RP. However, these studies with phosphodiesterase type 5 inhibitors are limited and demonstrate varied responses. Therefore, the benefit of these agents has yet to be proven, and they should not be used if the patient is taking nitrates.

6. Rho-kinase inhibition—Rho-kinases are implicated in cold-induced vasoconstriction by inducing α_{2c}-adrenoreceptors on smooth muscle cells of blood vessels. While agents that block this pathway in theory could be helpful, they are not yet tested or available.

7. Angiotensin-converting enzyme (ACE) inhibitors—Although controversial, some studies suggest that ACE inhibitors may be helpful in RP by increasing blood flow through increased kinin release. Captopril, a traditional ACE inhibitor, improved RP attacks in primary RP, but not RP secondary to SSc. A recent 3-year study of quinapril, however, did not demonstrate any benefit compared to placebo, strongly suggesting that ACE inhibitors are not useful for the treatment of RP. However, losartan, an angiotensin II receptor blocker, decreased the number and severity of RP attacks in both primary and secondary RP.

8. Selective serotonin reuptake inhibitors—Serotonin is a potent circulating vasoconstrictor. Its role in RP is not clearly defined; however, several reports have noted improvement in RP in patients treated with selective serotonin reuptake inhibitors. While the evidence is still preliminary, the use of selective serotonin reuptake inhibitors can be considered in complex cases, particularly if the patient's baseline blood pressure is low.

9. Anticoagulation—Anticoagulation therapy with aspirin (81 mg/d) is recommended in selected patients with severe secondary RP who are at risk for digital ulceration or larger-artery thrombotic events. Heparin may be used during an acute ischemic crisis to prevent further digital vessel thrombosis, but long-term anticoagulation with heparin or warfarin is not recommended unless there is evidence of a hypercoagulable disorder (eg, antiphospholipid syndrome, malignancy).

C. Surgical

Surgical sympathectomy may be used to ligate the sympathetic nerves that cause vasoconstriction. A chemical sympathectomy with a digital or wrist block using lidocaine or bupivacaine without epinephrine can rapidly reverse digital artery vasospasm. The risk of cervical sympathectomy, including neuralgia, decreased localized sweating, and Horner syndrome, is reduced by new scope-directed procedures. No controlled studies of surgical sympathectomy versus a control procedure exist and benefit of the procedure may be short-lived.

Botulinium toxin type A has also been shown to be effective in a small study of five patients with RP. There was a trend toward faster rewarming of the digits following cold provocation, but little change in final temperature after 20 minutes.

Case reports of a localized procedure of digital sympathectomy for RP demonstrate success. Among SSc patients, the complication rate is about 37% and amputation and recurrent ulceration still occurs during follow-up in up to 18% of patients. Sympathectomy can be very helpful in an acute digital ischemic crisis and it is best reserved for patients who have not responded to medical therapy and continue to have severe RP or ischemia threatening the digits. Most of the available evidence shows that RP attacks recur, often less severe, several weeks to months following either proximal or digital sympathectomy.

Complications

RP can vary from a mild inconvenience to recurrent ischemia and digital ulceration. Primary RP is not associated with critical ischemia or tissue ulcerations, but cold sensitivity, digital numbness, and discomfort can alter hand function. Emotional problems can occur from the social stigma of cold hands with unsightly skin color changes, especially in the adolescent population.

Digital tissue ischemia may occur in patients with secondary RP, leading to recurrent digital ulcerations, rapid deep tissue necrosis, and amputation. These patients, unlike patients with primary RP, have structurally abnormal digital vessels or disruption of the normal neurologic, hormonal, or rheologic regulation of regional blood flow. Pain so severe that the patient seeks medical attention or is positioning the hand downward to improve blood flow indicates critical ischemia and possible impending ulceration. This should be considered a medical emergency and hospitalization is indicated. Patients should be kept as warm as possible and at rest. Vasodilator therapy with a short-acting calcium channel blocker (eg, nifedipine 10–20 mg orally every 8 hours) should be started in combination with aspirin. If ischemia continues, a combination of vasodilators (eg, a calcium channel blocker plus a nitrate [topical nitrogylcerin], or in those not responding to oral agents, an intravenous vasodilator such as prostaglandin infusion [eg, epoprostenol]) may be used. A temporary chemical digital sympathectomy (eg, xylocaine) may rapidly reverse vasospasm if severe structural disease or vascular occlusion has not occurred. Anticoagulation (intravenous heparin or enoxaparin) for 48–72 hours should be considered if acute macrovascular occlusion disease is occurring. Long-term anticoagulation is not recommended unless a hypercoagulable state is discovered.

Surgical digital sympathectomy may be considered if ischemia persists despite vasodilator therapy.

Macrovascular disease may complicate the situation and present a surgically correctable lesion. Other complicating factors, such as a hypercoagulable disorder, embolic disease, or underlying vasculitis, need to be considered and treated if present. Early intervention with hospitalization and vasodilator therapy is the key to preventing irreversible vessel occlusion and breaking the cycle of vasospasm and digital ischemia.

Digital ulcerations from recurrent tissue ischemia may develop in patients who have secondary RP. These ulcers should be kept as clean as possible with soap and water and appropriate protective dressing in order to avoid infection. Topical or systemic antibiotics are used if an infection develops.

When to Refer

Patients with primary RP may be treated effectively by the primary care provider. Initial care is focused on preventive measures such as warm clothing and lessening emotional stress in order to avoid RP attacks. Patients with secondary RP due to a connective tissue disease or RP from an unknown cause should be referred to a specialist for further management. Any patient with critical digital ischemia should be referred for hospitalization for immediate management. A vascular surgeon should be consulted early in the hospitalization for chemical or surgical digital sympathectomy or vascular repair if the ischemia is unresponsive to oral or intravenous vasodilators.

Arthritis Foundation
    http://www.arthritis.org
Huisstede BM, Hoogvliet P, Paulis WD, et al. Effectiveness of interventions for secondary Raynaud's phenomenon: a systematic review. *Arch Phys Med Rehabil.* 2011;92(7):1166. [PMID: 21704799]
Scleroderma Foundation
    http://www.scleroderma.org
Scleroderma Research Foundation
    http://www.srfcure.org
Shenoy PD, Kumar S, Jha, LK, et al. Efficacy of tadalafil in secondary Raynaud's phenomenon resistant to vasodilator therapy: a double-blind randomized cross-over trial. *Rheumatology (Oxford).* 2010;49(12):2420. [PMID: 20837499]

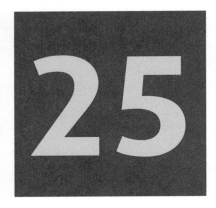

Scleroderma

Laura K. Hummers, MD
Fredrick M. Wigley, MD

ESSENTIALS OF DIAGNOSIS

▶ The most frequent symptoms are (in descending order) Raynaud phenomenon, gastroesophageal reflux with or without dysmotility, skin changes, swollen fingers, and arthralgias.

▶ Patients with Raynaud phenomenon and features atypical for primary Raynaud phenomenon should be evaluated for the possibility of scleroderma or another connective tissue disease.

▶ A negative antinuclear antibody test (by indirect immunofluorescence) makes the diagnosis of scleroderma very unlikely.

▶ The degree of skin involvement is highly variable. Many patients with limited scleroderma have only subtle cutaneous findings (eg, mild sclerodactyly).

▶ The current classification criteria do not include many patients with milder forms of scleroderma.

▶ Some patients may have overlapping clinical features with other systemic autoimmune rheumatic disorders such as polymyositis/dermatomyositis, Sjögren syndrome, systemic lupus erythematosus, and rheumatoid arthritis.

▶ General Considerations

Systemic sclerosis (scleroderma) is a chronic multisystem disease that belongs to the family of systemic autoimmune disorders. The word scleroderma literally means "hard skin" and describes the most dramatic clinical feature of the disease—namely, skin fibrosis. Scleroderma effects approximately 20 new patients per million per year and has an estimated prevalence of approximately 250 patients per million in the United States. As with many other autoimmune disorders, scleroderma is approximately 4–5 times more common in women than men. The average age at the time of diagnosis is approximately 50 years.

The prevalence and manifestations of scleroderma vary among racial and ethnic groups. For example, the disease is approximately 100 times more common among the Choctaw Native Americans in Oklahoma, in whom the disease is characterized by diffuse skin disease and pulmonary fibrosis. Milder, "limited" disease is more common among older white women, and African American patients are more likely to be younger and have severe lung disease. The finding of various subtypes of scleroderma among different ethnic or racial groups, the presence of familial clustering, and the appearance of specific autoantibodies that are associated with specific HLA types define genetic influences on disease expression. New genetic studies examining both candidate gene approaches and genome-wide association studies confirm genetic influence in disease susceptibility. Certain environmental factors are also thought to play etiologic roles. For example, characteristic antibodies and scleroderma disease manifestations can develop in workers exposed to high levels of silica dust (ie, coal miners, stone masons).

▶ Clinical Findings

Scleroderma is a rare disorder but is characterized by symptoms that occur frequently in the general population, such as Raynaud phenomenon, gastroesophageal reflux, fatigue, and musculoskeletal pain. Therefore, it is important for primary care practitioners to be aware of scleroderma because early recognition can reduce morbidity and detect treatable, life-threatening complications.

The American College of Rheumatology classification criteria for scleroderma include either thickened (sclerodermatous) skin changes proximal to the metacarpophalangeal joints or at least two of the following:

1. Sclerodactyly.
2. Digital pitting (loss of tissue on the finger pads due to ischemia).
3. Bibasilar pulmonary fibrosis.

A diagnosis of scleroderma may also be made if the patient has three or more features of the CREST (calcinosis, Raynaud phenomenon, esophageal dysmotility, sclerodactyly, telangiectasia) syndrome, although the term "limited scleroderma" is now preferred for this clinical subtype. Patients with definite Raynaud phenomenon who have abnormal nailfold capillary loops or the presence of autoantibodies known to be associated with scleroderma (see Laboratory Findings and Table 25–1) may be considered to have early scleroderma or a mild expression of the disease.

Although skin changes are usually the major diagnostic clue, scleroderma is a systemic disease that most commonly targets the peripheral circulation, muscles, joints, gastrointestinal tract, lung, heart, and kidney. Symptoms encountered in the early presentation of scleroderma include musculoskeletal discomfort, fatigue, weight loss, and heartburn associated with gastroesophageal reflux disease (GERD). When these symptoms are accompanied by the new onset of cold sensitivity or Raynaud phenomenon, then scleroderma should be considered and further diagnostic investigation is warranted.

A. Symptoms and Signs

1. Skin—Thickening of the skin is the most easily recognizable manifestation of scleroderma but is not prominent in all patients. Patients with scleroderma are typically classified based on the amount and location of skin involvement. Patients with "limited" cutaneous disease have skin

Table 25–1. Classic presentations of patients with limited and diffuse scleroderma.

Type of Scleroderma	Presentation
Limited	Long history of Raynaud phenomenon Gastroesophageal reflux and dysphagia Swelling or skin thickening of the fingers Infrequent systemic symptoms, such as arthralgias, weight loss, dyspnea
Diffuse	New onset of Raynaud phenomenon Rapid change in skin texture with new onset of edema, pruritus, pain Significant systemic symptoms with severe arthralgias, weight loss, tendon friction rubs Early evidence of internal organ involvement such as dyspnea, hypertension

changes on the face and distal to the knees and elbows. One subset of limited scleroderma, previously called the CREST syndrome, typically only involves the skin of the fingers (sclerodactyly) distal to the metacarpophalangeal joints (Plate 40). In contrast, diffuse scleroderma refers to the group of patients with proximal extremity or truncal skin thickening. The amount of skin thickening can be quantified by performing a "skin score," in which the skin is pinched between the examiner's thumbs in 17 specified areas of the patient's body, scoring the thickness of the skin from 0 (normal) to 3 (very thick). The skin score provides a systematic approach to longitudinal disease evaluations and is commonly used in clinical trials to assess treatment efficacy. This score, however, has limitations, including (1) high inter-observer variability, (2) not scoring the quality of the skin or level of disease activity, (3) and lacking sensitivity to change over short periods of time. However, epidemiologic studies indicate that higher skin scores and changes in skin scores correlate with greater degrees of internal organ involvement and worse overall prognosis.

Early in the course of diffuse scleroderma, the skin appears edematous and inflamed with erythema and pigmentary changes, and swelling in the fingers and hand may be confused with early rheumatoid arthritis. Hyperpigmented areas alternating with vitiligo-like areas of depigmentation impart to the skin a "salt and pepper" appearance. Diffuse hyperpigmentation develops in some patients, making them appear tanned. This early inflammatory phase is associated with pruritus and discomfort that usually lasts for weeks to months. In vitro studies show that dermal fibroblasts derived from patients with scleroderma overproduce extracellular matrix that leads to increased tissue collagen deposition in the skin. Collagen cross-linking then causes progressive skin tightening. In the later stages of the disease, the involved skin becomes atrophic, dry, and scaly because of sebaceous gland damage. These dry thickened areas of skin may be intensely pruritic, causing the patient to excoriate the skin, which leads to more damage and thickening (lichenification). Skin uclers can form over areas of joint contractures and local trauma. Digital ischemic ulcers form on the distal fingers in 30–50% of patients (Plate 41). Pitted areas on the distal finger and loss of digital pad is common, while a picture of pseudo-clubbing is a less common manifestation of underlying osteolysis due to microvascular disease. Patients often have other prominent skin changes, including marked telangiectasias (dilated capillaries) that occur on the skin of the face, the palmar surface of the hands (Plate 42), and the mucous membranes. Telangiectasias tend to be more numerous in those patients with other scleroderma related vascular disease (ie, pulmonary arterial hypertension). Telangiectasia increase in numbers and location with a longer disease duration. A small proportion of patients have subcutaneous calcinosis, primarily on the fingers and along the extensor surfaces of the forearms.

2. Vascular disease—Involvement of the vasculature is ubiquitous among patients with scleroderma. A widespread obliterative vasculopathy of peripheral arteries and the microcirculation is manifested pathologically by intimal thickening with marked luminal narrowing and evidence of local thrombi. Endothelial cell injury leads to abnormal vascular reactivity and altered tissue perfusion. Critical ischemia occurs in the tissues when vasoconstriction occludes these diseased vessels. Evidence suggests that this vascular disease is fundamental to organ damage and subsequent malfunction of the heart (cardiomyopathy), lung (pulmonary hypertension), kidney (scleroderma renal crisis [SRC]), and other organs in scleroderma (see below).

Raynaud phenomenon is the first manifestation of the disease in almost every patient. It tends to develop concurrently with other symptoms in those with diffuse disease and typically precedes other symptoms by years in those with limited skin disease. Stress and cold temperature induce an exaggerated vasoconstriction of the small arteries, arterioles, and arteriovenous shunts or thermoregulatory vessels of the skin of the digits. This is manifested clinically as pallor and cyanosis of the digits, followed by a reactive hyperemia after rewarming. Unlike episodes of uncomplicated primary Raynaud phenomenon, attacks of Raynaud phenomenon in patients with scleroderma are often painful and frequently lead to digital ulcerations, gangrene, or amputation.

Clinical features found to be predictive of an autoimmune rheumatic disease among patients with Raynaud phenomenon include the presence of antinuclear antibodies (ANA) and abnormal nailfold capillaries (see Special Examinations below). Patients over the age of 30 who develop new onset Raynaud phenomenon should be screened with an ANA test and nailfold capillary examination, particularly if they have severe, painful episodes of vasospasm, signs of digital ischemia or tissue damage, or any other systemic signs or symptoms of a secondary disease. Although patients with scleroderma almost always have a positive ANA, it is important to remember that the presence of a positive ANA does not, by itself, make the diagnosis of a connective tissue disorder (see Laboratory Findings below).

3. Lung involvement—Two main forms of lung disease occur in patients with scleroderma: inflammatory alveolitis leading to interstitial fibrosis and pulmonary vascular disease leading to pulmonary arterial hypertension (see Chapters 63 and 64). These two processes can occur independently or concomitantly. Active interstitial lung disease occurs typically in patients with early diffuse scleroderma in the first 4 years of illness, whereas pulmonary hypertension more commonly affects those with long-standing disease. Lung involvement (both types) usually presents as dyspnea on exertion but can be asymptomatic early in the course of the lung disease. Therefore, routine screening tests for lung disease (complete pulmonary function testing [PFTs] and echocardiograms) are important because early intervention may prevent progression. In the case of interstitial fibrosis, physical examination reveals fine crackles at the lung bases.

This finding, however, may not be present in early disease and its presence may indicate stable fibrosis and is not necessarily a sign of active disease. PFTs or high-resolution computed tomography (CT) scanning can detect very mild and early disease and are better indicators of disease activity (ie, change in forced vital capacity [FVC] over a short interval or ground glass opacities or fibrosis on CT). Approximately 80% of patients with scleroderma have restrictive ventilatory defects on PFTs, consistent with interstitial lung disease. However, only about 10–20% of these patients suffer from progressive severe interstitial lung disease. Predictors for progression of interstitial lung disease are the presence of diffuse skin disease, African American race, early decline in FVC, fibrosis on CT scan, and the presence of antitopoisomerase antibodies.

Pulmonary vascular disease with or without fibrosis can lead to pulmonary arterial hypertension and ultimately right heart failure. Estimates of the prevalence of pulmonary arterial hypertension among patients with scleroderma vary, but may be as high as 25%, although severe disease is only seen in roughly 10–15%. Typically, patients with isolated pulmonary arterial hypertension seek medical care complaining of dyspnea on exertion; however, signs of progressive, life-threatening right heart failure develop rapidly in later stages. Physical examination in these patients reveals systolic murmurs (from tricuspid regurgitation), a prominent P2 component of S2, right ventricular heaves, hepatomegaly and lower extremity edema.

4. Gastrointestinal involvement—Gastrointestinal disease in scleroderma usually involves both the upper and lower gastrointestinal tract but is highly variable in its clinical expression. Patients with measurable gastrointestinal involvement can be relatively asymptomatic (eg, mild constipation). Alternatively, they may have profound gastrointestinal tract dysfunction, with malnutrition and significant morbidity. The majority of patients with scleroderma have symptomatic GERD with dysphagia. Complaints include a sensation of food getting stuck in the mid or lower esophagus, atypical chest pain, or cough. Patients often complain that they must drink liquids to swallow solid food, particularly dry food such as meat or bread. Reflux and dysphagia occur because of dysmotility of the esophagus and stomach (gastroparesis). This type of organ dysfunction results from abnormal motility caused by atrophy of the gastrointestinal tract wall smooth muscle that occurs with or without pathologic evidence of significant tissue fibrosis or obvious vascular insult to the bowel. If GERD is left untreated, the upper gastrointestinal disease can cause esophagitis, esophageal ulceration with bleeding, esophageal stricture, or Barrett esophagus. Bleeding can also occur secondary to mucosal A-V malformations or telangiectasia in the wall of the stomach (gastric antral vascular ectasia or GAVE).

The small and large intestines can also be affected by smooth muscle atrophy of the bowel wall causing abnormal motility of the gut. The most common symptom is the combination of constipation alternating with diarrhea and patients frequently give a history compatible with irritable bowel syndrome. Severe disease causes recurrent bouts of pseudo-obstruction, bowel distention with leakage of air into the bowel wall (pneumatosis coli intestinalis), and even bowel rupture. Lower bowel dysmotility slows the movement of bowel contents severely, allowing bacterial overgrowth, diarrhea, and malabsorption. Fecal incontinence develops in a small subset of patients.

5. Renal involvement—Clinically important kidney disease occurs in only a minority of patients, but when it develops, renal disease poses a major threat to life. SRC develops in approximately 5% of patients. It is characterized by the sudden onset of malignant hypertension that, if untreated, can lead rapidly to renal failure and death. Prior to the discovery that angiotensin-converting enzyme (ACE) inhibitors can control hypertensive crises in scleroderma effectively, SRC was the leading cause of death. Despite the dramatic benefit of ACE inhibitors, significant morbidity or renal dysfunction can result from SRC. Patients in the early stages of diffuse scleroderma, particularly those treated with glucocorticoids and those who produce antibodies to RNA-polymerase III are at the greatest risk for SRC. Patients in whom SRC develops may have symptoms associated with the acute onset of severe hypertension, including headache, visual changes, or seizures. Some, however, are asymptomatic and have undetected hypertension and an abrupt rise in creatinine; therefore, patients at high risk (those with early, active diffuse skin involvement) must have their blood pressure monitored frequently. Renal biopsy specimens reveal changes similar to malignant hypertension, thrombotic thrombocytopenic purpura/hemolytic uremic syndrome, and eclampsia. There is intimal hyperplasia and vasospasm of cortical arteries. This leads to activation of the renin-angiotensin system and accelerated hypertension, proteinuria, microscopic hematuria, and thrombotic microangiopathy (schistocytes on peripheral blood smear).

6. Cardiac involvement—Cardiac involvement in scleroderma can frequently be demonstrated by objective testing (eg, echocardiography, thallium scan, or electrocardiogram) but is usually subclinical in the early stages of disease. Cardiovascular morbidity is seen primarily in the late stages of diffuse scleroderma. Ischemia-reperfusion injury secondary to small arterial disease of the myocardium leads to contraction band necrosis and tissue fibrosis. This process can result in arrhythmias, a cardiomyopathy with diastolic dysfunction, or overt symptoms of heart failure. Although pericardial effusions are frequently detected by echocardiography, they are usually clinically silent. Large pericardial effusions are associated with pulmonary arterial hypertension and confer a poor prognosis. Symptoms from scleroderma cardiac disease include chest pain from pericarditis, palpitations from arrhythmias, or dyspnea on exertion from heart failure.

7. Musculoskeletal involvement—Musculoskeletal symptoms range from mild arthralgias to frank erosive arthritis with synovitis resembling rheumatoid arthritis. The sclerosis of the skin of the fingers or limbs is often associated with contractures of the joints. Deeper tissue fibrosis can also involve the fascia and underlying muscle. If areas around the tendons are involved, active and passive range of motion of the joints are limited and painful. The physician can appreciate this on examination by feeling a "tendon friction rub" when placing the hand over the tendons as the patient flexes and extends the joint. Tendon friction rubs are found most commonly around the ankles, wrists, or knees in those patients with early diffuse scleroderma. The presence of tendon friction rubs is associated with disease activity and poor overall outcome.

Muscle weakness is a common complaint with a variety of causes including pain, prolonged muscle disuse, malnutrition, and a slowly progressive dysfunction of striated muscle that may be due to local fibrosis or a necrotizing myopathy. A true inflammatory myopathy is seen in a small subset of patients. Patients with "overlap" phenotypes who have scleroderma features (eg, Raynaud phenomenon, interstitial lung disease, and sclerodactyly) and a true inflammatory polyarthritis or polymyositis may be categorized as having mixed connective tissue disease (MCTD) that is associated with the presence of high-titer anti-U1-RNP antibodies.

8. Other symptoms—Sicca complex (dry eyes and dry mouth) are common in patients with scleroderma but are usually not as severe as in patients with primary Sjögren syndrome (see Chapter 26). Decreased saliva production, small oral aperature and gum recession leads to complex dental disease with risk for tooth loss. Pain is very common and usually is associated with digital ulcers, fibrosis of tendons, joint contractures, or musculoskeletal disease. Rarely, neuropathic pain is present secondary to carpal tunnel syndrome or trigeminal neuralgia. Studies suggest an unrecognized increase of neurosensory hearing loss, hypothyroidism, and osteolysis of bone among patients with scleroderma. Depression is frequent among patients with scleroderma but does not correlate directly with disease severity. Depression more likely reflects other factors such as degree of pain, personality traits, and lack of good social support systems.

Erectile dysfunction is very common among men with scleroderma and is often not detected or properly managed. Sexual dysfunction among women is also common; symptoms include vaginal dryness and dyspareunia secondary to a narrowed, fibrotic introitus. While infertility is not a manifestation of scleroderma, there is thought to be an increased risk for small gestational age newborns, pre-term delivery and, possibly, hypertension.

B. Laboratory Findings

There is no single laboratory study or test that confirms the diagnosis of scleroderma. The diagnosis is made by obtaining a careful history and performing a physical examination. However, autoantibodies are found in nearly every patient with scleroderma (sensitivity >95%) when performed by indirect immunofluorescence (ANAs performed by enzyme-linked immunosorbent assay may miss relevant scleroderma-associated autoantibodies). ANAs are the most frequently detected, but they are not specific for scleroderma. ANAs can be detected in other connective tissue diseases, other diseases associated with autoimmunity (eg, Hashimoto thyroiditis), chronic infections (such as hepatitis C), and up to 10% of healthy individuals (at low titers). Anticentromere antibodies are detected in approximately 20–40% of patients with scleroderma and are associated specifically with limited skin involvement and more severe digital ischemia and pulmonary arterial hypertension. Anticentromere antibodies are not specific to scleroderma and can also be found in patients with primary biliary cirrhosis and Sjögren syndrome. Antitopoisomerase I (anti-Scl-70) antibodies are also found in 20–40% of patients with scleroderma. Patients with antitopoisomerase I antibodies typically have diffuse skin changes, interstitial lung disease, and an overall worse prognosis. Antitopoisomerase I antibodies are highly specific for scleroderma. Antibodies to RNA polymerases I/III are associated with rapidly progressive diffuse skin changes and a much higher risk of renal involvement but lower risk for interstitial lung disease compared with those with Scl-70 antibodies. Antibodies to other nucleolar proteins are found in a small percentage of scleroderma patients, but assays for these are generally not commercially available (Th/To, Nor-90, Fibrillarin, Pm-Scl, B23). The more common scleroderma-associated autoantibodies are outlined in Table 25–2.

Table 25–2. Autoantibodies associated with scleroderma.

Autoantibody	Prevalence	Associated Clinical Features
Antinuclear antibody	>95%	–
Anti-Scl-70 (Antitopoisomerase I)	20–40%	Lung disease, diffuse skin involvement, African Americans, worse prognosis
Anticentromere	20–40%	CREST syndrome, digital ulcerations/digital loss
Anti-RNA polymerases	4–20%	Rapidly progressive diffuse skin involvement, scleroderma renal crisis, cardiac disease, lower risk for pulmonary fibrosis
Anti-Pm-Scl	2–10%	Limited cutaneous involvement, myositis
Anti-U3RNP (anti-fibrillarin)	8%	Lung disease, diffuse skin involvement, African American males
Anti-U1RNP	5%	Mixed connective tissue disease
Anti-Th/To	1–5%	Limited cutaneous involvement, pulmonary disease

CREST, calcinosis, Raynaud phenomenon, esophageal dysmotility, sclerodactyly, and telangiectasias.

C. Imaging Studies

Chest films are an insensitive method to diagnose scleroderma lung disease. High-resolution CT scans of the chest have an increased sensitivity and may provide some insight into disease activity and severity (eg, fibrosis or ground glass opacities). Radiographic testing for evaluation of upper gastrointestinal disease is not often required unless patients have atypical symptoms or do not respond to standard treatments. A cine esophagram, however, typically shows a dilated esophagus, lower esophageal dysmotility, and gastroesophageal reflux.

D. Special Tests

The use of specialized diagnostic testing depends on the organ system to be investigated. Every patient with scleroderma should be screened routinely at baseline and monitored for the development of pulmonary and cardiac disease. Patients should have PFTs (eg, spirometry, lung volumes, and diffusing capacity [DLCO]) performed at baseline and then every 4–12 months depending on symptoms and disease stage. PFTs provide the most sensitive measure for the development of interstitial lung disease, typically revealing a restrictive pattern with or without a reduction in diffusing capacity. PFTs can also suggest the presence of pulmonary arterial hypertension by the finding of an isolated reduction in DLCO or a reduction out of proportion to the degree of the decline in FVC. New studies suggest that changes in DLCO and elevations in natriuretic peptides may predict future development of pulmonary hypertension. The degree of pulmonary arterial hypertension can be estimated on a two-dimensional echocardiogram by measuring the right ventricular systolic pressure. Definitive diagnosis of pulmonary arterial hypertension can only be made with right heart catheterization documenting a mean pulmonary artery pressure of ≥25 mm Hg with a normal wedge pressure. Studies of the upper gastrointestinal tract are often unnecessary in a patient with scleroderma who has symptomatic gastroesophageal reflux alone. Patients with atypical symptoms, poor responses to proton pump inhibitors, or long-standing untreated symptoms warrant further studies such as a barium swallow or upper gastrointestinal endoscopy. The barium swallow is relatively insensitive to measure motility problems but is useful for the exclusion of other potentially treatable causes of dysphagia, such as a stricture. Any patient with long-standing reflux should be referred for endoscopy to evaluate for the complications of GERD, including Barrett esophagus.

E. Special Examinations

The capillaries of the skin can be visualized at the nailfold by using simple tools available in a typical examination room, thus giving insight into a patient's microvasculature. Nailfold capillary dropout and dilated capillary loops are seen in nearly every patient with scleroderma but are not specific for scleroderma because nailfold changes can also be seen in other connective tissue diseases (such as dermatomyositis and MCTD). To examine the nailfold capillaries, a drop of high resolve microscope immersion oil is placed on the nail bed and ideally viewed under a bifocal microscope. A bedside examination can be done using an ophthalmoscope, set at minus 20–40 diopters (40 green) to visualize the capillaries. Normally, the nailfold capillaries should be thin, linear, and uniform. In patients with scleroderma, these capillaries become dilated and areas of vessel dropout are apparent. Studies suggest that nailfold changes are dynamic and progressive changes correlate with systemic disease.

▶ Differential Diagnosis

Given the multisystem nature of systemic sclerosis, the differential diagnosis is broad. Scleroderma is a rare disease but a protean one. Often, the diagnosis only becomes obvious after several evaluations over time.

Patients with symptoms compatible with early scleroderma are encountered frequently in the primary care office. For this reason, primary care providers should be aware of this potentially life-threatening disease and be able to distinguish it from other disorders with similar features so that appropriate referrals can be made. The differential diagnosis includes other disorders that are associated with Raynaud phenomenon; those with similar skin changes; and those with other components of systemic autoimmune rheumatic diseases, such as arthralgias and positive autoantibodies (Table 25–3).

▶ Scleroderma Mimics

There are several diseases that are rare but have substantial overlapping features with systemic sclerosis and should be considered strongly in the differential diagnosis of a patient with thickened skin (Table 25–4).

A. Scleredema

1. Presentation—Scleredema is an uncommon cause of thickened skin that occurs in three distinct patient populations: poorly controlled type 1 or 2 diabetes mellitus, in association with monoclonal gammopathies, or as a postinfectious complication (classically streptococcal pharyngitis). The skin in scleredema can be somewhat similar in texture and appearance to scleroderma, but the pattern of skin involvement is distinct, which almost always begins in the upper back and more often involves proximal extremities and the midportion of the back (an area that is distinctly spared in scleroderma). The texture of the skin is indurated but typically slightly more mobile than in scleroderma. There are no clear internal organ complications of scleredema and autoantibodies should be absent.

Table 25–3. Differential diagnosis of scleroderma.

Clinical Feature	Differential Diagnosis

Raynaud phenomenon	Primary Raynaud phenomenon
	Systemic lupus erythematosus
	Vibration-Hand syndrome
	Medication-induced
	    Chemotherapy (cisplatin,
	        bleomycin, etc)
	    Sympathomimetics
	Thoracic outlet syndrome
	Cryoglobulinemia/cryofibrinogenemia/
	    cold agglutins
	Systemic vasculitis
	Chilblains

Skin thickening	Scleredema Scleromyxedema Eosinophilic fasciitis Eosinophilia-myalgia syndrome Localized scleroderma/morphea Nephrogenic fibrosing dermopathy Diabetic cheiroarthropathy POEMS syndrome Graft-versus-host disease
Overlapping clinical features	Systemic lupus erythematosus Sjögren syndrome Inflammatory myopathies Rheumatoid arthritis

POEMS, polyneuropathy, organomegaly, endocrinopathy, monoclonal gammopathy, and skin changes.

2. Management—Scleredema is notoriously treatment resistant, but there are cases of good response to a variety of treatments. Occasionally, it may respond to UVA-based treatment regimens (PUVA, UVA-1).

B. Nephrogenic Fibrosing Dermopathy/ Nephrogenic Systemic Fibrosis

1. Presentation—Nephrogenic fibrosing dermopathy/ nephrogenic systemic fibrosis is a nodular or plaque-like thickening of the skin associated with exposure to gadolinium-containing contrast materials in the setting of moderate to severe renal insufficiency. Typically, this is accompanied by a rapid progression of large joint contractures. The lesions are more commonly found on the extremities and form coalescing brawny plaques of induration and thickening. Fingers and face are usually spared. The presence of systemic manifestations is debated but may include muscle and cardiopulmonary involvement. Raynaud phenomenon and autoantibody production should be absent.

2. Management—Nephrogenic fibrosing dermopathy is notoriously treatment resistant. Imatinib has been used in some patients, with mixed success.

Table 25–4. Distinguishing features of scleroderma and its mimics.

	Distribution of Skin Changes	Skin Quality	Systemic Features	Laboratory Features/ Clinical Associations
Scleroderma	Hands and face common Mid-back spared Changes progress from distal to proximal on extremities	Thick, smooth, shiny induration	Raynaud phenomenon with ulcerations Gastroesophageal reflux, dysphagia Interstitial lung disease	Positive ANA Scleroderma specific autoantibodies Restriction on pulmonary function testing
Scleromyxedema	Scleroderma distribution Prominent findings around glabella, ears	Cobblestone induration with 2–3 mm waxy papules	Dysphagia Raynaud phenomenon Musculoskeletal pain Global CNS disturbances	Monoclonal gammopathy
Eosinophilic fasciitis	Extremities and trunk Hands and feet spared	Woody induration deeper than superficial dermis	Can overlap with plaque morphea	Peripheral eosinophilia Immune mediated cytopenias Hypergammaglobulinemia Elevated inflammatory markers
Nephrogenic fibrosing dermopathy	Extremities and trunk Face spared	Deep indurated plaques	Marked flexion contractures	Renal failure or insufficiency Exposure to gadolinium
Scleredema	Neck, upper back prominent Proximal upper > lower extremities	Doughy induration	Discomfort in areas of involvement	Poorly controlled diabetes Recent streptococcal infection Monoclonal gammopathy
Pansclerotic morphea	Extremities, face, feet Fingers and hands spared	Thick induration similar to that of diffuse scleroderma	Contractures No systemic features of scleroderma	

ANA, antinuclear antibodies; CNS, central nervous system.

C. Scleromyxedema

1. Presentation—Scleromyxedema is a very rare disorder of mucin deposition in the skin and internal organs that develops in the setting of a circulating monoclonal gammopathy. The distribution of skin disease may mimic scleroderma quite closely with fingers and face commonly involved but also commonly involves the mid-back, which is typically spared in scleroderma. Another distinction in distribution is the almost universal and prominent involvement of the glabella (the space between the eyebrows and above the nose) and the skin of the ears. Another distinguishing feature compared to scleroderma is the texture of the skin. Scleromyxedema is characterized by small flesh-colored papules that may coalesce and leads to a cobblestone texture of the skin. Systemic manifestations (including a myopathy, Raynaud phenomenon, pulmonary vascular disease, arthritis and, in rare cases, renal involvement) may also mimic scleroderma. In contrast to scleroderma, however, a major complication of scleromyxedema may be the presence of neurologic involvement, which occurs in about 10% of patients and includes seizures, global encephalopathy, and coma.

2. Management—Scleromyxedema has been successfully treated with a number of agents most notably intravenous immunoglobulin (IVIG) and thalidomide/thalidomide analogues.

D. Localized Scleroderma

1. Presentation—Typical plaque morphea is not often confused with systemic sclerosis, but some subtypes of localized scleroderma may have widespread skin involvement and may closely resemble diffuse scleroderma. In particular, pansclerotic morphea is a severe cutaneous variant of localized scleroderma with a distribution and texture that mimics scleroderma almost entirely but characteristically spares the fingers, hands, and face. These patients, however, should not have systemic manifestations including Raynaud phenomenon. The skin biopsy in these patients is virtually indistinguishable from the skin in systemic sclerosis but may have deeper fascial involvement and even an overlap with eosinophilic fasciitis.

2. Management—Localized forms of scleroderma may respond to UVA-based treatment regimens (PUVA, UVA-1).

E. Eosinophilic Fasciitis

1. Presentation—Eosinophilic fasciitis is distinguished from the other scleroderma mimics in that the involvement of tissue is deeper than the dermis and subcutis. This leads to a clear distinction in physical examination findings. The thickness is appreciated at a deeper level and is characteristically "woody" in nature. The skin overlying this induration is usually flexible and able to be pinched between the fingers. However, the inflammation occurring at the level of the fascia may lead to puckering of the skin as the subcutaneous and cutaneous tissue is tethered by the fascial involvement. This leads to the classic peau d'orange appearance of the skin and venous furrowing, most often notable in the upper arms when the shoulder is abducted to 90 degrees. Systemic features should be absent except for occasional occurrence of arthritis and Raynaud phenomenon. Laboratory investigation demonstrates eosinophilia in the majority but is not required for a diagnosis. There are often elevations of total immunoglobulins and other inflammatory markers. A full thickness biopsy, which includes the fascia to the level of the muscle, will distinguish this condition from other fibrosing skin disorders. MRI may be particularly useful in demonstrating fascial edema and in guiding biopsy location.

2. Management—Eosinophilic fasciitis often responds well to moderate doses of glucocorticoids, a treatment often avoided in scleroderma due to the increase in risk of renal crisis and lack of benefit.

▶ Treatment

A. General Principles

No single drug has been found to treat all of the manifestations of scleroderma, so no effective **disease-specific** therapy exists. Management, therefore, is based on the symptoms and disease manifestations of each individual patient and is often **organ-specific.** Recent therapeutic advances and improved screening tests have decreased the morbidity and mortality in scleroderma. For example, since the routine use of ACE inhibitors in the management of SRC, the incidence of end-stage renal disease and mortality from this once fatal complication has declined significantly.

Some important principles to keep in mind when treating patients with scleroderma follow:

- Each patient with scleroderma is unique with regard to disease features and prognosis (see below).
- No *proven* disease-modifying medication exists.
- Scleroderma skin disease tends to reach peak involvement over the first 18–24 months but then gradually improves with or without therapy.
- Routine screening and early intervention for internal organ manifestations may significantly reduce morbidity and mortality.

B. Fibrosis

Although the pathogenesis of fibrosis is understood better, this understanding has yet to translate into medications that treat cutaneous fibrosis effectively. Until new antifibrotic drugs are available, most experts believe that the immune process that triggers inflammation, tissue injury, and progressive fibrosis needs to be controlled rapidly. Once fibrosis is established, organ dysfunction may be irreversible. Therefore, various immunosuppressive agents are used early in the disease course of patients with diffuse skin involvement in an attempt to modify the course of skin fibrosis. Unfortunately, no convincing controlled trial using these agents is available to provide complete guidelines for their use. Agents that are currently used include glucocorticoids, methotrexate, mycophenolate mofetil, cyclophosphamide, antithymocyte globulin, and IVIG. The role of agents such as rituximab, tocilizumab, inhibitors of transforming growth factor beta, and tyrosine kinase inhibitors are under investigation. Each drug has unique toxicities and risks. Great care and expert guidance should be sought when prescribing these medications, since no one agent has proven effective and safe for overall disease control.

C. Vascular Disease

While the vascular insult is common to all patients with scleroderma, the clinical expression varies widely. Many patients have only mildly symptomatic Raynaud phenomenon, whereas others can have recurrent digital ulcerations that can progress to gangrene and digital loss. In addition, the scleroderma vasculopathy (intimal thickening and loss of lumen of arteries) is often a contributing factor in the internal organ involvement that is the major cause of morbidity and mortality. Episodes of critical ischemia are multifactorial and are a culmination of severe vasospasm (with ischemia-reperfusion injury), progressive vascular intimal proliferation with narrowing of the vessel lumen, and microvascular thrombosis. A combined therapeutic approach that addresses each of these processes is often used. The management of Raynaud phenomenon is discussed in detail in Chapter 24.

D. Inflammation

In early diffuse scleroderma, biopsy specimens of the skin reveal inflammatory infiltrates, and patients often complain of pain and swelling and stiffness of skin, joints, and periarticular structures. Inflammation can also be demonstrated in the lungs of some patients with interstitial lung disease (see below). It is postulated, therefore, that an early inflammatory insult leads to the downstream processes of fibrosis, atrophy, and loss of function. Because of this, a variety of immunosuppressive agents have been tried in the treatment of scleroderma. Regimens of intense immunosuppression are also currently being studied (bone marrow transplantation, immunoablative with high-dose cyclophosphamide) in patients with severe, early disease. These interventions carry the risk of significant adverse events, and their use should be limited to patients at high risk for significant morbidity and mortality. Patients with early, potentially modifiable disease, but features associated with poor prognoses, are the ideal candidates for these yet unproven aggressive therapies.

E. Organ-Specific Therapy

1. Scleroderma renal crisis (SRC)—Scleroderma patients considered to be at high risk for the development of renal crisis (those with early diffuse skin changes, prednisone use) should have their blood pressure monitored several times a week. A physician should promptly evaluate any unexplained rise in blood pressure, and renal function should be checked (urinalysis and creatinine). If there is persistently elevated blood pressure or signs of renal insufficiency, SRC should be suspected. In this setting, further diagnostic work-up (such as a renal biopsy) may be necessary. Prompt institution of ACE inhibitor therapy is needed to control blood pressure, with a target blood pressure of 130/80 mm Hg or lower. ACE inhibitors should be titrated upward to gain control of blood pressure as quickly as possible. If blood pressure remains high, patients may require hospitalization for the management of medications and close monitoring of blood pressure and renal function. Some data suggest that angiotensin II receptor blockers are as beneficial as ACE inhibitors in SRC. Despite the availability of effective therapy and aggressive management, approximately 40% of patients with SRC have poor outcomes (death within 6 months or permanent dialysis), likely due to underrecognition of renal vascular disease without early symptoms and signs.

2. Interstitial lung disease—All scleroderma patients should be monitored for the development of lung disease. Patients with a restrictive pattern on PFTs or interstitial fibrosis on high-resolution CT scanning should be treated with immunosuppression if there is evidence of progression. Bronchoalveolar lavage should be performed in selected patients to rule out infection or when other causes of lung disease are considered. There are now data from a multicenter, randomized, placebo-controlled trial that suggest daily oral cyclophosphamide is beneficial in those patients with evidence of an active alveolitis (decline in lung function or ground glass opacities on CT scan). Monthly intravenous cyclophosphamide also showed benefit in another trial and is an alternative mode of therapy. Other immunosuppressive drugs (mycophenolate, azathioprine) or targeted therapy with biologics may also be effective and are under study. Younger patients (under 60 years of age) with severe end-stage interstitial lung disease who do not respond to therapy should be considered for lung transplantation.

3. Pulmonary arterial hypertension—Isolated pulmonary arterial hypertension is more commonly seen in those patients with limited scleroderma. All patients with scleroderma, however, should be evaluated with echocardiograms to screen for elevated pulmonary pressures. Patients with isolated pulmonary hypertension usually have a reduction in the DLCO on PFTs. Patients are treated with traditional therapy for fluid overload and heart failure. Anticoagulation is

considered but is of unproven benefit, and there is an increase risk of gastrointestinal bleeding in patients with scleroderma.

In the past several years, new medications have been developed to treat patients with pulmonary hypertension. Currently approved therapies include epoprostenol and other analogues of prostacyclin, endothelin-1 antagonists, and phosphodiesterase inhibitors. Patients with mild to moderate pulmonary arterial hypertension (class II and III) can be treated with oral monotherapy (endothelin-1 inhibitor or phosphodiesterase inhibitor). These agents can improve signs and symptoms, such as a 6-minute walk, but have not significantly altered hemodynamic measures. If disease progression is seen, then both oral agents are used in combination. Prostaglandin therapy (delivered by continuous intravenous or subcutaneous infusion or intermittent inhalation) is currently used for the management of severe/refractory pulmonary hypertension. Intravenous epoprostenol and the other prostacyclin analogues treprostinil and iloprost are available. Iloprost and treprostinil are approved in the United States for delivery by inhalation. Treprostinil is also available for subcutaneous delivery. Oral prostacyclin analogues are used in Japan and are under study elsewhere. Recent data suggest that aggressive management of early pulmonary arterial hypertension with these agents may improve survival in scleroderma. However, more experience is necessary with these agents to define their long-term benefit in the management of scleroderma. Patients with severe pulmonary arterial hypertension should be considered candidates for lung transplantation (occasionally performed simultaneously with heart transplantation).

4. Gastrointestinal disease—The gastrointestinal involvement in scleroderma can be successfully managed in the majority of patients. The most frequent symptoms, gastroesophageal reflux and esophageal dysmotility, may be treated effectively with proton pump inhibitors (ie, omeprazole 20–40 mg once or twice daily). All patients with upper gastrointestinal symptoms should also be instructed in simple behavioral measures that can reduce symptoms:

- Eat small, frequent meals.
- Do not eat meals within 2-3 hours of bedtime.
- Keep the head of the bed elevated.
- Avoid aggravating factors (tobacco, alcohol, caffeine, etc).

Those with persistent symptoms may require the use of promotility agents, such as metoclopramide or domperidone. Any patient with severe dysphagia or symptoms unresponsive to the above measures should be referred to a gastroenterologist for an upper gastrointestinal endoscopy.

Lower gastrointestinal symptoms are less frequent but often more difficult to manage. Over-the-counter preparations such as loperamide or fiber supplements are used to treat mild symptoms. Persistent, frequent diarrhea may be a sign of bacterial overgrowth that requires treatment with antibiotics (eg, metronidazole). Promotility agents may also improve lower gastrointestinal symptoms (eg, octreotide). Severe dysmotility that is refractory to medical therapy and associated with either recurrent bouts of pseudo-obstruction or progressive weight loss and malnutrition is best treated with bowel rest and total parenteral nutrition.

Prognosis

The prognosis in scleroderma is highly dependent on the extent of major organ disease. This can be predicted to some extent by the degree of skin involvement. Patients with limited scleroderma have a normal life expectancy with approximately a 90% 5-year survival rate. Patients with diffuse skin disease have about a 70–80% 5-year survival rate. Clinical features that predict poor outcomes include high skin scores; progressive lung disease; tendon friction rubs; evidence of heart disease; and the presence of pulmonary arterial hypertension, anemia, and SRC. Aggressive management early in the course of the disease can improve quality of life and reduce morbidity. In the future, new therapies and better methods of recognizing disease complications early will improve the prognosis of patients with scleroderma. In the meantime, primary care physicians are encouraged to refer scleroderma patients to a rheumatologist or specialty scleroderma treatment centers.

[American College of Rheumatology]
http://www.rheumatology.org

Boin F, Hummers LK. Scleroderma-like fibrosing disorders. *Rheum Dis Clin North Am.* 2008;34:199. [PMID: 18329541]

Mathai SC, Hassoun PM. Pulmonary arterial hypertension associated with systemic sclerosis. *Expert Rev Respir Med.* 2011;5:267. [PMID: 21510736]

Nikpour M, Stevens WM, Herrick AL, Proudman SM. Epidemiology of systemic sclerosis. *Best Pract Res Clin Rheumatol.* 2010;24:857. [PMID: 21665131]

[Scleroderma Clinical Trials Consortium]
http://www.sctc-online.org

[Scleroderma Foundation]
http://www.scleroderma.org

[Scleroderma Research Foundation]
http://www.srfcure.org

Steen VD. The many faces of scleroderma. *Rheum Dis Clin North Am.* 2008;34:1. [PMID: 18329529]

Tan A, Denton CP, Mikhailidis DP, Seifalian AM. Recent advances in the diagnosis and treatment of interstitial lung disease in systemic sclerosis (scleroderma): a review. *Clin Exp Rheumatol.* 2011;29:S66. [PMID: 21586221]

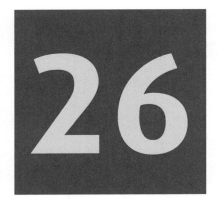

Primary Sjögren Syndrome

Manuel Ramos-Casals, MD, PhD
Pilar Brito-Zerón, MD, PhD
Antoni Sisó-Almirall, MD, PhD

ESSENTIALS OF DIAGNOSIS

▶ Sjögren syndrome (SjS) is a systemic autoimmune disease that presents with sicca symptomatology of mucosal surfaces.

▶ The main sicca features (xerophthalmia and xerostomia) are determined by specific ocular (rose bengal staining and Schirmer test) and oral (salivary flow measurement and parotid scintigraphy) tests.

▶ The histologic hallmark is a focal lymphocytic infiltration of the exocrine glands, determined by a biopsy of the minor labial salivary glands.

▶ The spectrum of the disease includes systemic features (extraglandular manifestations) in some patients, and may be complicated by the development of lymphoma.

▶ Patients with SjS present a broad spectrum of analytic features (cytopenias, hypergammaglobulinemia, and high erythrocyte sedimentation rate) and autoantibodies, of which antinuclear antibodies are the most frequently detected, anti-Ro/SS-A the most specific, and cryoglobulins and hypocomplementemia the main prognostic markers.

▶ General Considerations

Sjögren syndrome (SjS) is a systemic autoimmune disease that mainly affects the exocrine glands and usually presents as persistent dryness of the mouth and eyes due to functional impairment of the salivary and lacrimal glands. An estimated 2–4 million persons in the United States have SjS, of whom approximately 1 million have established diagnoses. The prevalence in European countries ranges between 0.60% and 3.3%. The incidence of SjS has been calculated as 4 cases per 100,000. SjS primarily affects white perimenopausal women, with a female:male ratio ranging from 14:1 to 24:1 in the largest reported series. The disease may occur at all ages but typically has its onset in the fourth to sixth decades of life. When sicca symptoms appear in a previously healthy person, the syndrome is classified as primary SjS. When sicca features are found in association with another systemic autoimmune disease, most commonly rheumatoid arthritis, systemic sclerosis, or systemic lupus erythematosus, it is classified as associated SjS.

Major clinical manifestations are summarized in Table 26–1. Although most patients present with sicca symptoms, there are various clinical and analytic features that may indicate undiagnosed SjS (Table 26–2). The variability in the presentation of SjS may partially explain delays in diagnosis of up to 10 years from the onset of symptoms. SjS is a disease that can be expressed in many guises depending on the specific epidemiologic, clinical, or immunologic features. The management of SjS is centered mainly on the control of sicca features, using substitutive and oral muscarinic agents. Glucocorticoids and immunosuppressive agents play a key role in the treatment of extraglandular features.

▶ Clinical Findings

A. Symptoms and Signs

1. Sicca features—Xerostomia, the subjective feeling of oral dryness, is the key feature in the diagnosis of primary SjS, occurring in more than 95% of patients. Other oral symptoms may include soreness, adherence of food to the mucosa, and dysphagia. Reduced salivary volume interferes with basic functions such as speaking or eating. The lack of salivary antimicrobial functions may accelerate local infection, tooth decay, and periodontal disease. Xerostomia can lead to difficulty with dentures and the need for expensive dental restoration, particularly in elderly patients. Various oral signs may be observed in SjS patients. In the early stages, the mouth may appear moist, but as the disease progresses, the usual pooling of saliva in the floor of the mouth disappears. Typically, the surface of the tongue becomes red and lobulated, with

Table 26–1. Major clinical manifestations of Sjögren syndrome.

Organ	Manifestations
Mouth	Oral dryness (xerostomia), soreness, caries, periodontal disease, oral candidiasis, parotid swelling
Eyes	Ocular dryness (xerophthalmia), corneal ulcers, conjunctivitis
Nose, ear, and throat	Nasal dryness, chronic cough, sensorineural hearing loss
Skin	Cutaneous dryness, palpable purpura, Ro-associated polycyclic lesions, urticarial lesions
Joints	Arthralgias, nonerosive symmetric arthritis
Lungs	Obstructive chronic pneumopathy, bronchiectasis, interstitial pneumopathy
Cardiovascular	Raynaud phenomenon, pericarditis, autonomic disturbances
Liver	Associated hepatitis C virus infection, primary biliary cirrhosis, type 1 autoimmune hepatitis
Nephro-urologic	Renal tubular acidosis, glomerulonephritis, interstitial cystitis, recurrent renal colic
Peripheral nerve	Mixed polyneuropathy, pure sensitive neuronopathy, mononeuritis multiplex, small-fiber neuropathy
Central nervous system	White matter lesions, cranial nerve involvement (V, VIII, and VII), myelopathy
Thyroid	Autoimmune thyroiditis
General symptoms	Low-grade fever, generalized pain, myalgias, fatigue, weakness, fibromyalgia, polyadenopathies

Table 26–2. Non-sicca manifestations suggestive of Sjögren syndrome.

Clinical features
  Chronic fatigue
  Fever of unknown origin
  Leukocytoclastic vasculitis
  Parotid/submandibular gland swelling (isolated
    submandibular gland swelling rare)
  Raynaud phenomenon
  Peripheral neuropathy
  Pulmonary fibrosis
  Mother of a baby born with congenital heart block
Laboratory features
  Elevated erythrocyte sedimentation rate
    (often with normal C-reactive protein)
  Hypergammaglobulinemia
  Leukopenia and thrombocytopenia
  Serum and/or urine monoclonal band
  Positive antinuclear antibodies or rheumatoid
    factor in an asymptomatic patient

partial or complete depapillation (Figure 26–1). In advanced disease, the oral mucosa appears dry and glazed and tends to form fine wrinkles. Angular cheilitis, erythematous changes of the hard palate, and a red tongue with atrophic papillae strongly suggest *Candida* infection.

The subjective feeling of ocular dryness is associated with sensations of itching, grittiness, soreness, and dryness, although the eyes have a normal appearance. Other ocular complaints include photosensitivity, erythema, eye fatigue, or decreased visual acuity. Environmental irritants such as smoke, wind, air conditioning, and low humidity may exacerbate ocular symptoms. Diminished tear secretion may lead to chronic irritation and destruction of corneal and bulbar conjunctival epithelium (keratoconjunctivitis sicca). In severe cases, slit-lamp examination may reveal filamentary keratitis, marked by mucus filaments that adhere to damaged areas of the corneal surface (Figure 26–2). Tears also have inherent antimicrobial activity and SjS patients are more susceptible to ocular infections such as blepharitis, bacterial keratitis, and conjunctivitis. Severe ocular complications may include corneal ulceration, vascularization, and opacification.

Reduction or absence of respiratory tract glandular secretions can lead to dryness of the nose, throat, and trachea resulting in persistent hoarseness and chronic, nonproductive cough. Likewise, involvement of the exocrine glands of the skin leads to cutaneous dryness. In female patients with SjS, dryness of the vagina and vulva may result in dyspareunia and pruritus, affecting their quality of life.

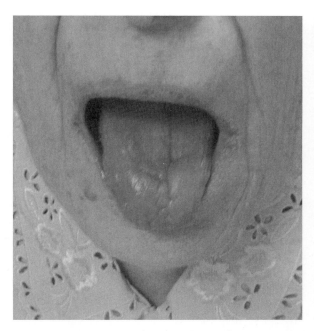

▲ **Figure 26–1.** Dry mouth in a patient with primary SjS: red tongue with depapillation.

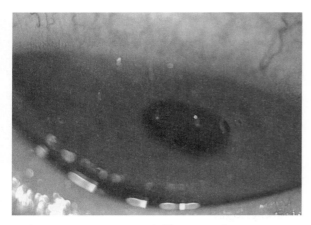

▲ **Figure 26–2.** Dry eye with filamentary keratitis.

Chronic or episodic swelling of the major salivary glands (parotid and submandibular glands) is reported in 10–20% of patients and may commence unilaterally, but often becomes bilateral (Figure 26–3).

2. Extraglandular manifestations

a. General symptomatology—Patients with primary SjS often have general symptomatology, including fever, polyadenopathies, generalized pain, fatigue, weakness, sleep disturbances, anxiety, and depression, which may have a much greater impact on the quality of life of patients than sicca features. Low-grade fevers may occur in SjS, usually in young patients with positive immunologic markers. Fatigue, generalized pain, and weakness are among the most debilitating clinical features of primary SjS. The coexistence of primary SjS with a defined fibromyalgia is reported often.

b. Joint and muscular involvement—Joint involvement, primarily generalized arthralgias, is seen in 25–75% of patients. Less frequently, joint disease presents as an intermittent symmetric arthritis primarily affecting small joints. Joint deformity and mild erosions are rare, except for those cases associated with rheumatoid arthritis. Clinical myopathy is rare but myalgias are frequently observed, and a recent study reported that subclinical muscular inflammation is often observed.

c. Skin—Although the main cutaneous manifestation of patients with primary SjS is skin dryness, a wide spectrum of cutaneous lesions may be observed, the most frequent of which is a small-vessel vasculitis, overwhelmingly leukocytoclastic. The skin findings include palpable purpura (Figure 26–4), urticaria, and erythematous macules or papules, and are associated with cryoglobulins in 30% of patients. Life-threatening vasculitis is also closely related to cryoglobulinemia.

Primary SjS patients may also have nonvasculitic cutaneous lesions. Some patients with anti-Ro/SS-A antibodies may present with polycyclic, photosensitive cutaneous lesions (Figure 26–5), clinically identical to the so-called annular erythema described in Asian SjS patients and subacute cutaneous lupus.

d. Lungs—Two types of pulmonary involvement, bronchial and interstitial, can complicate primary SjS. Bronchial/bronchiolar involvement is more common than pulmonary

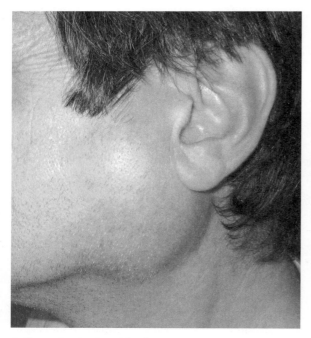

▲ **Figure 26–3.** Parotid enlargement.

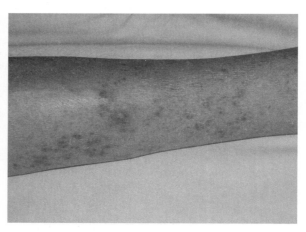

▲ **Figure 26–4.** Cutaneous purpura in the legs in a patient with SjS and cryoglobulinemia.

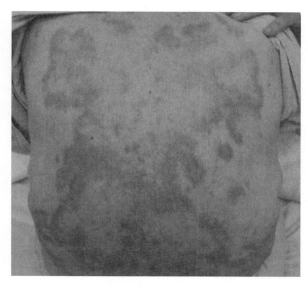

▲ **Figure 26–5.** Polycyclic, photosensitive cutaneous lesions in a 67-year-old woman with primary SjS and anti-Ro/SS-A antibodies.

fibrosis. The typical symptoms of patients with pulmonary involvement are chronic cough, dyspnea, and recurrent respiratory infections. Studies of respiratory tract involvement in primary SjS have demonstrated that the main underlying pathology in these patients is peribronchial infiltrates that lead to small airway disease. High-resolution computed tomography of the lungs reveals ground-glass pattern or thickened bronchial walls or both. Lymphocytic interstitial pneumonitis evolves only rarely. Interstitial lung disease can occur early in the course of SjS but rarely worsens over follow-up, and a conservative therapeutic approach is advised. Pleurisy is an extremely rare manifestation of primary SjS and often signals the presence of an additional autoimmune disease, particularly lupus.

e. Cardiovascular features—Raynaud phenomenon, with a prevalence of 10–20%, is probably the most common vascular feature observed in primary SjS. The clinical course of Raynaud phenomenon in primary SjS is milder than in other systemic autoimmune diseases such as systemic sclerosis. Vascular complications (eg, digital loss, digital pulp pitting, or fingertip infarctions) are uncommon, and pharmacologic interventions are required in only 40% of cases. Cardiac involvement is rarely observed, with pericardial effusions (usually mild and asymptomatic) being the most frequent feature. Recent studies have described autonomic cardiovascular disturbances.

f. Gut—Gastrointestinal involvement may include altered esophageal motility, chronic gastritis, and less frequently, malabsorption. *Helicobacter pylori* infection should be excluded in patients with gastritis because of the close association with gastric mucosa-associated lymphoid tissue lymphoma. Pancreatic involvement, usually asymptomatic, is demonstrated by altered pancreatic function tests. Some patients may have chronic pancreatitis. Liver function tests may be elevated in 10–20% of patients with primary SjS. After exclusion of potentially hepatotoxic drugs, the main causes are chronic hepatitis C viral infection (especially in geographic areas with a high prevalence) and primary biliary cirrhosis. Less frequently, SjS patients may present with type 1 autoimmune hepatitis, and even more rarely, autoimmune or sclerosing cholangitis.

g. Nephro-urologic involvement—Overt renal involvement was only found in 5% of the nearly 2000 patients included in the largest reported series. The main types of renal involvement described are interstitial renal disease and glomerulonephritis. Interstitial nephritis can be an early manifestation of SjS. This condition is usually subclinical, and manifested by a low urine specific gravity (hyposthenuria) and an alkaline urine pH (type I distal tubular acidosis). Nephrocalcinosis that presents with renal colic is a common clinical feature in these patients. Finally, interstitial cystitis, sometimes with severe symptoms, has recently identified as a frequent extraglandular SjS feature.

h. Neurologic involvement—Peripheral neuropathy is the most common neurologic involvement. A joint analysis of 1025 patients with primary SjS showed peripheral neuropathy in 18%. The most frequent types of neuropathy were mixed polyneuropathy, pure sensory neuronopathy, and mononeuritis multiplex. Of these, pure sensory neuronopathy is recognized as a characteristic neurologic complication of primary SjS, caused by damage to the sensory neurons of the dorsal root and gasserian ganglia. Dorsal root and gasserian ganglionopathies are associated with potentially devastating deficits in proprioception. Mixed polyneuropathy and multiplex mononeuritis are usually associated with vasculitis and often with concomitant cryoglobulinemia. Some patients with primary SjS present with small-fiber neuropathy. SjS patients may present cranial nerve involvement, mainly of the trigeminal (V), vestibulocochlear (VIII), and facial (VII) cranial pairs.

Although earlier studies described central nervous system involvement as a frequent extraglandular manifestation of primary SjS, clinically significant central nervous system involvement is actually very rare. The most frequently detected central nervous system feature in primary SjS is probably asymptomatic white matter lesions in magnetic resonance examinations. A recent study found that these lesions are overwhelmingly associated with concomitant cardiovascular risk factors, although isolated cases of SjS patients presenting with a multiple sclerosis–like disease have been reported. Some patients may present with myelopathy and optic neuritis, similar to neuromyelitis optica (NMO).

i. Other organs—Nearly one third of patients with primary SjS have thyroid disease. Subclinical hypothyroidism is the most frequent finding, especially in patients with antithyroid autoantibodies (suggesting previous Hashimoto thyroiditis). Although ear, nose, and throat involvement has been little studied in patients with primary SjS, some studies have described sensorineural hearing loss in nearly 25% of SjS patients. Psychiatric disorders, including depression and anxiety, have been described in many patients with SjS.

B. Laboratory Findings

The results of routine laboratory tests and immunologic markers in primary SjS are summarized in Table 26–3. The

Table 26–3. The laboratory evaluation in Sjögren syndrome.

Test	Typical Result
Complete blood cell count	• Normochromic, normocytic anemia. Isolated cases of hemolytic anemia • Mild leukopenia (3–4 × 10⁹/L); lymphopenia, neutropenia • Mild thrombocytopenia (80–150 × 10⁹/L)
Erythrocyte sedimentation rate (ESR) and C-reactive protein (CRP)	• Elevated ESR (>50 mm/h) in 20–30% of cases, especially in patients with hypergammaglobulinemia • Normal values of CRP
Serum protein	• Hypergammaglobulinemia • Monoclonal band
Liver function tests	• Raised transaminases (associated with hepatitis C virus or autoimmune hepatitis) • Raised alkaline phosphatase and/or bilirubin (associated with primary biliary cirrhosis)
Electrolytes and urinalysis	• Proteinuria (glomerulonephritis) • Hyposthenuria, low plasma bicarbonate, and low blood pH (renal tubular acidosis)
Antinuclear antibody test	• Positive in more than 80%
Rheumatoid factor	• Positive in 40–50% of patients, often leading to diagnostic confusion with rheumatoid arthritis
Anti-extractable nuclear antigens antibodies	• Positive anti-Ro/SS-A (30–70%) and anti-La/SS-B (25–40%)
Complement (C3, C4, and CH50)	• Complement levels are decreased in 10–20% of patients
Cryoglobulins	• Present in 10–20% of patients
Other autoantibodies	• Antimitochondrial antibodies (associated with primary biliary cirrhosis) • Antithyroid antibodies (associated with thyroiditis) • Anti-dsDNA (associated with systemic lupus erythematosus) • Anticentromere (associated with a limited form of systemic sclerosis)

most frequent analytic features are cytopenia, elevated erythrocyte sedimentation rate, and hypergammaglobulinemia (20–30%). The most frequent cytopenias detected are normocytic anemia, leukopenia, and thrombocytopenia. The differential leukocyte count has been studied in large series of patients with primary SjS; the most frequent abnormality was lymphopenia, closely followed by neutropenia. Cytopenias are found more commonly in patients with positive immunologic markers and are usually asymptomatic, but may be clinically overt in some cases. Erythrocyte sedimentation rate levels correlate closely with the percentage of circulating gamma globulins (hypergammaglobulinemia), while serum C-reactive protein levels are usually normal. Highly elevated serum C-reactive protein levels in a patient with primary SjS should raise the suspicion of an infection. Finally, circulating monoclonal immunoglobulins may be detected in nearly 20% of patients with primary SjS, with monoclonal IgG being detected most frequently.

C. Special Tests

1. Salivary gland biopsy—Minor salivary gland biopsy remains a highly specific test for the diagnosis of SjS, although it is an invasive technique that may be accompanied by local side effects when performed incorrectly. Focal lymphocytic sialadenitis, defined as multiple, dense aggregates of 50 or more lymphocytes in perivascular or periductal areas in the majority of sampled glands, is the characteristic histopathologic feature of SjS. The key requirements for a correct histologic evaluation are an adequate number of informative lobules (at least four) and the determination of an average focus score (a focus is a cluster of at least 50 lymphocytes). However, nonspecific sialadenitis is quite common in biopsy samples of minor salivary glands in healthy control populations. Although sialoadenitis is the key histopathologic feature of SjS, this finding in the absence of symptoms and markers suggestive of SjS should be interpreted with caution. Minor salivary gland biopsy is often essential in parsing the differential diagnosis in patients who present with sicca symptoms (eg, sarcoidosis, amyloidosis).

2. Assessment of oral involvement—Several methods to assess oral involvement have been proposed, such as measurement of the salivary flow rate, sialochemistry, sialography, or scintigraphy. Measurement of the salivary flow, with or without stimulation, is the simplest method in evaluating xerostomia, and is acceptable to patients and needs no special equipment, while the study of the degree of salivary gland dysfunction by parotid scintigraphy offers valuable clinical information on the prognosis and outcome of primary SjS. The other tests, though useful for the purposes of research, rarely have clinical applications. Ultrasonography is a noninvasive method that may provide useful information about the etiology of parotid enlargements.

3. Assessment of ocular involvement—The main ocular tests are the Schirmer test and rose bengal staining.

The Schirmer test for the eye quantitatively measures tear formation via placement of filter paper in the lower conjunctival sac. The test can be performed with or without the instillation of anesthetic drops to prevent reflex tearing. The test result is positive when less than 5 mm of paper is wetted after 5 minutes. Rose bengal scoring involves the placement of 25 mL of rose bengal solution in the inferior fornix of each eye and having the patient blink twice. Slit-lamp examination detects destroyed conjunctival epithelium due to desiccation.

4. Immunologic tests—The main immunologic markers found in primary SjS are antinuclear antibodies, anti-Ro/SS-A or anti-La/SS-B antibodies, rheumatoid factor, hypocomplementemia, and cryoglobulins (see Table 26–3). Antinuclear antibodies are the most frequently detected antibodies in primary SjS (in more than 80% of cases), and titers ≥1:80 play a central role in differentiating SjS from non-autoimmune causes of sicca syndrome. Anti-Ro/SS-A and La/SS-B antibodies, detected in 30–70% of patients, are closely associated with most extraglandular features, especially with cutaneous lesions, neurologic features, congenital heart block, and cytopenias. In nearly 50% of cases, patients with primary SjS also present with positive rheumatoid factor.

Hypocomplementemia and cryoglobulinemia (see Chapter 36) are two closely-related immunologic markers that have been linked with more severe SjS. Recent studies have associated low complement levels and cryoglobulins (usually type II, which are found in 10–20% of patients) with chronic hepatitis C viral infection, lymphoma development, and mortality. Serum monoclonal gammopathy often indicates the presence of an underlying type II mixed cryoglobulinemia.

Table 26–4. Classification of Sjögren syndrome (SjS): primary, associated, and mimicked SjS.

1. **Primary SjS**
2. **Associated SjS**
   Systemic autoimmune diseases
      Systemic lupus erythematosus
      Systemic sclerosis
      Rheumatoid arthritis
      Still disease
      Sarcoidosis
      Inflammatory myopathies
   Organ-specific autoimmune diseases
      Primary biliary cirrhosis
      Autoimmune thyroiditis
      Multiple sclerosis
      Diabetes mellitus
   Chronic viral infections
      Chronic HCV infection (Mediterranean countries)
      HTLV-1 I infection (Asian countries)
      HIV infection
3. **Mimicked SjS**
   Other diseases infiltrating exocrine glands
      Granulomatous diseases (sarcoidosis and tuberculosis)
      Amyloidosis
      Neoplasias (lymphoma)
      IgG4-related disease
      Type V hyperlipidemia
   Other processes
      Graft-versus-host disease
      Eosinophilia-myalgia syndrome
      Radiation injury
      Medication-related dryness

HCV, hepatitis C virus; HTLV, human T-cell lymphoma virus.

▶ Differential Diagnosis

The proven diagnosis of SjS requires not only documentation of sicca symptoms, but also objective evidence of dry eyes and mouth and analytic evidence of autoimmunity, as sicca syndrome has many causes. The most frequent cause of sicca features is the chronic use of medications leading to mucosal dryness (mainly antihypertensive, antihistamine, and antidepressant agents), especially in the elderly. After this cause is excluded, there are three main causes of sicca syndrome (Table 26–4). First, some processes may mimic the clinical picture of SjS through nonlymphocytic infiltration of the exocrine glands by granulomas (sarcoidosis and tuberculosis), amyloid proteins (amyloidosis), or malignant cells (hematologic neoplasia). A more recently recognized cause of salivary gland enlargement is IgG4-related disease (see Chapter 71). Second, extrinsic factors, mainly chronic viral infections such as hepatitis C virus or HIV, may induce a lymphocytic infiltration of exocrine glands. Third, patients may have primary SjS or SjS associated with other autoimmune diseases.

▶ Diagnosis

Sicca features are symptoms that usually receive little attention and may be considered trivial by both doctor and patient. Although often elusive, an early, accurate diagnosis of SjS can help prevent, or ensure timely treatment of, many of the complications associated with the disease. For example, early restoration of salivary function can relieve symptoms of dry mouth and may prevent or slow the progress of the oral complications of SjS, including dental caries, oral candidiasis, and periodontal disease. Untreated severe dry eye can result in corneal ulcers and further perforation, which may eventually lead to loss of the eye. An early diagnosis is also mandatory for the main extraglandular features, in order to prevent chronic organ damage by prompt recognition and treatment. Table 26–5 summarizes the current classification criteria.

▶ Complications

Primary SjS usually progresses very slowly, with no rapid deterioration in salivary function or dramatic changes in

Table 26–5. The American-European Classification Criteria for Sjögren syndrome.

I. Ocular symptoms: a positive response to at least one of the following questions:
   a. Have you had daily, persistent, troublesome dry eyes for more than 3 months?
   b. Do you have a recurrent sensation of sand or gravel in the eyes?
   c. Do you use tear substitutes more than three times a day?
II. Oral symptoms: a positive response to at least one of the following questions:
   a. Have you had a daily feeling of dry mouth for more than 3 months?
   b. Have you had recurrently or persistently swollen salivary glands as an adult?
   c. Do you frequently drink liquids to aid in swallowing dry food?
III. Ocular signs: objective evidence of ocular involvement defined as a positive result for at least one of the following two tests:
   a. Schirmer test, performed without anesthesia (5 mm in 5 minutes)
   b. Rose bengal score or other ocular dye score (4 according to the van Bijsterveld scoring system)
IV. Histopathology: In minor salivary glands (obtained through normal-appearing mucosa) focal lymphocytic sialoadenitis, evaluated by an expert histopathologist, with a focus score of 1, defined as a number of lymphocytic foci (which are adjacent to normal-appearing mucous acini and contain more than 50 lymphocytes) per 4 mm² of glandular tissue.
V. Salivary gland involvement: objective evidence of salivary gland involvement defined by a positive result for at least one of the following diagnostic tests:
   a. Unstimulated whole salivary flow (1.5 mL in 15 minutes)
   b. Parotid sialography showing the presence of diffuse sialectasias (punctate, cavitary, or destructive pattern), without evidence of obstruction in the major ducts
   c. Salivary scintigraphy showing delayed uptake, reduced concentration, and/or delayed excretion of tracer
VI. Antibodies to Ro/SS-A or La/SS-B antigens, or both

Patients are classified as having primary SjS when they fulfill four or more of the six classification criteria; either criterion IV (salivary gland biopsy) or criterion VI (anti-Ro/La antibodies) are mandatory.

sicca symptoms. The main exceptions to this benign course are the development of extraglandular manifestations and the high incidence of lymphoma.

Primary SjS patients are at higher risk for lymphoma than are healthy individuals (10- to 44-fold) and patients with other autoimmune diseases (7-fold in patients with systemic lupus erythematosus, 4-fold in patients with rheumatoid arthritis). The long-term risk of lymphoma for patients with primary SjS is often estimated to be 5%. Persistently hard enlargement of the lacrimal or parotid glands should alert the clinician to the possibility of a lymphoma. Lymphomas that develop in primary SjS patients are extranodal in 80% of cases, with the most common site being the parotid glands. Ninety percent of primary SjS patients in whom lymphoma

develops have histories of major salivary gland enlargement during the disease course. Lymphomas developing in SjS may also occur in the gastrointestinal tract or lungs. They often begin as B cell mucosa-associated lymphoid tissue (MALT) lymphomas or, in lymph nodes, as marginal zone lymphomas. After years of slow progression, these low-grade tumors may progress to rapidly-growing, high-grade lymphomas. Various studies have identified risk factors for lymphoma development (cryoglobulinemia, hypocomplementemia, CD4-lymphopenia, and palpable purpura). The few studies that have analyzed the causes and rates of mortality in these patients compared to the general population found that the overall mortality of patients with primary SjS increased only in patients with these adverse predictors.

The European League Against Rheumatism (EULAR) has recently promoted an international collaboration between primary SjS experts to develop consensus disease activity indexes. Two indexes have been developed: (1) a patient-administered questionnaire to assess subjective symptoms, called the EULAR Sjögren's Syndrome Patients Reported Index (ESSPRI), and (2) a systemic activity index to assess systemic complications, called the EULAR Sjögren's Syndrome Disease Activity Index (ESSDAI).

▶ Treatment

At present, there is no treatment capable of modifying the evolution of SjS. A recent systematic review highlights the limited evidence available for the drugs most frequently used in primary SjS and the difficulties of offering solid therapeutic recommendations.

Treatment of sicca manifestations is mainly symptomatic and is typically intended to limit the damage resulting from chronic involvement. Moisture replacement products can be effective for patients with mild or moderate symptoms. Frequent use of preservative-free tear substitutes are recommended, while ocular lubricating ointments are usually reserved for nocturnal use; controlled trials support the use of topical 0.05% cyclosporine twice daily for patients with moderate to severe dry eye disease. Patients with severe refractory ocular dryness may require the addition of topical nonsteroidal anti-inflammatory drugs or glucocorticoids, although these should only be prescribed by ophthalmologists for the minimum time necessary, because of adverse events associated with long-term use.

Saliva replacement products and sugar-free chewing gums may be effective for mild to moderate dry mouth. Alcohol and smoking should be avoided and thorough oral hygiene is essential. For patients with residual salivary gland function, oral pilocarpine and cevimeline are the treatment of choice. However, the efficacy of the two drugs has not been compared. The doses that best balance efficacy and adverse effects are 5 mg every 6 hours for pilocarpine and 30 mg every 8 hours for cevimeline. In patients with contraindications or intolerance to muscarinic agonists, N-acetylcysteine may be an alternative.

As a rule, the management of extraglandular features should be organ-specific, with glucocorticoids and immunosuppresive agents limited to potentially severe scenarios. Nonsteroidal anti-inflammatory drugs usually provide relief from the minor musculoskeletal symptoms of SjS, as well as from painful parotid swelling. Hydroxychloroquine may be used in patients with fatigue, arthralgias, and myalgias. For patients with moderate extraglandular involvement (mainly arthritis, extensive cutaneous purpura, and non-severe peripheral neuropathy), 0.5 mg/kg/d of prednisone may suffice. For patients with internal organ involvement (pulmonary alveolitis, glomerulonephritis, or severe neurologic features), a combination of prednisone and immunosuppressive agents (cyclophosphamide, azathioprine, or mycophenolate mofetil) is suggested.

With regard to biologic agents, evidence from controlled trials suggests the lack of efficacy of tumor necrosis factor inhibitors in primary SjS. B-cell targeted agents seem to be the most promising future therapy. Rituximab has shown improvement in some extraglandular features (vasculitis, neuropathy, glomerulonephritis, and arthritis) in recent controlled and uncontrolled studies. However, while awaiting the results of larger trials, rituximab may be considered as a rescue therapy in patients refractory to standard treatment. Agents that block BAFF (B cell–activating factor of the tumor necrosis factor family) may also be a promising therapy.

Arthritis Research Campaign: Sjögren's syndrome
www.arc.org.uk/about_arth/booklets/6041/6041.htm

Baimpa E, Dahabreh IJ, Voulgarelis M, Moutsopoulos HM. Hematologic manifestations and predictors of lymphoma development in primary Sjögren syndrome: clinical and pathophysiologic aspects. *Medicine (Baltimore).* 2009;88:284. [PMID: 19745687]

Brito-Zerón P, Ramos-Casals M, Bove A, Sentis J, Font J. Predicting adverse outcomes in primary Sjogren's syndrome: identification of prognostic factors. *Rheumatology (Oxford).* 2007;46:1359. [PMID: 17569749]

Dry.Org—Internet resources for Sjogren's syndrome
www.dry.org

International Patient Sjögren's Network
http://www.afgs-syndromes-secs.org/ (France)
http://www.sjogrens.org.au/ (Australia)
http://www.sjogrenscanada.org/ (Canada)
http://www.sjoegren-erkrankung.de/ (Germany)
http://www.animass.org/sjogren/ (Italia)
http://www.sjogrensyndrom.se/ (Sweden)
http://www.bssa.uk.net/ (UK)
www.aesjogren.org/publico/na_consejo.asp (Spain)

Ioannidis JP, Vassiliou VA, Moutsopoulos HM. Long-term risk of mortality and lymphoproliferative disease and predictive classification of primary Sjogren's syndrome. *Arthritis Rheum.* 2002;46:741. [PMID: 11920410]

Kassan SS, Moutsopoulos HM. Clinical manifestations and early diagnosis of Sjogren syndrome. *Arch Intern Med.* 2004;164:1275. [PMID: 15226160]

Ramos-Casals M, Brito-Zerón P, Font J. Lessons from diseases mimicking Sjögren's syndrome. *Clin Rev Allergy Immunol.* 2007;32:275. [PMID: 17992594]

Ramos-Casals M, Solans R, Rosas J, et al. GEMESS Study Group. Primary Sjögren syndrome in Spain: clinical and immunologic expression in 1010 patients. *Medicine (Baltimore).* 2008;87:210. [PMID: 18626304]

Ramos-Casals M, Tzioufas AG, Stone JH, Sisó A, Bosch X. Treatment of primary Sjögren syndrome: a systematic review. *JAMA.* 2010;304:452. [PMID: 20664046]

Seror R, Ravaud P, Mariette X, et al. EULAR Sjögren's Task Force. EULAR Sjögren's Syndrome Patient Reported Index (ESSPRI): development of a consensus patient index for primary Sjögren's syndrome. *Ann Rheum Dis.* 2011;70:968. [PMID: 21345815]

Sjogren's Syndrome - NHS Choices
www.nhs.uk/conditions/Sjogrens-syndrome

Sjogren's Syndrome Support: Sjogren's World
www.sjsworld.org

The Sjögren's Syndrome Foundation
www.sjogrens.org

Theander E, Manthorpe R, Jacobsson LT. Mortality and causes of death in primary Sjögren's syndrome: a prospective cohort study. *Arthritis Rheum.* 2004;50:1262. [PMID: 15077310]

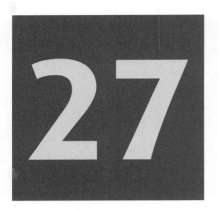

Dermatomyositis, Polymyositis, & Immune-Mediated Necrotizing Myopathy

Andrew L. Mammen, MD, PhD

Alex Truong, MD

Lisa Christopher-Stine, MD, MPH

ESSENTIALS OF DIAGNOSIS

▶ Symmetric proximal muscle weakness progressing over weeks to months.

▶ Elevated muscle enzymes, including creatine kinase (CK), aldolase, aspartate aminotransferase (AST), and alanine aminotransferase (ALT).

▶ An "irritable myopathy" shown by electromyography (EMG).

▶ MRI of affected muscles reveals evidence of edema or fasciitis or both.

▶ A heliotrope rash, Gottron sign/papules are pathognomonic for dermatomyositis.

▶ Muscle biopsy findings frequently reveal endomysial, perimysial, and perivascular lymphocytic infiltrates. Except for perifascicular atrophy, which is pathognomonic for dermatomyositis, muscle biopsy findings are variable and nonspecific.

▶ A careful family history, medication list review, physical examination, laboratory evaluation, and muscle biopsy are critical and help exclude an alternative diagnosis, such as an inherited muscle disease or toxic myopathy.

General Considerations

Polymyositis and dermatomyositis are a rare, heterogeneous group of autoimmune myopathies with an approximate incidence of 1 case per 100,000 per year. Although polymyositis is virtually unheard of in children, juvenile dermatomyositis is well-described and occurs most frequently between the ages of 10 and 15 years. In adults, the autoimmune myopathies can occur at any age but seem to peak between the ages of 45 and 60 years.

In polymyositis and dermatomyositis, muscle biopsies are characterized by lymphocytic infiltrates. Recently, however, a form of autoimmune muscle disease with prominent myofiber degeneration and necrosis with minimal, if any, inflammatory cells has also been recognized. This form of myositis, termed "immune-mediated necrotizing myopathy," has been included in the most contemporary diagnostic classification schemes of the autoimmune myopathies.

Although most patients with dermatomyositis have both skin and muscle involvement, patients occasionally have only the skin manifestations and are classified as having "dermatomyositis sine myositis" or amyopathic dermatomyositis. Conversely, in rare instances, the classic muscle biopsy features of dermatomyositis are observed in the absence of rash. These patients are said to have "dermatomyositis sine dermatitis" (Table 27–1).

▶ Clinical Findings

A. Symptoms and Signs

Symmetric proximal muscle weakness evolving over weeks to months is the presenting symptom in most patients. Typical complaints include difficulty rising from a low chair, walking up steps, and washing one's hair. In more severe cases, weakness of the neck flexors, pharyngeal weakness, and diaphragmatic weakness can cause head drop, dysphagia, and respiratory compromise, respectively. On physical examination, weakness of the proximal arm muscles, especially the deltoids, but often including the biceps and triceps, is expected. Hip flexors are the most commonly affected leg muscles but the hamstrings and quadriceps are also frequently weak. Subtle leg weakness can be detected by having the patient attempt to rise from a 6-inch high stool without using the arms.

As a general rule in the autoimmune myopathies, distal weakness should only occur in the presence of severe proximal muscle weakness. Isolated or even mild distal weakness should always raise doubts about the diagnosis of dermatomyositis, polymyositis, or immune-mediated necrotizing

Table 27–1. Classification of the autoimmune myopathies.

1. Polymyositis (PM)
2. Immune-mediated necrotizing myopathy (IMNM)
3. Dermatomyositis
   a. Dermatomyositis sine myositis (amyopathic dermatomyositis)
   b. Dermatomyositis sine dermatitis
   c. Juvenile dermatomyositis

myopathy. The examiner can test whether distal weakness is present by evaluating the strength of wrist flexors, wrist extensors, distal finger flexors, and finger extensors. In the lower extremities, ankle dorsiflexion and ankle plantarflexion strength should be assessed manually and by having the patient attempt to walk on their heels and toes. The presence of facial weakness or scapular winging (Plates 43 and 44) should be assessed, since these are extremely atypical in autoimmune myopathy and suggest the probability of an alternative diagnosis (see Differential Diagnosis section).

In addition to muscle weakness, arthralgias or frank arthritis, myalgias, severe fatigue, Raynaud phenomenon, or symptoms of another overlapping rheumatologic condition (such as lupus or scleroderma) may be present. Dyspnea may reflect diaphragmatic weakness or, especially in patients with the antisynthetase syndrome (see below), interstitial lung disease. The latter is often associated with a persistent dry cough, crackles on chest auscultation, and decreased oxygen saturation with exercise. Serious clinically significant cardiac manifestations occur, albeit rarely, in the autoimmune myopathies.

Patients with dermatomyositis may present with cutaneous manifestations either before or after the development of muscle symptoms. **Gottron papules** are raised violaceous lesions at the extensor surfaces of the metacarpophalangeal, proximal interphalangeal, and the distal interphalangeal joints (Figure 27–1). The **Gottron sign** is an erythematous rash involving these sites that can also be found at the extensor surfaces of the elbows and knees. The heliotrope rash is an often red or purplish discoloration of the eyelids (Figure 27–2); in blacks, this may appear hyperpigmented. Although both the heliotrope and Gottron rashes are pathognomonic for dermatomyositis, other less specific rashes may occur. These include an erythematous or poikilodermatous rash across the posterior neck and shoulders (the shawl sign) and a similar rash on the anterior neck and chest (the V-sign). In some patients, dermatomyositis-associated rashes are sun-sensitive. In some patients, particularly those with the antisynthetase syndrome (see below), hyperkeratotic skin thickening, often with painful cracking, on the radial surfaces of the fingers (mechanic's hands) or toes (mechanic's feet) may develop. In addition, periungual telangiectasias and nailfold capillary changes identical to those found in scleroderma may develop.

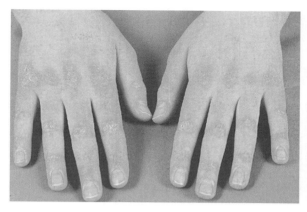

▲ **Figure 27–1.** Dermatomyositis. Gottron papules on the dorsa of the hands and fingers, especially over the metacarpophalangeal and interphalangeal joints. (Reproduced, with permission, from Wolff K, Johnson RA, Suurmond D. *Fitzpatrick's Color Atlas and Synopsis of Clinical Dermatology.* 6th ed. McGraw-Hill, 2009.)

In general, no definite environmental exposures have been associated with the development of polymyositis. While increased UV light exposure may predispose patients to dermatomyositis, a history of intense sun exposure is only occasionally elicited from patients with this condition. In contrast, there is emerging evidence that a distinct form of immune-mediated necrotizing myopathy may be triggered by statin use and is associated with autoantibodies recognizing HMG-CoA reductase, the pharmacologic target of statins (see below).

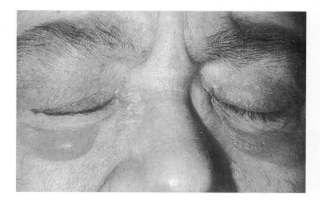

▲ **Figure 27–2.** Dermatomyositis. Heliotrope erythema of upper eyelids and edema of the lower lids. (Reproduced, with permission, from Wolff K, Johnson RA, Suurmond D. *Fitzpatrick's Color Atlas and Synopsis of Clinical Dermatology.* 6th ed. McGraw-Hill, 2009.)

B. Laboratory Findings

Creatine kinase (CK), aldolase, AST, ALT, and lactate dehydrogenase, are released from damaged muscle and elevated levels are often, but not always, found in patients with autoimmune myopathy. In some instances of dermatomyositis and polymyositis, the aldolase may be elevated in the presence of a normal CK level. Not infrequently, elevated AST and ALT levels are misinterpreted as evidence of liver disease in patients with myopathy. To rule out liver disease, a serum gamma glutamyl transferase (GGT) level can be measured; GGT is usually released along with AST and ALT in liver disease but not from damaged muscle.

As in other systemic autoimmune diseases, there is a strong association of autoantibodies against specific autoantigens with distinct clinical phenotypes. The term "myositis-specific autoantibody" has been used to describe those antibodies that are found in ~60–80% of patients with polymyositis, dermatomyositis, and immune-mediated necrotizing myopathy but not other rheumatic diseases or neuromuscular disorders (Table 27–2).

Autoantibodies recognizing one of the aminoacyl tRNA synthetases (eg, anti-Jo-1) are the most common of the myositis-specific autoantibodies and occur in ~30% of patients with polymyositis or dermatomyositis. In addition to an autoimmune myopathy, patients with antisynthetase autoantibodies may have one or more of the following features: interstitial lung disease, nonerosive arthritis, fevers, Raynaud phenomenon, and mechanic's hands. Patients with 1 of the antisynthetase autoantibodies and 2 or more of these features are said to have the antisynthetase syndrome. Interestingly, different antisynthetase antibodies appear to be associated with these features at different frequencies. For example, in patients with anti-Jo-1, 90% have muscle involvement and 50–75% have interstitial lung disease. In contrast, PL-12 positive patients have muscle involvement at a frequency of only 52%, but interstitial lung disease at a frequency of 90%.

Table 27–2. Myositis-specific autoantibodies.

Name	Antigen	Clinical Manifestation
Antisynthetase autoantibodies		
Anti-Jo-1	Histidyl t-RNA synthetase	PM or DM with ILD
Anti-PL-7	Threonyl t-RNA synthetase	PM or DM with ILD
Anti-PL-12	Alanyl t-RNA synthetase	ILD more often than Myo
Anti-EJ	Glycyl t-RNA synthetase	PM more often than DM with ILD
Anti-OJ	Isoleucyl t-RNA synthetase	ILD with PM/DM
Anti-KS	Asparaginyl t-RNA synthetase	ILD more often than Myo
Anti-Zo	Phenylalanyl t-RNA synthetase	ILD with Myo
Anti-Ha	Tyrosyl t-RNA synthetase	ILD with Myo
Nonsynthetase autoantibodies		
Dermatomyositis-specific autoantibodies		
Anti-Mi-2	DNA helicase	Dermatomyositis with rash > muscle symptoms, treatment responsive
Anti-MDA5 (anti CADM 140)	Melanoma differentiation-associated gene 5	DM: CAM, DM with rapidly progressive lung disease, pneumomediastinum
Anti-155/140	Transcriptional intermediary factor 1-gamma	CAM
Anti-140	Nuclear matrix protein (NXP-2)	Juvenile DM
Anti-SAE	Small ubiquitin-like modifier-activating enzyme	DM: CAM, DM with rapidly progressive lung disease, pneumomediastinum
Immune-mediated necrotizing myopathy–specific autoantibodies		
Anti-SRP	Signal recognition particle	Severe, acute, resistant necrotizing myopathy
Anti-HMGCR (anti 200/100)	HMG CoA Reductase	Necrotizing myopathy related to statin use in majority. Majority of patients received statin therapy but also reported in a minority of patients who did not receive statin therapy

CAM, cancer-associated myositis; DM, dermatomyositis; ILD, interstitial lung disease; JDM, juvenile dermatomyositis; myo, myositis (may be either PM or DM); PM, polymyositis; RP, Raynaud phenomenon.

A number of different autoantibodies are found exclusively in dermatomyositis. For example, antibodies recognizing the chromatin remodeling enzyme Mi-2 are found in as many as 20% of patients with dermatomyositis where they are associated with particularly fulminant initial cutaneous manifestations. However, these patients tend to have a good response to treatment and have a lower risk of associated malignancy. The anti-MDA5 antibodies have been reported only in patients with amyopathic dermatomyositis, especially in those with interstitial lung disease. Anti-small ubiquitin-like modifier 1 (SUMO-1) autoantibodies have also been reported in ~8% of patients with dermatomyositis. The so-called anti-p155/140 autoantibody is also found exclusively in patients with dermatomyositis; it is associated with an increased risk of malignancy. Unlike other autoantibodies, anti-p155/140 and anti-NXP-2 may also be found in children with dermatomyositis. Children with anti-p155/140 have especially severe skin disease and patients with anti-NXP-2 have an increased risk of developing subcutaneous calcium deposits. However, there was no increased risk of tumors in children with or without these autoantibodies.

Two different myositis-specific antibodies are particularly associated with immune-mediated necrotizing myopathy. Anti-SRP autoantibodies are found in ~5% of myositis patients and are associated with muscle biopsies showing predominantly myofiber degeneration and necrosis with minimal inflammation. These patients tend to have a rapidly progressive myopathy associated with very high CK levels, early muscle atrophy, dysphagia and, frequently, an incomplete response to immunosuppressive therapy. Patients with anti-HMGCR antibodies are found in ~5% of myositis patients and have a strong association with a necrotizing muscle biopsy and prior statin exposure; in patients over the age of 50 with these antibodies, 92% reported a prior statin exposure. In such patients, the myalgias and weakness that began during statin therapy persists and progresses for months or years after the statin is withdrawn. Significant improvement (and sometimes resolution) of the myopathy requires immunosuppressive therapy.

Antinuclear antibodies are found in more than half of patients with polymyositis or dermatomyositis and are associated with the presence of antibodies recognizing Mi-2 (a nuclear protein) or an autoantigen associated with one of the other connective tissue diseases. Examples include anti-PM-Scl and anti-Scl-70, autoantibodies found in patients with scleroderma-myositis overlap, and anti-RNP, which is found in patients with mixed connective tissue disease. The erythrocyte sedimentation rate and C-reactive protein are only markedly elevated in about 20% of myositis patients and are not particularly diagnostically useful.

C. Imaging Studies

Although neither conventional radiography nor radionuclide imaging have proved particularly useful in patients with muscle diseases, computer-based image analysis using

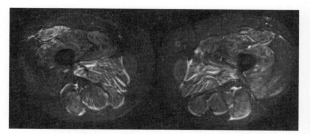

▲ **Figure 27–3.** Axial short tau inversion recovery (STIR) MRI through the midsection of the thighs of a patient with dermatomyositis. There is marked enhancement of the fascia and the quadriceps muscles of both thighs in a symmetric fashion.

ultrasonography, CT, and MRI can aid in diagnosis and assessment of disease activity. Of these, MRI with T2-weighted images and fat suppression or short tau inversion recovery (STIR) offers the best imaging of soft tissue and muscle (Figure 27–3). MRI plays an important role in the evaluation of management of autoimmune myopathy because of its ability to evaluate muscle edema (as an indicator of active inflammation) and fatty infiltration (as an indicator of chronic disease). MRI can detect early or subtle disease changes as well as patchy muscle involvement. Because of these capacities and the fact that it is noninvasive, MRI may prove superior to EMG in determining the site for muscle biopsy. Furthermore, MRI can be used to assess degree of fascial involvement as well as to semi-quantitatively grade muscle involvement and, therefore, can be used to monitor the response to therapy. This may be particularly useful when trying to differentiate between active myositis and glucocorticoid-induced myopathy. In such situations, the presence of edema in the muscle tissue is indicative of an ongoing inflammatory process. Use of MRI to guide biopsy may lower the rates of false-negative muscle biopsies, which range from 10% to 25%. Repeated MRIs can be used to monitor disease progression and response to therapy. However, treatment with immunosuppressive medications can result in decreased signal intensity on MRI, but histologically detected inflammation may not change significantly.

While its clinical use is currently limited, ultrasound provides some potential benefits over CT or MRI in evaluating autoimmune myopathy, such as its high spatial resolution and real-time imaging without the radiation exposure. Although there are subtle differences among the 3 different forms of immune-mediated muscle disease, conventional ultrasound is generally not sensitive enough to differentiate between them. Use of contrast-enhanced ultrasound does not seem to improve sensitivity or positive or negative predictive values.

CT scan with intravenous of radio-opaque contrast is useful in evaluation of muscle perfusion and mass. However, CT has lower contrast resolution than MRI and is less useful in evaluation of myositis. However, in the emergency department, it is helpful in the detection of calcification and diagnosis of pyomyositis.

Imaging may also be used to identify malignancies that are known to occur in close association with polymyositis, dermatomyositis, and immune-mediated necrotizing myopathy. While the utility of "pan-scanning" is currently unknown, most experts recommend imaging of the ovaries by transvaginal ultrasound due to the over-representation of ovarian carcinoma in dermatomyositis and polymyositis. In addition, colonoscopy is recommended for patients over the age of 50, and perhaps should be done in all adult patients (regardless of age) in whom immune-mediated myopathy was recently diagnosed. Finally, a CT scan of the chest is indicated to rule out pulmonary involvement and can also serve as malignancy surveillance when iodinated contrast is used.

D. Special Tests

Nerve conduction tests and EMG play a critical role in the evaluation of neuromuscular diseases and can aid in determining whether a patient with weakness has a defect of the anterior horn cell, nerve, neuromuscular junction, or muscle. In patients with only autoimmune myopathy, the sensory nerve tests should be normal and the motor nerve tests should be normal or, in very severe cases, notable only for decreased compound muscle action potentials. In patients with myopathy, EMG reveals the early recruitment of small polyphasic motor unit potentials. In those with active disease resulting in myofiber necrosis, abnormal insertional and spontaneous activity (ie, fibrillations and positive sharp waves) are frequently observed. When spontaneous activity occurs in the context of myopathic motor units, a patient is said to have an irritable myopathy. While classically found in dermatomyositis, polymyositis, and immune-mediated necrotizing myopathy, an irritable myopathy on EMG is not specific for autoimmune muscle disease and can be found in many other myopathic conditions.

Except perhaps in patients with the pathognomonic skin features of dermatomyositis, muscle biopsy should be performed in the initial evaluation of all patients in whom autoimmune myopathy is suspected. Ideally, the muscle selected for biopsy should be clinically affected, but not so weak that the study is likely to reveal only end-stage muscle. In general, a deltoid or biceps muscle with 4/5 strength would be well-suited to biopsy. One of the quadriceps muscles is also frequently selected for biopsy. Since the muscle pathology may be patchy and all of the quadriceps muscles may not be involved, muscle MRI may help guide biopsy to the rectus medialis, rectus femoris, or rectus lateralis muscles. In instances where MRI is not available, EMG may be used to guide muscle biopsy. However, the contralateral muscle should be selected given that biopsy of a recently needled muscle may show iatrogenic muscle damage, which could theoretically be mistaken for some other process.

Except for the presence of perifascicular atrophy, which is pathognomonic for dermatomyositis, the autoimmune myopathies do not have specific features on muscle biopsy. Nonetheless, muscle biopsies revealing perivascular inflammation and complement deposition on endomysial capillaries is suggestive of dermatomyositis. Similarly, in patients with polymyositis, muscle biopsies classically show non-necrotic muscle fibers surrounded and invaded by cytolytic CD8+ T cells (although this can also be seen in non–immune-mediated myopathies). The presence of myofibers expressing MHC I on cell surface is more specific for polymyositis, particularly if the fibers are found distant from sites of inflammation. In some patients with myopathy, the muscle biopsy reveals abundant regenerating, degenerating, and necrotic muscle fibers with scanty lymphocytic infiltration. These patients may have one of the immune-mediated necrotizing myopathies, polymyositis, or dermatomyositis in which the inflammation was missed due to sampling error, a toxic myopathy, or a muscular dystrophy.

Although the muscle biopsy may not by itself be used to definitively diagnose polymyositis or immune-mediated necrotizing myopathy, it is still essential for ruling out the presence of another myopathic process.

▶ Differential Diagnosis

Distinguishing patients with an autoimmune myopathy from those with a non-autoimmune process is crucial since only the former have muscle weakness that improves significantly with immunosuppression. Patients with proximal muscle weakness, Gottron sign, or a heliotrope rash are extraordinarily unlikely to have a disease other than dermatomyositis. However, in the absence of a classic dermatomyositis skin rash, the differential diagnosis for a myopathic process is extensive and includes muscular dystrophy, congenital myopathy, metabolic myopathy, mitochondrial myopathy, myotonic dystrophy, inclusion body myositis, and dermatomyositis without skin involvement (ie, dermatomyositis sine myositis). A diagnosis of polymyositis or immune-mediated necrotizing myopathy can only be entertained when the possibility of each of these other diseases has been excluded by careful consideration of the history, physical examination findings, laboratory results, EMG, and muscle biopsy findings.

A number of features from the patient's history should suggest the possibility of a diagnosis other than an autoimmune myopathy. First, patients who report a slowly progressive decline over years are unlikely to have immune-mediated disease, which tends to present over weeks to months. However, the converse is not necessarily true; some patients with long-standing muscle disease may not notice weakness until the disease reaches an advanced stage. Second, since autoimmune myopathy is not hereditary, a family history significant for another family member with "polymyositis" strongly suggests both subjects have one of the hereditary myopathies. Third, exercise-induced cramping should suggest the possibility of a metabolic myopathy. Finally, the lack of markedly improved muscle strength with aggressive immunosuppressive therapy should always raise doubts about a diagnosis of an autoimmune process. Importantly, improved CK levels should not be misinterpreted as a positive response since glucocorticoids may dramatically reduce serum CK levels even in patients with non–immune-mediated myopathies.

As discussed above, patients with one of the autoimmune myopathies usually have symmetric proximal muscle weakness. Unless the proximal muscle weakness is unusually severe, patients with autoimmune myopathy rarely have distal weakness; in general, a non–immune-mediated muscle disease should be suspected in patients with wrist and finger weakness or who cannot walk on their heels (requiring normal ankle dorsiflexion strength) or toes (requiring normal ankle plantar flexion strength). Similarly, a noticeable asymmetry in strength between the same muscle groups should raise doubts about a diagnosis of dermatomyositis or polymyositis. The facial muscles should be examined carefully, since these are not typically weak in the autoimmune myopathies. Finally, the presence of scapular winging should always be assessed and, if found, initiate a search for one of the genetic muscular dystrophies associated with this feature (Table 27–3).

The myositis-specific autoantibodies are found in ~60% of patients with an autoimmune myopathy and are rarely, if ever, found in patients with other neuromuscular conditions. Consequently, the presence of a myositis-specific antibody is diagnostically very useful. However, not all patients with an autoimmune process have a known myositis-specific antibody, tests for all of the myositis-specific antibodies are not readily commercially available, and it may take weeks to receive results of specialized autoantibody testing.

Electrophysiologic studies play a key role in distinguishing myopathic processes from neuropathic processes. In patients with active, untreated myositis, EMG usually reveals an irritable myopathy, but this is not specific for immune-mediated myopathies. Furthermore, many patients with

Table 27–3. Myopathies associated with scapular winging.

Dystrophies
Facioscapulohumeral dystrophy
Limb-girdle muscular dystrophy (LGMD)
LGMD2A (calpain-3)
LGMD 2E (α-sarcoglycan)
LGMD 2I (fukutin gene related peptide)
LGMD 2N (POMT2)
Emery-Dreifuss muscular dystrophy
Scapuloperoneal syndromes (eg, centronuclear myopathy)
Other neuromuscular conditions
Hereditary inclusion body myositis type 2
Distal spinal muscular atrophy type 4

Table 27–4. Myopathies that may have inflammation on muscle biopsy.

Autoimmune myopathies
Polymyositis
Dermatomyositis
Inclusion body myositis
Muscular dystrophies
Dystrophinopathies (eg, Duchenne and Becker muscular dystrophy)
Facioscapulohumeral dystrophy
Limb-girdle muscular dystrophy 2A (calpainopathy)
Limb-girdle muscular dystrophy 2B (dysferlinopathy)

partially-treated myositis have a non-irritable myopathy on EMG. Certain findings on EMG strongly suggest an alternative diagnosis. For example, the majority of patients with myotonic dystrophy have characteristic myotonic discharges.

In the absence of definitive dermatomyositis skin findings (ie, a heliotrope rash or Gottron sign), the muscle biopsy is an essential part of the diagnostic evaluation for any patient in whom an immune-mediated myopathy is suspected. When perifascicular atrophy is observed, a diagnosis of dermatomyositis sine dermatitis can be made even in the absence of rash. However, although inflammatory cell infiltrates are characteristic of polymyositis and dermatomyositis muscle biopsies, their presence is not specific for immune-mediated muscle disease. Rather, abundant inflammatory cells can be found in inclusion body myositis and several of the most common muscular dystrophies (Table 27–4). Certain features of the muscle biopsy (discussed below) should prompt an evaluation for a non–immune-mediated process.

A. Inclusion Body Myositis

Inclusion body myositis is a slowly progressive myopathic process that responds poorly, if at all, to immunosuppressive therapy. The typical pattern of muscle involvement includes prominent—and often *asymmetric*—weakness of the triceps, wrist flexors, distal finger flexors, quadriceps, and ankle dorsiflexors. Obicularis occuli weakness is rarely noticed by the patient but can frequently be detected by the careful examiner. Dysphagia is another typical feature of inclusion body myositis. Although hip flexor weakness can occur, deltoid weakness is less common and usually less profound than the triceps and finger flexor weakness.

Although the underlying pathologic mechanisms remain obscure, it is unlikely that inclusion body myositis is primarily an immune-mediated process. Rather, accumulating evidence suggests that inclusion body myositis may predominantly be a myodegenerative disease characterized by the abnormal intracellular accumulation of proteins such as beta amyloid, phosphorylated tau, and TDP-43.

Routine muscle biopsy classically reveals not only primary inflammation as seen in polymyositis, but red-rimmed vacuoles on the Gomori trichrome stain, which can be helpful in distinguishing inclusion body myositis from polymyositis. However, in many patients with clinical features of inclusion body myositis, no rimmed-vacuoles are found, even on repeat muscle biopsy. Indeed, a recent study showed that more than one third of patients with primary inflammation and no rimmed vacuoles had the typical clinical features of inclusion body myositis. Because of the overlapping biopsy features, inclusion body myositis is very frequently misdiagnosed and treated as polymyositis. Only a very careful physical examination allows the clinician to distinguish between inclusion body myositis and one of the immune-mediated myopathies for which aggressive immunosuppressive therapy may be warranted.

B. Facioscapulohumeral Dystrophy

Facioscapulohumeral dystrophy is an autosomal-dominant muscular dystrophy. With an incidence of about 4 per million and a prevalence of about 50 per million, facioscapulohumeral dystrophy is the second most common adult-onset muscular dystrophy and is roughly just as common as polymyositis or dermatomyositis in the general population.

Although it may go unnoticed, facial weakness is present in most patients by the age of 30. If asked, patients may admit to difficulty using straws, blowing up balloons, and whistling. On examination, a transverse smile is characteristic. In many cases, patients do not seek medical attention until they are disabled by weakness of the scapular or humeral (especially biceps) muscles. There is often asymmetric involvement and patients may complain that 1 arm became weak long before the other. On examination, scapular winging and relative sparing of the deltoids (observed when the scapula is manually fixed to the chest wall by the examiner) are typical. As the disease progresses, proximal and distal muscles (especially the tibialis anterior [used for walking on heels]) may become weak as well. Laboratory features include a CK in the normal to ~1000 international units/L range and a myopathic EMG. Because genetic testing can usually establish the diagnosis of facioscapulohumeral dystrophy, muscle biopsy is rarely necessary when patients see a clinician who is familiar with this disease. However, ~2–5% of patients with the facioscapulohumeral dystrophy phenotype may have an unusual mutation leading to a false-negative genetic test. When performed, muscle biopsies can sometimes reveal an inflammatory myopathy, occasionally leading to the misdiagnosis of polymyositis, especially when the genetic testing is normal. Unnecessary and potentially harmful treatment can be avoided by recognizing that the patient with a combination of facial weakness and scapular winging is exceedingly unlikely to have an autoimmune myopathy.

C. Limb-Girdle Muscular Dystrophy (LGMD)

The limb-girdle muscular dystrophies are a heterogenous collection of disorders that can be inherited in either an autosomal-dominant (LGMD 1A through LGMD 1H) or autosomal-recessive (LGMD 2A through LGMD 2N) fashion. Because they may present in early adulthood without a family history and with symmetric proximal muscle weakness, markedly elevated muscle enzymes, an irritable myopathy on EMG, and an inflammatory muscle biopsy, LGMD 2A (due to mutations in the gene for calpain-3) and LGMD 2B (due to mutations in the dysferlin gene) are frequently misdiagnosed as polymyositis. Indeed, a recent report showed that 25% of genetically confirmed cases of LGMD 2B were initially treated for polymyositis because of the presence of inflammatory infiltrates, sometimes in previously physically active patients with rapid progression. However, certain clinical characteristics should raise suspicion and lead to genetic testing for these forms of LGMD. This includes scapular winging, which is found in ~80% of LGMD 2A patients, and ankle plantar flexion weakness (difficulty standing on tiptoe), which is found in many patients with LGMD 2B. Finally, a diagnosis of LGMD should be considered in any patient with "refractory polymyositis."

D. Metabolic Myopathy

The metabolic myopathies are autosomal recessive and X-linked disorders that can be separated into abnormalities of carbohydrate, lipid, and adenine nucleotide metabolism.

1. Disorders of carbohydrate metabolism—There are 14 different enzyme mutations associated with disorders of carbohydrate metabolism (Table 27–5). Six of these present only in infancy or early childhood. Of the remainder, 3 can present in adulthood with exercise intolerance but are not associated with weakness. Three may present in adulthood with exercise-induced cramping and, rarely, static weakness; these include patients with defects in (1) amylo-1,4,-1 6-transglucosidase (ie, branching enzyme deficiency), (2) myophosphorylase (ie, McCardle disease), and (3) phosphorylase b kinase. Since fixed weakness is uncommon and muscle biopsies reveal characteristic glycogen accumulation without inflammation, these disorders are unlikely to be confused with the autoimmune myopathies. Patients with debranching enzyme deficiency may have generalized muscle weakness but more often also have significant distal muscle weakness; muscle biopsies reveal glycogen containing vacuoles with no inflammation. Each of these enzyme deficiencies can be detected by performing the appropriate commercially available enzyme analysis on frozen muscle specimens.

In patients with adult-onset acid maltase deficiency (Pompe disease), proximal muscle weakness, which can mimic one of the immune-mediated myopathies, develops. The diaphragm is often markedly affected and respiratory failure is the presenting feature in some patients with this disease. Although muscle biopsies may reveal glycogen-filled vacuoles, sometimes only nonspecific changes, such as necrotic and regenerating muscle fibers, are found. Therefore, when patients have an autoantibody-negative necrotizing myopathy, it is prudent to perform a dried bloodspot enzyme analysis to rule-out the possibility of Pompe disease. This is important not only to

Table 27–5. Disorders of carbohydrate metabolism.

	Enzyme Defect	Adult presentation?	Fixed weakness?
Type I	Glucose-6-phosphate	N	N
Type II (Pompe disease)	Acid α-1,4-glucosidase	Y	Y
Type III (Cori-Forbes disease)	Amylo-1,6-glucosidase (Debrancher)	Y	Y
Type IV (Anderson disease)	Amylo-1,4-1,6-transglucosidase (Brancher)	Y	Y
Type V (McCardle disease)	Myophosphorylase	Y	Y
Type VI	Liver phosphorylase	N	N
Type VII	Phosphofructokinase	N	Y
Type VIII	Phosphorylase b kinase	Y	Y
Type IX	Phosphoglycerate kinase	N	Y
Type X	Phosphoglycerate mutase	Y	N
Type XI	Lactate dehydrogenase	Y	N
Type XII	Aldolase	N	Y
Type XIII	Trioesphosphate isomerase	N	Y
Type XIV	β-enolase	Y	N

avoid unnecessary immunosuppressive treatment, but also because some patients with adult-onset Pompe disease may be eligible for enzyme replacement therapy.

2. Disorders of lipid metabolism—Defects affecting both lipid metabolism and the transport of long-chain fatty acids can cause myopathy as well as affecting other organ systems. **Carnitine transporter deficiency** can present in early adulthood with progressive proximal muscle weakness and cardiomyopathy. Muscle biopsy reveals abnormal lipid accumulation when the appropriate stain, such as Sudan black or an oil red O stain, is performed. In some patients, oral L-carnitine treatment may be beneficial.

Carnitine palmitoyltransferase 2 deficiency is an autosomal recessive disorder that can present in young adults with myalgias and exercise-induced myoglobinuria. CK levels, muscle strength, and routine muscle biopsies may be normal between episodes of rhabdomyolysis. In suspected cases, carnitine palmitoyltransferase 2 enzyme deficiency can be assessed in frozen muscle tissue and the presence of mutations confirmed by genetic testing.

Very-long chain acyl-CoA dehydrogenase deficiency can also present with exercise-induced myoglobinuria and muscle pain. CK is normal between attacks of rhabdomyolysis and muscle biopsies may be normal or show abnormal lipid deposits. The diagnosis can be confirmed by genetic testing.

E. Mitochondrial Myopathy

Defects in mitochondrial oxidative phosphorylation can cause muscle dysfunction but the clinical picture is frequently dominated by other organ systems including the central nervous system and heart. Patients with **myoclonic epilepsy and ragged red fibers** may present in adulthood with myopathy accompanied by myoclonus, seizures, ataxia, dementia, hearing loss, and optic atrophy. **Kearns-Sayre syndrome** occasionally presents in young adults with myopathy associated with progressive external ophthalmoplegia, pigmentary retinopathy, cardiomyopathy, or endocrinopathies. Sometimes **progressive external ophthalmoplegia** presents with limb weakness. **Mitochondrial neurogastrointestinal encephalopathy** can present with a variety of clinical manifestations, sometimes including distal greater than proximal muscle weakness. Muscle biopsies from each of these entities are characterized by evidence of mitochondrial dysfunction, including the presence of ragged red fibers on Gomori trichrome stain or increased staining for succinic dehydrogenase (encoded by nuclear DNA) in the context of reduced staining for cytochrome oxidase (encoded by mitochondrial DNA). Given the other organ system involvement and lack of inflammation on muscle biopsy, mitochondrial myopathies should rarely be misdiagnosed as one of the immune-mediated myopathies.

▶ Treatment

Given that the current understanding of the pathogenesis of the immune-mediated myopathies centers around an overactive immune system leading to inflammation that causes muscle damage, the mainstay of therapy focuses on control of inflammation through immunosuppression. Goals of therapy include increasing muscle strength, controlling pain, enabling patients to manage their activities of daily living, as well as improving their quality of life. Few randomized clinical trials exist on effective therapies, and current therapeutic regimens, especially in resistant disease, are based on expert opinion and clinical experience. Serum CK concentrations may decrease without parallel improvements in strength, and vice versa. Thus, improvement in strength, function, and skin manifestations (in the case of dermatomyositis) should be the primary goal of therapy. The usefulness of monitoring serum CK levels may be helpful as an indicator of possible flare, although trend in CK levels alone should not be used as the sole measure of the efficacy of therapy.

A. Glucocorticoids

Prednisone is generally used as the empiric first-line therapy. In general, prednisone should be started at 1–2 mg/kg/day (or equivalent dose is used) to control acute disease, and then it is tapered after 3–4 weeks, depending on level of clinical improvement. Tapering to the lowest effective dose is preferred in order to reduce comorbidities associated with glucocorticoid therapy. Retrospective studies have demonstrated effectiveness in reducing mortality, improving muscle strength and function with use of prednisone as well as short courses of intravenous methylprednisolone. Elevations in serum CK levels in addition to clinical deterioration in strength and function may indicate that glucocorticoids are being tapered too quickly or that additional immunosuppression should be used. Concomitant glucocorticoid-sparing immunosuppressive therapy is warranted in most adults with immune-mediated myopathy. Indicators that additional immunosuppressants are required include the following: (1) patients are experiencing complications from long-term glucocorticoid use, (2) the inability to taper glucocorticoid dose without precipitating a myositis flare, (3) ineffectiveness after 2–3 months of therapy, and (4) rapidly progressive disease with respiratory failure. Patients taking high-dose prednisone (ie, >20 mg/day) are at significantly increased risk for *Pneumocystis jiroveci* (previously called *Pneumocystis carinii*) infection and should receive prophylaxis until the glucocorticoid dose can be tapered. Vitamin D and calcium supplementation should be used in patients who are taking 5 mg of glucocorticoid therapy for more than 3 months to prevent bone loss, especially in postmenopausal women.

B. Glucocorticoid-Sparing Immunosuppressive Medications

Usually used in addition to glucocorticoids, immunosuppressive medications have been shown to be effective in some studies, although their use remains largely empiric. In general, methotrexate and azathioprine are the first-line of glucocorticoid-sparing drugs to be used.

C. Methotrexate

There have not been any randomized, prospective clinical trials of the use of methotrexate that have demonstrated effectiveness in myositis, but several retrospective trials suggest that a majority of patients with dermatomyositis and polymyositis have responded to treatment. One potential side effect of methotrexate therapy is pneumonitis, which may be difficult to differentiate from the interstitial lung disease seen in patients with antisynthetase syndromes; thus, methotrexate is used with caution in this subset of patients. Often, azathioprine is the preferred choice in this instance.

D. Azathioprine

One clinical trial of azathioprine in addition to prednisone showed no improvements in strength or histologic findings but showed a significant improvement in serum CK levels when compared with patients receiving prednisone alone. However, several retrospective studies suggest that azathioprine may be effective, with some beneficial response seen in 64% of patients with polymyositis and dermatomyositis, although complete response only occurred in 11% of patients. Patients who were previously responsive to glucocorticoids tend to respond better to the addition of azathioprine, when compared with those who had poor response to glucocorticoids alone.

E. Cyclophosphamide

Use of cyclophosphamide has shown mixed results, with some case reports indicating positive improvements in patients with severe polymyositis, although this could not be replicated in other studies. It is probably best reserved for severe interstitial lung disease or myopathy nonresponsive to other immunosuppressants. Interstitial cystitis occurs in up to one third of patients taking the drug orally. This complication can be reduced by administering cyclophosphamide intravenously; however, efficacy of this route of administration is unclear in the immune-mediated myopathies.

F. Mycophenolate Mofetil

Mycophenolate mofetil has shown some benefit in patients with polymyositis and dermatomyositis who have been resistant to other therapies. It has shown some benefit for dermatomyositis-related skin disease.

G. Rituximab

The monoclonal antibody rituximab has also been looked at as a potential option, although with mixed results. Rituximab appears to be helpful in dermatomyositis as well as resistant SRP-related myopathy.

H. Intravenous Immunoglobulin (IVIG)

One trial of IVIG in glucocorticoid-resistant polymyositis and dermatomyositis demonstrated significant improvements in strength, function, and CK levels. However, adverse reactions were seen in 43% of patients, although none required hospitalization. IVIG has been shown to be successful in mitigating the pathologic changes seen on repeated muscle biopsy as well as improving strength in patients with dermatomyositis.

I. Exercise and Supplements

While exercise was once discouraged, it has become increasingly clear that maintaining daily exercise is beneficial in all stages of the disease to help maintain and restore normal function. Patients may benefit from formal physical therapy. Isometric exercises are recommended, while heavy weight lifting is discouraged. When supplemented with creatine, exercise may further improve function over exercise alone. Thus, a moderate exercise routine can be beneficial in patients with polymyositis and dermatomyositis without increased rates of myositis flares or injury.

▶ Complications

Major complications that develop in patients with inflammatory muscle diseases are most often seen in patients in whom the diagnosis, and thus therapy, was delayed or in patients with refractory disease. Persistent or progressive muscle weakness can result in the permanent muscle damage leading to atrophy. These patients may become wheelchair-dependent. Patients with dysphagia or dysphonia are at risk for aspiration pneumonia. Those with interstitial lung disease may progress to respiratory failure due to worsening end-stage fibrosis. Cardiomyopathy with congestive heart failure can develop in the few patients with cardiac involvement.

Complications can also result from therapy. Most notable are the side effects and toxicities of glucocorticoid use. Although patients treated with these agents can manifest all of the features of iatrogenic Cushing syndrome (including central obesity, hypertension, hyperhidrosis, "moon facies," striae, and hirsutism), 2 of the more troubling complications are opportunistic infections and glucocorticoid-induced proximal muscle weakness. Opportunistic pulmonary infections such as *P jiroveci* pneumonia can be rapidly fatal.

Glucocorticoid-associated myopathy can be particularly frustrating because it can complicate the course of a patient who is getting stronger in response to therapy. Clinically, this is often observed in patients who show improvement with glucocorticoid therapy and then suddenly plateau or deteriorate. In this setting, it is difficult to determine whether the decrease in muscle strength is due to disease flare or glucocorticoid toxicity. Other well-known glucocorticoid-related toxicities include cataracts, acne, emotional lability, hyperlipidemia (especially hypertriglyceridemia), and osteopenia/osteoporosis. Finally, malignancy is a concern in long-term immunosuppression with all agents currently used to treat autoimmune inflammatory diseases, such the autoimmune myopathies.

Bushby K. Diagnosis and management of the limb girdle muscular dystrophies. *Pract Neurol.* 2009;9:314. [PMID: 19923111]

Greenberg SA. Theories of the pathogenesis of inclusion body myositis. *Curr Rheumatol Rep.* 2010;12:221. [PMID: 20425523]

Gunawardena H, Betteridge ZE, McHugh NJ. Myositis-specific autoantibodies: their clinical and pathogenic significance in disease expression. *Rheumatology (Oxford).* 2009;48:607. [PMID: 19439503]

[International Myositis Assessment and Clinical Studies Group] https://dir-apps.niehs.nih.gov/imacs/index.cfm

Mammen AL. Dermatomyositis and polymyositis: Clinical presentation, autoantibodies, and pathogenesis. *Ann N Y Acad Sci.* 2010;1184:134. [PMID: 20146695]

Mammen AL, Chung T, Christopher-Stine L, Rosen P, Rosen A, Casciola-Rosen LA.

Autoantibodies against 3-hydroxy-3-methylglutaryl-coenzyme A reductase (HMGCR) in patients with statin-associated autoimmune myopathy. *Arthritis Rheum.* 2010 Nov 19 [Epub ahead of print]. [PMID: 21104722]

[The Johns Hopkins Myositis Center] http://www.hopkinsmedicine.org/myositis/

[The Myositis Association] http://www.myositis.org

Tomasova Studynkova J, Charvat F, Jarosova K, Vencovsky J. The role of MRI in the assessment of polymyositis and dermatomyositis. *Rheumatology (Oxford).* 2007;46:1174. [PMID: 17500079]

[Washington University Neuromuscular Disease Center] http://www.neuro.wustl.edu/neuromuscular/index.html

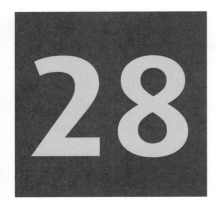

Relapsing Polychondritis

John H. Stone, MD, MPH

▶ Auricular chondritis (spares the earlobe).

▶ Inflammation in other cartilaginous areas (eg, the nose, joints, trachea, ribcage, and airways) and in tissues rich in proteoglycans, such as the eyes and heart valves.

▶ Frequently associated with an underlying disorder such as systemic vasculitis, connective tissue disease, or myelodysplastic syndrome.

▶ General Considerations

Relapsing polychondritis (RP) is an immune-mediated condition associated with inflammation in cartilaginous structures and other connective tissues throughout the body, including the ears, nose, joints, respiratory tract, and others. The incidence of RP is estimated to be approximately 3.5 cases/million people. Thirty percent of RP cases occur in association with another disease, usually some form of systemic vasculitis (particularly granulomatosis with polyangiitis [formerly Wegener granulomatosis]), connective tissue disorder (eg, rheumatoid arthritis or systemic lupus erythematosus), or a myelodysplastic syndrome. RP is often assumed to be "autoimmune" in nature, but the evidence for a true autoimmune pathogenesis is relatively weak. Some patients have been reported to have antibodies to type 2 collagen, but these assays are not widely available and their poor sensitivities and specificities make them inappropriate for general clinical use. In general, a cartilage biopsy is not required to make the diagnosis. Rather, the identification of cartilaginous inflammation in typical areas (auricular cartilage, nasal bridge, costochondral joints) and the exclusion of other possible causes suffice.

RP is associated with a broad range of clinical courses. One end of the disease spectrum includes intermittent bouts of auricular cartilage inflammation that respond quickly to treatment. The other end is characterized by widespread, aggressive cartilaginous inflammation that leads to serious end-organ complications. The greatest clinical challenge is identifying the presence of cartilaginous inflammation and instituting effective therapy before irreparable damage occurs in the involved organs.

▶ Clinical Findings

Table 28–1 lists the major clinical manifestations of RP.

A. Symptoms and Signs

1. Ears—Unilateral or bilateral auricular chondritis is often the first disease symptom (Figure 28-1). The onset of auricular inflammation is usually quite abrupt and not subtle. The inflammation may be confused with cellulitis of the ear or even sunburn in more minor cases. A major clue to the diagnosis of RP is confinement of the inflammation to the auricular part of the ear, with sparing of the earlobe. The cartilaginous portions of the ears are erythematous and tender to touch. Swelling of the external ear canal may cause conductive hearing loss. RP may also be associated with sensorineural hearing loss, the mechanism of which remains obscure (vasculitis is often implicated, without proof).

2. Nose—Inflammation of the nasal cartilage leads to tenderness of the nasal bridge and often to epistaxis. In severe cases, "saddle-nose" deformities develop through collapse of the nasal bridge (see Figure 32-1). This is usually preceded by the development of a nasal septal perforation.

3. Trachea—Subglottic stenosis results from tracheal inflammation and scarring inferior to the vocal cords. Early subglottic involvement often has minimal symptoms and may manifest itself as only subtle changes in voice. Thickening of the tracheal wall may be evident on computed tomography (CT) scanning. With time, however, substantial airway scarring may occur, leading to potentially life-threatening

Table 28–1. Major clinical manifestations of relapsing polychondritis.

Feature Data	Data
Mean age at diagnosis	47 years
Auricular chondritis	90%
Reduced hearing	37%
Nasal chondritis	60%
Saddle-nose deformities	25%
Laryngotracheal involvement	52%
Ocular inflammation	54%
Arthritis	69%
Skin involvement	25%
Aortic or mitral regurgitation	8%
Vasculitis	12%

Data from Molina JF, Espinoza LR. Relapsing polychondritis. *Baillieres Best Pract Res Clin Rheumatol.* 2000;14:97.

tracheal narrowing. In addition to the subglottic region, other parts of the tracheal wall may be softened by cartilaginous inflammation, leading to a tendency of the airway to collapse. Tracheal inflammation may be associated with tenderness to palpation of the anterior cervical trachea, the thyroid cartilage, and larynx.

4. Bronchi and airways—Cartilaginous inflammation may extend to the lower respiratory tract, with bronchial involvement. This manifestation, unlike the tracheal disease, may have a lengthy subclinical period but is usually detectable by investigations such as pulmonary function testing or CT scanning. RP may mimic bronchial asthma. Lower airway disease and its associated mucociliary dysfunction may heighten patients' susceptibility to infections.

5. Eyes—Nearly any part of the eye may be involved in RP. Scleritis causes photophobia and painful, often raised, scleral erythema. If unchecked, necrotizing scleritis may lead to scleral thinning (Plate 45), scleromalacia perforans, and visual loss. Peripheral keratitis may cause ulcerations on the margin of the cornea and lead to the syndrome of "corneal melt." Episcleritis and conjunctivitis are very common in RP. Extraocular involvement may include periorbital edema, chemosis, and proptosis.

6. Heart—Cartilaginous inflammation within the heart valve rings may lead to valvular dysfunction. The usual lesions are aortic and mitral regurgitation; aortic valve disease is more common. The proximity of the conduction system to some areas of valve ring inflammation may lead to cardiac conduction abnormalities. Pericarditis and rare cases of coronary arteritis have also been described in RP.

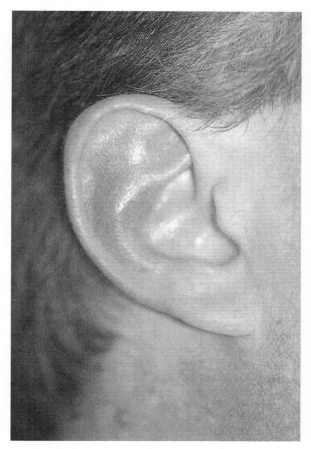

▲ **Figure 28–1.** Auricular chondritis in a patient with relapsing polychondritis. Note the sparing of the earlobe (a noncartilaginous portion of the ear).

7. Joints—Articular lesions are often the first nonspecific manifestation of RP. The pattern of joint involvement at presentation is typically an intermittent, migratory oligoarthritis, but symmetric polyarticular presentations are also seen. In general, the arthritis associated with RP is nondestructive, unless there is underlying rheumatoid arthritis. Joint symptoms tend to correlate well with activity of disease at other sites.

8. Skin—Patients with RP may demonstrate a panoply of cutaneous lesions, none of which is specific for the disorder. Cutaneous findings are particularly common in cases of RP that are associated with myelodysplasia but occur frequently in other cases as well. Among patients with primary RP, the most common skin findings are aphthous ulcers, nodules (erythema nodosum–like lesions), purpura, papules, and sterile pustules. The cutaneous lesions of RP may resemble those of Behçet syndrome. An overlap condition known as the MAGIC syndrome, comprising **m**outh **a**nd **g**enital ulcers with **i**nflamed **c**artilage, has been described.

9. Kidneys—Renal lesions in RP range from pauci-immune glomerulonephritis to mild mesangial expansion and cellular proliferation. Distinguishing RP from granulomatosis with polyangiitis is difficult in the setting of pauci-immune glomerulonephritis.

B. Laboratory Findings

There are no specific laboratory findings in RP. Mild normochromic, normocytic anemias, and mild degrees of thrombocytosis may be observed. Major cytopenias should trigger suspicion of myelodysplasia. Mild to moderate elevations of acute phase reactants are expected. Antinuclear antibodies and rheumatoid factor are usually negative, and complement levels are normal. In the setting of antineutrophil cytoplasmic antibody (ANCA) positivity, granulomatosis with polyangiitis must be suspected, particularly if the antibody specificity is to either proteinase-3 or myeloperoxidase.

C. Imaging Studies

CT scans are useful in the evaluation of airway disease. CT findings in RP include edema, wall thickening, granulation tissue, and fibrosis. Thin-cut CT scans of the trachea are sensitive means of evaluating subglottic stenosis. In some cases of subglotting narrowing, however, direct visualization with fiberoptic laryngoscopy is required to make the diagnosis.

D. Special Tests

1. Biopsy—Given the proper constellation of clinical symptoms and signs, tissue biopsy is rarely required to establish the diagnosis of RP. Biopsy may be important, however, in the exclusion of RP mimickers. In contrast to granulomatosis with polyangiitis, RP is not associated with granulomatous inflammation. Biopsy of the trachea or larynx should be performed only with great caution because acute airway narrowing may result from additional damage to already compromised tissues.

2. Pulmonary function tests—Full sets of pulmonary function tests, including inspiratory and expiratory flow-volume loops, are useful in RP. Patterns consistent with either extrathoracic or intrathoracic obstruction (or both) may occur in RP. Pulmonary function tests (flow-volume loops) provide a useful noninvasive means of quantifying and following the degree of extrathoracic airway obstruction.

▶ Differential Diagnosis

Aural chondritis is often confused initially with infectious processes, particularly cellulitis of the ear. Other infections in the differential diagnosis include tuberculous laryngitis, now rare in developed countries. The differential diagnosis

of nasal inflammation (often accompanied by saddle-nose deformity) is quite short, including granulomatosis with polyangiitis, Crohn disease, syphilis, leprosy, lymphoma, and leishmaniasis.

"Pure" RP must be distinguished from RP associated with an underlying condition because the complications of the underlying disorder may greatly affect the patient's prognosis. The major underlying disorders of concern are systemic vasculitides, connective tissue diseases, and myelodysplastic syndromes.

▶ Treatment

Glucocorticoids are the treatment of choice for reducing major inflammation in cartilaginous areas. In order to limit glucocorticoid exposure, dapsone, colchicine, and nonsteroidal anti-inflammatory drugs have all been used empirically. For patients with sustained disease, however, methotrexate is the most commonly used glucocorticoid-sparing agent. Cyclophosphamide is required for glomerulonephritis and other disease manifestations that are refractory to glucocorticoid alone.

In the case of airway disease, it is essential to distinguish dysfunction secondary to active cartilaginous inflammation from that caused by damage from previously active disease.

The management of upper airway problems in RP requires collaboration with an experienced otolaryngologist or pulmonologist or both. Some upper airway disease manifestations (eg, subglottic stenosis) respond better to mechanical interventions and glucocorticoid injections than to systemic therapies. Stenting may also be required for cases in which the tracheal or bronchial walls have lost their integrity, provided that the regions of tracheomalacia or bronchomalacia are not too long. Continuous positive airway pressure may help some patients during sleep.

▶ Complications

Prolonged or repeated bouts of aural chondritis may lead to deformation of the ear cartilage and "cauliflower ear" (Plate 46). Similarly, nasal chondritis may cause nasal septal perforation and "saddle-nose" deformities.

Tracheomalacia may lead to extrathoracic airway obstruction and sometimes requires tracheostomy. Collapsible airways may be associated with postobstructive infections. Cardiac valvular regurgitation in RP may lead to valve replacement.

Kemta Lekpa F, Kraus VB, Chevalier X. Biologics in Relapsing Polychondritis: A Literature Review. *Semin Arthritis Rheum.* 2011 Nov 7. [Epub ahead of print] [PMID: 22071463]

Marie I, Proux A, Duhaut P, et al. Long-term follow-up of aortic involvement in giant cell arteritis: a series of 48 patients. *Medicine (Baltimore).* 2009;88(3):182. [PMID: 19440121]

Introduction to Vasculitis: Classification & Clinical Clues

29

David B. Hellmann, MD, MACP

General Considerations

Vasculitis refers to a heterogeneous group of disorders that is characterized by inflammatory destruction of blood vessels. Inflamed blood vessels are liable to occlude or rupture or develop a thrombus, and thereby lose the ability to deliver oxygen and other nutrients to tissues and organs. Depending on the size, distribution, and severity of the affected vessels, vasculitis can result in clinical syndromes that vary in severity from a minor self-limited rash to a life-threatening multisystem disorder.

Because it often begins with nonspecific symptoms and signs and unfolds slowly over weeks or months, vasculitis is one of the great diagnostic challenges in all of medicine. Yet, physicians who know the general and specific clinical clues for vasculitis can often learn to suspect when vasculitis is present at the bedside. Establishing the diagnosis of vasculitis requires confirmation by laboratory tests, usually a biopsy of an involved artery but sometimes an angiogram or a serologic test.

Treating vasculitis has become as rewarding as establishing the diagnosis. In the absence of treatment, most patients with systemic vasculitis will suffer and die. With treatment, the vast majority of patients will improve, many will achieve remission, and a few will be cured.

Classification

Because the causes of most forms of vasculitis are not known, the vasculitides are classified according to their clinicopathologic features. Although no schema has been accepted universally, one frequently used classification system separates the vasculitides based first on whether the process is primary (ie, of unknown cause) or secondary to some other condition (eg, a connective tissue disease or infection). The vasculitides can then be further separated by the size of vessels usually affected—large-sized, medium-sized, or small-sized arteries (Table 29–1 and Figure 29–1). Finer distinctions among forms of vasculitis affecting the same size vessel can be made by other clinicopathologic characteristics. For example, Takayasu arteritis and giant cell arteritis are grouped together because they both can affect the aorta and other large arteries. However, they are distinguished from each other by their clinical differences, such as the age of onset. Takayasu arteritis is chiefly a disease of young women, while giant cell arteritis almost never occurs before age 50. To take another example, both granulomatosis with polyangiitis (formerly Wegener granulomatosis) and eosinophilic granulomatosis with polyangiitis (Churg-Strauss syndrome) affect small-sized vessels and are associated with antineutrophil cytoplasmic antibodies. But only Churg-Strauss syndrome is associated with asthma and striking levels of eosinophilia.

Although classification systems are useful in highlighting differences among the vasculitides, the arbitrary categories suggest neater lines of demarcation than nature always recognizes. Despite being classified as a form of primary, medium-vessel vasculitis, polyarteritis nodosa results from chronic hepatitis B or C infection in about 20% of cases and can affect small vessels. Until the causes of all forms of vasculitis are known, exceptions in the classification schema will be common.

Epidemiology

The epidemiology of individual forms of vasculitis is covered in the relevant chapters. In general, the vasculitides are relatively uncommon but not rare in Western countries: about 1 out of 2000 adults has some form of vasculitis, and each year vasculitis develops in approximately 1 in 7000 adults. In the United States, the most common forms of primary systemic vasculitis are giant cell arteritis, granulomatosis with polyangiitis (formerly Wegener granulomatosis), and microscopic polyangiitis (Table 29–2).

Table 29–1. Classification of the primary vasculitides: Major examples.

Large-artery vasculitis
  Giant cell arteritis
  Takayasu arteritis
  Cogan syndrome
Medium-vessel vasculitis
  Polyarteritis nodosa
  Primary central nervous system disease
  Buerger disease
Small-vessel vasculitis
  ANCA-associated small-vessel vasculitis
  • Granulomatosis with polyangiitis (formerly Wegener granulomatosis)
  • Microscopic polyangiitis
  • Churg-Strauss syndrome
  • Drug-induced ANCA-associated vasculitis
  Behçet disease
  Hypersensitivity vasculitis
  Urticarial vasculitis

ANCA, antineutrophil cytoplasmic antibody.

Table 29–2. Average annual incidence rates of different forms of vasculitis.

Form of Vasculitis	Incidence Per Million
Giant cell arteritis	170[a]
Granulomatosis with polyangiitis (formerly Wegener granulomatosis)	4-15
Polyarteritis nodosa	9
Microscopic polyangiitis	1-24
Takayasu arteritis	2

[a]Population 50 years of age or older.

▶ Pathophysiology

While the etiology of most forms of vasculitis is unknown, progress has been made in elucidating the humeral and cellular mechanisms that participate in inflammatory destruction of blood vessels. As is discussed in subsequent chapters, the pathogenic mechanisms vary among the different forms of vasculitis. For example, T cells appear important in the

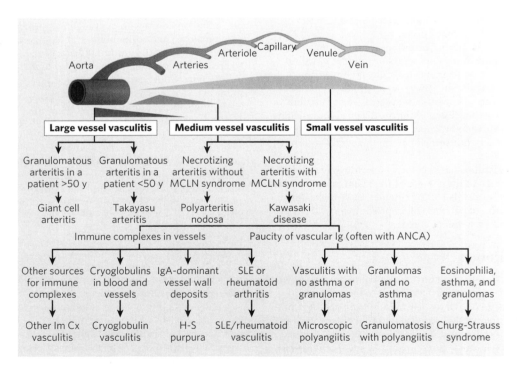

▲ **Figure 29–1.** Diagram illustrating the vascular distribution of major types of vasculitis. ANCA, antineutrophil cytoplasmic antibody; H-S purpura, Henoch-Schönlein purpura; Im Cx, immune complex; MCLN, mucocutaneous lymph node syndrome; SLE, systemic lupus erythematosus. (Modified, with permission, from Jennette JC, Falk FJ. Nosology of primary vasculitis. *Curr Opin Rheumatol.* 2007;19:10.)

pathogenesis of giant cell arteritis, complement activation in some forms of hypersensitivity vasculitis, and autoantibodies in vasculitis associated with antineutrophil cytoplasmic antibodies.

▶ Clinical Findings

Although the presenting manifestations of vasculitis are protean, they can be grouped into five categories of clinical clues (Table 29–3). The first general clue is that most forms of systemic vasculitis begin with constitutional symptoms (such as malaise, fever, sweats, fatigue, decreased appetite, and weight loss). These nonspecific symptoms, in the absence of more specific signs, usually effectively camouflage the vasculitic nature of the patient's illness. A second clue is that most forms of vasculitis unfold subacutely over weeks or months. In contrast to many patients with acute infections, patients with vasculitis usually cannot pinpoint the hour or the day that their illness began. More typically, patients with vasculitis struggle to define the month or the season in which their nonspecific symptoms accumulated sufficiently to become memorable. A corollary of the subacute course typical of vasculitis is that the initial diagnosis of vasculitis is rarely made (correctly) in the intensive care unit. Although pulmonary hemorrhage, bowel infarction, or other devastating complications of vasculitis frequently result in a patient being admitted to the intensive care unit, these catastrophic events usually develop late, weeks or months after other clinical clues have suggested or established the patient's diagnosis.

The tendency of most forms of vasculitis to produce striking signs of inflammation constitutes a third general clue. Manifestations of inflammation can include fever, arthritis, rash, pericarditis, anemia of chronic disease, or a markedly elevated erythrocyte sedimentation rate. Pain is a fourth common feature of the vasculitides and can originate from many different sources, such as arthritis; myalgia; or infarction of a digit, nerve, bowel, or testicle. The fifth general clinical clue is that vasculitis tends to cause multisystem disease. The skin, joints, nervous system, kidneys, lung, and gastrointestinal tract are especially favorite targets of many different forms of vasculitis. Although specific forms of vasculitis can defy generalization, most vasculitides start with constitutional symptoms that evolve over weeks and months to a painful disorder marked by signs of inflammation and multiorgan injury.

Table 29–3. General clinical clues suggesting the presence of systemic vasculitis.

1. Constitutional symptoms prominent
2. Subacute onset
3. Symptoms and signs of inflammation common
4. Pain common
5. Multisystem disease evident

A. Symptoms and Signs

The signs and symptoms of specific forms of vasculitis are detailed in the individual chapters. The signs and symptoms common to many forms of systemic vasculitis are found in Table 29–4.

In general, the skin and the peripheral nervous system signs are especially useful because they often develop early in the course of the disease and because they can be detected at the bedside. The onset of small-vessel vasculitis (eg, hepatitis C–associated vasculitis) is often heralded by palpable purpura, usually on the lower extremities, whereas medium-vessel diseases (eg, polyarteritis nodosa) more commonly produce nodules, ulcers, or digital gangrene.

The most characteristic nervous system manifestation of vasculitis is mononeuritis multiplex, which is defined as a distinctive peripheral neuropathy in which named peripheral nerves are infarcted one at a time. The nerve infarctions result from vasculitis of the vessels of the vasa nervorum, causing ischemia of a nerve. Clinically, the two features that characterize this neuropathy are the **asynchrony** and **asymmetry** of the symptoms and findings. These features are best illustrated by comparing mononeuritis multiplex with other peripheral neuropathies. With most forms of nonspecific neuropathy, the patient experiences numbness and tingling in a symmetric, stocking or glove distribution; these symptoms develop so slowly that the patient cannot accurately date the onset of the neuropathy. Examination of these patients usually fails to identify the involvement of large, named nerves. In sharp contrast, the onset of mononeuritis multiplex is strikingly memorable: The patient often recalls the day that his or her foot drop or wrist drop began. The patient also often vividly recalls how the neuropathy progressed asynchronously

Table 29–4. Organ- or tissue-specific manifestations of vasculitis.

Organ or Tissue	Manifestation
Skin	Livedo reticularis, palpable purpura, nodules, ulcers, gangrene
Peripheral nervous system	Mononeuritis multiplex, polyneuropathy
Central nervous system	Stroke, seizure, encephalopathy
Kidney	Hypertension, proteinuria, hematuria, renal failure
Heart	Myocardial infarction, cardiomyopathy, pericarditis, arrhythmia
Lung	Cough, chest pain, hemoptysis, breathlessness
Eyes	Blindness, scleritis
Gastrointestinal tract	Pain, bleeding, perforation
Genitals	Testicular infarction, ovarian mass

so that each month or so a new area of the body (usually an extremity) became involved. On examination, the damage from mononeuritis multiplex can be mapped to individual, named nerves (eg, the peroneal, tibial, ulnar, radial, or median nerves). Almost all patients have sensory abnormalities and about half have weakness as well. Although mononeuritis multiplex is often bilateral, the lesions are usually asymmetric. The right hand may demonstrate a median nerve infarct while the left hand has an ulnar nerve lesion.

Mononeuritis multiplex produces such a characteristic clinical picture that usually it can be diagnosed at the bedside. Occasionally, identifying mononeuritis multiplex becomes difficult late in the course when the infarctions of so many nerves can coalesce to produce an unusually symmetric pattern of deficits. In most cases, the early history of sequential peripheral nerve lesions supports the diagnosis of vasculitic neuropathy. In some cases, proof of mononeuritis multiplex requires electrodiagnostic studies.

Mononeuritis multiplex is one of the physical findings in medicine of great differential diagnostic value. In the absence of diabetes or multiple compression injuries, mononeuritis multiplex usually means the patient has some form of vasculitis. Polyarteritis nodosa, microscopic polyangiitis, eosinophilic granulomatosis with polyangiitis (Churg-Strauss syndrome), and granulomatosis with polyangiitis (formerly Wegener granulomatosis) are the forms of vasculitis most likely to cause mononeuritis multiplex.

B. Laboratory Findings

Laboratory abnormalities accompany virtually every form of vasculitis (Table 29–5). Some abnormalities, such as anemia and an elevated erythrocyte sedimentation rate, are very nonspecific and can be seen with many other diseases. Other findings, such as red blood cell casts in the urine (indicating vasculitis of the glomeruli) or antineutrophil cytoplasmic antibodies (associated with granulomatosis with polyangiitis [formerly Wegener granulomatosis]), have much greater specificity.

C. Imaging Studies

The role of imaging studies depends greatly on the form of vasculitis suspected. Plain radiographs rarely provide important clues except in granulomatosis with polyangiitis (formerly Wegener granulomatosis), where views of the sinuses and chest may yield findings (albeit usually not specific ones). CT scans of the chest are more sensitive in granulomatosis with polyangiitis (formerly Wegener granulomatosis). Angiograms—performed conventionally with CT or with MR—are especially helpful in supporting or establishing the diagnosis of Takayasu arteritis, polyarteritis nodosa, and primary central nervous system vasculitis.

D. Special Tests

Biopsy of involved tissues is the most common method for establishing definitively the diagnosis of vasculitis. Skin,

Table 29–5. Common laboratory tests in vasculitis.

Test	Laboratory Finding and Associated Disease
Hematocrit	Low in many forms
Erythrocyte sedimentation rate	Usually high, especially in giant cell arteritis
Creatinine	Elevated by renal forms of vasculitis
Urinalysis	Often abnormal, red blood cell casts caused by vasculitis of the glomeruli
Liver function tests	Abnormal in hepatitis B- or C-associated polyarteritis
Serum cryoglobulins	Present in cryoglobulinemia
Complement levels	Low in SLE, cryoglobulinemia
Immunoelectrophoresis	Monoclonal gammopathies common in hepatitis C-related vasculitis
Antineutrophil cytoplasmic	Positive in granulomatosis with polyangiitis,[a] microscopic polyangiitis,
Antibodies	Churg-Strauss syndrome

[a]Formerly known as Wegener granulomatosis.
SLE, systemic lupus erythematosus.

peripheral nerves, airways, arteries, kidney, and gut are the most commonly sampled tissues. In general, biopsies of symptomatic areas have a yield of about 66%, whereas biopsy of sites with no symptoms or findings have low yield. Special stains are sometimes required to reveal the degree of damage to particular arterial layers (such as the internal elastic lamina) or the extent of immune complex deposition.

▶ Differential Diagnosis

Specific diagnostic criteria have been established for most forms of vasculitis and are detailed in subsequent chapters. In general, the diagnosis of vasculitis requires a compatible clinical picture and a laboratory test—usually a biopsy but sometimes an angiogram or a specific serologic test (such as antineutrophil cytoplasmic antibodies for granulomatosis with polyangiitis [formerly Wegener granulomatosis]). It is also important to consider, and to exclude where appropriate, other diseases that can mimic primary systemic vasculitis. Cholesterol emboli, drug reactions, Whipple disease, syphilis, HIV, endocarditis, antiphospholipid antibody syndrome, and atrial myxoma are particularly common mimickers of primary vasculitis. Indeed, endocarditis and syphilis can cause vasculitis. In the appropriate setting, these conditions may need to be considered.

▶ Treatment

An important general principle in the treatment of vasculitis is to make sure that the intensity of treatment fits the severity of vasculitis. Although most forms of vasculitis require aggressive treatment to prevent morbidity and mortality, some do not. Minor vasculitis limited to the skin and caused by drug reactions requires no therapy other than stopping the offending drug. In contrast, rapid and intensive therapy is required to prevent blindness from developing in giant cell arteritis or renal failure from complicating granulomatosis with polyangiitis (formerly Wegener granulomatosis).

Another important principle of treatment is to limit the toxicity of therapy. When long-term prednisone is required, for example, appropriate measures to prevent osteoporosis should be initiated. If immunosuppression will result (as occurs with high-dose prednisone or immunosuppressive drugs), then prophylaxis against *Pneumocystis jiroveci* (formerly *Pneumocystis carinii*) pneumonia should be started. Other potential toxicities of therapies must be monitored closely.

González-Gay MA, García-Porrúa C. Epidemiology of the vasculitides. In: Stone JH, Hellmann DB, eds. *Rheumatic Disease Clinics of North America*. WB Saunders, 2001:729–749.

[Johns Hopkins Vasculitis Center] http://vasculitis.med.jhu.edu

Monach PA, Merkel PA. Genetics of vasculitis. *Curr Opin Rheumatol*. 2010;22:157. [PMID: 20051862]

Spira D, Kötter I, Ernemann U, et al. Imaging of primary and secondary inflammatory diseases involving large and medium-sized vessels and their potential mimics: a multitechnique approach. *Am J Roentgenol*. 2010;194:848. [PMID: 20173169]

Giant Cell Arteritis & Polymyalgia Rheumatica

David B. Hellmann, MD, MACP

Giant cell arteritis (GCA)—also known as temporal arteritis—is the most common form of systemic vasculitis in adults. GCA is a panarteritis that occurs almost exclusively in older people and preferentially affects the extracranial branches of the carotid artery. The most feared complication of GCA is blindness, which usually can be prevented by early diagnosis and treatment with glucocorticoids. Polymyalgia rheumatica (PMR) is an aching and stiffness of the shoulders, neck, and hip-girdle area that can occur with GCA, or more commonly, by itself.

ESSENTIALS OF DIAGNOSIS

GCA

▶ Headache, polymyalgia rheumatica, jaw claudication, visual symptoms, PMR.

▶ Temporal artery biopsy is the gold standard for diagnosis.

PMR

▶ Stiffness and aching of the shoulders, neck, and hip region.

▶ Diagnosis is clinical.

▶ Elevated erythrocyte sedimentation rate (ESR).

▶ General Considerations

Although the causes of PMR and GCA are unknown, the disorders share many risk factors and probably mechanisms of pathogenesis. Age is the greatest risk factor for developing either condition. Almost all patients who have GCA are older than 50 years (the average age of onset is 72). The incidence of GCA rises from 1.54 cases per 100,000 people in the sixth decade to 20.7 per 100,000 in the eighth decade.

PMR is 2–4 times more common than GCA, and its incidence also rises with age. Women are twice as likely as men

to have GCA or PMR. Both conditions develop most often in Scandinavians and in Americans of Scandinavian origin. GCA rarely develops in black men.

GCA and PMR are associated with the same human leukocyte antigen genes as those seen in patients with rheumatoid arthritis (ie, human leukocyte antigen-DR4 variants *0401 and *0404). The pathogenesis of GCA appears to be initiated by T cells in the adventitia responding to an unknown antigen, which prompts other T cells and macrophages to infiltrate all layers of the affected artery and to elaborate cytokines that mediate both local damage to the vessel and systemic effects (Figure 30–1). The differential expression of inflammatory cytokines may explain the clinical subsets seen in GCA. Patients with the highest levels of interleukin-6, for example, are more likely to have fever and less likely to experience blindness. MRI and ultrasonography show that PMR is caused by inflammation of the synovial lining of the bursa and joints around the neck, shoulders, and hips.

Although GCA may develop later in some patients with PMR, patients who have only PMR are not at risk for losing their vision and usually require small doses of prednisone (ie, <20 mg/day). In contrast, patients with GCA are at risk for losing their vision and require higher doses of prednisone (≥40 mg/day) to prevent blindness. Because patients who have GCA and PMR require treatment with glucocorticoids for months or years, it is important to minimize the likelihood of adverse effects from therapy (eg, osteoporosis, hypertension, and cataracts).

▶ Clinical Findings

A. Symptoms and Signs

The classic symptoms of GCA include headache, jaw claudication, PMR, visual symptoms, and malaise (Table 30–1). The onset may be gradual or sudden. The American College of Rheumatology has developed classification criteria for the diagnosis of GCA (Table 30–2).

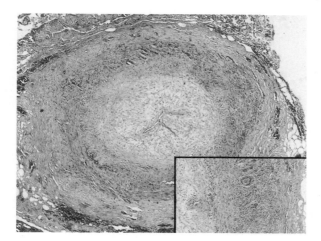

▲ **Figure 30–1.** Giant cell arteritis. Temporal artery biopsy showing endothelial proliferation, fragmentation of internal elastic lamina, and infiltration of the adventitia and media by inflammatory cells. Giant cells are especially well seen in the inset. (Reproduced, with permission, from Hellmann DB. Vasculitis. In: Stobo J, et al, eds. *Principles and Practice of Medicine.* Appleton & Lange; 1996.)

The most frequent finding during a physical examination is an abnormal temporal artery, which develops in only 50% of patients; thus a normal temporal artery does not exclude the diagnosis of GCA. The temporal artery may be enlarged, difficult to compress, nodular, or pulseless. About 15–20% of patients have axillary or subclavian disease, which manifests as diminished pulses, unequal arm blood pressures, or bruits heard above or below the clavicle or along the upper arm. Tongue ulcers, mass lesions of the breast and ovaries, and aortic regurgitation are other signs of GCA.

Table 30–1. Classic presenting manifestations of giant cell arteritis.

Symptoms	Percentage of Cases
Headache	70
Jaw claudication	50
Constitutional symptoms	50
Polymyalgia rheumatica	40
Visual loss	20
Abnormal temporal artery	50
Anemia	80
Erythrocyte sedimentation rate >50 mm/hour	90
Arthritis	15

Table 30–2. The American College of Rheumatology classification criteria for giant cell arteritis.

Criterion[a]	Definition
Age at disease onset ≥50 years	Development of symptoms or findings beginning at age 50 or older
New headache	New onset or new type of localized pain in the head
Temporal artery abnormality	Temporal artery tenderness to palpation or decreased pulsation, unrelated to arteriosclerosis of cervical arteries
Elevated erythrocyte sedimentation rate (ESR)	ESR ≥50 mm/hour by the Westergren method
Abnormal artery biopsy	Biopsy specimen with artery showing vasculitis characterized by a predominance of mononuclear cell infiltration or granulomatous inflammation, usually with multinucleated giant cells

[a]For purposes of classification, a patient is said to have giant cell (temporal) arteritis if at least 3 of these 5 criteria are present. Reproduced, with permission, from Hunder GG, Bloch DA, Michel BA, et al. The American College of Rheumatology 1990 criteria for the classification of giant cell arteritis. *Arthritis Rheum.* 1990;33:1125.

1. Headache—The intensity and location of the headache, the most common symptom, varies greatly from patient to patient. The headache is typically described as a dull, aching pain of moderate severity, localized over the temporal area, but variations in location, quality, and severity occur often. The most striking feature of the headache is that the patient notices that it is new or different. Even if the patient has had migraine or other headache problems in the past, features of the new headache are different. Patients frequently describe tenderness of the scalp, especially when they comb or brush their hair. Some patients localize the tenderness to the temporal arteries, which may be enlarged or nodular in only a minority of cases.

2. Jaw claudication—Jaw claudication, defined as pain in the masseter muscles associated with protracted chewing, develops when the oxygen demand of the masseter muscles exceeds the supply provided by narrowed and inflamed arteries. Typically, patients with jaw claudication notice pain when eating foods that require vigorous chewing, such as meats, and little or no pain when chewing soft foods. Of all the possible symptoms of GCA, jaw claudication is the most specific for this disease. Many patients do not provide such a classic description of jaw claudication, and instead report a vague sense of discomfort along the jaw or face, with or without protracted chewing. Atypical manifestations of jaw claudication include discomfort over the ear or around the nose.

Table 30–3. Diagnostic criteria[a] for polymyalgia rheumatica.

Criteria for Chuang and Colleagues
Age 50 years or older
Bilateral aching and stiffness for 1 mo or more and involving 2 of the following areas; neck or torso, shoulders or proximal regions of the arms, and hips or proximal aspects of the thighs
Erythrocyte sedimentation rate (ESR) >40 mm/hour
Exclusion of all other diagnoses except giant cell arteritis
Criteria of Healey
Pain persisting for at least 1 mo and involving 2 of the following areas: neck, shoulders, and pelvic girdle
Morning stiffness lasting >1 hour
Rapid response to prednisone (20 mg/day or less)
Absence of other diseases capable of causing musculoskeletal symptoms
Age older than 50 years
ESR >40 mm/hr

[a]For each of the criteria, all the findings must be present for polymyalgia rheumatica to be diagnosed.
Reproduced with permission from Salvarani C. Cantini F, Boiardi L, Hunder GG. Polymyalgia rheumatica and giant-cell arteritis. *N Engl J Med.* 2002;347:261.

3. PMR and joints—PMR is defined as pain and stiffness in the neck, shoulders, and hip-girdle area that are usually much worse in the morning. Criteria for the diagnosis of PMR have been developed (Table 30–3).

The shoulders are more commonly involved (70–95%) than the hips (50–70%). Shoulder pain in PMR may begin unilaterally but quickly becomes bilateral. Patients with PMR may report great difficulty getting out of bed, arising from the toilet, or brushing their teeth. People in whom GCA develops frequently describe feeling "old" for the first time at the onset of the disease. The stiffness is especially severe in the morning but may improve, usually a little but sometimes markedly, during the day. When asked to localize the pain, patients often say the pain is "in the flesh" rather than in the joints. Examination of the shoulders and hips is usually unremarkable except for decreased active and passive range of motion. Swelling, erythema, and heat are usually absent. However, some patients with PMR or GCA experience arthralgia or arthritis of the sternoclavicular joint, wrists, fingers, knees, or ankles. Rarely, pitting edema develops in the patient's hands or feet.

4. Visual symptoms—About one third of patients with GCA have visual symptoms, chiefly diplopia or visual loss. Visual hallucinations occur rarely. The visual loss may be transient or permanent or monocular or binocular. Visual loss is the most feared complication of GCA because it is usually irreversible. Blindness can develop abruptly but more often is preceded by episodes of blurred vision or amaurosis fugax. Rarely is visual loss the first manifestation of GCA; on average, visual loss develops 5 months after the onset of

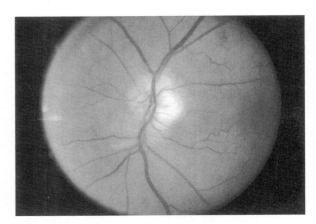

▲ **Figure 30–2.** Early funduscopic appearance in a patient with giant cell arteritis in whom blindness has developed.

other GCA symptoms. The direct cause of visual loss in GCA is usually occlusion of the posterior ciliary artery, a branch of the ophthalmic artery, which is a branch of the carotid artery. The posterior ciliary artery supplies blood to the optic nerve head. Interruption of that flow leads to anterior ischemic optic neuropathy.

When visual loss occurs, it usually is profound. Patients often cannot detect a hand waving directly in front of the affected eye. In the first few hours after infarction, the disc generally appears normal on funduscopic examination, even in the presence of profound visual loss. Later, disc pallor (Figure 30–2) and swelling, cotton-wool spots, and flame-shaped intraretinal hemorrhages may develop. Over weeks or months, the disc becomes atrophic. Most patients with visual loss also demonstrate a relative afferent pupillary defect, demonstrated by moving a shining light from the normal eye to the blind eye and noting that both pupils dilate. Not all patients with GCA have the same risk of developing blindness. Multiple studies reveal that those who experience fever or other manifestations of a strong inflammatory response are less likely to experience visual loss. Fever and other inflammatory features correlate with high serum levels of interleukin-6. About three-quarters of all blindness occurs before treatment is begun, and another quarter develops during treatment, usually within the first month. Blindness rarely develops thereafter.

5. Other features—Almost all patients with the classic features of GCA also have nonspecific manifestations such as malaise, fatigue, and loss of appetite. Weight loss of 2–10 kg is common. Some patients also experience depression.

B. Atypical Manifestations

GCA presents with atypical features in 40% of cases. Awareness of these atypical presentations (Table 30–4)

Table 30–4. Atypical manifestations of giant cell arteritis.

Fever of unknown origin
Respiratory tract symptoms
Dry cough
Throat pain
Tongue pain
Neurologic symptoms
Mononeuritis multiplex
Stroke
Transient ischemic attack
Dementia
Hallucinations
Large artery involvement
Claudication in arms or legs
Unequal arm blood pressures
Thoracic aortic aneurysm
Tumorlike lesions
Especially of the breasts and ovaries
Syndrome of inappropriate antidiuretic hormone secretion

maximizes the physician's chance of diagnosing GCA before blindness develops.

1. Fever of unknown origin—Fever develops in about 40% of patients with GCA; of those, 10–15% are fevers of unknown origin. Although GCA causes only 2% of all cases of fever of unknown origin, it accounts for 16% of all cases of fever of unknown origin in patients over the age of 65. Fevers in GCA may reach nearly 40°C, and average about 39°C. About two thirds of patients with fevers also have rigors and drenching sweats. Despite these manifestations of a robust inflammatory response, the white blood cell count is almost always normal (at least before prednisone is started).

2. Respiratory—Respiratory symptoms develop in 1 of 10 patients and constitute the presenting complaint in 1 of 25. The most common symptom is a dry cough, resembling that seen in some patients taking angiotensin-converting enzyme inhibitors. The cause of the cough is obscure because chest imaging studies are normal. The cough may reflect inflammation within the arteries adjacent to cough centers, which are distributed throughout various sites in the respiratory apparatus, including the diaphragm, the bronchi, and the mid-brain. Other respiratory or otolaryngeal manifestations include tongue pain, glossitis, dental pain, and posterior or anterior pharyngeal pain. These symptoms reflect ischemia caused by arteritis of nearby vessels; tongue ulceration and gangrene may also occur.

3. Neurologic—The most common neurologic manifestation of GCA is mononeuritis multiplex. Unlike mononeuritis multiplex in other forms of vasculitis, which most commonly affects the foot or the hand, mononeuritis multiplex in GCA most commonly affects the shoulder, producing sudden weakness and pain that mimics a C5 radiculopathy. Central nervous system disease, outside of the eye, also

occurs. Delirium, dementia, transient ischemic attacks, and cerebrovascular accidents have been reported. GCA preferentially affects the posterior circulation of the brain, whereas the ratio of anterior to posterior circulation cerebrovascular accidents is about 3:2 in the general population, the ratio is reversed in GCA. Intracranial disease does not occur in GCA, perhaps because arteries lose their elastic lamina almost as soon as they penetrate the dura. Therefore, transient ischemic attacks and cerebrovascular accidents complicating GCA are attributed to occlusion of extracranial vessels or to thromboemboli.

4. Large-artery disease—Clinically evident involvement of large arteries—the aorta and its major branches—develops in at least 25% of patients. Positron emission tomography scans reveal subclinical inflammation of large arteries in over 80% of patients. The most commonly affected vessels include the vertebral, carotid, subclavian, and axillary arteries, and the aorta. Involvement of large arteries in the lower extremities has also been described. Presenting symptoms may include transient ischemic attack, cerebrovascular accident, hand ischemia, and arm or leg claudication. Aortic involvement may lead to thoracic aortic aneurysm, which is increased 17-fold in patients with GCA. Thoracic aortic aneurysm develops an average of 7 years after the diagnosis of GCA. Thoracic aortic aneurysm may be asymptomatic or cause aortic regurgitation, myocardial infarction, or dissection. Abdominal aortic aneurysms, although less common than thoracic lesions, also occur. Involvement of the pulmonary or mesenteric arteries virtually never occurs.

5. Other atypical manifestations—The protean manifestations of GCA include tumor-like lesions localized to the breast or ovaries, mimicking cancer at those sites. Other manifestations include the syndrome of inappropriate antidiuretic hormone secretion and hemolytic anemia (see Table 30–4).

C. Laboratory Findings

The laboratory hallmarks of GCA and PMR are a markedly elevated ESR and anemia (see Table 30–1). An ESR >30 mm/hour is present in 96% of patients with GCA, and an ESR of >50 mm/hour is seen in 87% of patients with GCA. A normal ESR may be seen in a slightly higher percentage of patients with PMR. The ESR averages about 100 mm/hour in GCA and slightly lower in isolated PMR. The C-reactive protein is also usually elevated and may be more sensitive than the ESR in detecting flares. The anemia, typically normochromic and normocytic, is usually mild with a hematocrit often in the 32–35 range. Occasionally, the anemia may be profound with hematocrits in the 20s. Approximately 20% of patients with GCA demonstrate a mildly elevated alkaline phosphatase (of liver origin). The platelet count, often elevated nonspecifically by inflammatory disorders, is frequently increased in GCA and PMR.

D. Imaging Studies

Radiographs of shoulders and hips are invariably unhelpful. However, MRI and ultrasonography of shoulders and hips in patients with PMR show inflammation of the bursa and the synovium of nearby joints. Color duplex ultrasonography of affected temporal arteries can show a characteristic "halo" of edema or stenosis, but this technology is no more sensitive for the diagnosis of GCA than a careful physical examination of the temporal artery. Magnetic resonance angiography or CT angiography can provide noninvasive assessment of larger-artery disease. Positron emission tomography scanning can demonstrate occult large-vessel inflammation, but the practical value of this technique is not established.

▶ Diagnostic Criteria

The diagnosis of PMR rests almost entirely on clinical grounds, namely symptoms of proximal limb stiffness associated with an elevated ESR and a dramatic response to prednisone. While MRI and ultrasonographic images are abnormal in PMR, their sensitivity and specificity have not been established, and usually these studies are not obtained.

Classification criteria have also been proposed for GCA (Table 30–2), but their predictive value in clinical settings is not well established. Since GCA is uncommon, clinicians have to maintain a high index of suspicion for the diagnosis. Among its classic symptoms, only jaw claudication has been shown to increase the odds (by about 3-fold) that a patient in whom GCA is suspected actually has the disease (Table 30–5). The only physical finding with a high positive predictive value for diagnosing GCA is an abnormal temporal artery. Although a strikingly elevated ESR (eg, >100 mm/ hour) strongly suggests the diagnosis in the proper setting, moderate elevations of the ESR are quite nonspecific. A normal ESR substantially reduces the likelihood of GCA but does not eliminate it altogether.

Two guidelines may help determine when to suspect GCA. First, one should consider the composite clinical picture when trying to decide whether a patient could have GCA. A comprehensive review of systems may be especially helpful since most patients with GCA have multiple symptoms. For example, vasculitis should not be suspected in most patients with a dry cough, one of the atypical symptoms of GCA. However, GCA should be considered in a 72-year-old patient with a dry cough, PMR, headache, weight loss, fever, anemia, and an ESR of 105 mm/hour. Second, because many of the atypical symptoms involve some type of pain above the neck—headache, or vague discomfort around the jaw, throat, ear, tongue, or teeth—it may be prudent to consider the diagnosis of GCA in any patient over the age of 50 who has pain in any of these areas without another explanation. Thus, the elderly patient with ear pain and a normal ear examination does not benefit from a diagnosis of otitis media and antibiotics but may benefit from a comprehensive review of systems and an ESR.

Table 30–5. Likelihood ratios for symptoms, signs, and laboratory findings in giant cell arteritis.

Finding	Positive Likelihood Ratio (95% CI)	Negative Likelihood Ratio (95% CI)
Symptoms		
Jaw claudication	4.2 (2.8-6.2)	0.72 (0.65-0.81)
Diplopia	3.4 (1.3-8.6)	0.95 (0.91-0.99)
Weight loss	1.3 (1.1-1.5)	0.89 (0.79-1.0)
Any headache	1.2 (1.1-1.4)	0.7 (0.57-0.85)
Polymyalgia rheumatic	NS	NS
Fever	NS	NS
Visual Loss	NS	NS
Signs		
Beaded temporal artery	4.6 (1.1-18.4)	0.93 (0.88-0.99)
Tender temporal artery	2.6 (1.9-3.7)	0.82 (0.74-0.92)
Any temporal artery abnormality	2.0 (1.4-3.0)	0.53 (0.38-0.75)
Scalp tenderness	1.6 (1.2-2.1)	0.93 (0.86-1.0)
Laboratory results		
ESR abnormal	1.1 (1.0-1.2)	0.2 (0.08-0.51)
ESR >50 mm/hour	1.2 (1.0-1.4)	0.35 (0.18-0.67)
ESR >100 mm/hour	1.9 (1.1-3.3)	0.8 (0.68-0.95)
Anemia	NS	NS

CI, confidence interval; ESR, erythrocyte sedimentation rate; NS, not significant.
Data from Smetana GW, Shmerling RH. Does this patient have temporal arteritis? *JAMA.* 2002;287:92.

In practice, then, the diagnosis of GCA is suggested by the clinical picture combined with an elevated ESR, and proven by a positive temporal artery biopsy. Infrequently, large-artery involvement, such as subclavian disease, is diagnosed by MRI, CT angiography, or conventional angiography showing long, smooth arterial taperings uncharacteristic of atherosclerosis (Figure 30–3). Although some experts have proposed using color duplex ultrasonography of the temporal artery, experience with that technique is not sufficient for it to replace temporal artery biopsy as the gold standard for diagnosing GCA.

▶ Differential Diagnosis

It is important to distinguish patients who have PMR alone from those who have PMR plus GCA. Patients are classified as having PMR alone if they have no "above-the-neck" symptoms, namely headache, jaw claudication, scalp tenderness,

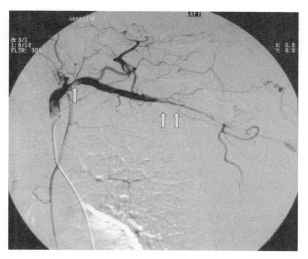

▲ **Figure 30–3.** Large-artery involvement in giant cell arteritis (GCA). Angiogram in a patient with GCA showing tight stenosis of the proximal left subclavian artery (*single arrow*) with diffuse, marked narrowing of the axillary artery (*double arrows*). (Used with permission from Dr. Elliott Levy.)

or visual symptoms. Although about 20% of patients with symptoms of PMR have positive temporal artery biopsy results, practice has shown that patients who have symptoms of PMR alone respond well to low-dose prednisone (see the following section on treatment).

Distinguishing PMR from rheumatoid arthritis in an older person can be difficult, especially in those patients with PMR who have distal polyarthritis. Severe erosive arthritis, rheumatoid nodules, and a positive rheumatoid factor make rheumatoid arthritis the more likely diagnosis. Because both conditions can respond well to low-dose prednisone, differentiating the two disorders may not be possible during the early months of treatment.

Polymyositis causes much more proximal weakness than pain. In contrast, patients with PMR always rate their pain greater than any weakness. The creatine kinase is usually elevated in polymyositis but normal in PMR. Proximal limb pain or stiffness can occur with a variety of endocrine disorders, including hypothyroidism and panhypopituitarism. PMR is usually easily distinguished from fibromyalgia, which is a condition of diffuse pain—both proximal and distal—typically occurring in young women in the absence of objective findings or abnormal laboratory tests. Solid tumors, especially renal cell carcinoma, can produce musculoskeletal pain that resembles PMR. However, patients with malignancy usually have some atypical feature such as pain that affects the distal limbs as much as the proximal portions, clubbing, or a requirement for more than 20 mg of prednisone per day.

Other conditions that can mimic PMR include early Parkinson disease, amyloidosis, late-onset systemic lupus erythematosus, endocarditis, myelodysplastic syndrome, and drug reactions (eg, myositis from statin drugs). Since absence of shoulder involvement is rare in PMR, patients thought to have "below the waist" PMR are more likely to have lumbar spinal stenosis, which can cause stiffness and pain restricted to the hip-girdle region.

Transient monocular loss of vision (amaurosis fugax) or permanent monocular blindness can also occur from atherosclerotic cerebrovascular or cardiovascular disease. The nonarteritis patients may be distinguished by their lack of other symptoms and a normal ESR. Both atherosclerosis and GCA can also cause upper or lower extremity claudication. Angiography can usually differentiate these conditions. GCA produces isolated long segments of smooth narrowing in the mid-portions of arteries, whereas atherosclerosis tends to be diffuse and favors branch points.

Some of the clinical features of GCA can be produced by other forms of systemic vasculitis. Granulomatosis with polyangiitis (formerly Wegener granulomatosis) and polyarteritis nodosa, for example, can cause jaw claudication. Takayasu arteritis can affect the large vessels as GCA does, but Takayasu arteritis is usually seen in young women. Multiple myeloma, Waldenström macroglobulinemia, and osteomyelitis can produce systemic features with markedly elevated ESRs. Endocarditis should also be considered in a patient with symptoms resembling GCA and a new heart murmur. Many patients with diabetes in whom proteinuria has developed feel poorly and have very high ESRs, as do patients with other forms of renal failure. For example, about 20% of all patients receiving hemodialysis have ESRs >100 mm/hour. Although many of these patients also suffer from malaise, they rarely have symptoms strongly suggestive of GCA. Those who do have symptoms suggesting GCA will require temporal artery biopsy. Other mimickers of GCA include myelodysplastic syndromes and systemic amyloidosis.

▶ Treatment

Prednisone (40–60 mg/day) should be given to any patient in whom GCA is strongly suspected. Then the patient should be referred for a temporal artery biopsy. Temporal artery biopsy has almost zero mortality and very low morbidity. It is the only test that can confirm the diagnosis of GCA, so it is recommended in all suspected cases. Although it is traditional to obtain the temporal artery biopsy quickly, evidence suggests that the pathologic features persist for at least 2 weeks after the start of glucocorticoid treatment. GCA does not involve arteries contiguously, so skip areas may occur. Consequently, the greatest yields will come from biopsies of large segments of artery (eg, 3–5 cm) that have multiple sections examined pathologically. Positive biopsy results demonstrate chiefly mononuclear cells infiltrating all the layers of the artery with varying degrees of intimal proliferation and disruption of the internal elastic lamina. About 50% of positive specimens show multinucleated giant cells. It is intuitively appealing to biopsy the temporal artery that is abnormal on physical examination or that corresponds to the side of the head with symptoms. Unilateral temporal artery biopsy is about 90% sensitive and bilateral biopsies are about 95% sensitive. These figures come from centers where GCA is studied frequently and percentages may not be as high in other communities. In any setting, some patients with a convincing picture of GCA may have a negative biopsy result.

Patients with suspected GCA who have experienced transient visual loss for a few hours should be admitted and given high-dose intravenous methylprednisolone (eg, 1000 mg/day) for 3–5 days; a few patients have recovered some vision with this regimen. Visual loss of more than 1 day duration is almost always permanent.

There is increasing evidence that optimal treatment of GCA includes not only prednisone but also low-dose aspirin (ie, 80–100 mg/day). Several retrospective studies have shown that the addition of aspirin reduces by 5-fold the risk of blindness or stroke in GCA.

Patients with PMR alone are usually treated with 10–20 mg/day of prednisone. Nonsteroidal anti-inflammatory drugs can help alleviate PMR symptoms but rarely obviate the need for glucocorticoids.

Patients with PMR or GCA respond dramatically to initial treatment. Some report improvement within hours of taking the first dose of prednisone, and most describe a "miraculous" improvement within 2 days. However, about 10% require a week of therapy before feeling better. Dividing the dose of prednisone into a morning and evening dose for the first 1–2 weeks helps some patients. If the patient does not improve within the first week, doubt should be cast on the diagnosis of PMR or of biopsy-negative GCA. Every-other-day prednisone is not effective initial treatment.

The best studied glucocorticoid-sparing drug for GCA or for PMR is methotrexate. The effectiveness of methotrexate (10–15 mg orally once per week) for GCA is controversial: two randomized, double-blind, controlled trials came to opposite conclusions about methotrexate's efficacy. The experience with using either azathioprine or cyclophosphamide as glucocorticoid-sparing treatment for GCA has been too small to be conclusive. Of the biologic therapies, infliximab has been best studied and appears ineffective for GCA or PMR. One study suggests that methotrexate is modestly glucocorticoid-sparing for isolated PMR.

To prevent osteoporosis, patients starting prednisone therapy should take 1500–1800 mg of calcium daily with 400–800 units of vitamin D. Bone density scans should be performed, and those with osteopenia or osteoporosis should be given bisphosphonates.

After the first month of treatment, almost all patients will have a normal ESR. At this point, the prednisone can begin to be tapered by 10% every week or two. The rate of prednisone tapering should be determined by the total clinical picture produced by the patient's symptoms (most important), physical findings, and some laboratory measure of inflammation, such as the ESR or C-reactive protein (least important). Once patients with GCA reach 15 mg of prednisone or patients with PMR reach 10 mg, decrements of 1 mg every 2 or so weeks may reduce the chance of flare.

▶ Complications

Unfortunately, 50–80% of patients with PMR or GCA relapse during the first year as prednisone is tapered. Flares are defined clinically; isolated elevations of ESR or C-reactive protein do not require alteration of therapy. The only exception to this rule is that very rare case when visual loss develops in a patient with biopsy-proven GCA in the absence of other symptoms. Patients who experience renewed symptoms usually respond to increasing the prednisone dose 5–10 mg above the last dose at which the patient was asymptomatic. Most patients are unable to completely taper off of prednisone for 1–2 years, and a substantial minority will require some prednisone—usually in the range of 5–10 mg—for longer periods.

Complications from prednisone therapy develop in most patients being treated for PMR or GCA (Table 30–6). For example, diabetes or osteoporosis is 2–5 times more likely to develop in patients treated with prednisone than in others of the same age not receiving therapy. Important measures for limiting the toxicity of prednisone therapy include slow but steady tapering of prednisone as suggested above, protecting against early osteoporosis, and avoiding manipulating the dose of prednisone because of an isolated ESR or C-reactive protein elevation.

Table 30–6. Possible side effects of long-term glucocorticoid therapy.

Weight gain
Diabetes
Cataracts
Insomnia
Fluid retention
Hypertension
Proximal weakness
Alopecia
Sweats
Osteoporosis
Infection
Psychiatric disturbance (eg, depression, mania, psychosis)
Easy bruising of the skin
Stress
Tremor
Peptic ulcer disease

Blockmans D, Bley T, Schmidt W. Imaging for large-vessel vasculitis. *Curr Opin Rheumatol.* 2009;21:19. [PMID: 19077714]

Gonzalez-Gay M, Vazquez-Rodriguez TR, Lopez-Diaz MJ, et al. Epidemiology of giant cell arteritis and polymyalgia rheumatica. *Arthritis Rheum.* 2009;61:1454. [PMID: 19790127]

[The Cleveland Clinic Foundation Center for Vasculitis]
http://www.clevelandclinic.org/arthritis/vasculitis/default.htm

[The Johns Hopkins Vasculitis Center]
http://hopkinsvasculitis.org

[The National Institute of Allergy and Infectious Diseases]
http://www.niaid.nih.gov/dir/general.htm

[Vasculitis Foundation]
http://www.vasculitisfoundation.org/

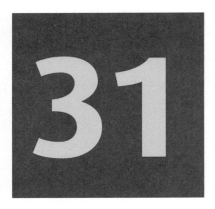

Takayasu Arteritis

David B. Hellmann, MD, MACP

Takayasu arteritis, named for the Japanese ophthalmologist who first described the ocular manifestations in 1908, is a large-vessel vasculitis of unknown cause that chiefly affects women during their reproductive years. The disease often presents two challenges. First, the diagnosis can be delayed for months or even years due to the rarity of the disease, the young age of the (typical) patient, and the protean presenting manifestations. Second, treatment is a challenge. Although Takayasu arteritis is a chronic disease, it usually pursues a waxing and waning course that requires careful monitoring to determine when the disease is active and medical therapy is needed. Treatment with glucocorticoids usually succeeds in halting progression of the vasculitis. Indeed, because of the advances in medical therapy and surgical treatment of vascular complications, such as aortic regurgitation, survival of patients with Takayasu arteritis has increased dramatically.

ESSENTIALS OF DIAGNOSIS

► Causes vasculitis of the aorta and its major branches.
► Preferentially affects young women.
► Often presents with absent pulse, bruit, claudication, hypertension, or fever of unknown origin.
► Erythrocyte sedimentation rate is usually elevated.
► Most patients respond to prednisone.

▶ General Considerations

Although Takayasu arteritis has been most extensively reported in Japan, Korea, China, Southeast Asia, and Mexico, cases have been described worldwide. In North America, the annual incidence is about 1–3 cases per million people. Takayasu arteritis affects women eight times more frequently than men. The average age of diagnosis is in the mid-20s but the disease may begin as early as age 7 or as late as

age 70. Symptoms develop before age 20 in nearly one third of patients and after age 40 in about 10%. The age of onset tends to be later in European countries.

▶ Pathogenesis

The cause of Takayasu arteritis remains elusive. The geographic clustering of cases suggests important genetic or environmental factors, but few have been identified. HLA associations have been found in Japanese patients (who preferentially express Bw52, DR2, Dw12, and DQw1), but not in other populations. The predominance of Takayasu arteritis in women of childbearing age suggests that female hormones may play a permissive role, as in systemic lupus erythematosus. An animal model of Takayasu arteritis has been produced with a herpes virus. In that model, the media of the aorta provides an immunoprivileged site for persistent herpes virus infection, which results in chronic inflammation (arteritis).

However initiated, Takayasu arteritis appears to be propagated by a T-cell–driven immune response that results in a granulomatous inflammation affecting all layers of the vessel. Indeed, the histopathology of Takayasu arteritis cannot be distinguished from that of temporal arteritis (also called giant cell arteritis; see Chapter 30). The inflammatory injury mediated by activated T cells, macrophages, and cytokines often results in proliferation of the intima and of smooth muscle cells in the media, leading to occlusion and stenosis of the artery. Transmural inflammation can also cause aneurysmal dilation of the vessel. Overproduction of inflammatory cytokines, such as interleukin-6, results in fever and other constitutional symptoms.

▶ Clinical Findings

A. Symptoms and Signs

Although the presenting features of Takayasu arteritis vary greatly, they can be categorized into two broad groups: those

Table 31–1. Clinical features of Takayasu arteritis.

Feature	At Presentation (%)	Ever Present (%)
Vascular	50	100
Bruit		80
Claudication (upper extremity)	30	62
Claudication (lower extremity)	15	32
Hypertension	20	33
Unequal arm blood pressures	15	50
Carotidynia	15	32
Aortic regurgitation		20
Central nervous system	30	57
Light-headedness	20	35
Visual abnormality	10	30
Stroke	5	10
Musculoskeletal	20	53
Chest wall pain	10	30
Joint pain	10	30
Myalgia	5	15
Constitutional	33	43
Malaise	20	30
Fever	20	25
Weight loss	15	20
Cardiac	15	38
Aortic regurgitation	8	20
Angina	2	12
Congestive heart failure	2	10

Data based on studying 60 patients reported by Kerr GS, Hallahan CW, Giordano J, et al. Takayasu arteritis. *Ann Intern Med*. 1994;120:919. With permission.

caused by vascular damage (ie, occlusion, stenosis, or dilation of blood vessels), and those caused by systemic inflammation (Table 31–1). The separation of these presenting features is not always neatly maintained; many patients have both vascular complications and constitutional symptoms, and others have a biphasic presentation, with constitutional symptoms dominating early and vascular features becoming more salient later.

Among the vascular manifestations, bruit, claudication, hypertension, light-headedness (associated with vertebral or carotid artery disease), unequal blood pressures in the extremities, carotidynia, aortic regurgitation, and loss of a pulse are most common. Bruits develop most frequently over the carotid arteries, but also often develop in

the supraclavicular or infraclavicular space (reflecting subclavian disease), along the flexor surface of the upper arm (from axillary artery disease), or in the abdomen (from renal or mesenteric artery vasculitis). Many patients have multiple bruits. Upper extremity claudication—commonly manifested in young women by fatigue and pain in the arm while exercising or blow-drying hair—develops more often than lower extremity claudication. A widened pulse pressure and diastolic murmur along the right sternal border may signal the aortic regurgitation that develops in 20% of patients. Other cardiac manifestations include angina (most commonly from stenotic lesions at or near the ostia of the coronary arteries), mitral regurgitation (secondary to left ventricular dilatation from aortic regurgitation), or congestive heart failure (early in the course caused by myocarditis or late in the course caused by chronic aortic with or without mitral regurgitation). Stroke affects a significant minority of patients. Glomerulonephritis is quite rare in this form of large vessel vasculitis; renal disease usually results from hypertension which in turns develops because of stenosis of the renal arteries.

The visual symptoms that were first described in 1908 occur rarely today. When present, visual symptoms chiefly result from retinal ischemia produced by narrowing or occlusion of the carotid arteries. Some patients may have such limited blood flow through their carotids and vertebral arteries that merely turning and tilting their head causes light-headedness, dizziness, or visual loss.

Almost half of patients experience constitutional or musculoskeletal symptoms. These constitutional and musculoskeletal features dominate the presentation in approximately one third of all cases of Takayasu arteritis. Asthenia, weight loss, fever, myalgia, and arthralgia occur commonly. Prominent back pain, especially in the thoracic region, develops in a few patients. This pain resembles that seen in older patients with thoracic dissection and probably results from stimulation of nociceptive nerve fibers along the inflamed aorta.

B. Laboratory Findings

Takayasu arteritis does not cause any specific blood test or urinary abnormalities but usually produces nonspecific findings of inflammation. Nearly 80% of patients have elevated erythrocyte sedimentation rates (ESR) or C-reactive protein (CRP) values, especially during phases of active disease. Unfortunately, no blood test accurately measures disease activity. For example, the ESR is normal in 30% of patients with active disease and is elevated in 40% of patients with inactive disease. Recent studies have suggested that pentraxin-3 may more accurately reflect disease activity than either ESR or CRP. Anemia develops in 50% of patients, with hematocrits typically in the high 20s or low 30s. Anemic patients commonly have slightly low mean corpuscular volume (eg, high 70s). Thrombocytosis, which develops in one-third of patients, is often mild but may exceed 800,000/mcL.

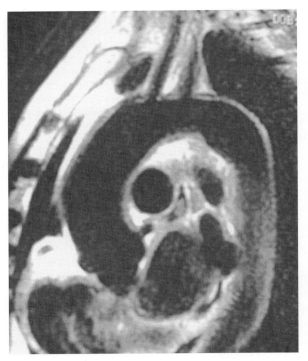

▲ **Figure 31–1.** Magnetic resonance image showing thickening of the wall of the ascending and descending thoracic aorta in a 26-year-old woman with Takayasu arteritis.

Less than 10% of patients with Takayasu arteritis have an elevated serum creatinine. About one quarter will have mild proteinuria or hematuria. Renal abnormalities usually result from hypertension; glomerulonephritis from Takayasu arteritis very rarely occurs.

C. Imaging Studies

Magnetic resonance imaging (MRI), computed tomography (CT), vascular ultrasonography, and conventional aortography are abnormal in virtually all patients with Takayasu arteritis. MRI appears most sensitive in that it can detect the inflammatory thickening of the aorta or its branches (Figure 31–1) that precedes changes in the caliber of the vessels' lumen. Conventional angiography, although unhelpful in determining the thickness of the vessel wall, provides the most detailed images of the stenoses, occlusions, dilatation, and other vascular wall irregularities characteristic of Takayasu arteritis (Figure 31–2). Advances in CT and three-dimensional image reconstruction have allowed CT angiography to replace the more invasive conventional angiograms.

The most frequently affected vessels are the aorta, subclavian arteries, and carotid arteries (Table 31–2). Involvement of the aorta above and below the diaphragm occurs most

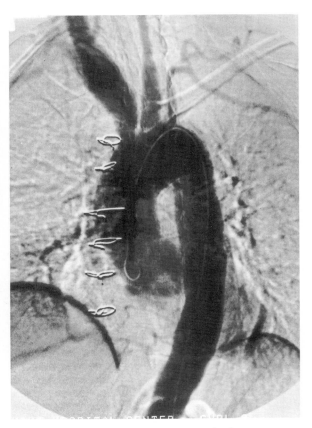

▲ **Figure 31–2.** Angiogram showing multiple changes of Takayasu arteritis, including dilatations of the ascending aorta (with surgical wires from aortic valve replacement surgery)and the brachiocephalic and proximal right common carotid arteries. The left common carotid artery is occluded distal to its origin. (Used with permission from Hellmann DB, Flynn JA. Clinical presentation and natural history of Takayasu's arteritis and other inflammatory arteritides. In: Perler BA, Becker GJ, eds. *Vascular Intervention. A Clinical Approach.* Thieme Medical; 1998:249–256.)

commonly. The distribution of vascular involvement varies in people from different countries: whereas disease of the ascending aorta and great vessels is most common in patients from Japan, involvement of the abdominal aorta and renal arteries is most common in patients from India and Korea. In the extra-aortic vessels, long segments of stenosis are more frequent than dilation or aneurysm. Takayasu arteritis is one of the few forms of vasculitis that can affect, albeit rarely, the pulmonary arteries. Positron emission tomography scanning offers the theoretical advantage of allowing quantification of the degree of vascular inflammation. Indeed, positron emission tomography scanning appears to be sensitive in

Table 31–2. Frequency of blood vessel involvement in Takayasu arteritis.

Blood Vessel	% Abnormal
Aorta	65
Aortic arch or root	35
Abdominal aorta	47
Thoracic aorta	17
Subclavian artery	93
Common carotid artery	58
Renal artery	38
Vertebral artery	35
Celiac axes	18
Common iliac artery	17
Pulmonary artery	5

Data based on studying 60 patients reported by Kerr GS, Hallahan CW, Giordano J, et al. Takayasu arteritis. *Ann Intern Med.* 1994;120:919. With permission.

Table 31–3. American College of Rheumatology classification criteria for Takayasu arteritis.[a]

1. Onset at age <40 years
2. Limb claudication
3. Decreased brachial artery pulse
4. Unequal arm blood pressures (>10 mm Hg)
5. Subclavian or aortic bruit
6. Angiographic evidence of narrowing or occlusion of the aorta or its primary branches, or large limb arteritis

[a]The presence of three or more of the six criteria was sensitive (91%) and specific (98%) for the diagnosis of Takayasu arteritis. Data from Arend WP, Michel BA, Bloch DA, et al. The American College of Rheumatology 1990 criteria for the classification of Takayasu Arteritis. *Arthritis Rheum.* 1990;33:1129.

detecting vascular inflammation in patients with Takayasu arteritis, but the cost and level of radiation exposure pose important limitations. No imaging technique has been proven to be reliable in measuring disease activity. The initial enthusiasm for the ability of MRI to measure disease activity has not been substantiated by long-term follow-up studies.

D. Specific Tests

Biopsies of the aorta or other actively affected arteries show a granulomatous vasculitis with giant cells.

▶ Differential Diagnosis

The biggest impediment to diagnosing Takayasu arteritis is that few physicians are familiar enough with this rare disease to recognize its presenting manifestations. The American College of Rheumatology has developed six criteria for classification of Takayasu arteritis (Table 31–3). In practice, the diagnosis of Takayasu arteritis requires demonstrating vasculitis of the aorta or its major branches by imaging tests (Figure 31–3; also see Figures 31–1 and 31–2) or biopsy, and excluding the diseases that can produce similar abnormalities (Table 31–4).

Of the other vasculitides, giant cell arteritis (see Chapter 30) is the form most likely to be confused with Takayasu arteritis. Both diseases cause a granulomatous panarteritis and an elevated ESR. In contrast to Takayasu arteritis, giant cell arteritis exclusively affects patients over the age of 50 and chiefly involves extracranial branches of the carotid artery (such as the temporal artery). Cogan syndrome is a rare disease characterized by vestibular-auditory abnormalities (often producing deafness and vertigo) and ocular inflammation (especially keratitis or inflammation of the cornea). A minority of patients with Cogan syndrome have medium- or large-vessel vasculitis, or both. A few other diseases can affect the aorta or its branches, but almost never do they convincingly mimic Takayasu arteritis (see Table 31–4). Relapsing polychondritis, which results in characteristic changes in cartilage, may also affect the aorta. Rheumatoid arthritis and ankylosing spondylitis rarely affect the thoracic root. Buerger disease—a form of medium-vessel vasculitis associated with smoking—may affect the femoral, brachial, and axillary arteries, as can ergotism. Syphilitic aortitis can be excluded by appropriate

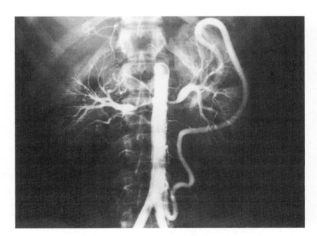

▲ **Figure 31–3.** Angiogram showing bilateral renal artery stenosis in Takayasu arteritis. A large left colic branch of the inferior mesenteric artery provides collateral circulation. (Used with permission from Hellmann DB, Flynn JA. Clinical presentation and natural history of Takayasu's arteritis and other inflammatory arteritides. In: Perler BA, Becker GJ, eds. *Vascular Intervention. A Clinical Approach.* Thieme Medical; 1998:249–256.)

Table 31–4. Differential diagnosis of Takayasu arteritis: other diseases that can affect the aorta.

Rheumatic diseases	Giant cell arteritis, Cogan syndrome, relapsing polychrondritis, ankylosing spondylitis, rheumatoid arthritis, systemic lupus erythematosus, Buerger disease, Behçet disease
Infectious disease	Syphilis
Other	Atherosclerosis, inflammatory abdominal aortic aneurysm, ergotism, radiation-induced damage, retroperitoneal fibrosis, inflammatory bowel disease, sarcoidosis, neurofibromatosis, congenital coarctation, Marfan syndrome

serologic studies. Neurofibromatosis and congenital coarctation may affect the abdominal aorta and mesenteric great vessels. Radiation-induced damage can affect any vessel including the aorta. Atherosclerosis of the aorta and major branches rarely develops before age 50 and does not produce the long, smoothly tapered and stenotic segments of arteries that are so characteristic of Takayasu arteritis. Inflammatory abdominal aortic aneurysm is an unusual form of atherosclerosis characterized by marked thickening of the abdominal aorta, often associated with retroperitoneal inflammation. Almost all of the patients with this disorder are smokers. Patients with inflammatory abdominal aortic aneurysm often have mild anemia and modest elevations of the ESR. Marfan syndrome does not produce inflammatory symptoms or signs. Aortitis, especially of the abdominal aorta, can also be a manifestation of IgG4-related systemic disease.

Patients with predominantly constitutional symptoms are often evaluated for other conditions. For example, a woman with a hematocrit of 28, a mean corpuscular volume of 78 (reflecting anemia of chronic disease), and a platelet count of 980,000/mcL (nonspecifically reflecting inflammation)—not uncommon findings in Takayasu arteritis—will often unproductively undergo evaluation for gastrointestinal hemorrhage, iron deficiency anemia, or another hematologic disorder. Fatigue and weight loss might erroneously suggest a diagnosis of depression. Transient ischemic attacks in a young woman can be wrongly attributed to migraine. Fever and aortic regurgitation may initially suggest bacterial endocarditis. Measuring blood pressure in both arms, carefully palpating pulses in all extremities, and listening for bruits in the abdomen and chest and along the carotids and supraclavicular and axillary areas provide the best clinical tools in early diagnosis of Takayasu arteritis.

▶ **Treatment**

Although glucocorticoid therapy for Takayasu arteritis has not been tested in controlled trials, it appears very effective in suppressing vascular inflammation. Initial therapy consists of prednisone (1 mg/kg) for 1 month and then tapered to 10 mg/d over 4–6 months. This treatment nearly universally succeeds in eliminating constitutional and musculoskeletal symptoms within days to a few weeks. Anemia, thrombocytosis, and elevated ESRs also usually respond promptly. Remission, defined as resolution of signs, symptoms, and laboratory markers of inflammation, as well as lack of progression of angiographic abnormalities, is seen in most patients who receive glucocorticoid therapy. Unfortunately, many patients with Takayasu arteritis experience relapses of symptoms or progression of vascular disease that necessitate restarting high-dose prednisone therapy. Open studies suggest that methotrexate plus prednisone or mycophenolate mofetil plus prednisone may be more effective than prednisone alone in some patients. Small open trials also suggest that infliximab, an inhibitor of tumor necrosis factor, is an effective glucocorticoid-sparing agent. Because of its toxicity, cyclophosphamide is rarely used to treat Takayasu arteritis. Rituximab has been reported to be effective in a few small series of patients.

Complications of Takayasu arteritis, such as hypertension, congestive heart failure, angina, or aortic regurgitation, may benefit from other forms of medical therapy. Treating hypertension is especially tricky in patients with extensive Takayasu arteritis who may have two or more arterial beds with substantially different blood pressures. Reducing blood pressure to achieve a "normal" blood pressure in the legs may aggravate or cause upper extremity claudication. Often the physician must accept compromises in blood pressures that sustain perfusion of critical organs or tissues. Other complications that can be prevented or treated include osteoporosis. Patients taking prednisone long term can guard against osteoporosis by performing weight-bearing exercises and taking 400–800 units of vitamin D and 1200–1800 mg of calcium daily; whether a bisphosphonate or other agent to prevent osteoporosis is added depends on the patient's menopausal status and overall risk of developing osteoporosis (see Chapter 58).

Interventional radiologists and surgeons also can play important roles in treatment. Surgery can be life-saving for treating aortic regurgitation, mitral regurgitation, severe coronary artery ostial lesions, and thoracic aortic aneurysms. Angioplasty and stenting have been successful in treating some cases of hypertension caused by renal artery stenosis. However, restenosis is common. Severely stenotic lesions of the subclavian or carotid arteries are often surprisingly well tolerated, especially when the patient is supported with effective medical therapy. For these vascular areas, the adage "less is more" often applies. Whenever possible, angioplasty or vascular surgery should be deferred until medical therapy has suppressed the inflammation.

▶ **Prognosis**

Most patients have a chronic relapsing and remitting course requiring careful monitoring and adjustment of suppressive therapy. Judging the level of inflammation can be difficult and requires monitoring symptoms, signs, and laboratory markers of inflammation (eg, hematocrit and ESR). Some experts advocate annual MRI of the aorta and its branches since some patients show progression in the absence of obvious symptoms or signs of active disease. Pregnancy appears surprisingly well tolerated if the patient has inactive disease, is taking low doses of prednisone (ie, <15 mg), and has normal renal function.

Almost all patients experience permanent morbidity from Takayasu arteritis. Because of the morbidity, only about half of the patients are able to work. Survival rates have increased greatly recently so that 10-year survival rates of 80–90% have become common. Advances in diagnosis, medical and surgical treatment, and monitoring augur even better prognosis in the near future. Mortality has been caused chiefly by renal failure, stroke, cardiac failure, or infectious complications of immunosuppressive treatment.

Dagna L, Salvo F, Tiraboschi M, et al. Pentraxin-3 as a marker of disease activity in Takayasu arteritis. *Ann Intern Med.* 2011;155:425. [PMID: 21969341]

Direskeneli H, Aydin SZ, Merkel PA. Assessment of disease activity and progression in Takayasu's arteritis. *Clin Exp Rheumatol.* 2011;29(1 Suppl 64):S86. [PMID: 21586201]

Johns Hopkins Vasculitis Center
http://vasculitis.med.jhu.edu

Ogino H, Matsuda H, Minatoya K, et al. Overview of the late outcome of medical and surgical treatment of Takayasu arteritis. *Circulation.* 2008;118(25):2738. [PMID: 19106398]

Vasculitis Foundation
http://www.vasculitisfoundation.org/

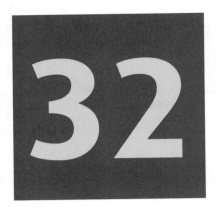

Granulomatosis with Polyangiitis (Wegener Granulomatosis)

32

John H. Stone, MD, MPH

ESSENTIALS OF DIAGNOSIS

▶ Three pathologic hallmarks: granulomatous inflammation, vasculitis, and necrosis.

▶ Classic clinical features are found in multiple organ systems:

- Nonspecific constitutional symptoms, such as fatigue, myalgias, weight loss, and fevers.
- Persistent upper respiratory tract and ear "infections" that do not respond to antibiotic therapy.
- Orbital pseudotumor, nearly always associated with chronic nasosinus conditions.
- Migratory pauciarticular or polyarticular arthritis.
- Nodular or cavitary lung lesions that are misdiagnosed initially as malignancies or infections.
- Rapidly progressive glomerulonephritis.

▶ Antineutrophil cytoplasmic antibody (ANCA) assays are helpful in diagnosis if positive by both immunofluorescence and enzyme immunoassay. A significant minority of patients with granulomatosis with polyangiitis are ANCA-negative, particularly those with "limited" disease.

▶ General Considerations

Granulomatosis with polyangiitis (GPA; formerly called Wegener granulomatosis) is one of the most common forms of systemic vasculitis, with a reported annual incidence of 10 cases per million. The disease involves small- to medium-sized blood vessels (small more often than medium). GPA affects both the arterial and venous circulations, in contrast to polyarteritis nodosa, a disorder in which only arteries and muscular arterioles are affected. The cause of GPA is not known, but the prominence of upper and lower airway involvement suggests a response to an inhaled antigen. The

disease is the prototype of conditions associated with ANCAs, an autoantibody generally believed to amplify rather than to initiate the inflammatory process. GPA occurs in people of all ethnic backgrounds but demonstrates a strong predilection for whites, particularly those of northern European ancestry. The male:female ratio is approximately 1:1. The mean age at diagnosis is 50 years. The elderly are often affected. The disease is less common but known to occur in children.

GPA typically presents in a subacute fashion. Patients complain of symptoms that appear to be innocuous at first, such as nasal stuffiness, "sinusitis," and decreases in hearing. During this "prodrome," attentive primary care providers may suspect and diagnose GPA before the onset of generalized disease. Such early recognition of GPA may prevent the disabling and disfiguring end-organ complications of this disorder, such as collapse of the nasal bridge, renal failure, diffuse alveolar hemorrhage, and widespread infarctions of peripheral nerves.

Therapies for GPA are associated with substantial treatment-induced morbidity in both the short- and long-term. Careful follow-up and monitoring of basic laboratory tests (eg, regularly obtaining complete blood cell counts) may prevent some adverse effects of treatment or minimize their impact. More widespread use of rituximab in lieu of cyclophosphamide may diminish some of the long-term side effects associated with GPA treatment, particularly infertility and malignancy.

Because of the remitting and relapsing nature of many GPA cases and the disease's tendency to recur during or after the taper of treatment, primary care providers play an important role in the early detection of disease flares.

▶ Clinical Findings

A. Symptoms and Signs

1. Nose, sinuses, and ears—Approximately 90% of patients with GPA have nasal involvement. This is often the first disease manifestation. The typical symptoms are

Table 32–1. Major clinical manifestations of granulomatosis with polyangiitis (formerly Wegener granulomatosis).

Organ	Manifestation
Nose	Persistent rhinorrhea; bloody, brown nasal crusts; nasal obstruction; nasal septal perforation; saddle-nose deformity
Sinuses	Sinusitis with radiologic evidence of bony erosions
Ears	Conductive hearing loss due to granulomatous inflammation in the middle ear; sensorineural hearing loss; mixed hearing loss common
Mouth	Strawberry gums; tongue or other oral ulcers; occasional purpuric lesions on palate
Eyes	Orbital pseudotumor; scleritis (often necrotizing); episcleritis; conjunctivitis; keratitis (risk of corneal melt); uveitis (anterior)
Trachea	Subglottic stenosis
Lungs	Nodular, cavitary lesions; nonspecific pulmonary infiltrates; alveolar hemorrhage; bronchial lesions
Heart	Occasional valvular lesions, usually not evident during life; pericarditis
Gastrointestinal	Mesenteric vasculitis uncommon; splenic involvement quite common but usually subclinical (detected as splenic infarcts on cross-sectional imaging)

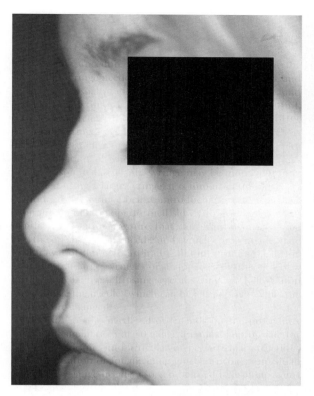

▲ **Figure 32–1.** Cartilaginous inflammation of the nose in granulomatosis with polyangiitis (Wegener granulomatosis) may lead to nasal septal perforation and ultimately to collapse of the nasal bridge ("saddle-nose" deformity).

persistent rhinorrhea, unusually severe nasal obstruction, epistaxis, and bloody or brown nasal crusts (Table 32–1). Cartilaginous inflammation may lead to perforation of the nasal septum and collapse of the nasal bridge (a "saddle-nose" deformity) (Figure 32–1). Bony erosions of the sinus cavities are characteristic of GPA but only develop after long-standing disease (months).

Both conductive and sensorineural forms of hearing loss occur in GPA. The usual pattern of auditory dysfunction is a mixed one, with the simultaneous occurrence of both conductive and sensorineural hearing loss. Conductive hearing loss results from granulomatous involvement of the middle ear, most often leading to serous otitis media. Granulomatous inflammation in the middle ear may also compress the seventh cranial nerve as it courses through the middle ear cavity, leading to a peripheral facial nerve palsy. (This is often misdiagnosed as Bell palsy or Lyme disease.) Sensorineural hearing loss results from inner ear (cochlear) involvement and may also be associated with vestibular dysfunction (eg, nausea, vertigo, tinnitus). However, the sensorineural hearing loss associated with GPA is seldom profound. Additional information about sensorineural hearing loss is found in Chapter 68.

2. Eyes—GPA may present with a variety of inflammatory lesions of the eye (Figure 32–2). Orbital pseudotumors in

the retrobulbar space may lead to proptosis and visual loss through optic nerve ischemia (compression of the nerve's blood supply by the space-occupying mass). Scleritis causes photophobia and painful, often nodular, scleral erythema. If unchecked, necrotizing scleritis may lead to scleral thinning, scleromalacia perforans, and visual loss. Peripheral keratitis may cause ulcerations on the margin of the cornea and lead to the syndrome of "corneal melt."

Episcleritis and conjunctivitis constitute less serious ocular complications of GPA but are very common. Their occurrence may be the presenting symptom of the disease or the first manifestation of a flare. Nasolacrimal duct obstruction leads to poor outflow of tears such that the eyes in a patient with GPA are characteristically wet. Anterior uveitis is rare in GPA in comparison to other rheumatologic conditions such as ankylosing spondylitis (see Chapter 17), Behçet disease (see Chapter 38), and sarcoidosis (see Chapter 54). Central retinal artery occlusions are a known complication of this disorder, but other retinal lesions and posterior uveitis are uncommon.

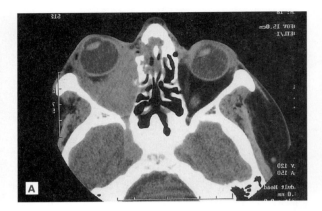

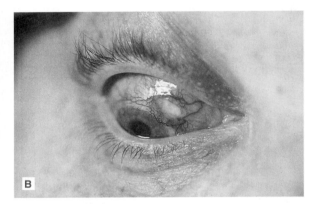

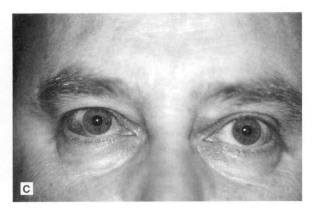

▲ **Figure 32–2.** **A:** CT scan of the orbit showing an orbital pseudotumor, leading to proptosis and visual loss. **B:** Scleritis with a marginal corneal ulceration. **C:** Painless erythema of the superficial surface of the eye—episcleritis—the most common ocular complication of granulomatosis with polyangiitis (formerly Wegener granulomatosis).

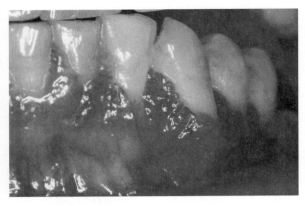

▲ **Figure 32–3.** Granulomatosis with polyangiitis (formerly Wegener granulomatosis) patient with intense inflammation of the gums, a physical finding known as "strawberry gums."

3. Mouth—Two classic mouth lesions of GPA are gum inflammation ("strawberry gums" [Figure 32-3]) and tongue ulcers. The gum inflammation of GPA, which derives its name from the resemblance of the dental papillae to strawberries, is quite distinctive among rheumatologic conditions. The oral ulcerations of GPA, caused by medium-vessel vasculitis, typically occur on the lateral sides of the posterior tongue. Strawberry gums and tongue ulcers, both quite painful, respond promptly to glucocorticoids.

4. Trachea—Subglottic stenosis, the result of tracheal inflammation and scarring below the vocal cords, is a potentially disabling manifestation that is largely specific to GPA (relapsing polychondritis can also cause this lesion). Subglottic involvement is often asymptomatic and may manifest itself only as a subtle hoarseness. With time, however, airway scarring and profound tracheal narrowing may occur. Pulmonary function tests with flow volume loops can show a fixed extrathoracic obstructive defect, but this may not become apparent until the process is advanced. Supraglottic disease, although substantially less common than subglottic stenosis, may also occur in GPA.

5. Lungs—Approximately 80% of patients with GPA have pulmonary lesions during the course of their disease. Pulmonary symptoms include cough, hemoptysis, dyspnea, and sometimes pleuritic chest pain. Lung lesions are often asymptomatic, however, and some are detectable only if chest imaging is performed. The most common radiologic findings are pulmonary infiltrates and nodules (Figure 32–4). The infiltrates, which may wax and wane, are often misdiagnosed initially as pneumonia. Single, large pulmonary nodules are often misdiagnosed as lung cancer. Nodules are usually multiple, bilateral, and often cavitary. Many nodules have peripheral locations and, if wedge-shaped, may be mistaken for pulmonary emboli.

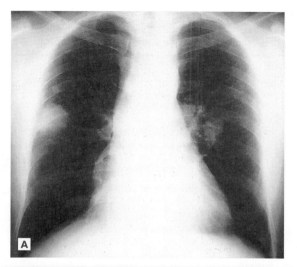

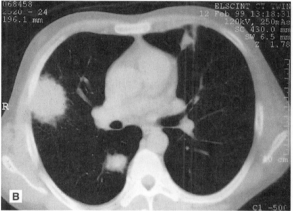

▲ **Figure 32–4.** Chest radiograph and computed tomography scan show multiple bilateral nodules. **A:** Posteroanterior view of the chest shows bilateral lung nodules. **B:** Computed tomography scan of the chest in the same patient shows additional lesions not evident of the radiograph.

Pulmonary capillaritis can lead to hemoptysis and rapidly changing alveolar infiltrates. Large airway disease leading to significant bronchial stenosis, similar to the findings found in subglottic stenosis, occurs in a minority of GPA patients. Large airway disease may be more common in pediatric than in adult GPA. Finally, venous thrombotic events (particularly deep venous thromboses) occur in a substantial proportion of patients, perhaps as a complication of the disease's propensity to involve the venous circulation. These events tend to occur in close association with periods of active disease. Pulmonary emboli should be considered in the GPA patient in whom dyspnea, pleuritic chest pain, or other compatible symptoms develop.

6. Kidneys—Renal disease, among the most ominous clinical manifestations of GPA, is often a marker for swift disease progression. Renal involvement, present in approximately 20% of patients with GPA at the time of diagnosis, develops eventually in a substantially higher portion of patients (up to 80%) during the course of the disease. The clinical presentation of renal disease in GPA is rapidly progressive glomerulonephritis: hematuria, red blood cell casts, proteinuria (usually non-nephrotic), and rising serum creatinine. Without appropriate therapy, loss of renal function can ensue within days or weeks. More subacute courses of renal diseases also develop in some patients with GPA, particularly those with anti-myeloperoxidase antibodies (MPO-ANCA) as opposed to PR3-ANCA. GPA is also known to present with renal mass lesions that mimic malignancy.

7. Other organs—Nonspecific arthralgias and frank arthritis often occur early in the course of GPA. The arthritis of GPA is migratory in nature and may assume a variety of joint patterns. The most common form of arthritis is a pauci- or monoarticular syndrome of lower or upper extremity joints that is often migratory in nature. Polyarthritis of the small joints of the hands can also occur. Digital ischemia and gangrene resulting from inflammation in medium-sized digital arteries are occasionally the presenting feature of GPA. The skin manifestations of GPA include the full array of findings associated with cutaneous vasculitis: palpable purpura, papules, ulcers, and vesiculobullous lesions.

Examination of the skin should include careful inspection for the nodular lesions of "Churg-Strauss granulomas" (cutaneous extravascular necrotizing granulomas). These nodules are located typically on the extensor surfaces of the elbows and other pressure points (Figure 32–5). Splinter

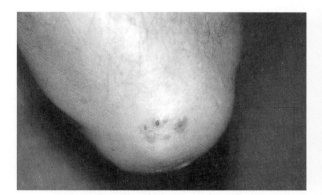

▲ **Figure 32–5.** The patient has granulomatosis with polyangiitis (formerly Wegener granulomatosis) and has a positive test result for rheumatoid factor. The nodule over the extensor surface of the elbow was initially misdiagnosed as a rheumatoid nodule instead of a "Churg-Strauss granuloma" (cutaneous extravascular necrotizing granuloma).

hemorrhages may occur in GPA, raising diagnostic confusion with endocarditis. Lesions resembling pyoderma gangrenosum but caused by a medium-vessel vasculitis may also occur. Although involvement of the brain parenchyma with GPA has been reported, meningeal inflammation (presenting as excruciating headaches and cranial neuropathies) is a more typical central nervous system disease manifestation. Mononeuritis multiplex can complicate GPA but is less characteristic of this disease than other forms of systemic vasculitis (eg, polyarteritis nodosa, microscopic polyangiitis, and eosinophilic granulomatosis with polyangiitis [the Churg-Strauss syndrome]).

B. Laboratory Findings

The results of routine laboratory tests and more specialized assays in GPA are shown in Table 32–2. All of these tests are appropriate at the initial evaluation of a patient with possible GPA. The exclusion of renal disease through the careful performance of a urinalysis is essential in the evaluation and follow-up of all patients with GPA. The erythrocyte sedimentation rate and serum C-reactive protein level are useful (albeit imperfect) biomarkers in the longitudinal evaluation of disease activity. The utility of ANCA testing is discussed below.

C. Imaging Studies

Up to one third of patients with GPA have asymptomatic pulmonary lesions on radiologic imaging. Computed tomography is superior to chest radiography in demonstrating the extent of pulmonary disease. Consequently, patients with confirmed or strongly suspected diagnoses of GPA should have CT scans of the chest as baseline studies. Virtually any finding (with the rare exception of hilar and mediastinal adenopathy) may be present on chest imaging in GPA, including pleural effusions and nonspecific infiltrates.

D. Special Tests

1. Biopsy—Because of the numerous potential mimickers of GPA and the frequent shortcomings of ANCA (see next section on ANCA testing), the diagnosis of GPA is most secure when established through biopsy of an involved organ. Among the organs commonly involved in GPA, those most likely to yield tissue that permits a diagnosis are (in descending order): lung, kidney, and upper respiratory tract (nose or sinuses). The tissue necrosis associated with GPA is frequently so extensive within diseased tissues that it is termed "geographic necrosis."

Even when all three pathologic hallmarks (granulomatous inflammation, vasculitis, and necrosis) are present, the diagnosis of GPA requires the careful integration of pathologic findings with clinical, laboratory, and radiologic data. Acid-fast and fungal pathogens must be excluded by special stains and cultures.

Biopsies of the upper respiratory tract (nose, sinuses, and subglottic region) are frequently nondiagnostic, yielding only

Table 32–2. The laboratory evaluation in granulomatosis with polyangiitis (formerly Wegener granulomatosis).

Test	Typical Result
Complete blood cell count	• Normochromic, normocytic anemia; acute, severe anemias possible in alveolar hemorrhage • Mild to moderate leukocytosis common, usually not exceeding 18×10^9/L • Moderate to pronounced thrombocytosis typical, ranging from platelet counts of 400×10^9/L to occasionally $>1000 \times 10^9$/L
Electrolytes	Hyperkalemia in the setting of advanced renal dysfunction
Liver function test	Hepatic involvement is quite unusual in GPA; when present, there can be elevations of transaminases (AST/ALT) in excess of 1000 mg/dL
Urinalysis with microscopy	• Hematuria (ranging from mild to so high that red blood cells are too numerous to count) • Red blood cell casts • Proteinuria (nephritic range proteinuria in a small minority)
Erythrocyte sedimentation rate/ C-reactive protein	Dramatic elevations of acute phase reactants are typical, generally with good correlation to disease activity
ANA	Negative
Rheumatoid factor	Positive in 40–50% of patients, often leading to diagnostic confusion with rheumatoid arthritis
C3, C4	Complement levels are normal to elevated in GPA, in contrast to systemic lupus erythematosus, cryoglobulinemia, and other diseases in which immune complexes appear to play major roles
ANCA	Positive in 60–90% of patients with GPA
Anti-GBM	A minority of patients with GPA also have anti-GBM antibodies

ANA, antinuclear antibody; ANCA, antineutrophil cytoplasmic antibody; anti-GBM, antiglomerular basement membrane antibody; AST/ALT aspartate aminotransferase/alanine aminotransferase; GPA, granulomatosis with polyangiitis.

nonspecific acute and chronic inflammation. Upper respiratory tract biopsies demonstrate the complete diagnostic triad in only about 15% of cases. However, these biopsies are generally safer than lung or kidney biopsies, and the finding of even parts of this triad in a nose or sinus biopsy may serve as compelling evidence for the diagnosis of GPA, provided that other manifestations of the disease are present elsewhere. Compelling if not diagnostic histopathologic findings may clinch the diagnosis if the patient's ANCA serologies are also consistent with GPA.

GPA finds its fullest pathologic expression in the lung, where the large amounts of tissue obtained at open or thoracoscopic lung biopsy may capture the entire spectrum of disease. Transbronchial and radiologically-guided needle biopsies usually fail to yield diagnostic tissue specimens. The leukocytoclastic vasculitis of GPA may involve arteries, veins, and capillaries, with or without granulomatous features. Vascular necrosis begins as clusters of neutrophils within the blood vessel wall (microabscesses) that degenerate and become surrounded by palisading histiocytes. Coalescence of such neutrophilic microabscesses leads to geographic necrosis.

Renal biopsy findings are not specific for GPA because other pauci-immune forms of glomerulonephritis can have identical histopathologic features. However, renal biopsy results are sufficiently characteristic to establish the diagnosis in appropriate clinical settings. The typical renal lesion of GPA is segmental necrotizing glomerulonephritis, with or without crescent formation. Thrombotic changes in the glomerular capillary loops are among the earliest histologic lesions. Immunofluorescence studies of renal biopsies in GPA confirm the "pauci-immune" nature of the renal involvement (ie, the relatively sparse immunoglobulin and complement deposition found in this disorder compared with such diseases as systemic lupus erythematosus, Henoch-Schönlein purpura, and Goodpasture syndrome).

2. Serologic testing for ANCA—ANCAs are directed against antigens that reside within the primary granules of neutrophils and monocytes. Positive ANCA assays are often instrumental in suggesting the diagnosis. In patients with multiple classic organ system features of GPA, a positive ANCA assay that has been confirmed by both immunofluorescence and enzyme immunoassay testing can preclude the need for biopsy. However, a small percentage of patients with disseminated GPA are ANCA-negative, so a negative ANCA assay does not exclude the diagnosis. Among patients with "limited" disease (see Treatment section), 30% or more may lack ANCA. Rises and falls in ANCA titers often demonstrate poor correlation with the timing of disease flares and should never be used as the sole guide to the use of immunosuppression.

The two types of ANCA tests now in common use are immunofluorescence assays and enzyme immunoassays. These two tests are complementary in the diagnosis of GPA. Both should be used in evaluating patients in whom this disease is suspected.

With immunofluorescence, three principal patterns are recognized: cytoplasmic (C-ANCA), perinuclear (P-ANCA), and atypical. Immunofluorescence testing alone has low specificity and a low positive predictive value for GPA. Hence, the diagnosis of GPA should never rest primarily on a positive immunofluorescence assay, regardless of whether the pattern is C-ANCA or P-ANCA. In patients with vasculitis, the C-ANCA pattern usually corresponds to the presence of antiproteinase-3 antibodies (PR3-ANCA),

detected by enzyme immunoassay. The combination of a C-ANCA pattern by immunofluorescence and a positive PR3-ANCA by enzyme immunoassay has a high positive predictive value for GPA.

The P-ANCA pattern usually corresponds to the presence of MPO-ANCA in patients with vasculitis. MPO-ANCA occur in approximately 10% of patients with GPA but are more typical of microscopic polyangiitis (see Chapter 33), eosinophilic granulomatosis with polyangiitis (the Churg-Strauss syndrome; see Chapter 34), and necrotizing crescentic glomerulonephritis (ie, renal-limited, ANCA-associated vasculitis).

Atypical immunofluorescence ANCA patterns, which may occur in association with a wide variety of diseases such as inflammatory bowel disease and connective tissue disorders, are not directed against either PR3 or MPO and do not imply the presence of a primary vasculitis. Atypical ANCA patterns of immunofluorescence are often misread by inexperienced laboratories as showing perinuclear immunofluorescence.

▶ Differential Diagnosis

The protean nature of GPA dictates that an all-inclusive differential diagnosis for the varied presentations of this disease is enormously broad. It encompasses sinusitis and pneumonia caused by microbial pathogens, other forms of vasculitis often associated with ANCA, and the confluence of several common medical problems in the same patient (eg, the simultaneous occurrence of pneumonia and interstitial nephritis caused by antibiotics). The major disease entities in the differential diagnosis of GPA are shown in Table 32–3.

GPA may smolder in the upper respiratory tract for months or even years before becoming a generalized, life-threatening illness. Recognition of the systemic disorder underlying the repeated "ear infections," allergies, musculoskeletal symptoms, and other complaints is often delayed. Patients with GPA frequently endure multiple courses of antibiotics, myringotomies, and other interventions that are largely ineffectual or provide only temporary relief before the correct diagnosis is made. GPA should be suspected when mundane complaints persist long enough to become unusual.

Limited GPA may pose difficult diagnostic problems. The destructive upper airway disease that occurs in limited GPA may also be caused by infection (eg, mycobacteria, fungi, actinomycosis, and syphilis), malignancy (eg, squamous cell carcinoma and extranodal lymphoma), or illicit drug use (eg, intranasal cocaine or smoking crack). Patients with cocaine-induced midline lesions that mimic GPA often have ANCA directed against human neutrophils elastase, another primary granule enzyme. Finally, the sinus destruction of GPA may be mimicked by nonvasculitic disorders such as "lethal midline granuloma," now known to be an angioproliferative T-cell lymphoma.

Table 32–3. Differential diagnosis of granulomatosis with polyangiitis (Wegener granulomatosis).

Other vasculitides
Polyarteritis nodosa
Microscopic polyangiitis
Churg-Strauss syndrome
Henoch-Schönlein purpura
Mixed cryoglobulinemia
Goodpasture syndrome
Giant cell arteritis
Infections
Mycobacterial diseases
Fungal infections (histoplasmosis,
blastomycosis, coccidioidomycosis)
Streptococcal pneumonia with glomerulonephritis
Malignancies
Nasopharyngeal carcinoma
Hodgkin disease
Non-Hodgkin lymphoma
Angiocentric lymphoma ("lymphomatoid granulomatosis")
Castleman disease
Granulomatous disorders
Sarcoidosis
Berylliosis
Systemic autoimmune conditions
Systemic lupus erythematosus
Rheumatoid arthritis
Relapsing polychondritis

Chronic infections such as those caused by mycobacterial and fungal pathogens are essential to exclude through special stains and cultures of tissue biopsies. Because granulomatous infections of the lung may also cause vasculitis and necrosis, special stains and cultures for infection should show negative results before the diagnosis of GPA is made. Infections are especially important to consider in patients with established diagnoses of GPA who have been treated with immunosuppressive medications.

Rheumatoid arthritis is a common misdiagnosis because arthritis is a frequent finding at presentation. Furthermore, approximately half of all patients with GPA have positive test results for rheumatoid factor, and Churg-Strauss granulomas often occur at precisely the most frequent sites for rheumatoid nodules—the elbows—further heightening the diagnostic confusion. (Patients are usually unaware of these lesions, as they may be unaware of rheumatoid nodules.) Other systemic inflammatory conditions associated with autoimmunity (eg, lupus) also affect multiple organ systems and must be distinguished from GPA. Sarcoidosis is an excellent mimicker of GPA because of the frequency with which it involves many of the same organs.

Finally, many other forms of systemic vasculitis are high on the differential diagnosis for GPA. Accurate distinction among GPA, polyarteritis nodosa, giant cell arteritis, Goodpasture syndrome, microscopic polyangiitis, eosinophilic granulomatosis with polyangiitis (Churg-Strauss syndrome), Henoch-Schönlein purpura, relapsing polychondritis, and cryoglobulinemia is essential because their complications, treatments, and prognoses vary widely. ANCA-associated vasculitis can also be induced by certain medications, particularly propylthiouracil and hydralazine (see Chapter 42). Cutaneous vasculitis is usually the predominant manifestation of drug-induced ANCA-associated vasculitis, and the type of ANCA typically found is MPO- rather than PR3-ANCA.

▶ Treatment

The management of GPA should be stratified according to whether the patient has severe or limited disease. Severe disease (defined as an immediate threat to either the function of a vital organ or to the patient's life) requires treatment with either rituximab or cyclophosphamide and high doses of glucocorticoids. A randomized, double-blind, placebo-controlled trial of rituximab versus cyclophosphamide for the induction of disease remission (the Rituximab in ANCA-Associated Vasculitis [RAVE] trial) concluded that rituximab was not inferior to cyclophosphamide followed by azathioprine in efficacy and might be preferable to the alkylating agent because of a potentially superior long-term side-effect profile. Rituximab is superior to cyclophosphamide for the treatment of relapsing GPA. The RAVE trial was conducted with a rituximab regimen consisting of 375 mg/m^2, administered weekly times four doses. In practice, however, many clinicians find it simpler to use a regimen of 1000 mg times two doses, separated by 15 days.

Rituximab has been approved by the US Food and Drug Administration for the induction of remission in GPA and is viewed widely as the standard of care. Long-term follow-up of the RAVE cohort indicates that one course of rituximab plus glucocorticoids is as effective as the standard remission induction and maintenance regimen (cyclophosphamide/azathioprine plus glucocorticoids) for at least 18 months. The most appropriate timing of re-treatment with rituximab (and decisions about which patients should be re-treated) requires further study.

The alternative to rituximab plus glucocorticoids for remission induction in GPA is the combination of cyclophosphamide (2 mg/kg/d for those with normal renal function) and glucocorticoids (1 mg/kg/d of prednisone, perhaps preceded by a 3-day intravenous "pulse" of methylprednisolone). This combination leads to excellent initial therapeutic responses in 90% or more of patients and to complete remission in 75%. In attempting to control the disease and avoid the side effects of long-term cyclophosphamide therapy, shorter courses (eg, 3–6 months) of induction treatment with cyclophosphamide are now used followed by longer-term treatment for the maintenance of remission with either azathioprine (up to 2 mg/kg/d) or methotrexate. More recent data suggest that the intermittent administration of intravenous cyclophosphamide is equally likely to lead to disease remission at a substantially lower cumulative cyclophosphamide dose and possibly a lower rate of adverse effects. However, the rate of disease flares following remission is higher in patients treated with intermittent as opposed to daily cyclophosphamide regimens.

By definition, limited disease includes all cases of GPA that are not severe. Because patients with limited GPA are more likely to have nasosinus disease, arthritis, nodular pulmonary lesions, cutaneous findings, minor ocular complications, and mild renal disease as their principal manifestations, they are likely to benefit from a less dangerous approach to therapy. Patients with limited GPA may respond to the combination of methotrexate (up to 25 mg/wk) and glucocorticoids, thus sparing patients the potential side effects of cyclophosphamide. Methotrexate is not an appropriate first-line treatment for patients with severe involvement of the kidney, lung, or other vital organs and should not be used in patients with significant renal dysfunction (eg, a serum creatinine of >2.0 mg/dL). The use of rituximab in patients with limited GPA requires further investigation, but this medication will likely be useful in a substantial proportion of patients with limited GPA.

Regardless of which remission induction approach is used, all patients with GPA should receive prophylaxis against *Pneumocystis jiroveci* pneumonia with single-strength trimethoprim-sulfamethoxazole, 100 mg/d of dapsone, or 1500 mg/d of atovaquone.

For the maintenance of remission, a variety of approaches are appropriate. Patients treated with rituximab may not require a remission maintenance agent, but the serial administration of rituximab to maintain B cell depletion and disease remission requires further study. Both azathioprine (1.0–2.5 mg/kg/d) and methotrexate (20–25 mg/wk) are appropriate as agents to follow the use of cyclophosphamide for remission induction.

Patients with subglottic stenosis comprise a unique subset of GPA. This disease complication often responds better to mechanical interventions than to immunosuppressive therapy (ie, to surgical dilatation accomplished through noninvasive approaches and glucocorticoid injections rather than to systemic immunosuppression). Laser techniques should be avoided during these procedures because they may exacerbate tissue injury. Otolaryngologists frequently use mitomycin C injections to help prevent the proliferation of scar tissue following dilatations of subglottic stenoses.

▶ Complications

Regimens of cytotoxic agents and glucocorticoids have converted this once nearly always fatal disease into one that responds well to treatment and, in most cases, enters remission for variable lengths of time. Unfortunately, GPA is marked by a pronounced tendency to flare during the tapering of medications or after the cessation of treatment. The requirement of treating disease flares with additional courses of therapy frequently leads to mounting treatment-related morbidity.

Under the original regimen established by the National Institutes of Health (NIH), patients were treated with cyclophosphamide for a mean period of approximately 2 years (for 1 full year after the achievement of remission). Although many patients had remissions that lasted for up to several years, less than 40% of the patients in the NIH series achieved "cures" following their initial courses of therapy. Repeated administration of these potentially toxic treatments to patients with disease recurrences led to substantial long-term morbidity. Forty-two percent of patients treated under the NIH regimen suffered permanent medication-induced morbidity. The major complications of treating GPA with cytotoxic agents (not including the multiple and often severe side effects of prolonged glucocorticoid treatment) follow:

- Bone marrow suppression
- Myelodysplastic syndromes
- Opportunistic infection
- Drug-induced injury to the lungs, bladder, and liver
- Infertility
- Long-term risk of malignancies, particularly lymphoma and bladder cancers

Remission induction regimens that use rituximab rather than cyclophosphamide appear likely to have fewer implications for patients' fertility and malignancy risks.

▶ When to Refer

The overall disease process frequently appears to accelerate once renal involvement becomes evident. Thus, the finding of an active urine sediment or a rise in serum creatinine in GPA signals a matter of utmost urgency.

Gross hematuria may indicate drug-induced cystitis in patients treated with cyclophosphamide. This complication may be associated with dysuria but not always. Cystoscopy is required to confirm the diagnosis in patients with drug-induced cystitis. Upon the diagnosis of cyclophosphamide-induced bladder injury, further treatment with this medication is contraindicated. Alternatively, gross hematuria is sometimes a presenting feature of active glomerulonephritis. The occurrence of hematuria months to years after a course of cyclophosphamide may indicate the development of bladder cancer and should prompt a cystoscopic evaluation by a urologist.

Hemoptysis, shortness of breath, rapidly changing pulmonary infiltrates, and abrupt declines in hematocrit may all indicate active pulmonary capillaritis. Hemoptysis may be an insensitive indicator of diffuse alveolar hemorrhage. This GPA complication requires rapid intervention with immunosuppressive medications (cyclophosphamide and glucocorticoids) and perhaps observation or management in an intensive care unit.

A fever in a patient who is receiving therapy for GPA signals a potential medical emergency, indicating the possibility of infection in immunocompromised patients.

The complaint of ocular pain, photophobia, or visual loss should prompt a swift referral to an ophthalmologist. Orbital pseudotumor, necrotizing scleritis, and marginal ulcers of the cornea may all lead quickly to vision-threatening ocular events.

Voice huskiness and subtle signs of stridorous breathing may indicate impending critical stenosis of the subglottic region. Some patients have subacute respiratory stridor. Severe cases may require tracheostomies. Pulmonary function tests (flow-volume loops) provide a useful noninvasive means of quantifying and following the degree of extrathoracic airway obstruction. However, thin-cut CT scans of the trachea are more sensitive for these lesions. In some cases, direct visualization with fiberoptic laryngoscopy is required to make the diagnosis.

De Groot K, Harper L, Jayne DR, et al. EUVAS (European Vasculitis Study Group). Pulse versus daily oral cyclophosphamide for induction of remission in antineutrophil cytoplasmic antibody-associated vasculitis: a randomized trial. *Ann Intern Med.* 2009;150:670. [PMID: 19451574]

Hoffman GS, Kerr GS, Leavitt RY, et al. Wegener's granulomatosis: an analysis of 158 patients. *Ann Intern Med.* 1992;116:488. [PMID: 1739240]

Hoffman GS, Specks U. Antineutrophil cytoplasmic antibodies. *Arthritis Rheum.* 1998;41:1521. [PMID: 9751084]

Jayne D, Rasmussen N, Andrassy K, et al. European Vasculitis Study Group. A randomized trial of maintenance therapy for vasculitis associated with antineutrophil cytoplasmic antibodies. *N Engl J Med.* 2003;349:36. [PMID: 12840090]

Seo P, Stone JH. The antineutrophil cytoplasmic antibody-associated vasculitides. *Am J Med.* 2004;117:39. [PMID: 15210387]

Stone JH, Merkel PA, Spiera R, et al. RAVE-ITN Research Group. Rituximab versus cyclophosphamide for ANCA-associated vasculitis. *N Engl J Med.* 2010;363:221. [PMID: 20647199]

Wegener's Granulomatosis Etanercept Trial (WGET) Research Group. Etanercept plus standard therapy for Wegener's granulomatosis. *N Engl J Med.* 2005;352:351. [PMID: 15673801]

[The Vasculitis Foundation]
   http://www.vasculitisfoundation.org/

Microscopic Polyangiitis

33

Geetha Duvuru, MD, MRCP
John H. Stone, MD, MPH

ESSENTIALS OF DIAGNOSIS

- ► Microscopic polyangiitis (MPA) is the most common cause of the pulmonary-renal syndrome of alveolar hemorrhage and glomerulonephritis.
- ► Usually includes combinations of two or more of the following:
  - Nonspecific constitutional symptoms, including fatigue, myalgias, weight loss, and fevers.
  - Migratory arthralgias or arthritis, either pauciarticular or polyarticular.
  - Palpable purpura, sometimes with skin ulcerations.
  - Sensorimotor mononeuritis multiplex.
  - Alveolar hemorrhage associated with hemoptysis and respiratory compromise.
  - Glomerulonephritis.
- ► Antineutrophil cytoplasmic antibodies (ANCAs) are often critical in making the diagnosis, but a significant minority of patients are ANCA-negative.
- ► The majority of patients with MPA who are ANCA positive have antibodies directed against myeloperoxidase (MPO-ANCA).
- ► ANCA titers are often elevated during disease flares but do not have a consistent temporal relationship with disease activity. Thus, ANCA titers are not reliable predictors of disease flares.

► General Considerations

Microscopic polyangiitis (MPA) is a form of systemic vasculitis that may affect many major organs with crippling or fatal effects. Seventy percent of patients with MPA have antineutrophil cytoplasmic antibodies (ANCAs). MPA is recognized

to be related to both granulomatosis with polyangiitis (GPA; formerly Wegener granulomatosis) and eosinophilic granulomatosis with polyangiitis (EGPA; the Churg-Strauss syndrome) (see Chapters 32 and 34). These disorders are sometimes considered together as the ANCA-associated vasculitides, but important differences exist among these three conditions and significant percentages of patients with these diagnoses do not have ANCA.

MPA has been recognized increasingly since the first Chapel Hill Consensus Conference on the nomenclature of systemic vasculitides, the results of which were published in 1994. Many cases before then were considered to be forms of polyarteritis nodosa (PAN), a disease with which MPA shares substantial overlap. Table 33–1 compares the features of MPA with those of GPA (Wegener) and PAN.

The term "polyangiitis" is preferred to "polyarteritis" for MPA because of the disease's tendency to involve veins as well as arteries. The first Chapel Hill Consensus Conference defined MPA as a process that (1) involves necrotizing vasculitis with few or no immune deposits; (2) affects small blood vessels (capillaries, arterioles, or venules) and possibly medium-sized vessels; and (3) demonstrates a tropism for the kidneys and lungs. With an estimated incidence of 4 cases per million per year, MPA is more common than classic PAN but somewhat less common than GPA (Wegener).

MPA occurs in people of all ethnic backgrounds. The male:female ratio is approximately 1:1. The typical patient is middle-aged to elderly, but the disease may affect people of all ages. The mean age at diagnosis for MPA patients (approximately 60 years) is about 10 years older than the mean age of GPA (Wegener) patients at diagnosis. Several epidemiologic studies have tried to elucidate environmental factors associated with the onset of vasculitis. Some authors have found associations with silica and solvent exposure.

The strongest link between an exposure and MPA relates to the use of propylthiouracil (PTU) for the treatment of hyperthyroidism (a handful of other drugs for other

Table 33–1. Comparison of the features of MPA, GPA, and PAN.

	MPA	GPA	PAN
Vessel size	Small to medium	Small to medium	Medium
Vessel type	Capillaries, venules, and arterioles; sometimes arteries and veins	Capillaries, venules, and arterioles; sometimes arteries and veins	Muscular arteries
Granulomatous inflammation	No	Yes	No
Lung involvement	Yes (pulmonary capillaritis)	Yes (pulmonary nodules, often cavitary)	No
Glomerulonephritis	Yes	Yes	No
Renin-mediated hypertension	No	No	Yes
ANCA-positive	75%	60–90%	No
Hepatitis B association	No	No	Yes (<10% of cases now)
Microaneurysms	Rarely	Rarely	Typically
Mononeuritis multiplex	Commonly (60%)	Occasionally	Commonly (60%)
Likelihood of disease recurrence	33%	>50%	≤10%

ANCA, antineutrophil cytoplasmic antibody; GPA, granulomatosis with polyangiitis (formerly Wegener granulomatosis); MPA, microscopic polyangiitis; PAN, polyarteritis nodosa.

indications have also been implicated, but not as strongly). Anti-MPO antibodies are detected frequently in PTU-treated patients, albeit overt vasculitis occurs in only a small minority (<5%). Drug-induced, ANCA-associated vasculitis is discussed further in Chapter 42).

▶ Clinical Findings

A. Symptoms and Signs

The interval between the onset of first disease symptoms and diagnosis in MPA is substantially shorter than for patients with GPA (Wegener). This is because of the tendency for GPA (Wegener) to smolder in the upper respiratory tract and cause apparently mundane symptoms for months before leading to medical attention. In contrast, the clinical presentation of MPA is usually more obvious at the time the patient becomes aware of symptoms: cutaneous vasculitis, vasculitis neuropathy, or alveolar hemorrhage. Nevertheless, subtle and subacute presentations of MPA are known to occur, and the range of organ system manifestations is extensive.

Although MPA is classified appropriately as a "pulmonary-renal syndrome," regarding this disorder exclusively as a disease that affects the kidneys and lungs is a major potential clinical error. The five most common clinical manifestations of MPA are glomerulonephritis (nearly 80% of patients), weight loss (>70%), mononeuritis multiplex (60%), fevers (55%), and cutaneous vasculitis (>60%). Alveolar hemorrhage, in contrast, occurs in only about 12% of patients. The major clinical manifestations of MPA are shown in Table 33–2.

Table 33–2. Major clinical manifestations of microscopic polyangiitis.

Organ	Manifestation
Constitutional	Weight loss, anorexia, fevers
HEENT	Rhinitis, tongue or other oral ulcers; occasional purpuric lesions on palate; ocular inflammation (eg, sclerouveitis) reported but rare
Lungs	Alveolar hemorrhage; nonspecific infiltrates; pulmonary fibrosis; pleural effusions
Gastrointestinal	Mesenteric vasculitis with microaneurysms in some patients
Kidneys	Glomerulonephritis (small-vessel vasculitis of the kidney); medium-vessel vasculitis occasionally evident on renal biopsy or demonstrated by cross-sectional imaging studies (renal infarcts)
Skin	Palpable purpura, ulcers, vesiculobullous lesions, splinter hemorrhages
Joints	Migratory pauciarthritis or polyarthritis or arthralgias; arthritis is nondestructive
Peripheral nerve	Sensory or motor mononeuritis multiplex
Central nervous system	True central nervous system vasculitis rare but reported

HEENT, head, eyes, ears, nose, throat.

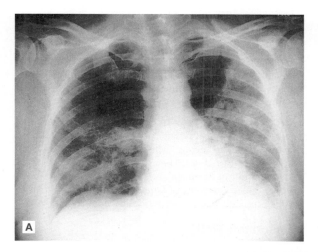

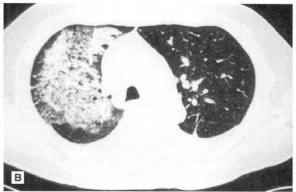

▲ **Figure 33–1.** Radiologic features of alveolar hemorrhage. **A:** Chest radiograph. **B:** Computed tomography scan of the chest.

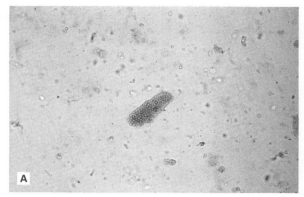

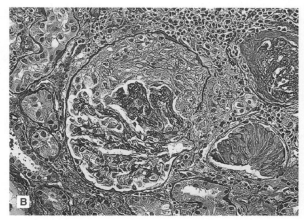

▲ **Figure 33–2.** Renal manifestations of microscopic polyangiitis. **A:** Red blood cell cast in a patient with glomerulonephritis secondary to microscopic polyangiitis. (Reproduced, with permission, from Stone JH, et al. Vasculitis. A collection of pearls and myths. *Rheum Dis Clin North Am.* 2001;27:677.) **B:** Glomerular crescent in a patient with microscopic polyangiitis.

1. Head, eyes, ears, nose, and throat—Some vasculitis experts regard the presence of any upper respiratory tract involvement as evidence that the diagnosis is GPA (Wegener), not MPA. Thus, HEENT involvement in MPA is limited generally to rhinitis or mild cases of nondestructive sinusitis. Serous otitis media may occur in MPA but unlike in GPA (Wegener), granulomatous inflammation is absent. Ocular lesions in MPA (eg, episcleritis, conjunctivitis, keratitis, and occasionally scleritis) have been reported but are less common and less severe than in GPA (Wegener).

2. Lungs—The principal pulmonary manifestation of MPA is capillaritis, which leads to alveolar hemorrhage and often to hemoptysis. Hemoptysis may be only a late indication of bleeding. The typical radiologic features of alveolar hemorrhage are shown in Figure 33–1. Alveolar hemorrhage is associated with a worse prognosis. Interstitial fibrosis and

pleuritis occur in some patients with MPA. Pulmonary fibrosis that resembles usual interstitial pneumonitis in clinical presentation is increasingly recognized as a disease manifestation of MPA. Many cases of pulmonary fibrosis are associated with previous alveolar hemorrhage, but the precise relationship between alveolar hemorrhage and fibrosis is not clear.

3. Kidneys—Renal involvement is seen in at least 80% of patients with MPA. The classic presentation of renal disease in MPA is a rapidly progressive glomerulonephritis reminiscent of GPA (Wegener) (Figure 33–2A). Some patients, however, have renal deterioration that progresses more slowly, over many months. Renal involvement may also present with urinary abnormalities such as proteinuria, microscopic hematuria, and red cell casts. Up to 40% of patients have 24-hour urinary protein excretion of more than 3 g. Proteinuria of this severity is regarded as a poor prognostic factor for renal outcome. The pathologic features of renal disease in MPA are indistinguishable from other forms of pauci-immune glomerulonephritis—namely, a necrotizing, crescentic lesion (Figure 33–2B). Compared with biopsies from patients with ANCA directed against proteinase 3, those with MPO-ANCA have a more chronic pattern of renal injury, with more glomerulosclerosis, tubular atrophy, and interstitial fibrosis.

4. Nervous system—Vasculitic neuropathy is a potentially devastating complication of MPA. The nerve involvement typically occurs in the pattern of a distal, asymmetric, axonal polyneuropathy (mononeuritis multiplex). The first symptoms of vasculitic neuropathy are usually sensory, with numbness, tingling, and dysesthesias. Muscle weakness and wasting follow the infarction of motor nerves (Figure 33–3). Because the named peripheral nerves are usually mixed nerves, bearing both sensory and motor fibers, patients with vasculitic neuropathy typically have both sensory and motor symptoms. Recovery from vasculitic neuropathy may take months; some patients have residual nerve damage after the disease is controlled. Although peripheral nerve lesions tend to dominate the neurologic features of MPA, central nervous system involvement by vasculitis is also described in this disease.

Small-fiber neuropathy has also been reported in MPA. In patients with small-fiber neuropathy, the predominant symptoms are pain and numbness rather than motor weakness. Electrodiagnostic studies in small-fiber neuropathy patients are normal because the involved fibers are below the resolution of nerve conduction velocity assessments. Diagnosis is made by biopsy of the skin and staining for the density of small nerve fibers.

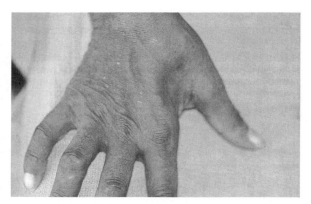

▲ **Figure 33–3.** Muscle wasting caused by vasculitic neuropathy (mononeuritis multiplex) associated with microscopic polyangiitis.

5. Skin—The skin manifestations of MPA include all of the cutaneous lesions associated with small-vessel vasculitis (palpable purpura, papules, vesiculobullous lesions, splinter hemorrhages). In the presence of medium-vessel involvement, nodules, ulcers, livedo reticularis (Plate 47), and digital gangrene may occur. As with most forms of cutaneous vasculitis, the lesions favor the lower extremities.

6. Musculoskeletal system—Nonspecific arthralgias and frank arthritis usually present early in the course of MPA and respond quickly to therapy. Musculoskeletal symptoms may also herald disease flares. The arthritis of MPA is migratory in nature and can assume a variety of joint patterns, from a pauci-articular syndrome of large joints to a polyarthritis of small joints. Destructive joint lesions do not occur in MPA.

B. Laboratory Findings

The results of routine laboratory tests and specialized assays in MPA are shown in Table 33–3. All of these tests are appropriate at the initial evaluation in patients who demonstrate features consistent with MPA. The exclusion of renal disease through the careful performance of a urinalysis is essential in the evaluation and follow-up of all patients with MPA. The erythrocyte sedimentation rate and serum C-reactive protein level are useful in the longitudinal evaluation of disease activity.

Positive ANCA assays are often instrumental in suggesting the diagnosis, but the titers of these antibodies correlate poorly in time with disease flares. Moreover, approximately 30% of patients with MPA diagnosed on a clinical basis are ANCA negative (see serologic testing, below). Thin-cut computed tomography scans are sensitive in the detection of lung disease in MPA.

C. Special Tests

1. Tissue biopsy—By definition, MPA involves small blood vessels: arterioles, venules, and capillaries. Glomerulonephritis is the renal equivalent of small-vessel vasculitis, akin to palpable purpura in the skin and capillaritis in the lung. Renal biopsy findings, although not specific for MPA, are sufficiently characteristic to establish the diagnosis in appropriate clinical settings. Immunofluorescence studies of renal biopsies in MPA confirm the "pauci-immune" nature of the renal involvement. MPA may also involve medium-sized arteries and veins, but the identification of medium-vessel involvement is not essential to the diagnosis.

MPA is high on the differential diagnosis of leukocytoclastic vasculitis within the small blood vessels of skin lesions. The presence of extracutaneous findings and ANCA increases the likelihood of MPA. If sufficiently deep, skin biopsies may also demonstrate the involvement of medium-sized vessels in the deep dermis subcutaneous tissue layer. The finding of medium-vessel involvement eliminates certain forms of cutaneous vasculitis limited to small-vessel disease, eg, hypersensitivity vasculitis (cutaneous leukocytoclastic angiitis) and

Table 33–3. The laboratory evaluation in MPA.

Test	Typical Result
Complete blood cell count	• Normochromic, normocytic anemia; acute, severe anemias possible in alveolar hemorrhage • Mild to moderate leukocytosis common, usually not exceeding 18×10^9/L • Moderate to pronounced thrombocytosis typical, ranging from platelet counts of 400×10^9/L to occasionally >1000×10^9/L
Electrolytes	Hyperkalemia in the setting of advanced renal dysfunction
Liver function tests	Hepatic involvement unusual in MPA When present, there can be elevations of transaminases (AST/ALT) in excess of 1000 mg/dL
Urinalysis with microscopy	• Hematuria (ranging from mild to so high that red blood cells are too numerous to count) • Red blood cell casts • Proteinuria (nephritic range proteinuria in a small minority)
Erythrocyte sedimentation rate/C-reactive protein	• Dramatic elevations of acute phase reactants are typical, generally with good correlation to disease activity
ANA	Negative
Rheumatoid factor	Positive in 40–50% of patients, often leading to diagnostic confusion with rheumatoid arthritis
C3, C4	Usually normal (or increased, because complement proteins are acute phase reactants)
ANCA	Positive in 70% of patients with MPA (and probably a higher percentage of patients with generalized disease)
Anti-GBM	A small number of patients have both ANCA and anti-GBM antibodies

ANA, antinuclear antibody; ANCA, antineutrophil cytoplasmic antibody; anti-GBM, antiglomerular basement membrane antibodies; AST/ALT, aspartate aminotransferase and alanine aminotransferase; MPA, microscopic polyangiitis.

Henoch-Schönlein purpura. Direct immunofluorescence of skin biopsy tissue is also important in the exclusion of immune complex-mediated processes such as cryoglobulinemia. The involvement of both veins and arteries distinguishes MPA from classic polyarteritis nodosa, which is confined to arterial lesions.

2. Nerve conduction studies—Nerve conduction studies are an important part of the evaluation for patients with neuropathic symptoms. Nerve conduction studies may reveal the characteristic asymmetric, axonal sensorimotor neuropathy. Nerves such as the sural nerve shown to be involved in this fashion are prime candidates for biopsy, with simultaneous sampling of adjacent muscle (eg, the gastrocnemius). The sural nerve is an excellent candidate for biopsy because, in contrast to most peripheral nerves, it contains only sensory fibers. In some cases, histopathology diagnostic of vasculitis is confined to the muscle as opposed to the nerve, or vice versa. As noted, nerve conduction studies may be negative in patients with small-fiber neuropathies.

Although lung involvement can be a florid manifestation of MPA, demonstration of vasculitis on thoracoscopic or open lung biopsy is often challenging; frank capillaritis may be difficult to detect. Nevertheless, lung biopsies are often essential to exclude other processes (eg, infections or malignancies) if no other tissue options exist for biopsy.

3. Serologic testing for ANCA—Three fourths of all patients with clinical diagnoses of MPA are ANCA-positive. A full discussion of ANCA is found in the chapter on GPA (Wegener) (see Chapter 32). In MPA, the classic pattern of serum reactivity upon immunofluorescence testing (with human neutrophils as the substrate) is perinuclear staining (P-ANCA). The P-ANCA pattern in MPA patients is usually caused by antibodies to MPO, a constituent of the primary granules of neutrophils. A variety of nonvasculitic conditions (Table 33–4) can also cause P-ANCA immunofluorescence, but these results are usually caused by antibodies to antigens not associated with vasculitis (eg, lactoferrin).

The combination of both a P-ANCA pattern on immunofluorescence testing and MPO-ANCA demonstrated by

Table 33–4. Differential diagnosis of microscopic polyangiitis.

Other vasculitides
   Polyarteritis nodosa
   Granulomatosis with polyangiitis (formerly Wegener granulomatosis)
   Eosinophilic granulomatosis with polyangiitis (Churg-Strauss syndrome)
   Henoch-Schönlein purpura
   Hypersensitivity vasculitis
   Mixed cryoglobulinemia
   Goodpasture disease
   Giant cell arteritis
   Drug-induced ANCA-associated vasculitis
Infections
   Endocarditis
Pulmonary conditions
   Interstitial pulmonary fibrosis
   Idiopathic pulmonary hemosiderosis
Systemic autoimmune conditions
   Systemic lupus erythematosus
   Rheumatoid arthritis
Miscellaneous nonvasculitic conditions associated with P-ANCA
   Inflammatory bowel disease
   Autoimmune hepatitis
   Sclerosing cholangitis

ANCA, antineutrophilic cytoplasmic antibody; P-ANCA, perinuclear antineutrophilic cytoplasmic antibody.

enzyme immunoassay has a high positive predictive value for ANCA-associated vasculitis, most commonly MPA. The other type of ANCA found in MPA is PR3-ANCA, directed against proteinase 3. This type of ANCA is usually associated with a cytoplasmic (C-ANCA) pattern of immunofluorescent staining. Despite advances in ANCA testing techniques, histopathology remains the cornerstone of diagnosis in MPA. When the diagnosis is unconfirmed, all reasonable attempts to obtain a tissue diagnosis should be pursued.

▶ Differential Diagnosis

The greatest mimickers of MPA are other forms of vasculitis (Table 33–4). Henoch-Schönlein purpura and hypersensitivity vasculitis (also known as cutaneous leukocytoclastic angiitis) can cause identical skin lesions, as can GPA (Wegener), EGPA (Churg-Strauss), mixed cryoglobulinemia, and PAN. The delineation of MPA from these disorders comes from the pattern recognition of extracutaneous involvement (kidneys, lung, nerve), the biopsy of involved organs, and ANCA testing. The difficulties of distinguishing MPA from GPA (Wegener) and PAN are illustrated in Table 33–1.

Since Goodpasture disease (anti-glomerular basement membrane disease) can present in a manner indistinguishable from MPA, such patients may benefit from plasma exchange in addition to glucocorticoids and cytotoxic agents. As discussed below, the potential benefits of plasma exchange in MPA are less clear than in Goodpasture disease.

MPA can lead to lymphoplasmacytic infiltrates within the adventitia and also cause severe headaches, thereby mimicking temporal (giant cell) arteritis both clinically and pathologically. In contrast to "true" temporal arteritis, MPA involving the temporal artery is not associated with giant cells. In addition, some medications, particularly propylthiouracil (used to treat thyroiditis), can cause a drug-induced, ANCA-associated vasculitis associated with high titers of antibodies to MPO.

A variety of pulmonary, renal, and peripheral nerve disorders must be distinguished from MPA by imaging studies, tissue biopsy, nerve conduction studies, and serologic testing. Systemic autoimmune conditions such as systemic lupus erythematosus and rheumatoid arthritis are also prone to imitating MPA because of their abilities to involve multiple organ systems and cause positive P-ANCA results on immunofluorescence testing of serum (see above).

▶ Treatment

The essentials of management for MPA are shown in Table 33–5. MPA is one of a handful of vasculitic conditions in which the conventional standard of care for many years called for combination therapy with both glucocorticoids and a cytotoxic agent. However, rituximab has been demonstrated to be as effective as cyclophosphamide in the induction of remission in ANCA-associated vasculitis (AAV)

Table 33–5. Essentials of MPA management.

- Because most patients with MPA have major organ involvement such as glomerulonephritis, alveolar hemorrhage, or vasculitic neuropathy, the combination of cyclophosphamide and glucocorticoids is the cornerstone of most treatment regimens.
- Cyclophosphamide may be administered on either a daily or intermittent basis.
- "Pulse" methylprednisolone (1 g/d for 3 days) may be considered for patients with severe organ involvement at diagnosis.
- Alternative medications such as azathioprine or methotrexate should be considered after 3-6 months of cyclophosphamide therapy.

MPA, microscopic polyangiitis.

(MPA and GPA [Wegener]). The induction of remission with rituximab is preferred to cyclophosphamide because of rituximab's potentially superior long-term side effect profile. Rituximab has a particular advantage over cyclophosphamide in the treatment of patients with relapsing (as opposed to newly-diagnosed) disease.

If rituximab cannot be given or if the patient has not responded to this regimen, cyclophosphamide is the treatment of choice. The combination of cyclophosphamide (2 mg/kg/d for those with normal renal function) and glucocorticoids (1 mg/kg/d of prednisone, perhaps preceded by a 3-day intravenous "pulse" of methylprednisolone) leads to excellent therapeutic responses if treatment is initiated early enough. Three- to 6-month courses of cyclophosphamide are used followed by longer-term treatment for the maintenance of remission with either azathioprine (up to 2 mg/kg/d) or methotrexate (20–25 mg/wk).

Both intravenous and oral daily administration regimens of cyclophosphamide are effective at inducing disease remission. The preferred route of administration is largely a function of practice style. The important points are that cyclophosphamide be used promptly when indicated and with appropriate cautions. All patients who are receiving treatment for MPA should be given a daily dose of single-strength trimethoprim-sulfamethoxazole, 100 mg/d of dapsone, or 1500 mg/d of atovaquone as prophylaxis against *Pneumocystis jiroveci* pneumonia.

The need for a remission maintenance regimen following rituximab-induced disease remissions is not clear and must be determined in longitudinal studies. Following the induction of remission by cyclophosphamide, patients may be switched to either azathioprine (up to 2 mg/kg/d) or methotrexate (up to 25 mg/wk, assuming that residual renal dysfunction does not preclude this medication). The optimal duration of these remission maintenance agents is not clear. In general, the continuation of azathioprine or methotrexate for a period of 1 year after the achievement of remission is a reasonable recommendation.

Once the inflammatory process has been controlled with immunosuppressive therapy, primary care clinicians may institute renal preservation therapies for patients with renal damage (blood pressure control, angiotensin-converting enzyme inhibition, and salt restriction).

▶ Complications

If MPA is diagnosed early and treated promptly, patients have a high likelihood (>90%) of achieving disease remissions. Approximately one third of patients suffer disease flares after the achievement of remission by conventional therapies (cyclophosphamide and prednisone). In general, MPA is considered less likely than GPA (Wegener) to flare. Unfortunately, significant damage frequently ensues before recognition of the disease. One study indicated that the 5-year renal survival for patients with this disease was only 55%. This prognosis may have improved somewhat since the widespread availability of ANCA testing.

The renal prognosis in MPA may be worse than that of GPA (Wegener), perhaps because of a greater likelihood of delay in diagnosis in MPA, attributable to the involvement of fewer organ systems. Another major disability associated with MPA results from nerve damage and consequent muscle weakness caused by vasculitic neuropathy. Finally, patients with AAV have a high risk of venous thrombotic events. Heightened suspicion for this complication, possibly caused by involvement of the veins by the vasculitic process, should be maintained.

Corral-Gudino L, Borao-Cengotita-Bengoa M, Del Pino-Montes J, Lerma-Marquez JL. Overall survival, renal survival, and relapse in patients with microscopic polyangiitis: A systematic review of current evidence. *Rheumatology (Oxford).* 2011;50:1414. [PMID: 21406467]

Jennette JC, Falk RJ, Andrassy K, et al. Nomenclature of systemic vasculitides. Proposal of an international consensus conference. *Arthritis Rheum.* 1994;37:187. [PMID: 8129773]

Kallenberg CG. Pathogenesis of ANCA-associated vasculitides. *Ann Rheum Dis.* 2011;70 (Suppl 1):i59-63. [PMID: 2139221]

Stone JH, Merkel PA, Spiera R, et al. RAVE-ITN Research Group. Rituximab versus cyclophosphamide for ANCA-associated vasculitis. *N Engl J Med.* 2010;363:221. [PMID: 20647199]

The Johns Hopkins Vasculitis Center
http://vasculitis.med.jhu.edu

Vasculitis Clinical Research Consortium
http://rarediseasesnetwork.epi.usf.edu/vcrc/

Eosinophilic Granulomatosis with Polyangiitis (Churg-Strauss Syndrome)

Philip Seo, MD, MHS
John H. Stone, MD, MPH

ESSENTIALS OF DIAGNOSIS

▶ Asthma, eosinophilia, and systemic vasculitis are the hallmarks of eosinophilic granulomatosis with polyangiitis (EGPA; Churg-Strauss syndrome).

▶ Classic clinical features include the following:

- Allergic rhinitis and nasal polyposis.
- Reactive airway disease.
- Peripheral eosinophilia (10–60% of all circulating leukocytes).
- Fleeting pulmonary infiltrates and occasional alveolar hemorrhage.
- Vasculitic neuropathy.
- Congestive heart failure.

▶ Approximately 50% of patients with EGPA have antineutrophil cytoplasmic antibodies (ANCAs), usually with a specificity for myeloperoxidase (MPO).

General Considerations

In 1951, Churg and Strauss reported a series of 13 patients with "periarteritis nodosa" (see Chapter 35) who demonstrated severe asthma and an unusual constellation of other symptoms: "fever...hypereosinophilia, symptoms of cardiac failure, renal damage, and peripheral neuropathy, resulting from vascular embarrassment...." The investigators termed this new disease "allergic angiitis and allergic granulomatosis," and specified three histologic criteria for the diagnosis: (1) the presence of necrotizing vasculitis, (2) tissue infiltration by eosinophils, and (3) extravascular granuloma.

In 1990, an American College of Rheumatology panel liberalized the criteria for the classification of this disease, dropping the requirements for histopathologically proven vasculitis and granuloma (Table 34–1). The Chapel Hill Consensus Conference on nomenclature of the vasculitides

subsequently defined the Churg-Strauss syndrome as a disorder characterized by eosinophil-rich, granulomatous inflammation of the respiratory tract and necrotizing vasculitis of small- to medium-sized vessels, associated with asthma and eosinophilia. In 2012, the Revised Chapel Hill Consensus Conference Nomenclature of Vasculitides recommended the term "eosinophilic granulomatosis with polyangiitis (EGPA)" for this disease. The purpose for this recommendation was twofold: (1) to emphasize certain cardinal features of the condition, and (2) for consistency with the names preferred for two related disorders, granulomatosis with polyangiitis (formerly Wegener granulomatosis)(see Chapter 32) and microscopic polyangiitis (see Chapter 33).

EGPA is a rare disease—significantly less common than the other forms of ANCA-associated vasculitis. The annual incidence of EGPA is approximately 2.4 cases per million individuals. The distribution of cases is roughly equal between men and women. In recent years, associations between the use of leukotriene antagonists and EGPA have been reported. Rather than causing the disease, however, it is more likely that these medications permit the tapering of glucocorticoids, thereby "unmasking" the vasculitic phase of EGPA.

Clinical Findings

A. Symptoms and Signs

After the diagnosis of EGPA has been made, three disease phases are often recognizable: the prodrome, eosinophilia/tissue infiltration, and vasculitis.

The **prodrome phase** is characterized by the presence of allergic disease (typically asthma or allergic rhinitis). This phase often lasts for several years.

During the **eosinophilia/tissue infiltration phase,** striking peripheral eosinophilia may occur. Tissue infiltration by eosinophils is observed in the heart, lung, gastrointestinal tract, and other tissues.

Table 34–1. American College of Rheumatology 1990 criteria for the classification of Churg-Strauss syndrome (eosinophilic granulomatosis with polyangiitis).[a]

Criterion	Definition
Asthma	History of wheezing or diffuse high-pitched rales on expiration
Eosinophilia	Eosinophilia >10% on white blood cell differential count
Mononeuropathy or polyneuropathy	Development of mononeuropathy, multiple mononeuropathies, or polyneuropathy (ie, stocking/glove distribution)
Pulmonary infiltrates, nonfixed	Migratory or transitory pulmonary infiltrates on radiographs
Paranasal sinus abnormality	History of acute or chronic paranasal sinus pain or tenderness, or radiographic opacification of the paranasal sinuses
Extravascular eosinophils	Biopsy including artery, arteriole, or venule, showing accumulations of eosinophils in extravascular areas

[a]To be classified as having Churg-Strauss syndrome (eosinophilic granulomatosis with polyangiitis), a patient must have at least four of these six criteria. Among patients with various forms of systemic vasculitis, the sensitivity of these criteria for the classification of an individual patient as having Churg-Strauss syndrome was estimated to be 85%. (Adapted from Masi AT, Hunder GG, Lie TT, et al. The American College of Rheumatology 1990 criteria for the classification of Churg-Strauss syndrome [allergic granulomatosi sand angiitis]. *Arthritis Rheum.* 1990;33:1094. With permission.)

In the third phase, **vasculitis,** systemic necrotizing vasculitis affects a wide range of organs, ranging from the heart and lungs to the peripheral nerves and skin (Figure 34–1).

1. Nose and sinuses—Upper airway disease in EGPA usually takes the form of nasal polyps or allergic rhinitis. A surprisingly high percentage of patients with EGPA have histories of nasal polypectomies, usually long before suspicion of an underlying disease is raised. Although pansinusitis occurs frequently, destructive upper airway disease is not characteristic of EGPA.

2. Ears—Middle ear granulation tissue with eosinophilic infiltrates occurs in some patients, leading to conductive hearing loss. Cases of sensorineural hearing loss (see Chapter 68) have also been reported.

3. Lungs—More than 90% of patients with EGPA have histories of asthma. Typically, the asthma represents either adult-onset reactive airway disease or, less commonly, a significant worsening of long-standing disease. Upon encroachment of the vasculitic phase of EGPA, patients' asthma may improve substantially, even before therapy for vasculitis has begun. Following successful treatment of the vasculitic phase,

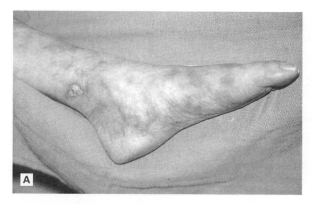

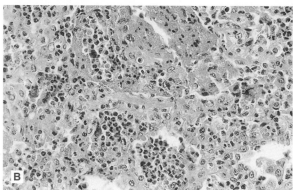

▲ **Figure 34–1. A:** Foot of a patient with eosinophilic granulomatosis with polyangiitis (EGPA; formerly Churg-Strauss syndrome) showing livedo reticularis and a cutaneous ulcer just superior to the medial malleolus. The patient's foot is held in extension because of a left foot drop (vasculitis neuropathy of the left peroneal nerve). **B:** Eosinophilic pneumonia in a patient with EGPA. Biopsy shows dense clusters of eosinophils within the lung parenchyma.

however, glucocorticoid-dependent asthma persists in many patients.

The pathologic features of lung disease in EGPA vary according to the disease phase. In the early phases, there may be extensive eosinophilic infiltration of the alveoli and interstitium. During the vasculitic phase, necrotizing vasculitis and granuloma may be evident. In the current era, when many patients with asthma are treated with systemic glucocorticoids, lung biopsy specimens showing all three histologic hallmarks of this disease are unusual.

4. Peripheral nerves—Mononeuritis multiplex occurs with a remarkable frequency in EGPA, with often devastating effects. Vasculitic neuropathy was evident in 74 (77%) of the 96 patients in one series. Nerve infarctions may appear several weeks after the start of appropriate treatment, but

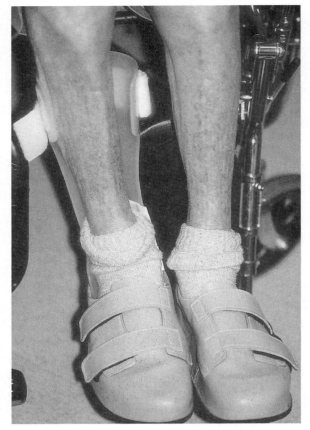

▲ **Figure 34–2.** The ravages of vasculitic neuropathy. Bilateral ankle-foot orthoses required because of bilateral foot drop. Note severe muscle wasting in both legs.

do not always indicate the need to intensify therapy, particularly if treatment with both high-dose prednisone and cyclophosphamide has already been initiated. This may be due to continued disease activity but is more likely secondary to thrombosis of vessels that have become severely compromised by previously active inflammation. Clinically, nerve infarctions are heralded by the abrupt occurrence of a foot drop, wrist drop, or some other focal nerve lesion. Muscle wasting secondary to nerve infarctions may continue to appear for weeks after the disease has been brought under control (Figure 34–2).

5. Heart—Cardiac involvement also occurs with a disproportionate frequency in EGPA, and is a common cause of death. Some form of cardiac involvement occurred in 12.5% of patients in one large series. Congestive heart failure is the most common cardiac manifestation, although coronary arteritis and valvular abnormalities have also been reported.

6. Skin—Skin disease in EGPA takes many forms, none of which is specific: Palpable purpura, papules, ulcers, and vesiculobullous lesions are common. Nodular skin lesions are usually "Churg-Strauss granuloma" (cutaneous extravascular necrotizing granuloma). These tend to occur on the extensor surfaces of the elbows and other pressure points. Skin biopsy specimens in EGPA reveal eosinophilic infiltration of blood vessel walls. Splinter hemorrhages, digital ischemia, and gangrene associated with inflammation in medium-sized digital arteries are often present at the time of diagnosis.

7. Kidneys—EGPA is less likely to cause end-stage renal disease than are other forms of ANCA-associated vasculitis. Acute kidney injury may be caused by an eosinophil-mediated interstitial nephritis. When glomerulonephritis does occur, however, the histopathologic findings are often indistinguishable from those of other forms of pauci-immune vasculitis (eg, granulomatosis with polyangiitis [formerly Wegener granulomatosis], microscopic polyangiitis, and renal-limited vasculitis).

8. Joints—Nonspecific arthralgias and frank arthritis often occur early in the course of EGPA. The arthritis of EGPA is migratory in nature and may assume a variety of joint patterns, from a pauciarticular syndrome of lower extremity joints to a polyarthritis of the small joints of the hands.

B. Laboratory Findings

Eosinophilia (before treatment) is a *sine qua non* of EGPA. Eosinophil counts may comprise as much as 60% of the total white blood cell count. Eosinophil counts are usually sensitive markers of disease flares, but generally respond very quickly to treatment with high doses of glucocorticoids. Most patients with EGPA also have elevated serum IgE levels. Serum complement levels are usually normal. Immune complexes are not believed to play a primary role in this disease. The erythrocyte sedimentation rate, serum C-reactive protein level, and eosinophil count can be useful in the longitudinal evaluation of disease activity. The reported percentages of EGPA patients with ANCA are variable, with most figures in the literature in the range of 50% (see Chapter 32 for a full discussion of ANCA). Antibodies to either proteinase-3 or MPO (but not to both) may be found. Of the two vasculitis-specific ANCAs, which include antibodies to MPO and proteinase-3, those to MPO are more common in EGPA. MPO-ANCAs usually produce a perinuclear-ANCA (P-ANCA) pattern on serum immunofluorescence testing. Patients who are ANCA-negative tend to have more cardiopulmonary complications, while patients who are ANCA-positive tend to have more of the classic vasculitic manifestations of this disease, although there is considerable overlap between these two groups.

C. Imaging Studies

Pulmonary infiltrates are evident in approximately one third of patients with EGPA. These lesions are usually migratory infiltrates that occur bilaterally. Pulmonary hemorrhage is unusual but has been reported. Nodular or cavitary lesions suggest the alternative diagnoses of granulomatosis with polyangiitis (formerly Wegener granulomatosis), infection, or malignancy. Among patients with cardiac involvement, echocardiography or cardiac MRI may confirm poor cardiac function consistent with cardiomyopathy or demonstrate findings compatible with regional myocardial fibrosis.

▶ Differential Diagnosis

The major disease entities in the differential diagnosis of EGPA are shown in Table 34–2. There are many diseases in which patients occasionally demonstrate mild eosinophilia (eg, a peripheral blood eosinophilia on the order of 10% or so in asthma or parasitic infections). Only a handful of diseases, however, can cause eosinophilia as high as 20–60%, as is occasionally observed with EGPA and its related conditions. *Strongyloides* infection, which can cause both high levels of eosinophilia and asthma, should be considered in endemic areas, which include the southeastern United States. EGPA must also be distinguished from other hypereosinophilic disorders: Löffler syndrome, chronic eosinophilic pneumonia, eosinophilic gastroenteritis, hypereosinophilic syndrome, eosinophilic fasciitis, IgG_4-related disease, and eosinophilic leukemia.

The fleeting pulmonary infiltrates of the Löffler syndrome and the peripheral infiltrates of chronic eosinophilic pneumonia may both mimic EGPA closely.

Differentiating EGPA from hypereosinophilic syndrome may be the biggest challenge, however. Clinically, hypereosinophilic syndrome is rarely associated with reactive airway disease. Laboratory tests for the F1P1L1-PDGFR gene translocation or elevated serum tryptase levels (both of which are associated with hypereosinophilic syndrome) may also be helpful in the evaluation of such patients.

Table 34-2. Differential diagnosis of eosinophilic granulomatosis with polyangiits (formerly Churg-Strauss syndrome).

Eosinophilic Disorders	Other Vasculitides
Löffler syndrome	Granulomatosis with polyangiitis (formerly Wegener granulomatosis)
Chronic eosinophilic pneumonia	Microscopic polyangiitis Polyarteritis nodosa
Eosinophilic gastroenteritis	Mixed cryoglobulinemia
Hypereosinophil syndrome	Goodpasture syndrome
Eosinophilic leukemia	
Eosinophilic fasciitis	

Many other forms of systemic vasculitis are high on the differential diagnosis for EGPA. Granulomatosis with polyangiitis, polyarteritis nodosa, microscopic polyangiitis, Goodpasture syndrome (antiglomerular basement membrane disease), cryoglobulinemia, and other vasculitic disorders have clinical features that overlap with those of EGPA. However, the finding of eosinophilia superimposed upon a history of allergy or asthma usually permits the clear distinction of EGPA from these other disorders.

▶ Treatment

In contrast to other forms of ANCA-associated vasculitis, many patients with EGPA may be treated effectively with glucocorticoids alone. Nevertheless, certain disease complications, particularly the presence of vasculitic neuropathy or glomerulonephritis, should trigger the use of cyclophosphamide (2 mg/kg/d orally, decreased in the setting of renal dysfunction or advanced age) as part of the remission induction strategy. Cyclophosphamide should also be considered with other complications of EGPA that pose immediate threats to the function of vital organs (eg, the heart). Appropriate cautions are paramount when using this medication (see Chapter 32). Whenever possible, the duration of cyclophosphamide therapy should be limited to 6 months or less. Milder cases may be treated with azathioprine (2 mg/kg/d), methotrexate (15–25 mg/wk), or mycophenolate mofetil (2–3 g/d in divided doses). For patients whose disease remains active despite the combination of glucocorticoids and a cytotoxic agent, interferon-α and rituximab have been used with some success in a limited number of cases. The bronchospastic component of this disease rarely responds to glucocorticoid-sparing agents, and should be managed with conventional bronchodilators (including leukotriene inhibitors) and, if necessary, glucocorticoids.

▶ Complications

Substantial morbidity and death may result from EGPA. The major sources of morbidity are the disease itself and its therapies. Because the disease begins with a long prodrome of comparatively mundane problems (eg, atopic symptoms and asthma), the diagnosis is often overlooked until the occurrence of significant damage. The complications of vasculitic neuropathy are particularly devastating in this regard. Crippling nerve dysfunction may occur to varying degrees in all four distal extremities, leading to enormous disabilities. The recovery of function in infarcted nerves generally requires months, and in many cases the return of function is minimal. Recovery is likely dependent partly on the age of the patient and on the severity and extent of nerve damage.

Treatment regimens for EGPA that include prolonged courses of high-dose glucocorticoids and (often) cyclophosphamide are associated with a high incidence of adverse effects, some of which may be permanent or fatal. Following the remission of vasculitis, many patients have persistent, glucocorticoid-dependent asthma. The long-term use of even moderately low-dose glucocorticoids brings many unwanted side effects. More dangerous, however, is the intensive immunosuppression associated with the combination of glucocorticoids and cytotoxic agents. Even with careful monitoring, opportunistic infections, myelosuppression, infertility, bladder toxicity, and (in the long term) an increased risk of certain malignancies are all major concerns.

Although clinical remissions may be obtained in more than 90% of patients with EGPA, disease recurrences are common upon cessation of therapy. In the largest series reported to date, flares were detected in more than 25% of the patients. In most cases, relapses are heralded by the return of eosinophilia. In an even higher percentage of patients, following the resolution of the vasculitic phase of EGPA, glucocorticoid-dependent asthma remains an issue requiring ongoing management.

Churg A. Recent advances in the diagnosis of Churg-Strauss syndrome. *Mod Pathol.* 2001;14:1284. [PMID: 11743052]

Sable-Fourtassou R, Cohen P, Mahr A, et al. French Vasculitis Study Group. Antineutrophil cytoplasmic antibodies and the Churg-Strauss syndrome. *Ann Intern Med.* 2005;143:632. [PMID: 16263885]

Jennette JC, Falk RJ, Bacon PA, et al. Revised Chapel Hill Consensus Conference Nomenclature of Vasculitides. (Submitted January 2012).

The Cleveland Clinic Foundation Center for Vasculitis
http://www.clevelandclinic.org/arthritis/vasculitis/default.htm

The Johns Hopkins Vasculitis Center
http://vasculitis.med.jhu.edu

Vasculitis Clinical Research Consortium
http://rarediseasesnetwork.epi.usf.edu/vcrc/

Polyarteritis Nodosa

John H. Stone, MD, MPH

ESSENTIALS OF DIAGNOSIS

▶ Subacute onset of constitutional complaints (eg, fever, weight loss, malaise, arthralgias), lower extremity nodules and ulcerations, mononeuritis multiplex, and intestinal angina (postprandial pain caused by the involvement of mesenteric vessels).

▶ Cutaneous polyarteritis nodosa (PAN) is a variant of the systemic disease in which vasculitis is limited to the skin, usually presenting as nodules that break down into ulcers.

▶ Angiogram or biopsy of an involved organ required for diagnosis.

▶ Angiography may reveal microaneurysms in the kidneys or gastrointestinal tract.

▶ Biopsies of the skin and peripheral nerves (with sampling of the adjacent muscle) are the least invasive ways of confirming the diagnosis histopathologically.

General Considerations

Classic PAN is characterized by necrotizing inflammation of muscular arterioles and medium-sized arteries that spares the smallest blood vessels (eg, capillaries). PAN is not associated with glomerulonephritis, although it can cause renovascular hypertension and renal infarctions through its involvement of the medium-sized intrarenal vasculature. Features that distinguish PAN from other forms of systemic vasculitis are confinement of the disease to the arterial as opposed to the venous circulation, the sparing of the lung, and the absence of granulomatous inflammation.

Reported annual incidence rates of PAN range from 2 to 9 cases per million people per year. A higher incidence (77 cases/million) was reported in an Alaskan area hyperendemic for hepatitis B virus (HBV). With the availability of the HBV vaccine, however, the percentage of cases associated

with HBV has declined substantially (now <10% of all cases in the developed world). PAN appears to affect men and women with approximately equal frequencies and to occur in all ethnic groups.

Clinical Findings

A. Symptoms and Signs

PAN can involve virtually any organ system with the exception of the lungs. The disease demonstrates a predilection for certain organs, particularly the skin, peripheral nerves, gastrointestinal tract, and kidneys. A nearly universal complaint among patients is some type of pain, caused by myalgias, arthritis, peripheral nerve infarction, testicular ischemia, or mesenteric vasculitis.

1. Constitutional symptoms—Fevers are a common feature of PAN. The characteristics of the fever vary substantially among patients, ranging from periods of low-grade temperature elevation to spiking febrile episodes accompanied by chills (patterns of low-grade fever are more common than are hectic fevers). Tachycardia with or without fever may be another feature of PAN. Malaise, weight loss, and myalgias are also common.

2. Skin and joints—Vasculitis of medium-size arteries may produce several types of skin lesions. These cutaneous findings include livedo racemosa (Plate 48), nodules, papules, ulcerations, and digital ischemia leading to gangrene. All of these findings or combinations of them may occur in the same patient. The livedo racemosa (often termed "livedo reticularis"), which may have a diffuse distribution over the extremities and buttocks, does not blanch with the application of pressure to the skin. Nodules, papules, and ulcers tend to occur on the lower extremities, particularly near the malleoli, in the fleshy parts of the calf, and over the dorsal surfaces of the feet. Nodules frequently evolve into ulcerations that have scalloped borders (Figure 35–1) and heal with scarring.

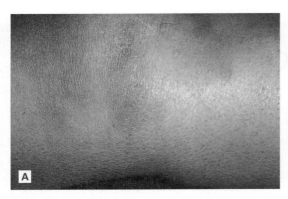
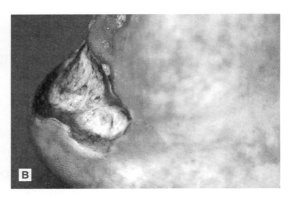

▲ **Figure 35–1.** Cutaneous manifestations of polyarteritis nodosa. **A:** A nodular lesion. **B:** An ulcer with scalloped borders. (Reproduced, with permission, from Stone JH, Nousari HC. Essential cutaneous vasculitis: what every rheumatologist should know about vasculitis of the skin. *Curr Opin Rheumatol.* 2001 Jan;13(1):23–34.)

Although the principal skin manifestations relate to disease caused by arteritis in medium-sized muscular arteries and arterioles, crops of purpura (caused by the involvement of smaller blood vessels) occur in a minority of patients. Digital ischemia, often accompanied by splinter hemorrhages, sometimes leads to tissue loss.

Arthralgias of large joints (knees, ankles, elbows, wrists) occur in up to 50% of patients; however, true synovitis is seen in substantially fewer patients.

3. Peripheral nerves—Mononeuritis multiplex, the infarction of named nerves by inflammation in the vasa nervorum, occurs in approximately 60% of patients with PAN. The most commonly involved nerves are the sural, peroneal, radial, and ulnar. Vasculitic neuropathy tends to involve the longest (ie, distal) nerves first and usually begins asymmetrically. Thus, the first motor symptoms of vasculitic neuropathy may be a foot or wrist drop (resulting from infarctions of the peroneal and radial nerves, respectively). In advanced stages, the neuropathy may mimic a confluent, symmetric polyneuropathy. Careful history taking, however, may unmask its initial asymmetry. Both sensory and motor findings are characteristic of vasculitic neuropathy because with the exception of the sural nerve (a pure sensory nerve), peripheral nerves typically have mixed sensory and motor fibers bundled within the same nerve.

4. Gastrointestinal tract—The gastrointestinal manifestations of PAN occur in approximately half of all patients and are among the most challenging symptoms to diagnose correctly because of their nonspecific nature. Postprandial abdominal pain ("intestinal angina") is common. Involvement of the mesenteric arteries in PAN may lead to the disastrous complications of mesenteric infarction or aneurysmal rupture, each of which is associated with a high mortality rate. Angiography of the mesenteric vessels reveals multiple microaneurysms (Figure 35–2A). These range in size from lesions that are barely visible to the naked eye to

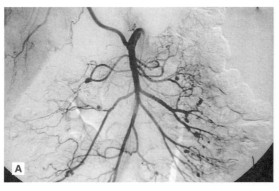
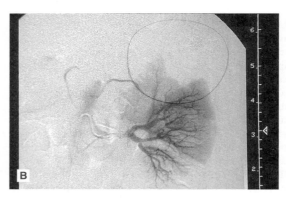

▲ **Figure 35–2.** Angiographic features of polyarteritis nodosa. **A:** Mesenteric angiogram showing multiple microaneurysms. **B:** A wedge-shaped renal infarction. (Reproduced, with permission, from Stone JH. Vasculitis: a collection of pearls and myths. *Rheum Dis Clin North Am.* 2007 Nov;33(4):691–739.)

several centimeters in diameter. Sometimes PAN is detected at cholecystectomy or appendectomy in the absence of other disease manifestations. In such cases, surgical removal of the involved organ may be curative.

5. Intraparenchymal renal inflammation—This major feature of PAN is found in 40% of patients. The inflammatory process targets the renal and interlobar arteries (the medium-sized, muscular arteries within the kidney) and occasionally also involves the smaller arcuate and interlobular arteries. Angiography may reveal microaneurysms within the kidney or large, wedge-shaped renal infarctions (Figure 35–2B). Renal artery involvement or involvement of intra-renal arterioles in PAN may lead to renin-mediated hypertension. Red blood cell casts on urinalysis imply glomerulonephritis and thus usually implicate another disease (eg, microscopic polyangiitis). However, both proteinuria and hematuria may be observed in PAN.

6. Cardiac symptoms—Tachycardia may reflect either direct cardiac involvement or a general inflammatory state. Congestive heart failure and myocardial infarction sometimes occur. Specific heart lesions are rarely diagnosed while the patient is alive; however, autopsy series indicate that cardiac involvement is present in a majority of patients with PAN. Patchy necrosis of the myocardium caused by subclinical arteriolar involvement is a common finding at autopsy.

7. Miscellaneous—Central nervous system involvement occurs in a small percentage of patients with PAN. The usual presentations are encephalopathy and strokes. Renin-mediated hypertension may contribute to both of these neurologic complications. Other unusual presentations of PAN include involvement of the eyes (scleritis), pancreas, testicles, ureters, breasts, and ovaries.

B. Laboratory Findings

Although the laboratory features of PAN are often strikingly abnormal and help characterize the disease process as inflammatory, they do not distinguish PAN from a host of other inflammatory diseases. Anemia, thrombocytosis, and elevation of acute phase reactants are typical (Table 35–1). The erythrocyte sedimentation rate and C-reactive protein are often useful in longitudinal evaluations of disease activity but are imperfect for this purpose.

One of the diagnostic challenges in PAN is the fact that the disorder is not associated with any of the autoantibodies found in other immune-mediated conditions. Assays for antinuclear antibodies and rheumatoid factor are generally negative in patients with PAN, albeit low titers of these antibodies are detected in a minority of patients. Patients with HBV-associated PAN are generally hypocomplementemic, regardless of whether they have demonstrable cryoglobulins. When associated with HBV, PAN usually develops within weeks to months of the acute viral infection.

Table 35–1. Laboratory and radiologic evaluation in PAN.

Test	Typical Results
Complete blood cell count	Normochromic, normocytic anemia. Mild to moderate leukocytosis common, usually not exceeding $18 \times 10^9/L$. Moderate to pronounced thrombocytosis typical, ranging from platelet counts of $400 \times 10^9/L$ to occasionally $>1000 \times 10^9/L$.
Renal function	Renal artery involvement may cause elevated serum creatinines, and occasionally, end-stage renal disease.
Serum hepatic transaminases	Hepatic artery involvement common in PAN. Can lead to mild to moderate elevations in serum hepatic transaminases.
Urinalysis with microscopy	Hematuria (ranging from mild to severe). Red blood cell casts suggest glomerulonephritis and are therefore atypical. Proteinuria (nephritic range proteinuria distinctly unusual).
ESR/CRP	Dramatic elevations of acute phase reactants are typical. ESRs in excess of 100 mm/h are frequently found.
ANA	Negative.
Antiprecipitin antibodies (anti-Ro, -La, -Sm, -RNP)	Negative.
Rheumatoid factor	Negative.
C3, C4	Low in patients with PAN associated with HBV. In patients with idiopathic PAN, serum complement levels may be elevated (as acute phase reactants).
ANCA	Occasionally positive on immunofluorescence testing (low titers of perinuclear [P-ANCA] immunofluorescence, but specific antibodies to serine proteinase-3 and myeloperoxidases are negative).
Hepatitis B and C serologies	Hepatitis B causes a minority of cases (<10% in the developed world).
Chest radiography	Normal. PAN spares the lungs.

ANA, antinuclear antibody; ANCA, antineutrophil cytoplasmic antibody; CRP, C-reactive protein; ESR, erythrocyte sedimentation rate; HBV, hepatitis B virus; PAN, polyarteritis nodosa.

When tested by immunofluorescence, the sera of some patients with PAN are positive for antineutrophil cytoplasmic antibodies (ANCAs). However, specific enzyme immunoassays for antibodies to proteinase-3 or myeloperoxidase (the two antigens known to be associated with systemic vasculitis) are negative. Thus, PAN is not considered to be a form of ANCA-associated vasculitis.

C. Special Tests

The diagnosis of PAN requires either a tissue biopsy or an angiogram that demonstrates microaneurysms.

1. Biopsy—In the skin, medium-sized arteries lie within the deep dermis and in the subdermal adipose tissue. Thus, the diagnosis of PAN can be made by obtaining biopsy specimens of the skin that capture lobules of subcutaneous fat. Biopsies of nodules, papules, and the edges of ulcers have higher yields than biopsies of livedo racemosa.

PAN is a panarteritis characterized by transmural necrosis and a homogeneous, eosinophilic appearance of the blood vessel wall (fibrinoid necrosis). The cellular infiltrate is pleomorphic, with both polymorphonuclear cells and lymphocytes present in varying degrees at different stages. Degranulation of neutrophils within and around the arterial wall leads to leukocytoclasis. During later stages, complete occlusion may occur secondary to endothelial proliferation and thrombosis. Throughout involved tissues, the coexistence of acute and healed lesions is typical.

2. Nerve conduction studies—Nerve conduction studies are useful in detecting the typical axonal pattern of nerve injury and identifying involved nerves for biopsy. Because muscle tissue is highly vascular and may harbor involved vessels even in the absence of symptoms or signs of muscle involvement, biopsies of adjacent muscle should be performed simultaneously (eg, the gastrocnemius, if the sural nerve is biopsied). Blind biopsies of asymptomatic organs such as the testicle, however, are rarely diagnostic.

3. Angiography—The vascular wall inflammation in PAN may be strikingly segmental, affecting only part of the circumference of a given artery. Segmental necrosis, in turn, leads to aneurysm formation. Lesions known as microaneurysms can occur throughout the mesenteric and renal vasculature. Even in patients without gastrointestinal symptoms, mesenteric angiography may demonstrate telltale microaneurysms.

Conventional, catheter-based angiography generally has a higher resolution than computed tomography or magnetic resonance angiograms and remains the gold-standard approach to the detection of microaneurysms. The interpretation of angiograms requires experience. Alternating areas of vascular narrowing and dilatation can be caused by a variety of non-vasculitic processes, including (most commonly) vasospasm. The finding of true microaneurysms, however, is diagnostic of PAN in the proper setting.

▶ Differential Diagnosis

Even when flagrant inflammation is present, PAN may elude diagnosis for weeks or months. Except for evidence obtained from angiography or biopsy, the disease has no individual features that are pathognomonic. Many connective tissue diseases must be considered in the differential diagnosis of PAN (Table 35–2). However, systemic lupus erythematosus, mixed connective tissue disease, and undifferentiated connective tissue disorders usually can be distinguished from PAN by the presence of specific autoantibodies (eg, anti-Ro/SS-A, anti-La/SS-B, anti-Sm, anti-RNP). These are absent in PAN. Less specific autoantibodies such as antinuclear antibodies and rheumatoid factor are often present in PAN but are nondiagnostic because of their poor specificities.

In its early phases, rheumatoid arthritis may mimic PAN, but the arthritis of PAN is usually migratory and always nondestructive. Rheumatoid vasculitis, which has features very similar to PAN, almost always occurs in patients with severe, long-standing, destructive joint disease, not simultaneously with or before the arthritis. Similarly, although the fever pattern of PAN recalls that of Still disease in a minority of patients, the evanescent, salmon-colored rash of Still disease does not occur in PAN. Moreover, diffuse polyarthritis develops in 95% of patients with Still disease within 1 year

Table 35–2. Differential diagnosis of polyarteritis nodosa.

Systemic disorders associated with autoimmunity
Systemic lupus erythematosus
Mixed connective tissue disease
Catastrophic antiphospholipid antibody syndrome
Rheumatoid arthritis (with rheumatoid vasculitis)
Still disease
Systemic vasculitides
Granulomatosis with polyangiitis (formerly Wegener granulomatosis)
Microscopic polyangiitis
Eosinophilic granulomatosis with polyangiitis (Churg-Strauss syndrome)
Cryoglobulinemia
Isolated vasculitis of peripheral nerves
Infections
Endocarditis
Deep fungal infections (histoplasmosis, coccidioidomycosis, blastomycosis)
Miscellaneous
Inflammatory bowel disease
Sarcoidosis
Erythema nodosum
Atrophie blanche
Cholesterol emboli
Fibromuscular dysplasia
Lymphoma

(or earlier) of disease onset. The catastrophic antiphospholipid syndrome, which causes digital ischemia, strokes, and other arterial thrombotic events, may be confused with PAN. However, venous events, which are even more common than arterial events in most patients with the antiphospholipid syndrome, are not characteristic of PAN.

The lack of pulmonary involvement in PAN helps distinguish it from most cases of ANCA-associated vasculitis. The occurrence of pulmonary lesions (pulmonary nodules, cavities, infiltrates, or alveolar hemorrhage) in combination with systemic vasculitis shifts the differential diagnosis in favor of other vasculitides, such as granulomatosis with polyangiitis (formerly Wegener granulomatosis), microscopic polyangiitis, and eosinophilic granulomatosis with polyangiitis (Churg-Strauss syndrome). In addition, features of small-vessel disease (eg, purpura) are generally absent in PAN. Isolated peripheral nervous system vasculitis, a form of vasculitis that involves the peripheral nervous system alone, may mimic PAN and require similar therapy. In addition, in a subset of cases, the predominant features of PAN imitate the presentation of giant cell arteritis (eg, headache, jaw claudication, fever, and polymyalgias). Findings of histopathologic features of PAN on temporal artery biopsy specimens have been reported.

The multiorgan system inflammatory nature of PAN may be mimicked by numerous bacterial, mycobacterial, or fungal infections. These must be excluded with great caution before beginning a treatment course for vasculitis. Finally, a host of other systemic or single-organ diseases may mimic PAN in their individual organ features. These include inflammatory bowel disease, sarcoidosis, erythema nodosum, cholesterol emboli, fibromuscular dysplasia, and malignancies (particularly lymphoma). PAN may occur as a complication of hairy cell leukemia.

Livedoid vasculopathy is a thrombotic process that involves small blood vessels in the skin. It may cause skin lesions that are very difficult to distinguish from those of PAN on the basis of clinical findings alone. Nodules and particularly ulcers involving the lower extremities are typical of livedoid vasculopathy. Skin biopsy is required to distinguish PAN from livedoid vasculopathy. The distinction is critical because treatment approaches to these two disorders are divergent: immunosuppression or antiviral therapies in PAN, as opposed to anticoagulation in livedoid vasculopathy.

Treatment

In patients with idiopathic PAN, glucocorticoids and cytotoxic agents remain the cornerstones of treatment. Approximately half of patients with PAN achieve remissions or cures with high doses of glucocorticoids alone. Cyclophosphamide (eg, 2 mg/kg/d orally or 0.6 g/m^2/mo intravenously, decreased in the setting of renal dysfunction)

is indicated for patients whose disease is refractory to glucocorticoids or who have serious involvement of major organs. Prophylaxis against *Pneumocystis jiroveci* pneumonia is an important consideration in patients treated with these medications.

Treatment of HBV-associated PAN with immunosuppressive agents has deleterious long-term effects on the liver. Fortunately, the availability of effective antiviral agents has revolutionized the treatment of HBV-associated cases in recent years. One effective strategy involves the initial use of prednisone (1 mg/kg/d) to suppress the inflammation. Patients begin 6-week courses of plasma exchange (approximately three exchanges per week) simultaneously with the start of prednisone. The doses of glucocorticoids are tapered rapidly (over approximately 2 weeks), followed by the initiation of antiviral therapy (eg, lamivudine 100 mg/d or entecavir 0.5–1.0 mg/d).

Complications

Advanced mononeuritis multiplex can be a severely disabling problem from which recuperation is measured in months or years, if at all. Residual nerve dysfunction in the form of muscle weakness or painful neuropathy is common. The patient's ultimate degree of recovery is difficult to predict. The occurrence of bowel perforation and rupture of a mesenteric microaneurysm are potentially catastrophic events in PAN, requiring emergency surgical intervention and associated with high mortality rates. Patients treated with levels of immunosuppression required for PAN are at substantial risk for opportunistic infection and other complications of treatment.

When to Refer

Appearance of symptoms suggesting mononeuritis multiplex may signal the need for cyclophosphamide and thereby trigger a prompt consultation with the neurologist (electrophysiologist) for diagnostic confirmation and with the rheumatologist for treatment.

Postprandial abdominal pain may be a symptom of intestinal angina. A period of bowel rest, hospitalization for the exclusion of other causes, surgical consultation, and consideration of intensified immunosuppression may be necessary.

Fever in a patient receiving or recently treated with high doses of glucocorticoids or cyclophosphamide or both is considered to be an infection until proven otherwise.

Prognosis

In contrast to the ANCA-associated vasculitides, which are more prone to recurrences, PAN is generally considered to be a "one-shot" disease. For patients with HBV-associated PAN, seroconversion to anti-HBe antigen antibody usually signals the end of the active phase of vasculitis. Among those with idiopathic PAN, disease recurrences are observed in perhaps 10% of cases.

de Menthon M, Mahr A. Treating polyarteritis nodosa: current state of the art. *Clin Exp Rheumatol.* 2011;29(1 Suppl 64):S110. [PMID: 21586205]

Guillevin L, Mahr A, Callard P, et al. French Vasculitis Study Group. Hepatitis B virus-associated polyarteritis nodosa: clinical characteristics, outcome, and impact of treatment in 115 patients. *Medicine (Baltimore).* 2005;84:313. [PMID: 16148731]

Stone JH. Polyarteritis nodosa. *JAMA.* 2002;288:1632. [PMID: 12350194]

[The Johns Hopkins Vasculitis Center] http://vasculitis.med.jhu.edu

[Vasculitis Clinical Research Consortium] http://rarediseasesnetwork.epi.usf.edu/vcrc/

Mixed Cryoglobulinemia

36

John H. Stone, MD, MPH

General Considerations

Cryoglobulins are immunoglobulins (Ig) that precipitate from the serum at low temperatures (see method of collection under Laboratory Findings). Cryoprecipitates are composed most commonly of IgG and IgM (either singly or, in the case of mixed cryoglobulinemia, together). Occasionally IgA may be associated with clinically relevant cryoglobulin syndromes, as well. **Cryoglobulinemia** is divided into three clinical subsets—Types I, II, and III (Table 36–1)—based on two features: the clonality of the IgM component and the presence of RF activity. RF activity, by definition, is the reactivity of an IgM component with the Fc portion of IgG. This chapter focuses on cryoglobulinemia types II and III. (Type I cryoglobulinemia is usually not "mixed," being associated with only a monoclonal IgG or IgM in the setting of a malignancy.)

Formerly referred to as "essential" MC, hepatitis C virus (HCV) infections are now known to be associated with approximately 90% of all cases of MC. Latency periods of up to 15 years between the occurrence of HCV infection and the development of clinical signs of MC have been reported. In some cases, the presentation of HCV may be the development of the clinical features of MC (usually palpable purpura). Cryoglobulins also occur in the setting of other types of infections as well as in connective tissue disorders (eg, Sjögren syndrome) and hematopoietic malignancies.

The presence of cryoglobulins is not always associated with clinical disease, but these proteins may result in a wide variety of immune complex–mediated complications. The term "mixed cryoglobulinemia" was coined to differentiate types II and III (both of which contain mixtures of both IgG and IgM) from type I (which contains only a single monoclonal antibody).

When an underlying infection, autoimmune disorder, or malignancy can be identified, the preferred treatment approach is to direct therapy toward the underlying condition. B cell depletion strategies are often coupled with antiviral therapies in patients with HCV-associated cryoglobulinemia. Occasionally, in patients with rampant systemic vasculitis, generalized immunosuppression or measures designed to remove immune complexes (ie, plasma exchange) may be required for limited periods.

Clinical Findings

The symptoms and signs of MC-associated vasculitis are caused by the vascular deposition of cryoprecipitate components. In type II MC, the cryoprecipitate contains polyclonal IgG, a highly restricted monoclonal IgM that has RF activity, low-density lipoprotein and, in cases of HCV-associated disease, HCV RNA. In general, the diagnosis of MC is made by some combination of the following: (1) recognition of a compatible clinical syndrome, accompanied nearly invariably by cutaneous vasculitis of small blood vessels (Figure 36–1); (2) isolation of cryoglobulins from serum; (3) detection of antibodies to HCV or HCV RNA; and (4) biopsy of other apparently involved organs as necessary to exclude other diagnoses. Because assays for cryoglobulins are not 100% sensitive and because HCV does not cause all cases of MC, all four of these conditions are not required.

Table 36–1. Types of cryoglobulinemia.

Subtype	Rheumatoid Factor Positivity	Monoclonality	Associated Diseases
Type I	No	Yes (IgG or IgM)	Hematopoietic malignancy (multiple myeloma, Waldenström macroglobulinemia)
Type II	Yes	Yes (polyclonal IgG)	Hepatitis C (other infection, Sjögren syndrome, monoclonal IgM, systemic lupus erythematosus)
Type III	Yes	No (polyclonal IgG and IgM)	Hepatitis C (other infection, Sjögren syndrome, systemic lupus erythematosus)

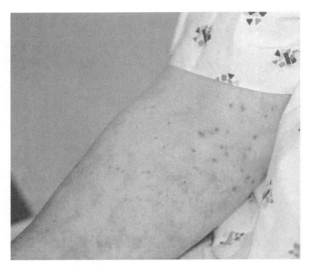

▲ **Figure 36–1.** Small- and medium-vessel vasculitis in a patient with mixed cryoglobulinemia. Palpable purpura, a feature of small-vessel vasculitis, coexists with florid livedo reticularis, a manifestation of medium-vessel disease.

A. Symptoms and Signs

1. Skin—A major hallmark of MC is a small-vessel vasculitis of the skin. Medium-vessel vasculitis may also be present, but this type of involvement generally does not occur without small-vessel disease. Biopsy of the skin with immunofluorescence studies shows an immune complex–mediated leukocytoclastic vasculitis, with deposition of IgG, IgM, C3, and other immunoreactants in and around the walls of small- and medium-sized vessels. Vascular thrombi are also prominent in many cases. Palpable purpura with a predilection for the lower extremities is the typical skin rash, but the rash is also found sometimes on the upper extremities, trunk, or buttocks. In addition, a host of other types of vasculitic rashes may be encountered, depending on the size of blood vessel involved. Such findings may include macules, papules, vesiculobullous lesions, urticarial lesions in the setting of small-vessel involvement, and ulcers above the malleoli—potentially extensive—in the context of medium-vessel disease.

2. Rheumatologic—Arthralgias are a prominent symptom in most cases of MC. The typically involved joints are the proximal interphalangeal and metacarpophalangeal joints and the knees. Frank arthritis, much less common than arthralgias, occurs in a small minority of patients. The arthritis of MC is nondeforming. Raynaud phenomenon and acrocyanosis may also complicate MC.

3. Peripheral nerve—In the peripheral neuropathy of MC, sensory involvement predominates over motor nerve disease. The typical presentation is an axonal sensory neuropathy, associated with pain and paresthesias for years before the development of motor deficits. Motor mononeuritis multiplex may also occur, but never in the absence of sensory symptoms. HCV-induced vasculitis of the vasa nervorum

is the pathogenetic mechanism of this peripheral nerve dysfunction.

4. Kidney—Renal involvement is present in up to 20% of patients at diagnosis. The most frequent manifestations are asymptomatic microscopic hematuria, proteinuria, and variable degree of renal insufficiency. A small proportion may present as acute nephrotic syndrome and acute nephritic syndrome. The most frequent histologic picture is membranoproliferative glomerulonephritis, which can mimic lupus nephritis. Three specific histologic findings serve to distinguish glomerulonephritis secondary to MC: intraluminal thrombi composed of precipitated cryoglobulins; diffuse IgM deposition in the capillary loops; and subendothelial deposits presenting a crystalloid aspect on electron microscopy. MC-related renal disease may lead to nephrotic-range proteinuria, but progression to end-stage renal disease is uncommon. Rapidly progressive glomerulonephritis occurs in only a small number of patients.

5. Liver—Although HCV is obviously a hepatotropic virus, the clinical manifestations of liver disease in MC are few. Moreover, correlations between clinical liver disease and histology are poor. Most patients with HCV-related MC have various degrees of periportal inflammation, fibrosis, and even cirrhosis on liver biopsy. The formation of lymphoid follicles in the liver is a characteristic histologic feature of chronic HCV infection. Within these follicles (and in the bone marrow), most of the IgM RF is formed. Immunophenotyping of mononuclear cells within liver biopsy specimens from patients with HCV-associated MC reveals that they are mostly B cells that express IgM.

6. Hematopoietic system—In addition to its hepatotropism, HCV also tends to infect lymphocytes, and in many cases, MC is truly a lymphoproliferative condition. Infection of lymphocytes often leads to lymphoproliferation and a type III (polyclonal) MC. If a dominant B-cell clone emerges, a type II (monoclonal) MC is produced. In some cases, the emergence of a dominant B-cell clone results from a genetic alteration that favors B-cell survival, eg, a *bcl-2* gene mutation (translocation of the *bcl-2* gene from chromosome 18 to chromosome 14). Such a mutation leads to overexpression of the antiapoptotic *bcl-2*. B-cell lymphoma is the most frequent form of malignancy complicating MC. Hepatocellular carcinoma is also found with an increased incidence among patients with MC, almost certainly related to the effects of underlying viral hepatitis infections in most cases.

7. Central nervous system (CNS)—CNS disease in MC usually results from hyperviscosity and symptoms secondary to "sludging" of blood within the brain. Hyperviscosity, a rare complication of types II or III MC, is more common in type I cryoglobulinemia, a condition in which the cryoglobulin levels are often substantially higher. The occurrence of a hyperviscosity syndrome is an indication for plasma exchange. In addition to hyperviscosity syndromes, true CNS vasculitis also occurs in a very small number of patients with MC.

8. Gastrointestinal tract—Clinically evident gastrointestinal tract involvement is uncommon, but patients with MC present occasionally with acute abdomen. Acute cholecystitis and mesenteric vasculitis secondary to MC have both been reported.

9. Miscellaneous organ involvement in MC—Pulmonary disease, consisting chiefly of interstitial lung lesions, has been described in MC. This manifestation remains poorly understood; cases are usually mild or even asymptomatic. Dryness of the mouth and eyes caused by lymphocytic salivary gland infiltration is not uncommon in MC. This type of organ involvement occurs in the absence of specific serologic evidence of Sjögren syndrome, ie, the finding of anti-Ro/SS-A or anti-La/SS-B antibodies. Bilateral parotid swelling and lymphadenopathy have also been described.

B. Laboratory Findings

MC is associated with a number of laboratory findings that offer clues to the diagnosis. These tests are of limited value in the assessment of disease activity, however, because in general their levels correlate very poorly with disease. An overview of laboratory test results is shown in Table 36–2.

1. Cryoglobulins—Assays for cryoglobulins are associated with a high false-negative rate, caused principally by insufficient care in handling. After phlebotomy, the blood sample must be transported to the laboratory at 37°C and allowed to clot at that same temperature. Specimens are then

Table 36–2. Laboratory and radiologic evaluation in possible mixed cryoglobulinemia.

Test	Typical Results
Complete blood cell count	Mild anemia common. Thrombocytopenia may be present if liver disease is advanced.
Renal and hepatic function	Renal function may be impaired in patients with glomerulonephritis. Hepatic dysfunction often subclinical but evident in most cases on liver biopsy. Liver transaminases may be normal.
Urinalysis with microscopy	Abnormal in cases with renal involvement. Proteinuria may reach nephrotic range.
Erythrocyte sedimentation rate/C-reactive protein	Moderate to severe elevations common, generally reflecting disease activity when very high.
ANA	Positive in the majority of cases.
Rheumatoid factor	Positive in types II and III.
C3, C4	Low, particularly C4 levels.
ANCA	Negative.
Hepatitis B and C serologies	Hepatitis C serologies positive in approximately 90% of patients.
Antiphospholipid antibodies	Negative rapid plasma reagin and anticardiolipin antibody assays. Normal Russell viper venom time (for lupus anticoagulant).
Blood cultures	Negative.

ANA, antinuclear antibody; ANCA, antineutrophil cytoplasmic antibody.

centrifuged at 37°C and stored at 4°C for up to 1 week. The presence of cryoglobulins is indicated by the development of a white precipitate at the bottom of the tube.

2. Cryocrit—The percentage of serum composed of cryoglobulins may be determined by the centrifugation of serum at 4°C. The **cryocrit** may then be measured in precisely the same fashion as a hematocrit. As with other laboratory indicators, the cryocrit correlates poorly with clinical status and treatment. Cryocrit levels should not dictate therapeutic decisions, which are driven more appropriately by patients' clinical condition.

3. Hypocomplementemia—Because complement proteins are involved in the formation of immune complexes, C3 and C1q are often found on specific immunofluorescence testing of biopsy specimens. Serum complement levels—C3, C4, and CH50—are also low in MC. The finding of a very low serum C4 level in the setting of a normal or only moderately reduced level of C3 is a strong clue to the presence of MC.

4. Rheumatoid factor positivity—Eighty percent of the monoclonal IgMs found in HCV-associated MC share a major complementarity region termed "WA." ("WA" refers to the initials of the patient in whom it was initially reported.) This cross idiotype has a high degree of RF activity. Virtually all patients with type II MC are RF positive.

5. Anti-HCV antibodies and quantification of HCV RNA—Anti-HCV assays are typically performed by enzyme immunoassay or immunoblotting. Levels of HCV RNA may be used to follow the treatment response to specific antiviral therapies. HCV genotyping may also be performed by polymerase chain reaction, but no specific viral genotype has been associated with a predisposition to the development of MC.

▶ Differential Diagnosis

MC develops in up to one third of patients with Sjögren syndrome, but manifestations of vasculitis are present in only a small subset of these patients. Clinical and laboratory features of MC and Sjögren syndrome also overlap. In both disorders, patients may have sicca symptoms of the eyes and mouth and have RF, antinuclear antibodies (ANAs), and hypocomplementemia. In general, patients with MC not associated with Sjögren syndrome do not have antibodies to the Ro- and La-antigens.

Patients with systemic lupus erythematosus (SLE) and patients with MC share tendencies for ANA positivity and hypocomplementemia, as well as the clinical features of Raynaud phenomenon, joint complaints, and an immune complex–mediated glomerulonephritis. The two disorders are usually distinguishable through the presence of other clinical and laboratory features (eg, specific antibody testing for antibodies to double-stranded DNA or precipitins). Some patients with SLE have positive test results for cryoglobulins, but the attribution of disease to these proteins in the setting of SLE is often difficult.

RF positivity and joint complaints among patients with MC often lead to the misdiagnosis of rheumatoid arthritis. True synovitis in MC is the exception, however, and when MC is associated with arthritis the joint disease is nondestructive.

Other forms of systemic vasculitis must also be distinguished from MC. There may be considerable overlap in the clinical features of polyarteritis nodosa (see Chapter 35), microscopic polyangiitis (see Chapter 33), granulomatosis with polyangiitis (formerly Wegener granulomatosis) (see Chapter 32), and Henoch-Schönlein purpura (see Chapter 39). The reader is referred to these specific chapters for further details.

▶ Treatment

Although certain laboratory tests (see above) are useful in making the diagnosis, there remain no laboratory values—apart from acute phase reactants such as the erythrocyte sedimentation rate and C-reactive protein levels—that are generally reliable in attempts to ascertain levels of disease activity.

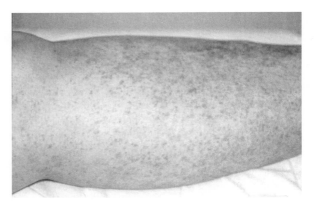

▲ **Figure 36–2.** Hyperpigmentation of the lower extremities resulting from recurrent bouts of purpura in a patient with mixed cryoglobulinemia.

As a rule, treatment decisions must be based on the presence of other clinical manifestations of the disease and on the determination by the physician that the symptoms or signs are the result of active disease rather than damage.

MC is characterized by periods of remission and exacerbation. There is also a wide range of disease severity, from mild purpura to severe necrotizing vasculitis. Consequently, all treatment decisions must be individualized, based on the patient's particular circumstances, considerations of organs at risk, and the potential for adverse effects of therapy. The tendency for cutaneous vasculitis to develop in dependent areas may be exacerbated by venous stasis. Support stockings may reduce the number of cutaneous vasculitis flares.

Under ideal circumstances, the treatment of MC is based on the identification and treatment of the underlying cause, such as a viral infection. For HCV, the sustained response rates to interferon-α are poor (15–20%) but improved somewhat by the addition of ribavirin. Pegylated preparations of interferon-α are more effective for the treatment of HCV and presumably, therefore, for HCV-associated MC, as well. Pegylated interferon-α and ribavirin currently comprise the optimal antiviral regimen for patients with HCV-associated MC who require therapy.

Antiviral strategies are commonly combined with B cell depletion approaches. The typical combination regimen involves the addition of rituximab (1 g times two doses, separated by 15 days) to the full complement of anti-HCV therapies. The combination of B cell depletion and antiviral regimens are synergistic in the treatment of HCV-associated MC. Intervention with interleukin-2 also appears to be a promising treatment strategy.

For patients with truly "essential" MC, ie, MC not associated with a primary cause such as HCV, B cell depletion with rituximab alone may be effective.

Complications

Hyperpigmentation over the involved areas of skin often develops in patients with long-standing, recurrent cutaneous vasculitis (Figure 36–2). Cutaneous ulcers may heal with scarring. End-stage renal disease results in glomerulonephritis in a small number of patients, particularly those who are not treated adequately. Vasculitic neuropathy may lead to permanent sensory or motor neurologic sequelae. In 10% or less of type II MC cases, the disease evolves into a malignant B-cell lymphoma. The portion of HCV-related non-Hodgkin lymphomas ranges widely in different studies, from 0% to 40%. Low-grade B-cell lymphomas may regress with effective treatment of the underlying HCV infection (ie, interferon), but high-grade malignancies require chemotherapy.

De Vita S, Quartuccio L, Isola M, et al. A randomized, controlled trial of rituximab for treatment of severe cryoglobulinemic vasculitis. *Arthritis Rheum.* 2012;64:843. [PMID: 22147661]

Ramos-Casals M, Stone JH, Cid MC, Bosch X. The cryoglobulinaemias. *Lancet.* 2012;379:348. [PMID: 21868085]

Saadoun D, Rosenzwaig M, Joly F, et al. Regulatory T-cell responses to low-dose interleukin-2 in HCV-induced vasculitis. *N Engl J Med.* 2011;365:2067. [PMID: 22129253]

[The Johns Hopkins Vasculitis Center]
http://vasculitis.med.jhu.edu

Hypersensitivity Vasculitis

John H. Stone, MD, MPH

▶ Small-vessel vasculitis of the skin, often accompanied by little or no apparent involvement of other organs.

▶ Known by a variety of other names, including cutaneous leukocytoclastic angiitis.

▶ Precipitants such as medications and infections are often identifiable, but approximately 40% of cases have no definable cause.

▶ Primary forms of vasculitis such as Henoch-Schönlein purpura, microscopic polyangiitis, and granulomatosis with polyangiitis (formerly Wegener granulomatosis) must be excluded. Similarly, well-recognized forms of secondary vasculitis such as mixed cryoglobulinemia caused by hepatitis C must also be eliminated from the differential diagnosis.

▶ Most cases are self-limited if the precipitant can be identified and removed. Glucocorticoids or other medications are required in other cases.

▶ General Considerations

Hypersensitivity vasculitis refers to small-vessel vasculitis that is restricted to the skin and not associated with any other form of primary or secondary vasculitis. Implicit in this definition is that the condition is not associated with medium- or large-vessel disease at other sites, nor with small-vessel disease in other organs (eg, the glomeruli or pulmonary capillaries). In many cases, an identifiable precipitant such as a drug or an accompanying infection is present—hence the term "hypersensitivity." In up to 40% of cases, however, no specific cause is identified.

The term "hypersensitivity vasculitis" has been associated with much confusion ever since it was incorporated into the first vasculitis classification scheme in the early 1950s. The condition's name derives from the fact that by the 1950s, both human and animal models of hypersensitivity to foreign antigens had been shown to cause small-vessel vasculitis involving the kidneys, lungs, and other organs besides the skin. Consequently, even microscopic polyangiitis (see Chapter 33), a disorder that commonly affects internal organs as well as the skin and is often associated with antineutrophil cytoplasmic antibodies (ANCAs), was grouped initially under the heading of hypersensitivity vasculitis. Because of the confusion surrounding its name, many clinicians have suggested that hypersensitivity vasculitis be replaced, but no entirely suitable alternative has been found. Terms used synonymously with hypersensitivity vasculitis have included **leukocytoclastic vasculitis, cutaneous leukocytoclastic angiitis, and cutaneous small-vessel vasculitis,** among others. In evaluating patients with small-vessel vasculitis of the skin, it is critical to remember that skin findings may only herald an underlying disorder involving other organs, as well. Extracutaneous involvement, which mandates reconsideration of the diagnosis, must be excluded with appropriate tests.

In most cases of hypersensitivity vasculitis, the problem is believed to have an immune complex–mediated pathophysiology. Histopathology generally shows a leukocytoclastic vasculitis, with features of necrosis in some cases but not granulomatous inflammation. Biopsies very early in the course of disease may show a lymphocytic predominance.

▶ Clinical Findings

Table 37–1 outlines the classification criteria for hypersensitivity vasculitis established in 1990 by the American College of Rheumatology.

A. Symptoms and Signs

1. Skin—The lesions of small-vessel vasculitis of the skin include purpura (either palpable or nonpalpable) (Figure 37–1), papules, urticaria/angioedema, erythema multiforme, vesicles, pustules, ulcers, and necrosis. The lesions typically occur first and most prominently in dependent

Table 37–1. American College of Rheumatology 1990 criteria for the classification of hypersensitivity vasculitis.[a]

1. Age at disease onset >16 years
2. Medication at disease onset
3. Palpable purpura
4. Maculopapular rash
5. Biopsy including arteriole and venule, showing granulocytes in a perivascular or extravascular location

[a]For purposes of classification, hypersensitivity vasculitis may be diagnosed if the patient meets at least three of these five criteria. Sensitivity = 71%; specificity = 83.9%.
Data from Calabrese LH, Michel BA, Bloch DA, et al. The American College of Rheumatology 1990 criteria for the classification of hypersensitivity vasculitis. *Arthritis Rheum.* 1990;33;1108.

Table 37–2. Laboratory and radiographic work-up of patients with possible hypersensitivity vasculitis.

Test	Typical Result
Complete blood cell count, with differential	Normal
Electrolytes	Normal
Liver function tests	Normal
Urinalysis with microscopy	Normal
Erythrocyte sedimentation rate/ C-reactive protein	Mild to moderate elevations in <50% of patients
ANA	Negative
Rheumatoid factor	Negative
C3, C4	Normal
ANCA	Negative
Antihepatitis B and C assays	Negative
Cryoglobulins	Negative
Chest radiography	Normal

ANA, antinuclear antibody; ANCA, antineutrophil cytoplasmic antibody.

regions, ie, the lower extremities or buttocks. The lesions tend to occur in cohorts or "crops" that are of the same age. The occurrence of the lesions may be asymptomatic but is usually accompanied by a burning or tingling sensation.

2. Joints—Hypersensitivity vasculitis is sometimes accompanied by arthralgias and even frank arthritis, with a predominance for large joints.

B. Laboratory Findings

The results of routine laboratory tests and more specialized assays in hypersensitivity vasculitis are shown in Table 37–2. All of these tests are appropriate at the time of initial patient evaluation, primarily for the purpose of excluding other forms of vasculitis that may mimic hypersensitivity vasculitis.

C. Special Tests

The pleomorphic lesions of cutaneous vasculitis and the large number of vasculitis mimickers make histopathologic confirmation of the diagnosis by skin biopsy important in most cases. A biopsy specimen of an active lesion (<48 hours old, if possible) usually demonstrates leukocytoclastic vasculitis of the postcapillary venules. Direct immunofluorescence (DIF) studies show variable quantities of immunoglobulin and complement deposition, with a nondiagnostic pattern. The performance of DIF studies, however, is an important (and often neglected) part of the work-up, critical for the exclusion of Henoch-Schönlein purpura, cryoglobulinemia, and other conditions.

▶ Differential Diagnosis

The differential diagnosis of hypersensitivity vasculitis is shown in Table 37–3. Hypersensitivity vasculitis must be distinguished primarily from other small-vessel vasculitides, from autoimmune inflammatory conditions associated with joint disease and rashes, and from other cutaneous reactions to medications.

▶ Treatment

Treatment strategies for hypersensitivity vasculitis are largely empiric. The type, intensity, and duration of therapy are based on the degree of disease severity in individual cases. For patients in whom a precipitant can be identified, removal of the offending agent usually leads to resolution of the vasculitis within days to weeks. Mild cases may

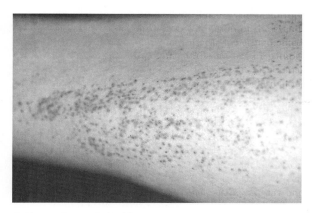

▲ **Figure 37–1.** Palpable purpura.

Table 37–3. Differential diagnosis of hypersensitivity vasculitis.

Other vasculitides
Henoch-Schönlein purpura
Microscopic polyangiitis
Eosinophilic granulomatosis with polyangiitis
(Churg-Strauss syndrome)
Granulomatosis with polyangiitis (formerly Wegener granulomatosis)
Mixed cryoglobulinemia
Polyarteritis nodosa
Systemic autoimmune conditions
Systemic lupus erythematosus (including urticarial vasculitis)
Rheumatoid arthritis
Miscellaneous
Acute hemorrhagic edema of infancy
Other types of drug eruptions

be treated simply with leg elevation and the administration of nonsteroidal anti-inflammatory drugs (or H_1 antihistamines). For persistent disease that does not lead to cutaneous ulcers or gangrene, colchicine (0.6 mg two or three times daily), hydroxychloroquine (200 mg twice daily), or dapsone (100 mg/d) may be used. For refractory or more severe cases, immunosuppressive agents may be indicated, generally beginning with a moderate dose of glucocorticoids (eg, prednisone 20–40 mg/d). When a patient cannot tolerate a glucocorticoid taper over weeks or even several months, the addition of an immunosuppressive agent may be necessary. Azathioprine (2 mg/kg/d) is used most commonly for this purpose.

▶ **Complications**

Most cases with a clearly identified precipitant resolve over 1 to 4 weeks, often with some residual hyperpigmentation or (in the case of ulcerated lesions) scars. Some patients, however, have recurrent disease that remains confined to the skin and requires prolonged therapy.

Carlson JA. The histological assessment of cutaneous vasculitis. *Histopathology.* 2010;56:3. [PMID: 20055902]

[The Cleveland Clinic Foundation Center for Vasculitis] http://www.clevelandclinic.org/arthritis/vasculitis/default.htm

[The Johns Hopkins Vasculitis Center] http://vasculitis.med.jhu.edu

Behçet Disease

38

David B. Hellmann, MD, MACP

ESSENTIALS OF DIAGNOSIS

► Recurrent attacks of oral aphthous ulcers, genital ulcers, uveitis, and skin lesions.

► Onset usually in young adults, aged 25–35 years.

► Prevalent in parts of Asia and Europe; rare in North America.

► Blindness, central nervous system disease, and large-vessel events are the most serious complications.

► Glucocorticoids, immunosuppressive drugs, or both are required for severe disease.

▶ General Considerations

Behçet disease, a form of vasculitis of unknown cause, is named for the Turkish dermatologist who in 1937 described the syndrome as a triad of recurrent oral aphthous ulcers, genital ulcers, and ocular inflammation. Although these features are often the most salient, Behçet disease can cause inflammation in almost any organ. Indeed, involvement of the central nervous system, gastrointestinal tract, and large vessels can be life-threatening. Except for eye disease, most of the manifestations of Behçet disease do not persist chronically but recur in attacks, which usually become less frequent over time. Disability stems most often from ocular inflammation, which causes blindness, and less often from central nervous system disease. Mortality results chiefly from major vascular events, including thrombosis, aneurysm, and rupture of large vessels.

▶ Epidemiology

One of the most striking features of Behçet disease is how common it is in countries along the ancient Silk Road and how rarely it develops elsewhere. Most prevalent in Turkey (up to nearly 400 cases per 100,000 people), Behçet disease also occurs frequently in Iran, Saudi Arabia, Greece, Japan, Korea, and China. In contrast, Behçet disease rarely develops in Western countries such as the United States, where the disease affects about 1 of every 170,000 people.

Behçet disease is chiefly a disease of young people; typically, patients are in their 20s or 30s when symptoms first develop. Although males are more commonly affected than females in the Middle Eastern countries, female patients predominate in Japan, the United States, and Europe.

▶ Etiology & Pathogenesis

Although the cause of Behçet disease is unknown, the distinct geographic clustering of cases suggests the importance of environment, genes, or both. Genetic studies have revealed a strikingly high prevalence of the HLA-B51 allele in patients living along the Silk Road, reaching nearly 80% of Asian patients. However, this allele is not associated with Behçet disease in Western countries.

Much of the damage in Behçet disease results from blood vessel inflammation, justifying the disease's classification as a form of vasculitis. Although Behçet disease typically affects the small- and medium-sized vessels, it is one of the rare forms of vasculitis capable of also affecting large arteries. Arterial inflammation can lead to occlusion, aneurysm, or rupture. Behçet disease joins granulomatosis with polyangiitis (formerly Wegener granulomatosis) and Buerger disease in being a form of vasculitis that has a predilection for involving veins and causing venous thrombosis.

Vasculitis does not appear to account for all of the pathologic changes in Behçet disease. Many of the pathologic changes—including ulceration of the mouth and gut—may be more attributable to an abnormal reactivity of neutrophils and lymphocytes.

▶ Clinical Findings

A. Symptoms and Signs

Oral ulceration is the hallmark of the disease, tends to be the earliest manifestation, and is required for the diagnosis of Behçet disease (Table 38–1). Oral ulcers are painful, shallow or deep, round or oval, with a white or yellow base and red halo (Figure 38–1). They vary in size from 1–20 mm. The ulcers most frequently affect the buccal mucosa, tongue, lips, gingivae, palate, tonsils, uvula, or pharynx. During an attack, patients usually have two to five lesions, but some patients may have a single ulcer or too many to count. The aphthae may be so painful that the patient has trouble eating or drinking. Usually the aphthous lesions heal without scarring over 10–20 days.

Genital aphthae occur slightly less often than oral ulceration (Table 38–1). However, genital ulcers tend to be larger and deeper, and often heal with scarring. In men, the ulcers develop most commonly on the scrotum and less commonly on the shaft of the penis, and in women ulcers affect the vagina and vulva. Genital lesions in men are often associated with epididymitis.

Cutaneous manifestations of Behçet disease, which develop in 60–90% of patients, are protean. Erythema nodosum occurs most commonly, especially in women. Erythema nodosum in Behçet disease tends to ulcerate and heal with scarring and hyperpigmentation, compared with erythema nodosum associated with sarcoidosis and inflammatory bowel disease, which does not ulcerate and heals without scarring. In men, pseudofolliculitis and acneiform nodules develop frequently over the neck and face. Pathergy—the phenomenon of developing an aseptic nodule or ulcer larger than 2 mm in diameter 24–48 hours following a sterile needle prick to the forearm—occurs frequently in Japanese and Turks but in only approximately one third of Americans with Behçet disease. Migratory thrombophlebitis also commonly occurs in Behçet disease.

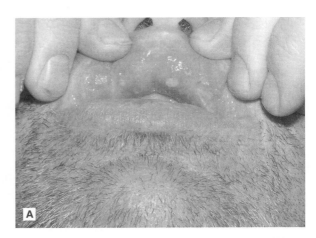

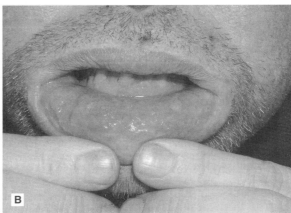

▲ **Figure 38–1.** **A** and **B:** Multiple aphthous ulcers behind the upper and lower lips of a man with Behçet disease.

Table 38–1. Frequency of clinical manifestations of Behçet disease.

Feature	Frequency (%)
Oral ulcers	100
Genital ulcers	75
Skin lesions	60–90
Arthritis	50
Gastrointestinal disease	25
Thrombophlebitis	20
Central nervous system disease	10–20
Epididymitis	5

Ocular inflammation, one of the hallmark manifestations of Behçet disease, tends to occur early in the course. Recurrent or persistent ocular inflammation frequently leads to visual loss, making eye inflammation one of the most common causes of disability in Behçet disease. Behçet disease is one of the few autoimmune diseases that can cause both anterior and posterior uveitis. Anterior uveitis typically presents with a red eye, intense photophobia, and blurred vision. The anterior uveitis may be so intense that a grossly visible layer of pus in the anterior chamber (hypopyon) develops. The posterior uveitis and vasculitis of the carotid and retina occur less commonly but pose a greater threat to vision.

Peripheral arthritis or spondylitis develops in approximately half of patients with Behçet disease. The peripheral arthritis may be monarticular or polyarticular, while the spondylitis usually presents as sacroiliitis (with low back or buttock pain). The peripheral arthritis is usually not deforming.

Gastrointestinal involvement develops in about one-quarter of patients. Although gastrointestinal involvement can appear at any time, it typically emerges several years after the onset of oral ulcers. Behçet disease of the gastrointestinal tract most commonly presents as aphthous ulcers affecting the ileum and cecum. However, any portion of the gut from the mouth to the anus can be involved. The most frequent manifestations of bowel involvement are pain, anorexia, rectal bleeding, vomiting, and diarrhea. In American patients, esophageal ulceration appears especially common. In addition, ischemia of the bowel may result from vasculitis of the medium- and large-sized mesenteric arteries. The unusual predilection for Behçet disease to involve veins explains why the Budd-Chiari syndrome develops in some patients.

Central nervous system disease, which develops in 10–20% of patients, resembles gastrointestinal involvement in following oral ulceration by 3–5 years. The neurologic features are variable and include headache and confusion (from recurrent sterile meningitis) and meningoencephalitis. Meningoencephalitis in Behçet disease most commonly affects the brainstem but can also affect the thalamus, basal ganglia, thalamus, cortex and white matter, spinal cord, or cranial nerves. Other complications are thrombotic or hemorrhagic hemispheric stroke, dural venous thrombosis, seizures, hearing and vestibular involvement, progressive dementia, and psychiatric disease including personality changes. Behçet disease rarely involves the peripheral nervous system.

Large-vessel vasculitis explains why bruits develop in some patients' chest or abdomen. The most commonly involved sites are the pulmonary, carotid, aortic, iliac, femoral, and popliteal arteries. Affected vessels—especially in the pulmonary and mesenteric circulation—may occlude, develop aneurysm swelling, or rupture. Hemoptysis and pulmonary nodules are common manifestations of lung involvement. Aneurysms of the proximal pulmonary arteries develop commonly in those with lung disease. The Hughes-Stovin syndrome, defined by pulmonary artery thrombosis and aneurysms occurring with peripheral thrombophlebitis, develops most commonly in patients with Behçet disease. Clinically important cardiac disease (most typically with coronary artery vasculitis) develops infrequently, and renal disease occurs rarely.

B. Laboratory Findings

Behçet disease produces no specific blood test abnormalities. Nonspecific markers of inflammation, such as anemia, mild leukocytosis, and an elevated erythrocyte sedimentation rate, are common during attacks of active inflammation. Patients with active Behçet disease also often show elevated levels of serum IgD. Cerebrospinal fluid analysis in patients with meningoencephalitis usually reveals elevations of protein and IgG and a pleocytosis of either polymorphonuclear cells or lymphocytes.

C. Imaging Studies

Patients with neurologic disease can have abnormalities evident on computed tomography (CT) scans or magnetic resonance imaging (MRI). The most frequent MRI abnormalities are seen with T2 weighting and consist of multiple high-intensity focal lesions that are widely distributed. Angiograms or magnetic resonance angiography can demonstrate large-artery thrombosis and aneurysm, typically seen in the chest or abdomen.

D. Special Tests

Biopsies of mucocutaneous lesions and gastrointestinal ulcers reveal a neutrophilic vascular reaction. True vasculitis is rare. The pathergy phenomenon is uncommon in Americans.

▶ Diagnosis & Differential Diagnosis

Since Behçet disease produces no pathognomonic laboratory finding, the diagnosis rests upon clinical criteria, which have been refined by an international study group (Table 38–2).

The differential diagnosis of recurrent oral and genital aphthous ulceration includes complex aphthosis (the label given to patients who suffer from almost constant mouth ulcers or recurrent oral and genital ulcers in the absence of Behçet disease), herpes simplex virus infection, Crohn disease, gluten-sensitive enteropathy, HIV disease, various vitamin or other nutrient deficiencies (including iron, zinc, folate, and vitamins B_1, B_2, B_6, or B_{12}), cyclic neutropenia, reactive

Table 38–2. Criteria for the diagnosis of Behçet disease.

Clinical Feature	Definition
Recurrent oral ulceration	Minor aphthous, major aphthous, or herpetiform ulcerations observed by physician or patient that recurred at least three times over a 12-month period
Plus two of the following criteria:	
Recurrent genital ulceration	Aphthous ulceration or scarring observed by patient or physician
Ocular lesions	Anterior uveitis, posterior uveitis, or cells in vitreous on slit lamp examination, or retinal vasculitis observed by ophthalmologist
Skin lesions	Erythema nodosum observed by patient or physician, pseudofolliculitis or papulopustular lesions, or acneiform nodules observed by physician in a postadolescent patient not taking glucocorticoids
Positive pathergy test	Interpreted by physician at 24–48 hours

Data from International Study Group for Behçet's Disease. Criteria for diagnosis of Behçet's Disease. *Lancet.* 1990;335:1078.

arthritis (formerly Reiter syndrome), and factitious disease. Medications, especially nonsteroidal anti-inflammatory drugs and methotrexate, can cause recurrent oral ulcerations. Another cause of recurrent oral lesions is systemic lupus erythematosus. The oral and pharyngeal lesions of granulomatosis with polyangiitis (formerly Wegener granulomatosis) and histoplasmosis are not usually recurrent. Stevens-Johnson syndrome, pemphigoid, and lichen planus can involve the mouth, genitals, and eye, but do not produce aphthous lesions.

Erythema nodosa has many causes besides Behçet disease, including sarcoidosis and inflammatory bowel disease. As noted, only erythema nodosa associated with Behçet tends to ulcerate. Some of the skin lesions in Behçet disease can mimic those of Sweet syndrome.

Syphilis and sarcoidosis are two diseases that, like Behçet disease, can cause both anterior and posterior uveitis. Anterior uveitis can also be caused by inflammatory bowel disease, ankylosing spondylitis, and reactive arthritis (formerly Reiter syndrome).

It can be virtually impossible to distinguish Behçet disease from Crohn disease unless the patient has bowel biopsies showing granulomatous lesions (supporting the diagnosis of Crohn disease).

Neurologic disease can sometimes mimic multiple sclerosis.

All patients with unexplained recurrent oral and genital ulcers should have the following tests performed or considered: cultures or polymerase chain reaction testing for herpes simplex virus infection; complete blood count with differential; comprehensive metabolic panel; erythrocyte sedimentation rate; urinalysis; HIV antibody test; serum levels of iron, folate, zinc, and vitamin B_{12}; antiendomysial or antigliadin antibodies; and antinuclear antibody. Patients with visceral symptoms may require imaging with MRI or CT, or invasive testing including lumbar puncture or upper and lower endoscopy. Consultation by a rheumatologist, gynecologist, ophthalmologist, neurologist, dermatologist, or gastroenterologist may also be helpful in establishing the diagnosis of Behçet disease or conditions that can mimic it.

▶ **Treatment**

Treatment—like the disease itself—runs the gamut in intensity and illustrates how important it is to ensure that the treatment fits the disease manifestation. Recurrent oral ulcers, although painful, can be treated with topical glucocorticoids or dapsone. Vision-threatening uveitis or life-threatening meningoencephalitis requires decisive intervention with the combination of high-dose systemic glucocorticoids and a tumor necrosis factor inhibitor such as infliximab or adalimumab. Tumor necrosis factor inhibitors have gained favor the past several years over traditional immunosuppressive agents such as cyclophosphamide and chlorambucil. Interferon-alpha is effective in treating refractory mucocutaneous manifestations but is often tolerated poorly. Standard anticoagulation therapies are used to treat venous thrombosis. Other treatments and their indications are listed in Table 38–3.

Table 38–3. Treatment for Behçet disease.

Treatment	Dose	Used as First-Line Therapy	Used as Alternative Therapy
Topical glucocorticoids			
Triamcinolone acetonide	Three times a day topically	Oral ulcers	
Betamethasone ointment	Three times a day topically	Genital ulcers	
Betamethasone drops	1–2 drops three times daily topically	Anterior uveitis, retinal vasculitis	
Dexamethasone	1–1.5 mg injected below tenon capsule for an ocular attack	Retinal vasculitis	
Systemic glucocorticoids			
Prednisone	5–20 mg/d orally		Erythema nodosum, anterior uveitis, retinal vasculitis, arthritis
	20–100 mg/d orally	Gastrointestinal lesions, acute meningoencephalitis, chronic progressive central nervous system lesions, arteritis	Retinal vasculitis, venous thrombosis
Methylprednisolone	1000 mg/d for 3 days intravenously	Acute meningoencephalitis, chronic progressive central nervous system lesions, arteritis	Gastrointestinal lesions, venous thrombosis

(continued)

Table 38–3. Treatment for Behçet disease. (*continued*)

Treatment	Dose	Used as First-Line Therapy	Used as Alternative Therapy
Other agents			
Tropicamide drops	1–2 drops once or twice daily topically	Anterior uveitis	
Tetracycline	250 mg in water solution once a day topically		Oral ulcers
Colchicine	0.5–1. 5 mg/d orally	Oral ulcers,[a] genital ulcers,[a] pseudofolliculitis,[a] erythema nodosum, anterior uveitis, retinal vasculitis	Arthritis
Thalidomide	100–300 mg/d orally		Oral ulcers,[a] genital ulcers,[a] pseudofolliculitis[a]
Dapsone	100 mg/d orally		Oral ulcers, genital ulcers, pseudofolliculitis, erythema nodosum
Pentoxifylline	300 mg/d orally		Oral ulcers, genital ulcers, pseudofolliculitis, erythema nodosum
Azathioprine	100 mg/d orally		Retinal vasculitis,[a] arthritis,[a] chronic progressive central nervous system lesions, arteritis, venous thrombosis
Chlorambucil	5 mg/d orally		Retinal vasculitis, acute meningoencephalitis, chronic progressive central nervous system lesions, arteritis, venous thrombosis
Cyclophosphamide	50–1000 mg/d orally		Retinal vasculitis, acute meningoencephalitis, chronic progressive central nervous system lesions, arteritis, venous thrombosis
	700–1000 mg/mo intravenously		Retinal vasculitis, acute meningoencephalitis, chronic progressive central nervous system lesions, arteritis, venous thrombosis
Methotrexate	7.5–1 5 mg/wk orally		Retinal vasculitis, arthritis, chronic progressive central nervous system lesions
Cyclosporine[b]	5 mg/kg of body weight/day orally	Retinal vasculitis[a]	
Interferon-α	5 million units/d intramuscularly or subcutaneously		Retinal vasculitis, arthritis
Indomethacin	50–75 mg/d	Arthritis orally	
Sulfasalazine	1–3 g/d orally	Gastrointestinal lesions	Arthritis
Warfarin[c]	2–10 mg/d orally	Venous thrombosis	Arteritis
Heparin[c]	5000–20,000 units/d subcutaneously	Venous thrombosis	Arteritis
Aspirin[d]	50–100 mg/d orally	Arteritis, venous thrombosis	Chronic progressive central nervous system lesions
Dipyridamole	300 mg/d orally	Arteritis, venous thrombosis	Chronic progressive central nervous system lesions
Surgery	—		Gastrointestinal lesions, arteritis, venous thrombosis

[a]The efficacy of this drug for this use has been reported in controlled clinical trials.
[b]Cyclosporine is contraindicated in patients with acute meningoencephalitis or chronic progressive central nervous system lesions.
[c]This drug should be used with caution in patients with pulmonary vascular lesions.
[d]Low-dose aspirin is used as an antiplatelet agent.
Data from Sakane T, Takeno M, Suzuki N, Inaba G. Behçet's Disease. *N Engl J Med.* 1999;341:1284.

► Course & Prognosis

Behçet is a chronic disease characterized by recurrent attacks. Most manifestations, except for eye disease and large-vessel inflammation, tend to burn out over 1–2 decades. Disability most commonly results from uveitis (causing blindness), central nervous system disease (causing stroke and dementia), and gastrointestinal disease. Mortality results from central nervous system disease, rupture of arterial aneurysms, and infectious and oncologic complications of immunosuppressive therapy.

Aguiar de Sousa D, Mestre T, Ferro JM. Cerebral venous thrombosis in Behçet's disease: a systematic review. *J Neurol.* 2011;258:719. [PMID: 21210139]

Alexoudi I, Kapsimali V, Vaiopoulos A, Kanakis M, Vaiopoulos G. Evaluation of current therapeutic strategies in Behçet's disease. *Clin Rheumatol.* 2011;30:157. [PMID: 20842513]

Borhani Haghighi A, Safari A, Nazarinia MA, Habibagahi Z, Shenavandeh S. Infliximab for patients with neuro-Behçet's disease: case series and literature review. *Clin Rheumatol.* 2011;30:1007. [PMID: 21431864]

Calamia KT, Schirmer M, Melikoglu M. Major vessel involvement in Behçet's disease: an update. *Curr Opin Rheumatol.* 2011;23:24. [PMID: 21124084]

Hello M, Barbarot S, Bastuji-Garin S, Revuz J, Chosidow O. Use of thalidomide for severe recurrent aphthous stomatitis: a multicenter cohort analysis. *Medicine (Baltimore).* 2010;89:176. [PMID: 20453604]

[The Johns Hopkins Vasculitis Center] http://vasculitis.med.jhu.edu

[The Vasculitis Foundation] http://www.vasculitisfoundation.org/

Henoch-Schönlein Purpura

39

Geetha Duvuru, MD, MRCP

John H. Stone, MD, MPH

ESSENTIALS OF DIAGNOSIS

▶ The sine qua non of Henoch-Schönlein purpura (HSP) is nonthrombocytopenic purpura, caused by inflammation in blood vessels of the superficial dermis.

▶ The pathologic hallmarks of HSP are a leukocytoclastic vasculitis and deposition of immunoglobulin (Ig) A in the walls of involved blood vessels.

▶ The tetrad of purpura, arthritis, glomerulonephritis, and abdominal pain is often observed. However, all four elements are not required for the diagnosis.

▶ More than 90% of cases occur in children. The disease is self-limited most of the time, resolving within a few weeks. Adult cases are sometimes more recalcitrant.

▶ Renal insufficiency develops in less than 5% of patients with HSP. The long-term renal prognosis depends mainly on the degree of initial damage to the kidney.

▶ HSP can be mimicked by other forms of systemic vasculitis that are more often life-threatening. For example, antineutrophil cytoplasmic antibody (ANCA)–associated vasculitides such as granulomatosis with polyangiitis (formerly Wegener granulomatosis) and microscopic polyangiitis (see Chapters 32 and 33, respectively) may also present with purpura, arthritis, and renal inflammation. Both of these disorders have the potential for serious involvement of other organs (eg, the lungs and peripheral nerves) and carry more dire renal prognoses.

▶ General Considerations

Henoch-Schönlein purpura (HSP) is the most common form of systemic vasculitis in children, with an annual incidence of 140 cases per million persons. The peak incidence is in the first and second decades of life (90% of patients are younger than 10 years of age), with a male to female ratio of 2:1. The incidence is significantly lower in adults, with a mean age at presentation of 50 years. Males and females are affected equally and although HSP affects all ethnic groups, it is reportedly less common among blacks. Some epidemiologic studies suggest that HSP is more prevalent in the winter months.

HSP may be misdiagnosed as another form of vasculitis—most commonly hypersensitivity vasculitis (see Chapter 37)—because of the frequent failure to perform direct immunofluorescence testing on skin biopsy specimens. In two thirds of the cases, the disease follows an upper respiratory tract infection, with onset an average of 10 days after the start of respiratory symptoms. Despite this association, no single microorganism or environmental exposure has been confirmed as an important cause of HSP. HSP can also be induced by medications, particularly antibiotics. The American College of Rheumatology 1990 criteria for the classification of HSP are shown in Table 39–1. The first Chapel Hill Consensus Conference on the nomenclature of vasculitides defined HSP as a form of vasculitis characterized by the following: (1) IgA-dominant immune deposits within vessel walls; (2) small-vessel involvement (ie, capillaries, venules, or arterioles); and (3) skin, gut, renal, and joint manifestation.

The skin histopathology of HSP shows a leukocytoclastic vasculitis of small blood vessels within the superficial dermis. Necrosis is often present, but features of granulomatous inflammation are not. Immunofluorescent staining of biopsy specimens shows coarse, granular IgA staining in and around small blood vessels. In the kidney, the renal inflammation is indistinguishable from IgA nephropathy. There is a predilection for IgA deposition within the mesangium. However, in HSP nephritis, capillary wall staining for IgA is more frequently found and may be even more prominent than IgA in the mesangium. Most patients have increased serum IgA levels and circulating immune complexes that contain IgA, as well as IgA deposition in inflamed blood vessels.

Table 39-1. American College of Rheumatology 1990 Criteria[a] for the classification of Henoch-Schönlein purpura (HSP).

1. Palpable purpura
2. Age at onset <20 years
3. Bowel angina
4. Vessel wall granulocytes on biopsy

[a]The presence of two criteria classified HSP with a sensitivity of 87% and specificity of 88% in a group of individuals with forms of systemic vasculitis.

▶ Clinical Findings

A. Symptoms and Signs

The classic full presentation includes the acute onset of fever, palpable purpura on the lower extremities (Figure 39–1) and buttocks, abdominal pain, arthritis, and hematuria. All components of this presentation are not required for the diagnosis, however. Conversely, even classic presentations are not diagnostic of this disorder. In adults, the diagnosis should be confirmed in most cases by biopsy (direct immunofluorescence as well as conventional hematoxylin and eosin staining). Pediatricians are more likely to rely on clinical diagnoses in the setting of classic presentations, which is reasonable given the relatively high incidence of HSP in children compared to adults.

1. Skin—The cutaneous findings of HSP include purpura (usually palpable, although sometimes not), urticarial papules, and plaques. Among adults, 60% of the patients have bullous or necrotic lesions (Figure 39–2), but these are

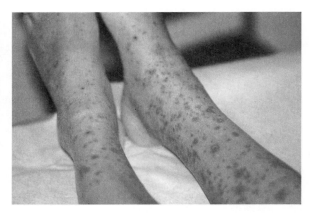

▲ **Figure 39–1.** Palpable purpura with some superficial ulcerations in a patient with Henoch-Schönlein purpura. Note also the presence of right ankle swelling due to arthritis.

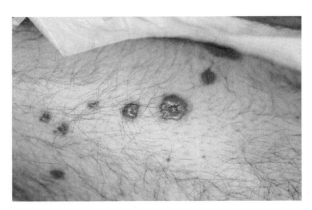

▲ **Figure 39–2.** A bullous lesion with a purpuric component in a patient with Henoch-Schönlein purpura.

uncommon in children. Lesions are concentrated over the buttocks and lower extremities and tend to involve the small blood vessels in the superficial dermis. Medium-sized vessels are rarely involved in HSP except in the rare cases of HSP associated with IgA paraproteinemia. Localized edematous swelling of the subcutaneous tissues of the lower extremities is frequently observed and does not correlate with the presence or degree of proteinuria. Persistent rash over a period longer than 1 month is a significant predictor of disease relapse and renal sequelae in children with HSP.

2. Joints—Joint disease, which occurs in more than 80% of patients with HSP, manifests itself as arthralgias or arthritis in large joints, especially the knees and ankles and, to a lesser degree, the wrists and elbows. Migratory patterns of joint involvement are common. Lower extremity involvement among patients with HSP and arthritis is nearly universal; up to one third of patients have upper extremity involvement as well. The pain associated with HSP arthritis may be incapacitating. The arthritis is nondeforming in nature.

3. Gastrointestinal tract—Approximately 60% of patients with HSP have abdominal pain and 33% have evidence of gastrointestinal bleeding. Abdominal symptoms result from edema of the bowel wall as well as hemorrhage induced by mesenteric vasculitis. Abdominal pain may precede the appearance of purpura by up to 2 weeks, leading often to diagnostic confusion and occasionally to invasive testing or even laparotomy. The abdominal pain is typically colicky and may worsen after eating (ie, intestinal angina). Some patients experience nausea, vomiting, and upper or lower gastrointestinal bleeding. Mesenteric ischemia in HSP rarely leads to gut perforation. Massive gastrointestinal hemorrhage occurs in only 2% or so of patients. Purpuric lesions may be seen on endoscopy, commonly in the descending duodenum, stomach, and colon.

Gastrointestinal involvement in children with HSP can cause intussusception, a rare complication in adults. In contrast to idiopathic intussusception, which typically is ileocolic, HSP-associated intussusception is usually ileoileal. Other rare complications include pancreatitis, cholecystitis, and a protein-losing enteropathy.

4. Kidney—Renal involvement is the most potentially debilitating complication of HSP. Forty percent of patients with HSP have renal disease. In general, renal involvement is more frequent and tends to be persistent in adults, who have a higher risk of developing end-stage renal disease than children. In a retrospective study of 134 children with HSP, age greater than 4 years, persistent purpura, and severe abdominal symptoms increased the likelihood of renal involvement.

In contrast to gastrointestinal disease and arthritis, both of which occasionally precede the onset of purpura, glomerulonephritis almost always appears after the development of skin manifestations. The occurrence of glomerulonephritis may be delayed by several weeks in up to 25% of all patients with this complication. The clinical hallmark of nephritis in HSP is hematuria, often macroscopic, but more typically microscopic. The hematuria can be transient, persistent, or recurrent. Proteinuria never occurs in the absence of hematuria in the acute setting. Even in cases in which the renal disease resolves spontaneously, many patients have persistent urinary abnormalities (eg, proteinuria).

The most common renal lesion (60% of cases) is a focal, proliferative endocapillary glomerulonephritis. Crescents are present in up to 40% of biopsies. Direct immunofluorescence studies characteristically demonstrate IgA deposition in the mesangium. Regardless of age, the degree of proteinuria, the presence of renal dysfunction at presentation, the number of crescents, and the degree of interstitial fibrosis on biopsy correlate with outcome. Histologic recurrences of HSP nephritis in renal allografts occur in 50% of patients who undergo renal transplantation. Allograft recurrences are associated with clinically significant disease in 20%, allograft failure in 12%, and allograft loss in 9% of cases.

5. Other organs—Pulmonary and central nervous system (CNS) complications of HSP have been described, but these are very rare. When present, the usual lung manifestation of the disease is alveolar hemorrhage. Seizures are the usual CNS manifestation of HSP; the precise mechanism is obscure. Testicular involvement occurs in up to 10% of boys with this disease and may mimic torsion.

B. Laboratory Findings

The results of routine laboratory tests and more specialized assays in HSP are shown in Table 39–2. All of these tests are appropriate at the initial evaluation of a patient with possible HSP. The exclusion of other forms of vasculitis that may mimic HSP in presentation is essential. Sixty percent of patients have an elevated serum IgA. Although there are two subclasses of IgA, HSP is associated with serum elevations and tissue deposits of IgA1 only. The reason for the preferential elevation of IgA1 is not clear.

Table 39–2. The laboratory evaluation in Henoch-Schönlein purpura (HSP).

Test	Typical Result
Complete blood cell count, with differential	Mild to moderate leukocytosis common, but otherwise the complete blood count is usually normal.
Electrolytes	Hyperkalemia in the setting of advanced renal dysfunction.
Liver function tests	Hypoalbuminemia can occur with nephrotic proteinuria. Otherwise, the liver function tests are normal.
Urinalysis with microscopy	Hematuria (ranging from mild to too numerous to count red blood cells). Red blood cell casts. Proteinuria (nephrotic range proteinuria in a small minority).
Erythrocyte sedimentation rate/ C-reactive protein	Modestly elevated acute phase reactants may be observed. Approximately one-third of patients have abnormal erythrocyte sedimentation rates.
Serum IgA level	60% of patients have an elevated serum IgA. Although there are two subclasses of IgA, HSP is associated with increases only in IgA1.
ANA	Negative
Rheumatoid factor	Negative
C3, C4	Even though immune complexes containing IgA are essential to the pathophysiology of HSP, serum complement levels are usually normal.
ANCA	Negative (both IgG and IgA ANCA)
Cryoglobulins	Negative

ANA, antinuclear antibody; ANCA, antineutrophil cytoplasmic antibody.

C. Imaging Studies

Chest radiography should be performed to rule out pulmonary lesions. The presence of pulmonary involvement, unusual in HSP, raises the possibility of other diagnoses that may require other treatment approaches (see Differential Diagnosis).

D. Special Tests

Direct immunofluorescence studies of skin biopsies can only be performed on fresh samples, and therefore must be planned at the time the biopsy is performed. The usual procedure is to biopsy one skin lesion for hematoxylin and eosin staining and another for immunofluorescence. Alternatively, a single biopsy sample can be split into different portions for the two types of studies.

▶ Differential Diagnosis

The differential diagnosis of HSP is shown in Table 39–3. HSP must be distinguished from other small-vessel vasculitides, from autoimmune inflammatory conditions associated with joint disease and rashes, and from infections. Other disorders may be associated occasionally with mild IgA deposition in blood vessels, but the process is rarely so florid as with HSP. IgA nephropathy is pathologically indistinguishable from the renal disease associated with HSP (including the preferential deposition of IgA1), but it has a typically chronic course and is not associated with disease in other organ systems.

A particularly crucial distinction is between HSP and the ANCA–associated conditions, primarily granulomatosis with polyangiitis (formerly Wegener granulomatosis) and microscopic polyangiitis. (Churg-Strauss disease may be distinguished more readily by the presence of eosinophilia.) The ANCA-associated vasculitides often present with purpura, migratory arthritis, and renal inflammation but, in contrast to HSP, do not typically have self-limited courses. Organ manifestations that are atypical for HSP, such as pulmonary involvement, symptoms or signs compatible with vasculitic neuropathy, or inflammatory eye disease, should broaden the differential diagnosis. Misdiagnoses of HSP because of failure to perform direct immunofluorescence testing on skin biopsies and ANCA assays on serum can lead to poor outcomes.

▶ Treatment

Nonsteroidal anti-inflammatory drugs may alleviate arthralgias but can aggravate gastrointestinal symptoms and should be avoided in any patient with renal disease. Dapsone (100 mg/d) may be effective in cases of HSP, perhaps through interference with the interactions of IgA and neutrophils. Although glucocorticoids have not been evaluated rigorously in HSP, they appear to ameliorate joint and gastrointestinal symptoms. Glucocorticoids do not appear to improve the rash, however, and their effectiveness in renal disease is controversial. Uncontrolled trials suggest that high-dose methylprednisolone followed by oral prednisone or high-dose prednisone combined with azathioprine or cyclophosphamide may help patients with severe nephritis (ie, nephrotic syndrome and >50% crescents).

▶ Complications

In most cases, HSP follows a self-limited course, resolves without substantial morbidity, and does not recur. The vast majority of cases resolve within 6–8 weeks. Recurrences, found in 33% of patients, usually develop within the first few months after resolution of the first bout. Even when associated with small ulcerations, the cutaneous lesions are usually so superficial that they heal without scarring. A small percentage of patients have progressive renal disease and long-term follow-up of all patients with severe renal symptoms at onset is needed.

Table 39–3. Differential diagnosis of Henoch-Schönlein purpura.

Other Vasculitides
Hypersensitivity vasculitis
Microscopic polyangiitis
Eosinophilic granulomatosis with polyangiitis
(Churg-Strauss syndrome)
Granulomatosis with polyangiitis
(formerly Wegener granulomatosis)
Mixed cryoglobulinemia
Polyarteritis nodosa
Systemic autoimmune conditions
Systemic lupus erythematosus
Rheumatoid arthritis
Renal disorders
IgA nephropathy
Infections
Acute viral or bacterial infections
Malignancies
Childhood leukemias
Miscellaneous
Acute hemorrhagic edema of infancy

Jauhola O, Ronkainen J, Koskimies O, et al. Renal manifestations of Henoch-Schönlein purpura in a 6-month prospective study of 223 children. *Arch Dis Child*. 2010;95:877. [PMID: 20852275]

Pillebout E, Alberti C, Guillevin L, Ouslimani A, Thervet E; CESAR study group. Addition of cyclophosphamide to steroids provides no benefit compared with steroids alone in treating adult patients with severe Henoch-Schönlein Purpura. *Kidney Int*. 2010;78:495. [PMID: 20505654]

Saulsbury FT. Henoch-Schönlein purpura. *Curr Opin Rheumatol*. 2010;22:598. [PMID: 20473173]

[The Johns Hopkins Vasculitis Center] http://vasculitis.med.jhu.edu

Vasculitis of the Central Nervous System

40

David B. Hellmann, MD, MACP

Central nervous system (CNS) vasculitis is not a single disease but a collection of conditions that cause inflammatory damage of blood vessels in the brain and spinal cord. About half of the cases have no known cause and are therefore classified as **primary** vasculitis of the CNS. The other half of the cases arise in the setting of some other disorder, often a rheumatic disease such as systemic lupus erythematosus, and are classified as **secondary** forms of CNS vasculitis. Primary vasculitis of the CNS has been referred to by many names. Bowing to tradition, this chapter will use the term "primary angiitis of the CNS" (PACNS).

CNS vasculitis presents a two-handed clinical challenge. On the one hand, clinicians need to recognize and treat those rare patients whose strokes and other neurologic deficits result from CNS vasculitis. On the other hand, clinicians need to avoid overdiagnosis of CNS vasculitis and must realize that the angiographic and magnetic resonance imaging (MRI) abnormalities observed in CNS vasculitis can be mimicked by infection, tumor, and other conditions.

ESSENTIALS OF DIAGNOSIS

- Common presentation includes headache, encephalopathy, and multiple strokes.
- Brain MRI sensitive but not specific.
- Most patients in whom PACNS is suspected have some other disorder.
- Angiographic abnormalities are suggestive but not specific.
- Definitive diagnosis requires brain biopsy.

General Considerations

PACNS is a disease of unknown cause characterized by vasculitis limited to the brain and spinal cord. PACNS is rare; at large medical centers, PACNS constitutes only about 1% of all cases of systemic vasculitis. The annual incidence is 2.4 cases per 1,000,000 person-years. Evidence suggests that PACNS is not one disease. Indeed, the clinical picture of PACNS that emerges from reviewing the literature depends a great deal on whether the analysis focuses on biopsy-proven cases (BP-PACNS) or cases defined by angiography (AD-PACNS) without biopsy proof. Some clinicians have speculated that AD-PACNS may be caused by spasm rather than by inflammation. The term "benign angiography of the CNS" or reversible cerebral vasoconstriction syndrome is sometimes applied to cases of AD-PACNS. Table 40–1 outlines the clinical pictures of both BP-PACNS and AD-PACNS.

Clinical Findings

A. Symptoms and Signs

The average age of onset in one study of 101 patients with BP-PACNS or AD-PACNS was 47 years (range 17–84). BP-PACNS chiefly affects middle-aged men. The initial presentation is typically headache and encephalopathy, and multifocal strokes develop later. BP-PACNS usually develops insidiously, unfolding with additive neurologic deficits over weeks or months before the diagnosis is suspected. Strokes in the absence of diffuse cortical dysfunction would be most unusual for BP-PACNS. However, the presentation of BP-PACNS is highly variable. Some patients may appear to have had one stroke, but PACNS is suspected after an MRI reveals multiple strokes of varying age. In other patients, headache may be the dominating feature. In some patients who have headache and what appear to be mass lesions on MRI, a brain tumor is suspected. Diffuse cortical dysfunction can manifest as either a decline in cognitive ability or an alteration in consciousness. The English teacher who can no longer spell accurately or the bank teller who cannot count change exemplifies how cognitive changes from diffuse cortical dysfunction may present. Seizure and brainstem or cranial

Table 40–1. Clinical and laboratory features of PACNS based on the method of diagnosis.[a]

Feature	BP-PACNS	AD-PACNS	P Value
Sex, no. (%)			
Males	78 (69.0)	17 (30.8)	<.001
Females	38 (31.0)	38 (69.1)	<.001
Age, mean ± SD	46 ± 17	33 ± 14	
Headache, no. (%)			
Yes	63 (55.8)	43 (78.2)	
No	50 (44.3)	12 (21.8)	
Stroke, no. (%)			
Yes	83 (86.5)	15 (32.6)	
No	13 (13.5)	31 (67.4)	<.008
Seizure, no. (%)			
Yes	29 (30.2)	11 (23.9)	
No	67 (69.8)	35 (76.1)	
Cerebral hemorrhage, no. (%)			
Yes	13 (11.5)	5 (9.1)	
No	100 (88.5)	50 (90.9)	
Diffuse neurologic dysfunction, no. (%)			
Yes	77 (68.1)	26 (47.3)	
No	36 (31.9)	29 (52.7)	<.009
Decreased cognition, no. (%)			
Yes	64 (83.1)	20 (76.9)	
No	13 (16.9)	6 (23.1)	
Days from symptom onset to diagnosis, mean ± SD	170 ± 261	46 ± 73	<.001
Abnormal CSF/total tested (%)	90	50	<.005

[a]An abnormal cerebrospinal fluid (CSF) sample had >5 cells/mcL or protein >55 mg/dL or both.
AD-PACNS, angiographically-defined PACNS; BP-PACNS, biopsy-proven PACNS; PACNS, primary angiitis of the central nervous system. Used, with permission, from Calabrese LH, Duna GF, Lie JT. Vasculitis in the central nervous system. *Arthritis Rheum.* 1997;40:1189.

nerve dysfunction develops in approximately one third of patients. Spinal cord involvement occurs less commonly. Isolated dementia is a very rare presentation of BP-PACNS. It is a common misconception that BPPACNS is associated with systemic symptoms such as fever, weight loss, or sweats. In reality, such symptoms develop in less than 10% of cases.

The clinical picture of AD-PACNS, also designated in some series as reversible cerebral vasoconstriction syndrome, differs in several important ways. AD-PACNS preferentially affects women four times more commonly than men. The average age of onset is 40, the onset is sudden, and the most prominent presenting symptom is a severe headache. Focal findings of seizure or stroke develop in approximately 60% of patients (see Table 40–1). Diffuse cortical abnormalities

develop less commonly. In AD-PACNS, as in BP-PACNS, systemic symptoms and signs are usually absent. As will be discussed in greater detail below, AD-PACNS patients also differ from BP-PACNS patients by having fewer cerebrospinal fluid abnormalities and responding to relatively short courses of glucocorticoids.

B. Laboratory Findings

In BP-PACNS, about one fifth of the patients have anemia (usually mild), one half have an elevated white blood cell count, and two thirds have an elevated erythrocyte sedimentation rate. The hematocrit and erythrocyte sedimentation rate are less frequently abnormal in AD-PACNS cases. The cerebrospinal fluid (CSF) is abnormal in nearly 90% of BP-PACNS cases and in about 50% of AD-PACNS cases. The most common abnormalities are an elevated CSF protein (with a mean of 177 mg/dL and a median of 100 mg/dL) and a CSF lymphocytosis (with a mean of 77 cells/mcL). A CSF cell count exceeding 250/mcL rarely occurs in PACNS. In AD-PACNS, the CSF abnormalities are typically very mild. CSF protein levels are usually below 60 mg/dL and the CSF white blood cell count is usually less than 10 cells/mcL. In one study of 48 patients with AD-PACNS, the median leukocyte count in the CSF was only 4 cells/mcL, and the medial total CSF protein was 54 mg/dL. Less than 10% of AD-PACNS patients have CSF with a protein >70 mg/dL or a white blood count >10/mcL.

C. Imaging Studies

MRI is the most sensitive imaging method for detecting PACNS, being abnormal in approximately 90% of cases. However, the abnormalities are not specific for vasculitis. On average, patients with PACNS have multiple lesions that are predominantly bilateral and supratentorial. The most commonly affected areas are the subcortical white matter, the deep gray matter, the deep white matter, and the cortex. The lesions appear most commonly as infarcts but can also appear as mass lesions or areas of signal change. Hemorrhagic lesions develop in approximately 15% of cases. Gadolinium enhancing lesions are present in approximately one third of patients; prominent gadolinium enhancement of the meninges is found in about 10%. MRI angiograms are normal in the vast majority of cases. Even though PACNS is classified as a vasculitis of medium-sized vessels, MRI angiography lacks the resolution to detect the size of arteries usually affected by PACNS.

Computed tomography of the brain is much less sensitive in PACNS, detecting abnormalities in only about two thirds of the cases. However, computed tomography is more sensitive than MRI at detecting hemorrhagic lesions.

Traditional angiography is abnormal in 50–90% of patients with PACNS. The classic finding in PACNS of "beading" of the small arteries (intracranial arteries, second division branches or smaller) is caused by dilations interspersed with normal areas of artery (Figure 40–1). Slow flow,

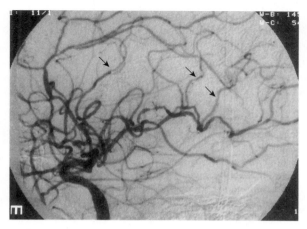

▲ **Figure 40–1.** Angiogram of intracranial arteries showing segmental narrowing typical of central nervous system vasculitis.

threadlike thinning of arteries, and occlusion are other angiographic (albeit nonspecific) abnormalities found in PACNS. Microaneurysms occur much less commonly in PACNS than in polyarteritis nodosa. The small branches of the middle anterior arteries and the posterior cerebral arteries are the most commonly affected. Angiographic abnormalities of large (intracranial internal carotid artery and proximal anterior, middle, and posterior cerebral) arteries occur less frequently. Angiographic abnormalities are usually bilateral and more widespread than the MRI lesions. None of the angiographic abnormalities are absolutely specific for PACNS. In patients in whom CNS vasculitis is suspected, angiography carries an 11.8% risk of transient neurologic deficit and a 0.8% risk of permanent stroke.

The role of positron emission tomography scanning in PACNS has not been defined.

D. Special Tests

Brain biopsy, which is required for definitive diagnosis of PACNS, carries a risk of serious morbidity of 0–2% and is diagnostic in only 50–70% of cases. The highest yield is obtained from biopsies that target an imaging abnormality and that include the leptomeninges. Biopsies should be processed for histologic examination and cultures and should be stained for bacteria, fungi, and viruses. PACNS affects chiefly small- and medium-sized arteries and arterioles of the brain and spinal cord. Histopathologic findings of positive biopsies vary. In some series, infiltration with lymphocytes is most common, but in other series, granulomatous inflammation is more frequently found. Acute necrotizing vasculitis occurs in about 15%. Thrombosis and rupture can lead to infarction and hemorrhage of the surrounding tissue.

E. Evaluation

Most patients in whom CNS vasculitis is suspected need to undergo a battery of tests. Since MRI is the most sensitive noninvasive imaging method overall, it is preferred over computed tomography unless hemorrhage is a concern. After MRI has excluded mass lesion, the patient should undergo lumbar puncture. The CSF analysis can help support the diagnosis of CNS vasculitis, as noted above, and can help exclude the many infections and tumors that can mimic CNS vasculitis (see below). Angiograms can be done to exclude other causes of the patient's symptoms and to add support to the diagnosis of vasculitis. However, repeated studies have emphasized that the classic beading pattern of angiographic changes is not specific for vasculitis. Indeed, in one series of 35 patients who had undergone angiography and leptomeningeal biopsy, none of the patients whose angiogram was considered positive for vasculitis had a brain biopsy positive for vasculitis. Conversely, the only patients with brain biopsies positive for vasculitis did not have classic angiographic changes. Whether all patients in whom PACNS is suspected should undergo brain biopsy is controversial. Few centers have a large experience with either PACNS or brain biopsy. It is reasonable to recommend brain biopsy for those who have a slow onset, severe neurologic impairment, and striking CSF abnormalities, or for others who have not responded to glucocorticoid therapy. Other laboratory evaluations depend on the patient's presentation and differential diagnosis (see below).

▶ Diagnostic Criteria

A definite diagnosis of PACNS requires the following:

1. Symptoms and signs of an acquired neurologic deficit consistent with the diagnosis of PACNS (eg, headache, confusion, and multiple strokes).

2. No evidence of a systemic vasculitis or another disorder that could cause the clinical picture, despite a thorough investigation.

3. A brain or spinal cord biopsy demonstrating vasculitis in the absence of infection.

The diagnosis of PACNS should be regarded as *possible* if, in the absence of a positive biopsy, the patient meets the first two criteria and has an angiogram with classic changes of vasculitis in multiple intracranial vessels.

▶ Differential Diagnosis

Since most patients in whom CNS vasculitis is suspected have some other disorder, the differential diagnosis should be reviewed meticulously (Table 40–2). Among the rheumatic diseases, systemic lupus erythematosus, polyarteritis nodosa, and granulomatosis with polyangiitis (formerly Wegener granulomatosis) are the disorders that most often

Table 40–2. Differential diagnosis of primary angiitis of the central nervous system.

Category	Examples
Rheumatic disorders	Systemic lupus erythematosus, granulomatosis with polyangiitis (formerly Wegener granulomatosis), polyarteritis nodosa, Takayasu arteritis, temporal arteritis, Behçet disease, Sjögren syndrome, Cogan syndrome
Infections	Bacteria (eg, endocarditis, bacterial meningitis, tuberculosis, syphilis, Lyme disease) Fungi (eg, histoplasmosis, *Aspergillus*) Viruses (eg, herpes zoster, HIV, hepatitis C)
Drugs	Cocaine, ephedrine, amphetamine, allopurinol, phenylpropanolamine, heroin
Vasculopathies	Atherosclerosis, antiphospholipid antibody syndrome, cerebral amyloid angiopathy, moya moya, radiation-induced vasculopathy, vasospasm associated with severe hypertension or hemorrhage, arterial fibromuscular dysplasia, cardiac myxoma, embolism, cholesterol embolism, pregnancy- and postpartum-associated vasculopathy, sickle cell anemia, thrombotic thrombocytopenic purpura, Susac syndrome
Malignancy	Vascular lymphoma, Hodgkin disease, small-cell lung cancer
Heritable disorders	Cerebral autosomal dominant arteriopathy with subcortical infarcts and leukoencephalopathy (CADASIL)
Other inflammatory disorders	Sarcoidosis, inflammatory bowel disease, celiac disease
Metabolic disorders	Pheochromocytoma

Compiled from Lie, JT. Vasculitis and the nervous system: classification and histopathologic spectrum of central nervous system vasculitis. *Neurol Clin.* 1997;15(4):805–819; Razavi M, Bendixen B, Maley JE, et al. CNS pseudovasculitis in a patient with pheochromocytoma. *Neurology.* 1999;52(5):1088–1090; Williamson EE, Chukwudelunzu, FE, Meschia JF, et al. The importance of family history. Distinguishing primary antiitis of the central nervous system from cerebral autosomal dominant arteriopathy with subcortical infarcts and leukoencephalopathy. *Arthritis Rheum.* 1999;42(10):2243–2248; Younger DS, Calabrese, LH, Hays AP: Granulomatous angiitis of the nervous system. *Neurol Clin.* 1997;15(4):821–834; Calabrese LH, Duna GF, Lie JT. Vasculitis in th ecentral nervous system. *Arthritis & Rheum.* 1997;40(7):1189–1201; Calabrese LH & Mallek JA. Primary angiitis of the central nervous system. Report of 8 new cases, review of the literature and proposal for diagnostic criteria. *Medicine.* 1987;67(1):20–39.

cause secondary CNS vasculitis. Rarely, however, are these conditions confused with PACNS. Almost all patients with those conditions have other organs involved (eg, skin in systemic lupus erythematosus) and have other characteristic laboratory abnormalities (eg, positive antineutrophil cytoplasmic antibodies in granulomatosis with polyangiitis [formerly Wegener granulomatosis]).

Infection can be more difficult to distinguish from PACNS. HIV, herpes zoster virus, syphilis, and histoplasmosis are among the infections that can closely mimic PACNS. Most patients affected are immunosuppressed by HIV, alcoholism, or cancer chemotherapy. Many of the infections, especially fungi, preferentially affect the base of the brain. Infection should also be considered whenever the number of cells in the CSF exceeds 250/mcL.

The possibility of herpes zoster virus–related vasculitis should be considered in a person who is immunosuppressed or who has had shingles in a V_1 distribution in the last few weeks. Angiographic abnormalities seen with infection can perfectly mimic the changes seen with PACNS. Because of the difficulty of recognizing when infection is causing vasculitis, CSF and brain biopsies should be cultured and stained for infection. Blood cultures, HIV testing, and CSF Venereal Disease Research Laboratory tests should also be routinely performed when evaluating a patient for PACNS. Special tests (eg, polymerase chain reaction assay) for other infections may be warranted if the patient is immunosuppressed.

Cocaine, amphetamines, and ephedrine derivatives are the drugs that most commonly produce CNS vasculopathy. There is some evidence that these drugs can produce vasculitis itself and not just a vasculopathy that imitates PACNS. Most patients with cocaine-induced vasculitis are men in their 20s. However, profiling for PACNS is an inexact science, so detailed drug histories and toxicology screens should be used routinely.

Atherosclerosis should always be considered because it is so common, especially if the patient is over the age of 50 and has hypertension, hypercholesterolemia, or diabetes mellitus. No angiogram should be interpreted as showing vasculitis if atherosclerosis is evident in the carotid siphon or other vessels. Cerebral amyloid should be considered if the patient is over the age of 65 and has cerebral hemorrhages. Other conditions that can resemble PACNS are listed in Table 40–2.

▶ **Treatment**

Patients with BP-PACNS should be treated with glucocorticoids. The role of immunosuppressive drugs such as cyclophosphamide is not yet established. Patients who have declined rapidly should be given methylprednisolone 1000 mg intravenously daily for 3–5 days, followed by prednisone (or equivalent) 1 mg/kg/d. Patients who have not progressed rapidly can begin treatment with prednisone. The rarity of PACNS means that no large, detailed studies are available to guide tapering. Prednisone should not be reduced until the patient has stabilized and after all manifestations of inflammation (erythrocyte sedimentation rate, hematocrit, and CSF abnormalities) have resolved. Typically, this takes a month. Thereafter, prednisone can be tapered by 10% every 1–2 weeks until 20 mg is reached, at which time the reduction schedule is slowed further. New symptoms or signs or new imaging abnormalities require an increase in prednisone dose. Cyclophosphamide or other immunosuppressive drugs should be considered if the patient has severe deficits or if the disease progresses despite glucocorticoid therapy.

Treatment of AD-PACNS is also not well defined. However, studies suggest that some cases result more from spasm of the arteries (and called reversible cerebral vasoconstriction syndrome) than from true inflammation. Spasm appears to be especially likely in young women who have an abrupt onset of headache and focal deficits and who have no or minimal abnormalities of the CSF. There is growing evidence that these patients infrequently require immunosuppressive drugs. Some experts advocate treating these cases with a calcium channel blocker such as verapamil (to reduce spasm) and prednisone (1 mg/kg/d). Following resolution of the acute illness, the prednisone is tapered over 6–12 weeks. Failure to demonstrate substantial angiographic improvement should cast doubt on spasm as a major component and should suggest true vasculitis that requires a slower tapering of prednisone. All patients with PACNS should be instructed to avoid drugs that cause vasoconstriction or thrombosis (such as birth control pills, ephedrine, nicotine, and cocaine). All patients who take prednisone for more than 2 months should be evaluated and treated to minimize the risks of osteoporosis.

▶ Prognosis

In the absence of treatment, almost all patients with BP-PACNS die of progressive neurologic deficits. Treatment has reduced mortality in the first year to 5%. The prognosis of AD-PACNS appears to be better. More than 90% of patients in whom spasm is suspected will recover. In a series of 101 patients with a mixture of BP-PACNS and AD-PACNS, approximately one quarter of patients relapsed. Relapse rates were higher in patients whose disease involved large arteries. In this series, mortality was higher than that expected for age- and sex-matched controls. Five-year survival was about 75%, and 10-year survival was 60%. Large-vessel involvement, focal neurologic deficits, cognitive impairment, and cerebral infarction conferred a higher risk of death. Conversely, patients with prominent gadolinium enhancing lesions or meninges had a better prognosis.

Birnbaum J, Hellmann DB. Primary angiitis of the central nervous system. *Arch Neurol.* 2009;66:704. [PMID: 19506130]

Hajj-Ali RA, Singhal AB, Benseler S, Molloy E, Calabrese LH. Primary angiitis of the CNS. *Lancet Neurol.* 2011;10:561. [PMID: 21601163]

Miller DV, Salvarani C, Hunder GG, et al. Biopsy findings in primary angiitis of the central nervous system. *Am J Surg Pathol.* 2009;33:35. [PMID: 18941399]

Salvarani C, Brown RD Jr, Calamia KT, et al. Angiography-negative primary central nervous system vasculitis: a syndrome involving small cerebral vessels. *Medicine (Baltimore).* 2008;87:264. [PMID: 18794709]

Salvarani C, Brown RD Jr, Calamia KT, et al. Primary central nervous system vasculitis: analysis of 101 patients. *Ann Neurol.* 2007;62:442. [PMID: 17924545]

Salvarani C, Brown RD Jr, Calamia KT, et al. Primary central nervous system vasculitis with prominent leptomeningeal enhancement: a subset with a benign outcome. *Arthritis Rheum.* 2008;58:595. [PMID: 18240248]

[The Johns Hopkins Vasculitis Center]
http://vasculitis.med.jhu.edu

[The Vasculitis Foundation]
http://www.vasculitisfoundation.org/

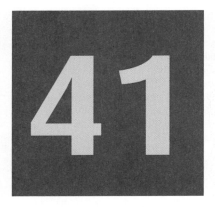

Buerger Disease

John H. Stone, MD, MPH

ESSENTIALS OF DIAGNOSIS

▶ Active tobacco use, typically moderate to heavy.

▶ Severe digital ischemia without evidence of internal organ involvement.

▶ Angiography reveals segmental involvement of medium-sized arteries, with abrupt vascular cut-offs and corkscrew collaterals.

▶ The major vessel involvement occurs at the levels of the ankle and wrist.

▶ General Considerations

In Buerger disease, also called thromboangiitis obliterans, the classic patient is a young male smoker. The mean age of onset is approximately 40 years, but the disease can occur in teenagers as well as in the elderly. Although the patients described initially were men, the disease may afflict women as well, probably in direct proportion to the number of women in any particular society who smoke. The precise mechanism underlying the relationship between Buerger disease and cigarette smoking is unknown; autoimmune reactions to constituents of tobacco have been postulated. Cases may present several years after the start of smoking, but Buerger disease does not occur in the absence of ongoing tobacco exposure.

There are four keys to the diagnosis of Buerger disease: (1) Recognition of clinical findings compatible with that condition; namely, digital ischemia without involvement of other organs. (2) Identification of the typical pattern of vascular involvement by angiography. (3) Exclusion of diseases that may mimic Buerger disease (Table 41–1). (4) Confirmation that the major risk factor, ongoing tobacco exposure, is present.

Because of difficulty in accessing medium-sized vessels for biopsy, the diagnosis is rarely confirmed by biopsy. The

exceptions to this rule are superficial thrombophlebitis, which seldom comes to medical attention, and amputation specimens, by which time medical attention is (at least in some senses) too late. When biopsy is possible, acute Buerger disease is characterized by a highly inflammatory thrombus, composed of a variety of cell types: lymphocytes, neutrophils, giant cells, and occasional microabscesses. Inflammation is typically more intense within the clot itself than within the walls of affected blood vessels. Fibrinoid necrosis, a hallmark of most systemic vasculitides, is absent in Buerger disease.

▶ Clinical Findings

A. Symptoms and Signs

1. Extremities—A major hallmark of Buerger disease is its confinement to the extremities. The initial symptoms may be nonspecific pains in the calf, foot, or toes. The progression of thrombosis and vasculitis can lead to horrific pain in the digits and limbs and ultimately to gangrene and tissue loss, through either autoamputation or elective amputation. For unknown reasons, however, other vascular beds (eg, the cardiac, pulmonary, renal, and mesenteric vasculature) are nearly always spared in Buerger disease.

Although Buerger disease has a predilection for the feet and toes, the hands and fingers may also be affected prominently. More than 60% of patients have abnormal Allen tests, indicating compromise of circulation to the hand; many demonstrate obliterations of the radial or ulnar artery pulses on physical examination. In contrast to atherosclerosis, which is a disease of the proximal vasculature, Buerger disease is characterized by inflammation and thrombosis of medium-sized, distal blood vessels (both arteries and veins), most intense at the levels of the ankles and wrists.

2. Skin—The earliest lesion may be a superficial thrombophlebitis. This complaint is often disregarded by the patient or misdiagnosed as deep varicosities. Histologic examination of

Table 41–1. Differential diagnosis of Buerger disease.

Cardiovascular conditions
  Atherosclerosis
  Cardiogenic emboli (eg, infective endocarditis)
Systemic disorders associated with autoimmunity
  Systemic lupus erythematosus
  Antiphospholipid antibody syndrome
  Systemic sclerosis (particularly limited scleroderma,
    or CREST syndrome)
  Mixed connective tissue disease
Systemic vasculitides
  Rheumatoid vasculitis
  Polyarteritis nodosa
  Granulomatosis with polyangiitis (formerly Wegener granulomatosis)
  Microscopic polyangiitis
  Eosinophilic granulomatosis with polyangiitis (Churg-Strauss syndrome)
  Cryoglobulinemia
Miscellaneous
  Paraproteinemia
  Ergotism

CREST, calcinosis, Raynaud phenomenon, esophageal motility, sclerodactyly, and telangiectasias.

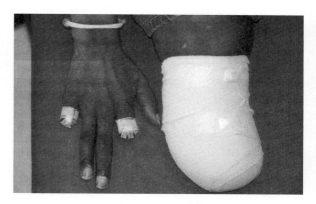

▲ **Figure 41–2.** As a consequence of failure to stop smoking, this patient required multiple amputations, including fingers on both hands and bilateral below-the-knee amputations.

these lesions reveals an acute thrombophlebitis with marked perivascular infiltration. This herald lesion is then followed by progressive occlusion of the deeper veins and arteries, leading the patient to seek medical attention. Patients with Buerger disease may have splinter hemorrhages, arousing suspicions of infective endocarditis. Most cutaneous features of disease are those of a process involving the medium-sized vessels exclusively (purpura, for example, a manifestation of small-vessel disease, is absent).

Gangrene occurs in the most distal tissues, ie, the toes and fingers, first (Figure 41–1). If the process remains undiagnosed or if the patient continues to smoke even after the diagnosis, larger portions of the extremities become compromised. In advanced cases, the major arterial supplies to the hands and feet may become occluded, leading to coolness and pain of the entire distal extremity, necessitating amputation (Figure 41–2).

3. Peripheral nerve—Early in the disease, nonspecific pains in the calf, foot, or toes may recall a primary neuropathic process. These sensory symptoms may result from thickening of the tissues immediately surrounding the veins and arteries, leading to connective tissue proliferation around the nerve bundles that are intimately connected with the vasculature. True vasculitic neuropathy, however, does not occur in Buerger disease.

4. Gastrointestinal tract and other organs—Extremely rare cases of Buerger disease involving the gastrointestinal tract and central nervous system have been reported.

B. Laboratory Findings

There is no single diagnostic test for Buerger disease. The demonstration of "corkscrew collaterals" (Figure 41–3) on angiography is highly characteristic but not pathognomonic. Such vessels may also be observed in polyarteritis nodosa and other forms of medium-vessel vasculitis. Laboratory and radiologic investigations are important in Buerger disease, both to identify the typical vascular lesions and to exclude conditions that require other approaches to management. Table 41–2 lists the results of routine laboratory tests and specialized assays that are done to rule out disorders masquerading as Buerger disease.

The erythrocyte sedimentation rate and C-reactive protein levels are generally lower than observed in many other types of diffuse systemic vasculitis, but most patients have at least moderate elevations of these acute phase reactants. Routine hematology, serum chemistry, and urinalysis studies are normal in Buerger disease; abnormalities in these tests suggest other diagnoses. Markers of hypercoagulable states

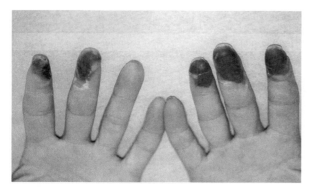

▲ **Figure 41–1.** Digital ischemia with gangrene in Buerger disease.

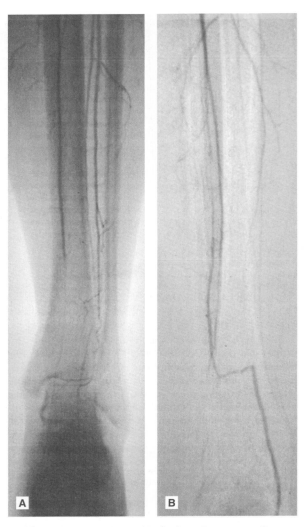

▲ **Figure 41–3.** Angiographic findings in Buerger disease. **A:** Attenuation of the anterior tibial artery in the mid-calf. This artery forms a collateral at the site of occlusion with the peroneal artery. The posterior tibial artery is occluded superiorly. **B:** Abrupt arterial cut-offs several centimeters above the ankle, with minimal blood flow distal to the cut-offs.

Table 41–2. Laboratory and radiologic evaluation in possible Buerger disease.

Test	Typical Results
Complete blood cell count	Normal. Mild elevations of the white blood cell and platelet count would not be unexpected.
Renal and hepatic function	Normal
Urinalysis with microscopy	Normal
Erythrocyte sedimentation rate (ESR)/C-reactive protein	Mild to moderate elevations in patients with severe digital ischemia. Dramatically elevated acute phase reactants (eg, an ESR >100 mm/h) unusual.
ANA	Negative
Rheumatoid factor	Negative
C3, C4	Normal
ANCA	Negative
Hepatitis B and C serologies	Negative
Antiphospholipid antibodies	Negative rapid plasma reagin and anticardiolipin antibody assays. Normal Russell viper venom time (for lupus anticoagulant).
Blood cultures	Negative
Echocardiography (or TEE)	No cardiac valvular vegetations. Normal aortic root.
Angiography	Corkscrew collaterals (see Figure 41–3). Abrupt cutoffs of medium-sized arteries at levels of the ankles and wrists, and often higher. Segmental areas of involvement, with diseased regions interspersed with normal-appearing arterial stretches.

ANA, antinuclear antibody; ANCA, antineutrophil cytoplasmic antibody; TEE, transesophageal echocardiography.

that may be associated with widespread arterial thromboses, eg, antiphospholipid antibodies, should be investigated.

C. Imaging Studies

Echocardiography (possibly including a transesophageal study) should examine the heart valves and aortic root. Comprehensive angiographic studies that define the vasculature of the extremities, proximal aorta, gastrointestinal tract, and renal arteries should be considered. Such studies are critical in identifying vascular involvement typical of Buerger disease and excluding atheroembolic sources as well as findings more typical of other vasculitides (eg, microaneurysms). The arterial involvement in Buerger disease is highly segmental, with abrupt vascular occlusions interspersed with regions of vessels that appear angiographically normal (Figure 41–3). In advanced cases, the thready appearance of vessels distal to the wrists and ankles may resemble a disorganized spider web. The most commonly involved vessels are the digital arteries of the fingers and toes as well as the palmar, plantar, tibial, peroneal, radial, and ulnar vessels.

▶ Differential Diagnosis

The major conditions in the differential diagnosis of Buerger disease are cardiovascular diseases, autoimmune disorders, and systemic vasculitides (see Table 41–1). Among the cardiovascular diseases, atherosclerosis and cardiogenic emboli are the principal considerations. Echocardiography (including transesophageal echocardiography) and angiography may be helpful in distinguishing Buerger disease from cardiovascular conditions. Careful imaging of the proximal aorta is essential. In contrast to Buerger disease, atherosclerotic disease characteristically affects the proximal vessels. Sources of cardiogenic emboli must be excluded by echocardiography and blood cultures.

Among the autoimmune disorders, systemic lupus erythematosus, the antiphospholipid syndrome, systemic sclerosis, and mixed connective tissue disease all may present with digital ischemia. Limited scleroderma (the CREST [calcinosis, Raynaud phenomenon, esophageal dysmotility, sclerodactyly, telangiectasias] syndrome; see Chapter 25) may pose special diagnostic challenges because of its propensity to cause digital loss, particularly when associated with anticentromere antibodies. Careful examination of the vasculature in the nailbeds, where dilated capillary loops appear in systemic sclerosis and other connective tissue disorders, may help distinguish these conditions from Buerger disease. Buerger disease, in contrast to connective tissue diseases, is not associated with a significant autoantibody response.

The systemic vasculitides commonly associated with distal ischemia and gangrene are rheumatoid vasculitis, polyarteritis nodosa, granulomatosis with polyangiitis (formerly Wegener granulomatosis), microscopic polyangiitis, eosinophilic granulomatosis with polyangiitis (Churg-Strauss syndrome), and cryoglobulinemia. In general, the lack of visceral involvement in Buerger disease helps distinguish Buerger disease from other vasculitides. For example, ulcerations of the shins, calves, and malleolar regions are atypical of Buerger disease but common among other forms of vasculitis listed above. Vasculitic neuropathy, often striking in the other forms of systemic vasculitis, does not occur in Buerger disease.

▶ Treatment

The only effective intervention in Buerger disease is complete smoking cessation. Despite the similarities of Buerger disease to systemic vasculitides that affect medium-sized blood vessels and to hypercoagulable states, there is no role for immunosuppressive interventions or anticoagulation in this condition. Moreover, because of the obliterative nature of the vascular inflammatory and thrombotic processes, the vasculature distal to the lesions generally offers no blood vessels large enough to sustain bypass grafts. Thrombolysis, which has not been studied in substantial numbers of patients, carries with it significant risks and perhaps a low likelihood of success, given the length of thromboses present in Buerger disease. Effective pain control is important during periods of intense pain from digital ischemia (without it, patients may only smoke more).

A variety of investigational therapies have been used, with reports of mixed success.

▶ Complications

Without smoking cessation, Buerger disease progresses inexorably through an obliterative vascular process, leading to coolness of the digits, hands, and feet; paresthesias; symptoms of intermittent claudication; skin ulcerations over the fingers and toes; and gangrenous infarctions of the extremities. Once established, the disease may be maintained by even small exposures to tobacco. Failure to stop smoking is associated with a dramatic increase in the risk of limb loss by amputation. Associations with second-hand smoking and smokeless tobacco have been reported but not confirmed. The angiogram often looks far worse than the patient does: The extent of vascular obliteration may appear to offer little hope for limb preservation, but complete tobacco abstinence can be remarkably successful in saving limbs.

Buerger L. Landmark publication from the American Journal of the Medical Sciences, 'Thrombo-angiitis obliterans: a study of the vascular lesions leading to presenile spontaneous gangrene'. 1908. *Am J Med Sci.* 2009;337:274. [PMID: 19365174]

Piazza G, Creager MA. Thromboangiitis obliterans. *Circulation.* 2010;121:1858. [PMID: 20421527]

[The Johns Hopkins Vasculitis Center] http://vasculitis.med.jhu.edu

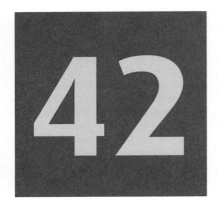

Miscellaneous Forms of Vasculitis

Philip Seo, MD, MHS
John H. Stone, MD, MPH

RHEUMATOID VASCULITIS

ESSENTIALS OF DIAGNOSIS

▶ Rheumatoid vasculitis usually occurs in patients with severe, long-standing, nodular, destructive rheumatoid arthritis, especially when the joint disease is "burnt out."

▶ Palpable purpura, cutaneous ulcers (particularly in the malleolar region), digital infarctions, and peripheral sensory neuropathy are common manifestations.

▶ Tissue biopsy helps establish the diagnosis of rheumatoid vasculitis. Nerve conduction studies can identify involved nerves for biopsy. Muscle biopsies should be performed simultaneously with nerve biopsies to increase the diagnostic yield of the procedure.

▶ General Considerations

Rheumatoid vasculitis (RV) is a medium-vessel vasculitis that occurs in patients with "burnt-out" but previously severe rheumatoid arthritis (RA). The typical patient has long-standing RA characterized by rheumatoid nodules, destructive joint disease, and high titers of rheumatoid factor. The diagnosis of RV should be considered in any patient with RA in whom new constitutional symptoms, skin ulcerations, serositis, digital ischemia, or symptoms of sensory or motor nerve dysfunction develop. RV resembles polyarteritis nodosa because it leads to multiorgan dysfunction in the skin, peripheral nerves, gastrointestinal tract, and other organs. Manifestations of RV, which resemble those of polyarteritis nodosa, include cutaneous ulcerations, digital ischemia, mononeuritis multiplex, and mesenteric vasculitis (see Chapter 35).

▶ Pathogenesis

Immune complex deposition and antibody-mediated destruction of endothelial cells both appear to contribute to RV. Certain HLA-DR4 alleles that predispose patients to severe RA may also heighten patients' susceptibility to RV. Cigarette smoking increases the risk of RV and has a synergistic interaction in this regard with antibodies to cyclic citrullinated peptides (anti-CCP antibodies). However, the inciting events leading to the development of RV among patients with previously destructive arthritis are not known. Factors in addition to vasculitis (eg, diabetes mellitus, atherosclerosis, and hypertension) likely play an important adjunctive role in promoting vascular occlusion, but the central issue in RV is necrotizing inflammation of blood vessels.

▶ Clinical Findings

A. Symptoms and Signs

1. Skin—Dermatologic findings, the most common manifestation of RV, may include palpable purpura, cutaneous ulcers (particularly in the malleolar region), and digital infarctions (Figure 42–1).

2. Nervous system—A peripheral sensory neuropathy is a common manifestation of RV. A mixed motor-sensory neuropathy or mononeuritis multiplex may also be seen. Central nervous system manifestations (such as strokes, seizures, and cranial nerve palsies) are considerably less common.

3. Eyes—Retinal vasculitis as a manifestation of RV is common but frequently asymptomatic. Necrotizing scleritis and peripheral ulcerative keratitis (Figure 42–2) pose threats to vision and require aggressive immunosuppressive therapy.

4. Serositis—Pericarditis and pleuritis may occur in association with RV. Other cardiopulmonary manifestations of RV are unusual.

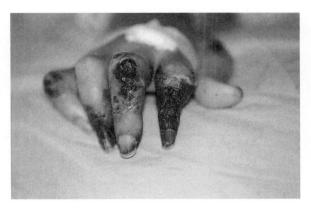

▲ **Figure 42–1.** Digital infarctions in rheumatoid vasculitis.

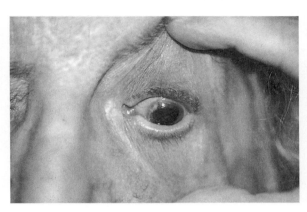

▲ **Figure 42–2.** Peripheral ulcerative keratitis in a patient with nodular, destructive rheumatoid arthritis and rheumatoid vasculitis.

B. Laboratory Findings

Most laboratory abnormalities in RV such as elevations in the erythrocyte sedimentation rate are nonspecific and merely reflect the presence of an inflammatory state. Hypocomplementemia, antinuclear antibodies (ANAs), atypical antineutrophil cytoplasmic antibodies (ANCAs) (by immunofluorescence testing but not enzyme immunoassay; see Chapter 32), and anti-endothelial cell antibodies are all detected more frequently in patients with RV than in those with RA alone. All of these tests, however, are nonspecific.

C. Imaging Studies

The presence of bony erosions is a risk factor for the development of RV, but plain radiographs and other imaging studies have no consistent role in the evaluation of this disorder.

D. Special Tests

Because the treatment implications for RV are so severe, the diagnosis must be established by tissue biopsy whenever possible. Deep skin biopsies (full-thickness biopsies that include some subcutaneous fat) taken from the edge of ulcers are very useful in detecting the presence of medium-vessel vasculitis. Nerve conduction studies help identify involved nerves for biopsy. Muscle biopsies (eg, of the gastrocnemius muscle) should be performed simultaneously with nerve biopsies.

▶ Differential Diagnosis

Patients with erosive RA are at increased risk for infections. When patients with RA seek medical attention for the new onset of nonspecific systemic complaints, the possibility of infection must be considered first. Cholesterol emboli may cause digital ischemia and a host of other signs and symptoms that mimic vasculitis. Diabetes mellitus is another major cause of mononeuritis multiplex, but multiple

mononeuropathies occurring over a short period of time are unusual in that condition. Many clinical features of RV mimic those of polyarteritis nodosa and other forms of necrotizing vasculitis.

▶ Treatment

Therapy must reflect the severity of organ involvement. Small, relatively painless infarctions around the nail bed develop in some patients with nodular RA (Figure 42–3). Such lesions, known as Bywaters lesions, do not herald the presence of a necrotizing vasculitis and require no adjustment in the patients' therapy. With other disease manifestations, however, such as cutaneous ulcers, vasculitic neuropathy, and inflammatory eye disease, glucocorticoids

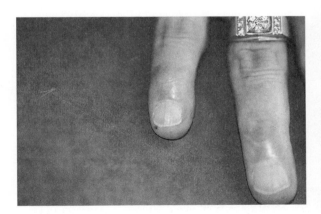

▲ **Figure 42–3.** Nail bed infarctions in a patient with rheumatoid arthritis. Such lesions do not necessarily herald the onset of rheumatoid vasculitis.

may be required. Glucocorticoids remain a cornerstone of therapy for RV but severe disease is treated generally with two agents, both for greater efficacy in controlling the vasculitis and for sparing of the potential adverse effects of high-dose glucocorticoids. Cyclophosphamide, used to treat many cases of RV, should be used with appropriate caution, given that many patients with RV suffer from substantial disabilities and the effects of previous immunosuppression at baseline. Tumor necrosis factor (TNF) inhibition and B cell depletion may both be effective strategies in RV and are likely safer than cyclophosphamide in most patients. For this reason, it is appropriate to use TNF inhibitors or rituximab before cyclophosphamide in patients who require more treatment than high-dose glucocorticoids alone.

▶ Prognosis

RV is a treatable condition but the development of this complication in patients who usually already have significant impairment is a poor prognostic indicator.

COGAN SYNDROME

ESSENTIALS OF DIAGNOSIS

► The hallmark of Cogan syndrome is the presence of ocular inflammation and audiovestibular dysfunction. These findings may be accompanied by evidence of a systemic vasculitis.

► Interstitial keratitis is the most common form of ocular involvement.

► Audiovestibular dysfunction may lead to the acute onset of vertigo, tinnitus, nausea, and vomiting.

► Vasculitis in Cogan syndrome may take the form of aortitis, renal artery stenosis, or occlusion of the great vessels.

▶ General Considerations

Cogan syndrome (CS), an immune-mediated condition that primarily affects young adults, is associated with ocular inflammation (usually interstitial keratitis) and audiovestibular dysfunction. This syndrome may be accompanied by a systemic vasculitis of large- and medium-sized arteries that may resemble Takayasu arteritis.

▶ Pathogenesis

The onset of CS is frequently preceded by an upper respiratory tract infection. Because many features of CS can be caused by known pathogens (eg, *Treponema pallidum*), CS may be the direct consequence of an unidentified pathogen

affecting the eyes, ears, and blood vessels. Alternatively, CS may be the indirect consequence of a pathogen that induces an immune response that continues to attack the host long after the pathogen has been eliminated (ie, molecular mimicry). Neither of these theories has been proved.

▶ Clinical Findings

A. Symptoms and Signs

1. Eye—The most common ocular manifestation of CS is interstitial keratitis, which is characterized by the abrupt onset of photophobia, lacrimation, and eye pain. CS may also be associated with inflammation in other parts of the eye. Scleritis (Figure 42–4), peripheral ulcerative keratitis, episcleritis, anterior uveitis, conjunctivitis, and retinal vascular disease are all possible.

2. Ear—Patients with CS frequently suffer the acute onset of vertigo, tinnitus, nausea, and vomiting. These symptoms may be enormously disabling. The audiovestibular symptoms may occur before or after the onset of ocular disease, and are often separated in onset by weeks or months. If not treated promptly and aggressively, permanent hearing loss may ensue. Recurrent attacks, which are common, may cause decremental loss of hearing. Ultimately, complete hearing loss occurs in as many as 60% of patients.

3. Large-vessel vasculitis—The most common manifestation of vasculitis in patients with CS is aortitis. Aortitis may lead to dilatation of the aorta and subsequent incompetence of the aortic valve. Involvement of aortic branches (Figure 42–5) may cause arm or leg claudication. Renal artery stenosis or occlusion of the great vessels may also occur. These manifestations may be accompanied by nonspecific constitutional symptoms, such as malaise, fever, or weight loss as well as arthralgias and frank arthritis.

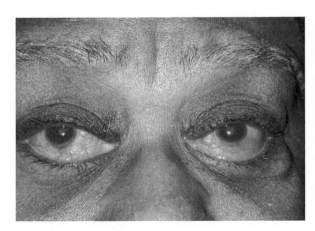

▲ **Figure 42–4.** Bilateral scleritis in a patient with Cogan's syndrome who had suffered the rapid onset of sensorineural hearing loss in both ears.

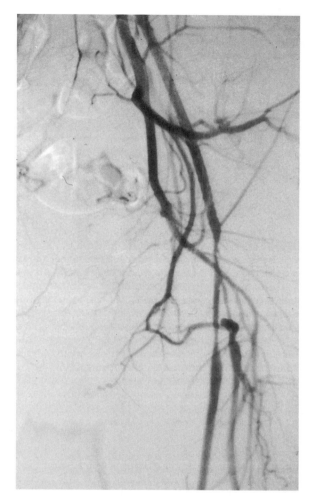

▲ **Figure 42–5.** Large-vessel vasculitis in Cogan syndrome. Femoral artery disease led to lower extremity claudication.

B. Laboratory Findings

Laboratory findings are nondiagnostic and generally reflect the presence of inflammation. An antibody against a 68-kD antigen has been identified in cases of autoimmune sensorineural hearing loss but is not found in patients with CS. Exclusion of syphilis with fluorescent treponemal antibody testing (ie, FTA-ABS, not just the rapid plasma reagin) is essential.

C. Imaging Studies

Gadolinium-enhanced T1-weighted magnetic resonance imaging (MRI) studies may demonstrate a hyperintensity in the membranous labyrinth secondary to vessel inflammation in the stria vascularis. This enhancement is not seen in

patients with inactive CS and may be useful in identifying the activity of the disease. Brainstem MRI studies are also essential to exclude tumors of the cerebellopontine angle, which may mimic the audiovestibular features of CS. Angiography may be useful to define the involvement of the great vessels (Figure 42–5). Magnetic resonance angiography is useful in evaluating vessel wall thickness and edema as well as the degree of luminal stenosis.

D. Special Tests

Formal audiometric testing is important early in the evaluation to distinguish conductive hearing loss from sensorineural hearing dysfunction. In CS, audiometry demonstrates sensorineural hearing loss that preferentially affects the low- and high-range frequencies. This may be a useful way to document response to therapy, although subsequent hearing loss is not always due to active disease.

▶ Differential Diagnosis

The differential diagnosis of immune-mediated inner ear disease (ie, sensorineural hearing loss with or without vestibular dysfunction) is shown in Table 42–1. Inflammatory eye disease may be caused by a variety of pathogens, including bacterial (eg, *Chlamydiae, Neisseriae*), spirochetal (eg, *Borrelia*

Table 42–1. Differential diagnosis of the audiovestibular complications of Cogan syndrome.

Alternate Diagnoses	Comments
Immune-mediated inner ear disease	Sensorineural hearing loss and vestibular dysfunction in the absence of eye inflammation.
Syphilis	Latent and tertiary forms of this disease. Ordering both rapid plasma reagin and FTA-ABS essential.
Other infections	Lyme disease, mumps
Acoustic neuroma	Performance of brainstem magnetic resonance imaging essential to exclude this tumor.
Ménière syndrome	Inner ear disturbances in Ménière syndrome are generally more intermittent, with a waxing/waning character.
Systemic vasculitides	Granulomatosis with polyangiitis (formerly Wegener granulomatosis), giant cell arteritis
Collagen vascular diseases	Sjögren syndrome
Other inflammatory conditions	Sarcoidosis, Susac syndrome
Barotrauma	Other etiologies of perilymph fistula formation
Medications	Aminoglycosides, loop diuretics, antimalarials

FTA-ABS, fluorescent treponemal antibody, absorption test.

burgdorferi), viral (eg, herpes simplex, varicella zoster), and mycobacterial (eg, *Mycobacterium tuberculosis, M leprae*).

Treatment

Some manifestations of CS respond well to symptomatic therapy. In general, the ocular manifestations are more amenable to therapy than the auditory complications. Interstitial keratitis may be treated with topical atropine or glucocorticoids. Sensorineural hearing loss in CS is analogous to rapidly progressive glomerulonephritis in other forms of systemic vasculitis: prompt treatment with immunosuppression is indicated. In addition to glucocorticoids, cyclophosphamide, azathioprine, methotrexate, and mycophenolate mofetil have all been used. The basis for choosing among these agents is largely empiric. The role for biologic agents, if any, has not been defined. For patients with advanced, irreversible hearing loss, hearing aids and cochlear implants may help. Vestibular retraining may be required for some patients with significant cochlear damage.

Complications

The prevention of complications depends directly on the rapid recognition of this diagnosis, and the equally swift institution of therapy. Permanent damage may result early in the course of immune-mediated inner ear disease, and hearing deficits will not respond to therapy if initiated too late. Therefore, a high index of suspicion for this diagnosis must be maintained when evaluating patients with compatible complaints.

Prognosis

Even if the initial event is recognized and responds to therapy, recurrent bouts of sensorineural hearing loss may cause the gradual loss of hearing. Up to 60% of patients experience some degree of permanent hearing loss. Some patients become completely deaf.

URTICARIAL VASCULITIS

ESSENTIALS OF DIAGNOSIS

▸ The lesions of urticarial vasculitis are frequently associated with burning or pain rather than pruritus and require more than 24 hours to resolve.

▸ Immunofluorescence on skin biopsy specimen is the critical test. Intense staining for immunoreactants (ie, IgG, IgM, C3, C4, C1q) not only in and around small blood vessel walls but also in a ribbon along the dermal/epidermal junction is pathognomonic of hypocomplementemic urticarial vasculitis.

General Considerations

Urticarial vasculitis (UV) is a leukocytoclastic vasculitis that presents as hives (often associated with pain or discomfort) that last longer than 24 hours. Although UV is occasionally seen in isolation, it most often appears in association with connective tissue disorders such as serum sickness, cryoglobulinemia, and systemic lupus erythematosus (SLE).

UV targets the capillaries and postcapillary venules in the skin, leading to the appearance of hive-like lesions. In evaluating patients with this problem, it is critical to distinguish cases associated with hypocomplementia from those in which the serum complement levels are normal.

Hypocomplementemic UV is associated with depressed serum levels of C3 and C4 and often with antibodies directed against the C1q component of complement. Such cases often overlap with known connective tissue disorders, particularly SLE. At the severe end of the spectrum of this disorder are patients with a distinct disorder known as the **hypocomplementemic urticarial vasculitis syndrome** (HUVS).

The normocomplementemic form is a subset of cutaneous leukocytoclastic angiitis (see Chapter 37) in which the leukocytoclastic vasculitis manifests clinically as urticaria. In general, these cases are secondary to "hypersensitivity" reactions (usually caused by a medication) and respond to discontinuation of the offending agent. This form of UV is not discussed further in this chapter.

Pathogenesis

Hypocomplementemic UV is mediated at least in part by immune complex deposition. In one model, following an unknown inciting event, the deposition of IgG and C3 leads to further complement activation. The complement cascade activates mast cells and eosinophils, both of which act to form the typical urticarial wheal. The eosinophils are gradually replaced by neutrophils, leading to the leukocytoclastic destruction of capillary walls. Antibodies to C1q are a marker of hypocomplementemic UV and likely contribute substantially to the finding of hypocomplementemia because they target an early component of the classical pathway of complement activation. The trigger(s) for anti-C1q antibodies remain unknown, and their full role in disease pathogenesis remains to be elucidated. Antibodies to C1q are not entirely specific for hypocomplementemic UV; they are also found in SLE.

Clinical Findings

A. Symptoms and Signs

The lesions of UV, typically between 0.5 and 2.0 cm in diameter (Figure 42–6), are frequently associated with burning or pain rather than pruritus. In contrast to common urticaria, UV lesions usually require more than 24 hours to resolve, and typically leave small amounts of hyperpigmentation in the skin, caused by red blood cell extravasation.

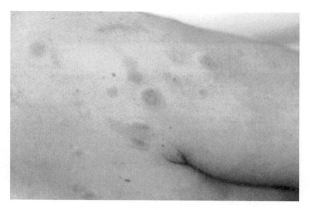

▲ **Figure 42–6.** Lesions of hypocomplementemic urticarial vasculitis.

Like SLE, hypocomplementemic UV may also be associated with malaise, arthralgias, fever, and glomerulonephritis. Unlike SLE, HUVS is characterized not only by recurrent or chronic UV, but also by angioedema. Moreover, severe chronic obstructive pulmonary disease (COPD) and uveitis—manifestations that are atypical of SLE—often complicate this condition. Jaccoud arthropathy has been noted in some patients with HUVS and possibly correlates with the presence of cardiac valvular lesions.

B. Laboratory Findings

Serum C3, C4, and CH50 levels are depressed. Hypocomplementemic UV is generally accompanied by the presence of anti-C1q autoantibodies. The presence of these antibodies is not pathognomonic, since they also may be found in patients with SLE who do not have UV. Patients with hypocomplementemic UV have ANAs and, if significant overlap with SLE is present, may also have other autoantibodies (eg, anti-dsDNA, anti-Ro/SS-A, anti-La/SS-B, anti-Sm, and anti-RNP).

C. Special Tests

Hematoxylin and eosin staining of skin biopsy specimens reveal a leukocytoclastic vasculitis in the superficial dermis. Older lesions may have a predominantly lymphocytic infiltrate. The critical test is the performance of immunofluorescence on the skin biopsy specimen, which reveals intense staining for immunoreactants (ie, IgG, IgM, C3, C4, C1q) not only in and around small blood vessel walls but also in a ribbon along the dermal/epidermal junction. These findings are pathognomonic of hypocomplementemic UV.

▶ Differential Diagnosis

The skin lesions of hypocomplementemic UV must be distinguished from common urticaria (which is characterized by pruritic lesions that resolve completely over 2–8 hours, leaving no traces of the original lesion), neutrophilic urticaria (a persistent, treatment-refractory form of urticaria not associated with vasculitis), and normocomplementic UV (see above).

▶ Treatment

UV may respond to therapies commonly used in SLE, such as low-dose prednisone, hydroxychloroquine, dapsone, or other immunomodulatory agents. There is anecdotal evidence that antihistamines, calcium channel antagonists, doxepin, methotrexate, indomethacin, colchicine, and pentoxifylline are effective in some cases.

HUVS is frequently a therapeutic challenge. Serious cases, particularly those presenting with glomerulonephritis or other organ involvement, may require treatment with high doses of glucocorticoids, cyclophosphamide, or cyclosporine. Dramatic anecdotal success has also been reported with infliximab, an inhibitor of TNF. Angioedema, COPD, and cardiac valvular abnormalities may all necessitate other specific interventions.

▶ Prognosis

Hypocomplementemic UV frequently reflects the presence of an underlying disorder, which may influence the prognosis substantially. HUVS may be associated with multiple complications (eg, severe COPD) that affect prognosis adversely.

ERYTHEMA ELEVATUM DIUTINUM

ESSENTIALS OF DIAGNOSIS

- ▶ New lesions come in the form of tender papules, associated with pruritus or a burning sensation.
- ▶ Lesions develop into red, reddish-brown, or purple papules or nodules.
- ▶ Lesions may coalesce to form large plaques, usually over the extensor surfaces of joints.

▶ General Considerations

Erythema elevatum diutinum (EED) is a chronic, recurring cutaneous vasculitis in which tender papules appear on the extensor surfaces of the extremities. The onset of these lesions is usually heralded by the presence of pruritus or stinging, followed by the development of tender papules or nodules that coalesce with others to form plaques. The skin findings are frequently located near joints, such as on the extensor surfaces of the hands and fingers.

Pathogenesis

The pathogenesis of EED is unknown but may involve recurrent immune complex deposition, followed by incomplete attempts at healing. Persistence of an antigen, with a subsequent increase in dendrocyte activity, may also play a role in its pathogenesis. There is an association between EED and multiple infections (including HIV, hepatitis B and C, tuberculosis, and streptococcal infections), autoimmune diseases (such as RA, relapsing polychondritis, and type 1 diabetes mellitus), and the paraproteinemias (such as multiple myeloma).

Clinical Findings

A. Symptoms and Signs

A new lesion is heralded by the presence of pruritus or a burning sensation in the skin, which then leads to the development of a red, reddish-brown, or purple papule or nodule. These lesions may coalesce to form large plaques, usually over the extensor surfaces of joints. With healing, the lesions often assume a yellowish or brown color, resembling xanthomata.

B. Laboratory Findings

Patients in whom EED is suspected should be screened for possible causes, including HIV infection, viral hepatitis, syphilis, cryoglobulinemia, and monoclonal gammopathy. When appropriate, patients may benefit from screening for associated autoimmune diseases as well.

C. Special Tests

Skin biopsy specimens usually show a nonspecific leukocytoclastic vasculitis with C3 deposition and are important for excluding non-vasculitis mimickers. In older lesions, the neutrophils are replaced by histiocytes, and there is marked granulation tissue and fibrosis.

Differential Diagnosis

Biopsy of lesions at various stages of development may demonstrate findings that are also consistent with a wide variety of diagnoses, including Sweet syndrome, pyoderma gangrenosum, drug reaction, erythema multiforme, fibrous histiocytoma, Kaposi sarcoma, xanthoma, and necrobiotic xanthogranuloma. The diagnosis can be established only by clinical judgment, supplemented by supportive findings on pathology.

Treatment

When a cause can be established, EED may respond to treatment of the underlying disorder. It is well established, for instance, that patients with EED as a consequence of HIV

infection experience a regression of the cutaneous lesions with institution of highly active antiretroviral therapy. Nonspecific therapies are less successful. Lesions may be suppressed by dapsone but tend to recur when the drug is stopped. Lesions may also respond to tetracycline, colchicine, chloroquine, and glucocorticoids (either topical or systemic).

Complications

Although recurrent and frequently unresponsive to therapy, EED is limited to the skin and does not lead to significant morbidity.

Prognosis

The prognosis associated with EED itself, even when unresponsive to therapy, is generally quite good. The overall prognosis for the patient, however, largely depends on the underlying disease process.

DRUG-INDUCED ANCA-ASSOCIATED VASCULITIS

 ESSENTIALS OF DIAGNOSIS

▶ Cutaneous eruptions, such as palpable purpura or a maculopapular rash limited to the lower extremities, are the most common manifestation of drug-induced ANCA-associated vasculitis.

▶ Frequently associated with very high titers of anti-myeloperoxidase ANCA.

▶ Tissue biopsy provides a definitive diagnosis.

General Considerations

Drug-induced, ANCA-associated vasculitis (AAV) is a form of vasculitis induced by certain medications in some patients. The majority of cases are associated with ANCA directed against myeloperoxidase, often in very high titers. Drug-induced AAV may resolve following discontinuation of the offending agent. Other cases, however, are indistinguishable from idiopathic AAV and require intensive therapy with glucocorticoids and cytotoxic agents.

Many cases of drug-induced AAV are associated with relatively minor symptoms (eg, constitutional symptoms, arthralgias or arthritis, and purpura). Propylthiouracil is a well-documented cause of drug-induced AAV. Other drugs implicated thus far include hydralazine, sulfasalazine, minocycline, D-penicillamine, ciprofloxacin, phenytoin, clozapine, allopurinol, and pantoprazole. Leukotriene inhibitors have been linked to the occurrence of the eosinophilic granulomatosis with polyangiitis (Churg-Strauss syndrome), but the true direct relationship (if any) between these medications and that condition remains unclear (see Chapter 34).

Pathogenesis

All of the events in the pathogenesis of drug-induced AAV remain undefined. Propylthiouracil is known to accumulate within neutrophil granules and alter myeloperoxidase, an event that may trigger the production of anti-myeloperoxidase ANCA. The presence of this human model of ANCA-associated disease forms one of the strongest arguments for a direct contribution of ANCA to the pathophysiology of other human disorders. Recent mouse models also strongly support the concept that ANCA may be pathogenic in humans.

Clinical Findings

A. Symptoms and Signs

Cutaneous eruptions are the most common manifestation of drug-induced AAV. These often present as palpable purpura or a maculopapular rash limited to the lower extremities. Unlike other AAV, the skin lesions in the drug-induced form frequently appear in "crops" (ie, simultaneously). Arthralgias and myalgias are common. The kidneys and upper respiratory tract may also be involved, as with the classic forms of AAV.

B. Laboratory Findings

In drug-induced AAV, very high titers of anti-myeloperoxidase antibodies are characteristic. Reports of cases associated with anti-proteinase 3 antibodies are rare. Even when the vasculitis resolves after discontinuation of the causative agent and initiation of immunosuppression, ANCA titers often remain elevated.

C. Special Tests

Tissue biopsy is usually necessary to provide a definitive diagnosis.

Differential Diagnosis

Drug-induced AAV is frequently slow to resolve after cessation of the offending agent and may be difficult to distinguish from the primary ANCA-associated vasculitides. In general, the manifestations of drug-induced AAV are mild and responsive to short courses of immunosuppression, although this is not always the case.

Treatment

The first step in treatment is the identification of the potential offending agents. Clinicians should take into account all exposures during the 6 months before the onset of symptoms, including nonprescription medications, herbal and dietary supplements, and illicit substances. Withdrawal of the offending agent may result in the resolution of the symptoms, although this may take months and may require the withdrawal of numerous agents simultaneously.

Patients with severe organ involvement may require aggressive immunosuppression with glucocorticoids and cytotoxic agents such as cyclophosphamide. The required length of therapy in drug-induced AAV may be shorter than that recommended for primary AAV.

Prognosis

Overall, the prognosis associated with drug-induced AAV is quite good. Organ involvement is frequently limited to the skin, and even systemic involvement frequently responds to lower doses of immunosuppressive agents administered for shorter periods of time than that required for primary AAV.

Bartels CM, Bridges AJ. Rheumatoid vasculitis: Vanishing menace or target for new treatments? *Curr Rheumatol Rep.* 2010;12:414. [PMID: 20842467]

Choi HK, Merkel PA, Walker AM, Niles JL. Drug-associated antineutrophil cytoplasmic antibody-positive vasculitis: prevalence among patients with high titers of antimyeloperoxidase antibodies. *Arthritis Rheum.* 2000;43:405. [PMID: 10693882]

Csernok E, Lamprecht P, Gross WL. Clinical and immunological features of drug-induced and infection-induced proteinase 3-antineutrophil cytoplasmic antibodies and myeloperoxidase-antineutrophil cytoplasmic antibodies and vasculitis. *Curr Opin Rheumatol.* 2010;22:43. [PMID: 19770659]

Gibson LE, el-Azhary RA. Erythema elevatum diutinum. *Clin Dermatol.* 2000;18:295. [PMID: 10856661]

Kroshinsky D, Stone JH, Nazarian RM. Case records of the Massachusetts General Hospital. Case 22-2011. A 79-year-old man with a rash, arthritis, and ocular erythema. *N Engl J Med.* 2011;365:252. [PMID: 21774714]

Myasoedova E, Crowson CS, Turesson C, Gabriel SE, Matteson EL. Incidence of extraarticular rheumatoid arthritis in Olmsted County, Minnesota, in 1995-2007 versus 1985-1994: a population-based study. *J Rheumatol.* 2011;38:983. [PMID: 21459933]

Stone JH, Francis HW. Immune-mediated inner ear disease. *Curr Opin Rheumatol.* 2000;12:32. [PMID: 10647952]

Stone JH, Nousari HC. "Essential" cutaneous vasculitis: what every rheumatologist should know about vasculitis of the skin. *Curr Opin Rheumatol.* 2001;13:23. [PMID: 11148712]

Osteoarthritis

43

David T. Felson, MD, MPH

ESSENTIALS OF DIAGNOSIS

▶ Joint pain brought on and exacerbated by activity and relieved with rest.

▶ Stiffness that is self-limited upon awakening in the morning or when rising from a seated position after an extended period of inactivity.

▶ Absence of prominent constitutional symptoms.

▶ Examination notable for increased bony prominence at the joint margins, crepitus or a grating sensation upon joint manipulation, and tenderness over the joint line of the symptomatic joint.

▶ Diagnosis supported by radiographic features of joint-space narrowing and spur (or osteophyte) formation.

General Considerations

Osteoarthritis is the leading cause of arthritis in the adult American population and affects an estimated 27 million people in the United States. Joint pain is a frequent symptom that often prompts a patient to seek medical attention; osteoarthritis figures prominently in the differential diagnosis. The challenge for clinicians is to identify correctly the cause of the patient's pain and to initiate appropriate therapy, both pharmacologic and nonpharmacologic. Synonymous with degenerative joint disease, osteoarthritis is characterized by joint pain related to use, self-limited morning stiffness, an audible grating sound or crepitus on palpation, the presence of tenderness over the affected joint on palpation, and frequently reduction in joint range of motion.

Characteristic sites of involvement in the peripheral skeleton include the hand (distal interphalangeal [DIP] joint, proximal interphalangeal [PIP] joint, and first carpometacarpal joint) (Figure 43–1), knee (Figure 43–2), and hip (Figure 43–3). Constitutional symptoms are absent. The diagnosis of osteoarthritis can usually be made easily and confidently based on the history and examination alone. The bedside diagnosis of osteoarthritis can be supported by plain radiography.

Epidemiology

At the population level, osteoarthritis results in substantial morbidity and disability, particularly among the elderly. It is the leading indication for several hundred thousand knee and hip replacement surgeries performed each year in the United States. Therefore, much effort has been invested in improving the understanding of the epidemiology of this disorder, including identifying the risk factors that predispose persons to osteoarthritis, especially ones that are reversible or modifiable.

Several factors heighten the risk of incident osteoarthritis, including age, gender, joint injury, and obesity. Although the clinical manifestations of osteoarthritis can begin as early as the fourth and fifth decades of life, the incidence of osteoarthritis continues to increase with each decade of age. Moreover, women in their 50s, 60s, and 70s have a greater prevalence of osteoarthritis in the hands and knees than do men. Osteoarthritis among blacks is more severe and has greater impact on disability than in whites. Genetics probably plays a role in increasing the vulnerability of some joints to disease. The influence of genetics on disease occurrence is significant and usually joint specific. For example, hip osteoarthritis runs in families but these families do not have an increased risk of osteoarthritis in other joints.

Trauma to a pristine joint such as a ruptured anterior cruciate ligament or torn meniscus increases the risk of later osteoarthritis at that joint site. Incidental and usually asymptomatic meniscal tears are common in middle aged and elderly men and women and increase the risk of knee osteoarthritis. Obese women and men are at high risk for knee osteoarthritis and have a modest increase in risk for hip osteoarthritis. This increase in risk is due mostly to the excess load across weight-bearing joints conferred by obesity and,

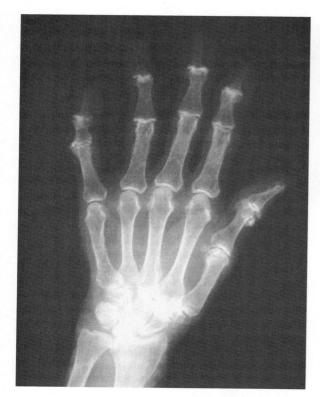

▲ **Figure 43–1.** Radiograph of a hand showing osteoarthritis of the distal interphalangeal (DIP), proximal interphalangeal (PIP), and first carpometacarpal (CMC) joints. Note the joint-space narrowing of the DIP and PIP joints compared to the metacarpophalangeal joints, as well as the bony sclerosis (eburnation) of all joints involved by the osteoarthritis process.

at least for women, the risk is proportional to the degree of overweight. For knee osteoarthritis, weight loss in middle age may lower this risk.

▶ Pathogenesis

Osteoarthritis is a disease in which most or all of the joint structures are affected by pathology. The defining tissue affected is the thin layer of hyaline articular cartilage interposed between the two articulating bones. This avascular tissue becomes worn away, especially in areas of injury. There is also degeneration of fibrocartilaginous structures like the meniscus, sclerosis of underlying bone, growth of osteophytes at the joint margin, weakness and atrophy of muscles that bridge the joint, ligamentous laxity and disruption and, in many joints, synovitis. With focal cartilage loss on one side of the joint and bony remodeling there, malalignment across the joint can develop, increasing focal transarticular loading and causing further damage to cartilage and underlying bone.

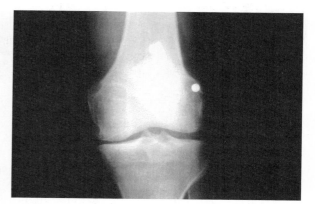

▲ **Figure 43–2.** Knee osteoarthritis with medial joint-space narrowing and osteophytes.

Both subtle chronic and flagrant acute injuries can start this disease process. Cartilage matrix turnover, spurred by daily loading across the joint, can replenish cartilage, but as a consequence of genetic abnormalities, age, and other metabolic factors not yet fully understood, some cartilage is especially vulnerable to loading that for normal cartilage, may be well tolerated.

▶ Prevention

At present, there are no proven preventive strategies.

Among women who participated in the Framingham Osteoarthritis Study, those who experienced a 5-kg or more weight reduction over 10 years had half the risk of developing symptomatic knee osteoarthritis. Such data support the claim that weight reduction can alter the risk of developing

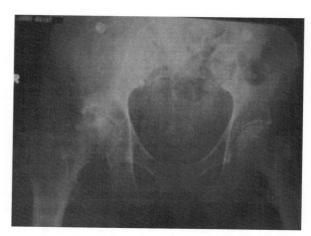

▲ **Figure 43–3.** Right hip osteoarthritis. Note the joint-space narrowing of the superior portion of the involved joint, compared to the same portion of the opposite joint.

osteoarthritis, and it stands to reason that weight loss may also delay disease progression.

Because major joint injury causes a large proportion of knee osteoarthritis in the community, avoiding major injuries may prevent disease. This is especially relevant to young women athletes who are at high risk for ACL tears, injuries associated with a high risk of subsequent knee osteoarthritis. Persons with knees that have already sustained major injuries are at high risk for subsequent injuries and should avoid athletic activities associated with high risk.

▶ Clinical Findings

A. Symptoms and Signs

The patient with osteoarthritis affecting a joint in the peripheral skeleton, such as the finger, knee, or hip, may initially experience relatively minor pain or discomfort with use of the involved joint (Table 43–1). For example, at the outset of osteoarthritis involving the hip joint, patients may have some difficulty crossing their legs to put on a pair of shoes or pants; however, once they are dressed and upright, bearing weight and ambulation are still well tolerated. As osteoarthritis progresses, a patient will gradually experience progressively severe joint discomfort and increasing difficulty with activities of daily living.

With further disease progression, such as at an osteoarthritic hand or finger, increasing difficulty with previously routine activities often follows. Thus, such tasks as gripping, holding, or writing with a pen or pencil; putting car keys in and turning the ignition switch; lifting a gallon of milk out of the refrigerator; or removing a pot of water from the stove become difficult tasks. At the extreme end of the disease spectrum, marked impairment in activity follows. Even walking from room to room in one's home may be unbearably painful when advanced osteoarthritis affects the hip or knee joint.

In patients with knee osteoarthritis, joint instability or "giving way" is common, sometimes leading to falling or near

Table 43–1. Signs, symptoms, and diagnostic features of osteoarthritis.

Joint pain that increases with activity
Morning stiffness that is relatively brief and self-limited
Crepitus (a grating sensation with motion)
Bony enlargement at the joint margin
Tenderness to palpation over the joint
Noninflammatory synovial fluid (<1000 WBC/mcL)
Erythrocyte sedimentation rate normal for age
Radiographic evidence of osteoarthritis (nonuniform joint-space narrowing, osteophyte [spur] formation, subchondral cysts, and eburnation [bony sclerosis])
Negative serologic tests for antinuclear antibody and rheumatoid factor

WBC, white blood count.

falling events. These pose substantial health risks to the elderly, and can contribute significantly to fear, frailty, and isolation.

B. Laboratory Findings

There is no specific laboratory test used in clinical practice to confirm a diagnosis of osteoarthritis. Instead, routine laboratory blood testing, including complete blood cell counts, acute phase reactants (erythrocyte sedimentation rate and C-reactive protein), and screening autoantibodies (rheumatoid factor and antinuclear antibody) are indicated if inflammatory arthritis such as rheumatoid arthritis is being considered. If joints affected are typical of osteoarthritis (eg, DIPs, PIPs, the first carpometacarpal joints) and symptoms in hands and other joints are related to activity, serologic evaluation is probably unnecessary. However, if the clinical presentation is consistent with rheumatoid arthritis (eg, if the wrists are affected or if prolonged morning stiffness—lasting >30–60 minutes—is present), blood tests may be of diagnostic value. Unlike most patients with osteoarthritis, those with inflammatory arthritis (including rheumatoid arthritis) will have elevated levels of acute phase reactants and may be anemic.

C. Imaging Studies

Radiographic imaging can confirm the diagnosis of osteoarthritis. In an older patient with bony enlargement on examination and activity-related pain, radiographs (which have imperfect sensitivity, sometimes being negative in the presence of disease), may not be indicated. The radiographic hallmarks of osteoarthritis, established more than 5 decades ago, are joint-space narrowing, osteophytes, subchondral cysts, and bony sclerosis (eburnation) (see Figure 43–1). Although MRI may reveal characteristic findings of osteoarthritis, such findings are universal in older persons, making MRI a test with poor discriminative power for the diagnosis of osteoarthritis.

D. Special Tests

An arthrocentesis can be a valuable test when encountering a patient with presumptive osteoarthritis. In osteoarthritis, synovial fluid cell WBC count is less than 2000 cells/mcL (typically less than 1000/mcL). Counts greater than 2000/mcL suggest the possibility of an inflammatory arthritis (see Chapter 4). In fluids from osteoarthritic joints, crystals visible by light microscopy are absent, but the presence of gout or pseudogout crystals provides diagnostic evidence of other forms of arthritis that occasionally are difficult to distinguish from osteoarthritis. This is particularly true for pseudogout.

▶ Differential Diagnosis

The challenge when evaluating a patient with joint pain is to use the history, physical examination, and sometimes a modicum of additional tests to arrive at the correct diagnosis in an efficient manner. Joint pain that is brought on by activity and relieved with rest suggests the existence of osteoarthritis. The

Table 43–2. Identifiable causes of osteoarthritis.

Congenital disorder (hip)
   Legg-Calvé-Perthes disease
   Acetabular dysplasia
   Slipped capital femoral epiphysis
Inborn error of connective tissue
   Ehlers-Danlos syndrome
   Marfan syndrome
Posttraumatic (knee)
   Anterior cruciate ligament tear
   Meniscus tear with or without prior meniscectomy surgery
Metabolic disorders
   Hemochromatosis
   Wilson disease
   Ochronosis (alkaptonuria)
   History of a septic joint
Postinflammatory
   Underlying rheumatoid arthritis
Generalized osteoarthritis
   Predilection for first CMC, DIP, PIP, knee, and hip joints

CMC, carpometacarpal; DIP, distal interphalangeal; PIP, proximal interphalangeal.

absence of constitutional signs and symptoms and the presence of bony enlargement and tenderness at the joint margin reinforce this clinical impression. Finally, the pattern of joint involvement is meaningful because osteoarthritis has a predilection for the knees, hips, and DIPs, PIPs, and first carpometacarpal joints of the hands. This distribution of joint involvement distinguishes osteoarthritis from such inflammatory forms of arthritis as rheumatoid arthritis, psoriatic arthritis, and gout, which have different sites of involvement.

It is also worth noting that a variety of secondary disorders represent identifiable causes of osteoarthritis. Several such disorders, including those resulting from inborn errors of metabolism and metabolic derangements, are listed in Table 43–2. Recognition of their distinct features, such as involvement of the second and third metacarpophalangeal joints in hemochromatosis-associated arthropathy, may identify the underlying cause of the joint pain. Finally, since osteoarthritis is extremely common, its presence does not exclude consideration of an alternate explanation for joint pain, such as an occult malignancy. Such diagnoses should be considered when there is a meaningful change in the pattern of joint pain.

If giving way (buckling) or locking of the knee occurs, this may indicate an internal derangement of the knee such as a tear of the anterior cruciate ligament or meniscus. Tears often occur abruptly and memorably.

► Treatment

The goals of medical therapy are to control pain, improve function, minimize disability, and enhance health-related quality of life. A further therapeutic priority is to minimize the risk of drug-associated toxicity, particularly that which may result from nonsteroidal anti-inflammatory drug (NSAID) therapy.

A. Nonpharmacologic

In patients with osteoarthritis, nonpharmacologic treatments are underutilized. They have demonstrated efficacy and can often help relieve pain and improve function. For example, an assistive device, such as a properly used cane or walker, can unload an affected knee or hip and diminish pain with walking. Similarly, quadriceps strengthening and aerobic exercise are effective in the management of osteoarthritis at the knee. For exercise therapy, referral to a physical therapist is often helpful, because the therapist can evaluate function and craft the right mix of exercises. Adherence to exercise is often poor, so it is helpful to reinforce the exercise regimen at each visit. A randomized trial demonstrated that neoprene sleeves reduce pain for patients with varus deformity due to knee osteoarthritis. If these do not work, fitted valgus braces, designed to decrease the varus malalignment across the knee, have been shown to decrease pain. Wedged insoles in the shoes help realign the knees but clinical trials of such insoles have mostly shown no effects on knee pain. Weight loss should be encouraged for all persons with knee or hip osteoarthritis.

B. Pharmacologic

A front-line approach to pharmacologic therapy for osteoarthritis includes use of acetaminophen. This drug improves pain and function and has a safer toxicity profile, particularly with regard to the gastrointestinal tract, than NSAIDs. For many years, NSAIDs have been widely used in the management of osteoarthritis and achieve symptomatic benefit through their inhibition of cyclooxygenase (COX), particularly the inducible isoform (COX-2), at sites of joint damage. Recent studies have demonstrated that NSAIDs are modestly more efficacious than acetaminophen for the pain of osteoarthritis. Patients are unlikely to respond to acetaminophen if they have already been treated with NSAIDs.

The gastrointestinal toxicity of NSAID therapy remains a major concern and such toxicity can be mostly avoided by using topical nonsteroidal drugs especially for superficial joints such as hands and knees. The following factors increase the risk of gastrointestinal toxicity from oral NSAIDs:

- Prior peptic ulcer disease.

- Age over 65 years.

- Concomitant tobacco and alcohol use.

- Coadministration of glucocorticoids or anticoagulation therapy.

- Comorbid *Helicobacter pylori* infection.

Ways to diminish NSAID toxicity include:

- Gastroprotective drugs. The two classes of drugs shown to be effective among NSAID users are proton pump

Table 43–3. Acute complications of osteoarthritis.

Microcrystalline arthropathy (knee and hand joints)
Gout
Pseudogout
Spontaneous osteonecrosis of the knee
Ruptured Baker cyst (pseudothrombophlebitis syndrome in the knee)
Bursitis
Anserine bursitis (knee)
Trochanteric bursitis (hip)
Symptomatic meniscal tear (knee)

inhibitors and misoprostol, although the latter frequently causes bloating and diarrhea.

- Administration of COX-2 isoenzyme inhibitors. Although COX inhibitors cause increased risks of heart disease and stroke, celecoxib may be less guilty of this, especially at doses under 400 mg/d.

The efficacy of glucosamine in the medical management of osteoarthritis is controversial. Glucosamine is a component of human articular cartilage that is administered orally. A multicenter National Institutes of Health (NIH) trial found no efficacy of glucosamine. Chondroitin sulfate (also commercially available) is similarly controversial. The same NIH trial failed to show efficacy either of chondroitin alone or combined glucosamine and chondroitin. Intra-articular hyaluronic acid is a controversial FDA-approved treatment for knee osteoarthritis. Meta-analyses evaluating placebo-controlled trials have reported significant but modest efficacy and have also reported publication bias suggesting that estimates of efficacy from published studies are inflated.

Complications

After a diagnosis of osteoarthritis has been firmly established, subsequent change in symptoms or course will not necessarily be directly attributable to this disease. If such changes occur, the clinician should search for other diagnoses as listed in Table 43–3. For example, the abrupt onset of heat, redness, and swelling in a known yet previously stable osteoarthritic knee may herald the onset of a superimposed microcrystalline arthritis or of a ruptured Baker (or popliteal) cyst. Alternately, new-onset joint locking or giving way may suggest the presence of a loose body or meniscal tear that warrants arthroscopic intervention. The development of new symptoms near the joint may be attributable to active inflammation of adjacent nonarticular tissues, including regional tendons and bursae.

Abramson SB. Attur M. Developments in the scientific understanding of osteoarthritis. *Arthritis Res Ther.* 2009;11:227. [PMID: 19519925]

[Arthritis Foundation]
http://www.arthritis.org

Felson DT. Clinical practice. Osteoarthritis of the knee. *N Engl J Med.* 2006;354:841. [PMID: 16495390]

Felson DT. Developments in the clinical understanding of osteoarthritis. *Arthritis Res Ther.* 2009;11:203. [PMID: 19232065]

[Johns Hopkins Arthritis Center]
http://www.hopkins-arthritis.org

Kirkley A, Webster-Bogaert S, Litchfield R, et al. The effect of bracing on varus gonarthrosis. *J Bone Joint Surg Am.* 1999;81:539. [PMID: 10225800]

Messier SP, Loeser RF, Miller GD, et al. Exercise and dietary weight loss in overweight and obese older adults with knee osteoarthritis: the Arthritis, Diet, and Activity Promotion Trial. *Arthritis Rheum.* 2004;50:1501. [PMID: 15146420]

[Osteoarthritis Research Society International]
http://www.oarsi.org

44

Gout

Christopher Burns, MD

Robert L. Wortmann, MD

ESSENTIALS OF DIAGNOSIS

▶ Caused by deposition of uric acid crystals and usually associated with hyperuricemia.

▶ Usually begins as an intermittent, acute monoarthritis, especially of the first metatarsophalangeal joint.

▶ Over time, attacks become more frequent, less intense, and involve more joints.

▶ Diagnosed by demonstrating uric acid crystals in joint fluid.

▶ Extra-articular manifestations include tophi and renal stones.

▶ Arthritis responds to nonsteroidal anti-inflammatory drugs or colchicine.

▶ General Considerations

The underlying basis for gout is an increased total body urate pool. This is generally manifested as hyperuricemia, which is defined as a serum urate concentration more than 6.8 mg/dL. The concentration of 6.8mg/dL is important because fluids with urate content greater than that are supersaturated with urate, a condition that favors urate crystal precipitation.

At least 10% of asymptomatic Americans manifest hyperuricemia on at least one occasion during adulthood. Hyperuricemia may be even more common in Europe and in countries in the Far East.

The likelihood of developing symptomatic gout and the age at which that occurs correlates with the duration and magnitude of hyperuricemia. In one study, persons with urate levels between 7.0 and 8.0 mL/dL had a cumulative incidence of gouty arthritis of 3%, while those with urate levels >9.0 mL/dL had a 5-year cumulative incidence of 22%. However, hyperuricemia alone is not sufficient for the diagnosis of gout, and asymptomatic hyperuricemia in the absence of gout is not a disease. It appears that clinical gout develops in fewer than 1 in 4 hyperuricemic persons at any point.

Gout presents predominantly in men with a peak age of onset in the fifth decade. The incidence of gout in women approaches that of men only after they have reached age 65 years. The onset of disease in men prior to adulthood or in women before menopause is quite rare and is almost always due to an inborn error of metabolism or congenital condition. The prevalence of self-reported gout is estimated to be 13.6 per 1000 men and 6.4 per 1000 women.

Hyperuricemia can result from increased urate production, decreased uric acid excretion by the kidneys, or a combination of the two mechanisms. Less than 5% of patients with gout are hyperuricemic because of urate overproduction. These persons can be recognized because they excrete more than 800 mg of uric acid in their urine during a 24-hour period. Those who excrete less uric acid than 800 mg are hyperuricemic because of impaired renal excretion. Defining individuals as "over-producers" or "underexcreters" is helpful in predicting whether the hyperuricemia is associated with a variety of acquired or genetic disorders (Table 44–1) and may be useful in some cases in determining the most appropriate treatment.

▶ Pathogenesis

Hyperuricemia, defined as a serum urate level of 6.8 mg/dL or greater, is the necessary precursor for the development of gout. When individuals are hyperuricemic, conditions exist such that urate crystals can precipitate in and around joint tissues. Without intervention, crystal precipitation continues forming larger and larger aggregates of crystals, termed "tophi." An attack of acute gout follows the ingestion of urate crystals by monocytes and synoviocytes. Uncoated urate crystals are endocytosed by and activate monocytes. Inside the cells, they are processed through Toll-like receptors with

Table 44–1. Classification of hyperuricemia.

Urate overproduction
Primary hyperuricemia
Idiopathic
Complete or partial deficiency of HGPRT
Superactivity of PRPP synthetase
Secondary hyperuricemia
Excessive purine consumption
Myeloproliferative or lymphoproliferative disorders
Hemolytic diseases
Psoriasis
Glycogen storage diseases: types 1, 3, 5, and 7
Uric acid underexcretion
Primary hyperuricemia
Idiopathic
Secondary hyperuricemia
Decreased renal function
Metabolic acidosis (ketoacidosis or lactic acidosis)
Dehydration
Diuretics
Hypertension
Hyperparathyroidism
Drugs including cyclosporine, pyrazinamide, ethambutol and
low-dose salicylates
Lead nephropathy
Overproduction and underexcretion
Alcohol use
Glucose-6-phosphatase deficiency
Fructose-1-phosphate-aldolase deficiency

HGPRT, hypoxanthine guanine phosphoribosyltransferase; PRPP,
5′-phosphoribosyl-1-pyrophosphate.

result of pre-IL-1 production. The NALP-3 inflammasomes are also activated resulting in caspace-1 formation and the conversion of pre-IL-1 to IL-1 and the generation of a variety of other cytokines, adhesion molecules and chemotactic agents. The result is a very acutely inflamed joint.

The acute inflammatory response resolves spontaneously over 10–14 days. As the monocytes mature into macrophages, they switch from producing pro-inflammatory cytokines to anti-inflammatory cytokines like transforming factor (TGF)-β. In addition, large proteins (such as apolipoprotein B) that normally do not have access to the synovial fluid can enter the joint space because of the vasodilation and increased vascular permeability of the acute inflammatory response. These proteins coat the crystals and have an anti-phlogistic effect.

In between attacks, the tophi continue to enlarge. They are surrounded by a mantle of macrophages that are releasing cytokines and enzymes. This chronic inflammatory response is responsible for eroding bone and cartilage and causes a secondary degenerative joint disease. With enough cartilage degeneration, chronic arthritis that is symptomatically identical to primary osteoarthritis develops.

► Clinical Findings

A. Symptoms and Signs

The natural history of gout can be divided into three distinct stages (Figure 44–1):

1. Asymptomatic hyperuricemia.

2. Acute and intermittent (or intercritical) gout.

3. Chronic tophaceous gout.

Although most untreated cases of gout progress to chronic tophaceous gout, the course varies considerably from one patient to another. Whereas some patients experience only one or two attacks of acute gouty arthritis during their lifetime, over 80% have a second flare within 2 years of the first. It is quite unusual for tophi to develop in a patient with no history of acute gouty arthritis.

The initial episode of acute gouty arthritis usually follows 10–30 years of asymptomatic hyperuricemia, and there is no evidence that damage occurs to any organ system during that time. Just why and when the first attack of gout occurs in susceptible persons remains a mystery. Although some patients experience prodromal episodes of mild discomfort, the onset of a gouty attack is usually heralded by the rapid onset of exquisite pain associated with warmth, swelling, and erythema of the affected joint (Figure 44–2). The pain escalates from the faintest twinges to its most intense level over an 8- to 12-hour period. Initial attacks usually affect only one joint, and in half the patients, the first attack involves the first metatarsophalangeal joint. Other joints frequently involved in the early stage of gout include the midfoot, ankle, heel, and knee. The wrist, fingers, and elbows are more typical sites of attacks later in the course of the disease. The intensity of the pain is such that patients cannot stand even the weight of a bed sheet on the affected part and most find it difficult or impossible to walk when the lower extremities are involved in an acute attack. The acute attack may be accompanied by fever, chills, and malaise. Cutaneous erythema associated with the attack may extend beyond the involved joint and

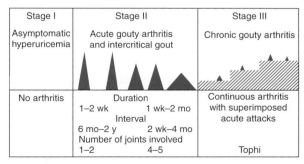

Stage I	Stage II	Stage III
Asymptomatic hyperuricemia	Acute gouty arthritis and intercritical gout	Chronic gouty arthritis
No arthritis	Duration 1–2 wk 1 wk–2 mo Interval 6 mo–2 y 2 wk–4 mo Number of joints involved 1–2 4–5	Continuous arthritis with superimposed acute attacks Tophi

▲ **Figure 44–1.** The natural history of gout progresses through three stages.

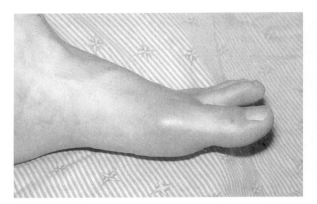

▲ **Figure 44–2.** Acute gouty attack of the first metatarsophalangeal joint.

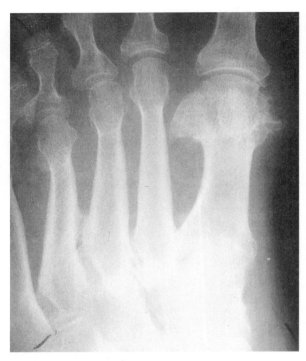

▲ **Figure 44–3.** Radiographic changes of gout.

resemble cellulitis. Desquamation of the skin may occur as the attack resolves.

Symptoms resolve quickly with appropriate treatment, but even untreated, an acute attack resolves spontaneously over 1–2 weeks. With resolution of the attack, patients enter an interval termed the "intercritical period" when they are again completely asymptomatic. Early in the intermittent stage, episodes of arthritis are infrequent and the intervals between the attacks vary from months to years. Over time, the attacks become more frequent, less acute in onset, longer in duration, and tend to involve more joints.

During the intercritical periods of acute intermittent gout, the previously involved joints are virtually free of symptoms. Despite this, monosodium urate crystal deposition continues and tophi increase in size. Urate crystals often can be identified in the synovial fluid despite the absence of symptoms and erosive changes indicative of bony tophi begin to appear on radiographs.

Although the reasons why acute gout develops when it does are not clear, attacks tend to be associated with rapid increases, and more often decreases, in the concentration of urate in synovial fluid. These concentrations mirror the fluctuations seen in the serum. Accordingly, a person may experience a sudden drop in the serum urate level leading to an acute attack, and therefore is found to be normouricemic when blood is tested at that time. Trauma, alcohol ingestion, and the use of certain drugs are known to trigger gout attacks as well. Gouty attacks not infrequently occur as a person is recovering from an alcoholic binge. Drugs known to precipitate attacks do so by rapidly raising or lowering serum urate levels. Candidate agents include diuretics, salicylates, radiographic contrast agents, and specific urate-lowering drugs (probenecid, allopurinol, febuxostat, and pegloticase). It is believed that these fluctuations in urate levels destabilize tophi in the gouty synovium. The sudden addition of urate to them may render them unstable, or the sudden lowering of the urate concentration may cause

partial dissolution and instability. As the microtophi break apart, crystals are shed into the synovial fluid and the gouty attack is initiated (see above).

As gout continues to progress, the patient gradually enters the stage of chronic gouty arthritis. This is the result of a macrophage-driven chronic inflammatory response that surrounds tophi (see above) and usually develops after 10 or more years of acute intermittent gout. The transition to chronic gout is complete when the intercritical periods are no longer pain-free. The involved joints are now persistently uncomfortable and may be swollen. Patients report stiffness or gelling sensations as well. Visible or palpable tophi may be detected on physical examination during this stage of gout, even though they may have been seen on radiographs prior to entry into this stage (Figure 44–3). The development of tophaceous deposits in individual patients varies; in general, they are a function of the duration and severity of the hyperuricemia, with a mean occurrence approximately 12 years after the onset of the first attack of gout in those not treated with urate-lowering drugs.

B. Laboratory Findings

Hyperuricemia remains the cardinal feature of gout. The usefulness of this laboratory finding in establishing the diagnosis of gout is limited. Whereas most patients with gout have an elevated serum urate (>6.8 mg/dL), levels may fall within the

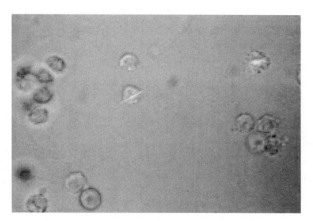

▲ **Figure 44–4.** Urate crystal ingested by a polymorphonuclear leukocyte in synovial fluid. This finding is pathognomonic for acute gouty arthritis.

normal range on occasion; in fact, levels in the normal range are not uncommon during acute attacks, as described above. In addition, during the acute attack, the complete blood cell count may show a leukocytosis with increased polymorphonuclear leukocytes on the differential and elevations of the erythrocyte sedimentation rate and C-reactive protein. The greatest utility of measuring serum urate is in monitoring the effects of urate-lowering therapy.

The 24-hour urine uric acid measurement is not required in all patients with gout but is useful for determining potential causes of hyperuricemia (see above) as well as determining whether uricosuric therapy can be effective, since this form of therapy is effective only in underexcreters.

During an acute attack, the synovial fluid findings are consistent with moderate to severe inflammation (see Chapter 2). The leukocyte count usually ranges between 5 and 80,000 cells/mcL with an average between 15,000 and 20,000 cells/mcL. The cells are predominantly polymorphonuclear leukocytes.

The definitive diagnosis of gout is made by examination of synovial fluid or tophaceous material with compensated polarized light microscopy and identifying the characteristic monosodium urate crystals in synovial fluid or aspirates of tophaceous deposits (Figure 44–4). These crystals appear as bright yellow needle-shaped objects when parallel to the axis of slow vibration on the first-order compensator. When these crystals are perpendicular to that axis, they are blue. Crystals are usually intracellular and needle-shaped during acute attacks but may be small, blunted, and extracellular as the attack subsides or during intercritical periods.

C. Imaging Studies

No radiographic abnormalities are present early in the disease course. In acute gouty arthritis, the only finding may be soft tissue swelling in the involved joint. Bony abnormalities indicative of deposition of urate crystals (microtophi) develop only after years of disease. These abnormalities are most frequently asymmetric and confined to previously symptomatic joints. The advanced bony erosions of advanced gout are often radiographically distinct. Typically, they are slightly removed from the joint space, have a rounded or oval shape, and are characterized by a hypertrophic calcified "overhanging edge." The joint space may be preserved or show osteoarthritic type narrowing (see Figure 44–3). Ultrasonography can also be used to make the diagnosis. The characteristic finding is a "double contour sign," a superficial, hyperechoic band on the surface of the articular cartilage.

MRI and CT scans are also sensitive methods of detecting tophi and erosions.

D. Special Tests

Patients with gout often suffer from hyperlipidemia, glucose intolerance, hypertension, coronary artery disease, and obesity. Accordingly, it is appropriate to measure serum lipids and fasting blood sugars in patients with gout. Because renal dysfunction develops in many patients with hypertension and gout, it is appropriate to monitor serum creatinine levels as well.

▶ Differential Diagnosis

The presumptive diagnosis of gout can be made by the presence of the characteristic triad of (1) hyperuricemia, (2) acute monoarticular arthritis, and (3) a gratifying clinical response to therapy with colchicine, defined as complete resolution of symptoms within 48 hours and no recurrence for 1 week. Clinicians may also use the criteria proposed by American College of Rheumatology for the diagnosis of gout (Table 44–2). Because gouty arthritis often occurs in

Table 44–2. Criteria for the diagnosis of acute gouty arthritis.

- Presence of characteristic urate crystals in joint fluid, or
- A tophus proved to contain urate crystals by chemical means or polarized light microscopy, or
- The presence of 6 of the following 12 clinical, laboratory, and radiographic phenomena listed below:
  1. More than one attack of acute arthritis
  2. Maximal inflammation developed within 1 day
  3. Attack of monoarticular arthritis
  4. Joint redness observed
  5. First metatarsophalangeal joint painful or swollen
  6. Unilateral attack involving first metatarsophalangeal joint
  7. Unilateral attack involving tarsal joint
  8. Suspected tophus
  9. Hyperuricemia
  10. A symptomatic swelling within a joint (radiograph)
  11. Subcortical cysts without erosions (radiograph)
  12. Negative culture of joint fluids for microorganisms during attack of joint inflammation

association with other diseases, those conditions in Table 44–1 should be considered in any person with gout. A variety of conditions can mimic or be confused with gouty arthritis. These include other crystal-induced diseases such as those related to the deposition of calcium pyrophosphate dihydrate crystals (pseudogout) or basic calcium phosphate crystals. The latter may cause a calcific tendinitis that is similar in presentation to gout. Septic arthritis can also mimic gout, although a gouty attack may coexist with an infected joint. The more common causes of septic arthritis are gonococcal, staphylococcal, or streptococcal infections. However, infections with fungi or mycobacteria may also be seen. A hemarthrosis or fracture in the joint line may be confused with a gouty attack. Finally, some conditions that are usually considered oligoarticular or polyarticular in presentation may involve only one joint early in the course and be confused with gout. This is particularly true with the peripheral arthritis associated with ankylosing spondylitis, reactive arthritis, psoriatic arthritis, and the arthritis of inflammatory bowel disease. Rarely, palindromic rheumatism may herald the onset of rheumatoid arthritis and begins with monoarticular arthritis.

Occasionally, chronic gouty arthritis and tophi are misdiagnosed as rheumatoid arthritis. The chronic symptoms are polyarticular and symmetric, and the tophaceous deposits mimic rheumatoid nodules. This problem is compounded by the fact that up to 25% of patients with gout have positive tests for rheumatoid factor although these are usually of low titer.

Complications

As described above, untreated and severe gout leads to visible and palpable tophaceous deposits and a destructive arthropathy. However, these complications are preventable with accurate diagnosis and appropriate therapy.

Nephrolithiasis develops in 10–25% of patients with gout at some time during the disease course. In 40% of these patients, the first episode of renal colic precedes the first attack of acute gouty arthritis. Most of these calculi are composed of uric acid; however, calcium-containing stones are 10 times more common in patients with gout than in the general population. The incidence of nephrolithiasis correlates with the serum urate level, but more strongly with the amount of uric acid excreted in the urine. The likelihood of developing a stone reaches 50% with either a serum urate level above 13.0 mg/dL or a 24-hour urinary uric acid excretion in excess of 1100 mg.

In the past, progressive renal failure has been common in patients with gout, with up to 25% of patients dying of renal disease. Today, this frequency is much less. Hypertension, diabetes, chronic lead exposure, and chronic atherosclerosis are the most important contributing factors to this complication. In fact, if blood pressure is rigorously controlled, it is very unusual for renal failure to develop in a patient with gout. Chronic urate nephropathy has been described and is a distinct condition caused by the deposition of monosodium urate crystals in the renal parenchyma and pyramids. Although chronic hyperuricemia is thought to be the cause of this urate nephropathy, this form of kidney disease is never seen in the absence of gouty arthritis. Furthermore, with appropriate management, urate nephropathy should easily be prevented.

Hyperuricemia and gout are frequently accompanied by obesity, alcoholism, glucose intolerance related to insulin resistance, and hyperlipidemia. In addition, a very high percentage of patients with gout have hypertension. These associated conditions should be managed aggressively.

Treatment

The management of gout includes the following:

1. Providing rapid and safe pain relief.
2. Preventing further attacks.
3. Preventing formation of tophi and destructive arthritis.
4. Addressing associated medical conditions.

The goal of treating the acute gout attack is to eliminate the pain and other symptoms caused by the intense inflammation as rapidly as possible. The choices in this situation include nonsteroidal anti-inflammatory drugs (NSAIDs), colchicine, and glucocorticoids. Effective management of the acute attack is not so much determined by which agent is used, but rather by how quickly that agent is initiated after the onset of the attack. If a single dose is given in the first minutes of an attack, it may eradicate the symptoms and terminate the attack. If, however, medication is not taken during the first 48 hours of symptoms, it will probably take at least 2 days before control is gained. Once symptoms have resolved, the particular agent used should be continued at a reduced dose for another 48–72 hours.

NSAIDs have become the most frequently used agents to treat gout because they are so well tolerated. Indomethacin is historically the NSAID of choice for acute gout, but other NSAIDs may be just as effective. The selected NSAID should be started at its recommended maximal dose. The dose may be lowered as symptoms resolve. NSAIDs should be avoided in patients with active or recent peptic ulcer disease and should be used with caution in patients with renal insufficiency or conditions associated with impaired renal blood flow (see Chapter 74).

Colchicine is effective but less well tolerated than NSAIDs. Colchicine is taken 1.2 mg orally and then 0.6 mg 1 hour later. This can be repeated every 24 hours as needed. Gastrointestinal side effects include gas, nausea, vomiting, diarrhea, and severe cramping abdominal pain.

Glucocorticoids are usually reserved for patients in whom colchicine or NSAIDs are contraindicated or ineffective. Anecdotal reports suggest early recurrence of gout after treating acute attacks with glucocorticoids, but recent studies have not confirmed that observation. The response time for glucocorticoids is comparable to that for NSAIDs and colchicine. Doses of prednisone of 20–40 mg/d have been used. The dosage is usually tapered over 1–2 weeks after symptoms resolve. Intramuscular or intravenous glucocorticoids provide alternatives for use in the hospitalized patient who can take nothing by mouth. Finally, intra-articular injections with 20–80 mg of methylprednisolone acetate or 10–40 mg of triamcinolone hexacetonide can also be used.

Most often the gout attack resolves with the use of one of these agents. However, when this does not occur or in the extremely severe case of gout, these agents may be used in combination. Potent analgesics, including opioids, may also be added to the regimen.

Once a patient has had an acute gouty attack, the likelihood of further attacks can be reduced by prophylactic therapy with low-dose colchicine or an NSAID on a daily basis. Prophylactic therapy, however, should not be prescribed unless a urate-lowering agent is added to the regimen. The use of prophylactic colchicine without controlling the hyperuricemia only allows tophi and destructive arthritis to continue to develop without the usual warning signs of recurrent acute gouty attacks. The prophylactic use of colchicine in doses of 0.6 mg once or twice a day reduces the frequencies of attacks by 75–85%. These small doses of colchicine rarely cause gastrointestinal side effects and appear to be relatively safe. Long-term colchicine use can cause neuromuscular complications in patients with decreased renal function, especially older patients. It is prudent to avoid using more than 0.6 mg of colchicine daily in a patient with a serum creatinine above 1.5 mg/dL. This toxicity manifests with proximal muscle weakness, painful paresthesias, elevated creatine kinase levels, and abnormalities on electromyograms. This axonal neuromyopathy resolves completely over several weeks after discontinuing the colchicine. Ultimately, specific urate-lowering drugs must be used to eliminate acute attacks and to prevent tophi from forming or cause them to disappear. Although dietary manipulation is essential for control of the comorbid conditions often found with gout, diet cannot reduce serum urate levels sufficiently.

The goal of treatment is to maintain the serum urate level at 6.0 mg/dL or less. Maintaining the serum level at this target allows precipitated crystals to dissolve and be cleared. If the urate level remains above 6.8 mg/dL, supersaturated conditions will persist and urate deposition will continue. In other words, lowering the serum urate from 10.0 mg/dL to 8.0 mg/dL will not reverse the disease; it will only allow it to continue to progress at a slower rate.

The xanthine oxidase inhibitor allopurinol is the agent of choice for most patients with gout. It can effectively lower serum urate levels in those patients with hyperuricemia due to underexcretion and is specifically indicated for those who overproduce urate. Patients with tophi, those with nephrolithiasis, and those who are intolerant of uricosuric therapy are also candidates for xanthine oxidase inhibition. Allopurinol may be used in the presence of renal insufficiency, but its dosage must be reduced to prevent toxicity. Allopurinol at a dose of 300 mg/d adequately controls the serum urate in 30-50% of patients with normal renal function. If the patient is already taking prophylactic colchicine (which is recommended), then allopurinol can be started at a dose of 300 mg/d. Otherwise, it is recommended that patients start with 100 mg/d for a week and gradually increase the dose until the lowest level of medication that keeps the serum urate level in the target range is reached. Most patients achieve the desired serum urate level of 6.0 mg/dL or less while taking 300–400 mg of allopurinol daily. The maximum recommended daily dose is 800 mg. Allopurinol must be used cautiously when the patient is also taking azathioprine or 6-mercaptopurine. Allopurinol reduces the catabolism of these agents, thereby greatly increasing their effective doses.

Side effects and toxicity of allopurinol include fever, headaches, diarrhea, dyspepsia, pleuritis, skin rashes, granulomatous hepatitis, and toxic epidermal necrolysis. The syndrome of allopurinol hypersensitivity is rare but serious with a mortality rate of 20–30%. Allopurinol hypersensitivity reactions are more common in older patients with impaired renal function taking diuretics. The development of a rash in patients taking allopurinol is an indication to stop the medicine.

Febuxostat is a potent xanthine oxidase inhibitor that appears to have certain benefits compared with allopurinol. First, it is metabolized by the liver so febuxostat may be used in patients with mild to moderate renal insufficiency (creatinine clearance of 30 mL/minute and above) without dose adjustment. Second, it can be used safely even in patients with mild to moderate hepatic insufficiency. To date, the use of febuxostat in patients with a history of allopurinol reactions has been safe, effective, and well tolerated. In clinical trials, a dose of 40 mg of febuxostat had similar effectiveness to 300 mg of allopurinol. It is also available in an 80 mg dose.

Uricosuric agents are also effective in lowering serum urate levels. The patients in whom they are most effective are those who have good renal function (glomerular filtration rate above 60 mL/minute), those who have no history of nephrolithiasis, those who can avoid all salicylate ingestions, and those under 65 years of age. Salicylate use in doses in excess of 81 mg/d interferes with the effectiveness of uricosuric agents. These agents should be avoided in patients with a history of nephrolithiasis because stone formation is more likely due to the flooding of urine with uric acid. Finally, uricosuric agents require good renal function to be effective. Probenecid is started at a dosage of 500 mg twice a day and advanced slowly up to a maximum dosage of 2.5 g a day or until the target urate level is reached. The most common side effects of this agent are rash and

---

Gout is Like Matches

The following paragraph is an analogy that can be used to explain gout to patients.

Gout is caused by uric acid. Everyone has uric acid in their blood but some people have too much of it, and some of those people get gout. In those who get gout, the uric acid accumulates around the joints and acts like matches. When you get a gout attack, one of the matches strikes and catches the joint on fire. When that happens, you should take your indomethacin (or nonsteroidal anti-inflammatory drug of choice). It is important to take it right away. If not, more matches will catch fire and the attack will worsen. Taking indomethacin does not cure the gout because it only puts out the fire. The matches are still there and can light again. A urate-lowering drug will remove the matches. If there are no matches, you cannot get gout. But until the urate-lowering drug has time to work, you can still get gout. Therefore you should take colchicine, one pill twice a day. Colchicine is very good at preventing gout attacks. You can think of colchicine as something that makes the matches damp and harder to strike.

Data from Wortmann RL. Effective management of gout: an analogy. *Am J Med.* 1998;105:513.

---

gastrointestinal upset. Benzbromarone, an agent available in Europe, is more potent and may be effective in the face of moderate renal insufficiency.

The most recently approved specific urate-lowering agent is pegloticase, a pegylated mammalian (porcine-like) recombinant uricase. The dosage is 8 mg intravenously every 2 weeks, and it has dramatic effects on serum urate levels. This agent should be reserved for those with severe gout with abundant tophaceous deposits. Its use may be limited by hypersensitivity reactions and the development of blocking antibodies.

Unfortunately, the treatment of gout is complicated by poor compliance. This is probably related to the difficulty people have in remembering how to take three different medicines on three different schedules. Frequently, they become confused about which medicines to take in what situations. An analogy has been developed that may help patients

understand and better remember how to take their medications (see the box: Gout is Like Matches).

Hyperuricemia alone is rarely an indication for treatment with specific urate-lowering drugs. Therefore, use of a xanthine oxidase inhibitor or uricosuric agent is not recommended in the treatment of asymptomatic hyperuricemia. On the other hand, the identification of asymptomatic hyperuricemia should not be ignored. First, the cause should be determined (see Table 44–1), and any associated problems, such as hypertension, obesity, alcoholism, diabetes, or hyperlipidemia, should be addressed rigorously.

▶ Prognosis

For patients that receive appropriate urate-lowering therapy and maintain their serum urate levels below 6.8 mg/dL (and preferably below 6.0 mg/dL), the prognosis is excellent with regards to eliminating gout flares. Tophaceous deposits can completely disappear, unless they have calcified. Unfortunately, if secondary osteoarthritis has developed as a result of the chronic inflammatory response to tophi, it will only progress.

Ernst ME, Fravel MA. Febuxostat: a selective xanthine oxidase/xanthine dehydrogenase inhibitor for the management of hyperuricemia in adults with gout. *Clin Ther.* 2009;31:2503. [PMID: 20109996]

Malik A, Schumacher HR, Dinnella JE, Clayburne GM. Clinical diagnostic criteria for gout: comparison with the gold standard of synovial fluid crystal analysis. *J Clin Rheumatol.* 2009;15:22. [PMID: 19125136]

Perez-Ruiz F, Dalbeth N, Urresola A, de Miguel E, Schlesinger N. Imaging of gout: findings and utility. *Arthritis Res Ther.* 2009;11:232. [PMID: 19591633]

Terkeltaub R. Update on gout: new therapeutic strategies and options. *Nat Rev Rheumatol.* 2010;6:30. [PMID: 20046204]

Wortmann RL, Schumacher HR Jr. Monosodium urate deposition arthropathy part I: review of the stages and diagnosis of gout. *Adv Stud Med.* 2005;5:133.

Wortmann RL, Schumacher HR Jr. Monosodium urate deposition arthropathy part II: treatment and long term management of patients with gout. *Adv Stud Med.* 2005;5:183.

Pseudogout: Calcium Pyrophosphate Dihydrate Crystal Deposition Disease

45

Jeffrey S. Alderman, MD
Robert L. Wortmann, MD

ESSENTIALS OF DIAGNOSIS

▶ Calcium pyrophosphate dihydrate (CPPD) crystal deposition disease can mimic gout, rheumatoid arthritis, or osteoarthritis.

▶ Pseudogout causes an intermittent monoarthritis, often of the knee or wrist.

▶ Diagnosis of pseudogout established by demonstrating CPPD crystals in joint fluid.

▶ CPPD crystal deposition disease is associated with other diseases, especially hemochromatosis and hyperparathyroidism.

General Considerations

Calcium pyrophosphate dihydrate (CPPD) deposition disease can be asymptomatic or may result in a variety of clinical presentations (Table 45–1). Although the term "pseudogout" is often used to represent the entire spectrum of CPPD, it accurately describes the acute gout-like attacks of inflammation that occur in some patients with CPPD crystal deposition disease. In fact, the name pseudogout was coined when it was discovered that a subset of patients believed to have gout actually had CPPD crystals in their synovial fluid, instead of uric crystals. CPPD deposition may give rise to clinical presentations that mimic septic arthritis, polyarticular inflammatory arthritis, or osteoarthritis (Table 45–1). In addition, CPPD crystals may coexist in synovial fluid with urate or basic calcium phosphate crystals in inflammatory and osteoarthritic-like diseases, as well as in Charcot joints.

Although the cause of CPPD crystal deposition is unknown, recent identification of mutations in the *ANKH* gene on chromosome 5p has been associated with familial chondrocalcinosis, probably through disordered inorganic pyrophosphate (PPi) transport mechanisms. Low ratios of inorganic phosphate (Pi) to inorganic pyrophosphate (PPi) favor CPPD crystal deposition in joints. Research also shows that the immune system may influence the development of pseudogout, through the secretion of interleukin-1 and other cytokines that facilitate local tissue inflammation.

Several risk factors for pseudogout have been identified. Perhaps the most important factor is aging. CPPD deposition will probably occur in everyone if they live long enough. Genetic factors also influence crystal formation, given that numerous familial cases of CPPD deposition have been described in many nationalities. Interestingly, the pattern of clinical manifestation differs from family to family. For example, disease may occur in some families at an early age that mimics a spondyloarthropathy. In other families, presentation occurs in later years with sporadic joint distribution. What is notable is the prevalence of CPPD deposition is greater in people who have suffered orthopedic trauma; symptoms may persist despite attempts to repair affected joints. Finally, several metabolic and endocrine conditions have been associated with an increased frequency of CPPD disease, including hyperparathyroidism, hemochromatosis, hypothyroidism, amyloidosis, hypomagnesemia, acromegaly, and hypophosphatasia.

Clinical Findings

A. Symptoms and Signs

Approximately 25% of patients with CPPD deposition disease exhibit the pseudogout pattern of disease. Signs and symptoms are characterized by acute, typically monoarticular inflammatory arthritis lasting for several days to 2 weeks. These self-limited attacks may vary in intensity but can occur just as abruptly as an acute gout attack. Between episodes, patients are usually asymptomatic. Nearly half of all attacks involve the knees, although pseudogout can affect other joints, including the first metatarsophalangeal joint, which is the most common site of gouty inflammation. However, attacks of pseudogout may occur spontaneously or be provoked by

Table 45–1. Conditions that may mimic CPPD crystal deposition disease.

Gout
Septic arthritis
Rheumatoid arthritis
Osteoarthritis
Spondyloarthritis
Meningitis

trauma, surgery, or severe medical illness. Differentiation of pseudogout from joint infection may be difficult and requires arthrocentesis with examination of synovial fluid for crystals and culture. Without appropriate analysis of synovial fluid, it may be impossible to differentiate pseudogout from septic arthritis.

Symptoms that mimic rheumatoid arthritis develop in nearly 5% of patients with CPPD deposition disease. These patients have low-grade inflammation in multiple, symmetric joints. Moreover, morning stiffness, fatigue, synovial thickening, joint contractures, and elevated erythrocyte sedimentation rate frequently accompany this form of arthritis. Fever and other constitutional symptoms may also be possible. Given these misleading findings, this particular variant of pseudogout is often misdiagnosed as rheumatoid arthritis. Making matters more confusing, a small percentage of patients with CPPD deposition have low titers of circulating rheumatoid factor.

Nearly half of patients with CPPD deposition have a progressive, degenerative disease termed "pseudo-osteoarthritis." Although there is some overlap with the pattern of joint involvement in primary osteoarthritis, the distribution of joint degeneration with CPPD deposition may differ. The knees are most commonly affected, followed by the wrists, metacarpophalangeal joints, hips, shoulders, elbows, and ankles. While symmetric involvement is typical, deformities and flexion contractures of affected joints are not uncommon. Several cases have been reported of severe derangement and destruction, mimicking the findings seen in Charcot joint. Valgus deformity of the knees is especially suggestive of underlying CPPD crystal deposition, as is disease localized to the patellofemoral joint. Patients with this pseudo-osteoarthritic pattern may have intermittent episodes of acute joint inflammation of varying severity, superimposed on their baseline disease state.

Rarely, CPPD crystal deposition occurs in the axial skeleton, which may potentially lead to acute neck pain. The ligamentum flavum has been the most regularly reported site of CPPD crystal deposition in the spine. At times, neck pain may be accompanied by stiffness and fever, mimicking meningitis. Crystal deposits, ligament hypertrophy, and cartilage metaplasia contribute to encroachment of the spinal cord. Infrequently, lumbar spine involvement may produce an acute radiculopathy or neurogenic claudication resulting from spinal stenosis. Thus, signs and symptoms of neurologic long tract disease, directly resulting from CPPD deposition and its related changes, may develop in some patients.

That being said, many patients with CPPD crystal deposits lack joint symptoms. Even patients with classic osteoarthritic symptoms in some joints may have other joints with crystal deposition that are completely asymptomatic and clinically normal.

B. Laboratory Findings

The critical laboratory feature of any form of CPPD crystal deposition disease is the demonstration of CPPD crystals. These are most commonly recognized in synovial fluid (Figure 45–1). Their identification requires the use of compensated polarized light microscopy. CPPD crystals are generally rhomboid-shaped and positively birefringent. They appear blue when parallel to the long axis of the compensator and yellow when perpendicular.

Arthrocentesis of patients with pseudogout (and pseudo-rheumatoid presentations) generally yields cloudy fluid with low viscosity; the white blood cell count typically ranges between 5000 and 25,000 cells/mcL. However, white blood cell counts greater than 100,000 cells/mcL have been observed, a finding that is more typically associated with septic arthritis. The white blood cells in the synovial fluid in pseudogout (or the pseudoseptic presentation) are most commonly polymorphonuclear leukocytes. Meanwhile, the fluid seen in the pseudo-osteoarthritic form is clear, viscous, and has a very low white blood cell count (generally less than 300 cells/mcL). Inflammatory presentation of CPPD crystal deposition disease may be accompanied by a peripheral blood leukocytosis with a shift to the left shift on the differential, along with an elevated erythrocyte sedimentation rate and C-reactive protein.

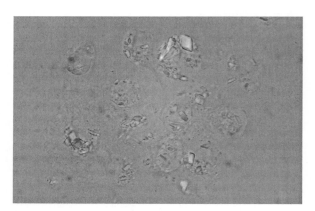

▲ **Figure 45–1.** Positive birefringent calcium pyrophosphate dihydrate crystals.

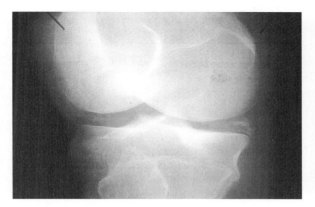

▲ **Figure 45–2.** Chondrocalcinosis of the knees.

C. Imaging Studies

The radiographic findings of punctate and linear densities in hyaline articular cartilage or fibrocartilaginous tissues are diagnostic of CPPD crystal deposition (Figure 45–2). Other radiographic features include degenerative changes in an uncommon site along with subchondral cyst formation. Radiographs most often demonstrate sites of CPPD crystal deposition in the knees, wrist (triangular cartilage of the radiocarpal joint) (Figure 45–3), and the synthesis pubis. The finding of isolated patellofemoral joint-space narrowing or degenerative change in the wrist may provide helpful clinical clues to the presence of CPPD deposition-related arthropathy.

When the deposits are typical or unequivocal, the radiographic appearance of pseudogout can be viewed as specific. However, the presence of atypical or calcific deposits can be difficult to interpret, since these changes may be confused with coexisting degenerative findings. Pseudogout can produce severe radiographic changes, marked by subchondral collapse, bone fragmentation, and intra-articular radiodense bodies.

Changes in the metacarpophalangeal joints, such as squaring of the bone ends, subchondral cysts, and hook-like osteophytes, are characteristic features of the arthritis associated with hemochromatosis. However, these changes can also be observed in patients with CPPD crystal deposition alone or related to another metabolic disorder, such as Wilson disease.

A patient can be screened for CPPD crystal deposition with four radiographs. These include an anterior-posterior view of the knees, anterior-posterior view of the pelvis, and a posterior-anterior view of both hands to include the wrists. If these views show no evidence of crystal deposition, it is unlikely that further study will be fruitful. Tomographic views may be required to identify CPPD deposits surrounding the odontoid process.

D. Specific Tests

Because of the recognized association between CPPD deposition and various metabolic diseases, the evaluation of a patient

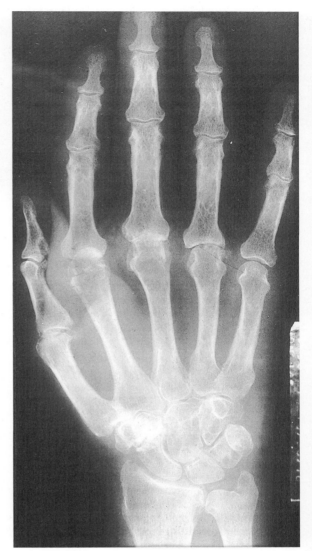

▲ **Figure 45–3.** Chondrocalcinosis of the radiocarpal triangular cartilage.

with newly diagnosed CPPD deposition should include tests of serum calcium, phosphorus, magnesium, alkaline phosphatase, thyroid-stimulating hormone levels, and possibly ferritin levels. The serum ceruloplasmin levels should also be assessed if Wilson disease is suspected. Hypophosphatasia and Wilson disease need not be considered in patients who become symptomatic after the age of 60 years.

▶ Diagnosis & Differential Diagnosis

The diagnosis of CPPD crystal deposition disease is made through the identification of CPPD crystals in tissue or

Table 45–2. Diagnostic criteria for CPPD crystal deposition disease.

Criteria

1. Demonstration of CPPD crystals and tissue or synovial fluid by definitive means (for example, characteristic x-ray defraction or chemical analysis)

2A. Identification of monoclinic or triclinic crystals showing no or weakly positive birefringence by compensated polarized light microscopy

2B. Presence of typical radiographic calcifications

3A. Acute arthritis, especially of the knees or other large joints

3B. Chronic arthritis, especially of the knee, hip, wrist, carpus, elbow, shoulder or metacarpophalangeal joint, especially if accompanied by acute exacerbations. The chronic arthritis shows the following features helpful in differentiating it from osteoarthritis:

  • **Uncommon site**—wrist, metacarpophalangeal, elbow, or shoulder joint
  • **Radiographic appearance**—radiocarpal or patellofemoral joint-space narrowing, especially if isolated (patella "wrapped around" the femur)
  • **Subchondral cyst formation for severity of degeneration**—progressive with subchondral bony collapse and fragmentation with formation of intra-articular radiodense bodies
  • **Osteophyte formation**—variable and inconstant
  • **Tendon calcification**—especially triceps, Achilles, obturators

Categories

Definite disease: Criteria for 1 or 2A must be fulfilled
Probable disease: Criteria for 2A or 2B must be fulfilled
Possible disease: Criteria for 3A or 3B should alert the clinician to the possibility of underlying

CPPD, calcium pyrophosphate dehydrate.

synovial fluid. These are definitively identified by the means of polarized light microscopy or x-ray defraction. The radiographic finding of chondrocalcinosis (calcium-containing radiodensities) in articular cartilage is also considered an indication of CPPD deposition. A criteria scheme for the diagnosis of these diseases is outlined in Table 45–2.

Because CPPD crystal deposition disease may present in many different ways, the differential diagnosis can be quite extensive. Acute monoarticular attacks of pseudogout can be misdiagnosed as gout, acute basic calcium phosphate crystal arthritis, or periarthritis. Septic arthritis must also be strongly considered in the differential diagnosis. Polyarticular or oligoarticular inflammatory presentations mirror rheumatoid arthritis and other inflammatory joint diseases. The polyarticular presentation may be difficult to distinguish from primary or posttraumatic osteoarthritis. Uncommonly, an acute inflammatory response to CPPD deposition of the ligament flavum or cervical spine can mimic meningitis.

Treatment

The recommendations for the management of acute attacks of pseudogout are exactly those that are recommended for the treatment for acute gouty arthritis (see Chapter 44). Therefore, therapeutic options include nonsteroidal anti-inflammatory drugs (NSAIDs), oral colchicine, intravenous colchicine, and intravenous or intra-articular glucocorticoids in patients who cannot tolerate oral medications.

Oral colchicine (0.5–0.6 mg once to three times daily) is useful in the patient with frequent bouts of pseudogout. However, this prophylactic therapy seems less effective in pseudogout than it is in classic gout. Nevertheless, regular colchicine can decrease the frequency of painful attacks in some patients. The management of the pseudo-osteoarthritic form of CPPD deposition disease is similar to that for the management of other forms of osteoarthritis, especially when acute attacks occur infrequently. Activity planning and pacing, assistive devices, analgesic medication (eg, NSAIDs and intra-articular glucocorticoid injections), and eventually surgery have all been proven to be effective tools. Several case studies have shown that resistant cases of pseudogout may respond to modulators of the immune system, including methotrexate and anakinra.

Unfortunately, there is no equivalent to allopurinol or a uricosuric agent for the treatment of CPPD deposition disease. Until the specific cause of this condition is determined, there will unlikely be a specific medicine that removes the crystals from joints. However, in patients with an associated metabolic condition, such as hyperparathyroidism, hemochromatosis, or hypothyroidism, treatment of the underlying disease may decrease the number of attacks but does not result in resorption of crystals.

Complications

The development of CPPD crystal deposition disease can lead to progressive degenerative damage of the joint. Findings may be severe with joint collapse and Charcot-like degeneration. Fortunately, abnormalities this severe are unusual.

Flares of pseudogout can follow general anesthesia and surgery, occurring most notably after parathyroidectomy. The sudden decline in calcium may precipitate a flare of polyarticular inflammation with fever and mental confusion.

When to Refer

Primary care clinicians can manage most cases of CPPD crystal deposition disease, if they are confident in making the diagnosis. However, patients with a puzzling clinical picture should be considered for referral to a rheumatologist, especially when symptoms of polyarticular inflammatory arthritis present in the setting of chondrocalcinosis. Moreover, patients with intractable pain from the degenerative forms of CPPD deposition should be considered for referral to an orthopedic surgeon for possible joint replacement surgery.

Canhão H, Fonseca JE, Leandro MJ, et al. Cross-sectional study of 50 patients with calcium pyrophosphate dihydrate crystal arthropathy. *Clin Rheumatol.* 2001;20:119. [PMID: 11346223]

Derfus BA, Kurian JB, Butler JJ, et al. The high prevalence of pathologic calcium crystals in pre-operative knees. *J Rheumatol.* 2002;29:570. [PMID: 11908575]

Lioté F, Ea HK. Recent developments in crystal-induced inflammation pathogenesis and management. *Curr Rheumatol Rep.* 2007;9:243. [PMID: 17531179]

McGonagle D, Tan AL, Madden J, Emery P, McDermott MF. Successful treatment of resistant pseudogout with anakinra. *Arthritis Rheum.* 2008;58:631. [PMID: 18240249]

Pay S, Terkeltaub R. Calcium pyrophosphate dihydrate and hydroxyapatite crystal deposition in the joint: new developments relevant to the clinician. *Curr Rheumatol Rep.* 2003;5:235. [PMID: 12744817]

Pons-Estel BA, Gimenez C, Sacnun M, et al. Familial osteoarthritis and Milwaukee shoulder associated with calcium pyrophosphate and apatite crystal deposition. *J Rheumatol.* 2000;27:471. [PMID: 10685816]

Reuge L, Van Linthoudt D, Gerster JC, et al. Local deposition of calcium pyrophosphate crystals in evolution of knee osteoarthritis. *Clin Rheumatol.* 2001;20:428. [PMID: 11771528]

Rosenthal AK, Mandel N. Identification of crystals in synovial fluids and joint tissues. *Curr Rheumatol Rep.* 2001;3:11. [PMID: 11177766]

Thouverey C, Bechkoff G, Pikula S, Buchet R. Inorganic pyrophosphate as a regulator of hydroxyapatite or calcium pyrophosphate dihydrate mineral deposition by matrix vesicles. *Osteoarthritis Cartilage.* 2009;17:64. [PMID: 18603452]

Disseminated Gonococcal Infection

46

Khalil G. Ghanem, MD, PhD

ESSENTIALS OF DIAGNOSIS

▶ Sexually active young person without prior joint disease.

▶ Typical presentation is triad of polyarthritis, tenosynovitis, and dermatitis.

▶ Synovial fluid Gram stain and culture are often negative.

▶ Urethral, cervical, pharyngeal, and rectal testing for *Neisseria gonorrhoeae* in aggregate are positive in up to 90% of cases.

General Considerations

Disseminated gonococcal infection (DGI) remains the most common cause of acute septic arthritis in young sexually active persons in the United States and affects persons without prior joint disease. Dissemination of *Neisseria gonorrhoeae* occurs in 0.5–3% of cases of untreated genital gonococcal infections. Women are affected with DGI 2–3 times more commonly than men, with dissemination of *N gonorrhoeae* observed most frequently within 7 days of menses, during pregnancy, or in the postpartum period.

Pathogenesis

The joint and skin manifestations of DGI are mediated by both circulating immune complexes and the direct effects of microbial proliferation. Mucosal infection with *N gonorrhoeae* always precedes the development of DGI, although this herald infection may be asymptomatic in the majority of cases. Inherited deficiencies in either the terminal complement components (C5–C9) or in properdin synthesis result in inefficient outer membrane attack of *Neisseria* species and predispose patients to dissemination of *N gonorrhoeae* from localized sites of infection.

▶ Clinical Findings

A. Symptoms and Signs

The time from sexual contact to the onset of DGI varies from 1 day to 2 months. Only 25% of patients with DGI manifest genitourinary or pharyngeal symptoms of the precedent mucosal infection.

DGI usually presents with the clinical triad of polyarthritis, tenosynovitis, and dermatitis. *N gonorrhoeae* accounts for only 20% of cases of monoarticular septic arthritis in young adults, since the most common joint presentation of DGI involves an oligoarthritis or polyarthritis. The initial symptoms include fevers, chills, and migratory symptoms of polyarthralgias, which usually progress to frank monoarthritis or polyarthritis in the knees, ankles, or wrists. Migratory symptoms of tenosynovitis occur in two thirds of patients and are most often present over the dorsum of the hand, the wrist, the ankle, or the knee. Skin lesions are seen in approximately two thirds of patients with DGI, although they are usually painless and patients may be unaware of them. Biopsy of these skin lesions demonstrates perivascular inflammation, leukocytoclastic vasculitis, intra-epidermal neutrophilic infiltration, and microthrombi; *N gonorrhoeae* can be cultured from biopsy specimens of the skin lesions approximately 10% of the time.

Unusual clinical manifestations of DGI include pericarditis, meningitis, aortitis, endocarditis, myocarditis, pyomyositis, and osteomyelitis.

B. Physical Examination

Gonococcal suppurative arthritis usually involves one or two joints, with the knees, wrists, ankles, and elbows being involved with decreasing frequency. The physical examination of these joints resembles that of septic nongonococcal arthritis. When tenosynovitis is present, there is tenderness to palpation in the periarticular regions of the wrists, fingers, toes, and ankles. The skin lesions of DGI may be asymptomatic

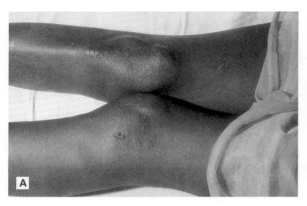
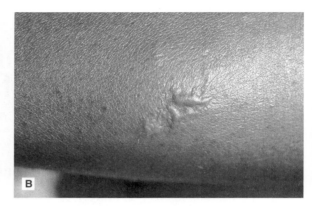

▲ **Figure 46–1. A:** Skin lesions and joint involvement in disseminated gonococcal infection (DGI). **B:** Close-up view of a pustular DGI lesion on the skin of a patient's arm. (Courtesy of Dr. Thomas F. Sellers, Public Health Image Library, CDC.)

and require careful inspection for their detection. A tender necrotic pustular lesion on an erythematous base is the classic skin lesion (Figure 46–1). However, macules and papules also occur. The rash is typically found on the distal extremities (including digits) in a relatively sparse distribution (10–25 lesions are usually found in total). Hemorrhagic bullae, erythema multiforme, and vasculitic lesions have also been reported.

C. Laboratory Findings

1. Blood cultures—Blood cultures are positive in only 20–30% of patients.

2. Synovial fluid analysis

- *Cell count and differential*: The synovial fluid cell count in gonococcal septic arthritis ranges between 30,000 and 60,000 white blood cells/mcL.

- *Gram stain for organisms*: The Gram stain for gonococcal organisms in synovial fluid is positive in less than 25% of persons with DGI (Figure 46–2).

- *Culture*: The culture for *N gonorrhoeae* in synovial fluid is positive in only 20–50% of cases, compared to 70–90% in nongonococcal septic arthritis. Reasons for this low yield of positive synovial cultures in DGI include its pathogenesis, which can involve circulating immune complexes rather than direct infection, and the fastidious growth requirements of the organism. Optimal growth conditions for the gonococcus involve the immediate plating of synovial fluid at the bedside on chocolate or Thayer-Martin media with incubation at 5–10% CO_2 concentration. *N gonorrhoeae* organisms may take more than 48 hours of incubation to grow, so the laboratory should be alerted to hold these cultures if DGI is suspected. As these stringent procedures of collection and incubation are not always followed, the yield of recovering *N gonorrhoeae*

from any culture site is usually lower than could be optimally achieved. Synovial fluid in DGI is more likely to be positive for gonococcus when the fluid has a high white blood cell count.

3. Molecular diagnostics—If DGI is suspected, urethral, cervical, pharyngeal, and rectal specimens should be collected. Nucleic acid amplification tests of genital and extragenital (rectal and pharyngeal) mucosal sites are the most sensitive diagnostic tests. They are positive in up to 90% of untreated persons. Nucleic acid amplification testing of rectal and pharyngeal specimens is not cleared by the US Food and Drug Administration, but laboratories that conduct in-house

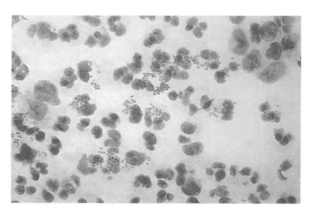

▲ **Figure 46–2.** Gram stain of purulent fluid sample showing the small intracellular gram-negative diplococci of *Neisseria gonorrhoeae* with surrounding polymorphonuclear cells. (Public Health Image Library, CDC.)

Table 46–1. Sensitivity and specificity of various nonculture-based tests for detection of *Neisseria gonorrhoeae* in genitourinary sites.

Method	Sensitivity (%)	Specificity (%)
Antigen detection	70–85	94–99
Nucleic acid amplification tests	94–100	96–100
Culture	80–95	98–100

Table 46–2. Recommended antibiotic therapy for treatment of gonococcal arthritis.

Antibiotic	Comments
Parenteral third-generation cephalosporin	• Ceftriaxone 1 g intravenously/intramuscularly every 24 hours is the first-line agent • Ceftizoxime (1 g intravenously every 8 hours) or cefotaxime (1 g intravenously every 8 hours) are second-line agents
Cefixime	• Can continue with oral therapy to complete 7–10 days (400 mg orally twice daily)

validation studies routinely provide testing of specimens from these sites. Nucleic acid amplification testing of joint fluid in DGI has been shown to be more sensitive than culture in detecting *N gonorrhoeae* but it is not routinely available (Table 46–1).

D. Imaging Studies

Imaging is usually not needed in diagnosing DGI. Radiographs almost never demonstrate abnormalities other than joint swelling, which is usually evident on physical examination. Although MRI and ultrasound may be more sensitive than physical examination in detecting tenosynovitis that is common in DGI, these imaging techniques are almost never needed for diagnosis.

▶ Differential Diagnosis

The differential diagnosis for DGI includes nongonococcal polyarticular septic arthritis, bacterial endocarditis, viral arthritis, and meningococcemia. Up to 40% of cases of meningococcemia have articular symptoms; meningococcus-associated arthritides are almost always sterile and present either as monoarticular or polyarticular disease. Postinfectious forms of arthritis (acute rheumatic fever and reactive arthritis) also can be difficult to differentiate from DGI early in their course. Both can begin abruptly and be associated with fever; tenosynovitis is often prominent in reactive arthritis, as it is in DGI.

▶ Treatment

A. Drainage

After the initial aspiration procedure to diagnose gonococcal infection in the joint, closed drainage of purulent effusions in DGI is usually only required once or twice given the brisk response of the organism to antibiotics alone. Open drainage of suppurative joints is rarely required except for joints that are difficult to drain percutaneously.

B. Antibiotics

Cephalosporins are the only class of antibiotics that are recommended as first-line agents for gonorrhea. Penicillin, tetracyclines, and fluoroquinolones are no longer recommended because of widespread resistance to these classes. Early reports of resistance to cephalosporins with concomitant clinical failures have been reported from the Far East and Western Europe. Table 46–2 lists the currently available options for initial intravenous or oral therapy for DGI. The initiation of antibiotics for DGI usually results in very rapid improvement (over 24–48 hours) in signs and symptoms, which can be a clue to the diagnosis. Unless complicated by systemic manifestations such as carditis, meningitis, endocarditis, or osteomyelitis, the duration of treatment for DGI is only 7–10 days. Intravenous therapy is usually given for 2–4 days, followed by oral therapy lasting 7–10 days. Given the high prevalence of concurrent chlamydial infections in patients with *N gonorrhoeae* infections, management of DGI usually requires additional treatment for *Chlamydia trachomatis* (eg, azithromycin or doxycycline). Sex partners of persons with DGI should be treated.

▶ Prognosis

The prognosis of arthritis in DGI is much more favorable than that of nongonococcal septic arthritis, with complete recovery in virtually all patients after the institution of appropriate antibiotic therapy.

Mathews CJ, Weston VC, Jones A, Field M, Coakley G. Bacterial septic arthritis in adults. *Lancet.* 2010;375:846. [PMID: 20206778]

Zimmerli W, Widmer AF, Blater M, Frei R, Ochsner PE. Role of rifampin for treatment of orthopedic implant-related staphylococcal infections: a randomized controlled trial. Foreign-Body Infection (FBI) Study Group. *JAMA.* 1998;279:1537. [PMID: 9605897]

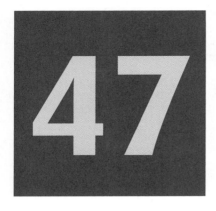

Septic Arthritis

Monica Gandhi, MD, MPH

Richard A. Jacobs, MD, PhD

Chris E. Keh, MD

SEPTIC BACTERIAL ARTHRITIS

ESSENTIALS OF DIAGNOSIS

- ▶ The classic presentation is acute onset of painful, warm, and swollen joint, usually monoarticular and affecting large weight-bearing joints.
- ▶ Synovial fluid white blood cell counts usually >50,000 cells/mcL with over 80% neutrophils.
- ▶ Positive synovial fluid culture.
- ▶ *Staphylococcus aureus* is the most common cause of septic arthritis in native joints.

▶ General Considerations

The reported incidence of septic arthritis varies from 2–10 per 100,000 per year in the general population, with substantially higher rates in patients with rheumatoid arthritis (RA) or joint prostheses (both ~30–70 cases per 100,000 per year). The incidence of bacterial arthritis is significantly higher among children than adults.

Septic (bacterial) arthritis is a medical emergency, and delay in diagnosis and treatment can lead to irreversible joint destruction and an increase in mortality. Even with the advent of better antimicrobial agents and techniques of joint incision and drainage, the rate of permanent joint damage from septic arthritis is 25–50%. The case fatality rate for monoarticular bacterial arthritis also remains high at 11%, with increased mortality rates seen in the setting of polyarticular septic arthritis (as high as 50%), underlying RA, and in immunocompromised states. Risk factors for the development of bacterial arthritis include chronic arthritic syndromes, prosthetic joints, parenteral drug use, extremes of age, diabetes mellitus, and immunocompromised conditions (Table 47–1).

▶ Pathogenesis

Bacterial pathogens reach the joint spaces by hematogenous spread (>50% of cases), direct inoculation, or spread from adjacent bony or soft-tissue infections. The lack of a limiting basement membrane and high vascularity of the synovium allows for easy bacterial access. Although skin infections are the most common predisposing infections to joint infections, transient bacteremia from respiratory, gastrointestinal, or genitourinary infections can also lead to septic arthritis. Bacteria enter the closed joint space, and within hours the synovium becomes infected, leading to synovial membrane proliferation and infiltration by polymorphonuclear and other inflammatory cells. This inflammatory response in turn leads to enzymatic and cytokine-mediated degradation of the articular cartilage, neovascularization, and the eventual development of granulation tissue. Without appropriate treatment, irreversible subchondral bone loss and cartilage destruction occur within a few days of the initial infection.

▶ Clinical Findings

A. Symptoms and Signs

The classic presentation of bacterial arthritis is the abrupt onset of a painful, warm, and swollen joint. More indolent presentations are seen in patients with preexisting rheumatic illnesses or immunocompromised states. An obvious joint effusion, moderate to severe joint tenderness to palpation, and marked restriction of both passive and active motion are common signs of septic arthritis.

A patient with an acute monoarticular arthritis should be considered to have septic arthritis until proven otherwise. Nongonococcal bacterial arthritis is monoarticular in 80–90% of cases, with polyarticular involvement (10–20%) carrying a poorer chance of survival. Polyarticular septic arthritis is more likely to occur in patients with RA or other systemic connective tissue diseases or in the syndrome of overwhelming sepsis. Infectious monoarthritis typically involves

Table 47–1. Risk factors and mechanisms of infection in bacterial arthritis.

Risk Factor	Mechanism of Infection	Comments
Rheumatoid arthritis (RA)	• Local and systemic factors play a role • Damaged joint serves as nidus for infection • Immunosuppressive medications predispose to infection, especially previous use of oral or intra-articular glucocorticoids	• RA is complicated by septic arthritis in 0.3–3% of patients • Polyarticular septic arthritis in RA has >50% mortality rate • *Staphylococcus aureus* most likely organism
Prosthetic joint	• Foreign body serves as nidus for infection, especially for pathogens that lay down biofilms or glycocalyx layer (eg, *Staphylococcus epidermidis*) • No microvasculature in artificial joint	• Rates of infection have decreased over the past 30 years • Higher incidence in revision arthroplasty (see text for details)
Injection drug use; indwelling lines; chronic skin infections	• Recurrent bacteremia with subsequent hematogenous seeding of joints • Patients receiving long-term hemodialysis, with chronic indwelling lines, with repeated skin injections (eg, insulin), or with chronic skin infections are susceptible	• The knee is the most commonly infected joint in injection drug users, but also see axial joint infections, including sternoclavicular and sacroiliac joint involvement • *S aureus* (often methicillin-resistant) most common cause in injection drug users • *Pseudomonas aeruginosa* seen in ~10% of cases
Crystal-induced arthritis (gout, pseudogout)	• Local factors • Joint damage from crystals • Synovial fluid acidosis in crystal-induced synovitis promotes cartilage damage	• Crystal-induced arthritis can cause high synovial WBC counts without infection • Presence of crystals does not rule out infection • Infection-mediated destruction of articular cartilage can rarely elicit crystals in synovial space
Severe osteoarthritis, Charcot joint, hemarthroses	• Joint disorganization, chronic synovitis, and blood within synovial space can provide a nidus for infection	• Always send a bloody synovial effusion for culture to exclude infection
Chronic, systemic disease (eg, lupus, cancer, diabetes mellitus, other immunosuppressive conditions, including extremes of age [children <5 or adults >65])	• Impaired host defenses from chronic illness, including phagocytic deficiencies • Medications for chronic illnesses (eg, glucocorticoids in lupus) predispose to infection	• *S aureus* and gram-negative bacilli most common organisms • In lupus, functional hyposplenism may occur, leading to susceptibility to encapsulated organisms (eg, *Neisseria gonorrhoeae, Salmonella, Proteus*)
Intra-articular injection (or arthrocentesis)	• Direct inoculation of the offending organism	• Most common agents are skin flora, including *S epidermidis* and *S aureus*
HIV infection	• Immunosuppression and an increased tendency to develop bacteremia with localized infections	• Even in asymptomatic HIV infection, underlying risk factors for acquiring HIV, such as injection drug use or hemophilia, can predispose
Sexual activity	• Predisposes to localized gonococcal infection, which may disseminate to cause joint and skin disease	• DGI 2–3 times more common in women than men, especially after menses or in postpartum period • Terminal complement deficiencies also predispose to DGI

DGI, disseminated gonococcal infection; WBC, white blood cell.

the knee (40–50%), hip (13–20%), shoulder (10–15%), wrist (5–8%), ankle (6–8%), elbow (3–7%), and the small joints of the hand or foot (5%). Bursitis, especially olecranon and prepatellar, may be the first manifestation of septic arthritis in patients with RA.

Septic arthritis manifests with fever in 60–80% of cases, although the temperature elevation is not usually pronounced. Twenty percent of patients with fever have shaking chills that usually correspond to waves of bacteremia. Cough, gastrointestinal symptoms, or dysuria may represent symptoms of the antecedent infection. Indeed, a preceding source

of infection, such as pneumonia, otitis, bronchitis, pharyngitis, or cutaneous, gastrointestinal, or genitourinary infection, can be identified in up to 50% of septic arthritis cases.

B. Physical Examination

The initial physical examination for septic arthritis should determine whether the source of inflammation and pain is articular or periarticular (specifically, localized to skin, bursae, or tendons). Septic arthritis produces warmth, swelling, and tenderness of the involved joint, and attempts at passive and active motion of the joint usually produce considerable discomfort. Similar findings occur in noninfectious forms of severe inflammatory arthritis, such as acute gout. In contrast, cellulitis and inflammation of bursae and tendons do not cause joint effusions, and passive motion of the adjacent joint usually does not elicit severe pain unless there is stretching of an inflamed tendon. Because septic arthritis can involve more than one joint, all joints should be examined for warmth, swelling, deformity, range of motion, pain on motion, and tenderness.

Septic arthritis of the sacroiliac (SI) joint is often difficult to distinguish from infection in the hip because both present with fever and pain upon ambulation and because examination of the SI joints is difficult (see Chapter 1). Moreover, findings of SI septic arthritis can be subtle and can be mistaken for the syndrome of a protruded disk or a paraspinous muscular strain. Similarly, infection of the shoulder joint is often difficult to identify given the usual lack of a visible effusion. Adults with shoulder infections tend to be elderly, with multiple risk factors for the development of septic arthritis. Infections of the sternoclavicular joint most often occur in injection drug users; an abscess of the chest wall or mediastinitis will develop in 20% of patients with septic arthritis of the sternoclavicular joint. Septic olecranon bursitis is distinguished from infection of the elbow joint by the presence of swelling and erythema overlying the olecranon process and the absence of joint pain with passive extension of the elbow. Infection of the olecranon bursa often follows minor trauma to the region, which leads to inoculation of organisms (usually S aureus) into the bursal space.

C. Laboratory Findings

1. Peripheral counts and cultures—Peripheral white blood cell (WBC) counts are elevated in bacterial arthritis approximately two thirds of the time. The erythrocyte sedimentation rate and C-reactive protein are usually elevated and may be useful to monitor during treatment, however, they can also be elevated in other noninfectious arthropathies. Approximately 40–50% of patients with septic arthritis have associated bacteremia, so blood cultures should be obtained prior to the administration of antibiotics. Targeted cultures from extra-articular sites, such as respiratory, cutaneous, gastrointestinal, or genitourinary sites, should also be collected after a careful history and physical examination.

2. Synovial fluid analysis—Synovial fluid analysis is critical for the definitive diagnosis of septic arthritis. Synovial fluid is usually obtained by emergent arthrocentesis, with fluoroscopic, computed tomographic (CT), or ultrasonographic guidance if necessary (see Chapter 2). An open surgical procedure may be required to obtain synovial fluid and biopsies of the synovial membrane for the diagnosis of bacterial arthritis, especially in suspected sternoclavicular, hip, or shoulder infections or in the presence of prosthetic joints. Of note, arthrocentesis is contraindicated if the needle must pass through an area of cellulitis, heavily colonized skin lesions (eg, psoriatic plaques), or infection of any kind because of the risk of introducing bacteria into the joint space. Bacteremia is also a relative contraindication for the performance of arthrocentesis.

Once synovial fluid has been collected, the following analyses should be performed (see Chapter 2):

- *Appearance*: Look for color and clarity of the fluid, since purulence or turbidity or both suggest a septic process.

- *Cell count and differential*: The joint fluid in nongonococcal septic arthritis has more than 50,000 WBC/mcL in 50–70% of cases. Low synovial fluid cell counts may be seen early in the process of infectious arthritis, in the setting of partially treated infections, or in immunosuppressed patients. The majority of WBCs in infected synovial fluid are neutrophils (usually >80% polymorphonuclear cells).

- *Gram stain for organisms*: A positive Gram stain is diagnostic for septic arthritis (highly specific), but a Gram stain that is negative for bacteria does not rule out an infected joint. The Gram stain is positive 50–75% of the time in nongonococcal bacterial arthritis, with grampositive bacterial arthritis more likely to stain positive than gram-negative bacterial arthritis. The Gram stain should be used to guide presumptive therapy.

- *Culture*: Bacterial culture of the synovial fluid is positive in 70–90% of cases of nongonococcal arthritis, depending on the organism. Inoculating synovial fluid into blood culture bottles rather than solid media increases the yield of culture growth and decreases the contamination rate.

- *Microbiology*: Table 47–2 shows the typical pathogens of nongonococcal bacterial arthritis and risk factors for their acquisition. S aureus is the most common cause of septic monoarthritis in native joints (60–70%) (Figure 47–1). The remaining causes of septic arthritis include streptococcal species, gram-negative rods, and anaerobes in relatively constant proportions. Hematogenous infection can result from transient bacteremia secondary to a remote infection or a surgical procedure, including dental work or respiratory, gastrointestinal, or genitourinary manipulations. Group A streptococci are often isolated from the infected joint after procedures in the oral cavity, whereas gastrointestinal procedures can lead to bacteremia with non–group A streptococcal species, gram-negative bacilli, or anaerobes.

D. Imaging Studies

1. Plain radiographs—Plain radiographs are of little diagnostic usefulness in acute septic arthritis but are often

Table 47–2. Major bacterial organisms implicated in nongonococcal septic arthritis and the percentage of adult infections attributable to each pathogen.

Organism	% of Adult Infections	Comments
Staphylococcus aureus	60–70%	• Most common pathogen in native joints and late prosthetic joint infections • Rates of MRSA are increasing in injection drug users and in the community
Streptococcal species	15–20%	• Group A streptococci most common streptococcal species implicated in septic arthritis • Usually preceded by primary skin or soft-tissue infection • Incidence is increasing of non-group A β-hemolytic streptococci (eg, groups B, C, and G streptococci), especially in immunocompromised persons or following gastrointestinal or genitourinary infections • *S pneumoniae* infectious arthritis is rare
Gram-negative bacilli	5–25%	• Most common in neonates, infants younger than 2 months, the elderly, injection drug users, and the chronically ill (diabetes mellitus, cancer, sickle cell anemia, connective tissue disorders, and renal transplant recipients and other immunosuppressed conditions) • Begin as urinary tract or skin infections, with subsequent hematogenous spread to a single joint • *Haemophilus influenzae* arthritis has decreased markedly since routine *H influenzae* type b childhood vaccination
Anaerobes	1–5%	• Common species include *Bacteroides, Propionibacterium acnes* (skin flora), and various anaerobic gram-positive cocci • 50% of anaerobic arthritis is polymicrobial • Predisposing factors: diabetes mellitus, immunocompromise, or postoperative wound infections, especially following total joint replacement or joint arthroplasty • Suspect if synovial fluid is foul smelling or air is present in the joint space radiologically • Collect cultures under anaerobic conditions and incubate for at least 2 weeks
Staphylococcus epidermidis	Rare in native joints	• Common in postoperative prosthetic joint infections • Forms glycocalyx layer over foreign surface • Organism often difficult to eradicate without joint removal
Brucella species	Rare	• *B melitensis* most common *Brucella* species implicated • Uncommon in the United States but more prevalent worldwide • Risk factors: ingestion of unpasteurized milk or cheese or occupational exposures (eg, farmers and meat packers) • Causes monoarthritis or an asymmetric peripheral oligoarthritis • Sacroiliitis and spondylitis also common • Diagnose with scintigraphy, CT scan, polymerase chain reaction, or positive blood or joint cultures • Treatment courses lengthy and involve antimicrobial combinations
Mycoplasma		• More common in children than adults • Seen in immunocompromised patients, particularly those with agammaglobulinemia

MRSA, methicillin-resistant *Staphylococcus aureus*.

obtained as a baseline and to exclude contiguous osteomyelitis. Radiographs usually reveal only soft-tissue swelling; in cases of infection with *Escherichia coli* or anaerobic organisms, however, radiographs may demonstrate gas formation within an untapped joint. In late septic arthritis (at least 8–10 days after infection), films may show subchondral bone destruction, periosteal new bone formation, joint-space narrowing, or osteoporosis.

2. Computed tomography—Because the hip, shoulder, sternoclavicular, and SI joints are difficult to palpate and to aspirate, evaluation of these joints usually requires CT or MRI. CT is preferred for the sternoclavicular joint. CT scans may demonstrate early bone erosions; reveal soft-tissue extension and detect effusions; and facilitate arthrocentesis of the hip, shoulder, sternoclavicular, and SI joints.

3. Magnetic resonance imaging—MRI scans demonstrate adjacent soft-tissue edema or abscesses and may be especially helpful in detecting septic sacroiliitis. MRI can also detect the early bone erosions of incipient contiguous osteomyelitis.

4. Scintigraphy—Scintigraphy makes use of various agents, such as labeled WBCs, technetium colloid, or immunoglobulin, to highlight areas of infection. The drawback of this

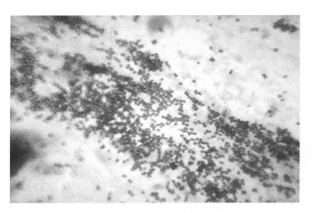

▲ **Figure 47–1.** Gram stain of an inflammatory exudate showing the clustered gram-positive cocci of *Staphylococcus aureus*. (Courtesy of Dr. Thomas F. Sellers, Public Health Image Library, CDC.)

imaging technique in the diagnosis of septic arthritis is the rate of false-positives with contiguous soft-tissue infections; scintigraphy cannot reliably differentiate septic from aseptic joint inflammation. False-positive scans can also result from underlying fracture or a recent operation. Given this low specificity, scintigraphy is rarely used as the imaging study of choice for the diagnosis of septic arthritis.

5. Gallium scan—Gallium accumulates where there is an extravasation of serum proteins and leukocytes and is better than scintigraphy in distinguishing infection from mechanical damage. Gallium scans have shown increasing usefulness in the diagnosis of septic arthritis and the identification of concurrent osteomyelitis.

▶ Differential Diagnosis

Septic arthritis usually presents as acute monoarthritis, and occasionally as an acute oligoarthritis or a polyarthritis. The differential diagnoses of these syndromes are reviewed in Chapter 4, but several points warrant emphasis here. The cause of acute monoarthritis is presumed to be infection unless proved otherwise. Differentiating infection from crystal-induced arthritis can be particularly difficult, since acute flares of pseudogout or gout can also cause fever, peripheral leukocytosis, and markedly elevated synovial cell counts. Bacterial superinfection can complicate crystal-induced arthritis, although this is rare. A history of recurrent monoarthritis, typical podagra, or radiologic evidence of chondrocalcinosis are all suggestive of crystal-induced arthritis. However, only arthrocentesis with culture of the synovial fluid and analysis for crystals can definitively distinguish septic arthritis from crystal-induced arthritis.

▶ Treatment

Early diagnosis is the key to successful treatment of septic arthritis; delay in instituting appropriate antibiotic therapy and débridement measures almost invariably leads to poor outcomes. The two mainstays of treatment are drainage and intravenous antibiotic therapy. Progressive joint mobilization also helps prevent some of the long-term complications of septic arthritis.

A. Drainage

The management of septic nongonococcal arthritis requires hospitalization for drainage of the infected joint. The joint must be thoroughly drained to decrease the number of inflammatory cells, which produce cytokines and proteolytic enzymes that cause permanent joint damage. Early arthroscopic lavage, débridement, and drain insertion have largely replaced the standard procedure of performing daily aspirations of the joint. Response to therapy can be gauged by monitoring the synovial fluid cell counts and culture results over the subsequent days of hospitalization.

Open surgical drainage and débridement (arthrotomy) may be required for the following indications:

- Failure to respond to more conservative therapy in 5–7 days.
- Coexistent osteomyelitis that needs surgical intervention.
- Involvement of joints that are difficult to drain using more conservative approaches, such as hips, shoulders, or SI joints.
- Involvement of a prosthetic joint (see section on prosthetic joint infections, below).
- Difficulty in performing adequate drainage of the joint with needle aspiration or arthroscopic manipulations.
- Refusal of the patient to accept repeated needle aspirations or catheter drainage (eg, young children).
- Open drainage is the initial procedure of choice in children with septic arthritis of the hip.

B. Antibiotics

After the initial diagnostic joint aspiration, intravenous antibiotics should be immediately administered. Empiric antibiotic therapy is based on either the initial Gram stain results or the clinical situation (Table 47–3) in suspected bacterial arthritis. The duration of antibiotic therapy has not been studied in controlled trials, but most patients are treated for at least 4 weeks. Initial therapy is administered intravenously. Once there has been improvement, transition to oral therapy can be considered if the organism is sensitive to drugs with good oral bioavailability (eg, fluoroquinolones, trimethoprim-sulfamethoxazole) and the patient is likely to be compliant. For difficult to treat organisms (*Pseudomonas*) and for *S aureus* infections associated with bacteremia, the

Table 47–3. Initial antibiotic therapy for septic arthritis based on synovial Gram stain or clinical situation.

Synovial Fluid Gram Stain or Clinical Situation	Antibiotic Therapy
Gram-positive cocci	• Use intravenous vancomycin initially due to increasing rates of MRSA in the community (dosing: 10–15 mg/kg per dose administered every 12 hours or every 8 hours; typical regimen is 1 g intravenously every 12 hours initially with doses subsequently adjusted to keep serum vancomycin troughs in the 15–20 mcg/mL range) • Switch to nafcillin 2 g intravenously every 4 hours or cefazolin 2 g intravenously every 8 hours if MSSA; if penicillin-sensitive streptococcal species, can use penicillin 12–18 million units daily in divided doses or ampicillin 2 g intravenously every 4 hours; if penicillin-resistant streptococcal species, use ceftriaxone 1–2 g intravenously every 12 hours or vancomycin • Oral options: ciprofloxacin (750 mg orally twice daily) plus rifampin (450 mg orally twice daily); combination provides bactericidal intra-articular concentrations, but these should be used only for prosthetic joint infections (see text); increasing data are available on linezolid (600 mg orally twice daily) in MRSA joint infections
Gram-negative bacilli	• Initial therapy with high-dose third-generation cephalosporin specific for gram-negative organisms (eg, ceftazidime 2 g intravenously every 8 hours, cefepime 2 g intravenously every 8 hours). Also consider piperacillin/tazobactam 4.5 g intravenously every 6 hours if concern for hospital-associated infection • If directed toward *Pseudomonas*, intravenous therapy with an aminoglycoside (eg, gentamicin 1 mg/kg intravenously every 8 hours or tobramycin 1.5 mg/kg intravenously every 8 hours) in synergistic combination with an antipseudomonal penicillin (eg, ticarcillin 4 g intravenously every 4 hours or piperacillin 4 g intravenously every 4 hours) or third-generation cephalosporin • If sensitive enteric gram-negative bacteria, can use ceftriaxone or fluoroquinolone
Injection drug use	• Initial therapy with vancomycin for MRSA, as well as single or combination therapy for *Pseudomonas* as listed for gram-negative bacilli • Tailor subsequent therapy based on culture results
Immunocompetent patient	• Initial therapy with intravenous vancomycin alone • Tailor subsequent therapy based on culture
Chronically ill or immunocompromised patient	• Initial therapy with broad coverage for gram-positive organisms (eg, vancomycin), gram-negative organisms, and anaerobes if clinically suspected; anaerobic coverage can involve adding a β-lactamase inhibitor to the antipseudomonal penicillin (eg, ticarcillin/clavulanate 3.1 g intravenously every 4 hours or piperacillin/tazobactam 3.375 g intravenously every 6 hours) or adding metronidazole 500 mg intravenously every 8 hours • Tailor subsequent therapy based on culture results
Young adults with negative smear	• Ceftriaxone 1 g intravenously every 24 hours for suspected gonococcal infection
Neonates and children <2 months old	• Broad-spectrum initial coverage for *Haemophilus influenzae* (assume ampicillin resistance, so use a third-generation cephalosporin with the doses given above), *S aureus* (vancomycin as above if MRSA; nafcillin if MSSA), group B streptococci (best covered by penicillin, although sensitive to vancomycin, ceftriaxone, and ceftizoxime) and gram-negative bacilli • Combination of vancomycin, an extended-spectrum penicillin (eg, ticarcillin or piperacillin), and an aminoglycoside (eg, gentamicin or tobramycin) often used • Tailor subsequent therapy based on culture results

MRSA, methicillin-resistant *Staphylococcus aureus;* MSSA, methicillin-sensitive *S aureus.*

entire course of therapy is usually administered parenterally. Intra-articular antibiotic instillation has not been shown to be beneficial and may lead to a chemical synovitis.

C. Mobilization

Management of septic arthritis also includes passive motion exercises to prevent formation of adhesions and to enhance the clearance of purulent exudates after the acute inflammatory response has subsided. Passive mobilization is gradually followed by active strengthening of periarticular structures to help prevent joint contractures.

▶ Complications

The major complications of septic arthritis include osteomyelitis, persistent or recurrent infection, a marked decrease in joint mobility, ankylosis, or persistent pain. Between 70% and 85% of patients with group A streptococcal infections recover without residual symptoms. Up to 50% of patients with septic arthritis secondary to *S aureus* or gram-negative rods, however, have residual joint damage. Patients with RA and polyarticular infection have a guarded prognosis, with a survival rate <50%.

PROSTHETIC JOINT INFECTIONS

ESSENTIALS OF DIAGNOSIS

▶ Prosthetic joints are at increased risk for developing infectious arthritis.

▶ Prosthetic joint infections that occur <4 weeks after the initial implantation or that are due to hematogenous seeding present with fever, pain, warmth, and swelling.

▶ Infections due to low-virulence organisms introduced at the time of surgery typically present >4 weeks after implantation with the insidious onset of pain, often without other signs of infection.

▶ Early prosthetic joint infections can usually be treated with prosthesis salvage; late infections may require replacement of the joint.

▶ General Considerations

Septic arthritis in prosthetic joints has unique characteristics in terms of incidence, risk factors, and management. The rate of prosthetic joint infection fell from 10% in the 1960s to <1% by 1990 due to improvements in surgical technique and equipment and the use of preoperative antibiotics. However, prosthetic joint infection is 5–10 times more likely with a revision arthroplasty. Prosthetic joint infections can be categorized as "early" or "late," depending on the temporal relationship to the surgical joint replacement. Early postoperative infections reflect contamination of the wound in the perioperative period from skin flora, contaminated equipment, operating room personnel, or airborne bacteria. Risk factors for early postoperative infections include prolonged duration of surgery; an inexperienced primary surgeon; and patient factors such as advanced age, underlying chronic illnesses, RA, or a perioperative nonarticular infection.

Late infections, which occur more than 1 month after the joint replacement, result from hematogenous seeding of the foreign body and damaged native tissue within the prosthetic joints or are due to low-virulence organisms (eg, coagulase-negative staphylococci, *Propionibacterium acnes*, or diphtheroids) introduced at the time of surgery. Prosthetic joint infections are often caused by microorganisms that grow in biofilms (Figure 47–2). For instance, pathogens such as *Staphylococcus epidermidis* excrete a polysaccharide ("glycocalyx") layer that covers the foreign material, creating a protected environment for further replication. Furthermore, the lack of microvasculature in the prosthetic material limits the penetration of antibiotics and host immune mediators into the joint. As a result, infections in a prosthetic joint require a much lower inoculum of microorganisms than those in a normal joint and eradication of infection is much more difficult.

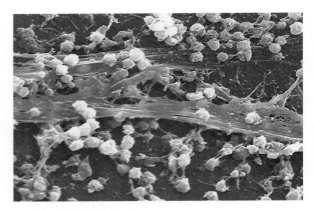

▲ **Figure 47–2.** Electron micrograph showing *Staphylococcus aureus* bacteria and development of biofilm. (Courtesy of Dr. Rodney Donlan and Janice Carr, Public Health Image Library, CDC.)

▶ Clinical Findings

A. Symptoms and Signs

Prosthetic joint infections have varying clinical presentations depending on the duration since orthopedic implant. Such infections can present early (≤4 weeks after joint replacement) or late (≥1 month after surgery). Furthermore, prosthetic joints are more susceptible to infection from hematogenous spread than normal joints throughout their lifetime because of the presence of a foreign body. Early prosthetic joint infections and those late infections due to hematogenous seeding are usually due to virulent organisms and typically present with the classic symptoms of acute bacterial arthritis with fever as well as pain, erythema, effusion, and warmth in the joint persisting beyond the postoperative period. Late infections due to less virulent organisms introduced at the time of surgery usually present with a more indolent course of increasing joint pain, implant loosening, or both, sometimes accompanied by joint drainage, but usually without concurrent fever or peripheral leukocytosis.

B. Physical Examination

The physical examination of early prosthetic joint infection or infection due to hematogenous seeding resembles that of acute suppurative arthritis, with warmth, effusion, and erythema in the joint, along with elicitation of pain with passive or active range of motion and fever. Overlying cellulitis and the formation of a sinus tract with purulent discharge may occur in early infections. The physical examination of late prosthetic joint infection is less dramatic and may reveal moderate pain with movement or joint instability.

C. Laboratory Findings

1. Peripheral counts and cultures—Peripheral WBC count may be elevated in early prosthetic joint infections but can remain normal in late indolent infections. The C-reactive protein level is elevated postoperatively from the surgery itself and should return to normal within weeks if an early postoperative infection does not occur. A combination of a normal erythrocyte sedimentation rate and C-reactive protein has been shown to be a good indicator for the absence of infection.

Blood cultures are rarely positive in late indolent infections, although they may be positive in early infections. If hematogenous spread from an extra-articular infection is suspected, targeted cultures of the involved site should be obtained. Cultures of a superficial wound or sinus tract overlying the prosthetic joint are often contaminated by skin flora and should therefore not be performed.

2. Synovial fluid analysis

- *Cell count and differential*: A synovial fluid WBC count of more than 1700 WBC/mcL has a sensitivity of 94% and a specificity of 88% for infection in a prosthetic joint in patients without underlying inflammatory joint disease. Alternatively, a neutrophil percentage >65% has 97% sensitivity and 98% specificity for infection in a prosthetic joint.

- *Gram stain for organisms*: As with septic arthritis in a normal joint, a positive Gram stain in a prosthetic joint is diagnostic for the infectious agent (highly specific), but a negative Gram stain does not rule out infection. Gram stains are less frequently positive in prosthetic joints than normal joints because frank infection can occur with a lower organism burden in the former.

- *Culture*: Cultures in aspirated synovial fluid of prosthetic joints are more frequently positive in early postoperative infections than late infections.

- *Microbiology*: The microbiology of early postoperative infections involves mainly *S aureus* and the coagulase-negative staphylococci introduced at the time of surgical repair. Late prosthetic joint infections that present at least a month after surgery usually evolve from a pathogen of low virulence or of low inoculum introduced at the time of the procedure. These pathogens include skin flora such as coagulase-negative staphylococci, *P acnes,* or diphtheroids, although anaerobes and *S aureus* can also be involved. Hematogenous infection in a prosthetic joint, as in a normal joint, can result from transient bacteremia secondary to a remote infection or a surgical or other invasive procedure and typically involves *S aureus,* streptococci, and gram-negative rods.

3. Histopathologic and microbiologic studies—Since most prosthetic joint infections need an open procedure for either débridement and retention of components or removal of the foreign material prior to replacement, tissue is often available for microscopic examination for inflammatory cells, Gram stain, or culture.

Neutrophilic infiltration on tissue specimens can be predictive of acute inflammation and infection; however, this is limited by adequate sampling. Tissue should be sent from areas with the most inflammatory changes; sensitivity reaches 80%, while specificity exceeds 90%. Alternatively, an infiltration of lymphocytes and macrophages may be indicative of chronic inflammation.

Cultures of periprosthetic tissue are the most reliable method of detecting the pathogen, with sensitivities reaching 95%. At least three intraoperative tissue specimens should be collected and testing using Gram stain and culture. Reasons for negative cultures include prior use of antimicrobials, a low organism count, fastidious organisms, or incorrect specimen handling procedures. Given that most late prosthetic joint infections are low grade, antimicrobial therapy should be discontinued 10 days to 2 weeks before tissue specimens are collected.

D. Imaging Studies

1. Plain radiographs—Plain radiographs help detect prosthetic joint infections when they are performed serially over time after implantation. New subperiosteal bone growth and transcortical sinus tracts are relatively specific for infection. Radiographs may also show zones of radiolucency at the bone-cement interface to suggest joint loosening, although loosening due to infection is difficult to distinguish from aseptic mechanical loosening.

2. Computed tomography—Prosthetic joints often have distorted joint architecture and CT imaging is better at distinguishing normal from abnormal tissue, but radiologic artifacts caused by metal implants limits its use.

3. Magnetic resonance imaging—MRI scans can only be performed in patients with implants made of safe metals, such as titanium or tantalum. Most of the newer implants are constructed of MRI-safe materials.

4. Scintigraphy—A technetium bone scan can remain positive for more than a year after uncomplicated arthroplasties because of periprosthetic bone inflammation and remodeling. Hence, nuclear scintigraphy is more useful for diagnosing late prosthetic joint infections than early infections.

▶ Differential Diagnosis

Early prosthetic joint infections are usually not subtle, but late prosthetic joint infections can manifest simply as persistent joint pain without any systemic signs of infection. Because joint pain and loosening can occur both in infection and aseptic failure of the joint, it may be difficult to distinguish late prosthetic joint infection from mechanical failure. A diagnosis of prosthetic joint infection may not be made until surgical exploration and cultures reveal purulence and a pathogen.

Treatment

Therapy of prosthetic joint infections varies by the temporal relationship of the infection to the surgical procedure. It is possible to manage infections occurring in the acute postoperative period (≤4 weeks after surgery) with surgical débridement and prolonged antibiotic therapy alone, without subsequent prosthesis removal. This treatment course has been labeled "prosthesis salvage" and has demonstrated up to a 70% success rate for early infections. Infections occurring in the late postoperative period and through hematogenous spread usually require removal of the prostheses for successful cure, although management of late prosthetic joint infections with débridement and prolonged antibiotics alone is becoming more common.

A randomized controlled trial looked at patients with stable orthopedic implants who had culture-proven staphylococcal infection and short durations of infectious symptoms (0–3 weeks). These patients all underwent surgical débridement of the joint without prosthetic material removal, followed by prolonged oral antibiotic therapy (3 months for fracture stabilization devices and prosthetic hips; 6 months for prosthetic knees) with either oral ciprofloxacin alone or a combination of oral ciprofloxacin and rifampin. The group treated with the oral antibiotic combination had a higher cure rate (100%) than the group treated with ciprofloxacin alone (58%), presumably because of rifampin's superior ability to penetrate tissues and biofilms. Factors associated with cure included stability of the orthopedic implant, a short duration of infections prior to débridement, immediate surgical débridement, and the addition of rifampin to the antibiotic regimen. Monotherapy with rifampin should never be used because resistance develops rapidly. A recent retrospective study of outcomes of treating prosthetic joint infection with débridement and retention of components followed by prolonged antibiotic therapy demonstrated that the presence of a sinus tract and a prolonged duration of symptoms prior to débridement (≥8 days) predicted treatment failure.

If surgical replacement of the device is necessary, two-stage procedures may be more successful than one-stage exchange. One-stage exchange combines removal of the infected implant, débridement, and replacement of the joint in one operation, followed by prolonged courses of antibiotics. However, management most often involves a two-stage procedure. First, the infected joint prosthesis is removed (with concomitant débridement and collection of appropriate diagnostic cultures), often with placement of a temporary cement spacer, and appropriate antibiotics are administered for at least 6 weeks. Second, revision arthroplasty is performed. Pooled data from small studies show a better cure rate with the use of antibiotic-impregnated cement than with regular cement, although randomized controlled trial data on its efficacy are lacking. Other surgical options include resection arthroplasty with permanent removal of the prosthesis and thorough débridement, as well as amputation. As with the management of septic arthritis in native joints, progressive mobilization during and after treatment helps prevent joint contractures.

Complications

The major complication of prosthetic joint infections is failure of the prosthesis and recurrent infection. Even if the patient initially does well with débridement and retention of prosthetic components and does not develop a recurrent infectious process, the joint will most likely require revision arthroplasty sooner than a joint that fails from routine wear and tear. The same risk factors that predispose to poor clinical outcomes in native joints can affect outcomes with prosthetic joint infections, including age and immune status of the patient, preceding joint disease such as RA, the virulence and susceptibilities of the organism, and the particular joint infected.

Marculescu CE, Berbari EF, Hanssen AD, et al. Outcome of prosthetic joint infections treated with debridement and retention of components. *Clin Infect Dis.* 2006;42:471. [PMID: 16421790]

Mathews CJ, Weston VC, Jones A, Field M, Coakley G. Bacterial septic arthritis in adults. *Lancet.* 2010;375:846. [PMID: 20206778]

Trampuz A, Zimmerli W. Diagnosis and treatment of implant-associated septic arthritis and osteomyelitis. *Curr Infect Dis Rep.* 2008;10:394. [PMID: 18687204]

Lyme Disease

48

Linda K. Bockenstedt, MD

ESSENTIALS OF DIAGNOSIS

▶ Lyme disease should be considered in individuals who have a reasonable risk of exposure to *Borrelia burgdorferi*-infected ticks and who have the characteristic complex of signs and symptoms.

▶ Classic clinical features occur in stages:

- Early localized disease (3–30 days after tick bite): a single hallmark skin lesion erythema migrans (EM), occasionally associated with fever, malaise, headache, arthralgias, and myalgias; less commonly, these latter symptoms can occur in the absence of EM.

- Early disseminated disease (weeks to months after tick bite): multiple EM lesions and associated fever, migratory arthralgias, and myalgias; acute pauciarticular arthritis; carditis manifested primarily as atrioventricular (AV) nodal block; neurologic features, including cranial nerve (especially facial nerve) palsies, lymphocytic meningitis, and radiculoneuropathies.

- Late disease (several months to years after tick bite): primarily neurologic features, especially peripheral neuropathies and chronic mild encephalopathy; arthritis, including monoarticular and migratory pauciarticular arthritis.

▶ Supporting serologic evidence of exposure to *B burgdorferi* is present in most cases but can be absent in early infection.

▶ General Considerations

Lyme disease is a multisystem disorder caused by infection with spirochetes of the genus *Borrelia burgdorferi* sensu lato: *B burgdorferi* sensu stricto, *B garinii*, and *B afzelii*. Hard-shelled ticks of the *Ixodes* family, primarily *I scapularis* and *I pacificus* in the United States and *I ricinus* in Europe, serve as vectors for infection. In the United States, the disease first came to medical attention in 1975 in the region around Lyme, Connecticut, where a clustering of children with presumed juvenile arthritis was observed. Lyme arthritis, as it was initially termed, was soon found to be one manifestation of systemic infection with *B burgdorferi*. Beginning with a characteristic skin lesion, erythema migrans (EM), early infection was either confined to the skin or disseminated to other sites, with disease most commonly found in the skin, heart, joints, and nervous system. Lyme disease is not a new entity; in Europe, EM had been associated with *I ricinus* tick bites since the early 20th century, and the skin disease was treated successfully with penicillin after spirochetes were visualized in biopsy specimens in the mid-1900s. Other systemic manifestations were occasionally present, especially neurologic disease (Bannwarth syndrome), but the broad clinical spectrum was not fully appreciated until the late 1970s.

Since its emergence in the United States 40 years ago, Lyme disease has become the most common vector-borne infection in this country. In 2008, 28,921 confirmed and 6277 probable cases of Lyme disease were reported to the Centers for Disease Control and Prevention (CDC) (see http://www.cdc.gov/osels/ph_surveillance/nndss/casedef/lyme_disease_2008.htm for the 2008 revised case definition of Lyme disease). More than 86% of confirmed cases originated from only 9 states: New York, Massachusetts, Pennsylvania, New Jersey, Connecticut, Maryland, Wisconsin, New Hampshire, and Minnesota. Delaware, Maine, and Virginia have experienced an increase in case reporting, accounting for an additional 8% of total confirmed cases in 2008. Cases of Lyme disease have been reported from 49 states and the District of Columbia, and also occur in other areas of North America as well as in Europe and Asia. In the latter two continents, other *B burgdorferi* sensu lato members—*B garinii* and *B afzelii*—are the main etiologic pathogens.

Lyme disease begins when humans serve as incidental bloodmeal hosts for *B burgdorferi*-infected ticks. Although all three forms of ticks—larvae, nymphs, and adults—can harbor *B burgdorferi*, nymphs are more likely to transmit infection to humans because of their promiscuous feeding patterns and small size (see CDC website for description of vector life cycle and image of ticks). *Ixodes* ticks feed only once per developmental stage, so that the incidence of Lyme disease follows the seasonal feeding patterns of nymphs (late spring, summer, and early fall). Larvae are rarely, if ever, vectors for the disease because they must first acquire infection by feeding on a reservoir host. Nymphs feed for 3–8 days, during which time spirochetes migrate from the tick midgut to the salivary gland and egress into the host through salivary secretions. Transmission of infection generally requires 24–48 hours of tick feeding, so that tick surveillance and early removal of embedded ticks is a primary preventive strategy in areas endemic for Lyme disease. Spirochetes first establish infection in the skin, where local immune responses give rise to EM, a hallmark of early, localized infection. This rash is present in up to 80% of cases and typically appears within the first month after tick bite. Thereafter, spirochetes can disseminate hematogenously to all areas of the body, but disease primarily manifests in other areas of the skin, the heart, the joints, and the nervous system.

The diagnosis of Lyme disease relies on a characteristic clinical presentation and can be supported by serologic tests showing the presence of antibodies to *B burgdorferi*. Patients may have negative test results early in the course of their treatment or, rarely, when they have been treated early with antibiotics. Most patients with Lyme disease can be treated successfully with antibiotics, with few long-term sequelae. Misdiagnosis of other conditions as Lyme disease remains the most common reason that patients do not respond to conventional therapy. Oral antibiotics for 2–4 weeks are appropriate initial therapy for all patients except those with severe cardiac or neurologic involvement, who should receive intravenous therapy. One exception may be patients with isolated Bell palsy because they respond equally well to oral antibiotics. Patients with chronic residual signs and symptoms after treatment for Lyme disease may have irreversible tissue damage, a post-Lyme fibromyalgia syndrome, or possibly infection-induced autoimmunity. Extended courses of oral or intravenous antibiotics have not been shown to provide benefit over placebo for this patient population and should be avoided unless clear objective evidence of active infection is present.

Pathogenesis

B burgdorferi survive in nature through alternating infection with ticks and reservoir hosts, including mammals and birds. Ticks feed only once per developmental stage and can lay dormant for years. Thus, spirochetes require that their vertebrate hosts survive in order to increase the probability of transmission back to ticks. In mammals, spirochetes cause disease as they initially infect and disseminate within the host, but inflammation generally resolves even if the organism is not cleared. In humans, *B burgdorferi* is difficult to culture from infected tissues except for EM lesions, but rare positive cultures have been reported at all stages of the disease, including from blood, cerebrospinal fluid (CSF), heart biopsies, and joint fluid. Recently, improved detection of *B burgdorferi* infection by large volume culture of human plasma has been reported but only in individuals with early signs of Lyme disease, such as EM, suggesting that the bloodborne phase of *B burgdorferi* infection is likely brief. In animal models, few spirochetes can be seen in infected tissues, yet an exuberant inflammatory response arises and then resolves, with spirochetes persisting in tissues. Despite transient sightings of spirochetes within cells, no intracellular phase of *B burgdorferi* infection has been documented. *B burgdorferi* uses several immune evasion mechanisms that are common to extracellular pathogens. Spirochete lipoproteins, which are expressed on internal and surface-exposed pathogen membranes, incite acute inflammation by activating innate immune cells through Toll-like receptor pattern recognition receptors. Downregulation of lipoprotein expression as spirochetes adapt to persist in the host may impede their clearance by innate immune cells and by borrelicidal antibodies targeting specific lipoproteins. Antigenic variation, particularly of the VlsE lipoprotein, has been demonstrated, providing another mechanism whereby the spirochete can evade protective antibodies. *B burgdorferi* also possesses a family of lipoproteins that bind host Factor H to impede lysis by complement. Antibiotic therapy may release internally sequestered lipoproteins from dead spirochetes and contribute to the Jarisch-Herxheimer reaction, a febrile response and transient exacerbation of symptoms noted by up to 15% of patients with Lyme disease at the start of therapy. Delayed clearance of spirochete inflammatory products may also contribute to lingering symptoms after antibiotic treatment for Lyme disease.

Prevention

The best way to prevent Lyme disease is to reduce the risk of human exposure to *B burgdorferi*-infected ticks through personal preventive behavior and environmental controls. Avoiding physical contact with common tick habitats, such as wooded areas, stone fences, woodpiles, tall grass and brush, helps limit exposure risk of individuals in areas endemic for Lyme disease. Environmental controls such as the removal of tall grass and brush, clearance of woodpiles and the application of area insecticides, can reduce the risk of human contact with infected ticks. If entry into tick habitats is anticipated, wearing protective, light-colored clothing such as long-sleeved shirts and long pants tucked into socks allows for ticks to be readily seen and reduces their access to exposed skin. Insect repellants containing diethyltoluamide (DEET) applied to the clothing and exposed skin surfaces provide added protection. Permethrin can also be sprayed on clothing and kills ticks directly.

Daily tick checks are essential for persons with exposure risk to ticks. Prompt removal of ticks embedded in the skin can effectively reduce the incidence of Lyme disease in endemic communities. Attached ticks should be removed by grasping the mouthparts with tweezers and pulling steadily up. Use of alcohol, heat, or vaso-occlusive substances will not promote tick detachment. A single 200 mg dose of doxycycline administered within 72 hours of tick bite has been shown to prevent Lyme disease. However, the risk of infection after tick-bite is low (~1.4% even in endemic areas), making the routine use of prophylactic antibiotics in individuals bitten by ticks unwarranted. Such persons should be observed for 30 days for the development of a rash at the site of tick bite or for unexplained fever, which may be indicative not only of Lyme disease but of other tick-borne infections as well.

One effective method for prevention of Lyme disease is vaccination. Two vaccines using the spirochete lipoprotein Osp A were developed and tested in humans for safety and efficacy. Although immune responses to Osp A that arise after natural infection have been associated with chronic arthritis (see below), the incidence of arthritis in patients undergoing Osp A vaccination did not differ from those receiving placebo. One of the two Osp A vaccines, LYMErix, was approved by the Food and Drug Administration; 76% of adults (aged 18–75) who received three doses of LYMErix were protected from symptomatic Lyme disease. However, limited demand for the vaccine and public concern over potential vaccine-related sequelae led to its discontinuation by the manufacturer.

▶ Clinical Findings

Lyme disease typically occurs in stages that reflect the in vivo biology of the spirochete. After establishing infection in the skin at the site of tick feeding, spirochetes that escape initial immune destruction disseminate through the skin, the blood, and the lymphatics to infect virtually any organ system. The clinical manifestations of Lyme disease thus depend on the stage of the illness at which the patient presents—early localized infection, early disseminated disease, or late disease.

A. Symptoms and Signs

1. Early localized infection—The most common early manifestation of Lyme disease is the skin rash EM, present in up to 80% of patients. EM appears within a month after exposure to *B burgdorferi*, with a median of 7–10 days, and first appears at the site of tick bite. Ticks may initially bind to clothing or exposed skin, but typically choose skin folds or creases and areas where clothes are particularly confining (eg, near elastic bands). In adults, the most common sites for EM are the popliteal fossa, gluteal fold, trunk, and axilla; in children, EM often arises near the hairline.

The most characteristic feature of EM is its morphology: a flat, macular erythematous lesion that expands rapidly, 2–3 cm/d, and which can enlarge to more than 70 cm

in diameter. The lesion should be >5 cm in diameter to fulfill diagnostic criteria. Although central clearing to produce a target or bull's-eye rash can occur in up to 40% of cases, especially when the lesion is large, more often it presents with uniform erythema. Occasionally, the center can be intensely erythematous, vesicular, or even necrotic. Despite its appearance, EM itself rarely produces much in the way of local symptoms other than tingling. Rarely, the lesion is intensely pruritic or painful. Systemic "flu-like" symptoms may be present, including low-grade fever, malaise, neck pain or stiffness, arthralgias, and myalgias; these are particularly severe in individuals with coinfection with another tick-borne pathogen, such as *Babesia microti* or *Anaplasma phagocytophilum*, the pathogen of human granulocytic ehrlichiosis. In about 18% of cases, Lyme disease can also manifest with a summer flu-like syndrome, without respiratory or gastrointestinal involvement, in the absence of EM.

2. Acute disseminated disease—Within weeks to months of initial infection, spirochetes can disseminate widely throughout the host. At this stage, infection can be present in multiple tissues but disease most commonly arises in four organ systems: the skin, the heart, the musculoskeletal system, and the nervous system. Patients are generally ill-appearing and complain of debilitating fatigue and malaise. While specific localizing signs and symptoms may be intermittent, persistent fatigue is a hallmark of untreated disseminated Lyme disease.

a. Skin—Multiple EM lesions are a sign of dissemination and arise in about 50% of patients with untreated early, localized infection. Secondary lesions have a random distribution, are smaller than the primary lesion, and less often necrotic or vesicular, although they may exhibit central clearing.

b. Musculoskeletal—A variety of musculoskeletal signs and symptoms may be present in disseminated Lyme disease. Migratory pains in muscles, joints, and periarticular structures (especially tendons and ligaments) that last only hours to days are seen in early localized infection as well as in acute disseminated disease. True inflammatory arthritis usually involves a single joint, particularly the knee, and presents with a large effusion (>50–100 mL) accompanied by stiffness and only mild pain. Other joints involved in order of frequency include the shoulder, ankle, elbow, temporomandibular joint, and wrist. It is rare for Lyme arthritis to involve more than five joints at any time. Acute Lyme arthritis is usually episodic, with attacks of monoarticular or oligoarticular arthritis lasting only weeks and decreasing in frequency with time. In most patients, the arthritis resolves completely within 5 years, even without antibiotic therapy. In a minority of patients arthritis can become chronic (see below).

c. Nervous system—Central or peripheral nervous system disease (or both) occurs in about 15% of patients with early, disseminated Lyme disease. The classic triad consists of aseptic meningitis with cranial neuropathy, especially involving the VIIth nerve, and painful peripheral radiculoneuropathy.

Central nervous system (CNS) involvement most commonly presents as aseptic meningitis, although meningoencephalitis with subtle cognitive deficits can occur. In comparison to other forms of meningitis, headache may be waxing and waning and neck stiffness is generally mild, so that a high index of suspicion may be required to make the diagnosis. Cranial neuropathy occurs in about 50% of patients with early neuroborreliosis and most often affects the facial nerve. CSF abnormalities may be present in cases of facial palsy and reflect asymptomatic CNS involvement. Although usually unilateral, bilateral facial nerve palsies occur in nearly 30% of patients with VIIth nerve involvement. Peripheral radiculoneuropathy is a mixed motor and sensory neuropathy that presents with sharp, lancinating pain in the distribution of the affected nerves and, later, hyporeflexia. Often, multiple nerves and nerve roots are involved in an asymmetric fashion. Acute radiculoneuritis is rarely seen in the United States but is common in Europe where it is also known as Bannwarth syndrome. In untreated patients, neurologic signs and symptoms can have a relapsing, remitting course over many months. Rarely, Lyme disease can be a cause of transverse myelitis.

d. Heart—Lyme carditis is relatively rare, occurring in <10% of patients with disseminated Lyme disease. Conduction system abnormalities with varying degrees of AV block are the most common cardiac manifestation, with symptomatic third-degree AV block occurring in about 50% of such patients. Occasionally, myocarditis with heart muscle dysfunction and pericarditis can also occur, but valvular disease is not found. Because Lyme carditis is usually self-limited, cardiac involvement in disseminated Lyme disease may be overlooked, especially if it remains clinically asymptomatic in comparison to other features.

e. Other organ system involvement—A variety of other organs can exhibit pathology with disseminated *B burgdorferi* infection. These include the eye (keratitis), the ear (sensorineural hearing loss), the liver (hepatitis), the spleen (necrosis), skeletal muscle (myositis), and subcutaneous tissue (panniculitis). In general, other more classic manifestations of Lyme disease are present concurrently or have been present in the recent past to suggest the diagnosis.

3. Late persistent disease—Less than 10% of patients with acute Lyme disease develop chronic manifestations of the disorder, most often in the skin, joints and nervous system. In Europe, infection with *B afzelii* is associated with the late skin lesion **acrodermatitis chronica atrophicans.** It first appears as an erythematous, hyperpigmented lesion that evolves to a chronic stage of hypopigmentation and atrophic, cellophane-like skin. Antibiotic treatment during the inflammatory phase of this lesion can lead to resolution. Chronic cardiomyopathy has been attributed to Lyme disease in Europe, but this late manifestation has not been documented in the United States.

Late neurologic manifestations include subtle cognitive dysfunction, meningoencephalitis, sensorimotor neuropathies,

and rarely, leukoencephalitis. Chronic encephalomyelitis is more commonly found in Europe where the neurotropic spirochete *B garinii* is endemic and is best documented by CSF examination and neuropsychology testing.

A small percentage of patients with acute intermittent Lyme arthritis (<10%) may subsequently evolve a pattern of chronic arthritis, usually involving a single joint and often the knee. These patients may not respond to antibiotics, particularly if polymerase chain reaction (PCR) of synovial fluid is negative for *B burgdorferi* DNA. Such "treatment-resistant" Lyme arthritis occurs primarily in patients who possess the HLA-DRB1*0401 or *0101 alleles and who have T lymphocyte and antibody responses to the spirochete lipoprotein Osp A. It has been postulated that synovitis can be perpetuated by immune responses to Osp A that cross-react with a human protein (LFA-1), which is expressed in inflamed joints, even though the spirochete itself has been eliminated. Animal studies have not supported LFA-1 as a relevant autoantigen, however. Chronic arthritis may also be due to the immune response to poorly degraded spirochete debris or to persistent infection with multiple antigenic variants transmitted by the tick.

B. Laboratory Findings

1. Routine studies (Table 48–1)—Results of laboratory studies of patients with Lyme disease depend on the stage and organ system involved. Routine laboratory tests are nonspecific, with some patients exhibiting a mild elevation in the white blood cell (neutrophil) count, erythrocyte sedimentation rate, and modest abnormalities of liver function tests. The synovial fluid from patients with acute arthritis is inflammatory. Cell counts range from 2000–100,000/mcL

Table 48–1. Laboratory tests in Lyme disease.

Test	Finding
Complete blood count	White blood cell count normal or slightly elevated (neutrophil predominance)
Erythrocyte sedimentation rate	Elevated in 50% of cases
Liver function tests	Mild elevation in GGT and ALT
ANA, rheumatoid factor	Negative
Synovial fluid	Inflammatory, cell counts ranging from 2000 to 100,000, (neutrophil predominance) Normal or elevated protein Normal glucose
Cerebrospinal fluid	Lymphocytic pleocytosis Elevated protein Normal glucose Negative oligoclonal bands

ANA, antinuclear antibody; GGT, gamma-glutamyl transpeptidase, ALA, alanine transminase.

with a predominance of neutrophils. The synovial fluid protein and glucose levels are usually normal. Serum antinuclear antibody and rheumatoid factor tests should be negative. Patients with neurologic Lyme disease, including isolated facial palsy, may have abnormalities within the CSF. A lymphocytic pleocytosis accompanied by elevated protein and normal glucose is consistent with CNS infection, but not specific for Lyme neuroborreliosis. It is debated whether all patients with isolated facial palsy should have a lumbar puncture to exclude CNS involvement, since these patients appear to respond well to oral antibiotics.

2. *B burgdorferi*-specific tests

a. Culture—In contrast to other infectious diseases for which isolation of the causative organism is a viable tool for diagnosis, it is rare to culture *B burgdorferi* from tissues and body fluids of patients with Lyme disease. EM provides an exception, with spirochetes readily cultivated from biopsies of the leading margin of the lesion. The morphologic features of EM, however, are sufficiently distinct to make this skin manifestation virtually diagnostic for Lyme disease so that biopsy and culture are rarely performed. While recovery of *B burgdorferi* from the plasma of patients is greatest early in infection when EM is present, the variability of culture medium lots for growing the spirochete make routine use of culture of any blood or tissue specimen impractical other than for research purposes.

b. Serologic tests—Serologic tests that measure antibodies to *B burgdorferi* provide evidence of exposure to the pathogen and can be used to support a clinical diagnosis of Lyme disease. A two-tiered approach to serologic testing uses an enzyme-linked immunosorbent assay (ELISA) with *B burgdorferi* antigens as a screening tool for IgM and IgG reactivity to *B burgdorferi*. IgM responses appear within the first 2–3 weeks of infection, whereas IgG responses can usually be detected after 1 month. IgM responses should be used to support a diagnosis of Lyme disease only in patients with ~4 weeks of suggestive signs and symptoms. For individuals with a clinical history of longer duration, IgG responses alone should be considered. A persistently positive IgM ELISA over many months without an IgG response suggests a false-positive test result. An immunoblot (Western blot), in which individual proteins of *B burgdorferi* are separated by molecular weight, should be used to confirm specificity of antibodies for all positive or equivocal ELISA tests, but should not be routinely performed on negative ELISA samples. Criteria for positive IgM and IgG immunoblots are listed in Table 48–2. The most commonly detected antigen, the 41 kd protein flagellin, is not unique to *B burgdorferi* and patients may have detectable antibodies because of past exposure to other bacteria with homologous proteins. Patients with early Lyme disease may initially be seronegative, but the majority will seroconvert after 1 month even with the use of antibiotics. Rarely, patients who receive inadequate antibiotic treatment for early Lyme disease may remain

Table 48–2. Criteria for Western blot interpretation in the serologic confirmation of Lyme disease.

Isotype Tested	Criteria for Positive Test
IgM	Two of the following 3 bands are present: 23 kDa (OspC), 39 kDa (BmpA), and 41 kDa (Fla)
IgG	Five of 10 bands are present: 18kDA, 21 kDa, 28 kDa, 39 kDa, 41 kDa, 45 kDa, 58 kDa (not GroEL), 66 kDa, and 93 kDa

Adapted from Centers for Disease Control and Prevention. Recommendations for Test Performance and Interpretation from the Second National Conference on Serologic Diagnosis of Lyme Disease. *MMWR.* 1995;44:590–591.

seronegative. False-positive test results are far more frequent than false-negatives, especially among patients whose pretest probability of having the disorder is low. Repetitive testing of an individual when initial acute and convalescent serologies were negative should be avoided, since this increases the risk of obtaining a false-positive result. A history of previous vaccination for Lyme disease, including participation in vaccine trials, should be obtained from patients prior to testing because standard Lyme ELISA and immunoblot tests may be positive in such individuals. Some laboratories offer modified Lyme ELISA and immunoblot tests that have eliminated the vaccine antigen, Osp A, from the assays so that infection-induced antibodies can be distinguished from those related to vaccination.

In patients with suspected neuroborreliosis, *B burgdorferi*-specific antibody testing of paired serum and CSF samples can demonstrate the production of intrathecal antibodies. If present, intrathecal *B burgdorferi*-specific antibody production is highly suggestive of CNS involvement in Lyme disease.

A peptide-based ELISA has been developed that measures antibodies to a conserved region (C6) of the VlsE protein of *B burgdorferi*. The C6 peptide ELISA has a high specificity (99%) and sensitivity (ranging from 74% in acute Lyme disease to 100% in late Lyme disease), and can be used to distinguish infection-induced antibodies in patients who have received Lyme vaccination. Recent studies suggest that the combination of Lyme ELISA (IgM and IgG) and C6 peptide ELISA may be superior to the currently recommended two-tiered approach, particularly in early infection.

Once present, antibodies to *B burgdorferi* can persist indefinitely and serologic titers should not be used to assess efficacy of antibiotic therapy. In this regard, it should be emphasized that serologic tests at best confirm exposure to the pathogen at some time in the past and are not by themselves indicative of active infection with *B burgdorferi*.

c. DNA tests—The PCR has widespread use in the diagnosis of many infectious diseases, especially for pathogens that are difficult to culture or when rapid diagnosis is critical for management. This technique has been used to detect *B burgdorferi* DNA in synovial fluid and CSF specimens from patients with Lyme disease with variable success. Up to 85% of synovial fluid samples may test positive whereas less than 40% of CSF samples from patients with Lyme meningitis yield positive results. The lower sensitivity is believed to be due, in part, to the preference of spirochetes for connective tissue rather than body fluids.

d. Other laboratory tests—A Lyme urine antigen test has been purported to detect *B burgdorferi* proteins in the urine of patients with chronic symptoms after Lyme disease, and some physicians have used this test to monitor response to treatment. This test, however, has been discredited because of its inconsistent results and marked interlaboratory variability. Currently there is no *B burgdorferi*–specific test that can be used to monitor efficacy of treatment.

C. Imaging Studies

Radiographic studies have limited use in establishing the diagnosis of Lyme disease and serve primarily to eliminate other diagnoses. Plain radiographs of inflamed joints may be normal or show only soft-tissue swelling and effusion. In contrast to septic arthritis due to other bacterial pathogens in which radiographic evidence of infection can be present early, overt changes with periarticular osteoporosis, cartilage loss, and bony erosions are relatively late findings in Lyme arthritis.

MRI scans of the brains of patients with CNS Lyme disease are generally normal, but 25% of patients with encephalopathy will have white matter lesions that may or may not enhance with gadolinium. Most patients with Lyme encephalopathy have multifocal abnormalities in cerebral blood flow on single photon emission computed tomography (SPECT) scans. These findings are not specific for Lyme encephalopathy, however, and can be seen in normal individuals. Abnormalities on SPECT scans alone should not be used as evidence of Lyme disease in the absence of suggestive clinical history and supportive serologic tests.

D. Special Tests

Specialized tests for Lyme disease are primarily used to evaluate the extent of cardiac and nervous system involvement. The electrocardiogram can show evidence of conduction system disease (especially varying degrees of AV block and escape rhythms) or, less commonly, more diffuse myocardial involvement with changes consistent with myocardial dysfunction and pericarditis. Electrophysiologic studies reveal a predilection for the AV node, but any part of the conduction system can be affected.

Patients with radicular symptoms should have nerve conduction testing and electromyography to document changes consistent with axonal polyradiculopathy. For patients with cognitive complaints, neuropsychological tests are useful to evaluate for depression and to provide objective evidence of memory loss.

▶ Differential Diagnosis

Lyme disease has been called "the new great mimicker" because its protean manifestations resemble those of other diseases. This label is misleading, however, because Lyme disease typically follows a characteristic presentation and clinical course. Accurate diagnosis requires that the patient have an appropriate clinical history and a reasonable risk of exposure to *B burgdorferi*–infected ticks. The hallmark skin lesion EM is a diagnostic criterion for early Lyme disease, but other more common skin disorders can be mistaken for EM (Table 48–3). The seasonal occurrence of EM in late spring and summer months, the size and number of lesions, and the paucity of associated cutaneous symptoms such as itch or pain are useful distinguishing features. Recently, an EM-like rash has been associated with the bite of the soft-shelled tick *Amblyomma americanum*, which is prevalent in the southeast and south central United States. The etiology of Southern Tick Associated Rash Illness (STARI) is unclear, but the disease appears localized to the skin. A noncultivatable spirochete named *Borrelia lonestari* has been found in *A americanum*, but individuals with STARI do not develop positive Lyme serology as would be expected with infection with a *B burgdorferi*-related spirochete. One patient was described in whom *B lonestari* DNA was detected in a skin biopsy of the STARI rash and in the biting tick. A subsequent study of 30 Missouri patients with STARI, however, failed to detect *B lonestari* or *B burgdorferi* DNA in biopsies of the rash.

Although early Lyme disease can less commonly present as a summer "flu-like" illness, headache, myalgia, and arthralgia are nonspecific symptoms of a variety of viral pathogens. Presence of upper respiratory symptoms or gastrointestinal complaints is unusual in Lyme disease. Patients with fibromyalgia and chronic fatigue syndrome often have debilitating fatigue and musculoskeletal complaints in the absence of objective findings or laboratory abnormalities. These syndromes are more insidious in onset than Lyme disease and patients may be symptomatic for many months or years before diagnosis. History of a sleep disturbance and the presence of trigger points on physical examination should suggest a diagnosis of fibromyalgia. Acute Lyme arthritis can mimic other causes of monoarticular or pauciarticular arthritis, including reactive arthritis and other seronegative spondylarthropathies, juvenile arthritis, and systemic lupus erythematosus. Low back pain and spine involvement is commonly seen in the seronegative spondyloarthropathies but is rare in patients with Lyme disease. Lyme arthritis patients generally have strong antibody responses to *B burgdorferi* and negative test results for rheumatoid factor and antinuclear antibodies. Presence of high titer rheumatoid factor and antinuclear antibodies can lead to false-positive ELISA tests for *B burgdorferi*, emphasizing the need to confirm ELISA results by immunoblot analysis. Other causes of acute monoarthritis, such as septic arthritis and crystal-induced disease, can usually be distinguished by

Table 48–3. Differential diagnosis of erythema migrans.

Differential Diagnosis	Seasonal Occurrence	Associated Symptoms	Location	Size	Evolution	Morphology
Erythema migrans	Yes	Mild systemic symptoms Paucity of pain or itch	Skin folds, central	Large	2–3 cm per day	See text
Tinea corporis	No	Itch	Variable	Variable	Slow progression	Ringlike; may have satellite lesion; scaling much more common
Cellulitis	No	Systemic symptoms Painful	Typically acral	Variable but rarely large except on legs	Grows more in typical cases	Usually a homogeneous erythema; tender to touch
Hypersensitivity to insect or tick bite	Yes	No	Variable	Small	Variable	Can be uniform erythema, often with tick still attached
Contact dermatitis	No	Itchy	Variable	Variable	Slow progression	Often linear (rhus) or in an area that suggests the diagnosis
Spider bite	Yes	Painful bite	Acral	Variable	Can develop dependent edema but spreads centrifugally	Often necrotic with eschar
Urticaria	No	Itch	Variable	Individual lesions vary	Individual lesions wax and wane over hours	Raised, multiple, often serpiginous around edges
Pityriasis rosea	More in spring and fall	Mild to moderate itch	Diffuse; usually not on face	Herald patch may be confused with erythema migrans	Tends to stay same day to day when it is expressed	Oval lesions, slightly scaly, with long axis oriented with skin cleavage lines
Fixed drug eruption	No	Variable, but often a burning sensation; recent drug ingestion	Fixed, often in genitals, hands, feet, and face	Variable	Tends to stay fixed	Plaque with deep violaceous hue and well-demarcated borders
Granuloma annulare	No	No	Acral	Several centimeters	Fixed over weeks to months	Tend to spread peripherally; can have central clearing
Erythema multiforme	No	Variable (may be associated with viral syndrome or medication)	Usually diffuse; often palms, soles, mucosa	Most lesions small without a single large one	Slow enlargement or stagnant over days	Target lesion is classic, but these lesions are usually much smaller than erythema migrans; often there is an obvious precipitant

Reproduced, with permission, from Edlow JA. Erythema migrans. *Med Clin North Am.* 2002;86:252.

the severity of pain and by examination of joint fluid for infectious microorganisms and crystals.

Even in areas endemic for Lyme disease, isolated facial palsy is more often found to be idiopathic in origin than due to *B burgdorferi* infection. Only a few conditions are common causes of bilateral facial palsy—Guillain-Barre syndrome, HIV infection, sarcoidosis and other causes of chronic meningitis—and these are readily distinguished from Lyme disease. Acute meningitis due to *B burgdorferi* infection resembles viral meningitis, but most patients

at this stage should have positive serologic tests for Lyme disease. The radiculoneuropathy of Lyme disease must be distinguished from neuropathy associated with disk disease or diabetes mellitus, and other infections, such as herpes zoster. Chronic encephalopathy can be confused with multiple sclerosis when the MRI scan of the brain shows evidence of white matter disease. Oligoclonal bands are generally not found in CSF of patients with Lyme disease, and multiple sclerosis patients have negative serologic tests for Lyme disease. Subtle neurocognitive deficits due to

Table 48–4. Recommended antimicrobial regimens for treatment of patients with Lyme Disease.

Drug	Dosage for Adults	Dosage for Children
Preferred oral regimens		
Amoxicillin	500 mg three times daily[a]	50 mg/kg/d in three divided doses (maximum, 500 mg per dose)[a]
Doxycycline	100 mg twice daily[b]	Not recommended for children younger than 8 years
		For children 8 years and older, 4 mg/kg/d in two divided doses (maximum, 100 mg per dose)
Cefuroxime axetil	500 mg twice daily	30 mg/kg/d in two divided doses (maximum, 500 mg per dose)
Alternative oral regimens		
Selected macrolides[c]	For recommended dosing regimens, see footnote 4 in Table 48–5	For recommended dosing regimens, see footnote 4 in Table 48–5
Preferred parenteral regimen		
Ceftriaxone	2 g intravenously once daily	50–75 mg/kg/d intravenously in a single dose (maximum, 2 g)
Alternative parenteral regimens		
Cefotaxime	2 g every 8 hours[d] intravenously	150–200 mg/kg/d intravenously in three or four divided doses (maximum, 6 g/d)[d]
Penicillin G	18–24 million units/d intravenously, divided every 4 hours[d]	200,000–400,000 units/kg/d divided every 4 hours[d] (not to exceed 18–24 million units/d)

[a]Although a high dosage given twice daily might be equally effective, in view of the absence of data on efficacy, twice-daily administration is not recommended.
[b]Tetracyclines are relatively contraindicated in pregnant or lactating women and in children younger than 8 years.
[c]Because of their lower efficacy, macrolides are reserved for patients who are unable to take or who are intolerant of tetracyclines, penicillins, and cephalosporins.
[d]Dosage should be reduced for patients with impaired renal function.
Modified, with permission, from Wormser GP, et al. The Clinical Assessment Treatment and Prevention of Lyme Disease, Human Granulocytic Anaplasmosis, and Babesiosis: Clinical Practice Guidelines by the Infectious Diseases Society of America. *Clin Infect Dis.* 2006;43:1089–1134.

chronic fatigue syndrome, fibromyalgia, or aging are often incorrectly attributed to chronic Lyme encephalopathy. As for any chronic encephalopathy, toxic-metabolic causes should be excluded.

Cardiac manifestations of Lyme disease can resemble those of acute rheumatic fever, except that valvular heart disease is absent. Coronary atherosclerotic disease, structural defects within the heart, and certain medications (especially β-blockers, calcium channel blockers, and digoxin) can lead to conduction system abnormalities characteristic of Lyme carditis. When patients have myocardial dysfunction, other infectious causes should be considered, such as infection with *coxsackievirus* A and B, *echovirus*, *Yersinia enterocolitica*, and *Rickettsia rickettsii*, the causative organism of Rocky Mountain spotted fever.

▶ Treatment

Practice guidelines for the treatment of Lyme disease have been established by the Infectious Disease Society of America (Tables 48–4 and 48–5). Because many of the manifestations of Lyme disease can resolve without specific therapy, the goal of antibiotic treatment is to hasten resolution of signs and symptoms and to prevent later clinical manifestations due to ongoing infection. This is

particularly true for facial palsy, in which the rate of recovery is the same as for untreated patients, and for cardiac involvement. Patients with localized or early disseminated disease without neurologic involvement or third-degree AV block can be treated with oral antibiotics. Although the ideal duration of antibiotics has not been firmly established, administration of oral doxycycline or amoxicillin for 14–28 days is effective therapy for EM, isolated facial palsy, first- or second-degree heart block, and acute arthritis. For isolated EM, a 10–21 day course of doxycycline may be sufficient. Doxycycline has the advantage of also being effective against *A phagocytophilum* (see below). Parenteral antibiotics should be reserved for patients with other forms of neurologic involvement (central or peripheral), recurrent arthritis after oral antibiotic therapy, or third-degree heart block. This latter group of patients should be hospitalized and monitored by telemetry for the need for temporary pacemaker insertion. The rationale for intravenous therapy for high degree heart block is that intense and prolonged inflammation may lead to irreversible cardiac damage. However, no study has directly addressed whether parenteral therapy is more effective than oral therapy in this setting, or whether other means for suppressing inflammation provide added benefit. In this regard, the use of glucocorticoids to limit cardiac inflammation may

Table 48–5. Recommended therapy for patients with Lyme disease.

Indication	Treatment	Duration, days (range)
Tick bite in the United States	Doxycycline, 200 mg in a single dose[a]; (4 mg/kg in children 8 years of age and older) and/or observation	—
Erythema migrans	Oral regimen[b,c]	14 (14–21)[d]
Early neurologic disease		
Meningitis or radiculopathy	Parenteral regimen[b,e]	14 (10–28)
Cranial nerve palsy[f]	Oral regimen[b]	14 (10–21)
Cardiac disease	Oral regimen[b,g] or parenteral regimen[b,h]	14 (14–21)
Borrelial lymphocytoma	Oral regimen[b,c]	14 (14–21)
Late disease		
Arthritis without neurologic disease	Oral regimen[b]	28
Recurrent arthritis after oral regimen	Oral regimen[b] or parenteral regimen[b]	28 / 14 (14–28)
Antibiotic-refractory arthritis[h]	Symptomatic therapy[i]	—
CNS or peripheral nervous system disease	Parenteral regimen[b]	14 (14–28)
Acrodermatitis chronica atrophicans	Oral regimen[b]	21 (14–28)
Post-Lyme disease syndrome	Consider and evaluate other potential causes of symptoms; if none is found, then administer symptomatic therapy	—

Note: Regardless of the clinical manifestations of Lyme disease, complete response to treatment may be delayed beyond the treatment duration. Relapse may occur with any of these regimens; patients with objective signs of relapse need a second course of treatment.

[a]A single dose of doxycycline may be offered to adult patients and to children >8 years of age when *all* of the following circumstances exist: (1) the attached tick can be reliably identified as an adult or nymphal *Ixodes scapularis* tick that is estimated to have been attached for ≥36 h on the basis of the degree of engorgement of the tick with blood or of certainty about the time of exposure to the rick, (2) prophylaxis can be started within 72 h after the time that the rick was removed, (3) ecologic information indicates that the local rate of these ricks with *Borrelia burgdorferi* is ≥20% *and* (4) doxycycline is not contraindicated. For patients who do not fulfill these criteria, observation is recommended.

[b]See Table 48–4.

[c]For adult patients intolerant of amoxicillin, doxycycline, and cefuroxime axetil, azithromycin (500 mg/d orally for 7–10 days), clarithromycin (500 mg twice daily orally for 14–21 days, if the patient is not pregnant), or erythromycin (500 mg four times daily orally for 14–21 days) may be given. The recommended dosages of these agents for children are as follows: azithromycin, 10 mg/kg/d (maximum, 500 mg/d; clarithromycin, 7.5 mg/kg twice daily (maximum, 500 mg per dose); and erythromycin, 12.5 mg/kg four times daily (maximum, 500 mg per dose). Patients treated with macrolides should be closely observed to ensure resolution of the clinical manifestations.

[d]Ten days of therapy is effective if doxycycline is used; the efficacy of 10-day regimens with the other first-line agents is unknown.

[e]For nonpregnant adult patients intolerant of β-lactam agents, doxycycline (200–400 mg/d orally [or intravenously, if the patient is unable to take oral medications]) in two divided doses may be adequate. For children ≥8 of age, the dosage of doxycycline for this indication is 4–8 mg/kg/d in two divided doses (maximum daily dose of 200–400 mg).

[f]Patients without clinical evidence of meningitis may be treated with an oral regimen. Parenteral antibiotic therapy is recommended for patients with both clinical and laboratory evidence of coexistent meningitis. Most of the experience in the use of oral antibiotic therapy is for patients with VIIth cranial nerve palsy. Whether oral therapy would be as effective for patients with other cranial neuropathies is unknown. The decision between oral and parenteral antimicrobial therapy for patients with other cranial neuropathies should be individualized.

[g]A parenteral antibiotic regimen is recommended at the start of therapy for patients who have been hospitalized for cardiac monitoring; an oral regimen may be substituted to complete a course of therapy or to treat ambulatory patients. A temporary pacemaker may be required for patients with advanced heart block.

[h]Antibiotic-refractory Lyme arthritis is operationally defined as persistent synovitis for at least 2 months after completion of a course of intravenous ceftriaxone (or after completion of two 4-week courses of an oral antibiotic regimen for patients who are unable to tolerate cephalosporins); in addition polymerase chain reaction of synovial fluid specimens (and synovial tissue specimens, if available) is negative for *B burgdorferi* nucleic acids.

[i]Symptomatic therapy might consist of nonsteroidal anti-inflammatory agents, intra-articular injections of glucocorticoids, or other medications; expert consultation with a rheumatologist is recommended. If persistent synovitis is associated with significant pain or if it limits function, arthroscopic synovectomy can reduce the period of joint inflammation.

CNS, central nervous system.

Modified, with permission, from Wormser GP, et al. The Clinical Assessment Treatment and Prevention of Lyme Disease, Human Granulocytic Anaplasmosis, and Babesiosis: Clinical Practice Guidelines by the Infectious Diseases Society of America. *Clin Infect Dis.* 2006;43:1089–1134.

be considered for patients with severe disease who do not respond rapidly to antibiotic therapy.

Pregnant patients and children <8 years of age can be treated in similar fashion to adult patients, except that tetracyclines should be avoided.

A puzzling feature of Lyme disease is that patients may experience a delay in resolution of symptoms after antibiotic treatment. This is particularly true for disseminated disease with neurologic abnormalities or arthritis, which may take several months to resolve. For patients with persistent arthritis, a second course of oral antibiotics (generally of 4 weeks duration) or a single 2–4 week course of parenteral therapy is reasonable after several months of observation. Repeat treatment is not recommended for chronic neurologic abnormalities unless objective signs of relapse are present.

Complications

Ixodes ticks can carry multiple pathogens simultaneously, some of which are also infectious for humans. These include *B microti*, a protozoan, and *A phagocytophilum*, the agent of human granulocytic ehrlichiosis. *B microti* infection presents as a malaria-like illness with fever, drenching sweats, and severe constitutional symptoms, especially myalgias, along with hemolytic anemia. Examining the peripheral blood smear for the characteristic "ring"-like organisms within red blood cells can make the diagnosis. *A phagocytophilum* infects granulocytes and leads to leukopenia and thrombocytopenia. The presence of morulae within granulocytes can establish a diagnosis, but PCR of peripheral blood for *A phagocytophilum* DNA or antibody testing is more sensitive. Coinfection with these pathogens should be suspected when severe constitutional symptoms and hematologic abnormalities are present in patients with Lyme disease from endemic areas. In one study of patients with *B microti* infection, 20% also tested positive by serology for exposure to *B burgdorferi*. Coinfection can increase the morbidity associated with Lyme disease; a fatality associated with Lyme carditis was reported in a patient with concomitant *Babesia* infection.

Maternal-fetal transmission of *B burgdorferi* has been reported, but earlier concerns that Lyme disease can cause congenital abnormalities appear unwarranted. Several prospective studies have failed to document an increased prevalence in adverse fetal outcomes (spontaneous abortion, premature delivery, or congenital abnormalities) among pregnant women who were treated with standard therapy for Lyme disease.

Adverse reactions from antibiotic usage occur at a frequency comparable to that seen in other infectious diseases. Cholestasis has been reported with intravenous ceftriaxone therapy, so its use should be limited to patients with disseminated disease as described above. About 15% of patients with Lyme disease may experience a Jarisch-Herxheimer reaction (see Pathogenesis above) within 24–48 hours of initiation of antibiotic therapy for Lyme disease. This condition is self-limited; supportive care with reassurance and nonsteroidal anti-inflammatory agents helps relieve symptoms.

Prognosis

Overall, most patients with Lyme disease respond to antibiotic therapy with few adverse sequelae. Complete resolution of clinical signs and symptoms may take several months, however, especially in individuals with arthritis or nervous system involvement. In some cases, permanent damage may result in residual deficits that do not improve with antibiotic therapy. A chronic arthritis unresponsive to antibiotic therapy may develop in a small percentage of patients, especially those with HLA-DRB1*0401 or *0101 genotype or Osp A antibodies. These patients are believed to be genetically predisposed to prolonged arthritis initiated by the immune response to *B burgdorferi* infection. As for other forms of chronic arthritis, treatment regimens directed toward suppression of the inflammatory response are effective. Arthroscopic synovectomy can achieve clinical remission in 80% of patients.

Patients who receive recommended treatment for Lyme disease can have persistent subjective complaints such as fatigue, memory loss, myalgias, and arthralgias. In such cases, evaluation to exclude entities other than persistent *B burgdorferi* infection should be considered. Rarely, coinfection with *B microti* or *A phagocytophilum* may explain unresolved symptoms of patients who acquired Lyme disease from areas in which ticks harbor multiple pathogens. More commonly, fibromyalgia can be seen as a consequence of Lyme disease. A clinical trial evaluating the efficacy of extended courses of antibiotics for patients with chronic unexplained symptoms after standard treatment for Lyme disease failed to show benefit over placebo. Alternative therapeutic approaches should be considered.

When to Refer

Primary care physicians who are knowledgeable about the disorder and who follow the recommended evaluation and treatment guidelines can care for most cases of early Lyme disease. Referral to a specialist is appropriate when the diagnosis is uncertain, when other tick-transmitted pathogens or pregnancy complicate *B burgdorferi* infection, or if patients do not respond to a standard course of antibiotics for presumed Lyme disease. Individuals with complications from disseminated infection should be monitored jointly by relevant subspecialists for optimum management and to exclude other disorders that have features in common with Lyme disease.

[ACP-ASIM Online - Initiative on Lyme Disease]
http://www.acponline.org/clinical_information/resources/lyme_disease/

Aguero-Rosenfeld ME, Wang G, Schwartz I, Wormser GP. Diagnosis of lyme borreliosis. *Clin Microbiol Rev.* 2005;18:484. [PMID: 16020686]

[Centers for Disease Control and Prevention: Caution regarding testing for Lyme disease]
http://www.cdc.gov/mmwr/preview/mmwrhtml/mm5405a6.htm

[Centers for Disease Control and Prevention: Lyme disease]
http://www.cdc.gov/ncidod/dvbid/lyme/index.htm

[Centers for Disease Control and Prevention: Southern tick associated rash illness]
http://www.cdc.gov/ncidod/dvbid/stari/index.htm

Feder HM Jr. Lyme disease in children. *Infect Dis Clin North Am.* 2008;22:315. [PMID: 18452804]

Feder HM Jr, Johnson BJ, O'Connell S, et al. A critical appraisal of "chronic Lyme disease". *N Engl J Med.* 2007;357:1422. [PMID: 17914043]

Halperin JJ, Shapiro ED, Logigian E, et al. Practice parameter: treatment of nervous system Lyme disease (an evidence-based review): report of the Quality Standards Subcommittee of the American Academy of Neurology. *Neurology.* 2007;69:91. [PMID: 17522387]

Klempner MS, Hu LT, Evans J, et al. Two controlled trials of antibiotic treatment in patients with persistent symptoms and a history of Lyme disease. *N Engl J Med.* 2001;345:85. [PMID: 11450676]

Marques A. Chronic Lyme disease: a review. *Infect Dis Clin North Am.* 2008;22:341. [PMID: 18452806]

[MEDLINEplus: Lyme Disease]
http://www.nlm.nih.gov/medlineplus/lymedisease.html

Stanek G, Strle F. Lyme disease: European perspective. *Infect Dis Clin North Am.* 2008;22:327. [PMID: 18452805]

Steere AC, Coburn J, Glickstein L. The emergence of Lyme disease. *J Clin Invest.* 2004;113:1093. [PMID: 15085185]

[The American Lyme Disease Foundation]
http://www.aldf.com

Wormser GP, Dattwyler RJ, Shapiro ED, et al. The clinical assessment, treatment, and prevention of Lyme disease, human granulocytic anaplasmosis, and babesiosis: clinical practice guidelines by the Infectious Diseases Society of America. *Clin Infect Dis.* 2006;43:1089. [PMID: 17029130]

Mycobacterial & Fungal Infections of Bone & Joints

Henry F. Chambers, MD

John B. Imboden, MD

INFECTIONS WITH *MYCOBACTERIUM TUBERCULOSIS*

Musculoskeletal infection with *M tuberculosis* accounts for 1–5% of cases of tuberculosis (TB) and can produce spondylitis (Pott disease), arthritis, osteomyelitis, tenosynovitis, bursitis, and pyomyositis. In developing countries, where the prevalence of TB is high, musculoskeletal TB remains an important source of morbidity and mortality, particularly among children. In the developed world, musculoskeletal TB is uncommon and largely affects adults. Immigrants from countries where TB is prevalent account for a substantial proportion of musculoskeletal TB in the United States and Europe. Musculoskeletal infection has been reported in HIV-infected persons and in patients whose TB reactivated in the setting of anti-tumor necrosis factor therapy. Tuberculosis is a reportable disease and suspected or proven cases should be reported to local public health authorities.

1. Spinal Tuberculosis (Pott Disease)

ESSENTIALS OF DIAGNOSIS

▶ Back pain.

▶ Radiographic evidence of spondylitis or spondylodisciitis.

▶ Identification of *M tuberculosis* in aspirates or biopsy specimens of skeletal lesions.

▶ General Considerations

Tuberculosis of the spine accounts for approximately 50% of musculoskeletal TB. The thoracic and lumbar vertebrae are most often affected; the cervical spine is involved in less than 10% of cases. Organisms reach the vertebrae either by hematogenous spread (at the time of initial infection or during reactivation) or through lymphatic spread from renal, pleural, or other foci of disease. Most patients do not have active TB at sites outside the skeleton. Pulmonary TB, which is the most common form of concomitant extraskeletal disease, occurs in less than 20% cases.

Infection usually begins within the body of a vertebra and then extends to involve adjacent vertebrae and disks; however, "skipping" to noncontiguous vertebrae is not rare. Soft-tissue involvement is common, and paravertebral cold abscesses develop in about 75% of cases. Isolated involvement of the posterior elements is unusual (5% in one large series).

▶ Clinical Findings

A. Symptoms and Signs

The most common presenting complaint is pain localized to the spine. The pain typically is not relieved by rest and may be present for months or longer before the patient seeks medical attention. In contrast to pulmonary TB, constitutional symptoms (weight loss, fever, and night sweats) occur in only 50% of cases.

Radicular pain is common. Approximately 50% of patients have lower extremity weakness at presentation; these figures are higher in case series from the developing world. Compression of either the cauda equina or the spinal cord by an inflammatory mass or abscess is the leading cause of neurologic compromise. Meningitis and meningomyelitis are less common. Severe spinal instability can lead to compression or ischemia of the cord. Destruction of the anterior vertebral body can result in severe angular kyphosis: the gibbus deformity of Pott disease. Paravertebral cold abscesses can track from the lumbar vertebrae along the psoas muscle and present as inguinal masses or can extend from the thoracic spine into the pleural space. Fistulae occur in a small number of patients. In a small percentage of cases, bone can become superinfected with pyogenic organisms.

B. Laboratory Findings

Routine laboratory investigations are of little diagnostic help. Patients may or may not manifest a peripheral leukocytosis. There usually is a moderate elevation in the erythrocyte sedimentation rate (ESR), but in 10% of cases the ESR is <20 mm/hour.

C. Imaging Studies

Plain radiographs can be normal early in the course of disease but then demonstrate evidence of spondylitis, including osteolysis, a combination of lytic and sclerotic lesions, and bony destruction that classically is confined to the vertebral body. Although initially there may be relative preservation of the intervertebral disk, disk narrowing is common later in the disease course. CT and MRI reveal changes earlier than plain radiography, provide greater detail of the extent of bony involvement, and can reveal paraspinal abscesses not suspected on clinical grounds. MRI permits prompt detection of compression of the spinal cord or cauda equina and is the preferred imaging technique in cases with signs or symptoms of neurologic compromise.

D. Special Tests

Most patients (75–90%) have a positive reaction to purified protein derivative (PPD). In one recent series from India, the sensitivity of an interferon-gamma release assay for TB was 84%. Cultures of material obtained by percutaneous needle aspiration of paraspinal abscesses, percutaneous needle biopsy of spinal lesions, and open surgical biopsy are positive for *M tuberculosis* in 70–90% of reported cases. Smears of biopsy material reveal acid-fast bacilli in a lower percentage (20–25%) than do smears of aspirates of paraspinal abscesses (60%). Biopsies reveal characteristic caseating granulomas in 70%. These percentages on the yields of culture, staining, and histopathology may be inflated by the relatively strict case definitions of the studies. The bacillary burden in spinal TB is low, and some writers with extensive clinical experience in endemic areas estimate that the false-negative rates of aspirates and biopsies approach 50%. Nucleic acid amplification tests may facilitate earlier diagnosis but have only been studied in small numbers of patients with spinal TB, and these tests are not approved by the Food and Drug Administration for diagnosis of extrapulmonary tuberculosis. In patients with extraspinal disease suggestive of tuberculosis, identification of *M tuberculosis* at another site is sufficient to establish the diagnosis of spinal TB.

▶ Differential Diagnosis

Pyogenic or fungal osteomyelitis or neoplasm can cause disease that is clinically indistinguishable from tuberculous spondylitis. Pyogenic vertebral osteomyelitis generally has a more acute presentation and is more often associated with fever and clinical toxicity than spinal TB. Blood cultures are positive for *Staphylococcus aureus*, streptococci, or enteric Gram-negative organisms in approximately 50% of cases of pyogenic vertebral osteomyelitis; but in up to 25% of cases, routine bone and blood cultures will not yield an organism. Imaging studies cannot reliably differentiate pyogenic and tuberculous spondylitis. Noncaseating granulomas, which occasionally are the only histologic evidence of spinal TB, can be seen on biopsy specimens of vertebral osteomyelitis due to *Brucella* or fungi (either of which can mimic spinal TB clinically). Certain imaging features, such as the presence of paravertebral abscesses, can help distinguish spinal TB from neoplastic disease, but these are not always present.

▶ Treatment

Antimicrobial therapy is the cornerstone of treatment for spinal TB. Unless there is strong suspicion of resistance to first-line drugs, most authorities recommend a 6- to 9-month course of therapy with isoniazid, rifampin, pyrazinamide, and ethambutol for 2 months followed by isoniazid and rifampin for 4–7 months.

When cultures and histopathologic studies fail to yield a definitive diagnosis, empiric therapy for tuberculosis should be considered, especially for foreign-born individuals from areas where *M tuberculosis* is endemic, those with evidence of past tuberculosis, or individuals who test positive for tuberculin skin tests or interferon-gamma release assays for TB.

The role for surgical intervention is controversial. Uncomplicated cases generally respond well to antituberculous therapy alone. A randomized trial conducted by the Medical Research Council found no additional benefit of surgery over medical therapy alone, but critics of these studies point out that there was a trend toward greater spinal instability in the medically treated groups and that patients with extensive disease were excluded. Surgery is indicated for patients with persistent neurologic deficits and spinal cord compression, with severe spinal instability, or with ongoing infection despite appropriate antibacterial therapy. A neurosurgeon or orthopedist should evaluate all patients with signs or symptoms of neurologic compromise or with spinal instability or deformity.

▶ Complications

Complications of spinal TB include destruction of vertebral bodies and disks with consequent spinal deformities and instability; paraparesis or paraplegia; and tracking of paravertebral cold abscesses to distant sites in the chest, abdomen, groin, and neck.

2. Tuberculous Arthritis

ESSENTIALS OF DIAGNOSIS

▶ Usually monoarticular with predilection for hip or knee.

▶ Periarticular abscesses and sinus tracts in late stages of disease.

▶ Culture of *M tuberculosis* from synovial fluid or biopsy.

▶ Demonstration of caseating granulomas on synovial biopsy.

▶ General Considerations

Tuberculous arthritis is the second most common form of musculoskeletal TB. Tuberculous arthritis is seen mostly in children and young adults who live in developing countries. In nonendemic regions, tuberculous arthritis tends to affect older persons. The hip is most often involved, followed by the knee. Any joint may be infected, however, and infection of non–weight-bearing joints and the sacroiliac joints were prominent in a recent European series. The great majority of cases (85%) of tuberculous arthritis are monoarticular; oligoarticular TB is an uncommon but well-recognized condition.

Tuberculous arthritis usually develops from adjacent TB osteomyelitis but also can be initiated by hematogenous spread directly to the synovium. Because *M tuberculosis* does not produce collagenases, joint destruction is more insidious than in septic arthritis due to pyogenic organisms.

▶ Clinical Findings

A. Symptoms and Signs

The classic presentation is that of a monoarthritis with pain, stiffness, and gradual loss of function over weeks to months. Some patients seek medical attention after years of symptoms. Approximately 15%, however, have an acute presentation that mimics septic arthritis or microcrystalline disease.

Constitutional symptoms such as fever, night sweats, and weight loss are present in only 50% of patients. Most patients do not have active TB elsewhere, and the chest radiograph may be normal.

On examination, there is swelling with or without warmth of the affected joint. Pain limits motion, particularly when the hip is involved. Cold abscesses and draining sinus tracts may be present in those with long-standing disease.

B. Laboratory Findings

A mild anemia is common. Peripheral leukocytosis is variable. Most patients have an elevated ESR.

C. Imaging Studies

The classic radiographic changes of tuberculous arthritis are juxta-articular osteopenia, bony erosions at the periphery of the joint, and gradual narrowing of the joint space (Phemister triad). CT and MRI detect changes earlier than plain radiography and can better visualize the extent of bony destruction. MRI is superior to CT for the detection of para-articular abscesses, sinus tract formation, and other soft-tissue abnormalities.

D. Special Tests

The great majority (>90%) of patients have a positive reaction to PPD, but false-negative tests can occur in immunocompromised patients. Synovial fluid analysis reveals inflammatory fluid; cell counts vary but usually are in the range of 10,000–20,000 cells/mcL with a predominance of neutrophils. Smears of synovial fluid reveal acid-fast bacilli in only 20% of cases, but 80% of cultures of synovial fluid grow *M tuberculosis*. Synovial biopsies yield positive cultures (>90%) and compatible histopathology (>90%) and are the test of choice when there is clinical suspicion of tuberculous arthritis and smears of synovial fluid are unrevealing. The sensitivity and specificity of nucleic acid amplification tests are not yet known for tuberculous arthritis.

▶ Differential Diagnosis

Infection with *M tuberculosis* should be suspected in any patient with an unexplained, chronic inflammatory monoarthritis. Fungal infections and non-tuberculous mycobacterial infections can have a similarly indolent course. The chronic nature of the infection may cause confusion with the spondyloarthropathies, particularly when there is sacroiliac joint involvement or in the unusual patient with oligoarticular involvement. Conversely, acute presentations of tuberculous arthritis can lead to a misdiagnosis of septic arthritis or crystal-induced arthritis. Noncaseating granulomas can be observed in synovial biopsy specimens from patients with sarcoidosis, Crohn disease, foreign body reactions, gout (rarely), brucellosis, and infections due to fungi or atypical mycobacteria.

▶ Treatment

Antimicrobial therapy is the primary treatment. Six- to 9-month regimens of isoniazid, rifampin, pyrazinamide, and ethambutol for 2 months followed by isoniazid and rifampin for 4–7 months are recommended for tuberculosis of bone and joint (see http://www.thoracic.org/statements/). Drainage or joint lavage is necessary if there is thick purulent material in the joint. Occasionally, surgical intervention is required for debridement of extensive foci of osseous infection or for drainage of cold abscesses. Arthroplasty has been successful for patients with joint destruction.

► Complications

Untreated infection leads to pannus formation that erodes cartilage and subchondral bone, eventually destroying the joint. Para-articular cold abscesses and draining sinus tracts develop in long-standing disease; the latter can be superinfected with pyogenic organisms.

3. Other Forms of Musculoskeletal TB

Spinal TB and tuberculous arthritis account for the great majority of cases of musculoskeletal TB. Although TB can cause tenosynovitis of the hand and wrist, olecranon bursitis, and trochanteric bursitis, infections of tenosynovium and bursae are more common with non-tuberculous mycobacterial species than with *M tuberculosis*. Tuberculous osteomyelitis of the phalanges can produce dactylitis, particularly in children.

Poncet disease is a polyarthritis seen with extra-articular TB. The failure to isolate *M tuberculosis* from involved joints led to the concept that Poncet disease is a reactive arthritis, but this hypothesis has been questioned.

Primary tuberculous myositis is rare and typically affects the psoas muscle. Muscle also can be infected secondarily by sites in joints or bone.

Blumberg HM, Burman WJ, Chaisson RE, et al. American Thoracic Society, Centers for Disease Control and Prevention, and the Infectious Diseases Society. American Thoracic Society/Centers for Disease Control and Prevention/Infectious Diseases Society of America: treatment of tuberculosis. *Am J Respir Crit Care Med.* 2003;167:603. [PMID: 12588714]

[Joint statement by the Centers for Disease Control and Prevention, the American Thoracic Society, and the Infectious Diseases Society of America on the treatment of tuberculosis.] http://www.thoracic.org/statements/

Kumar R, Das RK, Mahapatra AK. Role of interferon gamma release assay in the diagnosis of Pott disease. *J Neurosurg Spine.* 2010;12:462. [PMID: 20433293]

Malaviya AN, Kotwal PP. Arthritis associated with tuberculosis. *Best Pract Res Clin Rheumatol.* 2003;17:319. [PMID: 12787528]

NONTUBERCULOUS MYCOBACTERIA

Nontuberculous mycobacteria can cause bursitis, tenosynovitis, arthritis, and osteomyelitis. The disease is chronic, slowly progressive and indolent with a presentation that is similar to that of tuberculosis except that typically there is a history of surgery, a wound, an injection, or other local trauma leading to direct inoculation of the organism with subsequent infection. Bone or joint infection as a result of hematogenous dissemination is rare except in HIV-infected patients or other immunocompromised individuals. While virtually any nontuberculous mycobacterial species can cause bone or joint infection, *Mycobacterium marinum* and *M avium* complex are most frequent (Plate 49). Rapid growers (*M abscessus, M chelonei,* and *M fortuitum*) more typically cause cutaneous infection, which rarely can extend to contiguous bone or joint.

► Treatment

Infections caused by nontuberculous mycobacteria respond very slowly, and often poorly, to antimicrobial therapy. Chemotherapy and surgical excision or drainage are often used in combination. Because susceptibilities and, therefore, drugs of choice, vary from species to species, establishing a microbiologic diagnosis and susceptibility testing are essential for proper management. Clarithromycin is a particularly useful agent for *M avium* infection as one component of a three-drug combination regimen that is administered for 6–12 months. Consultation with an individual experienced in the treatment of mycobacterial infections is recommended when designing a chemotherapeutic regimen.

FUNGAL INFECTIONS

Fungal infections of bones and joints are uncommon in the United States. Histoplasmosis, coccidioidomycosis, blastomycosis, and cryptococcosis are acquired through inhalation. The primary infection is usually asymptomatic but may be associated with transient arthralgias or arthritis, probably on the basis of a hypersensitivity reaction to the pulmonary infection. Osteomyelitis and joint infection are the sequelae of disseminated infection; the clinical presentation is usually that of an indolent process and may mimic skeletal TB. Diagnosis is based on histologic demonstration of organisms on biopsy specimens of affected synovium or bone or on smears and cultures of synovial fluid and biopsy material.

1. Histoplasmosis

Primary infection with *Histoplasma capsulatum*, a soil fungus endemic in the midwestern and southeastern United States, can produce a self-limited syndrome of erythema nodosum or erythema multiforme with polyarthralgias or polyarthritis. Disseminated disease is uncommon, and infection of bone and joints is rare. In contrast, African histoplasmosis, due to *H capsulatum* var *duboisii*, frequently leads to osteomyelitis.

2. Coccidioidomycosis

Coccidioides immitis is endemic in the southwestern United States. Primary infection is usually asymptomatic but, in a minority of cases, it may result in self-limited arthralgias or arthritis, often in association with erythema nodosum or erythema multiforme. Disseminated disease, which can occur in otherwise healthy persons, commonly produces osteomyelitis and arthritis, due either to direct seeding of synovium or to extension from adjacent infected bone. The clinical presentation can be very similar to that of tuberculosis.

3. Blastomycosis

Blastomyces dermatitidis is endemic in the central and southeastern United States. Polyarthralgias may accompany the primary lung infection. Osteomyelitis develops in most patients with disseminated disease and can lead to cold abscesses and sinus tracts. Vertebral involvement can mimic spinal TB. Arthritis is uncommon and usually due to extension of infection from adjacent osteomyelitis.

4. Cryptococcosis

Cryptococcus neoformans is ubiquitous. Disseminated disease occurs in immunocompromised persons and leads to osteomyelitis, particularly of the vertebra, in 5–10% of cases. Cryptococcal arthritis is rare. Documentation of cryptococcal antigenemia strongly suggests the diagnosis.

McGill PE. Geographically specific infections and arthritis, including rheumatic syndromes associated with certain fungi and parasites, *Brucella* species and *Mycobacterium leprae. Best Pract Res Clin Rheumatol.* 2003;17:289. [PMID: 12787526]

Rheumatic Manifestations of Acute & Chronic Viral Arthritis

50

Dimitrios Vassilopoulos, MD

HEPATITIS C VIRUS

ESSENTIALS OF DIAGNOSIS

▶ Diagnosis by positive anti–hepatitis C virus (HCV) antibody confirmed by a sensitive, qualitative HCV RNA assay.

▶ Arthralgias and rarely a nonerosive arthritis are seen in patients with chronic HCV infection, with or without associated cryoglobulinemia.

▶ Coexistent rheumatoid arthritis (RA) and HCV infection can create diagnostic and therapeutic problems.

▶ General Considerations

Chronic hepatitis C is second only to hepatitis B (see next section) among the common chronic viral infection worldwide, with an estimated 170 million people infected. In the United States, chronic HCV infection affects 4.1 million people, represents the leading cause of liver transplantation and death from liver disease, and has surpassed HIV infection as a cause of death.

HCV, an RNA virus, is transmitted by the parenteral route. The most common causes of HCV transmission are injection drug use and transfusion of blood or blood-derived products before 1992. Infrequent modes of transmission include accidental exposures at work (eg, health care workers), sex, and childbirth. In a number of cases, no identifiable risk factor can be found. There is currently no vaccine available for HCV. Screening of blood products has almost eliminated the risk of post-transfusion hepatitis C. The persons at greatest risk for HCV now are injection drug users and persons with high-risk sexual behavior (multiple sexual partners).

Less than 20% of patients with acute HCV infections are symptomatic at the time of infection. Most cases of HCV, however, are associated with transition to chronicity (55–85%). The natural history of chronic HCV infection is variable. Between 5% and 20% of chronically infected HCV patients develop cirrhosis within several decades. Among cirrhotic patients, within 10 years 30% develop end-stage liver disease and 10–20% develop hepatocellular carcinoma. Factors associated with more rapid disease progression include older age, alcohol abuse, coinfection with HIV (see Chapter 51), and the presence of hepatic steatosis.

Chronic HCV infection is uniquely associated with a number of extrahepatic rheumatic manifestations including arthralgias, arthritis, sialadenitis (Sjögren-like), and cryoglobulinemic vasculitis.

▶ Pathogenesis

HCV replicates predominantly in hepatocytes after entrance into the circulation. Following acute infection, HCV RNA can be detected in the serum within 1 week. Alanine aminotransferase elevation occurs 2–3 months later. Anti-HCV antibodies can be found 1–2 months after acute infection. Acute HCV infection is not associated with rheumatic complaints (in contrast to acute hepatitis B), and many patients do not know that they are infected.

HCV exhibits tropism for hepatocytes, B lymphocytes, and salivary and lachrymal gland epithelial cells. Monoclonal and polyclonal B-cell expansions have been found in the liver and bone marrow of chronically infected patients. In approximately half of patients with chronic HCV infections, circulating cryoglobulins can be detected. However, only a minority of these patients (<5%) develop the syndrome of mixed cryoglobulinemia (see Chapter 36). Deposition of immune complexes containing cryoglobulins in different organs is the presumed disease mechanism in mixed cryoglobulinemia, characterized by purpura, arthralgias (or more rarely, arthritis), glomerulonephritis, and polyneuropathy.

HEPATITIS C–ASSOCIATED ARTHRALGIAS & ARTHRITIS

 ESSENTIALS OF DIAGNOSIS

▶ Chronic HCV infection diagnosed by positive anti-HCV antibody and confirmed by a sensitive, qualitative HCV RNA assay.

▶ Usually manifests as polyarthralgias, less often as a nonerosive arthritis.

▶ Coexisting RA and HCV infection can create diagnostic and therapeutic problems.

▶ Clinical Findings

A. Symptoms and Signs

Polyarthralgias without detectable joint swelling occur in approximately 20% of patients with chronic HCV infection. An inflammatory oligoarthritis or polyarthritis develops in between 2% and 5% of HCV-infected patients. The arthritis associated with HCV infection is relatively benign and does not lead to juxta-articular erosions or joint destruction. The majority of cases (~80%) of HCV-associated arthritis have polyarticular involvement of small joints in a RA-like distribution; a minority have monoarticular or oligoarticular involvement of large joints. Morning stiffness is present in two thirds of patients.

B. Laboratory Findings

Diagnosis of HCV infection is made initially by the detection of anti-HCV antibodies by enzyme immunoassays. A positive test should be confirmed by a qualitative assay designed to detect serum HCV RNA (by polymerase chain reaction or branched-DNA assays).

Unselected patients with chronic HCV infection display a number of autoantibodies including rheumatoid factor (40–65%), cryoglobulins (40–55%), antinuclear antibodies (10%), and antithyroid antibodies (<10%). None of these abnormalities distinguish those with articular symptoms from those without. Patients with HCV-associated arthralgias and arthritis do not have antibodies against cyclic citrullinated peptides (anti-CCP) and do not develop radiographic erosions or other findings. In patients with HCV-associated mixed cryoglobulinemia, rheumatoid factor positivity (virtually 100%) and low C4 levels (50–85%) are characteristic laboratory findings.

▶ Differential Diagnosis

It should always be kept in mind that since chronic HCV infection is not uncommon in the general population (~2%), any rheumatic condition can coexist with HCV infection. Differentiating between the arthritis associated with HCV and RA that has developed in a HCV-infected individual can be particularly difficult because the patterns of joint involvement are similar and both can have positive tests for serum rheumatoid factor. The presence of anti-CCP antibodies (present in 70% of RA patients) or erosive changes on radiographs of the hand or foot radiographs point to coexisting RA. If antinuclear antibodies are present, the differential diagnosis should include systemic lupus erythematosus.

▶ Treatment

The treatment of arthritis in the context of HCV infection is always a challenge. Patients with HCV-associated arthritis in the absence of cryoglobulinemia have been treated successfully with nonsteroidal anti-inflammatory drugs, hydroxychloroquine, and low-dose prednisone. Administration of antiviral treatment (interferon-α) has not been associated with significant improvement, and in certain cases has exacerbated the articular symptoms.

The treatment of RA in patients with coexisting HCV infection is also problematic. In mild cases, hydroxychloroquine can be tried first with or without low-dose prednisone (<7.5 mg/d). Disease-modifying drugs such as methotrexate and leflunomide are potentially hepatotoxic and should be used with extreme caution, if at all. Tumor necrosis factor-α inhibitors have also been used in patients with HCV infection without significant short-term side effects.

▶ Prognosis

The prognosis of HCV-associated inflammatory arthritis is good. According to a recent study of a large population of patients with HCV-associated cryoglobulinemia, mild disease activity is seen in half of the patients, whereas one third follow a moderate to severe course. Non-Hodgkin lymphomas can develop in some patients.

Vassilopoulos D, Manolakopoulos S. Rheumatic manifestations of hepatitis. *Curr Opin Rheumatol*. 2010;22:91. [PMID: 19864952]

Vitali C. Immunopathologic differences of Sjögren's syndrome versus sicca syndrome in HCV and HIV infection. *Arthritis Res Ther*. 2011;13:233. [PMID: 21888688]

HEPATITIS B VIRUS

 ESSENTIALS OF DIAGNOSIS

▶ Symmetric, self-limited polyarthritis accompanied by rash developing during the pre-icteric phase of acute hepatitis B.

▶ Diagnosis by hepatitis B surface antigen and IgM anti–hepatitis B core antigen.

General Considerations

Hepatitis B virus (HBV) infection is currently the most common chronic viral infection worldwide. It is estimated that 2 billion people have been exposed to the virus and 350 million are chronically infected. Every year 1 million people die of HBV-related complications, including end-stage liver disease and hepatocellular carcinoma.

HBV is an enveloped DNA virus that is transmitted parenterally, sexually, or vertically (during either childbirth or early childhood). HBV infection during the perinatal and early childhood period, though usually asymptomatic, is associated with a high rate of transition to chronicity (30–90%). In contrast, exposure to HBV during adolescence or adulthood leads to the syndrome of acute hepatitis B, followed by clearance of the virus in >95% of the cases (immunocompetent persons).

During the pre-icteric phase of acute hepatitis B, a symmetric polyarthritis accompanied by skin rash may occur. Joint complaints subside when the symptoms and signs typical of acute hepatitis (eg, jaundice) develop. Polyarthritis has been rarely reported during the course of chronic HBV infection, although it is difficult to establish a clear pathogenetic role for HBV in these cases. Polyarteritis nodosa (see Chapter 35) is a vasculitis affecting medium-sized vessels that can develop during the first few months of acute HBV infection, or more rarely during chronic HBV infection.

Pathogenesis

Both rheumatic syndromes associated with HBV infection are considered to be immune complex–mediated. The composition of the pathogenic immune complexes is a matter of controversy. Circulating HBV antigens (hepatitis B surface antigen and hepatitis B e antigen), their respective antibodies (anti–hepatitis B surface antigen and anti–hepatitis B e antigen), and complement have been detected in joints and involved blood vessels. The reason for the development of polyarteritis nodosa in some patients remains unclear.

Prevention

Through vaccination programs, HBV infection is a preventable disease. Since vaccination of infants is currently used in most countries worldwide and screening of blood and blood-derived products is a routine procedure, the most important target groups for hepatitis B prevention are those with high-risk behaviors or occupations (adolescents, injection drug users, men who have sex with men, individuals with multiple sex partners, and health care workers). HBV vaccination is generally very safe.

HEPATITIS B–ASSOCIATED ARTHRITIS

 ESSENTIALS OF DIAGNOSIS

► Symmetric, self-limited polyarthritis accompanied by rash developing during the pre-icteric phase of acute hepatitis B.
► Diagnosis by hepatitis B surface antigen and IgM anti–hepatitis B core antigen.

Clinical Findings

A. Symptoms and Signs

Exposure to HBV is followed by a long incubation period prior to the development of symptoms (6–20 weeks). HBV DNA can be detected by sensitive methods approximately 1 month after infection. During this same period, hepatitis B surface antigen and IgM anti-HBc appear in the circulation (Figure 50–1). Ten to 15 weeks after infection, serum alanine aminotransferase reaches its higher levels and typical symptoms of acute hepatitis develop.

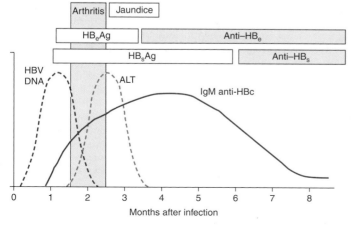

▲ **Figure 50–1.** The natural history of resolving acute hepatitis B is shown. During the pre-icteric phase, arthritis accompanied by rash can develop. The appearance of the different hepatitis B virus antigens (HB$_s$ Ag and HB$_e$ Ag) and their respective antibodies (anti-HB$_s$ and anti-HB$_e$) are also illustrated. ALT, alanine aminotransferase; IgM anti-HBc, IgM antibody against the hepatitis B virus core.

In a number of cases, 2–3 weeks prior to the onset of jaundice (the pre-icteric phase), acute polyarthritis may develop (see Figure 50–1). In the majority of cases, young adults are affected. The arthritis is characterized by its acute onset and involvement of multiple joints. The proximal interphalangeal joints, knees, and ankles are most commonly affected. An additive or rarely a migratory pattern of involvement is observed.

In 40% of cases, a rash can be detected in a urticarial, maculopapular, or (more rarely) petechial form. Other nonspecific symptoms include myalgias, malaise, and fever. There have been rare case reports of arthropathy developing during the course of chronic HBV infection, although a direct causal association cannot be proven.

B. Laboratory Findings

Most patients with HBV-associated arthritis have normal white blood cell counts and erythrocyte sedimentation rates. Rheumatoid factor has been detected in approximately 25% of the cases. Low C3 or C4 (or both) can be found in up to 40% of the cases. The diagnosis of acute hepatitis B is made by the highly elevated serum alanine aminotransferase levels and the presence of hepatitis B surface antigen and high titers of IgM anti-HBc in the circulation. Serum HBV DNA and hepatitis B e antigen may be also detected, although in many cases these have disappeared by the time of diagnosis.

▶ Differential Diagnosis

Serum sickness, other forms of viral infection associated with arthritis (erythrovirus [parvovirus], rubella, and HIV), systemic lupus erythematosus, and early RA should be included in the differential diagnosis.

▶ Treatment

Once the diagnosis has been made, no specific therapy is needed. Simple analgesics may be used for pain and fever control while nonsteroidal anti-inflammatory drugs should be avoided. There is usually no need for antiviral treatment in patients with acute hepatitis B. The decision to use antiviral treatment should be made in coordination with a hepatologist. Antiviral therapy can be used either as prophylactic treatment when immunosuppressive medications are administered, or as the main therapy when chronic hepatitis B is diagnosed (defined by elevated aminotransferase levels and moderate to severe hepatitis on liver biopsy). Lamivudine is the only agent that has been used so far as prophylactic treatment in patients receiving immunosuppression. Lamivudine is started a few weeks prior to the initiation of immunosuppressive therapy and is continued for several months after treatment discontinuation. For patients with chronic hepatitis B, currently available agents include lamivudine, adefovir, and interferon-α. Interferon-α should be used with extreme caution since it can precipitate or exacerbate autoimmune manifestations.

▶ Complications

There are no long-term sequelae of acute hepatitis B–associated arthritis. Close monitoring of liver function is needed for the rare possibility of fulminant hepatitis B (0.5–1%).

▶ Prognosis

Less than 5% of patients with acute icteric hepatitis B undergo transformations to chronic HBV infection. The overall prognosis for the joint disease associated with acute hepatitis B is excellent, with no long-term sequelae.

Inman RD. Rheumatic manifestations of hepatitis B virus infection. *Semin Arthritis Rheum.* 1982;11:406. [PMID: 7048532]

Ferri C, Govoni, M, Calabrese L. The A, B, Cs of viral hepatitis in the biologic era. *Curr Opin Rheumatol.* 2010;22:443. [PMID: 20386453]

ERYTHROVIRUS (PARVOVIRUS B19)

ESSENTIALS OF DIAGNOSIS

▶ In children, erythrovirus (parvovirus B19) is the cause of erythema infectiosum (fifth disease), the classic finding of which is the "slapped-cheek" facial rash. Only a minority of children with erythema infectiosum develop joint complaints.

▶ In adults, acute erythrovirus (parvovirus B19) infection is associated with a self-limited, symmetric polyarthritis that strongly resembles RA during its acute phase.

▶ Diagnosis is confirmed by the detection of serum anti-B19 IgM antibody.

▶ General Considerations

Human erythrovirus (parvovirus) infection is caused by erythrovirus (parvovirus B19), a small, nonenveloped, single-stranded DNA virus. Erythrovirus (parvovirus B19) infects only humans through binding to its specific receptor, blood group P antigen (globoside or Gb4). This receptor is expressed mainly on erythrocytes and erythroid precursors but also on the following cells and tissues: megakaryocytes, platelets, placental and endothelial cells, synovium, liver, lung, kidneys, and heart. Personal contact, through aerosol or respiratory secretions, is the major mode of virus transmission. Transmission through contaminated blood products (blood or clotting factor concentrate transfusion) and vertical transmission (via pregnancy) has been also documented.

Cyclic outbreaks of erythrovirus (parvovirus B19) infection occur worldwide, especially during the winter and

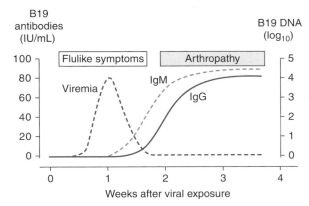

▲ **Figure 50–2.** The appearance of flulike symptoms and arthritis during the course of acute erythrovirus (parvovirus B19) infection is depicted. The timing of serum viremia and detection of IgM and IgG antibodies against erythrovirus (parvovirus B19) is also shown.

spring seasons. Children represent the major source of transmission and community epidemics. Before the age of 11, <20% of children are seropositive for IgG antibodies to erythrovirus (parvovirus B19). In contrast, 40–70% of the adult population has been exposed to the virus (as demonstrated by serum IgG anti-B19 positivity). Workers at schools or day care facilities (teachers, nurses, and day care staff) who have not been exposed previously represent the population at risk.

The time interval between viral exposure and onset of symptoms is approximately 1 week (Figure 50–2). The majority of infections during childhood remain asymptomatic. Erythrovirus (parvovirus B19) infection has been associated with a number of clinical manifestations including erythema infectiosum or fifth disease (mainly in children), arthropathy, pregnancy complications (fetal anemia, spontaneous abortion, and hydrops fetalis), transient aplastic crisis (in patients with chronic hemolytic anemias such as hereditary spherocytosis and sickle cell disease), and chronic anemia in immunocompromised hosts. Other manifestations such as vasculitis, myocarditis, hepatitis, and glomerulonephritis have been reported infrequently.

▶ Pathogenesis

Following the entrance of erythrovirus (parvovirus B19) through the respiratory tract, infection of erythroid precursors occurs. Entry into the cells is accomplished through binding to the P antigen or Gb4. Co-receptors such as $\alpha 5$ $\beta 1$ integrin and the Ku80 antigen may be also involved. Erythrovirus (parvovirus B19) replicates rapidly in the nucleus of these actively dividing cells, leading to high levels

of viremia (10^{10}–10^{12} copies/mL). The viremic phase lasts for approximately 5 days and is usually accompanied by flulike symptoms (see Figure 50–2).

The appearance of IgM antibodies marks the onset of the late viremic phase and disappearance of erythrovirus (parvovirus B19) from the circulation. IgG antibodies appear 2 weeks after exposure to the virus and indicate the transition to the antibody-response phase (see Figure 50–2). The co-appearance of IgM/IgG antibodies and the characteristic rash and arthropathy of infected individuals are consistent with an immune complex–mediated disease process. Although, the receptor for erythrovirus (parvovirus B19) is expressed in synovial cells, active replication in synovium has not been demonstrated to date.

Long-lasting protection from reinfection is mediated mainly by IgG antibodies. Sustained CD8+ T-cell responses may also contribute to this protective effect.

ARTHRITIS ASSOCIATED WITH ERYTHROVIRUS (PARVOVIRUS B19) INFECTION

▶ Clinical Findings

A. Symptoms and Signs

Joint manifestations such as arthralgias or arthritis occur in approximately 8% of children and 50–60% of adult patients with acute erythrovirus (parvovirus B19) infection. The typical arthropathy of erythrovirus (parvovirus B19) infection occurs 2 weeks after viral exposure and 1 week after the onset of flulike symptoms. Females are affected more often than males (60%). Joint manifestations of erythrovirus (parvovirus B19) comprise an acute symmetric polyarthritis that involves the hands and feet and knees and wrists in a distribution that is typical of RA. Joint pain rather than joint swelling dominates the clinical picture. The classic "slapped-cheek" facial appearance occurs in less than 20% of patients, although skin rash is common (~75%). The majority of joint symptoms subside in 2–3 weeks. Rarely, joint symptoms (arthralgias) can persist but without evidence of joint destruction.

The role (if any) of erythrovirus (parvovirus) infection in RA is highly debatable. Although erythrovirus (parvovirus B19) DNA has been found in synovial tissues of patients with chronic arthritis, this has been the case also for healthy seropositive individuals. Furthermore, most epidemiologic studies of patients with early inflammatory arthritides failed to identify erythrovirus (parvovirus B19) infection as an important etiologic factor. Erythrovirus (parvovirus) infection has been implicated in the pathogenesis or exacerbation of a variety of rheumatic disorders including vasculitis (of small, medium, and large vessels), Raynaud phenomenon, systemic lupus erythematosus, juvenile rheumatoid arthritis, and fibromyalgia. Except for some well-documented cases of small-vessel vasculitis, the evidence for the other diseases is weak.

CHAPTER 50

B. Laboratory Findings

Although cytopenias (anemia, leukopenia, thrombocytopenia, and pancytopenia) are commonly encountered during acute erythrovirus (parvovirus B19) infection, in the majority of cases of erythrovirus (parvovirus B19)–associated arthropathy, blood cell counts are normal. The erythrocyte sedimentation rate and C-reactive protein are usually normal. Antinuclear antibodies and rheumatoid factor are absent. In one study, C4 levels were decreased in one third of the cases. Transient detection of a number of autoantibodies including antinuclear antibodies, rheumatoid factor, and antibodies against double-stranded DNA or β_2-glycoprotein I have been reported during the course of acute erythrovirus (parvovirus) infection.

Diagnosis of erythrovirus (parvovirus) infection is based on the detection of specific erythrovirus (parvovirus B19) antibodies (IgM and IgG) and B19 DNA in the serum. Acute infection is documented by the detection of erythrovirus (parvovirus B19)–specific IgM antibodies. These antibodies appear 1 week after acute infection and persist for up to 6 months. Almost all patients with acute erythrovirus (parvovirus B19)–associated arthritis demonstrate these antibodies in their serum.

IgG B19 antibodies can be detected simultaneously with the IgM antibodies at the time of arthritis diagnosis. These antibodies are detected also in a large proportion of the general population (40–70%), indicating past infection.

Serum erythrovirus (parvovirus B19) DNA can be detected with various techniques with a sensitivity that ranges between 10^2 (direct DNA hybridization technique) to 10^6 genome copies per milliliter (polymerase chain reaction). During acute infection, serum B19 DNA is usually detected in association with IgM antibodies. The persistence of B19 DNA in the absence of B19 antibodies could indicate chronic erythrovirus (parvovirus B19) infection. This occurs more commonly in immunocompromised persons (patients receiving chemotherapy or long-term immunosuppression and those with HIV infection), and is usually manifested as chronic anemia. The usefulness of these methods, however, is limited by the frequent detection of B19 DNA in healthy immunocompetent individuals, making the differentiation between acute and past infection problematic. Detection of B19 DNA in tissues such as the synovium, bone marrow, and skin is not diagnostic for acute infection, since this can occur also in healthy individuals with past infection.

Differential Diagnosis

Other diseases that can present with an acute symmetric inflammatory polyarthritis involving the small joints with or without a skin rash should be included in the differential diagnosis. These include RA, systemic lupus erythematosus, other virus-associated arthritides (HCV, HBV, HIV, and rubella), and serum sickness.

Treatment

Given the self-limited course of the disease, only symptomatic therapy is recommended (eg, simple analgesics or nonsteroidal anti-inflammatory drugs). In patients with chronic courses and persistent viremia, intravenous immune globulin at a dose of 0.4 g/kg/d for 5 days can be given. There is no indication for intravenous immune globulin administration during the acute infection or in chronic cases without viremia.

Complications

Erythrovirus (parvovirus B19)–associated arthritis is a nonerosive arthropathy. No long-term complications are expected.

Prognosis

For cases with erythrovirus (parvovirus B19)–associated arthropathy the prognosis is good, without long-term sequelae.

Oiwa H, Shimada T, Hashimoto M, et al. Clinical findings in parvovirus B19 infection in 30 adult patients in Kyoto. *Mod Rheumatol.* 2011;21:24. [PMID: 20680378]

Young NS, Brown KE. Parvovirus B19. *N Engl J Med.* 2004;350:586. [PMID: 14762186]

OTHER VIRUSES

1. Alphaviruses

Alphaviruses are RNA viruses that are transmitted by mosquitoes in several areas around the world, leading to specific clinical syndromes characterized by fever, rash, and arthritis. Major Alphavirus epidemics have occurred in different areas of the world. There are 26 members of the Alphavirus genus, but only the ones that have been related to specific articular syndromes are shown in Table 50–1.

Table 50–1. Alphaviruses and arthritis.

Virus	Clinical Syndrome	Main Geographic Distribution
Sindbis	Ockelbo disease Karelian fever Pogosta disease	Norway, Sweden Russia Finland
Chikungunya	Polyarthritis, rash, fever	Africa, Southeast Asia
O'nyong-nyong	Polyarthritis, rash, fever	Africa
Mayaro	Polyarthritis, rash, fever	South America
Ross River	Epidemic polyarthritis	Australia, South Pacific
Igbo-ora	Polyarthritis, rash, fever	Ivory Coast
Barmah Forest	Polyarthritis, rash, fever	Australia

After an incubation period that lasts from 2–10 days, the typical clinical syndrome caused by these Alphaviruses begins with general complaints such as fever, myalgias, headache, and nausea. Some of these viruses (Chikungunya, O'nyong-nyong, and Mayaro) can also cause hemorrhagic phenomena such as petechiae, gastrointestinal bleeding, and epistaxis. The rash appears concomitantly or a few days after the constitutional symptoms and lasts for a week. Usually it starts from the trunk and spreads to the extremities and is maculopapular or vesicular. In some cases, itching can be a prominent feature. Desquamation is common when the rash resolves.

Articular symptoms are prominent and incapacitating in patients with Alphavirus infections. Typically, migratory polyarthralgias of the small joints of the hands and feet and wrists and ankles are accompanied by prolonged morning stiffness. In most cases, articular or periarticular swelling is prominent. Although articular symptoms can last only a few weeks, in many cases prolonged debilitating arthralgias lasting for many months or even years are observed. Serologic tests with the isolation of specific IgM antibodies against these viruses are utilized for diagnosis. There is no specific vaccine for these infections. Treatment is symptomatic.

Laine M, Luukkainen R, Toivanen A. Sindbis viruses and other alphaviruses as cause of human arthritic disease. *J Intern Med.* 2004;256:457. [PMID: 15554947]

2. Rubella Virus

Rubella virus is a togavirus that is transmitted mainly by nasopharyngeal secretions. With the introduction of the live attenuated rubella vaccine, postnatally acquired rubella infections has become very rare. Most cases involved young adults who present with malaise, fever, lymphadenopathy (posterior auricular, occipital, and cervical), and maculopapular rash. The rash begins on the face and spreads to the body. A symmetric polyarthritis involving hands, knees, and ankles can be observed in association with the appearance of the rash, particularly in female patients. Arthritis can last for several weeks. Diagnosis is made by the detection of specific IgM antibodies or by a fourfold increase in serum IgG antibodies obtained in the acute and convalescent period. Prevention of rubella infection is accomplished through administration of the live attenuated vaccine. Postvaccination arthritis has been occasionally described and in the majority of cases is mild and self-limited.

3. Human T-Lymphotropic Virus Type I

Human T-lymphotropic virus type I (HTLV-I) is a human retrovirus endemic in Japan. It is the cause of two distinct clinical syndromes: adult T-cell leukemia and HTLV-I–associated myelopathy (HAM, also known as tropical paraparesis). Furthermore, it has been implicated in a number of rheumatic/autoimmune disorders including an RA-like arthritis, a Sjögren-like syndrome, uveitis, vasculitis, and polymyositis. In certain cases, an HTLV-I–associated arthropathy has been described. Patients present with symmetric, polyarticular involvement characterized by prominent synovial proliferation. Most patients are rheumatoid factor positive and demonstrate elevation of the acute phase reactants (erythrocyte sedimentation rate and C-reactive protein). Erosive changes are present on radiographs of involved joints.

The virus is transmitted is transmitted in three ways: (1) perinatally from the infected mother to the child through breastfeeding, (2) through sexual activity, and (3) through infected blood or contaminated syringes. Diagnosis is made by serologic assays for HTLV-I (enzyme-linked immunosorbent assay) and confirmed by specific Western blot or polymerase chain reaction techniques. There is currently no treatment for HTLV-I infection. For HTLV-I associated arthropathy, treatment regimens include nonsteroidal anti-inflammatory drugs, glucocorticoids, and disease-modifying drugs.

Manns A, Hisada M, La Grenade L. Human T-lymphotropic virus type I infection. *Lancet.* 1999;353:1951. [PMID: 10371587]

Nishioka K, Sumida T, Hasunuma T. Human T lymphotropic virus type I in arthropathy and autoimmune disorders. *Arthritis Rheum.* 1996;39:1410. [PMID: 8702452]

Evaluation of Rheumatic Complaints in Patients with HIV

Khalil G. Ghanem, MD, PhD

Dimitrios Vassilopoulos, MD

Kelly A. Gebo, MD, MPH

The human retrovirus HIV infects an estimated 33 million people worldwide. Other retroviruses (eg, human T-lymphotropic virus type I) have been reported to be associated with inflammatory arthropathies, so it is not surprising that a number of rheumatologic manifestations have been described in HIV-infected persons (Table 51–1). These include various arthropathies, muscle diseases, bone disorders, symptoms and signs mimicking Sjögren syndrome, and systemic vasculitis. For some of these disorders, a clear pathophysiologic association with HIV has been established. For others, true relationships remain speculative. Geographic predisposition among HIV-infected persons to certain rheumatologic conditions is suggested by a number of studies.

ESSENTIALS OF DIAGNOSIS

▶ Diagnosis of HIV infection is made by serologic tests (enzyme-linked immunosorbent assay) and confirmed by Western blot.

▶ HIV causes nonspecific B-cell activation resulting in a polyclonal hypergammaglobulinemia and a high frequency of false-positive autoantibody tests.

▶ Rheumatologic manifestations include arthralgias, increased severity (and possibly increased incidence) of seronegative spondyloarthropathies, musculoskeletal infections, osteopenia/osteoporosis, and avascular bone necrosis.

▶ Myalgias with minimal laboratory evidence of muscle damage are consistent with several conditions, including fibromyalgia, the HIV wasting syndrome, and antiretroviral toxicity.

▶ Limited data suggest that highly active antiretroviral therapy (HAART) may be associated with several rheumatologic complications including arthralgias, myopathies, and abnormalities in bone mineralization.

▶ Concomitant use of HAART and immunosuppressive agents requires careful consideration of drug interactions, heightened toxicities, and difficulty in monitoring certain clinical HIV-related parameters.

General Considerations

Patients with HIV have heightened activation of the B-cell compartment and a high prevalence of polyclonal hypergammaglobulinemia. Partly as a consequence of this, the frequency with which autoantibody production is detected in patients with HIV is increased compared with healthy persons. The interpretation of positive autoantibody assays (eg, antinuclear antibodies, rheumatoid factor, and antineutrophil cytoplasmic antibodies) may be complicated in patients with HIV. Correlation between the laboratory and clinical findings is important.

Pathogenesis

HIV infection may modulate the host immune response contributing to the development of various rheumatic manifestations. Painful articular syndrome and HIV-associated arthritis represent distinct clinical syndromes that develop during the course of HIV infection, suggesting a direct role for HIV. The role of HIV in reactive arthritides, undifferentiated spondyloarthropathies, and musculoskeletal infections is most likely indirect, either by increasing susceptibility or influencing the clinical course of these diseases in susceptible patient groups. A unique spectrum of rheumatic manifestations has been recently recognized among HIV-infected persons treated with highly active antiretroviral therapy (HAART). Immune reconstitution after such therapy may be responsible for some of these manifestations.

Table 51–1. Musculoskeletal manifestations of HIV infection.

Arthralgias
Painful articular syndrome
HIV-associated arthritis
Spondyloarthropathies
Reactive arthritis
Psoriatic arthritis
Undifferentiated spondyloarthropathy
Musculoskeletal infections
Osteonecrosis
Osteopenia/osteoporosis
Rheumatic manifestations of HAART-associated IRIS
Myalgias
Noninflammatory myopathies
NRTI myopathy
HIV-associated myopathy
Nemaline rod myopathy
Inflammatory myopathies
Idiopathic polymyositis
Pyomyositis

HAART, highly active antiretroviral therapy; IRIS, immune reconstitution inflammation syndrome; NRTI, nucleoside reverse transcriptase inhibitor.

JOINT COMPLAINTS: ARTHRALGIAS, ARTHRITIS, & SPONDYLOARTHROPATHIES

1. HIV Painful Articular Syndrome

This syndrome is characterized by debilitating arthralgias that are often sufficiently severe to precipitate emergency department visits. Painful articular syndrome has been reported to occur in up to 10% of HIV-infected persons. Symptoms last from 2–24 hours and usually resolve spontaneously. The joint complaints are usually oligoarticular and asymmetric. The affected joints—most commonly the knees, but elbows and shoulders may also be affected—are free of any signs of inflammation on examination. Radiographs often reveal nonspecific findings such as periarticular osteopenia. Targeting symptoms using nonsteroidal anti-inflammatory drugs or opioids and reassurance is usually successful. If symptoms do not improve within 1–2 days, reconsidering the diagnosis is mandatory.

2. HIV-Associated Arthritis

A subacute asymmetric oligoarthritis that usually affects the large joints (most commonly the knees, but ankles and wrists may also be involved) may occur in patients with more advanced HIV infection. This form of arthritis usually has a self-limited course ranging from 1 week up to 6 months. The prevalence has been reported in the range of 3–25% of HIV-infected patients, the higher prevalence coming from a

cohort in Zambia, suggesting a possible geographic predisposition. The HIV has been detected in synovial fluid, which is consistent with (but not diagnostic of) an etiologic role for the virus itself. Suppression of viral replication using HAART may be beneficial for the treatment of this disorder, but controlled trials are lacking. Treatment has centered on nonsteroidal anti-inflammatory drugs, and some reports note benefit from low-dose glucocorticoids and hydroxychloroquine. The incidence of this condition appears to have decreased following the introduction of HAART.

3. HIV-Associated Acute Symmetric Polyarthritis

Acute symmetric polyarthritis affects the small joints of the hands, and its manifestations resemble rheumatoid arthritis. Findings include periarticular osteopenia, joint-space narrowing, swan-neck deformity, and ulnar deviation. Rheumatoid factor is usually negative. Studies have reported therapeutic success with the use of gold.

4. Adhesive Capsulitis

An association between the use of protease inhibitors and the development of subacute progressive shoulder pain with limited range of motion has been suggested (Table 51–2).

Table 51–2. Rheumatologic manifestations reported with antiretroviral medications.[a]

Medications	Class	Manifestation
Zidovudine Stavudine	NRTI	Myopathy, myalgias, rhabdomyolysis
Zalcitabine	NRTI	Arthralgias
Tenofovir	NRTI	Osteopenia
Lamivudine Emtricitabine	NRTI	Arthralgias, myalgias, rhabdomyolysis
Efavirenz	NNRTI	Arthralgias, myopathy, myalgias
Nevirapine	NNRTI	Arthralgias
Nelfinavir Lopinavir Atazanavir	PI	Osteopenia, osteoporosis, aseptic necrosis of bone
Saquinavir Ritonavir	PI	Myalgias, arthralgias, arthritis, cramps, osteopenia, osteoporosis
Indinavir	PI	Adhesive capsulitis of the shoulder, temporomandibular pain syndrome, osteopenia, osteoporosis, aseptic necrosis of bone
Enfuvirtide	FI	Myalgias

[a]The reported association between antiretroviral and the development of bone abnormalities is tenuous.
FI, fusion inhibitor; NNRTI, non-nucleoside reverse transcriptase inhibitor; NRTI, nucleoside reverse transcriptase inhibitor; PI, protease inhibitor.

Typically, symptoms begin a year after the medications are started and usually resolve within 7–12 months. Because radiographic findings are usually lacking, the diagnosis is clinical. Physical therapy, nonsteroidal anti-inflammatory drugs, and the judicious use of intra-articular glucocorticoids (see Chapter 2) have been successfully used to treat this condition. Although the association with protease inhibitors is far from convincing, physicians may consider switching the HAART regimen to a non–protease inhibitor class (eg, nonnucleoside reverse transcriptase inhibitors). If that is not an option, the data suggest that symptoms tend to resolve despite persistent use of protease inhibitors.

5. Psoriatic Arthritis

Psoriasis and psoriatic arthritis may be the initial presentation of underlying HIV infection. Prevalence estimates of psoriasis among HIV-infected patients range from 1–32%, with a tendency for appearance or exacerbation in more advanced stages of HIV infection. Arthritis develops in as many as 30% of HIV patients who have cutaneous psoriasis. The pattern of psoriatic arthritis—polyarticular, asymmetric involvement with dactylitis and enthesopathy—differs from that seen in individuals without HIV in that sacroiliac and axial skeleton involvement initially seems less common. As the natural history of HIV has been altered by new treatments, the axial bony changes commonly seen in persons with psoriasis who are not HIV-infected have been observed among patients living longer than 5 years with psoriatic arthritis. These include unilateral sacroiliitis and bulky spondylitis that skips adjacent vertebral bodies. HIV-associated psoriasis may be refractory to traditional therapy. Guidelines for the treatment of psoriasis in HIV-infected persons have been published by the National Psoriasis Foundation.

Menon K, Van Voorhees AS, Bebo BF Jr, et al. National Psoriasis Foundation. Psoriasis in patients with HIV infection: from the medical board of the National Psoriasis Foundation. *J Am Acad Dermatol*. 2010;62:291. [PMID: 19646777]

6. Reactive Arthritis & Other Spondyloarthropathies

Spondyloarthropathies in the setting of HIV infection may present with the typical form of reactive arthritis or may have atypical features classified as undifferentiated spondyloarthropathy. The characteristic clinical findings are those of a peripheral arthritis involving the lower extremities and prominent enthesopathy (eg, Achilles tendinitis and plantar fasciitis). Extra-articular manifestations, including eye inflammation, urethritis, and mucocutaneous lesions, are also common. Axial involvement is typically infrequent. The clinical course is unpredictable, although a severe form of erosive polyarthritis has been reported in black patients.

Studies from the late 1980s suggested an increased risk of reactive arthritis in HIV-positive patients. Data from several subsequent cohorts found no change in prevalence between HIV-infected and uninfected patients, suggesting that reactive arthritis was not due to HIV per se but due to the prevalence of high-risk sexual behaviors leading to postvenereal reactive arthritis. Data from sub-Saharan African patients, however, suggest a more complicated relationship. The prevalence of spondyloarthropathies has clearly risen with the increase in HIV infections, with no apparent change in triggers for reactive arthritis. In contrast to seronegative patients, these HIV-positive patients are predominantly HLA-B27 negative and have a more aggressive course of arthritis.

7. Other Rheumatic Conditions Associated with HIV

Septic arthritis and **malignancies** are not directly caused by HIV infection, but should be considered when evaluating HIV-infected patients with rheumatologic complaints.

Given the frequency of injection drug use as the primary risk factor for HIV infection, the high incidence of joint infections is not surprising in this subset of patients. As the CD4+ T-cell count drops below 200 cells/mcL, the risk of musculoskeletal infections rises. *Staphylococcus aureus* is the most common joint pathogen described. Mycobacterial arthritis mainly cause by *Mycobacterium avium intracellulare* has been reported among patients with a CD4 cell count less than 50 cells/mcL.

Rarely, lymphoma may present as arthritis of a large joint. Data suggest a decreased incidence of lymphoma after the introduction of HAART.

Restrepo CS, Lemos DF, Gordillo H, et al. Imaging findings in musculoskeletal complications of AIDS. *Radiographics*. 2004;24:1029. [PMID: 15256627]

DISORDERS OF BONE

The HIV population is aging due to effective antiretroviral therapy. This is resulting in more complex management of conditions related to bone. Recent data suggest that HIV infection has a significant effect on bone metabolism. Whether this is a direct result of HIV, or an indirect effect (eg, of HAART or injection drug use) is unclear. There are several biologic mechanisms that support a direct effect of HIV, including HIV-induced increases in osteoclastic activity. There are also data implicating HAART-mediated mechanisms, including changes in osteoblast activity, osteoclast differentiation, and vitamin D metabolism.

1. Osteopenia & Osteoporosis

A number of recent studies have indicated higher rates of osteopenia, osteoporosis, and fracture in the HIV-infected population than would be expected in age- and sex-matched seronegative adults. Persons living with HIV have several potential risk factors for low bone mineral density, including injection drug use, smoking, physical inactivity, glucocorticoid use, weight loss, hypogonadism, malabsorption, and vitamin D deficiency. Recent longitudinal studies suggest that antiretroviral therapy induces a loss of bone mineral density ranging from 2% to 6%. The initiation of tenofovir-containing antiretroviral regimens has been shown to lead to an initial, modest bone loss that subsequently stabilizes with time. There are conflicting data regarding the use of protease inhibitors and their effect on bone mineral density. Some studies have shown greater declines in bone mineral density after 1 year of antiretroviral therapy with regimens containing protease inhibitors than those regimens that did not include protease inhibitors; however, several other longitudinal studies have not supported this finding. Other medications used to treat HIV-related complications, including pentamidine, foscarnet, and human growth hormone, have resulted in abnormalities in calcium metabolism while other medications commonly used in people living with HIV and AIDS including glucocorticoids and ketoconazole, have been shown to accelerate bone loss.

At this time, there is no reason to modify the antiretroviral therapy based on bone mineral density considerations. Although not specifically validated for HIV-infected adults, many providers use the new World Health Organization Fracture Risk Assessment Tool (FRAX) to estimate the 10-year probability of fracture based on clinical risk factors and the bone mineral density at the femoral neck. An expert panel suggested that HIV infection should be considered a risk factor for osteoporosis and recommended dual-energy x-ray absorptiometry scans for all HIV-infected postmenopausal women and men aged 50 years or older. Treatment of osteoporosis in the HIV-infected older adult does not differ from those without HIV infection and should include both lifestyle changes (such as tobacco cessation, weight-bearing exercise, vitamin D therapy) and potentially medication. Pharmacologic therapy for HIV-infected patients should be considered. However, most data on the use of bisphosphonates are in postmenopausal women not HIV-infected younger persons, and the generalizability of the data is currently unknown. However, most experts advocate for therapy in persons living with HIV who have suffered a nontraumatic fracture.

2. Osteonecrosis

Osteonecrosis has been reported in both the pre-HAART and the HAART eras. One report of 339 HIV-infected persons showed a prevalence of hip osteonecrosis of 4.4%. The femoral head is the most common site of involvement, but studies from the pre-HAART and current HAART eras have also demonstrated involvement of knees, shoulders, and elbows. Among persons with AIDS, osteonecrosis is frequently bilateral. Studies conflict on the number of involved sites present concurrently as well as the correlation of disease with HIV stage. Initially, protease inhibitors were thought to be causative. More recent evidence suggests that traditional risk factors for osteonecrosis—trauma, smoking, alcohol abuse,

glucocorticoid use, and pancreatitis—are also important in HIV-associated osteonecrosis. Evaluation with MRI is essential for patients with strongly suggestive clinical histories and physical examination findings (eg, pain with internal rotation of the hip) but normal plain films. Prompt diagnosis at an early stage may allow successful core decompression (see Chapter 59). Late-stage disease is treated most effectively with joint replacement.

3. Osteomyelitis

Although osteomyelitis is relatively rare among patients with HIV (with a prevalence of less than 1%), the onset of persistent discomfort that localizes to the skeleton should raise suspicion for this disease. Although the risk factors for osteomyelitis are similar among HIV-infected and uninfected individuals, specific pathogens merit consideration in the setting of HIV. In addition to *S aureus, Salmonella* is a commonly encountered pathogen in patients with advanced immunosuppression. As the CD4 count declines to <100 cells/mL, the clinician must consider bone infections with atypical mycobacterial organisms (eg, *Candida,* and *Sporothrix),* which rarely cause such problems in immunocompetent patients.

4. Malignancy

Both Kaposi sarcoma and lymphoma may present as bone lesions. Evidence of periosteal reactions and destruction as well as soft tissue masses are not uncommon. The frequent difficulty in distinguishing the presentations of these diseases from infection highlights the importance of obtaining tissue for diagnostic purposes.

McComsey GA, Tebas P, Shane E, et al. Bone disease in HIV infection: a practical review and recommendations for HIV care providers. *Clin Infect Dis.* 2010;51:937. [PMID: 20839968]

DISORDERS OF MUSCLE

Although muscle weakness in HIV/AIDS patients can be the result of severe muscle wasting from infection, nutritional deficiency, or nervous system involvement, skeletal muscle disease occurs in the setting of HIV infection. The most common muscle disorders in HIV patients include nucleoside reverse transcriptase inhibitor (NRTI) myopathy, HIV myopathy, and muscle infections. Other muscle disorders including rhabdomyolysis, non-Hodgkin lymphomas, and myasthenia gravis have also been reported.

▶ Clinical Findings

The distinction between muscle pain and muscle weakness is an important initial step in the evaluation of patients with muscle complaints. Symptoms of acute HIV seroconversion include fever, arthralgias, and myalgias. In the current era of HAART, chronically infected patients who have discontinued antiretroviral medications are at risk for the development of symptoms consistent with HIV seroconversion syndrome as the viral load rebounds. This can occur as early as 1 week after cessation of HAART.

Patients with long-standing HIV infections may have muscle symptoms secondary to autoimmune phenomena, infections, or adverse drug effects. Muscle pain in the setting of elevated levels of serum muscle enzymes should prompt an evaluation of all medications. Statins are a common cause of myositis in HIV patients.

▶ Differential Diagnosis

A. Myalgias

Complaints of muscle pains of varying duration have been reported in as many as 30% of HIV-infected patients in several cohorts. The pathophysiology is unclear. At times these myalgias can be localized. Analgesics are often quite useful. Some clinicians recommend strategies similar to those for patients without HIV who have fibromyalgia.

B. Muscle Weakness

While weakness due to central or peripheral nerve involvement is always possible in the setting of HIV, weakness due to involvement of muscle tissue should not be overlooked. Muscle weakness or evidence of muscle damage identified by elevated serum creatinine kinase may have numerous causes in HIV patients. Biopsy of affected muscles is an important part of the evaluation. The myopathies may be divided into those with biopsy-proven inflammation and those with tissue necrosis accompanied by minimal inflammatory infiltrates.

1. Noninflammatory myopathy—NRTI myopathy was initially described as a complication of zidovudine therapy. This condition resembles HIV myopathy and idiopathic polymyositis. In addition to weakness, patients may first complain of myalgias, muscle tenderness, and proximal muscle weakness. Patients have generally been receiving NRTI therapy for months prior to symptom onset. Creatine kinase levels are elevated up to 10-fold. Electromyographic studies may be normal or demonstrate mild myopathic changes. Histopathologic studies indicate that NRTIs disrupt skeletal muscle mitochondrial function, yielding characteristic "ragged-red" fibers on biopsy. The quantity of ragged fibers present correlates loosely with the clinical severity of weakness.

All nucleoside analogues preferentially inhibit reverse transcriptase. Some of these medications also inhibit other DNA polymerases, including mitochondrial DNA polymerases. This type of mitochondrial toxicity can be the cause of myopathy, as well as other drug-induced complications such as a demyelinating polyneuropathy (similar to Guillain-Barré

syndrome) and hepatic steatosis. When NRTI myopathy is diagnosed, cessation of therapy leads to normalization of serum creatine kinase levels within several weeks, presaging return of power to affected muscles in subsequent months. If there is no response to discontinuation of the drug, it is likely that HIV myopathy (see below) is present. For acute symptoms, nonsteroidal anti-inflammatory drugs may help relieve the myalgias. Although there has been some evidence to suggest that carnitine may prevent the development and progression of NRTI myopathy, the clinical efficacy of this treatment is unknown.

2. HIV-associated myopathy—HIV-associated myopathy may resemble idiopathic polymyositis. Typical presentations include myalgias, muscle tenderness, and symmetric proximal muscle weakness, particularly in the lower extremities. Although this myopathy may be the presenting symptom of HIV, it does not appear to be related to the level of immunosuppression; it has been described both early and late in the course of HIV infection. Differentiating between HIV myopathy and NRTI-associated myopathy can be difficult because the clinical presentations of these 2 disorders (including elevation of muscle enzymes up to 10-fold) are similar. Electromyography and muscle biopsy demonstrate myopathic changes (ie, increased insertional activity, fibrillation, and polyphasic potentials characteristic of membrane irritability). Histologic changes on biopsy include a mononuclear cell infiltrate accompanied by some perivascular and interfascicular accumulation of inflammatory cells. Some clinicians have posited a causative role for malnutrition, with HIV simply exacerbating the dietary deficiency. A similar biopsy pattern has been described in patients experiencing clinical signs of HIV-associated wasting syndrome. The prognosis of HIV myopathy is generally better than polymyositis with some cases resolving spontaneously. Several case studies have demonstrated therapeutic benefit from glucocorticoids. Generally, therapy is initiated with prednisone at 1 mg/kg/d. Normalization of muscle enzymes and improvement in strength generally occur in 1–2 months. Upon full recovery, prednisone is gradually tapered and the patient is closely monitored for signs and symptoms of recurrent disease. Alternative diagnoses and glucocorticoid myopathy should be considered in patients who do not respond to glucocorticoids. In patients who are truly nonresponsive to glucocorticoids, other therapies, including intravenous immune globulin, methotrexate, and azathioprine, have all been tried.

3. Nemaline rod myopathy—Finally, the rare condition known as nemaline rod myopathy has been observed in HIV-infected patients as well as in individuals without HIV. Both congenital and acquired forms of this disease exist. Presenting symptoms and signs include a slowly progressive proximal myopathy; mildly elevated creatine kinase; and a biopsy revealing type 1 muscle fiber atrophy and small, punctate rods and vacuoles within myocytes. Inflammatory changes, if present, are generally mild. A clear therapeutic strategy for this condition has not been defined, although in some cases a response to glucocorticoids in doses similar to those used for HIV myopathy has been observed.

4. Inflammatory myopathies—An inflammatory muscle disease clinically indistinguishable from polymyositis in HIV-negative persons has been described in HIV-infected persons. Thus, the picture of progressive proximal muscle weakness, either subtle or dramatic, with minimal myalgias should prompt consideration of polymyositis. Inflammation-induced necrosis yields elevated serum muscle enzymes. Electromyographic evaluations demonstrate patterns of muscle dysfunction identical to those of idiopathic inflammatory myopathy (see Chapter 27). Confirmation of the diagnosis by muscle biopsy is important because therapy involves pharmacologic immunosuppression. The electromyogram can direct the clinician to biopsy muscle groups most affected, thus lowering the risk of false-negative results due to sampling bias. On biopsy, myositis manifests predominantly as a CD8+ lymphocytic infiltrate among myofibrils of varying states of destruction and regeneration.

Regardless of the person's state of HIV-induced immunosuppression, immunotherapy with glucocorticoids is a cornerstone of therapy. Patients with CD4 counts <200 cells/mL should receive prophylaxis against *Pneumocystis jiroveci* (formerly *carinii*) when using any immunosuppressive agent. Some patients may require adjunctive therapy either to control symptoms or to facilitate tapering the glucocorticoid regimen. In these cases, methotrexate or azathioprine are the agents used most often. Patients with HIV infection are susceptible to bone marrow suppression and may require hematologic growth factors while undergoing immunosuppression.

An infectious myositis (pyomyositis) presents as a deep muscle abscess caused by pyogenic bacteria. Patients complain of focal myalgias, swelling, and tenderness, localizing to the region of the affected muscle, frequently associated with fevers. True weakness is relatively uncommon. Muscle enzymes may not be elevated depending on the volume of muscle involved, but leukocytosis is typical. Persistence of localizing symptoms merits further evaluation with ultrasonography or MRI. *S aureus* is the most common etiology of pyomyositis, although other bacteria such as *Salmonella, Streptococcus pyogenes, Mycobacterium tuberculosis,* and *Nocardia* have also been described. Surgical incision and drainage or drainage by percutaneous interventional radiology often is necessary as an adjunct to parenteral antibiotics.

5. Non-Hodgkin lymphoma—Non-Hodgkin lymphoma may present as a painful muscle mass that needs to be distinguished from other localized muscle masses including pyomyositis and deep venous thrombosis. MRI may be useful in distinguishing infections from neoplasms. A hyperintense ring around a mass on T1-weighted images favors infection due to pyomyositis.

OTHER RHEUMATOLOGIC CONDITIONS

1. Vasculitis Syndromes

▶ General Considerations

Since the beginning of the HIV epidemic, a wide variety of vascular inflammatory diseases have been described in HIV-infected patients. Given the prevalence of HIV in the general population, it is not surprising that there are case reports of nearly every vascular inflammatory disease in the setting of HIV. In addition, HIV is associated with a number of other coinfections, including hepatitis B, hepatitis C, and cytomegalovirus, which can predispose patients to vascular inflammatory syndromes. Currently, there is no clear consensus on whether any distinct vasculitis forms exist in the setting of HIV.

Due to the low prevalence of vasculitis in the general population, extremely large epidemiologic studies would be required to thoroughly evaluate its association with HIV. Because of the prohibitive costs associated with this, most data are obtained from smaller studies. In terms of the primary forms of systemic vasculitis, there are no convincing data suggesting that HIV infection increases the risk of developing any of these diseases. In fact, some evidence indicates that HIV may diminish the chance of developing certain forms of vasculitis, such as polyarteritis nodosa (with or without hepatitis B; see Chapter 35) or the types of vasculitis associated with antineutrophil cytoplasmic antibodies. Several groups, however, have described clear examples of tissue-confirmed polyarteritis nodosa. Polyarteritis nodosa has been described in patients at all stages of disease and at all CD4 cell count levels.

Secondary vasculitis may result from infection from bacteria, viruses, mycobacteria, fungi, and parasites. Given the immunosuppression that occurs in HIV and the resulting higher susceptibility to infections, HIV-infected patients may have higher rates of secondary vasculitis than the general population. Clinicians should perform an extensive evaluation for treatable pathogens that may mediate direct vascular inflammation in HIV-infected patients. Cases of cryoglobulinemia secondary to hepatitis C have been well documented in HIV patients, with cutaneous, neurologic, and renal pathology suggestive of vasculitis. Of note, despite the strong association of hepatitis B infection and development of polyarteritis nodosa and hepatitis C infection with cryoglobulinemic vasculitis, the prevalence of these vasculitides in HIV appears exceedingly low.

Finally, there does appear to be growing clinical, epidemiologic, and pathologic evidence that several distinctive forms of vascular inflammatory disease occur in certain settings. These include aneurysmal disease of the large arteries of the brain occurring in children, and a large-vessel aneurysmal disease primarily affecting the aorta and its branches in young HIV-infected patients from sub-Saharan Africa.

Further study of these disorders is necessary to identify specific epidemiologic features and pathogenesis.

Clinical Findings

A. Laboratory Findings

The evaluation should include urinalysis with careful attention to the presence of protein, blood, and red blood cell casts. Serum complement levels are often depressed in the setting of immune complex–mediated processes, such as the cryoglobulinemic vasculitis associated with hepatitis C. Comprehensive hepatitis B and C serologies should be obtained. If the partial thromboplastin time is prolonged, antiphospholipid antibodies should be excluded through appropriate serologic testing (see Chapter 23).

B. Imaging Studies

In the patient with chronic active hepatitis B, complaints of abdominal pain may ultimately require selective mesenteric artery angiography to confirm polyarteritis nodosa.

Differential Diagnosis

Among the true systemic vasculitides, the most commonly described in HIV patients is a small-vessel vasculitis typically induced by medications (see Chapter 37). Palpable purpura is the most common manifestation, with skin biopsy yielding the nonspecific description of leukocytoclastic vasculitis. These lesions may be accompanied by arthritis of wrists, fingers, knees, or ankles as well as low-grade fevers. Abacavir, β-lactam antibiotics, and sulfa-based medications are the most common offenders in causing hypersensitivity vasculitis in the setting of HIV. Abacavir hypersensitivity, observed in 3–5% of patients before the availability of HLA testing, most often presents with a combination of flulike symptoms, fever, rash (usually urticarial or maculopapular), fatigue, and gastrointestinal upset. Symptoms worsen progressively during continued therapy and improve substantially within 24–48 hours of discontinuation. Patients being considered for abacavir therapy should have HLA-B5701 testing prior to initiation to rule out the risk of hypersensitivity reaction. A patient with a presumed abacavir hypersensitivity reaction should never be rechallenged with abacavir due to the possibility of a fatal reaction. Ordinarily, cessation of the drug is sufficient for improvement, which occurs over the ensuing several days to weeks. An identical clinical condition can occur in the weeks following streptococcal infections or subacute bacterial endocarditis, with the sensitizing antigen being a bacterial epitope rather than a medication.

Finally, when the diagnosis of vasculitis is entertained in the HIV patient, the numerous potential mimickers of vasculitis must also be considered. Case reports describe examples of cutaneous and neurologic pathology from infectious pathogens, including the herpesviruses (herpes simplex, varicella-zoster, and cytomegalovirus) and parasites such as *Toxoplasma gondii* and *P jiroveci*. Similarly, hypercoagulable states such as the antiphospholipid syndrome can mimic vasculitis by causing multiorgan system dysfunction. Antiphospholipid antibodies, such as the lupus anticoagulant, occur with increased frequency in patients with HIV, but the clinical significance is not always clear.

2. Sicca Syndrome

Clinical Findings

A. Symptoms and Signs

A significant number of patients with HIV complain of dry eyes and dry mouth. These are often assumed to be HAART-related symptoms, yet only indinavir (5% of patients who take the drug), efavirenz, ritonavir, saquinavir, and didanosine (all <2%) are associated with xerostomia. Mycobacterial infections should also be considered but are usually not subtle in presentation. Concurrent symptoms with evidence of a systemic process (eg, arthritis and shortness of breath) may indicate Sjögren syndrome or diffuse infiltrative lymphocytosis syndrome, a condition that occurs exclusively in HIV (see below).

B. Laboratory Findings

A biopsy of the minor salivary gland has a very low risk of morbidity and may contribute significantly to the work-up. However, histology may be normal in persons receiving HAART.

C. Imaging Studies

Gallium scintigraphy reveals significant signal enhancement in the affected salivary glands. When biopsy is normal, confirmatory gallium scintigraphy may be helpful.

Differential Diagnosis

A. Granulomatous Processes

Chronic granulomatous processes, such as mycobacterial infections or sarcoidosis, should be considered. Systemic symptoms are expected to accompany mycobacterial infections, but the presentation may be complicated in the setting of HIV. Sarcoidosis, although rare in HIV, has been reported in patients experiencing immune reconstitution. Medication changes may be considered after other conditions have been excluded.

B. Diffuse Infiltrative Lymphocytosis Syndrome

First described in the late 1980s, the prevalence of diffuse infiltrative lymphocytosis syndrome has been reported in 3–7% of outpatient HIV cohorts. Characterized by painless parotid gland swelling with concurrent asymmetric salivary gland enlargement, 60% of patients also experience sicca symptoms. Tissue biopsy of the minor salivary gland reveals prominent infiltrate of CD8+ lymphocytes, distinctly different from the inflammatory process of Sjögren syndrome. Extraglandular infiltrates also cause visceral organ disease with up to 50% of affected patients experiencing lymphocytic interstitial pneumonitis. Neurologic deficits can include cranial nerve VII palsies, likely secondary to parotid gland compression, and occasionally peripheral neuropathies. Additional extraglandular manifestations include renal tubular acidosis, polymyositis, and hepatitis. The primary treatment is HAART with or without the addition of glucocorticoids.

Guillevin L. Vasculitides in the context of HIV infection. *AIDS.* 2008;22 (suppl 3):S27. [PMID: 18845919]

RHEUMATOLOGIC MANIFESTATIONS OF HAART

The introduction of HAART in the mid-1990s has led to significant improvements in overall mortality among HIV-infected persons. In some studies, the incidence of reactive arthritis and psoriatic arthritis has declined significantly following the introduction of HAART. Whether HAART increases the risk for certain rheumatologic diseases is unclear. Table 51–2 summarizes the reported rheumatologic associations of the various agents used to treat HIV infection; for example, myopathy associated with zidovudine therapy is well documented. Most NRTIs (eg, zidovudine, stavudine, zalcitabine, didanosine, and lamivudine) have been associated with mitochondrial toxicity leading to lactic acidosis, muscle wasting, myalgias, and myopathies. The correlation between HAART and bone disease is still controversial. Whether the use of antiretroviral agents leads to bone demineralization or osteonecrosis is unclear. Longitudinal data are still needed to verify the associations listed in Table 51–2.

1. The Immune Reconstitution Inflammatory Syndrome

One important diagnosis to consider in the patient who has initiated HAART within the past few months is the immune reconstitution inflammatory syndrome (IRIS). This syndrome is caused by an improved capacity of the patient to mount an inflammatory response against persistent microbial antigens or self-antigens. Diagnostic criteria proposed include the following: a preexisting diagnosis of AIDS, increased CD4 cell counts and HIV RNA suppression following HAART initiation, and inflammatory symptoms that cannot be explained by an alternate diagnosis. The manifestations of IRIS are diverse. In addition to inflammatory responses to microorganisms, cases of autoimmune diseases (eg, Graves autoimmune thyroiditis, sarcoidosis, systemic lupus erythematosus, and rheumatoid arthritis) have been reported in patients with IRIS.

Following the institution of HAART, suppression of the viral load permits the release of memory CD4+ cells early after the initiation of HAART followed by the release of naïve T-cells. Cytokine production shifts from a Th-2 profile to a Th-1 profile with increases in interferon-γ and interleukin-2, resulting in aggressive immune responses occurring at specific tissue sites. Cessation of HAART is rarely necessary. Short courses of glucocorticoids mitigate symptoms and may be used in more severe cases.

2. HAART & Immunosuppressive Medications

The use of immunosuppressive agents in HIV-infected patients receiving HAART is challenging. There are no published data that offer guidance. The potential for drug interactions must be considered. Several antiretroviral agents have well-documented effects on the cytochrome P450 system. These effects may alter the metabolism of concomitantly administered immunosuppressive agents. The potential for synergistic toxicities, such as hepatotoxicity and bone marrow toxicity, should also be addressed. Efavirenz, for example, a non-NRTI, is well known to increase the risk of hepatotoxicity. Zidovudine has bone marrow suppressive effects. Because these 2 common side effects are shared by several immunosuppressive agents, antiretroviral regimens may require tailoring in order to minimize the potential for heightened toxicity when used in combinations with immunosuppressive agents. Recent small case series suggest that the use of TNF-blocking agents in persons infected with HIV who do not have advanced immunosuppression appears to be safe and well-tolerated.

The use of immunosuppressive medications may make it difficult to assess the immunologic response to HAART. Usually, when a patient starts an effective HAART regimen, suppression of the HIV viral load is followed by an increase in the CD4 count. Immunosuppressives may blunt a CD4 count increase. If feasible, the initiation of HAART prior to the initiation of immunosuppression may make it easier to achieve adequate virologic control. Once the immunosuppressives are added, the HIV viral load should remain undetectable; however, the CD4 count response may be blunted. Finally, it is imperative that prophylaxis against opportunistic infections be initiated should the CD4 cell counts decline. To improve outcomes, close collaboration between the rheumatologist and the HIV-care provider is essential.

[AIDS*info*]
http://aidsinfo.nih.gov/

Cepeda EJ, Williams FM, Ishimori ML, Weisman MH, Reveille JD. The use of anti-tumour necrosis factor therapy in HIV-positive individuals with rheumatic disease. *Ann Rheum Dis.* 2008;67:710. [PMID: 18079191]

Nguyen B, Reveille J. Rheumatic manifestations associated with HIV in the highly active antiretroviral therapy era. *Curr Opin Rheum.* 2009;21:404. [PMID: 19444116]

Rheumatic Fever

Preeti Jaggi, MD

Stanford T. Shulman, MD

Acute rheumatic fever (ARF) is a systemic, immune-mediated disease that is triggered by pharyngeal infection with group A streptococci (GAS). Fever, migratory polyarthritis, and carditis are the most common clinical manifestations. ARF is most frequent among 5–15 year olds with a declining incidence in adults. It is extremely rare in children under age 3, prompting speculation that more than one GAS infection is needed before ARF can develop. ARF is not considered a sequela of cutaneous GAS infection.

The pathogenesis of ARF is not clearly understood but appears to involve an immune response to group A streptococcal antigens that then cross-reacts with human tissue through molecular mimicry. Strains of GAS differ in their ability to trigger ARF, and changes in the prevalence of rheumatogenic strains can affect the incidence of ARF. Recent evidence supports the conclusion that ARF has declined in the United States over the past decades largely because of a decline in rheumatogenic types of GAS causing pharyngitis.

The reported attack rate of ARF among patients with untreated GAS pharyngitis is 0.4–3% in epidemic circumstances, with a much lower rate endemically. Genetic factors appear to influence the person's susceptibility to ARF. Observational studies in the 19th century recognized familial tendencies to develop ARF, and in the early 1940s, studies showed familial clustering of the disease, with greatest risk occurring in children if both parents had rheumatic heart disease. Genetic susceptibility to develop ARF has been characterized as autosomal recessive or autosomal dominant with variable penetrance and has been linked with HLA types. Significant increases in the frequency of DRB1*0701, DR6, and DQB1*0201 confer susceptibility to rheumatic fever in several international studies. Monozygotic twins, however, are not usually concordant for ARF, indicating that there are also important environmental factors involved in the pathogenesis of the disease.

▶ Clinical Findings

A. Diagnostic Criteria

In 1944, Dr. T. Duckett Jones developed diagnostic criteria for ARF—the "Jones criteria"—based on his observations of hundreds of patients. The Jones criteria have been revised several times, most recently in 1992 (Table 52–1), and continue to form the basis for the clinical diagnosis of ARF. Exceptions to these criteria include patients who present with chorea or indolent carditis; these patients often do not fulfill the requirement for evidence of antecedent GAS infection because their antistreptococcal antibody levels usually have returned to normal at the time of presentation.

1. Major clinical criteria—Arthritis occurs in approximately 75% of patients with ARF. The arthritis is migratory, which is in contrast to poststreptococcal reactive arthritis, and polyarticular. The arthritis usually affects the larger joints, especially knees, ankles, wrists and elbows, and less commonly involves the smaller joints of the hands and feet. The axial skeleton is rarely affected. Inflamed joints are often red, hot, swollen, and exquisitely tender—to the point that even minimal contact with the affected joint can cause exquisite pain. Left untreated, inflammation of an individual joint resolves spontaneously over days, but the polyarthritis persists for 1–4 weeks. The arthritis of ARF responds dramatically to salicylates. This response is so characteristic that the lack of response to salicylate therapy within 48 hours should prompt the clinician to doubt the diagnosis of ARF and to consider other possibilities.

Carditis occurs in approximately 50–60% of ARF cases and accounts for significant morbidity and even mortality. When ARF affects the heart, it usually involves the endocardium, myocardium, and pericardium to varying degrees. Endocarditis leading to mitral or aortic valvulitis (or both) is most characteristic and occurs most frequently; the tricuspid

Table 52–1. Modified Jones criteria for diagnosis of acute rheumatic fever.[a]

Major criteria
- Carditis
- Polyarthritis
- Chorea
- Erythema marginatum
- Subcutaneous nodules

Minor criteria
- Fever
- Arthralgia
- Elevated acute phase reactant (C-reactive protein or erythrocyte sedimentation rate)
- Prolonged PR interval on electrocardiogram

Supporting evidence of antecedent group A streptococcal infection
- Positive throat culture or rapid antigen test
- Elevated or rising streptococcal antibody titer

[a]Diagnosis requires two major criteria or one major and two minor criteria, plus supporting evidence of antecedent group A streptococcal infection.

and pulmonary valves are rarely affected. The revised Jones criteria for ARF require auscultation of a new valvular murmur in order to meet the criterion of "carditis"; echocardiography findings of valvular regurgitation without a murmur do not fulfill either major or minor criteria. When chronic rheumatic heart disease results, valvular regurgitation can be replaced by valvular stenosis. Myocarditis manifests as tachycardia that is disproportionate to the degree of fever and is persistent even in sleep. Pericarditis is the least common finding in rheumatic carditis. It usually manifests as a pericardial effusion or friction rub. The presence of myocarditis or pericarditis in the absence of valvular involvement is unlikely to be due to ARF, and other diagnoses should be explored in this circumstance.

Sydenham chorea (St. Vitus dance), which occurs in 10–15% of patients, is usually a later manifestation of ARF. The characteristic features of chorea are purposeless involuntary movements, incoordination, facial grimacing, and emotional lability. Chorea is a self-limited illness, and full recovery takes several months. Rarely, symptoms can occur over years and are exacerbated by stress, pregnancy, oral contraceptives, and intercurrent illnesses. Chorea is thought to be due to antibodies that cross-react with basal ganglia neurons.

Erythema marginatum occurs in less than 2% of patients. It is an erythematous, flat, serpiginous macular rash with pale central clearing. The rash usually occurs on the trunk and extremities and characteristically spares the face. The rash waxes and wanes and may be transient.

Subcutaneous nodules develop in less than 1% of cases of ARF, most often in those with severe carditis. The nodules are firm, nontender, and usually less than 2 cm in diameter. They are typically located over bony prominences or tendon sheaths. Nodules usually resolve spontaneously without permanent sequelae.

2. Minor clinical criteria—The fever in ARF is usually >39.0°C. It is commonly present at the onset of illness and resolves even without treatment over several weeks. In the absence of frank arthritis, arthralgia fulfill a minor criterion in the revised Jones criteria. Arthralgia may be migratory, and the pain may be severe, even without objective signs of arthritis.

B. Diagnostic Tests

Approximately one third of patients with ARF have no history of a recent symptomatic pharyngeal infection and, therefore, it is necessary to find laboratory evidence of a recent GAS infection. This can be done either by obtaining a throat culture or a rapid antigen test for GAS from a throat swab, or by documenting an elevated, or rising, serum antistreptococcal antibody titer. It is important to recognize that antistreptococcal antibody levels in the normal population vary by patient age, geographic location, and season of the year.

The antistreptolysin O (ASO) titer is the most commonly used streptococcal antibody test to establish a recent streptococcal infection. An ASO titer of 240 Todd units or higher in adults or 320 Todd units or higher in children is considered modestly elevated. ASO titers above 500 Todd units are uncommon in healthy individuals and therefore would serve as evidence of a recent streptococcal infection.

Because ASO titers can be normal in approximately 20% of ARF patients, other streptococcal antibody tests can be used to establish a recent GAS infection; these include antideoxyribonuclease B (anti-DNase B), antistreptokinase, and anti-hyaluronidase.

C. Special Tests

Aspiration of involved joints of ARF patients with polyarthritis reveals sterile inflammatory synovial fluid, typically with 10,000–100,000 white blood cells/mcL and a neutrophil predominance.

The nonclinical minor criteria of the revised Jones criteria include an increased PR interval on electrocardiogram and elevated acute phase reactants (C-reactive protein or erythrocyte sedimentation rate or both). Acute phase reactants are almost always elevated in patients with polyarthritis or acute carditis but are often normal in patients with chorea alone.

▶ Differential Diagnosis

Like ARF, juvenile rheumatoid arthritis, systemic lupus erythematosus (SLE), gonococcal arthritis, reactive arthritis, and serum sickness can cause fever and acute polyarticular arthritis in children. Choreiform movements can occur in SLE, neoplasms involving the basal ganglia, Wilson disease, and Huntington disease. Chorea can occasionally be encountered in pregnancy ("chorea gravidarum").

▶ Treatment

Treatment of ARF requires prevention of future streptococcal infections, anti-inflammatory treatment, and symptomatic care (Table 52–2). Upon diagnosis and irrespective of the results of throat cultures for GAS, a dose of benzathine penicillin or 10 days of oral penicillin or erythromycin is recommended. Anti-inflammatory treatment includes oral salicylates (50–100 mg/kg/d) in four daily doses. This is continued for 2–4 weeks then is gradually tapered over 4–6 weeks. Glucocorticoid treatment should be reserved for those patients with congestive heart failure or at least moderate cardiomegaly on chest radiograph. Glucocorticoids are tapered slowly over several weeks; during taper of glucocorticoids, salicylates are added. For patients with Sydenham chorea, haloperidol or phenobarbital may be of some benefit.

Prevention of GAS infection is of utmost importance and prevents recurrent attacks of ARF that can be associated with increased severity of cardiac disease or with development of cardiac disease not previously present. All patients with ARF should receive antimicrobial prophylaxis with intramuscular benzathine penicillin G every 4 weeks or twice daily oral penicillin or sulfadiazine (erythromycin if allergic to penicillin and sulfa). The recommendations for the duration of

Table 52–3. Recommendations of duration of antimicrobial prophylaxis in patients with acute rheumatic fever.

Clinical Condition	Recommendation
Patients with rheumatic fever with carditis and residual heart disease	At least 10 years after last episode and at least until age 40, sometimes lifelong prophylaxis
Rheumatic fever with carditis but no residual heart disease (no valvular disease)	10 years or well into adulthood, whichever is longer
Rheumatic fever without carditis	5 years or until age 21 years, whichever is longer

secondary prophylaxis of streptococcal infection are based on likelihood of recurrence and the numbers of years since the last ARF episode (Table 52–3).

▶ Prognosis

The long-term manifestation of ARF is rheumatic heart disease, and the prognosis of patients with ARF is generally attributable to the degree of cardiac involvement and the recurrence of GAS infection. Rheumatic heart disease may subsequently develop in patients with chorea or polyarthritis if they have recurrent ARF, thus emphasizing the importance of prophylactic antibiotics.

POSTSTREPTOCOCCAL REACTIVE ARTHRITIS

Patients who do not fulfill the diagnostic criteria for ARF but who have arthritis following streptococcal infection are deemed to have poststreptococcal reactive arthritis (PSRA). This arthritis is predominantly associated with GAS infections. PSRA also has been reported with group C and G streptococci but the significance of infection with nongroup A streptococci remains unclear. There appears to be a bimodal age distribution of PSRA, with peak incidence at ages 8–14 years and 21–37 years. In whites, PSRA is associated with the class II HLA antigen DRB1*01.

▶ Clinical Findings

A. Symptoms and Signs

PSRA is generally acute and nonmigratory and predominantly affects the large joints of the lower limbs. The arthritis may be monoarticular or polyarticular and symmetric or asymmetric. The axial skeleton is affected in about 20% of patients. Tenosynovitis occasionally occurs. During the antecedent GAS infection, fever and a scarlatiniform rash may be present, but they are not usually present during the time of arthritis. The incubation between the streptococcal infection and the onset of arthritis is generally shorter than that of ARF

Table 52–2. Treatment of acute rheumatic fever.

Anti-inflammatory treatment	
Mild or no carditis	Aspirin 50–100 mg/kg/d in four divided doses for 2–4 weeks, then taper over 4–6 weeks
Moderate or severe carditis	Prednisone 2 mg/kg/d in two doses for 2–4 weeks, then taper with addition of aspirin when prednisone is ≤0.5 mg/kg/d.
Primary antistreptococcal therapy	1.2 million units of benzathine penicillin G intramuscularly or penicillin or erythromycin orally for 10 days
Prophylaxis of GAS infection	1.2 million units benzathine penicillin G intramuscularly every 4 weeks or sulfadiazine 500 mg orally twice daily (≤27 kg) or 1 g orally twice daily (≥27 kg) or penicillin V 250 mg orally twice daily
Medications to control cardiac symptoms (if needed)	Diuretic, angiotensin-converting enzyme inhibitor, and/or cautious use of digoxin
Medications to control chorea (if needed)	Haloperidol or phenobarbitol
Bacterial endocarditis prophylaxis	As recommended by the American Heart Association

GAS, group A streptococci.

Table 52–4. Proposed criteria for diagnosis of poststreptococcal reactive arthritis.

A. Characteristics of arthritis
1. Acute in onset, symmetric or asymmetric, usually nonmigratory
2. Persistent or recurrent symptoms
3. Lack of a dramatic response to nonsteroidal anti-inflammatory drugs
B. Evidence of an antecedent group A streptococcal infection (by throat culture or rapid antigen test or by elevated or rising antistreptolysin O and/or anti- deoxyribonuclease B titers)
C. Does not fulfill the modified Jones criteria for acute rheumatic fever

Data from Ayoub EM, Ahmed S. *Curr Prob Pediatr.* 1997;27:90.

(onset usually 3–14 days after infection). The symptoms of PSRA resolve slowly within a few weeks to several months (mean duration of symptoms is 2 months). Recurrences have been reported following a subsequent episode of streptococcal pharyngitis. The most concerning potential sequela is late-onset carditis, which in the original description developed in 31% of patients 1 to 18 years after PSRA. Subsequent studies, however, have indicated much lower rates of possible cardiac sequelae. Other extra-articular manifestations of PSRA are uncommon and include glomerulonephritis (which is very rare with ARF) and uveitis. PSRA patients have a much slower response to nonsteroidal anti-inflammatory drug (NSAID) therapy than ARF patients, who typically have a dramatic and prompt response to NSAIDs.

B. Diagnostic Criteria

The diagnostic criteria for PSRA are not clearly defined, but the proposed criteria are detailed in Table 52–4.

▶ Treatment

Although the response is less dramatic than in ARF, aspirin or other NSAIDs are used to treat symptoms of arthritis. Some experts recommend both a baseline echocardiogram and a follow-up echocardiogram 1 year later because of the concern for possible occult carditis. The American Heart Association currently recommends that patients with PSRA should receive antistreptococcal prophylaxis for 1 year, that they should be monitored for 1 year to assess for evidence of cardiac involvement, and that treatment should be discontinued after 1 year if no evidence of carditis is found. Penicillin is recommended as first-line therapy, and erythromycin is appropriate for penicillin-allergic patients. Some experts suggest that the same prophylaxis recommendations for ARF patients should also apply to PSRA because the onset of documented carditis in PSRA is widely variable, but this recommendation has not been endorsed by the American Heart Association or other organizations.

Ayoub EM, Ahmed S. Update on complications of group A streptococcal infections. *Curr Prob Pediatr.* 1997;27:90. [PMID: 9099534]

Gerber M, Baltimore R, Eaton C, et al. Prevention of rheumatic fever and diagnosis and treatment of acute Streptococcal pharyngitis: a scientific statement from the American Heart Association Rheumatic Fever, Endocarditis, and Kawasaki Disease Committee of the Council on Cardiovascular Disease in the Young, the Interdisciplinary Council on Functional Genomics and Translational Biology, and the Interdisciplinary Council on Quality of Care and Outcomes Research: endorsed by the American Academy of Pediatrics. *Circulation.* 2009;119:1541. [PMID: 19246689]

Mackie SL, Keat A. Poststreptococcal reactive arthritis: what is it and how do we know? *Rheumatology.* 2004;43:949. [PMID: 15150434]

Special Writing Group of the Committee on Rheumatic Fever, Endocarditis, and Kawasaki Disease of the Council on Cardiovascular Diseases in the Young of the American Heart Association. Guidelines for the diagnosis of rheumatic fever. Jones criteria, 1992 update. *JAMA.* 1992;268:2069. [PMID: 1404745]

Shulman ST, Stollerman G, Beall B, Dale JB, Tanz RR. Temporal changes in streptococcal M protein types and the near-disappearance of acute rheumatic fever in the United States. *Clin Infect Dis.* 2006;42:441. [PMID: 16421785]

Stollerman GH. Rheumatic fever in the 21st century. *Clin Infect Dis.* 2001;33:806. [PMID: 11512086]

53

Whipple Disease

Gaye Cunnane, MB, PhD, FRCPI

▶ Weight loss, diarrhea, and abdominal discomfort are present in 85–90% of patients at time of diagnosis.

▶ An intermittent, migratory oligoarthritis occurs early in the disease course, preceding gastrointestinal symptoms by an average of 6–8 years.

▶ Inflammatory polyarthritis and sacroiliitis can develop in the chronic phase of disease.

▶ Neurologic involvement is present in 90% of cases.

▶ Diagnosis is based on demonstration of characteristic periodic acid–Schiff (PAS)–positive intracellular inclusions and identification of *Tropheryma whipplei* by polymerase chain reaction (PCR) in biopsies of involved tissues or in fluids.

General Considerations

Whipple disease, a chronic multisystem disease caused by infection with *T whipplei,* was first described in 1907 by George H. Whipple who noted the presence of rod-shaped organisms in the vacuoles of foamy macrophages in the intestinal tissue of a 36-year-old man during autopsy. Over 40 years later, these cells were found to stain positively with PAS and, in 1961, electron microscopy facilitated the recognition of bacterial components in these tissues. Identification of the bacillus was reported in 1992 with the aid of the PCR technique, which enabled the amplification of specific gene segments. In 2000, the organism *T whipplei* was successfully cultivated in vitro, thereby facilitating developments in the pathogenesis, diagnosis, and treatment of this disease.

Whipple disease is rare, with an estimated incidence of 1 per million. It has been most commonly reported in middle-aged white men with an occupational exposure to soil, animals, or sewage. There are two recognized phases of Whipple disease. In the initial stage, symptoms and signs are nonspecific and are marked predominantly by fatigue and joint pains, with or without synovitis. In the later phase, weight loss, diarrhea, and neurologic or psychiatric symptoms may prevail. Although the average interval between these stages is 6–8 years, the initiation of immunosuppressive treatment for presumed inflammatory arthritis may unmask the diagnosis by allowing proliferation of the organism, resulting in more acute symptoms.

T whipplei can be found in the general environment, in sewage plant effluent, and in the stool in asymptomatic human carriers. It has also been isolated from the saliva, blood, stool and duodenal samples from healthy individuals, although it is unclear if this represents environmental contamination, preclinical infection, or the inconsequential presence of commensal organisms. No link with specific genetic factors has been identified.

There is a striking absence of inflammation in tissues infected with *T whipplei.* The organism does not provoke a local cytotoxic reaction, and large numbers of bacilli accumulate at areas of infection. These observations suggest that aberrations of the host immune response may contribute to the clinical manifestations of disease.

The diagnosis of Whipple disease requires evidence of infection with *T whipplei.* The test of choice usually is upper gastrointestinal endoscopy and the acquisition of multiple biopsies from the duodenum and jejunum. The tissue should be stained with PAS, which yields a 78% positivity rate for detection of characteristic intracellular inclusions in patients with untreated Whipple disease. PCR analysis is recommended for confirmation. If gastrointestinal biopsies are negative, other symptomatic areas should be examined, such as synovial fluid, pleural fluid, skin, and lymph nodes. Examination of the cerebrospinal fluid is recommended in all confirmed cases to investigate for asymptomatic neurologic involvement.

Clinical Findings

Because of the systemic nature of Whipple disease, the wide variety of possible clinical presentations, and the chronicity of the illness, a high index of suspicion is essential in order to make the diagnosis in a timely manner before the onset of permanent or life-threatening sequelae. Approximately 15% of patients with Whipple disease have atypical signs. However, the presence of gastrointestinal symptoms with or without neurologic features on the background of an unusual seronegative arthropathy should trigger appropriate investigations. Ideally, however, the diagnosis should be made in the prodromal stage of unexplained, intermittent oligoarthritis or polyarthritis.

A. Symptoms and Signs

1. Articular manifestations—Articular symptoms occur in up to 90% of patients with Whipple disease. Joint involvement is characteristically an intermittent, migratory oligoarthritis, predominantly affecting the large joints, such as the knees, wrists, and ankles. Less frequently, the hips, elbows, and shoulders may be symptomatic. It is rare for small joints to be involved. Attacks usually last several hours to a few days and resolve spontaneously with complete remission between episodes. The average duration of joint symptoms is 6–8 years before the diagnosis of Whipple disease is made.

Chronic polyarthritis is less common but has been described in association with Whipple disease. It tends to show the features of an inflammatory arthritis, with prolonged early morning stiffness. Joint damage does not develop in most patients, but ankylosis of the wrists, ankles, and spine may occur in a minority. Furthermore, sacroiliitis and the radiographic changes of hypertrophic osteoarthropathy have been reported in patients with Whipple disease.

2. Gastrointestinal manifestations—The most common gastrointestinal symptom of Whipple disease is profound weight loss. Diarrhea is a frequent complaint and abdominal pain may be present. In advanced cases, evidence of chronic malabsorption is present, with edema, ascites, and muscle wasting. However, 10–15% of patients have no gastrointestinal symptoms at diagnosis. During upper gastrointestinal endoscopy, pale yellow mucosa punctuated with erosions may be observed.

3. Skin lesions—A variety of skin lesions have been described in association with Whipple disease. The most common of these is hyperpigmentation or melanoderma that develops in up to 46% of patients in the later stages of the illness. Other characteristic skin abnormalities include subcutaneous nodules; erythema nodosum–like lesions; and inflammatory rashes that may mimic cutaneous lupus, dermatomyositis, psoriasis, or eczema. Urticaria and vasculitic lesions have also been reported. Consequences of severe malnutrition may also affect the skin, leading to petechiae, purpura, and edema.

4. Central nervous system and eye disease—Neurologic involvement is common, particularly in long-standing disease and may be present in up to 90% of cases. Whipple disease causes a broad spectrum of symptoms, including cognitive impairment, psychiatric illness (such as depression), headaches, seizures, and ataxia. A pathognomonic sign of Whipple disease is oculomasticatory myorhythmia, where involuntary blinking occurs when the patient is talking or eating. Approximately 50% of patients have evidence of supranuclear ophthalmoplegia at presentation. Symptoms of hypothalamic involvement, such as insomnia, polydipsia, and hyperphagia develop in one third of patients. The most common ocular manifestation is anterior or posterior uveitis, which is often bilateral. Optic neuritis has also been described.

5. Cardiac manifestations—Up to 55% of patients with Whipple disease have cardiac involvement. Pericarditis is the most common manifestation and occurs in more than 50% of patients. Myocarditis may present with unexplained heart failure or sudden death. Blood culture–negative endocarditis, often involving native heart valves, has been described, typically occurring in middle-aged men with a preceding history of joint pains. Fever and a history of valvular heart disease are frequently absent in these cases, contributing to a delayed diagnosis.

6. Other presentations—Uncommonly, patients with Whipple disease may have fever and lymphadenopathy. Intra-abdominal adenopathy is more common than involvement of the peripheral lymph nodes. Kidney disease, hepatosplenomegaly, pleural effusions, pulmonary infiltrates, epididymitis, and orchitis have been reported in Whipple disease.

B. Laboratory Findings

1. Routine laboratory testing—A neutrophil leukocytosis may be present and, rarely, eosinophilia. A normocytic or macrocytic anemia is a common finding because of disease chronicity or nutritional deficiency. Ferritin levels may be elevated, in keeping with the underlying inflammatory process. There usually is a robust acute phase response, with erythrocyte sedimentation rates typically >100 mm/hour. Evidence of malabsorption may include hypoalbuminemia, clotting abnormalities, and low levels of vitamin B_{12} and folate. Serologic tests for rheumatoid factor, antibodies to cyclic citrullinated peptides, and antinuclear antibodies are usually negative. An absence of the normal circadian rhythm that characterizes cortisol, growth hormone, melatonin, and thyroid-stimulating hormone may suggest hypothalamic dysfunction.

2. Examination of fluid and tissue—Fluid aspiration or tissue biopsy is recommended to confirm the diagnosis of Whipple disease. If the initial area of examination is negative, further samples from other regions should be obtained if possible. Synovial fluid shows a predominance of neutrophils and mononuclear cells, with a cell count ranging from 4000–100,000/mcL. Cerebrospinal fluid examination is recommended, even in the absence of symptoms, since a positive PCR result influences both treatment and prognosis.

3. Histologic examination—Examination of involved tissue may demonstrate a mild inflammatory cell infiltrate and occasional noncaseating granuloma formation. The characteristic histologic finding in Whipple disease is the presence of PAS-positive macrophages in the involved tissue. The PAS-positive intracellular inclusions correspond to the bacterial cell wall of *T whipplei*. Multiple biopsies should be obtained in order to avoid sampling errors. Although PAS-positive cells are classically found in the duodenum, they may also be present in cerebrospinal fluid, brain tissue, synovial fluid, synovial tissue, lymph nodes, muscles, skin, bone marrow, and other involved areas. However, false-positive results may occur in tissues infected with mycobacteria, *Histoplasma*, and *Actinomyces*. Immunohistochemistry using specific antibodies directed against *T whipplei* is more sensitive than PAS staining and can be used in cases where added confirmation is required.

4. Polymerase chain reaction—The identification of the nucleotide sequence of *T whipplei* has facilitated the use of PCR in the detection of the organism. PCR is highly sensitive and specific and may help confirm the diagnosis when the PAS staining is negative. However, false-positive results may arise from environmental contamination or the presence of another bacterium with a similar genome sequence.

5. Cultivation of *T whipplei* from fluid or tissue—In specialized laboratories, *T whipplei* may be cultured from involved tissue and has been isolated from blood, cerebrospinal fluid and tissue derived from the joint, heart, duodenum, and lymph node, suggesting active infection of these areas.

C. Imaging Studies

Plain radiography of symptomatic joints is frequently normal. However, in some cases, marked articular damage occurs with subchondral cyst formation and ankylosis of involved areas. Sacroiliitis and syndesmophyte formation of the spinal column have been described in patients with Whipple disease who are HLA-B27 negative. Changes of hypertrophic osteoarthropathy are rare.

Because of the presence of chronic inflammation and malabsorption, low bone mineral density scores are commonly found on dual x-ray absorptiometry scanning.

Computed tomography (CT) of the thorax and pelvis may reveal enlarged lymph nodes, particularly in the mesenteric area. Mediastinal adenopathy has also been described. In patients with central nervous system involvement, single or multiple enhancing lesions in the brain or spinal cord may be observed on CT or MRI.

▶ Differential Diagnosis

A. Joint Diseases

Whipple disease is the prototypic disease-mimicker and a high index of suspicion is essential for diagnosis. The intermittent inflammatory nature of the joint involvement may be suggestive of a crystal arthropathy, such as gout or pseudogout. However, in gout, more than 90% of cases involve the first metatarsophalangeal joint in the initial stages, while microscopic examination of joint fluid demonstrates characteristic uric acid crystals. In pseudogout, large joints may be involved, associated with chondrocalcinosis and occasional underlying metabolic abnormalities, including hemochromatosis, hyperparathyroidism, hypomagnesemia, hypophosphatasia, and hypothyroidism. Examination of synovial fluid under polarized microscopy reveals the positively birefringent crystals of calcium pyrophosphate dihydrate, which are diagnostic.

Palindromic rheumatism, a condition that occasionally precedes the onset of rheumatoid arthritis is associated with recurrent episodes of joint pain or swelling (or both), with complete resolution between flares. Typically, these flares become more prolonged and the diagnosis reveals itself with time. In some patients, small joint disease and the presence of subcutaneous nodules may prompt the diagnosis of rheumatoid arthritis. However, nodular rheumatoid arthritis is usually associated with positivity for rheumatoid factor and anti-cyclic citrullinated antibodies, unlike Whipple disease where these serologic tests tend to be negative. In adult-onset Still disease, large joint involvement occurs in association with fever and leukocytosis, but ferritin levels are characteristically very high. Seronegative spondyloarthropathy may be suggested by the presence of large joint disease, sacroiliitis, and gastrointestinal symptoms. However, rapid weight loss and profound malabsorption are atypical features of this disorder and should trigger further diagnostic tests. Proliferative syndesmophyte formation along the spine is a classic finding of diffuse idiopathic skeletal hyperostosis, a condition in which there are no associated systemic features and inflammatory markers are usually normal.

B. Other Systemic Diseases

Lymphadenopathy and weight loss frequently lead to investigation for lymphoma or other forms of malignant disease. Celiac disease may present with musculoskeletal symptoms and gastrointestinal complaints or weight loss. However, upper gastrointestinal endoscopy and biopsy shows characteristic changes of intra-epithelial lymphocytosis, crypt hyperplasia, and villous atrophy. In addition, serologic testing for anti-tissue transglutaminase antibodies and IgA-endomysial antibodies helps confirm this diagnosis. Inflammatory bowel disease may be associated with large joint inflammation, but findings on endoscopy and biopsy are characteristic. Löfgren syndrome is a subset of sarcoidosis that typically presents with lower limb joint pain or swelling (or both) in addition to erythema nodosum and intrathoracic lymph node enlargement. Tissue biopsy demonstrates the presence of noncaseating granulomas that are PAS and PCR negative. Several endocrinopathies may present in a similar manner to Whipple disease. Addison disease may be suggested by the development of hyperpigmentation, diarrhea, and weight loss. Although musculoskeletal symptoms may also occur in this disorder, joint inflammation is rare and measurement of diurnal cortisol and corticotropin levels confirms the diagnosis. In patients with hyperthyroidism, weight loss, diarrhea, and joint and muscle pain occur. Testing for thyroid hormones and thyroid-stimulating hormone is diagnostic.

C. Neurologic Diseases

There is a wide differential diagnosis for the neurologic manifestations of Whipple disease, which may mimic central nervous system tumors, vasculitis, multiple sclerosis, atherosclerotic disease, and dementia. Associated psychiatric illness, particularly depression, is common. Oculomasticatory myorhythmia is pathognomonic. PCR examination of cerebrospinal fluid for *T whipplei* is helpful in these cases.

D. Infectious Diseases

Several infections should be considered in the differential diagnosis of Whipple disease. Tuberculosis may cause weight loss and lymphadenopathy in the absence of overt pulmonary disease. Although *Mycobacterium avium* may cause PAS-positive stains on histologic examination, PCR for *T whipplei* is negative in these cases. Lyme disease may result in lower limb synovitis, particularly involving the knee, in addition to neurologic and cardiac symptoms. A careful history to search for possible exposure to tick bites or the classic erythema migrans rash encourages appropriate serologic testing. However, in chronic, undiagnosed Lyme disease, a high index of suspicion is required.

► Treatment

A. Antibiotics

Prolonged antibiotic treatment is essential in order to eradicate the organism. For patients with confirmed or suspected neurologic involvement, parenteral treatment for a period of 2 weeks with ceftriaxone 2 g daily or penicillin G 2–4 million units every 4 hours is recommended in order to attain high cerebrospinal fluid levels. Thereafter, a maintenance regimen of co-trimoxazole (trimethoprim 160 mg with sulfamethoxazole 800 mg) should be taken by mouth twice daily for at least 1 year. Alternatively, doxycycline 100 mg twice daily may be used. It is usually prescribed in combination

with hydroxychloroquine 200 mg three times per day, which increases its bactericidal capacity. If there is no evidence of neurologic involvement, and in particular if cerebrospinal fluid PCR is negative, the parenteral induction regimen may be omitted. However, because central nervous system disease is frequently irreversible and may be initially asymptomatic, the full treatment regimen is recommended for all patients.

B. Glucocorticoids

Glucocorticoids are used to reduce the manifestations of central nervous system involvement in conjunction with antibiotics. They are also helpful in decreasing the signs of immune reconstitution inflammatory syndrome where persistent fever may develop after the initiation of antibiotics in patients with a heavy bacterial load.

► Prognosis

Prior to the availability of antibiotics, Whipple disease was invariably fatal. Early recognition and treatment greatly improves the outcome. For patients without central nervous system involvement, rapid improvement of symptoms occurs after initiation of antibiotic therapy. Diarrhea often resolves within 1 week, while joint symptoms remit within 1 month. The course of neurologic involvement is less predictable and long-standing neurologic deficits tend to be irreversible. Central nervous system infection is associated with a mortality rate of 25% within 4 years of diagnosis, while a further 25% remain significantly impaired.

Older treatment regimens using tetracycline alone were associated with a relapse rate of up to 30%. A much lower recurrence rate of 2% has been observed with co-trimoxazole–based regimens.

Fenollar F, Puéchal X, Raoult D. Whipple's disease. *N Engl J Med.* 2007;356:55. [PMID: 17202456]

Jones J, Vellend H, Detsky AS, Mourad O. Clinical problem-solving. *N Engl J Med.* 2007;356:68. [PMID: 17202458]

Puéchal X, Fenollar F, Raoult D. Cultivation of *Tropheryma whipplei* from the synovial fluid in Whipple's arthritis. *Arthritis Rheum.* 2007;56:1713. [PMID: 17469186]

Puéchal X. Whipple disease and arthritis. *Curr Opin Rheumatol.* 2001;13:74. [PMID: 11148719]

Schneider T, Moos V, Loddenkemper C, Marth T, Fenollar F, Raoult D. Whipple's disease: new aspects of pathogenesis and treatment. *Lancet Infect Dis.* 2008;8:179. [PMID: 18291339]

Sarcoidosis

54

Edward S. Chen, MD

David R. Moller, MD

ESSENTIALS OF DIAGNOSIS

- ▶ Systemic disease due to noncaseating epithelioid granulomatous inflammation in affected organs.
- ▶ Most frequently affected organs are lung, lymph nodes, eyes, skin, joints, liver, muscles, central and peripheral nervous system, upper airway, heart, and kidneys.
- ▶ Clinically apparent organ involvement is typically restricted to a few organs, usually defined early in the course of disease.
- ▶ In the United States, sarcoidosis is more common and severe in blacks.
- ▶ Diagnosis requires a compatible clinical picture and a biopsy with typical noncaseating granulomas, excluding diseases that can cause similar granulomatous reactions.

▶ General Considerations

A. Epidemiology

Sarcoidosis is found worldwide with a prevalence ranging from 10 to 80 cases per 100,000 in North America and Europe. Higher regional prevalence has been reported in Scandinavia and the southeast coastal United States. In the United States, one study from a Midwest city estimated that the lifetime risk of developing sarcoidosis was 2.7% in black women, 2.1% in black men, 1% in white women, and 0.8% in white men. Worldwide, there is a slight female predominance. Although all ages can be affected, most cases occur between the ages of 20 and 40 years, with a second peak incidence in women over age 60.

B. Genetics

A genetic predisposition to sarcoidosis is supported by familial clustering in approximately 5–10% of cases of sarcoidosis.

A recent multicenter study on the etiology of sarcoidosis in the United States (A Case-Control Etiologic Study of Sarcoidosis [ACCESS]) suggests that the familial relative risk is approximately 5.0 among first-degree relatives, and this risk is higher in white families compared with black families.

The strongest associations between genotype and sarcoidosis risk have been identified within the major histocompatibility (MHC) locus on chromosome 6. Two recent genome-wide linkage analyses identified an association with the butyrophilin-like 2 gene (BTNL2) (located within the MHC locus) in both whites and blacks with sarcoidosis.

C. Etiology

The cause of sarcoidosis is uncertain. The genetic pattern of inheritance suggests that susceptibility to sarcoidosis is polygenic and interacts importantly with environmental factors. Geographic differences in disease prevalence and reports of time-space clustering of cases have also suggested that sarcoidosis may be associated with an environmental, likely microbial, exposure. The large, multicenter study ACCESS found no evidence for a single dominant environmental or occupational exposure associated with an increased risk of developing sarcoidosis. Multiple regression analyses found positive associations with modest odds ratios of approximately 1.5 for exposures to molds and mildews, insecticides, or musty odors at work. The ACCESS data supported a negative association of tobacco use or tobacco smoke exposure among sarcoidosis patients.

Since the first description of sarcoidosis, many experts have speculated that a potential microbial cause of sarcoidosis exists. Recent studies using polymerase chain reaction (PCR) have associated mycobacterial and propionibacterial organisms as possible etiologic factors for sarcoidosis. A recent meta-analysis concluded that 26% of sarcoidosis tissues contained mycobacterial nucleic acids, with an odds-ratio of 9- to 19-fold higher chance of finding mycobacterial nucleic acids in sarcoidosis compared with control tissues. Recently, a limited proteomic approach identified the mycobacterial catalase-peroxidase protein (mKatG) as a candidate pathogenic antigen. This and other studies from the United States and Europe have demonstrated immunologic responses to mKatG and other mycobacterial proteins in a subgroup of sarcoidosis patients, supporting a mycobacterial etiology of sarcoidosis. In Japan, a subgroup of sarcoidosis patients has been demonstrated to have immunologic responses to *Propionibacterium acnes*. No studies have demonstrated the presence of live organisms from sarcoidosis tissues, distinguishing sarcoidosis from active infections. How these microbial organisms trigger sarcoidosis remains unknown.

Table 54–1. Clinical features of sarcoidosis.

Clinically Evident Organ System Involvement (%)	Major Clinical Features
Pulmonary (70–90%)	Bilateral hilar adenopathy, restrictive and obstructive disease, reticulonodular infiltrates, fibrocystic disease, bronchiectasis, mycetomas
Ocular (20–30%)	Anterior and posterior uveitis, optic neuritis, chorioretinitis, conjunctival nodules, glaucoma, keratoconjunctivitis, lacrimal gland enlargement
Cutaneous (20–30%)	Erythema nodosum, lupus pernio, cutaneous and subcutaneous nodules, plaques, alopecia, dactylitis
Hematologic (20–30%)	Peripheral lymphadenopathy, splenomegaly, hypersplenism, anemia, lymphopenia, thrombocytopenia, hypergammaglobulinemia
Musculoskeletal/joints (10–20%)	Arthralgias, bone cysts, myopathy, heel pain, Achilles tendinitis, sacroiliitis
Hepatic (10–20%)	Hepatomegaly, pruritus, jaundice, cirrhosis
Salivary and parotid gland (10%)	Sicca syndrome, Heerfordt syndrome
Neurologic (5–15%)	Cranial neuropathy, aseptic meningitis, mass brain lesion, hydrocephalus, myelopathy, polyneuropathy, mononeuritis multiplex
Sinuses and upper respiratory tract (5–10%)	Chronic sinusitis, nasal congestion, saddle-nose deformity, hoarseness, laryngeal or tracheal obstruction
Cardiac (5–10%)	Arrhythmias, heart block, cardiomyopathy, sudden death
Gastrointestinal (<10%)	Abdominal pain, gastrointestinal tract dysmotility, pancreatitis
Endocrine (<10%)	Hypercalcemia, hypopituitarism, diabetes insipidus, epididymitis, testicular mass
Renal (<10%)	Interstitial nephritis, glomerulonephritis, nephrolithiasis, hypercalciuria, nephrocalcinosis

D. Pathophysiology

There are certain immunologic hallmarks of sarcoidosis regardless of the potential etiologic trigger. There is usually an accumulation of CD4+ dominant T cell infiltration at sites of granulomatous inflammation, with fewer CD8+ T cells usually surrounding the granulomas. These CD4+ T cells have biased expression of specific T cell receptor genes, consistent with oligoclonal expansion of antigen-specific T cells. The antigen-specific T cell response is highly polarized toward a T helper 1 response with expression of interferon-gamma (IFN-γ) and the Th1 immunomodulatory cytokines, interleukin-12 (IL-12), and IL-18. Along with Th1 cytokines, pro-inflammatory cytokines such as tumor necrosis factor (TNF), IL-1, IL-6, and a Th1-associated chemokines together orchestrate the local granulomatous response. Dysregulated expression of Th1 immunomodulatory cytokines has been hypothesized to central to the development of granulomatous inflammation in sarcoidosis.

▶ Clinical Findings

There is tremendous heterogeneity in the clinical manifestations of sarcoidosis. Pulmonary involvement is documented in >90% of patients. Nonpulmonary manifestations are present in many patients with or without pulmonary involvement (Table 54–1).

An initial diagnostic evaluation should consist of tests to evaluate the presence and extent of pulmonary involvement and screening for common extrathoracic involvement (Table 54–2). Specialized testing is indicated when symptoms or signs suggest extrapulmonary involvement.

Table 54–2. Recommended tests for an initial evaluation of sarcoidosis.

Chest radiograph or chest CT scan
Pulmonary function tests
Spirometry (with flow-volume loops if upper airway obstruction is suspected)
Diffusion capacity
Lung volumes
Ophthalmologic examination
Blood work
Comprehensive metabolic panel (renal function, liver function, serum calcium level)
Complete blood count with differential
Electrocardiogram
Screen for tuberculosis exposure with purified protein derivative (PPD) skin test
Additional organ-specific tests may be indicated in patients with specific extrapulmonary symptoms. For example:
Cardiac: echocardiogram, Holter monitor, cardiac MRI, cardiac positron emission tomography
Neurologic: contrast MRI, nerve conduction study, lumbar puncture

A. Symptoms and Signs

1. Acute sarcoidosis (Löfgren syndrome)—This syndrome of acute sarcoidosis is characterized by erythema nodosum, bilateral hilar adenopathy, and often polyarthritis and uveitis (Figure 54–1). Löfgren syndrome is common among Scandinavians and Irish women but occurs in less than 5% of black patients with sarcoidosis. Acute sarcoidosis without erythema nodosum may also occur, often with disabling arthritis.

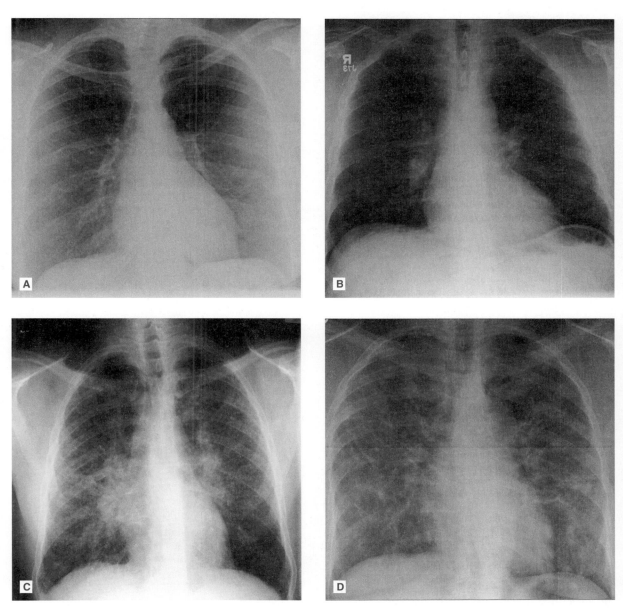

▲ **Figure 54–1.** Pulmonary sarcoidosis. Posteroanterior chest radiographs illustrating pulmonary sarcoidosis categorized as stage 0 (normal chest film), stage I (bilateral hilar adenopathy alone), stage II (adenopathy plus interstitial infiltrates), stage III (interstitial infiltrates alone), and stage IV (fibrocystic). Thoracic disease (lung and lymph node involvement) represent the most common manifestations of sarcoidosis affecting over 70% of all patients. Bronchscopy remains the most common method of confirming a diagnosis of sarcoidosis.

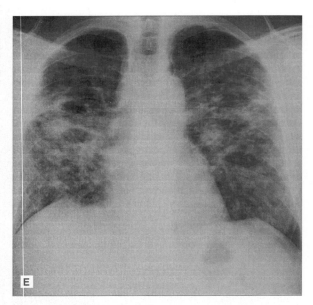

▲ **Figure 54–1.** (*Continued*)

2. Pulmonary sarcoidosis—The most common symptoms are progressive shortness of breath, nonproductive cough, and chest discomfort (Table 54–1). Chronic sputum production and hemoptysis are more frequent in advanced fibrocystic disease (chest radiograph stage IV, Figure 54–1). Typically, there are few physical findings of pulmonary sarcoidosis, with lung crackles heard in less than 10% of patients. Clubbing is rare. Airway obstruction is usually fixed (unresponsive to bronchodilators) and observed in a minority of patients. Bronchial hyperreactivity with occasional frank wheezing is found in 5–30% of patients.

Pulmonary hypertension or **cor pulmonale** is seen in >80% patients with advanced fibrocystic sarcoidosis with pulmonary fibrosis. Rarely, a granulomatous pulmonary vasculitis results in pulmonary hypertension with little evidence of interstitial lung disease. Dyspnea out of proportion to pulmonary function test results should prompt a search for pulmonary hypertension. Other causes of pulmonary hypertension, such as sleep disordered breathing or chronic thromboembolic disease, must be excluded. Severe pulmonary hypertension in patients with advanced lung disease is associated with higher rates of mortality while awaiting lung transplantation.

3. Ocular manifestations—Uveitis is the most common eye lesion in sarcoidosis and may be the initial presenting manifestation. The uveitis is more commonly anterior, may be unilateral or bilateral, and is frequently associated with bilateral hilar adenopathy. Chronic uveitis occurs in as many as 20% of patients with chronic sarcoidosis and is more common in the black population. **Granulomatous conjunctivitis**

appears as a granular or cobblestone-like appearance of the conjunctivae. Conjunctival nodules are also a common finding. **Optic neuritis** or **retinitis** may manifest dramatically with blindness. Severe chorioretinitis occurs uncommonly.

4. Chronic cutaneous sarcoidosis—Sarcoidosis commonly involves the skin (20–30%) and may be severe, especially in black patients. Cutaneous nodules, plaques and subcutaneous nodules, typically located around the hairline, eyelids, ears, nose, mouth, and extensor surfaces of the arms and legs, are common. **Lupus pernio** is a particularly disfiguring form of cutaneous sarcoidosis of the face with violaceous plaques and nodules covering the nose (Figure 54–2), nasal alae, malar areas, and around the eyes.

5. Hematologic sarcoidosis—Peripheral lymph node enlargement occurs in 20–30% of patients as an early manifestation of sarcoidosis but then typically undergoes spontaneous remission. Persistent, bulky lymphadenopathy occurs less than 10% of the time. Splenomegaly, occasionally massive, occurs in less than 5% of cases and is often associated with hepatomegaly and hypercalcemia. Polyclonal hypergammaglobulinemia is present in 25% or more of patients. Anemia and peripheral lymphopenia are relatively common while leucopenia and thrombocytopenia are rare. A clinical association exists between sarcoidosis and common variable immunodeficiency (CVID); CVID should be suspected in

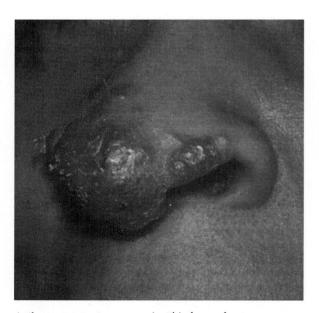

▲ **Figure 54–2.** Lupus pernio. This form of cutaneous eruption in sarcoidosis is typified by violaceous plaques and nodules that involve the nose, nasal alae, malar areas, nasolabial folds, around the eyes, scalp, and along the hairline. (© Bernard Cohen, MD, Dermatlas; http://www.dermatlas.org.)

patients with sarcoidosis who develop increased frequency of infections or hypogammaglobulinemia.

6. Musculoskeletal sarcoidosis—Systemic constitutional symptoms such as fever, malaise, and weight loss are seen in over 20% of patients and may be disabling. **Arthralgias** are common in active multisystem sarcoidosis, although joint radiographs are usually normal. Acute, often incapacitating polyarthritis involving the ankles, feet, knees, and wrists is commonly seen in patients with Löfgren syndrome; usually the polyarthritis regresses within weeks to several months with or without therapy. Persistent joint disease is found in less than 5% of patients with chronic sarcoidosis. Pain, swelling, and tenderness of the phalanges (sausage digit) of the hands and feet are most common.

Although random muscle biopsies in autopsy series often demonstrate muscle granulomas in patients with sarcoidosis,

symptomatic myopathy with weakness and tenderness is uncommon. Rarely, sarcoidosis can present as a polymyositis with profound weakness and elevated serum creatine kinase and aldolase levels.

Radiographic skeletal findings are most typically noted as incidental findings and observed in <10% of all patients. These typically present as cystic and lytic lesions of varying sizes and may have associated sclerotic margins (Figure 54–3). Most commonly involved areas include bones of the skull, vertebrae, hands, and feet. The use of other imaging modalities (CT, MRI with gadolinium, technetium bone scan) has not been proven to be useful for judging the activity of such lesions or differentiating them from infection or malignancy.

Fibromyalgia may be associated with sarcoidosis and causes considerable morbidity in such patients. This cause of pain does not respond to immunosuppressive therapy.

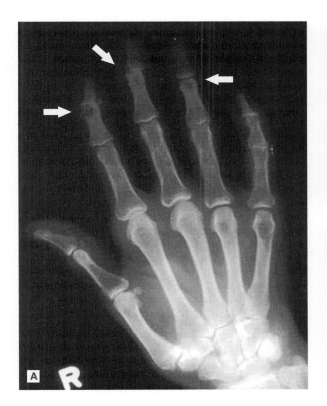

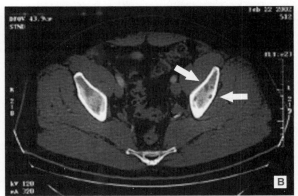

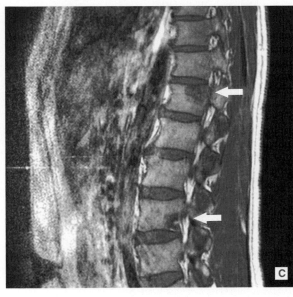

▲ **Figure 54–3.** Bone involvement in sarcoidosis. Multiple focal "punched-out" lesions (*arrows*) on a plain radiograph of the hand (Used, with permission, from William Herring, MD; http://www.learningradiology.com), CT of the pelvis (*arrow*), and MRI of the spine that are compatible with skeletal manifestations of sarcoidosis.

7. Gastrointestinal sarcoidosis—Although a liver biopsy demonstrates granulomatous inflammation in over 50% of patients, clinically significant liver involvement is documented in only 10–20% of patients and is rarely the sole manifestation of this disease. Active hepatic inflammation may be associated with fever, tender hepatomegaly, and pruritus. Characteristically, the serum alkaline phosphatase and γ-glutamyltransferase are elevated disproportionately higher than the transaminases or bilirubin. This is often part of a constellation of hepatic, spleen, and bone marrow involvement with or without hypercalcemia, sometimes referred to as "abdominal sarcoidosis." Elevated serum liver function tests frequently revert to normal spontaneously or after treatment with glucocorticoids. Progressive cirrhosis may occur if severe, persistent granulomatous hepatitis is not treated.

Symptomatic gastrointestinal involvement in sarcoidosis is rare, and other causes, such as Crohn disease or ulcerative colitis, must be excluded.

8. Neurosarcoidosis—This manifestation occurs in 5–10% of patients with sarcoidosis. The most common manifestation is cranial neuropathy with bilateral or unilateral seventh nerve (Bell) palsy or less commonly, glossopharyngeal, auditory, oculomotor, or trigeminal palsies. The palsies may resolve spontaneously or with glucocorticoid therapy but may recur years later. Optic neuritis can result in blurred vision, field defects, and blindness. Other manifestations include mass lesions, aseptic meningitis, obstructive hydrocephalus, and hypothalamic-pituitary dysfunction. Seizures, headache, change in mental status, confusion, and diabetes insipidus can be initial manifestations of sarcoidosis. Spinal cord involvement is rare, but paraparesis, hemiparesis, and back and leg pains may occur. Peripheral neuropathies account for about 15% of cases of neurosarcoidosis, often presenting as mononeuritis multiplex or a primary sensory neuropathy. Recently, small fiber neuropathy has been associated with a pain syndrome in sarcoidosis; a few case reports suggest TNF inhibitors may be helpful in treating this debilitating condition.

9. Sarcoidosis of the upper respiratory tract (SURT)—This manifestation occurs in 5–10% of patients, usually in those with long-standing disease. Severe nasal congestion and chronic sinusitis usually are unresponsive to decongestants and topical (intranasal) glucocorticoids. Chronic disease or surgical intervention may result in destruction of the nasal septum and a "saddle-nose" deformity. Laryngeal sarcoidosis may present with severe hoarseness, stridor, and acute respiratory failure secondary to upper airway obstruction. Often, SURT is associated with chronic skin lesions, particularly lupus pernio (see Figure 54–2).

10. Cardiac sarcoidosis—Although myocardial sarcoidosis is diagnosed in less than 10% of patients in the United States and Europe, autopsy series suggest that the histologic presence of sarcoidosis in the heart may be as high as 25%.

In Japan, cardiac sarcoidosis occurs in nearly 50% of sarcoidosis patients. Arrhythmia, heart block, dilated cardiomyopathy, or sudden death can be the presenting clinical manifestations. Endomyocardial biopsies fail to demonstrate granulomatous inflammation in 80% of cases due to sampling inefficiencies in the setting of patchy inflammatory involvement and the lack of involvement of the right ventricle. A diagnosis of cardiac sarcoidosis can be inferred from a combination of biopsy-proven systemic sarcoidosis and a compatible myocardial imaging study, such as thallium or sestamibi scan, cardiac MRI with gadolinium enhancement, or cardiac positron emission tomography (PET) scan (Figure 54–4).

11. Salivary, parotid, and lacrimal gland sarcoidosis—Parotid or lacrimal gland enlargement or sicca syndrome can occasionally be the dominant clinical manifestations of sarcoidosis. Heerfordt syndrome, or uveoparotid fever, is an uncommon acute presentation of sarcoidosis manifesting as fever, parotid and lacrimal gland enlargement, uveitis, bilateral hilar adenopathy, and often cranial neuropathies.

12. Endocrine abnormalities in sarcoidosis—In patients with neurosarcoidosis, disturbances to the hypothalamic-pituitary axis may result in diabetes insipidus and other manifestations of hypopituitarism. There is a higher association of autoimmune thyroid disease and sarcoidosis compared to control populations. Pancreatic sarcoidosis manifesting as a mass is a rare manifestation and must be distinguished from cancer.

13. Renal involvement in sarcoidosis—Sarcoidosis may be associated with hypercalcemia, and more commonly, hypercalciuria. The abnormalities are caused by the increased conversion of inactive 25-OH vitamin D_3 to the active $1,25(OH)_2$ vitamin D_3 by epithelioid macrophages within tissue granulomas. Primary care physicians must be aware that a low serum 25-OH vitamin D level (the standard serum vitamin D test) usually does not represent vitamin D deficiency in sarcoidosis patients, but rather is a result from this increased conversion to active $1,25(OH)_2$ vitamin D. Vitamin D supplementation in this instance may precipitate hypercalcemic crisis in untreated sarcoidosis patients. Vitamin D supplementation should only be based on serum levels of active $1,25(OH)_2$ vitamin D (which requires special ordering) in patients with sarcoidosis. Nephrocalcinosis may cause renal failure in sarcoidosis. Direct granulomatous involvement of the kidneys causing chronic interstitial nephritis or membranous glomerulonephritis is rare.

14. Psychosocial abnormalities—As many as 30–60% of patients with sarcoidosis report symptoms of depression. One study found this to be associated with female sex, lower socioeconomic status, poor access to health care and increased disease severity, but not race.

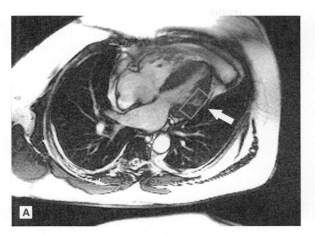

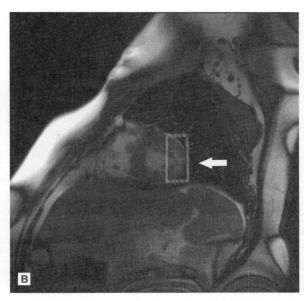

▲ **Figure 54–4.** Cardiac sarcoidosis. Cardiac MRI demonstrates gadolinium enhancement in the submyocardial region (*arrows*) in a patient with cardiac sarcoidosis and nonsustained ventricular tachycardia.

B. Laboratory Studies

Recommended initial studies for all patients with presumed or biopsy-proven sarcoidosis include the following:

- A comprehensive metabolic panel is useful to assess abnormalities of renal function, calcium level, and liver function.

- The complete blood cell count is usually either normal or demonstrates peripheral lymphopenia. Pancytopenia may be caused by hypersplenism or bone marrow infiltration with granulomas.

C. Imaging Studies

Chest radiographs are abnormal in 90% or more of patients with sarcoidosis and can be categorized by stage or type by international convention (Figure 54–1). **Stage 0** indicates a normal chest radiograph (ie, seen in extrapulmonary sarcoidosis). **Stage I** shows bilateral hilar adenopathy. **Stage II** shows bilateral hilar adenopathy plus interstitial infiltrates. **Stage III** demonstrates interstitial infiltrates only. **Stage IV** demonstrates fibrocystic lung disease.

Uncommon findings associated with pulmonary sarcoidosis include large, well-defined nodular infiltrates, miliary disease, a pattern of patchy air space consolidation with air bronchograms, termed "alveolar sarcoidosis," or the presence of mycetomas. Differential diagnoses include mycobacterial or fungal infection, malignancy, or granulomatosis with polyangiitis (formerly Wegener granulomatosis). Pleural effusions and pneumothoraces are unusual in sarcoidosis.

Chest CT typically demonstrates reticulonodular infiltrates that follow bronchovascular distribution. Occasionally, ground-glass infiltrates, well-defined nodules, mass-like infiltrates, alveolar consolidation, or honeycombing are seen. Pleural effusions are rarely secondary to sarcoidosis inflammation.

Nuclear medicine studies, such as 67-gallium scanning and positron emission tomography using 18-fluorodeoxyglucose (FDG-PET), have been used to detect active inflammatory sites in sarcoidosis, potentially aiding in choosing sites for biopsy. FDG-PET uses less radiation exposure while offering better resolution and has largely replaced gallium scanning. Classic findings using gallium or PET scanning are uptake in the bilateral hilar and right paratracheal lymph node region ("lambda" sign) of the lungs, and uptake in the parotids or lacrimal and salivary glands ("panda" sign). The combination of signs (lambda-panda) is suggestive of sarcoidosis.

Joint radiographs may demonstrate "punched out" lesions with cystic changes and marked loss of trabeculae but without evidence of erosive chrondritis. Cystic lesions of the long bones, pelvis, sternum, skull, and vertebrae rarely occur (Figure 54–4).

MRI with gadolinium contrast enhancement has an important role in the evaluation of neurosarcoidosis, particularly in cases of suspected brain, cranial nerve, or spinal cord involvement.

D. Pulmonary Function Testing

Pulmonary function tests may show restrictive, obstructive, or combined impairment with a parallel reduction in diffusing capacity for carbon monoxide (DLCO). Resting gas exchange is usually preserved until extensive fibrocystic changes are evident, although oxygen desaturation with exercise occurs in less advanced disease.

E. Other Tests

A well-recognized feature of sarcoidosis is the impaired cutaneous response to common antigens that elicit delayed-type hypersensitivity reactions, seen in 30–70% of patients. Since anergy to purified protein derivative (PPD) testing is common in sarcoidosis, active tuberculosis must be strongly considered in any patient in whom a positive tuberculin skin test develops.

An electrocardiogram is routinely performed to screen for conduction abnormalities, which may signal the presence of early cardiac sarcoidosis. When cardiac sarcoidosis is suspected on the basis of symptoms or electrocardiographic abnormalities, Holter monitoring, and cardiac imaging is indicated. Two-dimensional echocardiography is useful as a screening tool but is insensitive to mild cardiac abnormalities. Radionuclide imaging with gated 201-thallium scanning, cardiac MRI, or cardiac PET are more sensitive studies to detect myocardial abnormalities related to sarcoidosis (Figure 54–4). Electrophysiologic testing may be indicated to exclude arrhythmias undetected by routine studies.

In patients with suspected neurosarcoidosis, MRI with gadolinium enhancement of the brain or spine is indicated. The characteristic inflammatory lesions by contrast MRI have a propensity for periventricular and leptomeningeal areas. These findings are nonspecific and can be produced by infectious (tuberculosis, fungal disease) or malignant (lymphoma, carcinomatosis) disease. A normal scan does not exclude neurosarcoidosis, particularly for cranial neuropathies, peripheral neuropathies, or in the presence of glucocorticoid therapy.

In neurosarcoidosis, the cerebrospinal fluid may demonstrate lymphocytic pleocytosis or elevated protein levels, providing supportive evidence of central nervous system or spinal cord inflammation. A diagnosis of neurosarcoidosis is usually confirmed by biopsy of a non–central nervous system site, generally by bronchoscopic or lymph node biopsy. Rarely, brain or spinal cord biopsy is needed to exclude infectious or malignant disease. In suspected cases of peripheral neuropathy or myopathy, electromyography or nerve conduction studies are often indicated.

F. Diagnostic Examinations

Identifying the extent of specific organ involvement requires a careful review of localizing symptoms in the setting of biopsy-confirmed granulomatous inflammation. Biopsy of the easiest, most accessible abnormal tissue site is used for confirmation of the diagnosis and to exclude infection,

malignancy, or other diseases that have similar clinical manifestations. Biopsy by fiberoptic bronchoscopy is frequently used to diagnose pulmonary sarcoidosis because of its relative safety and high yield. Endobronchial or transbronchial needle aspiration biopsies may increase the yield further. Bronchoalveolar lavage fluid in sarcoidosis is typically characterized by increased proportions and numbers of activated CD4+ alveolar lymphocytes reflective of enhanced cell-mediated immune processes at sites of granuloma formation. These findings are not specific for sarcoidosis and do not predict clinical outcome.

Mediastinoscopy or surgical lung biopsy (open-lung, thoracoscopic) should be considered in cases where lymphoma or other intrathoracic malignancy cannot be reasonably excluded. Biopsy of a skin nodule, superficial lymph node, nasal mucosa, conjunctiva, or salivary gland (lip biopsy) sometimes can establish a diagnosis. Biopsy of the liver or bone marrow is nonspecific and should be used to support a diagnosis of sarcoidosis only after malignancy, infectious granulomatous diseases, or other organ-specific diagnoses are excluded. In rare cases, biopsy of critical organs may be necessary to exclude malignancy, such as when sarcoidosis presents as a mass lesion in the brain. Biopsy confirmation of sarcoidosis is usually not necessary in Löfgren syndrome except in regions where histoplasmosis is endemic, and fungal infection must be excluded before initiating glucocorticoid therapy.

▶ Differential Diagnosis

A diagnosis of sarcoidosis is based on a compatible clinical picture, histologic evidence of noncaseating granulomas, and the absence of other known causes of this pathologic response, such as tuberculosis, fungal diseases, and chronic beryllium disease.

▶ Treatment

There is consensus on the following indications for treatment (Table 54–3):

- Persistent, symptomatic, or progressive pulmonary disease.

- Threatened organ failure, such as severe ocular, central nervous system, or cardiac disease.

- Persistent hypercalcemia or renal or hepatic dysfunction.

- Posterior uveitis or anterior uveitis not responding to localized glucocorticoid therapy.

- Myopathy.

- Significant splenomegaly or evidence of hypersplenism such as thrombocytopenia.

- Severe fatigue and weight loss.

- Disfiguring skin disease or symptomatic lymphadenopathy.

Table 54–3. Evidence-based recommendations, summarizing consensus guidelines from the British/ Australian/New Zealand/Irish Thoracic Societies.

- Because of high rates of remission within first 2–3 years, no treatment is recommended for asymptomatic patients with only lymphadenopathy (stage I), or asymptomatic patients with lung infiltrates (stage II or III) and stable but mildly abnormal lung function.
- Oral glucocorticoids are first-line therapy in patients with progressive disease determined by lung function, significant symptoms, or extrapulmonary sarcoidosis.
- Given the duration of glucocorticoid treatment for sarcoidosis, bisphosphonates should be used to prevent accelerated bone loss.
- Inhaled glucocorticoids are not beneficial for treating progressive pulmonary sarcoidosis; however, inhaled glucocorticoids can be used to control cough or airway hyperreactivity in a subgroup of patients.
- Non-glucocorticoid immunosuppressant medications have limited role as primary therapy for sarcoidosis but should be considered in patients when reasonable doses of glucocorticoids alone (prednisone ≤20 mg daily) are not controlling the disease, or if glucocorticoid side effects are intolerable.
- Methotrexate is the preferred non-glucocorticoid, steroid-sparing medication for patients with progressive disease. Azathioprine is often used when methotrexate is contraindicated or not tolerated.
- Lung transplantation should be considered for end-stage pulmonary sarcoidosis.

There is consensus that patients with sarcoidosis and no evidence of end organ impairment (eg, normal pulmonary function tests with or without abnormal chest radiograph) with minimal respiratory symptoms should not be treated. Patients with limited cutaneous disease that is nondisfiguring can be considered for local intralesional glucocorticoid injections.

A. Medical

Currently, there are no medications approved by the US Food and Drug Administration for the treatment of sarcoidosis. Glucocorticoids remain the mainstay of treatment because of their effectiveness in reversing nonfibrotic organ impairment (at least over the short term), and relative safety.

1. Glucocorticoids—This class of drugs is the cornerstone of therapy for serious progressive pulmonary or extrapulmonary sarcoidosis (Table 54–3). Guidelines for when to initiate therapy with glucocorticoids and proper dosing have been formulated from extensive clinical experience without being subjected to prospective randomized control trials. Controversy exists regarding their overall effectiveness in altering the long-term course of the disease. However, clinical experience indicates that glucocorticoids provide prompt symptomatic relief and reverse organ dysfunction in almost all patients with active inflammation. The optimal dose and duration of glucocorticoid treatment have not been

established by rigorous clinical studies. Topical glucocorticoids are usually ineffective except for specific cases of ocular sarcoidosis. Most studies find inhaled glucocorticoids for pulmonary sarcoidosis to be ineffective, and only a minority of patients with airway obstruction demonstrate meaningful responses to bronchodilators.

In general, initial treatment with glucocorticoids should be planned for a period of 8–12 months, except for Löfgren syndrome. One well-designed study by the British Thoracic Society demonstrated that in patients with active pulmonary sarcoidosis with interstitial infiltrates, a stable maintenance regimen of low-dose glucocorticoids is more effective at preserving lung function than symptomatic use of glucocorticoids followed by repeated tapering regimens.

For patients who require maintenance therapy for chronic sarcoidosis, glucocorticoid therapy often results in significant adverse effects such as weight gain, diabetes, and osteoporosis. Thus, when these adverse effects become intolerable, glucocorticoid-sparing drugs are often considered. However, all glucocorticoid-sparing drugs show variable effectiveness and have adverse risk profiles that warrant careful dosing and monitoring in the absence of controlled clinical comparison trials.

2. Glucocorticoid-sparing agents

a. Hydroxychloroquine—This agent is used for dominant skin, nasal mucosal, and sinus sarcoidosis but has not been consistently effective for pulmonary or systemic disease. Hypercalcemia and laryngeal, bone, and joint involvement have been reported to respond to hydroxychloroquine. Serial ophthalmologic evaluations should be performed every 6 months during hydroxychloroquine therapy. Chloroquine may have greater effectiveness but is rarely used because of the higher risk of ocular toxicity. When chloroquine is used for treatment recalcitrant mucosal or skin disease, it is given for 6 months followed by a 6-month drug holiday; ophthalmologic follow-up should be scheduled every 3 months.

b. Minocycline and doxycycline (synthetic tetracycline derivatives)—These agents have anti-inflammatory properties. The relatively safe side-effect profile of these medications make them a reasonable choice for non-threatening manifestations of sarcoidosis, such as skin lesions, but clinical experience suggests that these drugs usually are not effective in pulmonary or non-skin multiorgan sarcoidosis.

c. Cytotoxic therapy—Methotrexate is usually the first cytotoxic therapy tried as a potent glucocorticoid-sparing drug. Studies suggest an approximate 60% response rate, which may take 4–6 months or longer for effect. Azathioprine and mycophenolate mofetil are alternative immunosuppressants that have been used in smaller series to treat severe extrapulmonary sarcoidosis and pulmonary sarcoidosis. These agents may require 2–3 months or more of therapy to demonstrate clinical effectiveness. Routine monitoring for renal, liver, and bone marrow toxicities are standard.

3. Biologic agents—Laboratory experiments demonstrate that TNF plays an important role in granuloma formation. There is evidence supporting the effectiveness of select TNF inhibitors in sarcoidosis. A large, randomized multicenter prospective study found that a 24-week course of treatment with infliximab was associated with an improvement in lung function. A separate study also showed infliximab was associated in improvement in nonpulmonary sarcoidosis. The humanized TNF inhibitor adalimumab has not been studied by controlled clinical trials, but small case series suggest this therapy may also be beneficial in some patients with skin sarcoidosis and peripheral neuropathy. Etanercept, a TNF receptor antagonist, failed to show benefit in small clinical trials and cannot be recommended for sarcoidosis. All TNF inhibitors are associated with significant risk of severe infections, reactivation of latent tuberculosis, and potential risk for malignancy and autoimmune phenomena. Given these risks, anti-TNF agents are reserved for patients in need of potent glucocorticoid-sparing therapy and who have not tolerated a trial of cytotoxic therapy. The use of other biologic agents to treat sarcoidosis targeting T cells (alefacept), B cells (rituximab), and other cytokines such as IL-2 (basiliximab) are under study.

B. Surgical

Successful lung, heart-lung, and liver transplantations have been performed in a small number of patients with advanced organ insufficiency. Noncaseating granulomas may develop in the transplanted organs in some lung and heart transplant patients but do not seem to have a significant impact on overall survival.

► Prognosis

Although sarcoidosis can potentially involve any part of the body, the extent of significant organ system involvement is usually evident within the first 2 years after diagnosis. The ACCESS study found that at 2-year follow-up, evidence for new organ system involvement developed in less than 25% of the study participants.

Studies suggest that approximately 50–70% of patients may undergo remission, which is usually evident within the first 2–3 years following diagnosis. Acute sarcoidosis (Löfgren syndrome) has a remission rate of greater than 70%. Monitoring of patients for several years after presumed remission is recommended to ensure stability of organ function. Patients with fibrocystic pulmonary sarcoidosis, lupus pernio, or nasal or sinus sarcoidosis, neurosarcoidosis, cardiac sarcoidosis or who have multisystem disease for greater than 2–3 years usually have unremitting, progressive (if not treated) disease. A waxing and waning course of sarcoidosis is unusual except in patients with ocular, neurologic, peripheral lymph node, or cutaneous involvement.

No biomarkers have been found to be useful in predicting outcomes or to assist in treatment decisions. Serum angiotensin-converting enzyme levels are elevated in 30–80% of patients with clinically active disease. The test has positive and negative predictive values of less than 70–80%, and serum angiotensin-converting enzyme levels do not predict clinical course. Thus, most clinicians agree this test is of limited usefulness in the management of sarcoidosis.

Major causes of death from sarcoidosis include respiratory insufficiency and cor pulmonale, massive hemoptysis, complications from cardiac sarcoidosis, neurosarcoidosis, or uremia from chronic renal failure. Several centers in the United States and Great Britain suggest that race is an important prognostic indicator, with blacks from Africa and West Indian patients more likely to have chronic persistent disease and suffer from increased morbidity and mortality. Hospital statistics suggest that sarcoidosis is the direct cause of death in 1–5% of persons admitted with this disease.

► When to Refer

A patient should be considered for referral to a specialist in sarcoidosis in the following situations:

- Uncertainty of the diagnosis or clinical course.
- Uncertainty whether treatment is indicated.
- Disease that is not responding as expected to therapy.
- Severe extrapulmonary involvement, such as cardiac, neurologic, skin, or sinus involvement.
- Unsure about the use of glucocorticoid-sparing or alternative medications.

Baughman RP, Lower EE. Novel therapies for sarcoidosis. *Semin Respir Crit Care Med.* 2007;28:128. [PMID: 17330197]

Bradley B, Branley HM, Egan JJ et al. British Thoracic Society Interstitial Lung Disease Guideline Group, British Thoracic Society Standards of Care Committee; Thoracic Society of Australia; New Zealand Thoracic Society; Irish Thoracic Society. Interstitial lung disease guideline: the British Thoracic Society in collaboration with the Thoracic Society of Australia and New Zealand and the Irish Thoracic Society. *Thorax.* 2008;63:v1 (suppl). [PMID: 18757459]

Chapelon-Abric C, de Zuttere D, Duhaut P, et al. Cardiac sarcoidosis: a retrospective study of 41 cases. *Medicine (Baltimore).* 2004;83:315. [PMID: 15525844]

Chen ES, Moller DR. Etiology of sarcoidosis. *Clin Chest Med.* 2009;28:365. [PMID: 18539232]

Drent M, Costabel U. Sarcoidosis. In: European Respiratory Society Monograph Series. Wouters E, editor. Volume 10, Monograph 32. Wakefield, UK: The Charlesworth Group; 2005. p. 341.

[Foundation for Sarcoidosis Research] http://www.stopsarcoidosis.org/

Gupta D, Agarwal R, Aggarwal AN, Jindal SK. Molecular evidence for the role of mycobacteria in sarcoidosis: a meta-analysis. *Eur Respir J.* 2007;30:508. [PMID: 17537780]

Iannuzzi MC, Rybicki BA, Teirstein AS. Sarcoidosis. *N Engl J Med.* 2007;357:2153. [PMID: 18032765]

Johns CJ, Michele TM. The clinical management of sarcoidosis. A 50-year experience at the Johns Hopkins Hospital. *Medicine (Baltimore).* 1999;78:65. [PMID: 10195091]

Moller DR. Treatment of sarcoidosis—from a basic science point of view. *J Intern Med.* 2003;253:31. [PMID: 12588536]

[National Heart, Lung, and Blood Institute (NHLBI): Sarcoidosis] http://www.nhlbi.nih.gov/health/dci/Diseases/sarc/sar_whatis.html

Newman LS, Rose CS, Bresnitz EA, et al. ACCESS Research Study Group. A case control etiologic study of sarcoidosis: environmental and occupational risk factors. *Am J Respir Crit Care Med.* 2004;170:1324. [PMID: 15347561]

[Sarcoid Networking Association] http://www.sarcoidosisnetwork.org

Statement on Sarcoidosis. Joint Statement of the American Thoracic Society (ATS), the European Respiratory Society (ERS), and the World Association of Sarcoidosis and Other Granulomatous Disorders (WASOG) adopted by the ATS Board of Directors and by the ERS Executive Committee, February 1999. *Am J Respir Crit Care Med.* 1999;160:736. [PMID: 10430755]

Stern BJ. Neurological complications of sarcoidosis. *Curr Opin Neurol.* 2004;17:311. [PMID: 15167067]

[World Association of Sarcoidosis and Other Granulomatous Disorders (WASOG)] http://www.wasog.org

Endocrine & Metabolic Disorders

Jonathan Graf, MD

Sarah Beckman Gratton, MD

Endocrine disorders commonly cause musculoskeletal symptoms and may even present with rheumatic syndromes before the nature of the underlying endocrinopathy is apparent (Table 55–1). On occasion, endocrine disorders can mimic rheumatic diseases and be a source of diagnostic error (Table 55–2). Rheumatic manifestations of endocrine diseases are usually a consequence of the hormonal abnormalities but, in the case of autoimmune thyroid disease, also can be a result of the underlying autoimmune process.

DIABETES MELLITUS

Patients with either type 1 or type 2 diabetes mellitus frequently have musculoskeletal complaints. Although relatively little is understood about the pathophysiological effects of hyperglycemia on bones, joints, tendons, and muscles, there are well-established associations between diabetes and certain musculoskeletal syndromes (Table 55–3).

1. Diabetic Cheiropathy (Limited Joint Mobility Syndrome)

 ESSENTIALS OF DIAGNOSIS

▶ Most commonly seen in hands.

▶ Limited flexion and extension of finger joints.

▶ Skin becomes progressively puffy and appears shiny and waxy.

▶ "Prayer sign" is simple diagnostic maneuver.

▶ General Considerations

Diabetic cheiropathy, or limited joint mobility syndrome, usually develops after 10 or more years of diabetes (type 1 or 2), particularly when glycemic control has been suboptimal, and likely is due to abnormal glycosylation of connective tissues. Although most frequently recognized and encountered in the hands, this condition can involve the shoulders, knees, and feet.

▶ Clinical Findings & Treatment

The limited mobility results from a generalized palmar fasciitis and from progressive thickening and tightening of the skin. In many instances, the skin becomes progressively puffy, shiny, and waxy in appearance, mimicking sclerodactyly. In a simple diagnostic maneuver, referred to as the **prayer sign,** the patient places his or her hands together, as if in prayer. Patients with limited mobility syndrome are unable to make complete contact between the palmar surfaces of their fingers (Figure 55–1). Improved glycemic control as well as physical and occupational therapy may help slow the progression of diabetic cheiropathy.

2. Flexor Tenosynovitis of the Hand

 ESSENTIALS OF DIAGNOSIS

▶ Presents with an isolated nodule on one of the flexor tendons of the hand, most commonly of the long or ring fingers.

▶ Nodules become symptomatic when they impede tendon motion.

▶ Dupuytren contractures may develop with chronic tenosynovitis of the flexor tendons.

▶ Clinical Findings

Flexor tenosynovitis of the hand, which develops in 12–15% of patients with diabetes, also may be due to abnormal glycosylation of collagen. Early in its course, this condition presents with an isolated nodule on one of the flexor tendons of

Table 55–1. Rheumatic manifestations associated with endocrine disorders.

Rheumatic Disorder	Endocrinopathy
Carpal tunnel syndrome	Diabetes Hypothyroidism Acromegaly
Flexor tenosynovitis	Diabetes Hypothyroidism
Chondrocalcinosis/pseudogout	Diabetes Hypothyroidism Hyperparathyroidism Acromegaly
Osteopenia/osteoporosis	Diabetes Hyperthyroidism Hyperparathyroidism Hypoparathyroidism
Destructive arthropathy	Diabetes Hypothyroidism Hyperparathyroidism
Premature/unusual osteoarthritis	Chondrocalcinosis Charcot arthropathy Acromegaly
DISH	Diabetes
Myopathy	Diabetes Hypothyroidism Hyperthyroidism Hyperparathyroidism Acromegaly

DISH, diffuse idiopathic skeletal hyperostosis.

Table 55–2. Early manifestations of endocrine disorders that can mimic rheumatic diseases.

Manifestation	Endocrine Disorder	Mimics
Myalgias, arthralgias, fatigue	Hyperthyroidism Hypothyroidism Hyperparathyroidism	Fibrositis SLE
Proximal muscle weakness	Hyperthyroidism Hypothyroidism Hyperparathyroidism Acromegaly Cushing syndrome	Polymyositis
Shoulder girdle pain and stiffness	Hyperthyroidism	Polymyalgia rheumatica
Degenerative arthritis	Acromegaly Hypothyroidism	Osteoarthritis
Distal soft-tissue swelling and periostitis	Graves disease (thyroid acropathy)	Hypertrophic osteoarthropathy
Synovitis with ANA	Hashimoto thyroiditis	SLE, RA
CPPD, pseudogout	Hyperparathyroidism Hypothyroidism Acromegaly	Idiopathic CPPD

ANA, antinuclear antibodies; CPPD, calcium pyrophosphate deposition disease; RA, rheumatoid arthritis; SLE, systemic lupus erythematosus.

3. Adhesive Capsulitis of the Shoulder

 ESSENTIALS OF DIAGNOSIS

► Loss of the range of motion of the shoulder is significant and develops rapidly.
► Plain radiographs reveal few abnormalities of the glenohumeral joint.

the hand, most commonly of the long or ring fingers. These nodules become symptomatic when they impede tendon motion, locking the finger in flexion or creating a racheting sensation when the finger is flexed and then extended. The nodules can be palpated just distal to the palmar crease of the affected finger. Local glucocorticoid injections into the tendon sheath usually reduce the size of the nodule and alleviate symptoms (see Chapter 6).

Chronic tenosynovitis of the flexor tendons can progress to Dupuytren contractures. These contractures most commonly involve the fourth finger and can result in significant disability when the affected fingers become locked in flexion. The fibrotic tendon is usually palpable as it courses through the palm proximal to the palmar crease.

► Treatment

Glucocorticoid injections have little efficacy, but there may be benefit from injections of collagenase. The standard recommendation for surgical referral is contracture at the metacarpophalangeal joint of at least 30 degrees or any contracture at the proximal interphalangeal joint.

Table 55–3. Rheumatic manifestations of diabetes.

Articular
  Charcot arthropathy
  DISH
  Chondrocalcinosis
Bone
  Osteopenia
Soft-tissue
  Carpal tunnel syndrome
  Flexor tendon nodule
  Dupuytren contracture
  Cheiropathy
  Adhesive capsulitis

DISH, diffuse idiopathic skeletal hyperostosis.

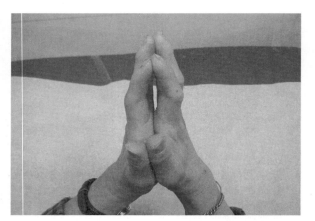

▲ **Figure 55–1.** Prayer sign in a patient with diabetic cheiropathy.

▶ Clinical Findings & Treatment

Adhesive capsulitis, commonly referred to as "frozen shoulder," occurs in up to 12% of patients with diabetes. Relatively rapid and significant loss of the range of motion of the shoulder develops in affected individuals. Some patients have antecedent calcific tendinitis, peritendinitis, or bursitis of the affected shoulder. Plain radiographs reveal few abnormalities of the glenohumeral joint, despite the degree of immobility. Early and aggressive physical therapy must be used to preserve range of motion and minimize the time of immobility.

4. Carpal Tunnel Syndrome

ESSENTIALS OF DIAGNOSIS

▶ Numbness or paresthesias in a distribution consistent with median nerve involvement.

▶ Can progress from an irritating sensory neuropathy to weakness and wasting of the thenar muscles of the hand.

▶ Clinical Findings

Diabetes and carpal tunnel syndrome are prevalent, and the frequent coexistence of these disorders has led many to believe that diabetes predisposes to carpal tunnel syndrome. Patients with carpal tunnel syndrome usually complain of numbness or paresthesias in a distribution consistent with that innervated by the median nerve (see Chapter 6). These symptoms are often exacerbated at night and may awaken a patient from sleep. Carpal tunnel syndrome can progress from an irritating sensory neuropathy to weakness and wasting of the thenar muscles of the hand. Provocation of paresthesias in a median nerve distribution by either a Phalen maneuver or Tinel sign can help confirm the diagnosis. Nerve conduction studies localize the site of the nerve compression to the wrist and differentiate carpal tunnel syndrome from other types of neuropathy.

▶ Treatment

Initial treatment focuses on conservative measures. Patients are asked to wear wrist splints, particularly at night, and refrain from various activities that may exacerbate the condition. Local glucocorticoid injection into the carpal tunnel or surgical decompression should be used if symptoms persist or motor signs develop.

5. Charcot (Neuropathic) Arthropathy

ESSENTIALS OF DIAGNOSIS

▶ The usual presentation is a single, painless (or relatively painless), swollen, and deformed joint, but bilateral disease also occurs.

▶ The metatarsophalangeal, tarsal, and talar joints are most commonly involved.

▶ Radiographs confirm the diagnosis.

▶ General Considerations

Diabetes mellitus is the leading cause of neuropathic arthropathy, which was first described by Jean Martin Charcot in patients with tabes dorsalis. A common complication of diabetes is a progressive sensory neuropathy that preferentially affects axons with the greatest length (ie, those innervating the extremities) and produces the classic "stocking and glove" distribution of paresthesias and numbness. The neurotraumatic hypothesis of joint damage postulates that the sensory neuropathy impairs normal protective mechanisms of the regional joints, particularly those of the foot and ankle. The lack of proprioceptive protection leads to progressive microfractures and subsequent destruction of the joint with little or no pain or recognition of what is developing. The neurovascular hypothesis of Charcot arthropathy proposes that an aberrant sympathetic tone results in increased blood flow to the bones with subsequent bone resorption and susceptibility to bone structural damage.

▶ Clinical Findings

A. Symptoms and Signs

Patients usually have a single, painless (or relatively painless), swollen, and deformed joint, but bilateral disease also occurs. There may be overlying warmth and erythema. The metatarsophalangeal, tarsal, and talar joints are most commonly affected (Figure 55–2), but the knees, spine, and shoulders

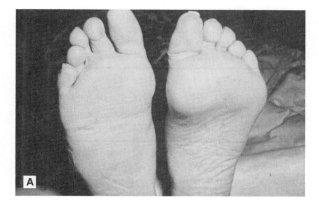

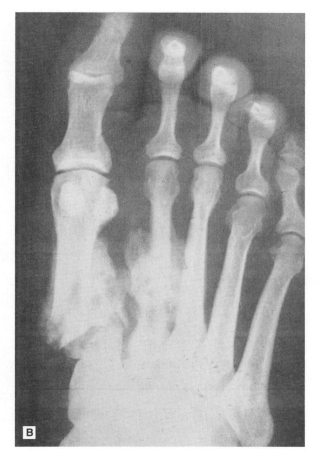

▲ **Figure 55–2.** Charcot arthropathy. **A:** Deformity of the left foot of a patient with chronic diabetes mellitus and long-standing peripheral neuropathy. **B:** Radiograph of Charcot arthropathy involving the first and second metatarsals. (Used with permission, from Dr. Carl Grunfeld, San Francisco Department of Veterans Affairs Medical Center, University of California, San Francisco.)

may also be involved. There are signs of a sensory neuropathy on neurologic examination.

B. Imaging Studies

Radiographs confirm the diagnosis. Classic radiographic findings of Charcot arthropathy include subluxation, fracture, bony fragmentation, exuberant sclerosis, and destruction of the joint (Figure 55–2). Sometimes there is dramatic osteolysis of the bones of the feet, with involvement ranging from areas of patchy osteopenia to marked distal bone resorption. The destruction can be so dramatic as to cause concern for osteomyelitis or a septic joint, especially when there is a contiguous diabetic ulcer. The radiographic appearance sometimes mimics severe osteoarthritis, leading to the admonition to consider Charcot arthropathy when a radiograph reveals "degenerative arthritis times ten." The combination of an unusually destructive degenerative disease in a location not usually affected by osteoarthritis (eg, the tibiotalar, subtalar, and glenohumeral joints) should raise the suspicion of a Charcot joint.

▶ Treatment & Prognosis

Unfortunately, the treatment of Charcot joints, particularly those below the knee, remains suboptimal once the destructive process has become advanced. If detected early, the progress of disease can be somewhat slowed by various protective measures, including the limitation of weight-bearing on the affected joint and the use of specially crafted orthotic supports for the surrounding joint structures.

6. Diffuse Idiopathic Skeletal Hyperostosis

 ESSENTIALS OF DIAGNOSIS

▶ Most commonly affects the spine, but can occur in extraspinal sites.
▶ Causes ossification and calcification of the anterior longitudinal spinous ligament.
▶ Usually asymptomatic.
▶ In advanced cases, large bony overgrowths can cause spinal rigidity and impingement of nearby structures and nerves.

▶ General Considerations

Diffuse idiopathic skeletal hyperostosis (DISH) is a disorder of excessive calcification along spinal ligaments and of new bone formation at insertion sites of tendons and ligaments. Although not uncommon in the general population, DISH is found with a higher prevalence among patients with diabetes, particularly those with type 2 diabetes mellitus.

▶ Clinical Findings

DISH most commonly affects the spine, particularly the midthoracic spine, and causes ossification and calcification of the anterior longitudinal spinous ligament (Figure 55–3). Despite the presence of large, osteophyte-like projections, patients with DISH are rarely symptomatic, and the diagnosis comes to light as an incidental finding on radiographs. In advanced cases, however, the large bony overgrowths can cause spinal rigidity and impingement of nearby structures and nerves; exuberant calcification of the anterior longitudinal ligament in the neck can lead to dysphagia. DISH also can occur in extraspinal sites with prominent bony reactions at ligamentous and tendinous insertions, particularly in the pelvis, greater trochanter, patella, and calcaneus.

The following three radiographic findings establish the diagnosis of DISH: (1) flowing ligamentous calcifications involving at least four contiguous vertebral levels, (2) minimal loss of disk space, and (3) absence of sacroiliitis. DISH can be confused with degenerative disk disease and with ankylosing spondylitis. The absence of disk-space narrowing, of end plate sclerosis, and of facet joint degenerative disease helps distinguish DISH from degenerative spondylitis (although these two entities can coexist). In contrast to ankylosing spondylitis, DISH does not cause inflammatory types of symptoms (eg, morning pain and stiffness in the back) or sacroiliitis.

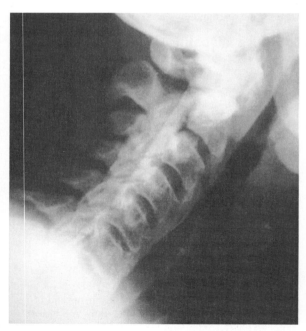

▲ **Figure 55–3.** Diffuse idiopathic skeletal hyperostosis (DISH).

▶ Treatment

The treatment of DISH is symptom-based and generally limited to analgesia as needed. Rarely, surgical removal of impinging bone bridges is undertaken when critical functions, such as swallowing, are compromised.

7. Osteopenia

Type 1 diabetes mellitus appears to be associated with reduced bone mineral density whereas type 2 diabetes mellitus may be associated with higher bone mineral density, perhaps due to its link with obesity. Both types of diabetes confer a higher risk of fracture, especially of the femoral neck. This fracture risk may be due to poor bone quality as well as to an increased risk of falls due to peripheral neuropathy and visual impairment.

8. Diabetic Muscle Infarction

ESSENTIALS OF DIAGNOSIS

▶ Acutely painful swollen thigh or calf (or both).
▶ Occasionally, a palpable mass.
▶ Biopsy can be diagnostic.

▶ Clinical Findings

Diabetic muscle infarction, or diabetic myonecrosis, is a rare complication of long-standing, poorly-controlled diabetes and likely is due to microvascular disease. The most common presentation is an acutely painful, swollen thigh or calf (or both), occasionally with a palpable mass. Serum levels of creatine kinase are often, but not always, elevated. MRI can point to the correct diagnosis. Invasive surgical measures are avoided if possible but, if the diagnosis is in question, a biopsy can be diagnostic and may be necessary to exclude alternative diagnoses, such as necrotizing fasciitis and myonecrosis.

▶ Treatment & Prognosis

Treatment is supportive. Some recommend using antiplatelet or anti-inflammatory medications. There is a significant recurrence rate, and overall prognosis, due to other diabetic comorbidities, is poor.

HYPERTHYROIDISM (TABLE 55–4)

1. Myopathy

The spectrum of muscular involvement in hyperthyroidism varies greatly, ranging from minor aches and pains to a profound and usually painless proximal myopathy that can mimic polymyositis.

Table 55–4. Rheumatic manifestations of hyperthyroidism.

Articular
    Arthralgias
    Periarthritis
    Thyroid acropachy
Bone
    Osteopenia/osteoporosis
Muscular
    Proximal myopathy

With milder muscular involvement, the patient may complain of weakness or easy fatigability but generally demonstrates minimal findings on physical examination. In its most extreme presentation, the myopathy can cause debilitating proximal muscle weakness with marked muscle wasting. However, hyperthyroid-associated myopathy, unlike inflammatory myopathies, causes no, or only minimal, elevations of serum levels of muscle enzymes. Hyperthyroid myopathy usually responds to restoration of the euthyroid state.

2. Arthralgias & Myalgias

Hyperthyroidism is associated with arthralgias, particularly of the shoulders, which can mimic polymyalgia rheumatica. It also can cause a generalized musculoskeletal pain syndrome that resembles fibrositis and manifests as fatigue, proximal myalgias, and arthralgias. These symptoms usually improve with correction of the hyperthyroidism.

3. Osteopenia

Both overt and subclinical hyperthyroid states cause increased bone turnover and reductions in bone mineral density that can progress to osteopenia and osteoporosis. Subclinical hyperthyroidism is a potentially treatable cause of osteoporosis and should be considered in patients with low bone mineral density.

4. Thyroid Acropachy

Thyroid acropachy, a complication of Graves disease, is a proliferative dermopathy that tends to occur in patients who also have ophthalmic involvement and pretibial myxedema. It manifests as distal soft-tissue swelling, clubbing, and periostitis, most commonly of the metacarpal bones (Figure 55–4). These abnormalities are thought to be due to effects of circulating thyroid-stimulating autoantibodies rather than of elevated thyroid hormone levels. Indeed, thyroid acropachy may progress, or even begin, after establishment of a euthyroid state due to the persistence of thyroid-stimulating autoantibodies. In some instances, removal of the target antigens via thyroid ablation may diminish the levels of the circulating pathogenic autoantibodies.

HYPOTHYROIDISM

The rheumatic manifestations of hypothyroidism are protean (Table 55–5). Many of these are due to the metabolic abnormalities of hypothyroidism. However, autoimmune

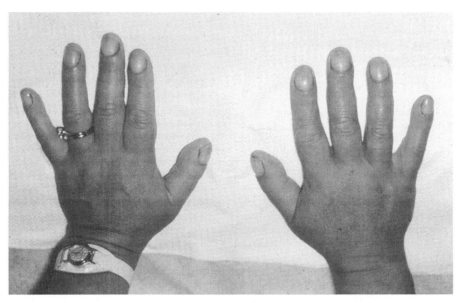

▲ **Figure 55–4.** Thyroid acropachy in a patient with Graves hyperthyroidism. Note swelling of digits and marked clubbing.

Table 55–5. Rheumatic manifestations of hypothyroidism.

Articular
    Inflammatory synovitis associated with thyroiditis
    Noninflammatory joint effusions
    Arthralgias
    Fibromyalgia
    Chondrocalcinosis
    Erosive osteoarthritis
    Charcot-type arthropathy
Bone
    Avascular necrosis
    Epiphyseal dysplasia
Muscular
    Myopathy
Soft-tissue
    Carpal tunnel syndrome
    Flexor tenosynovitis

thyroid disease (Hashimoto thyroiditis) is the most common cause of hypothyroidism, and the autoimmune process, although primarily directed against the thyroid gland, can affect other tissues as well, mimicking several rheumatic diseases. Moreover, rheumatoid arthritis, Sjögren syndrome, mixed connective tissue disease, and systemic lupus erythematosus (SLE), can coexist with autoimmune thyroid disease, complicating diagnosis.

1. Articular Manifestations

Hypothyroidism can produce a generalized musculoskeletal pain syndrome and should be included in the differential diagnosis of fibromyalgia.

Myxedematous arthropathy is a noninflammatory arthritis that affects large, peripheral joints, particularly the knees. Other patterns of myxedematous arthropathy include involvement of the elbows, wrists, and metacarpophalangeal joints together with a flexor tenosynovitis of the hands. Joint effusions are common and are characterized by generous quantities of viscous, noninflammatory synovial fluid.

Calcium pyrophosphate crystals and **chondrocalcinosis** have been identified in the joints of patients with hypothyroidism, but it is not certain whether the prevalence of calcium pyrophosphate deposition disease or pseudogout is increased in hypothyroidism.

2. Bony Abnormalities

Many studies suggest a link between hypothyroidism and the development of osteonecrosis. There appears to be a peculiar predilection for the tibial plateau, but osteonecrosis has been reported to involve bones ranging in size from the femoral heads to the carpal lunate bones. Other reported bony abnormalities in hypothyroid patients include decreased bone turnover (reversed with hormone replacement), a Charcot-like destructive process, and epiphyseal dysplasia.

3. Hypothyroid Myopathy

Patients who are hypothyroid frequently have muscle symptoms and a myopathy that varies in its severity. Elevations of muscle enzymes, often mild and without associated weakness, are common. However, profound muscle weakness and marked elevations in creatine kinase also occur. Hypothyroidism should always be included in the differential diagnosis of polymyositis and other causes of muscle weakness with an elevated serum level of creatine kinase.

4. Soft-Tissue Manifestations

The deposition of mucopolysaccharides in connective tissue may explain many of the soft-tissue manifestations of hypothyroidism. Carpal tunnel syndrome is encountered regularly. Patients with bilateral carpal tunnel syndrome, particularly those with no other known risk factors, should be screened for hypothyroidism. Flexor tenosynovitis of the hand and generalized sensory neuropathy, both associated with hypothyroidism, can mimic this diagnosis as well.

5. Hashimoto Thyroiditis & Immune-Mediated Rheumatic Syndromes

 ESSENTIALS OF DIAGNOSIS

▶ Nonerosive synovitis that is usually a small-joint, symmetric polyarthritis.
▶ Antinuclear antibodies frequently present.

▶ Clinical Findings

An overt synovitis that is probably immune mediated can develop in patients with Hashimoto thyroiditis. The synovitis is usually a small-joint, symmetric, polyarthritis that mimics rheumatoid arthritis in its pattern but is nonerosive. Large-joint oligoarthropathies, however, are not rare. Antibodies against thyroid antigens are almost always present. Rarely, Hashimoto thyroiditis causes urticarial vasculitis and glomerulonephritis that have been attributed to circulating immune complexes.

Diagnosis often is not straightforward. Depending on the stage of the autoimmune thyroiditis, patients with articular complaints can be euthyroid, hyperthyroid, or hypothyroid. Antibodies against thyroperoxidase and thyroglobulin have specificity for Hashimoto thyroiditis. However, patients also frequently have antinuclear antibodies, and it can be difficult to distinguish autoimmune thyroid disease with rheumatic manifestations from the coexistence of autoimmune thyroid disease and an ANA-positive systemic disease.

▶ Treatment

Thyroid replacement alone is often not enough to treat the rheumatic symptoms of these patients, and other medications such as nonsteroidal anti-inflammatory drugs, antimalarials, glucocorticoids, and methotrexate are sometimes used.

6. Associations Between Hashimoto Thyroiditis & Rheumatic Diseases

Hashimoto thyroiditis also occurs in association with well-defined rheumatic diseases. Ten percent to 15% of patients with rheumatoid arthritis, for example, suffer from autoimmune thyroid disease, while as many as 15% of patients with Hashimoto thyroiditis may have 1 or more additional autoimmune diseases, such as Sjögren syndrome and SLE. There is an association between Hashimoto thyroiditis and specific HLA alleles, particularly HLA-DR3 and HLA-B8.

HYPERPARATHYROIDISM

Primary hyperparathyroidism, the most common cause of asymptomatic hypercalcemia, is usually the result of an autonomously functioning parathyroid adenoma. Chronic renal insufficiency induces secondary and even tertiary parathyroid gland hyperplasia and hormone oversecretion. All forms of hyperparathyroidism can produce rheumatic symptoms.

1. Chondrocalcinosis & Pseudogout

Primary hyperparathyroidism is a cause of calcium pyrophosphate deposition disease. The presence of either chondrocalcinosis or of pseudogout should prompt determination of serum calcium (see Chapter 45).

The most common effect of primary hyperparathyroidism on bone is asymptomatic osteopenia and osteoporosis. Even in subclinical hyperparathyroidism, there is a decline in cortical bone that can be prevented by parathyroidectomy. The classic skeletal effects of long-standing hyperparathyroidism include subperiosteal resorption of bone (especially the phalanges and distal clavicle), osteoporosis circumscripta (generalized bone loss of the skull), osteitis fibrosa cystica (cystic lytic lesions of bones), and "rugger jersey" spine (intense sclerosis of the vertebral end plates alternating with marked osteopenia of the vertebral bodies) (Figure 55–5).

2. Myalgias & Arthralgias

Fatigue and myalgias are frequent complaints in hyperparathyroidism. Patients also may complain of proximal muscle weakness, particularly the lower extremities; there is little or no elevation of muscle enzymes. Arthralgias are more typical in large joints. Erosions can develop and may be confused with rheumatoid arthritis.

3. Metastatic Calcification & Calciphylaxis

Advanced renal disease and associated secondary hyperparathyroidism can cause metastatic calcification of soft-tissues and muscles, a process which, by itself or through the induction of inflammation, can produce various muscle and soft-tissue symptoms. Calciphylaxis, which usually occurs in the setting of end-stage renal failure and severe secondary hyperparathyroidism, results in diffuse calcification of skin as well as subcutaneous tissue and other soft-tissues, leading to painful skin erythema and ulcerations, vascular thromboses, and digital infarctions that can resemble vasculitis.

HYPOPARATHYROIDISM & PSEUDOHYPOPARATHYROIDISM

Hypoparathyroidism is most often the result of surgical damage to, or removal of, the parathyroid glands; autoimmune destruction of the parathyroid glands occurs but is uncommon. Muscle fatigue and weakness usually parallel the degree of hypocalcemia. Neuromuscular irritability and tetany can result from low levels of ionized calcium. Interestingly, some patients have ectopic soft-tissue, which rarely can cause calcification of the paraspinous ligaments and result in a restrictive process resembling a spondyloarthropathy.

Pseudohypoparathyroidism, which is due to resistance to parathyroid hormone action, is an inherited disorder that causes low serum calcium levels with elevated levels of parathyroid hormone. Pseudohypoparathyroidism can be associated with distinct skeletal deformities, particularly shortening of the fourth metacarpals bilaterally (Figure 55–6). Examination of the clenched fist reveals a characteristic depression where the knuckle of the fourth metacarpal should be located.

X-LINKED HYPOPHOSPHATEMIC RICKETS

The musculoskeletal manifestations and radiographic abnormalities of X-linked hypophosphatemic rickets can mimic those of a spondyloarthropathy, particularly ankylosing spondylitis. X-linked hypophosphatemic rickets is due to the inactivation of the gene encoding a phosphaturic hormone (PHEX or *ph*osphate regulatory gene with homology to *e*ndopeptidase on *X* chromosome), which in turn causes an increase in fibroblast growth factor 23, decreased phosphate reabsorption in the renal tubules, and decreased 1-α-hydroxylase activity for 1,25-OH2-vitamin D synthesis. Patients have normal serum calcium, low serum phosphate, low serum 1,25-hydroxy-vitamin D, and osteomalacia. X-linked hypophosphatemic rickets can present in early adulthood with decreased range of motion of the spine. The radiographic findings include those that resemble the abnormalities of spondyloarthropathies: exuberant entheseal bony

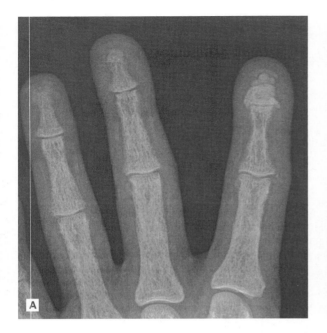

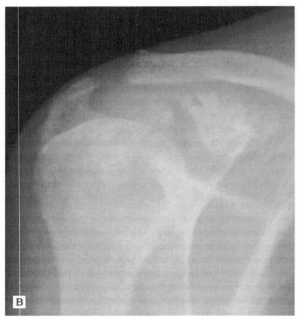

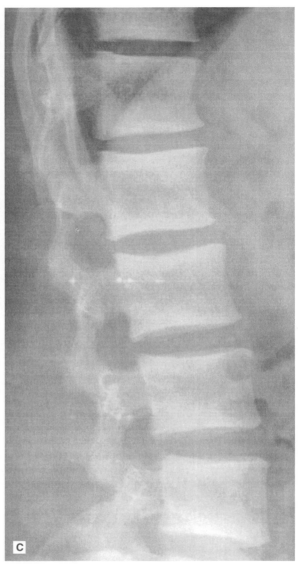

▲ **Figure 55–5.** Skeletal changes of hyperparathyroidism. **A:** Subperiosteal resorption of the phalanges and calcification of the digital arteries. **B:** Erosion of the distal clavicle and soft-tissue calcification. **C:** "Rugger jersey" spine.

proliferation, squaring of vertebral bodies, and abnormalities of the sacroiliac joints (widening or fusion). X-linked hypophosphatemic rickets, however, does not cause erosions of the sacroiliac joints and often has findings such as short stature and radiographic pseudofractures ("Looser zones") not seen in spondyloarthropathies.

ACROMEGALY

Acromegaly has multiple effects on bone and soft-tissues. The anabolic effects of excess growth hormone can cause marked proliferation of bone, cartilage, synovium, and other soft-tissues. Rheumatic symptoms are common

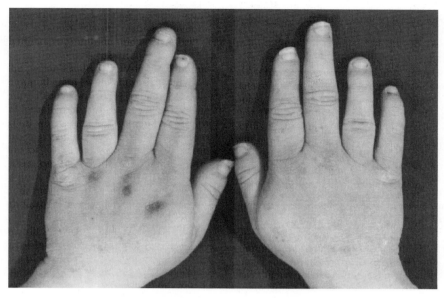

▲ **Figure 55–6.** Pseudohypoparathyroidism. Shortening of the fourth and fifth metacarpals results in brachydactyly. (Used, with permission, from Dr. Michael Levine, The Cleveland Clinic.)

in acromegaly and frequently predate recognition of the underlying disorder. The progression of acromegaly is insidious and, therefore, attention to the rheumatic manifestations may point to the diagnosis before advanced disease becomes evident.

1. Degenerative Arthritis

 ## ESSENTIALS OF DIAGNOSIS

▶ Progressive degenerative arthropathy that may be monoarticular or polyarticular.

▶ May affect a variety of joints.

▶ Clinical Findings

A. Symptoms and Signs

Initially, cartilage overgrowth leads to joint space widening, but this overgrowth involves haphazard deposition of matrix, resulting in its fissuring and degeneration. In addition, overgrowth and hypertrophy of joint capsules can cause progressive ligamentous laxity and hypermobility. Premature osteoarthritis ensues, particularly involving the weight-bearing joints, and invariably results in marked joint-space narrowing and osteophytosis characteristic of all forms of degenerative joint disease. In addition, acromegaly has been linked to calcium pyrophosphate dihydrate deposition

disease, a process that can further exacerbate any ongoing degenerative changes.

Up to 50% of patients with acromegaly have back pain. Patients can have widened disk spaces, large osteophytes, kyphosis or loss of lordosis, and ligamentous laxity of the spine. In one series of patients, duration of disease correlated with the height of vertebral bodies and intervertebral spaces, and concomitant DISH was diagnosed in 20% of patients. The degenerative changes in the spine can lead to radiculopathies, and bony overgrowth can impinge on the spinal canal.

Acromegaly should be suspected when precocious degenerative joint disease occurs. Particular attention should be paid to those patients who demonstrate excessive hypermobility or laxity of their joints, a finding that would appear to be in contradiction to the degree of degenerative disease encountered.

B. Imaging Studies

Early in disease, radiographs of the hands demonstrate increased soft-tissue of the hands, joint space widening, and spade-like deformities of the distal phalangeal tufts. Later, the changes observed radiologically resemble those seen in most forms of advanced osteoarthritis.

▶ Treatment

If treated early enough, most of the rheumatic manifestations of acromegaly respond to removal of the pituitary adenoma or pharmacologic suppression of growth hormone secretion.

However, once advanced degenerative changes have taken place, symptomatic relief is usually provided through conservative measures, including nonsteroidal anti-inflammatory medications. Severe disease may be amenable to surgical correction once the underlying metabolic abnormality has been successfully corrected.

2. Carpal Tunnel Syndrome

Acromegalic patients often have coarsely enlarged fingers and hands characteristic of the soft-tissue, bone, and fibrous proliferation associated with excess growth hormone secretion. As a result of this tissue overgrowth, crowding of the carpal tunnel occurs, leading to carpal tunnel syndrome. This condition is often bilateral and can be the initial clue to the diagnosis of acromegaly.

3. Myopathy

A painless, proximal myopathy has been reported in patients with acromegaly. Serum muscle enzyme levels are usually normal in this disorder.

HYPERCORTISOLISM

Cushing syndrome due to either pituitary or adrenal causes frequently causes a myopathy that manifests clinically as proximal muscle weakness and atrophy in the absences of elevated serum levels of muscle enzymes. The deleterious effects of Cushing syndrome on bone include osteonecrosis, osteopenia, and osteoporosis with an increased rate of vertebral fracture. Even patients with subclinical, mild chronic hypercortisolism due to an adrenal "incidentaloma" can have decreased bone mineral density.

HYPOADRENALISM

Myalgias, arthralgias, and back pain are common musculoskeletal manifestations of adrenal insufficiency and, in some cases, are the presenting complaints. The diagnosis should be considered especially in patients with other evidence of adrenal insufficiency such as hypotension, skin hyperpigmentation, gastrointestinal symptoms, and electrolyte abnormalities.

Biro E, Szekanecz Z, Czirjak L, et al. Association of systemic and thyroid autoimmune diseases. *Clin Rheumatol.* 2006;25:240. [PMID: 16247581]

Cagliero E, Apruzzese W, Perlmutter GS, Nathan DM. Musculoskeletal disorders of the hand and shoulder in patients with diabetes mellitus. *Am J Med.* 2002;112:487. [PMID: 11959060]

Carnevale V, Romagnoli E, D'Erasmo E. Skeletal involvement in patients with diabetes mellitus. *Diabetes Metab Res Rev.* 2004;20:196. [PMID: 15133750]

Chiodini I, Torlontano M, Carnevale V, Trischitta V, Scillitani A. Skeletal involvement in adult patients with endogenous hypercortisolism. *J Endocrinol Invest.* 2008;31:267. [PMID: 18401211]

Lee L, Blume PA, Sumpio B. Charcot joint disease in diabetes mellitus. *Ann Vasc Surg.* 2003;17:571. [PMID: 14508661]

Meier C, Beat M, Guglielmetti M, Christ-Crain M, Staub JJ, Kraenzlin M. Restoration of euthyroidism accelerates bone turnover in patients with subclinical hypothyroidism: a randomized controlled trial. *Osteoporos Int.* 2004;15:209. [PMID: 14727010]

Rubin MR, Bilezikian JP, McMahon DJ, et al. The natural history of primary hyperparathyroidism with or without parathyroid surgery after 15 years. *J Clin Endocrinol Metab.* 2008;93:3462. [PMID: 18544625]

Scarpa R, DeBrasi D, Pivonello R. Acromegalic axial arthropathy: A clinical case-control study. *J Clin Endocrinol Metab.* 2004;89:598. [PMID: 14764768]

Rheumatic Manifestations of Malignancy

56

John B. Imboden, MD

Rarely, tumor-like lesions, benign tumors, and malignancies involve joints directly, producing arthritis. More commonly, malignancies cause paraneoplastic syndromes with musculoskeletal manifestations. Certain paraneoplastic syndromes have rheumatic presentations that are distinctive and, therefore, warrant investigation of an underlying malignancy when recognized. Other paraneoplastic syndromes can mimic idiopathic rheumatic diseases, such as rheumatoid arthritis, and can be a source of diagnostic error.

BENIGN TUMORS & TUMOR-LIKE LESIONS OF THE SYNOVIUM

1. Pigmented Villonodular Synovitis

ESSENTIALS OF DIAGNOSIS

▶ Insidious onset of pain, swelling, and limited motion of a single joint, usually the knee or other large joint.
▶ Bloody synovial fluid in approximately 75% of cases.
▶ Characteristic histologic findings.

▶ General Considerations

Pigmented villonodular synovitis (PVNS) is a rare benign neoplasm of the synovium that typically develops in the knee or other large joint during the third or fourth decade of life but can occur in any synovial-lined joint at any age.

▶ Clinical Findings & Treatment

Involvement of the synovium is usually diffuse, producing boggy swelling that can be massive and disproportionate to the degree of discomfort. Rarely, PVNS is focal within the joint and presents with locking symptoms. The grossly thickened synovium has friable villi that bleed, leading to diffuse hemosiderin staining of the synovium and bloody or xanthochromic synovial fluid in most, but not all, cases. Plain radiographs do not show specific changes but may reveal erosions and cystic changes in adjacent bone, usually with preserved joint space. MRI is the preferred imaging method and may point to the correct diagnosis, but definitive diagnosis requires histologic examination of involved tissue. The treatment of choice for most patients is surgical excision.

2. Giant Cell Tumors of Tendon Sheaths

Giant cell tumors of tendon sheaths closely resemble PVNS histologically. They present as painless finger nodules that can mimic ganglia and foreign-body granulomas. Radiographs show erosion of the underlying bone in a minority of cases. Fine-needle aspiration can be diagnostic; surgical excision is usually curative.

3. Synovial Chondromatosis

ESSENTIALS OF DIAGNOSIS

▶ Chronic noninflammatory swelling of a single joint.
▶ Multiple calcified loose bodies on radiographs in later stages.
▶ Locking symptoms and secondary osteoarthritis.

▶ Clinical Findings & Treatment

Synovial chondromatosis is a rare tumor-like condition in which metaplastic synovial lesions develop into cartilaginous islands that in turn produce multiple chondroid loose bodies, which eventually calcify. The process is monoarticular and indolent; the typical presentation is chronic swelling

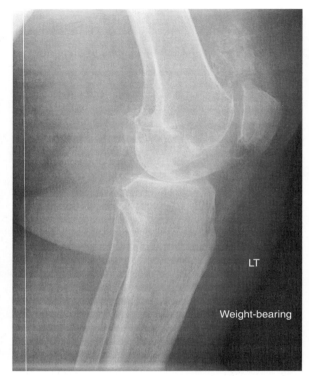

LT

Weight-bearing

▲ **Figure 56–1.** Synovial chondromatosis of the knee. There are multiple calcified loose bodies in the suprapatellar bursa.

of a knee, hip, or shoulder. In the early phases, radiographs may be unremarkable but, in the later stages, calcified loose bodies—sometimes numbering in the hundreds—are visible (Figure 56–1). Synovial chondromatosis is self-limited but can produce painful locking and secondary osteoarthritis. Surgical removal of loose bodies and synovectomy are usually effective.

ARTHRITIS DUE TO DIRECT INVOLVEMENT BY MALIGNANCY

1. Synovial Sarcoma

 ESSENTIALS OF DIAGNOSIS

▶ Rapidly growing, eccentric mass associated with a joint, tendon, or tendon sheath in an extremity.

▶ Deep, radiating pain.

▶ Characteristic histologic and cytogenetic findings.

▶ Clinical Findings & Treatment

Synovial sarcomas typically present as an enlarging mass in an extremity during the third to fifth decades of life. The mass is associated with tendon, tendon sheath, or joint capsule but rarely is truly intra-articular. In 20–40% of cases, plain radiographs of the mass reveal amorphous calcification that points to the diagnosis. MRI can delineate the extent of the lesion. Treatment consists of wide surgical excision. The 5-year survival rates range from 25% to 60%, and tumor size is an important prognostic factor.

2. Secondary Tumors

Leukemic and lymphomatous infiltration of synovium can produce an oligoarthritis or a polyarthritis. Metastatic carcinomatous arthritis, arthritis due to direct extension into a joint from a contiguous malignant bone lesion, and synovitis as a reaction to a juxta-articular malignancy are well-recognized but uncommon entities. Metastatic disease to the shoulder and pelvic girdles can produce a syndrome of atypical polymyalgia rheumatica.

RHEUMATIC SYNDROMES THAT SUGGEST A PARANEOPLASTIC PROCESS

These distinctive syndromes have known associations with malignancy. In most cases, their appearance should prompt a search for an underlying cancer.

1. Hypertrophic Pulmonary Osteoarthropathy

 ESSENTIALS OF DIAGNOSIS

▶ Triad of polyarthritis, clubbing, and periostitis.

▶ Rapid progression of symptoms.

▶ Association with intrathoracic malignancies.

▶ Clinical Findings & Treatment

Hypertrophic pulmonary osteoarthropathy may exist in a primary form or in a secondary form associated with infectious diseases (eg, lung abscess) or malignancy. This syndrome is associated most commonly with intrathoracic malignancies (eg, adenocarcinoma of the lung, mesotheliomas, lymphomas) but has also been described in association with other cancers. It may appear several months prior to detection of the associated neoplasm.

Hypertrophic pulmonary osteoarthropathy is characterized by painful polyarthritis, clubbing of the fingers and toes, and periostitis of the long bones. Rapidly progressive symptoms are a feature of paraneoplastic hypertrophic pulmonary osteoarthropathy. The polyarthritis can resemble rheumatoid arthritis in its joint distribution but elicits noninflammatory synovial effusions. The periostitis commonly causes severe pain and tenderness of the long bones of the legs, usually in association with characteristic radiographic and scintigraphic findings. Nonsteroidal anti-inflammatory drugs may improve joint pain. Treatment of the underlying neoplasm often leads to remission of the syndrome.

2. Palmar Fasciitis-Polyarthritis Syndrome

The development of polyarthritis and rapid progression of palmar fasciitis with flexion contractures of the hands is clearly linked with ovarian cancer but also has been described in patients with gastric, lung, colon, and pancreatic cancer. The syndrome is refractory to treatment, and the prognosis is poor.

3. Remitting Seronegative Symmetric Synovitis with Pitting Edema (RS3PE)

RS3PE is characterized by the presence of a symmetric synovitis of the small joints of the hands in association with pitting edema of the hands and feet. Serum rheumatoid factor is negative. Treatment with low-dose systemic glucocorticoids is usually effective. Although there are idiopathic forms of the syndrome, RS3PE can herald the development of hematologic malignancies or a variety of solid tumors. Treatment of the underlying neoplasm with surgery or chemotherapy can lead to resolution of RS3PE.

4. Panniculitis-Arthritis Syndrome

Patients with pancreatitis or with pancreatic cancer can present with the combination of arthritis and panniculitis. The arthritis is inflammatory and ranges from a monoarthritis to a polyarthritis. The panniculitis begins as tender red subcutaneous nodules, usually on the lower extremities, that initially mimic erythema nodosum but that later liquify and may drain a yellowish material. Release of pancreatic lipase likely plays a role in the pathogenesis of the syndrome.

5. Erythromelalgia

Erythromelalgia manifests as recurrent attacks of pain and erythema involving the feet and, sometimes, the hands. The reversible acral erythema bears a resemblance to Raynaud phenomenon, but the effect of ambient temperature is the converse of that of Raynaud phenomenon: heat exacerbates and cold ameliorates the symptoms of erythromelalgia. Erythromelalgia can be idiopathic but a substantial minority have an underlying myeloproliferative disorder, particularly essential thrombocytosis and polycythemia rubra vera. Approximately 50% of patients with essential thrombocytosis have erythromelalgia.

6. Atypical Polymyalgia Rheumatica

Renal cell carcinoma, other solid tumors, and multiple myeloma can cause a pain syndrome that resembles polymyalgia rheumatica but that fails to respond promptly to low doses of glucocorticoids. Other features that point to a paraneoplastic syndrome rather than true polymyalgia rheumatica include unilateral symptoms, distal extremity pain, and the presence of clubbing.

7. Dermatomyositis & Polymyositis (See Chapter 27)

Compared with the general population, the incidence ratio of malignancy has been reported to be as high as 6.2 for dermatomyositis and 2.4 for polymyositis at the time of diagnosis. Although the incidence of malignancy appears to be highest at the time of diagnosis, an increased risk of malignancy may be present for 2–5 years after the diagnosis has been made. A number of clinical features correlate with the presence of malignancy in association with inflammatory myositis. These include older age, fever, substantial weight loss (greater than 5%), and rapid onset of disease (defined as diagnosis within 2 months of symptoms). Dermatomyositis with cutaneous necrosis of the trunk is also associated with malignancy.

Although the distribution of malignancies seen with the inflammatory myopathies is similar to the general population, there are several specific associations with dermatomyositis and polymyositis. Cancer of the ovaries, lungs, and the gastrointestinal tract is reported most frequently in association with dermatomyositis. Non-Hodgkin lymphoma and cancer of the lung as well as bladder cancer are frequently described in patients with polymyositis. Asian patients with inflammatory myositis have a high incidence of nasopharyngeal cancer.

At a minimum, age-appropriate cancer screening is indicated for patients with dermatomyositis and polymyositis. Although no guidelines exist, some clinicians advocate additional screening, at least in certain circumstances. For example, transvaginal ultrasonography and CA-125 are warranted in women with dermatomyositis, given the high incidence of ovarian cancer. Because the risk of ovarian cancer may be elevated for up to 5 years, some experts argue that screening should continue annually during this time.

PARANEOPLASTIC SYNDROMES THAT MIMIC RHEUMATIC DISEASES

Certain paraneoplastic syndromes have manifestations that mimic rheumatic diseases (Table 56–1). When the appearance of the paraneoplastic syndrome antedates detection of the associated neoplasm, it may be very difficult to distinguish the paraneoplastic syndrome from its more common rheumatic counterpart. Older age, rapid onset of symptoms, prominent constitutional symptoms, and refractoriness to treatment can be clues to the presence of a paraneoplastic process.

Table 56–1. Paraneoplastic syndromes that mimic rheumatic disease.

Syndrome	Malignancy
Cancer-associated polyarthritis	Solid tumors
Jaccoud-like arthropathy	Carcinoma of the lung
Amyloid arthropathy	Myeloma
Adult-onset Still-like syndromes of fever and rash	Various, especially lymphomas and Hodgkin disease
Secondary gout	Leukemias; lymphomas; myeloma; polycythemia rubra vera; essential thrombocythemia
Lupus-like syndromes	Thymoma; Hodgkin disease; carcinoma of the lung, breast, ovary
Small-vessel vasculitis	Myeloproliferative and lymphoproliferative disorders
Medium-vessel arteritis	Hairy cell leukemia
Severe Raynaud phenomenon and digital necrosis	Various
Reflex sympathetic dystrophy	Various
Erythema nodosum	Lymphoproliferative disorders
Scleroderma-like skin changes	Carcinoma of stomach, lung, breast; melanoma; myeloma; POEMS[a] syndrome
Eosinophilic fasciitis	Myeloproliferative and lymphoproliferative disorders

[a]POEMS is an acronym for polyneuropathy, organomegaly, endocrinopathy, monoclonal protein, and skin changes.

1. Cancer-Associated Polyarthritis

 ESSENTIALS OF DIAGNOSIS

▶ May precede or follow the diagnosis of malignancy.

▶ Asymmetric oligoarthritis or polyarthritis, often in the elderly and with abrupt onset.

▶ Frequent sparing of the wrists and hands.

▶ Usually negative for rheumatoid factor and antibodies to cyclic citrullinated peptides.

▶ Clinical Findings & Treatment

Cancer-associated polyarthritis is an uncommon paraneoplastic syndrome reported in association with carcinoma of the breast, carcinoma of the lung, and other solid tumors. There is a close temporal relationship between the development of the arthritis and detection of malignancy (usually within 12 months). Characteristic features of cancer-associated polyarthritis include the abrupt onset of an asymmetric arthritis in an elderly patient (age greater than 65). The arthritis often involves the lower extremities with sparing of the small joints of the hands and wrists. Rheumatoid nodules are absent. Less commonly cancer-associated arthritis presents as a symmetric polyarthritis similar in appearance to rheumatoid arthritis. Serum rheumatoid factor is usually absent, and radiographs do not reveal erosions. Typically, cancer-associated polyarthritis responds poorly to nonsteroidal anti-inflammatory drugs. Treatment of the underlying malignancy often results in resolution of the arthritis.

2. Vasculitis

Small vessel vasculitis, usually presenting as palpable purpura with biopsy findings of leukocytoclastic vasculitis, can occur in association with myeloproliferative and lymphoproliferative disorders and, less commonly, with various carcinomas. Hairy cell leukemia is associated with a medium vessel arteritis that resembles polyarteritis nodosa. Angiocentric T cell lymphomas can cause destructive lesions of the nasopharynx, which mimic granulomatosis with polyangiitis (formerly Wegener granulomatosis).

Fam AG. Paraneoplastic rheumatic syndromes. *Baillieres Best Pract Res Clin Rheumatol.* 2000;14:515. [PMID: 10985984]

Naschitz JE, Rosner I, Rozenbaum M, Zuckerman E, Yeshurun D. Rheumatic syndromes: clues to occult neoplasia. *Semin Arthritis Rheum.* 1999;29:43. [PMID: 10468414]

Szendroi M, Deodhar A. Synovial neoformations and tumours. *Baillieres Best Pract Res Clin Rheumatol.* 2000;14:363. [PMID: 10925750]

Amyloidosis

57

Shanique R. Palmer, MD
Paul S. Mueller, MD, MPH
Morie Gertz, MD, MACP

Amyloidosis is not a single disease but a heterogeneous group of diseases that share in common the extracellular deposition of insoluble fibrillar proteins in tissues and organs. These protein deposits derive from diverse and unrelated serum precursor proteins, yet have similar beta-pleated sheet structural conformations. Furthermore, all forms of amyloid display apple-green birefringence when stained with the cotton-wool dye Congo red and viewed under polarized light. Indeed, this observation (via tissue biopsy) remains the primary means of establishing the diagnosis of amyloidosis. Accumulation of amyloid deposits leads to tissue and organ dysfunction, which in turn causes clinical symptoms and, for some patients, death.

Amyloid diseases are classified by the biochemical composition of the serum precursor proteins that form the amyloid fibrils and deposits. Indeed, once amyloid deposition has been identified, it is important to identify the precursor protein because the prognoses and treatments of the various amyloid diseases depend on the underlying cause. To date, more than 20 amyloid fibril precursor proteins and their associated diseases have been identified. Of these, the most common amyloid diseases are (1) primary or immunoglobulin light-chain protein–related (AL) amyloidosis; (2) secondary (AA) amyloidosis associated with chronic inflammatory disease; (3) dialysis-associated β_2-microglobulin (β_2-m) amyloidosis; and (4) hereditary amyloidosis. Notably, the clinical manifestations of these forms of amyloidosis are not identical (Table 57–1). Hence, each is discussed in detail.

AL AMYLOIDOSIS

ESSENTIALS OF DIAGNOSIS

▶ AL amyloidosis should be suspected in all patients with unexplained heart failure, nephrotic syndrome, neuropathy, and hepatomegaly.

▶ Approximately 98% of patients with AL amyloidosis have detectable serum or urine monoclonal immunoglobulin light-chain protein. However, this finding alone is insufficient to establish the diagnosis of AL amyloidosis.

▶ AL amyloid, like all forms of amyloid, displays apple-green birefringence when viewed under polarized light after staining with Congo red.

▶ Bone marrow examination almost always reveals a monoclonal population of plasma cells.

▶ Tissue immunohistochemical analysis or protein sequencing by mass spectroscopy is necessary to identify the light-chain origin of AL amyloid fibrils. If inconclusive, other diagnostic testing (eg, ultrastructural fibril characterization) should be done.

▶ General Considerations

AL amyloidosis is a plasma cell dyscrasia associated with multisystem involvement, rapid progression, and short survival. It is a rare disease with an incidence of 8 patients per 1 million persons per year. It usually affects people older than 40 years and men (65%) more than women. Amyloid fibrils derive from the N-terminal region of immunoglobulin light-chains (λ more often than κ) produced by a monoclonal population of plasma cells in the bone marrow. Notably, 5% of patients with multiple myeloma have AL amyloidosis, and it is unusual for patients with AL amyloidosis to develop multiple myeloma. AL amyloidosis affects most organs and the vascular system.

▶ Clinical Findings

A. Symptoms and Signs

The symptoms and signs of AL amyloidosis are nonspecific. For example, the most common symptoms are fatigue and involuntary weight loss. Other symptoms and signs of AL

Table 57–1. Organ systems commonly involved clinically by various forms of amyloidosis.

Organ System	Primary (AL) Amyloidosis	Secondary (AA) Amyloidosis	Dialysis-Associated β₂-Microglobulin (β₂-m) Amyloidosis	Hereditary Amyloidosis[a]
Heart	X			X
Kidney	X	X		X
Vascular	X			
Peripheral nerves	X			X
Autonomic nerves	X			X
Liver	X			
Gastrointestinal tract	X	X		
Joints	X		X	

[a]Organ involvement varies according to the specific amyloid precursor protein mutation.

amyloidosis reflect the organs and tissues involved. Hence, clinicians should suspect AL amyloidosis when seeing patients with syndromes associated with the disease. The syndromes associated most commonly with AL amyloidosis are nephrotic syndrome, congestive heart failure, idiopathic peripheral neuropathy, carpal tunnel syndrome, and hepatomegaly.

One third to one half of patients with AL amyloidosis have symptoms related to kidney involvement. Nephrotic syndrome (urinary excretion of more than 3 g of protein in 24 hours) with hypoalbuminemia and edema is the most frequent initial manifestation of kidney involvement. Symptomatic cardiac involvement affects up to 40% of patients with AL amyloidosis. Amyloid involvement of the myocardium, intramural coronary arteries, and conduction system may cause congestive heart failure, ischemic syndromes (eg, angina, myocardial infarction), and rhythm disturbances. Nearly 20% of patients with AL amyloidosis have neuropathy. These patients usually have lower extremity paresthesias. Pain and temperature senses are lost before light touch and vibratory senses. Motor neuropathy is rare. Patients may also have autonomic neuropathy, the manifestations of which include diarrhea, bladder control problems, erectile dysfunction, and orthostatic hypotension. Fifteen percent of patients have hepatomegaly.

Rheumatic manifestations also develop in some patients with AL amyloidosis. For example, one quarter of patients have carpal tunnel syndrome. Sensory abnormalities caused by amyloid neuropathy may lead to neuropathic joint destruction (Charcot joint). Joint disease resembling rheumatoid arthritis (RA) develops in some patients with AL amyloidosis. These patients have bilateral symmetric arthritis of the large and small joints characterized by pain, stiffness, swelling, and palpable nodules. However, unlike patients with RA, those with amyloid arthropathy do not experience fevers, joint tenderness on palpation, or evidence of inflammation on synovial fluid analysis. Patients with muscle involvement (amyloid myopathy) complain of stiffness, weakness, and enlargement of muscles (pseudohypertrophy). Amyloid

involvement of joints, muscles, and nerves may also lead to debilitating contractures. Finally, AL amyloidosis may masquerade as giant cell arteritis. Symptoms suggestive of giant cell arteritis (eg, jaw claudication) are present. However, rather than revealing giant cell arteritis, temporal artery biopsy reveals amyloid involvement of the temporal artery.

In fact, most patients with AL amyloidosis have vascular involvement, and for some, this involvement may be symptomatic (eg, angina pectoris, orthostatic hypotension, and purpura). Pathologic enlargement of the tongue (macroglossia), commonly associated with amyloidosis, is actually an uncommon finding, seen in less than 20% of patients.

B. Laboratory Findings

No laboratory findings are pathognomonic of AL amyloidosis. Instead, laboratory abnormalities reflect the organs and tissues involved. For example, renal insufficiency, hypoalbuminemia, hyperlipidemia, and proteinuria suggest kidney involvement. Hematologic abnormalities are relatively uncommon. However, peripheral blood smear may reveal Howell-Jolly bodies suggestive of hyposplenism, which is caused by amyloid infiltration of the spleen.

Immunoelectrophoresis of the serum or urine detects a monoclonal immunoglobulin light-chain protein in 90% of patients with AL amyloidosis. Use of the immunoglobulin free light chain (FLC) ratio raises the sensitivity to 98%. For those who do not have detectable monoclonal light chain in the serum or urine (nonsecretory AL amyloidosis), bone marrow examination usually reveals a monoclonal population of plasma cells. Patients with AL amyloidosis usually have increased plasma cells (approximately 5%) in the bone marrow.

C. Imaging Studies

In general, imaging studies do not reveal findings specific for AL amyloidosis. Some patients with kidney involvement may have enlarged kidneys when viewed by ultrasonography, but most have normal-sized kidneys. Echocardiography usually reveals wall thickening due to amyloid infiltration of the myocardium, evidence of diastolic dysfunction, and a misleadingly normal left ventricular ejection fraction. Reported radiographic findings in patients with AL amyloidosis include osteoporosis, pathologic fractures, osteonecrosis, soft tissue nodules and swelling, subchondral cysts and erosions, joint contractures, and neuropathic osteoarthropathy.

Quantitative scintigraphy with radiolabeled serum amyloid P (SAP) component is useful in determining the extent and total body burden of amyloid deposits in patients with AL amyloidosis. Serial studies reveal uptake of the radiolabeled SAP component that correlates with regression or progression of disease. This test, however, is not widely available.

Cardiac involvement is frequent in AL amyloidosis but can be diagnostically challenging. Echocardiography is frequently used but has limitations, especially if hypertrophy from other causes is present. There are also limitations with the use of other noninvasive modalities, such as electrocardiography and quantitative scintigraphy. The gold standard for diagnosis is cardiac biopsy but cardiovascular MRI has been evaluated in cardiac amyloidosis and has a very high positive predictive value (95%) for the diagnosis of cardiac amyloid involvement. This may be used as an alternative to the invasive method of cardiac biopsy to assess for cardiac involvement. The cornerstone of diagnosis using cardiac MRI is the presence of late gadolinium enhancement, related to the expansion of the interstitial compartment by the infiltrating amyloid protein, which is seen histologically.

D. Tissue Biopsy

Tissue biopsy is necessary to establish the diagnosis of amyloidosis. All forms of amyloid display apple-green birefringence when viewed under polarized light after staining with Congo red. The least invasive method is aspiration of subcutaneous abdominal fat, which reveals amyloid in 70–80% of patients with AL amyloidosis. Bone marrow biopsy (usually done to evaluate a monoclonal protein) reveals amyloid in one-half of patients. Together, fat aspirate and bone marrow biopsy reveal amyloid in 85% of patients. If analyses of aspirated subcutaneous fat and bone marrow do not reveal amyloid, yet suspicion for amyloidosis remains high, other tissue must be obtained. An effective approach is to obtain tissue specimens from organs suspected of having amyloid involvement (eg, kidney, heart, liver). The presence of a monoclonal light-chain protein in a patient with biopsy-proven amyloidosis strongly suggests AL amyloidosis, but it is not sufficient to establish the diagnosis. For example, monoclonal gammopathies are not uncommon in the general population, and detecting a monoclonal protein in a patient with a form of amyloidosis other than AL amyloidosis (eg, hereditary amyloidosis) may be misleading. Rarely, patients with AL amyloidosis do not have a detectable monoclonal protein. Hence, tissue immunohistochemical analysis is necessary to identify the light-chain origin of AL amyloid fibrils. If the diagnosis remains inconclusive, other testing (eg, electron microscopy or immunoelectrophoresis) may be necessary.

▶ Treatment

A major goal of treating AL amyloidosis is the reduction or elimination of the monoclonal plasma cells that produce the amyloidogenic proteins. Therapeutic options have evolved from the use of melphalan and prednisone in the 1960s, to high-dose chemotherapy and stem cell transplantation in the late 1980s and 1990s, to the introduction of small novel molecules within the past decade.

The standard treatment of AL amyloidosis is the combination of melphalan and prednisone. This combination is superior to placebo and colchicine. Compared with placebo, treatment with melphalan and prednisone increases median survival time from 6 months to 12 months. This treatment, however, is less effective if the disease involves the heart or kidneys. While high-dose melphalan followed by autologous stem cell support results in higher response rates than that of conventional chemotherapy alone, this strategy is associated with high treatment-associated mortality (10–25%) and therefore must be used only in selected patients (eg, those without significant amyloid cardiomyopathy or involvement of three or more other major organs). However, of the patients who can tolerate this treatment, many experience the disappearance of monoclonal light chains from the serum and urine and the normalization of the number of bone marrow plasma cells. Furthermore, the function of organs involved with amyloid may improve (eg, reduced proteinuria). The treatment options for patients with severe amyloid cardiomyopathy or involvement of three or more other major organs include standard melphalan and prednisone or high-dose dexamethasone (with or without melphalan).

More recently, within the past decade, the management of the monoclonal gammopathies, including AL amyloidosis, has seen the introduction of targeted therapies. These include thalidomide, lenalidomide, and bortezomib. Thalidomide has been shown to be a feasible and effective treatment option. Lenalidomide has also been reported to be active, especially when combined with dexamethasone. Bortezomib is a reversible proteasome inhibitor that may be used in the treatment of AL amyloidosis, with or without dexamethasone. It has been shown to induce responses in 68% of pretreated patients and in 64% of patients with disease refractory to previous therapy. Bortezomib with dexamethasone has also been shown to be active in previously untreated patients with high-risk features. Furthermore, responses were rapid (median of 28 days), compared with those in dexamethasone- or thalidomide-based regimens (median, 2–4 months). Further trials have been proposed to compare the combination of bortezomib, melphalan, and dexamethasone to the current standard of melphalan and dexamethasone in patients with newly diagnosed AL amyloidosis.

In addition to treatment directed at the specific form of amyloidosis, most patients with amyloidosis, including those with AL amyloidosis, require supportive treatment (Table 57–2). The aims of supportive treatment are to relieve symptoms caused by amyloid involvement of various organ systems and to prolong survival. Organ transplantation (eg, heart) has been used successfully to treat organ failure in selected patients with AL amyloidosis. Organ transplantation, however, does not prevent amyloid deposition in other organs or in the transplanted organ.

▶ When to Refer

Patients with AL amyloidosis should be referred to a hematologist who has experience managing this uncommon disease. Managing organ failure caused by amyloidosis can be challenging and often requires the assistance of a subspecialist (eg, nephrologist, cardiologist). Furthermore, many patients with amyloidosis have daunting psychosocial and spiritual challenges. Under these circumstances, referral to an appropriate allied health colleague (eg, social worker, chaplain) or support group may be helpful.

Table 57–2. Supportive measures for all forms of amyloidosis.

Organ System	Symptom	Treatment
Heart	Congestive failure	Salt restriction Diuretics ACE inhibitors Heart transplantation Avoidance of digoxin, calcium channel blockers, and β-blockers
	Heart block	Pacemaker
Kidney	Nephrotic syndrome	Salt restriction Elastic stockings Adequate dietary protein ACE inhibitors
	Kidney failure	Dialysis Kidney transplantation
Autonomic neuropathy	Orthostatic hypotension	Salt Elastic stocking Fludrocortisone, midodrine
	Gastroparesis	Small, frequent meals low in fat Metoclopramide Jejunostomy tube
Peripheral neuropathy	Sensory neuropathy	Pain control (eg, amitriptyline, gabapentin) Avoidance of trauma Proper foot care
	Motor neuropathy	Physical therapy Braces, other devices
Gastrointestinal tract	Diarrhea	Psyllium Loperamide Somatostatin analogues Dietary changes Total parenteral nutrition
	Macroglossia	Maintenance of airway
Blood	Bruising Factor X deficiency Hyposplenism	Avoidance of trauma Factor replacement before surgery and other invasive procedures Vaccination Splenectomy for massive splenomegaly

ACE, angiotensin-converting enzyme.
Modified, with permission, from Skinner M. Amyloidosis. In Lichtenstein LM, Fauci AS (editors): *Current Therapy in Allergy, Immunology, and Rheumatology,* 6th ed. Mosby, 2004.

Prognosis

Prognosis in AL amyloidosis is highly variable, as there are several factors that may individually predict survival. These include the number of organ systems involved and degree of involvement, level of bone marrow plasmacytosis, circulating plasma cells in the peripheral blood and β_2-m level, among others. Integrating all these parameters to accurately predict survival is challenging and is limited by subjectivity. The presence and severity of cardiac involvement has been found to be the most important determinant of prognosis in patients with AL amyloidosis. There have been several proposed definitions of cardiac involvement, including reduction in the left ventricular ejection fraction, increased interventricular septal wall thickness, hypotension, presence of cardiac failure and cardiac rhythm disturbances. Each of these parameters can be assessed individually. However, studies have shown that cardiac biomarkers provide the strongest prognostic information. Using two simple measurements, namely serum troponins and N-terminal pro brain natriuretic peptide (NT-proBNP), survival in patients with AL amyloidosis can be accurately stratified into three risk groups. Patients are stratified to stage I if both markers are less than a defined threshold value, stage II if either marker is above threshold, and stage III if both are above threshold. This corresponds with median survivals of 26, 11, and 4 months, respectively (Figure 57–1). This staging system does not directly supply information about other organ involvement, but it is an accurate predictor of survival because cardiac involvement is the primary determinant of prognosis.

The other major determinant of survival in AL amyloidosis is the response to therapy as measured by the FLC assay. Given that AL amyloid deposits are derived from circulating monoclonal immunoglobulin light chains, it is not surprising that the FLC response to therapy is a key determinant of outcome. Indeed, the main goal of therapy is suppression of FLC production. It has been shown that reduction in amyloidogenic FLC concentration by more than 50% portends better prognosis, with associated regression of amyloid and a survival advantage. In one study, 5-year survival was 88% in patients whose abnormal FLC concentration fell by more than 50% following therapy, compared with only 39% among those whose FLC did not fall by at least half.

Monitoring

Plasma cell burden is usually low in patients with AL amyloidosis, which makes monitoring difficult. Clinicians should assess the level of organ dysfunction, but apart from measuring troponins and NT-proBNP, there is no consensus regarding the ideal parameters to follow for continued assessment of each involved organ system. The development of the FLC assay has also been a major advance in this regard and has been shown to be the single most important parameter for monitoring the hematologic response in patients with AL amyloidosis. Typical monitoring during therapy includes

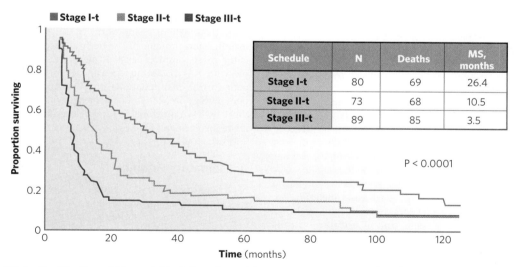

Schedule	N	Deaths	MS, months
Stage I-t	80	69	26.4
Stage II-t	73	68	10.5
Stage III-t	89	85	3.5

P < 0.0001

▲ **Figure 57–1.** Stratification of AL amyloidosis into three risk groups—stages I, II, and III—based on serum troponin and N-terminal pro brain natriuretic peptide (NT-proBNP) measurements. Patients are considered to be in stage I if both markers are within the normal range; stage II if either marker is above its respected threshold for normal; and stage III if both are above normal. These stages correspond to median survival lengths of 26, 11, and 4 months, respectively. (Used with permission from Dispenzieri A, Gertz MA, Kyle RA, et al. Serum cardiac troponins and N-terminal pro-brain natriuretic peptide: a staging system for primary systemic amyloidosis. *J Clin Oncol.* 2004;22(18):3751–3757. [PMId: 15365071]) measurement of FLCs after each treatment cycle (often monthly) to document response.

AA AMYLOIDOSIS

▶ AA amyloidosis should be suspected in all patients with chronic inflammatory conditions in whom renal insufficiency, nephrotic syndrome, gastrointestinal tract symptoms, or other symptoms and signs of amyloidosis develop.

▶ AA amyloid, like all forms of amyloid, displays apple-green birefringence when viewed under polarized light after staining with Congo red.

▶ Tissue immunohistochemical analysis identifies the serum amyloid A precursor protein from which AA amyloid fibrils derive. A monoclonal protein is generally absent.

▶ General Considerations

AA amyloidosis is an uncommon complication of chronic inflammatory diseases, including rheumatic conditions, infectious diseases, malignancies, and others. Amyloid fibrils derive from the acute-phase reactant serum amyloid A (AA) protein. The liver produces serum AA protein in response to inflammation. Serum levels of this protein, which is involved in chemotaxis, cell adhesion, cytokine production, and other immune processes, correlate with disease activity. In fact, serum AA protein levels may increase 1000-fold during an inflammatory response. Chronically elevated serum AA protein levels precede AA amyloid fibril formation. Treating the underlying inflammatory disease suppresses the acute-phase response, normalizes serum AA protein levels, and prevents the development of AA amyloidosis. Indeed, the incidence of AA amyloidosis in the developed world has fallen in recent decades as a result of effective treatment of chronic infections (eg, tuberculosis) and other inflammatory diseases.

Of the cases of AA amyloidosis seen today, about two thirds are caused by chronic rheumatic diseases, including RA, psoriatic arthritis, ankylosing spondylitis, reactive arthritis, adult-onset Still disease, juvenile chronic arthritis, systemic lupus erythematosus, Behçet syndrome, Takayasu arteritis, polymyalgia rheumatica, hypersensitivity vasculitis, polymyositis, retroperitoneal fibrosis, and the hereditary inflammatory diseases (eg, familial Mediterranean fever, familial cold urticaria, and Muckle-Wells syndrome). Malignancies associated with AA amyloidosis include Hodgkin disease, renal cell carcinoma, hepatoma, and astrocytoma. Other chronic inflammatory diseases associated with AA amyloidosis include inflammatory bowel disease, primary biliary

cirrhosis, bronchiectasis, cystic fibrosis, osteomyelitis, psoriasis, eosinophilic granuloma, and decubitus ulcers. The time from diagnosis of the underlying inflammatory disease to the diagnosis of AA amyloidosis is usually 10–20 years. Because chronic inflammatory illnesses afflict persons of all ages, AA amyloidosis may occur at any age.

Two diseases that cause AA amyloidosis, RA and familial Mediterranean fever, warrant special attention. RA is the most common rheumatic cause of AA amyloidosis (75% of cases). However, AA amyloidosis does not develop in most patients with RA. The 15-year incidence of AA amyloidosis in RA is about 10%. Patients in whom AA amyloidosis develops have had RA longer than those in whom amyloidosis does not develop. Furthermore, continuously active RA or inadequately treated RA are risk factors for developing AA amyloidosis. Familial Mediterranean fever is characterized by recurrent attacks of fever, arthritis, pleuritis, peritonitis, or erysipelas-like erythema lasting 24–48 hours. Familial Mediterranean fever begins in childhood and usually affects persons of Mediterranean origin. AA amyloidosis develops in one-quarter of patients with familial Mediterranean fever. Renal failure due to amyloid deposition usually occurs in the fifth decade of life.

▶ Clinical Findings

A. Symptoms and Signs

The clinical manifestations of AA amyloidosis differ from those of AL amyloidosis in a number of ways. For example, renal and gastrointestinal tract manifestations are common. More than 90% of people with AA amyloidosis have renal insufficiency, proteinuria, or both. Indeed, AA amyloidosis is the most common cause of nephrotic syndrome in people with RA. Gastrointestinal involvement affects 20% of patients; the manifestations include nausea, diarrhea, and poor energy intake. Unlike patients with AL amyloidosis, those with AA amyloidosis rarely have cardiac or peripheral nerve involvement. Macroglossia is not a feature of AA amyloidosis.

B. Laboratory Findings

No laboratory findings are pathognomonic of AA amyloidosis. Laboratory abnormalities reflect amyloid involvement of organs and tissues. For example, kidney involvement is common and is suggested by renal insufficiency and proteinuria.

C. Imaging Studies

Imaging studies usually do not reveal findings specific for AA amyloidosis. Instead, they usually reveal findings associated with the underlying inflammatory condition (eg, RA). As with AL amyloidosis, however, quantitative scintigraphy with radiolabeled SAP component can be used in determining the extent and total body burden of amyloid deposits in patients with AA amyloidosis, as well as regression and progression of disease. However, this test is not widely available.

D. Tissue Biopsy

Tissue biopsy is required to make the diagnosis of AA amyloidosis. Like other forms of amyloidosis, AA amyloid displays apple-green birefringence when viewed under polarized light after staining with Congo red. Aspiration of subcutaneous abdominal fat reveals amyloid in 60–70% of patients with AA amyloidosis. If the fat aspirate does not reveal amyloid yet suspicion remains high, other tissue must be obtained. Notably, because AA amyloidosis commonly involves the kidney and gastrointestinal tract, kidney and gastric mucosa biopsy specimens almost always reveal amyloid. Tissue immunohistochemical analysis of the specimen identifies the serum AA precursor protein.

▶ Treatment

The treatment of AA amyloidosis consists of treating the underlying inflammatory disease. This treatment results in reduced levels of serum AA protein and prevents AA amyloid fibril formation and deposition. Treatment may also reverse organ dysfunction caused by amyloid deposits and improve survival. For example, increased use of disease-modifying agents for RA reduces the need for dialysis and the number of deaths caused by AA amyloidosis. Remissions of nephrotic syndrome caused by AA amyloidosis with azathioprine and the combination of methotrexate and prednisolone also have been reported. Colchicine, the drug of choice for treatment of familial Mediterranean fever, prevents inflammatory attacks and the development of AA amyloidosis. Oral chlorambucil has been reported to stabilize amyloid deposits and reverse nephrotic syndrome in a patient with psoriatic arthritis complicated by AA amyloidosis.

A number of reports have described the efficacy of tumor necrosis factor (TNF) antagonists (eg, etanercept and infliximab) in patients with AA amyloidosis due to rheumatic diseases. TNF antagonists induce rapid and sustained clinical remission for a number of rheumatic diseases, including RA. In patients with AA amyloidosis due to RA, ankylosing spondylitis, psoriatic arthritis, and other rheumatic conditions, TNF antagonists used alone or in combination with other agents (eg, nonsteroidal anti-inflammatory drugs, glucocorticoids, and methotrexate) reduces serum acute phase reactants (including serum AA protein), reduces proteinuria, and improves kidney function. TNF induces hepatic production of serum AA protein, whereas TNF antagonists inhibit this process thereby reducing the potential for AA amyloid deposition.

The kidney is the most common organ affected in AA amyloidosis, and it therefore deserves special mention. Ongoing deposition of AA amyloid in the kidney results in proteinuria and progressive loss of renal function. At the molecular level, it is thought that the amyloid fibrils associate with other moieties, such as glycosaminoglycans, forming deposits that disrupt the structure and function of tissues and organs. Interactions between amyloidogenic proteins and glycosaminoglycans promote fibril assembly and stabilization of amyloid deposits in tissues. Eprodisate is a negatively charged molecule that is structurally similar to the glycosaminoglycan heparin sulfate. It can therefore be used to interfere with interactions between amyloidogenic proteins and glycosaminoglycans, thereby inhibiting polymerization of amyloid fibrils and deposition of the fibrils in tissues. It has been used successfully in the management of renal AA amyloid disease, reducing the risk of a doubling of serum creatinine and the risk of a 50% reduction in creatinine clearance, compared with placebo. However, eprodisate has not been found to affect proteinuria, which is thought to result from glomerular toxicity of the serum amyloid A protein precursor, which is not affected by this drug. Eprodisate has not yet been studied in other types of amyloidosis but may be potentially applicable.

Depending on the organs and tissues involved, patients with AA amyloidosis may require supportive treatment (Table 57–2).

▶ When to Refer

Treating the underlying inflammatory disease may prevent or reverse AA amyloidosis. This treatment may require the assistance of a subspecialist (eg, rheumatologist). Treating the manifestations of AA amyloidosis (eg, kidney failure) may also require the assistance of a subspecialist (eg, nephrologist).

▶ Prognosis

Having AA amyloidosis reduces survival. For example, RA patients without AA amyloidosis live nearly 8 years longer than RA patients with AA amyloidosis. Compared with AL amyloidosis, however, AA amyloidosis progresses slowly, and survival is often longer than 10 years. Factors associated with poorer prognosis include older age, reduced serum albumin concentration, end-stage renal disease at baseline, and the degree by which the serum AA concentration was elevated during follow-up. High serum AA level has been found to be the most powerful risk factor for end-stage renal disease and death. However, levels may be suppressed with the use of anti-inflammatory agents. The target for treatment is the achievement of a serum AA concentration in the low-normal range (<4 mg/L). However, decreased production of serum AA protein, with levels below 10 mg/L, is associated with more favorable renal outcome, stabilization or regression of amyloid deposits, and prolonged survival. In summary, treating the underlying inflammatory disease improves survival of patients with AA amyloidosis. In addition, treating organ failure caused by amyloid involvement may improve survival. For example, dialysis or kidney transplantation improves survival of patients with AA amyloidosis in whom kidney failure develops.

DIALYSIS-ASSOCIATED β_2-M AMYLOIDOSIS

ESSENTIALS OF DIAGNOSIS

▶ β_2-m amyloidosis should be suspected in all patients treated with long-term dialysis in whom rheumatic symptoms and signs, especially carpal tunnel syndrome, develop.

▶ Like all forms of amyloid, β_2-m amyloid displays apple-green birefringence when viewed under polarized light after staining with Congo red.

▶ Aspiration of subcutaneous abdominal fat is of little value in detecting amyloid in patients with dialysis-associated β_2-m amyloidosis; hence, other tissue (eg, synovium) must be obtained to establish the diagnosis.

▶ Tissue immunohistochemical analysis identifies β_2-m precursor protein from which β_2-m amyloid fibrils derive.

▶ General Considerations

β_2-m amyloidosis is a frequent complication of long-term dialysis (hemodialysis or peritoneal dialysis). In fact, β_2-m amyloidosis is a major cause of skeletal morbidity in dialysis-dependent patients. Amyloid fibrils derive from β_2-m, which is part of the class I major histocompatibility complex antigen. Patients with renal failure have chronically elevated serum β_2-m levels because 95% of this protein is eliminated via glomerular filtration. Indeed, β_2-m levels can be elevated 60-fold in anuric patients. Furthermore, β_2-m is only partially cleared during dialysis. Chronically elevated levels of this protein lead to the development of amyloidosis. In fact, β_2-m amyloidosis develops in nearly all patients treated with dialysis for more than 15–20 years. Notably, this form of amyloidosis may also develop in patients with chronic renal insufficiency not treated with dialysis.

▶ Clinical Findings

A. Symptoms and Signs

β_2-m amyloidosis has a striking predilection for affecting the joints, especially synovial membranes. Although β_2-m amyloid deposits can be widespread, β_2-m amyloidosis has primarily rheumatic manifestations, including carpal tunnel syndrome, trigger finger, tendon rupture, arthritis, spondyloarthropathy, and cystic bone lesions.

Carpal tunnel syndrome, caused by deposition of β_2-m amyloid in the synovium of the carpal tunnel, is the most common (and usually the first) manifestation of dialysis-associated β_2-m amyloidosis. Indeed, there is a direct relationship between development of this complication and duration of dialysis. In some patients, carpal tunnel

syndrome develops after only 5 years of dialysis. The prevalence of carpal tunnel syndrome after 10 years of dialysis is 20%; after 15 years, it is 30–50%; and after 20 years, it is 80–100%.

Roughly one-half of patients treated with dialysis for more than 10 years experience persistent joint effusions accompanied by mild discomfort. Joint involvement is bilateral and includes large joints (eg, shoulders, knees, wrists, hips). Spondyloarthropathy is caused by destruction of the intervertebral disks and perivertebral erosions. Juxta-articular bone erosions and cystic defects have been described involving the femoral head, acetabulum, humerus, tibia, vertebral bodies, and carpal bones. These defects are not true cysts but rather eroded cavities. Furthermore, they are prone to pathologic fracture. Although β_2-m amyloid deposits have been found in visceral tissues and organs, this deposition usually does not manifest itself clinically.

B. Imaging Studies

Imaging studies usually do not reveal findings specific for dialysis-associated β_2-m amyloidosis. The diagnosis is strongly suggested, however, in long-term dialysis patients who have rheumatic symptoms and have juxta-articular bone erosions or cystic defects on radiography or other imaging studies (eg, computed tomography).

C. Tissue Biopsy

Aspiration of subcutaneous abdominal fat is of little value in detecting amyloid in patients with dialysis-associated β_2-m amyloidosis, unlike AL and AA amyloidosis. Hence, other tissue must be obtained to establish the diagnosis (usually from joints, carpal tunnel tissue, and synovial membranes). β_2-m amyloid displays apple-green birefringence when viewed under polarized light after staining with Congo red. Tissue immunohistochemical analysis identifies the β_2-m precursor protein.

▶ Treatment

The treatment of dialysis-associated β_2-m amyloidosis is largely symptomatic. Rheumatic manifestations are treated with nonsteroidal anti-inflammatory drugs and local glucocorticoids (eg, intra-articular injections). Surgery (eg, carpal tunnel release, stabilization of areas of bone destruction) may be necessary.

Dialysis technology that clears β_2-m is improving. For example, high-flux hemodialysis with bicarbonate-buffered dialysate improves β_2-m clearance, is associated with reduced manifestations of β_2-m amyloidosis, and may improve survival. Kidney transplantation prevents and halts the progression of β_2-m amyloidosis. Serum β_2-m levels normalize and rheumatic symptoms lessen within days following transplantation. It is unclear, however, if kidney transplantation results in mobilization of β_2-m amyloid deposits.

When to Refer

Because this disease is associated with chronic renal failure and dialysis, nephrologists are almost always involved in the care of patients with dialysis-associated β_2-m amyloidosis. Rheumatic manifestations of this disease are common as well, and the assistance of other specialists (eg, rheumatologist, orthopedist) may be necessary.

Prognosis

Most patients treated with long-term dialysis develop β_2-m amyloidosis. Hence, the prognosis of this disease is determined, in part, by the underlying kidney disease and its cause (eg, diabetes mellitus). Rheumatic manifestations of this disease (eg, destructive spondyloarthropathy) may negatively affect survival.

HEREDITARY AMYLOIDOSIS

ESSENTIALS OF DIAGNOSIS

▶ Hereditary amyloidosis should be suspected in all patients with unexplained neuropathy, cardiomyopathy, or renal insufficiency, especially if there is a family history of these problems.

▶ Hereditary amyloidosis, like all forms of this condition, displays apple-green birefringence when viewed under polarized light after staining with Congo red.

▶ DNA analysis of blood and tissue immunohistochemical analysis can be used to identify the mutant precursor protein.

General Considerations

Hereditary amyloidosis consists of a group of autosomal dominant diseases in which amyloid fibrils derive from mutant serum proteins, including transthyretin, apolipoprotein A-I, lysozyme, and fibrinogen A α-chain. Mutations (eg, amino acid substitution) of these proteins render them amyloidogenic. Amyloid fibrils form (with consequent symptoms and signs) in midlife. Not surprisingly, a detailed family history may yield clues to the diagnosis of familial amyloidosis.

Notably, many patients with hereditary amyloidosis are mistakenly assumed to have AL amyloidosis. Monoclonal gammopathies are not uncommon in the general population, and detecting a monoclonal protein in a patient with hereditary amyloidosis may be misleading. Hence, it is important for clinicians to be certain of the origin of amyloid precursor protein in all patients with amyloidosis.

Clinical Findings

A. Symptoms and Signs

Peripheral neuropathy is the most common manifestation of the hereditary amyloidoses. Indeed, the term "familial amyloidotic neuropathy" was once used for these diseases. Cardiac involvement is also common, whereas kidney involvement is less common.

Transthyretin is the most commonly involved protein in hereditary amyloidosis. This protein is synthesized by the liver and choroid plexus and transports thyroxine and retinol-binding protein. More than 80 mutations (single amino acid substitutions) of transthyretin have been identified that cause amyloidosis. Peripheral and autonomic neuropathy is the most common manifestation of transthyretin-associated amyloidosis. Cardiac involvement is common but varies among the different transthyretin mutations. However, compared with AL amyloidosis, heart failure is less common and the prognosis is better. In addition, renal involvement is less common and macroglossia does not occur.

Patients with hereditary amyloidosis caused by apolipoprotein A-I, lysozyme, and fibrinogen A α-chain mutations usually have kidney disease. However, neuropathy does not develop in these patients.

B. Laboratory Findings

No laboratory finding is pathognomonic of hereditary amyloidosis. Instead, laboratory abnormalities reflect amyloid involvement of organs and tissues.

C. Imaging Studies

Imaging studies usually do not reveal findings specific for hereditary amyloidosis. Like other forms of amyloidosis, quantitative scintigraphy with radiolabeled SAP component can be used to assess patients with transthyretin-associated amyloidosis. This test is not widely available, however.

D. Tissue Biopsy

Amyloid deposits caused by the hereditary amyloidoses display apple-green birefringence when viewed under polarized light after staining with Congo red. DNA analysis of blood and tissue analysis identify the mutant precursor protein.

Treatment

Liver transplantation has been used successfully to treat hereditary amyloidosis caused by mutant proteins synthesized by the liver. For example, liver transplantation to treat hereditary amyloidosis caused by mutations of transthyretin may result in disappearance of the mutant protein from the blood and improvement of neuropathy. Other manifestations of hereditary amyloidosis (eg, kidney failure) are treated with supportive measures (Table 57–2).

When to Refer

Relatives of patients affected by hereditary amyloidosis should undergo genetic counseling. Since liver transplantation has been used successfully to treat hereditary amyloidosis caused by mutant proteins synthesized by the liver, referral to a liver transplant subspecialist is warranted. Treating other manifestations of hereditary amyloidosis (eg, kidney failure) may also require the assistance of a subspecialist (eg, nephrologist).

Prognosis

Patients with hereditary amyloidosis caused by mutant proteins synthesized by the liver who undergo liver transplantation experience improved symptoms and prolonged survival, especially if transplantation is done before irreversible organ failure has occurred. The rate of progression of hereditary amyloidosis caused by apolipoprotein A-I, lysozyme, and fibrinogen A α-chain mutations is usually slow. Patients with these forms of hereditary amyloidosis have kidney involvement and usually respond to supportive measures and, if necessary, kidney transplantation.

[Amyloidosis Foundation]
http://www.amyloidosis.org/

Dember LM, Hawkins PN, Hazenberg BP, et al. Eprodisate for AA Amyloidosis Trial Group. Eprodisate for the treatment of renal disease in AA amyloidosis. *N Engl J Med.* 2007;356:2349. [PMID: 17554116]

Dispenzieri A, Gertz MA, Kyle RA, et al. Serum cardiac troponins and N-terminal pro-brain natriuretic peptide: a staging system for primary systemic amyloidosis. *J Clin Oncol.* 2004;22:3751. [PMID: 15365071]

Fernandez-Nebro A, Tomero E, Ortiz-Santamaria V, et al. Treatment of rheumatic inflammatory disease in 25 patients with secondary amyloidosis using tumor necrosis factor alpha antagonists. *Am J Med.* 2005;118:552. [PMID: 15866260]

Floege J, Ketteler M. Beta2-microglobulin-derived amyloidosis: an update. *Kidney Int Suppl.* 2001;78:S164. [PMID: 11169004]

Kastritis E, Wechalekar AD, Dimopoulos MA, et al. Bortezomib with or without dexamethasone in primary systemic (light chain) amyloidosis. *J Clin Oncol.* 2010;28:1031. [PMID: 20085941]

Lachmann HJ, Booth DR, Booth SE, et al. Misdiagnosis of hereditary amyloidosis as AL (primary) amyloidosis. *N Engl J Med.* 2002;346:1786. [PMID: 12050338]

Lachmann HJ, Goodman HJ, Gilbertson JA, et al. Natural history and outcome in systemic AA amyloidosis. *N Engl J Med.* 2007;356:2361. [PMID: 17554117]

Maceira AM, Joshi J, Prasad SK, et al. Cardiovascular magnetic resonance in cardiac amyloidosis. *Circulation.* 2005;111:186. [PMID: 15630027]

[Mayo Clinic]
http://www.mayoclinic.org/amyloidosis/index.html

Merlini G, Westermark P. The systemic amyloidoses: Clearer understanding of the molecular mechanisms offers hope for more effective therapies. *J Intern Med.* 2004;255:159. [PMID: 14746554]

Mollee P. Current trends in the diagnosis, therapy and monitoring of the monoclonal gammopathies. *Clin Biochem Rev.* 2009;30:93. [PMID: 19841691]

Neben-Wittich MA, Wittich CM, Mueller PS, Larson DR, Gertz MA, Edwards WD. Obstructive intramural coronary amyloidosis and myocardial ischemia are common in primary amyloidosis. *Am J Med.* 2005;118:1287.e1-1287.e7. [PMID: 16271914]

Ruberg FL, Appelbaum E, Davidoff R, et al. Diagnostic and prognostic utility of cardiovascular magnetic resonance imaging in light-chain cardiac amyloidosis. *Am J Cardiol.* 2009;103:544. [PMID: 19195518]

Osteoporosis & Glucocorticoid-Induced Osteoporosis

58

Dolores Shoback, MD

OSTEOPOROSIS

Osteoporosis is a systemic skeletal disorder characterized by low bone mass, disruption of the microarchitecture of bone tissue, and compromised bone strength that leads to an increased risk for fracture.

Osteoporosis is common among menopausal women but is usually clinically silent until a fragility fracture occurs. Hip fractures are the most devastating of these in terms of medical, psychosocial, and financial consequences. The lifetime probability of sustaining a hip fracture for a 50-year-old white woman is 14%. The overall percentage of white women at age 50 or older who will sustain an osteoporotic fracture in their remaining lifetime is ~40%. Osteoporosis is being recognized with increasing frequency in older men, who account for about one third of all hip fractures in the United States. The 1-year mortality of men after a hip fracture approaches 30%. Finally, patients receiving long-term glucocorticoid therapy are at increased risk for osteoporosis and should have prevention and treatment approaches implemented.

1. Postmenopausal Osteoporosis

ESSENTIALS OF DIAGNOSIS

▶ Reduced bone mineral density.
▶ Decreased bone strength.
▶ Fragility fractures.

▶ General Considerations

Bone loss in women begins before the onset of menopause, typically in the late third and early fourth decades, and then accelerates for the 5–10 years after the menopause.

Postmenopausal osteoporosis is thought to result from an estrogen-deficiency–induced imbalance between bone formation and resorption such that resorption predominates over formation. Following the increased rate of bone loss immediately surrounding the menopause, a less aggressive phase of bone loss ensues that continues into the eighth and ninth decades. Estrogen deficiency and factors related to aging (reduced osteoprogenitor population, nutritional deficiencies, and malabsorption) play a role in this later phase of bone loss.

Clinically, osteoporosis is diagnosed when **bone mineral density** (BMD) is reduced or when fragility fractures occur. Such fractures are operationally defined as occurring after little or no trauma such as falling from a standing height. The most common osteoporosis-related fractures involve the thoracic and lumbar spine, hip, and distal radius.

Bone densitometry by dual energy x-ray absorptiometry (DXA) is the best standardized technique for diagnosing osteoporosis and monitoring responses to therapy. DXA assessments have been used by the World Health Organization (WHO) to define **osteopenia** and **osteoporosis.** Their criteria are based on a large body of data on postmenopausal white women (Table 58–1).

In addition to age and BMD, there are other risk factors associated with an increased incidence of osteoporotic fractures; the National Osteoporosis Foundation (NOF) has categorized these as modifiable and nonmodifiable (Table 58–2). As described below, all treatment and prevention strategies for osteoporosis begin with risk factor assessment and modification.

Until recently, there was no validated instrument for combining clinical risk factor assessments with BMD measurements to obtain absolute fracture risk estimates. In 2008, the WHO released its fracture risk calculator called FRAX (www.sheffield.ac.uk/FRAX). The FRAX tool combines gender and ethnicity together with several clinical risk factors (age, prior fracture history, parental hip fracture,

Table 58–1. WHO definition of osteoporosis for postmenopausal women based on DXA measurements.

	Definitions
T-score	Number of SD above or below peak bone mass ("young normal") according to race or ethnicity
Z-score	Number of SD above or below age-matched bone mass according to gender and race or ethnicity
Normal	BMD T-score ≥ −1
Low bone mass (osteopenia)	BMD T-score < −1 and > −2.5
Osteoporosis	BMD T-score ≤ −2.5
Severe osteoporosis	BMD T-score ≤ −2.5 with one or more fragility fractures

BMD, bone mineral density; DXA, dual-energy x-ray absorptiometry; SD, standard deviation; WHO, World Health Organization.

current smoking, long-term use of glucocorticoids, rheumatoid arthritis, and excessive alcohol consumption) in combination with femoral neck or total hip BMD to generate two probabilities: (1) 10-year absolute risk of hip fracture, and (2) 10-year absolute risk of major osteoporotic fracture (hip, spine, wrist, and humerus). The clinical risk factors used in FRAX calculation can be easily ascertained

Table 58–2. Risk factors for osteoporotic fractures in women independent of bone density.

Nonmodifiable
  History of fracture as an adult
  Presence of fracture (especially of hip) in first-degree relative
  White race
  Advanced age
  Dementia and frailty
  Immobilization
Modifiable
  Alcohol and tobacco use
  Low body weight (<127 lb for white, <100 lb for Asian)
  Premature menopause
  History of amenorrhea
  Low dietary calcium intake
  Frequent falls and poor eyesight
  Low level of physical activity
  Use of glucocorticoids
  Vitamin D deficiency

Data from National Osteoporosis Foundation, *Physician's Guide to Osteoporosis.* Accessible at http://www.nof.org/physguide/index.htm. 1998; and Kanis JA. Excerpta Medica, Diagnosis of osteoporosis and assessment of fracture risk. *Lancet.* 2002;359:1929.

Table 58–3. National Osteoporosis Foundation recommendations for the diagnosis, management, and prevention of osteoporosis in women and men.

1. Counsel on the risk of osteoporosis in susceptible individuals
2. Consider and eliminate secondary etiologies for osteoporosis
3. Provide sufficient calcium through diet and supplements (at least 1200 mg elemental calcium per day and vitamin D, 800–1000 international units per day) for patients 50 years and older
4. Advice for weight-bearing exercise to reduce falls and prevent fractures
5. Avoid tobacco smoking and excessive alcohol intake
6. Start therapy in patients with hip or vertebral (clinical or morphometric) fractures
7. Treat patients with BMD T-score ≤ −2.5 at femoral neck or spine by DXA
8. Treat postmenopausal women and men aged 50 and older who have low bone mass (T-score between −1.0 and −2.5, osteopenia) at the femoral neck or spine and a 10-year hip fracture probability of ≥3% or a 10-year major osteoporosis-related fracture probability of ≥20% based on the FRAX model (www.shef.ac.uk/FRAX)
9. Pharmacologic options include bisphosphonates, calcitonin, estrogens, progestin, teriparatide, and raloxifene
10. Monitor BMD after initiating therapy in 2 years and every 2 years thereafter with more frequent testing if the clinical circumstance dictates

BMD, bone mineral density; DXA, dual-energy x-ray absorptiometry. Data from *Clinician's Guide to Prevention and Treatment of Osteoporosis* (updated January, 2010) accessed at http://nof.org/professionals/Clinicians_Guide.htm

during the initial evaluation of the patient. NOF adapted FRAX for use in US women and men of different ethnicities (white, black, Hispanic, Asian) and set new treatment thresholds based on absolute fracture risk and cost-effectiveness analysis. Since its introduction, FRAX has been modified and updated. Their recommendations are summarized in Table 58–3. Recommendations for the use of BMD testing in postmenopausal women and for patients receiving glucocorticoids are in Table 58–4.

▶ Clinical & Laboratory Evaluation

The evaluation of perimenopausal or postmenopausal women with osteoporosis or a low BMD begins with the clinical assessment. At least 10–20% of postmenopausal women have an additional secondary cause for their bone loss beyond the estrogen deficiency of menopause. When taking the medical history, the practitioner should pay careful attention to medication use (especially glucocorticoids), smoking, alcohol intake, dietary calcium intake, and family history of osteoporosis and fractures. The physical examination focuses on height loss, the presence of bone pain or deformity, and signs of anemia, hyperthyroidism, hypercortisolism, malnutrition,

Table 58–4. Indications for BMD testing and Medicare reimbursement.

National Osteoporosis Foundation guidelines[a]
Women ≥65 years and men ≥age 70 regardless of risk factor status
Younger women after time of menopause and men aged 50-69 years with a risk factor:
    Prior fragility fracture (before age 50) or use of a high-risk medication
    Positive family history for osteoporosis
    Diagnosis of rheumatoid arthritis or other disorders associated with bone loss
    Use of glucocorticoids in a daily dose ≥5 mg prednisone or its equivalent for ≥3 months
    Current smoking
    Low body weight (<127 lb)
    Individuals initiating therapy for osteoporosis, receiving long-term therapy for osteoporosis, or discontinuing hormone therapy
US Preventive Services Task Force[b]
Women ≥65 years should be screened
    No upper age limit was recommended, instead clinical circumstances should be used as the guide to whether or not to screen elderly patients
    Women of all racial and ethnic groups were included in the recommendation
Women under 65 years (age 50-64) if their 10-year fracture risk is equal to or greater than the risk of a 65-year-old white woman who has no additional risk factors
    The 10-year fracture risk of a 65-year-old white woman without other risk factors is 9.3% calculated according to the FRAX algorithm (www.shef.ac.uk/FRAX/)
Current evidence is insufficient for making any recommendations for screening of men
Medicare coverage of BMD testing[c]
Postmenopausal women at risk for osteoporosis
Patients with vertebral abnormalities
Patients receiving glucocorticoids long term (prednisone ≥7.5 mg/d)
Patients with primary hyperparathyroidism
Patients receiving approved therapy to monitor response
American College of Rheumatology 2010 recommendations for the prevention and treatment of glucocorticoid-induced osteoporosis[d]
    (See detailed treatment recommendations in Tables 58-10, 58-11 and 58-12.)
Obtain baseline BMD measurement when initiating long-term (≥3 months) glucocorticoid therapy at any dose
Assess patients for prevalent fragility fractures when initiating long-term (≥3 months) glucocorticoid therapy at any dose
Consider assessing for prevalent vertebral fractures for those starting or continuing glucocorticoids (prednisone ≥5 mg/d or equivalent)
Consider repeat serial BMD testing for patients receiving glucocorticoids for ≥3 months (interval of testing not established)
Monitor patients receiving therapy for osteoporosis (interval of testing not established)

[a]Modified, with permission, from National Osteoporosis Foundation. *Clinician's Guide to the Prevention and Treatment of Osteoporosis* (updated January 2010).
[b]Modified, with permission, from US Preventive Services Task Force. Screening for osteoporosis: U.S. Preventive Services Task Force recommendation statement. *Ann Intern Med.* 2011;154:356.
[c]Modified, with permission, from Medicare Program: Medicare coverage of and payment for bone mass measurements. *Fed Regist.* 1998;63:34320.
[d]Modified, with permission, from Grossman JM, Gordon R, Ranganath VK, et al. American College of Rheumatology 2010 recommendations for the prevention and treatment of glucocorticoid-induced osteoporosis. *Arth Care Res.* 2010;62:1515.
BMD, bone mineral density.

and other disorders that cause secondary forms of osteoporosis (Table 58–5).

There is no consensus about the appropriate and cost-effective laboratory work-up for postmenopausal women with low BMD or osteoporosis. At a minimum, however, laboratory evaluation should include a complete blood cell count, serum chemistry panel, liver function tests, and serum thyroid-stimulating hormone and calcium determinations. Consideration should be given to assessing vitamin D status at the outset, and this is done by measuring 25-hydroxyvitamin D levels.

Postmenopausal women as a group are commonly affected by primary hyperparathyroidism (prevalence ~3 per 1000). Serum calcium and albumin determinations adequately screen for this disorder. In addition, multiple myeloma can be relatively silent clinically and present with osteoporosis, bone pain, pathologic fractures, or anemia. This diagnosis should be considered if BMD is remarkably low for age (ie, a low Z-score) or if low BMD is accompanied by an unexplained anemia or an elevated erythrocyte sedimentation rate. Multiple myeloma can be detected by serum and urine protein electrophoreses.

Table 58–5. Secondary causes of osteoporosis in men and women.

Rheumatologic disorders	Rheumatoid arthritis Ankylosing spondylitis
Connective tissue disorders	Marfan syndrome Ehlers-Danlos syndrome Osteogenesis imperfecta
Endocrine disorders	Primary hyperparathyroidism Hyperthyroidism Cushing syndrome Hypogonadism Anorexia nervosa with amenorrhea Hyperprolactinemia with amenorrhea or hypogonadism Insulin-dependent diabetes
Hematologic disorders	Multiple myeloma Systemic mastocytosis Lymphoma Leukemia Disseminated carcinoma
Gastrointestinal disorders	Malabsorption Celiac sprue Short bowel syndrome Crohn disease Chronic liver disease (especially cirrhosis) Primary biliary cirrhosis Postgastrectomy
Other conditions	Chronic obstructive pulmonary disease Posttransplantation Malnutrition
Drug therapy	Glucocorticoids Anticonvulsants Excessive thyroxine replacement Anticoagulants (heparin) Gonadotropin-releasing hormone agonists

Measurements of serum 25-hydroxyvitamin D and urinary calcium excretion can be very helpful. Subtle vitamin D deficiency is relatively common in elderly patients and contributes to bone loss because it interferes with the absorption of calcium and phosphorus and thus the mineralization of bone matrix. Low urinary calcium excretion can be caused by vitamin D deficiency, but it can also be due to underlying malabsorption or an extremely low calcium intake. Subtle forms of calcium malabsorption (eg, secondary to celiac sprue) are more common than previously thought. High levels of urinary calcium excretion suggest idiopathic hypercalciuria, which can be associated with renal stones or low BMD or both. Urinary calcium measurements in a patient taking calcium supplements can be informative as to absorption and the adequacy of therapy.

▶ Imaging Evaluation

The study of choice to assess BMD in a postmenopausal woman is DXA of the lumbar spine and hip. DXA reports often include both T- and Z-scores (Figure 58–1). A **T-score** relates the BMD of the patient to peak bone mass for race and gender. A **Z-score** relates the BMD of the patient to persons of the same age, gender, and race. The T-score is the more useful determination clinically. Operationally, the lower of the two T-scores (spine or hip) is used for making the diagnosis. Typically, there is concordance between T-scores at both sites. Discordance can be due to artifactual elevation of the spinal measurement as a result of degenerative arthritis, disk disease, or aortic calcification; in such cases, only measurements of the hip and femoral neck should be used.

Obtaining a BMD measurement allows the clinician not only to grade the severity of osteoporosis but also to assess fracture risk. Several studies have confirmed that the relative risk of fracture approximately doubles with each standard deviation below peak BMD (ie, a negative T-score) that a patient demonstrates.

The combination of BMD measurement and the patient's age is an even more powerful predictor of fracture risk. The 10-year risk of several types of osteoporotic fractures is strongly related to age and BMD T-score, and age is a powerful risk factor in the FRAX calculator of absolute fracture risk (Figure 58–2). Advanced age (over 70 years) dramatically increases the risks of vertebral and hip fractures.

▶ Disease Course & Complications

Postmenopausal osteoporosis can progress silently over years to a dangerously low BMD levels thereby reducing bone strength such that fracture threshold is reached. At this stage, fragility fractures can occur with minimal impact. Fractures

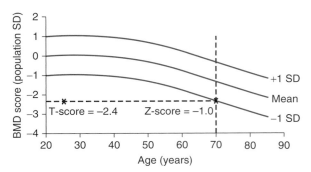

▲ **Figure 58–1.** This graph shows the mean ± 1 standard deviation for bone mineral density (BMD). For a given femoral neck BMD value in a 70-year-old woman, her Z-score is −1 and her T-score (extrapolated back to the age of 20) is −2.4. (Used, with permission, from Orwoll ES, Bliziotes M. *Osteoporosis: Pathophysiology and Clinical Management.* Humana Press, 2003:109.)

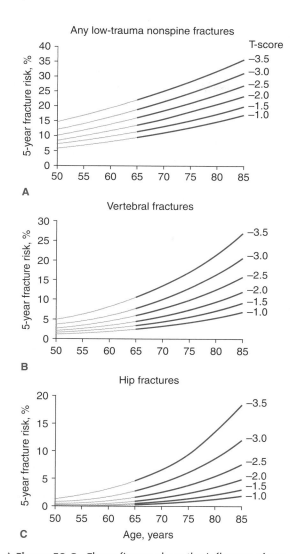

▲ Figure 58–2. These figures show the influence of age and bone mineral density (BMD) on the 5-year fracture risk for any low-trauma non-spinal fracture (**A**), vertebral fractures (**B**), and hip fractures (**C**). At approximately age 65, there is a steep increase in fracture risk at T-scores of −2.0 or −2.5 or greater in panels B and C. (Used, with permission, from Cummings SR, Bates D, Black DM. Clinical uses of bone densitometry: scientific review. *JAMA.* 2002;288:1889.)

are the dreaded complication of osteoporosis. Fractures of the spine cause pain that is generally self-limited. Multiple vertebral fractures can lead to loss of height, reduced thoracic expansion capacity and difficulty with breathing, progressive thoracic kyphosis, poor functional status, and ultimately increased frailty. Frailty itself is a risk factor for fractures, thereby setting up a vicious cycle.

Hip fractures have a more dramatic course, and prognosis in the elderly osteoporotic patient is guarded. These fractures require hospitalization and surgery. Because of the underlying frailty of most of these patients, their comorbid conditions and advanced age, and the prolonged immobilization and rehabilitation required, patients who fracture their hips have decreased life expectancy. Overall, mortality in the first year after a hip fracture (men and women combined) is approximately 20%.

In addition to the medical and financial consequences of hip fractures, there are substantial long-term human consequences. Hip fractures are life-altering events. It is estimated that 50% of patients who sustain a hip fracture do not live independently afterwards. Therefore, it is important to recognize osteoporosis early and to intervene with treatment strategies that reduce fracture risk.

2. Male Osteoporosis

 ESSENTIALS OF DIAGNOSIS

▶ Usually presents later in life than postmenopausal osteoporosis.

▶ Fragility fractures, height loss.

▶ Most patients have one or more secondary cause of bone loss.

▶ General Considerations

The diagnosis of osteoporosis in men is usually delayed relative to that of postmenopausal osteoporosis and often is made only after the patient presents with fractures, height loss, or obvious stigmata of the secondary causes for bone loss.

In contrast to women, men do not experience a clear-cut, easily defined cessation of gonadal function that raises awareness of risks for bone loss. Testosterone production declines with age, but there is controversy as to what the normal or accepted ranges of testosterone are for elderly men and how age-related declines in testosterone contribute to age-related declines in BMD. It is clear, however, that replacing testosterone does not restore BMD to "normal" even in hypogonadal men and that there are many determinants of low BMD and fractures in men beyond hypogonadism.

Differences in the peak bone mass and the rate of bone loss influence the differential clinical expression of osteoporosis in men and women. Men achieve higher peak bone mass than do women, and men lose bone mass at different rates than do postmenopausal women. In women, once the early rapid phase of postmenopausal bone loss ends, the rate of bone loss slows. Thereafter, the rates of bone loss in men and women are roughly comparable (Figure 58–3). Because

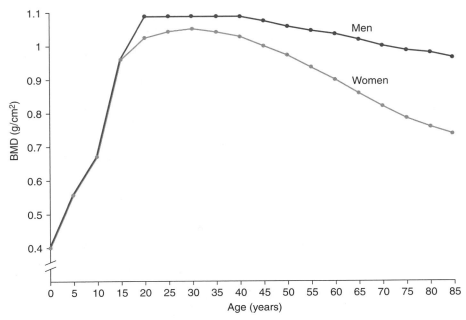

▲ **Figure 58–3.** Mean bone mineral density (BMD) in men versus women from age 5 to 85 demonstrating the lower peak BMD values for women versus men, the rapid perimenopausal rates of bone loss in women, and the slow continuous phase of bone loss that continues into the eighth decade. (Used, with permission, from Southard RN, Morris JD, Mahan JD, et al. Bone mass in healthy children: measurement with quantitative DXA. *Radiology.* 1991;179:735; and from Kelly TL. Bone mineral reference databases for American men and women. *J Bone Miner Res.* 1990;5(Suppl 2):702.)

of the early rapid phase of menopause-related bone loss and the lower peak bone mass attained by women, women have lower BMDs than men of the same age. This leads to an earlier onset of the typical osteoporotic fractures (hip, vertebral, and Colles fractures) in women compared with men (Figure 58–4). Men with low BMD experience most of the same fractures, but these fractures occur later—approximately 10 years later on average—than they do in women. Osteoporotic fractures therefore tend to occur in men at stages in their lives when they are more likely to be

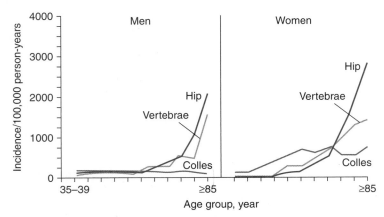

▲ **Figure 58–4.** The incidence of three common osteoporotic fractures in men and women over decades. (Used, with permission, from Cooper C, Melton LJ III. Epidemiology of osteoporosis. *Trends Endocrinol Metab.* 1992;314:224.)

Table 58–6. Determinants of low bone mineral density in men.

Advanced age
Frailty
Low body weight
Alcohol intake
Smoking
Caffeine intake
Use of glucocorticoids
History of hyperthyroidism
History of peptic ulcer disease
History of chronic lung disease
History of rheumatoid arthritis
History of fracture after the age of 50
Height loss since age 20

Data from Orwoll ES, Bevan L, Phipps KR. Determinants of bone mineral density in older men. *Osteoporos Int.* 2000;11:815.

frail and are less able to cope physically and emotionally with the loss of independence and the risks of fracture repair surgery. Hence, the morbidity and mortality of hip fractures are much greater in men than in women.

At least 80% of men with osteoporosis have one or more secondary causes of bone loss (Tables 58–5 and 58–6). Only 10–20% of men with low BMD have primary osteoporosis. These men are often middle-aged and present with height loss and multiple fractures. Whether they have intrinsic abnormalities in bone remodeling—defects in formation or resorption—is unknown.

Considerable effort has been directed toward identifying additional clinical risk factors for BMD loss and fractures in men as they age. An analysis from the MrOS study, a prospective cohort of 5995 elderly men (≥65 years old) from

Table 58–7. Risk factors for fracture in older men from the MrOS study.

Risk Factor	Hazard Ratio (HR) from Multivariable Analysis with 95% Confidence Interval (CI)
Depression	1.72 (95% CI, 1.00–2.95)
Tricyclic antidepressant use	2.36 (95% CI, 1.25–4.46)
Previous fracture (>age 50)	2.07 (95% CI, 1.62–2.65)
Inability to do a narrow walk trial	1.70 (95% CI, 1.23–2.34)
Experienced a fall in the prior year	1.59 (95% CI, 1.23–2.05)
Age ≥80 years	1.33 (95% CI, 1.01–1.76)

Data from Lewis CE, et al. Predictors of non-spine fracture in elderly men: the MrOS study. *J Bone Miner Res.* 2007;22:211.

six US cities followed over 4.1 years at the time of the report is summarized in Table 58–7. Investigators found that six clinical risk factors were significantly associated with risk of hip fracture independent of hip BMD by DXA. Having three or more of these risk factors increased a man's risk of fracture approximately 5-fold. Adding a low BMD to the risk factor profile—three or more risk factors plus being in the lowest BMD tertile—led to a 15-fold greater risk than the reference group (men without risk factors in the highest BMD tertile). There have been studies in countries outside the United States (Sweden, China, and so forth) that extend this type of prospective cohort analysis in men, but much still remains to be learned about susceptibility to fracture in men.

▶ Clinical & Laboratory Evaluation

Because of the prominence of secondary forms of osteoporosis, the clinical and laboratory investigation of men with low BMD and fractures must be thorough. The history and physical examination should pay attention to possible underlying pulmonary, gonadal, adrenal, gastrointestinal, and hematologic disorders. Habits (alcohol and tobacco use) are important risk factors to pursue in men together with the signs and symptoms of the disorders listed in Table 58–5. Men with a history of prostate cancer should be asked about past (or current) use of long-acting gonadotropin-releasing hormone agonists and androgen blockers. These men lose bone at an accelerated rate and treating them to prevent bone loss is effective. Such treatment suppresses turnover, halts loss, and reduces future fractures.

The complete, cost-effective laboratory evaluation of men with osteoporosis is unknown. Most would agree that the initial evaluation should include a complete blood cell count; liver function tests; determinations of serum chemistries, testosterone, thyroid-stimulating hormone, calcium, phosphate, and 25-hydroxyvitamin D; and 24-hour urinary calcium excretion.

If anemia is present and no other cause for osteopenia or osteoporosis has been identified, serum and urine protein electrophoreses should be performed to exclude multiple myeloma. This diagnosis should always be considered in older black men with unexplained bone loss because of its predilection for that population. Men with low testosterone levels should be referred to an endocrinologist for evaluation for primary or secondary forms of hypogonadism.

While primary hyperparathyroidism is a key consideration in women with low BMD, it is less prominent as a cause of accelerated bone loss in men. Nonetheless, because it is relatively common, it should be considered if there is a history of renal stones or if the serum calcium value is even marginally elevated.

Hypercortisolism is rare, but bone loss may be the very first clinical clue that cortisol excess is present. Cushing syndrome is easily excluded by a 24-hour urinary cortisol determination or overnight dexamethasone suppression testing.

Imaging Evaluation

DXA scanning of the spine of elderly men is often affected by the presence of degenerative arthritis, disk disease, and aortic calcifications. Instant vertebral assessment (IVA), a DXA-based determination of vertebral compressions and abnormalities, can be helpful in assessing the presence of early deformities and fractures. Determining the onset of the abnormalities is often very difficult. It is important to remember that men experience more traumatic fractures than do women (including fractures of the spine) at young ages.

A critical issue when using DXA T-scores in men to diagnose low bone mass and osteoporosis is that the data sets for men are much smaller compared to those for postmenopausal women. The WHO classification of osteoporosis and osteopenia (see Table 58–1) was developed based on data from postmenopausal white women. Although it is somewhat of an extrapolation to apply the same DXA T-score cut-points to define osteoporosis and osteopenia in men, this is widely done. Trials of drugs to treat osteoporosis in men (summarized below) usually use a T-score of ≤–2 or –2.5 or fractures to enroll patients. This further supports using similar DXA T-scores in making management decisions in men.

GLUCOCORTICOID-INDUCED OSTEOPOROSIS

General Considerations

Osteoporosis is among the most serious and disabling side-effects of glucocorticoid therapy. Adverse skeletal events occur in approximately 50% of patients receiving long-term glucocorticoid therapy. These patients are subject to an increased risk of fractures in the spine, hip, and other sites. It has been suggested that glucocorticoid-treated patients fracture at higher BMDs than other groups of patients due to the suppressive effects of glucocorticoids on osteoblastic function and on the ability of bone cells to repair tissue microdamage.

There is debate about the minimum dose of glucocorticoid required to induce deleterious effects on bone, but most evidence supports the conclusion that long-term therapy with oral doses of ≥7.5 mg of prednisone daily (or its equivalent) is associated with an increased risk of both vertebral and hip fractures. Most patients receiving glucocorticoids take these drugs orally. Other routes of administration (inhaled, intranasal, or topical) are far less likely to have deleterious skeletal consequences, unless particularly high doses of long-acting glucocorticoid preparations are used.

The pathogenesis of glucocorticoid-induced osteoporosis is complex. In the first few weeks of therapy, there is an increase in bone resorption, and patients can lose considerable bone mass during this initial phase. This period of enhanced resorption continues for approximately 6 months during long-term therapy. Thereafter, the predominant skeletal effect is that of suppressed bone formation. In addition, glucocorticoids antagonize the actions of the active metabolite of vitamin D (1,25-dihydroxyvitamin D), especially in the intestine, leading to reduced calcium absorption, and these agents promote calcium excretion by the kidney, producing marked hypercalciuria in some cases. These actions limit the amount of calcium available to form bone matrix properly. Glucocorticoids also act on the pituitary to suppress gonadotropin production, rendering patients functionally hypogonadal. Long-term glucocorticoid therapy promotes apoptosis (programmed cell death) of osteoblasts, which form new bone, and osteocytes, which are involved in mechanosensing and in maintaining bone's structural integrity. Therefore, ongoing bone resorption is not answered by increased bone formation, and the sensing of normal mechanical forces and physical loading may be impaired. Overall, an imbalance in bone remodeling is favored, and in the end, resorption predominates.

When glucocorticoids are discontinued, bone cells replace some but usually not all of the bone tissue that was lost. It is difficult to rebuild bone microarchitecture. Hence, the prevention of bone loss should be the primary strategy.

Not all patients taking high doses of glucocorticoids suffer adverse skeletal consequences. As noted above, only 50% of patients receiving long-term glucocorticoid therapy experience bony complications. What protects the other patients remains unknown. Men and women of all ages and children can lose bone while taking long-term glucocorticoid therapy. Children also experience stunting of linear growth. The most vulnerable patients, however, are postmenopausal women. Women who require long-term glucocorticoid therapy often have secondary amenorrhea that contributes to bone loss. Many of the diseases for which they receive glucocorticoids long-term (eg, rheumatoid arthritis) are themselves deleterious to bone.

Clinical, Laboratory, & Imaging Evaluation

Patients who are to receive long-term glucocorticoid therapy should be carefully assessed for relevant skeletal risk factors. The menstrual or menopausal status of women should be recorded. The initial laboratory evaluation should include serum chemistries, serum calcium and 25-hydroxyvitamin D levels, and measurement of 24-hour urinary calcium excretion.

The urinary calcium determination is used in much the same way as described above for postmenopausal women and men with osteoporosis. Because of the propensity of glucocorticoids to interfere with vitamin D action and enhance renal calcium excretion, this is a critical parameter to assess in patients treated with glucocorticoids long-term. In addition, a serum testosterone level should be obtained in men due to the effects of glucocorticoids on pituitary release of gonadotropins. Many men taking glucocorticoids long-term will not complain of the typical symptoms of hypogonadism but will have frankly low testosterone levels.

BMD measurements are essential for the evaluation of patients taking glucocorticoids long-term and should inform therapeutic decisions. T-scores that suggest that considerable bone loss has already occurred are usually a signal to treat aggressively.

DIFFERENTIAL DIAGNOSIS OF LOW BONE MINERAL DENSITY

The differential diagnosis of a low BMD measurement is narrow: it is either due to osteoporosis or osteomalacia. Any primary or secondary form of osteoporosis described in this chapter could cause this picture. Osteomalacia causes low bone mass or low BMD because the mineralization of the matrix is defective. Mineral content of the skeleton (not the protein content) is reduced in osteomalacia. A host of different conditions cause osteomalacia. These need to be considered seriously if there is any abnormality in the levels of serum calcium, phosphorus, alkaline phosphatase, or 25-hydroxyvitamin D. Patients with osteomalacia may also have bone pain, pathologic fractures, muscle weakness, and difficulty walking, especially when osteomalacia is moderate or severe and the diagnosis has been delayed. Because the disease is difficult to detect early in its course, the astute clinician must be aware of the manifestations of this less common bone disease and should not ignore subtle clinical and laboratory features that hint at the presence of osteomalacia.

TREATMENT OF OSTEOPOROSIS

1. Lifestyle Modifications

Lifestyle modifications should be implemented in all patients in whom the prevention of bone loss is desired and in whom the goals are stopping bone loss and reducing fractures. Initial efforts are directed at increasing the safety of the patient's immediate environment to prevent falls and fractures, eliminating habits that are deleterious to skeletal integrity and that can contribute to falls, and improving the calcium and vitamin D status of the patient. The latter strategy is absolutely essential if the pharmacologic therapies discussed below are to be successful.

The desired lifestyle modifications are straightforward in concept but not always in implementation. Patients should be encouraged to discontinue smoking and alcohol consumption. Both habits are injurious to bone. Patients should be prescribed a weight-bearing exercise program that emphasizes regular participation (five times weekly if possible for at least 30 and preferably 45 or 60 minutes each) and that is suitable for even frail elderly patients. Regular walking can provide benefits to the frail osteoporotic patient beyond positive changes in BMD. Exercise improves well-being and neuromuscular coordination, which can help condition reflexes to respond better to falls. In addition, although there is some controversy as to efficacy, hip protectors are a simple intervention that can help reduce the incidence of hip fractures in the frail elderly patient who is at risk for falls and is ambulatory.

In patients with inflammatory diseases who are receiving long-term glucocorticoid therapy and are at risk for osteoporosis, an exercise and physical therapy program is imperative. Such patients often suffer from glucocorticoid-induced myopathy as well as the disuse and deconditioning attendant to the joint pains, myalgias, and systemic inflammation caused by their underlying disorders (rheumatoid arthritis, systemic lupus erythematosus, and so forth).

2. Nutritional Interventions: Calcium Supplements & Vitamin D

Several studies support the ability of calcium and vitamin D supplements alone to prevent fractures in the elderly to a modest extent. This is especially true for individuals whose calcium intake is below recommended allowances. Every fracture trial done in recent years has included calcium—and usually vitamin D supplementation as well—in both the placebo and treatment groups.

Nutritional interventions for osteoporosis should assure that the diet plus supplements provide at least 1200 mg of elemental calcium per day in patients with postmenopausal or glucocorticoid-induced osteoporosis (Tables 58–3 and 58–8). Measurements of 24-hour urinary calcium excretion can be used to assure adequate absorption and to avoid hypercalciuria.

Other than nutritional supplements, there are two major sources of vitamin D. In the United States, milk is fortified with vitamin D and is the main dietary source of this vitamin. The second source of vitamin D is dermal synthesis, which is influenced by latitude and exposure to sunlight. For a variety of reasons, elderly patients and those who are chronically ill, including those with rheumatologic disorders, are often deficient in dairy intake and sunlight exposure. That vitamin D insufficiency is a substantial problem is strongly supported by a survey of 1526 postmenopausal women in North America who take prescription drug therapy for osteoporosis. Approximately 50% of these women had 25-hydroxyvitamin D levels below the desired target of 30 ng/mL.

Vitamin D is universally recommended to preserve bone health. The Institute of Medicine of the National Academy of Sciences in their 2011 report recommended a daily allowance of 400–800 international units depending on age, gender, and individual clinical circumstances (see Table 58–9). This level of intake is expected to maintain the serum levels of 25-hydroxyvitamin D at 20 ng/mL or more in ≥97.5% of the healthy population. The NOF recommended slightly more vitamin D per day (800 to 1000 international units, Table 58–3) for individuals at risk for bone loss and with established osteoporosis. The definition of vitamin D sufficiency is controversial. 25-Hydroxyvitamin D is the metabolite made by the liver and stored in fat, is the best indicator of overall vitamin D status in an individual. Estimates of optimal levels of 25-OH vitamin D to achieve skeletal and nonskeletal benefits range from 20–30 ng/mL (50–75 nmol/L) or higher.

Table 58–8. Management of postmenopausal, male and glucocorticoid-induced osteoporosis.

Management Strategy	Recommendation
Lifestyle modifications	Discontinue tobacco Discontinue alcohol intake Wear hip protector Exercise regularly
Nutritional interventions	Increase calcium intake to 1000 mg elemental calcium per day for prevention of osteoporosis in premenopausal women and to at least 1200 mg elemental calcium per day for postmenopausal women, men, and patients taking glucocorticoids long term; vitamin D intake: 800–1000 international units/d for men and postmenopausal women, and for patients taking glucocorticoids long-term

Pharmacologic therapies	**Bisphosphonates**
	  Alendronate 5 mg/d or 35 mg/wk orally for prevention of osteoporosis; 10 mg/d or 70 mg/wk orally for treatment of postmenopausal, male, and glucocorticoid-induced osteoporosis
	  Risedronate 5 mg/d, 35 mg/wk, or 150 mg/mo orally for prevention and treatment of postmenopausal and glucocorticoid-induced osteoporosis
	  Ibandronate 150 mg/mo orally for prevention and treatment and 3 mg/3 mos for treatment of postmenopausal osteoporosis
	  Zoledronic acid 5 mg/year intravenously for prevention and treatment of postmenopausal osteoporosis and for treatment of male and glucocorticoid-induced osteoporosis
	Parathyroid hormone (PTH)
	  Teriparatide (PTH 1-34) 20 mcg subcutaneous injection per day for postmenopausal, male and glucocorticoid-induced osteoporosis, especially in patients at high risk for fractures
	SERMs
	  Raloxifene 60 mg/d orally
	Calcitonin
	  Nasal spray calcitonin 200 international units intranasally daily
	RANK-ligand inhibitor
	  Denosumab 60 mg by subcutaneous injection every 6 months for treatment of postmenopausal women at high risk for fracture, men receiving androgen deprivation therapy for nonmetastatic prostate cancer, and women at high risk for fracture receiving adjuvant treatment with aromatase inhibitors for breast cancer

SERMs, selective estrogen response modulators; RANK-ligand, receptor activator of nuclear factor kappa B ligand.

Table 58–9. Recommended calcium and vitamin D reference intakes by age in adults from the 2011 Report of the Institute of Medicine.

Age, Gender, Circumstances	Calcium, RDA (mg/d)	Calcium, Upper Limit of Safety (mg/d)[a]	Vitamin D, RDA (International Units/d)[b]	Vitamin D, Upper Limit of Safety (International Units/d)[a]
14–18 yrs (M + F)	1300	3000	600	4000
19–50 yrs (M + F)	1000	2500	600	4000
51–70 yrs (M)	1000	2000	600	4000
51–70 yrs (F)	1200	2000	600	4000
71 + yrs (M + F)	1200	2000	800	4000
Pregnant or Lactating (F)				
14–18 yrs	1300	3000	600	4000
19–50 yrs	1000	2500	600	4000

[a]Upper limits of safety below which adverse events are unlikely to occur.
[b]Projected to produce a level of 25 hydroxyvitamin D of 20 ng/mL which is deemed sufficient for healthy individuals.
F, females; M, males; RDA, recommended daily allowance.
Adapted, with permission, from Ross AC, Manson JE, Abrams SA, et al. The 2011 report on dietary reference intakes for calcium and vitamin D from the Institute of Medicine: what clinicians need to know. *J Clin Endocrinol Metabol.* 2011;96:53.

3. Pharmacologic Therapies

Drug therapies have been intensively researched in recent years. Agents that are effective for treating osteoporosis and approved in the United States include (1) bisphosphonates, (2) selective estrogen response modulators, (3) calcitonin, and (4) teriparatide (parathyroid hormone [PTH] 1-34). Hormone therapy (HT) (conjugated estrogen with or without progestin) has also been shown to reduce fractures in the Women's Health Initiative (WHI) trial. This occurred, however, at the expense of increased cardiovascular events and breast cancer risk in the combined HT arm. Both adverse events were considered unacceptable for postmenopausal women. This has profoundly discouraged the use of HT regimens in osteoporosis prevention and treatment. A summary of treatment and prevention strategies is outlined in Table 58–8.

The skeletal status of young women of child-bearing age must be evaluated and managed with circumspection. Bisphosphonates accumulate in the skeleton and may alter fetal skeletal development should pregnancy occur, theoretically even several years after discontinuing bisphosphonate treatment. None of the medications, especially bisphosphonates, are approved for use in pregnant or lactating women.

▶ Bisphosphonates

A. Guidelines for Use

Four drugs in this class are approved for the prevention and treatment of osteoporosis in the United States: alendronate, risedronate, ibandronate, and zoledronic acid. Alendronate, risedronate, and zoledronic acid are approved for postmenopausal, glucocorticoid-induced, and male osteoporosis. Monthly oral ibandronate and quarterly intravenous ibandronate are approved to treat postmenopausal osteoporosis. Both glucocorticoid-treated men and women experience statistically significant increases in lumbar spine and hip BMD by DXA measurements compared with placebo. Overall, drugs of the bisphosphonate class are the most frequently prescribed medications for the treatment of osteoporosis.

The ability of oral (alendronate, risedronate, and ibandronate) and intravenous (zoledronic acid) bisphosphonates to reduce major morbidity from typical osteoporotic fractures has been well-demonstrated in several large, double-blind, placebo-controlled trials. These trials led to the registration and approval in the United States of all four agents for postmenopausal osteoporosis treatment as well as a variety of other indications (male and glucocorticoid-induced osteoporosis and prevention of postmenopausal bone loss), depending on the agent and the characteristics of the individuals studied in the trials. Dosing and approved indications for these agents are shown in Table 58–8.

Alendronate has been studied extensively in early postmenopausal women, women with established osteoporosis, men with osteoporosis, and patients taking glucocorticoids.

It is approved for the treatment of all four groups of patients based on trials showing reductions in spinal, hip, and nonvertebral fractures (patients with established osteoporosis), reductions in spinal fractures (glucocorticoid-treated persons), and significant increases in BMD compared to placebo at spine and hip sites (all groups).

Risedronate, available in three oral formulations (5 mg daily, 35 mg weekly, 150 mg monthly), has been shown to be effective at increasing spinal and hip BMD in women with postmenopausal osteoporosis and in preventing spinal, hip, and nonvertebral fractures in this high-risk population. These observations are based on two large multinational trials with fractures as their end points (VERT and HIP). Risedronate has been studied in patients starting glucocorticoid therapy as well as in those receiving long-term maintenance glucocorticoid therapy. This agent is highly effective at preventing reductions in spinal and hip BMD seen in placebo-treated patients who are treated with glucocorticoids. Risedronate has been studied in men with osteoporosis and is also effective in enhancing BMD at both spinal and hip sites.

Ibandronate is approved for the treatment of postmenopausal osteoporosis as an oral monthly agent (150 mg/mo) and a quarterly intravenous infusion (3 mg/3 mo). The monthly oral preparation is also approved for the prevention of postmenopausal osteoporosis. Ibandronate has been shown to be effective at reducing the risk of vertebral fractures in postmenopausal women with osteoporosis, compared to placebo, but has not demonstrated nonvertebral or hip fracture reduction in the studies thus far conducted.

Zoledronic acid, administered as an annual intravenous infusion (5 mg), has been extensively evaluated in postmenopausal, male, and glucocorticoid-induced osteoporosis. In the latter two populations, zoledronic acid has been compared to active therapy with an oral daily bisphosphonate. Zoledronic acid has also been compared to placebo in patients post-hip fracture. In the placebo-controlled trial that led to the approval of zoledronic acid for the treatment of postmenopausal osteoporosis, there were significant reductions in all the major osteoporotic fractures: hip (41%), nonvertebral (25%), clinical vertebral (77%), and any clinical (33%).

B. Adverse Effects

1. Esophageal, musculoskeletal, ocular, dental, renal— Much is known about the clinical tolerability of the bisphosphonates as a group. When bisphosphonates are given orally, esophageal irritation, esophagitis, and pain can occur. Some, but not all, of the recent epidemiology analyses have suggested an association between bisphosphonate use and esophageal cancer. The absolute number of cases is very small; the duration of bisphosphonate use before onset of the cancer is short; and data on compliance with drug therapy are lacking. All of these issues lead one to question the association.

Musculoskeletal pains and uveitis are rarely seen. In the doses used to treat osteoporosis, the complication of osteonecrosis of the jaw (painful or painless exposed bone) is very rare, occurring at a frequency of ~1/10,000–1/100,000. This oral lesion, often but not invariably, presents after a dental procedure, heals slowly, and can progress to infection and fistula formation along with loss of oral function in the most severe cases. An acute-phase reaction characterized by fever, myalgias, arthralgias, and fatigue can also occur (~10% of patients) particularly after the first intravenous dose of a bisphosphonate. It is essential that patients receiving these agents, especially intravenously, be vitamin D replete prior to therapy to avoid hypocalcemia due to the acute suppression of bone resorption. Renal function should be checked prior to each intravenous dose of a bisphosphonate and periodically during oral therapy with these agents. Product labeling generally recommends against the use of bisphosphonates in patients with estimated glomerular filtration rates less than 30 mL/min or 35 mL/min (depending on the specific agent).

2. Skeletal—Considerable attention has focused recently on atypical femur fractures seen in association with bisphosphonate treatment of osteoporosis. *Atypical* in this context refers to the location, which is subtrochanteric (5 cm distal to the lesser trochanter of the femur) or in the shaft of the femur. These fractures are non-comminuted and frequently bilateral and often present with the prodrome of thigh pain for weeks to months before the fracture presents clinically. Whether bisphosphonates play a causal role in these fractures is uncertain, but they typically occur in patients who have been treated for 5 years or longer with these agents.

▷ Raloxifene

Raloxifene belongs to the class of drugs called selective estrogen response modulators (SERMs), which differ from estrogen biochemically and structurally but can act as estrogen agonists or antagonists depending on the specific target tissues. Raloxifene was developed with the goal of capitalizing on the benefits of estrogen in bone and eliminating or strongly diminishing the impact of estrogen-like compounds on cardiovascular and breast cancer risks.

The MORE (Multiple Outcomes of Raloxifene Evaluation) study compared the efficacy of raloxifene to placebo in postmenopausal women with osteoporosis. After 3 years of therapy, women treated with raloxifene (60 or 120 mg/d) demonstrated modest (2.1–2.7%) but significant increases in lumbar spine and femoral neck BMD. The occurrence of vertebral fractures was significantly reduced by 30–50% compared with the placebo group. However, the overall incidence of nonvertebral fractures was unchanged by raloxifene, and there was no significant impact on hip fractures.

Raloxifene was not associated with an increased risk of endometrial carcinoma, vaginal bleeding, or mastalgia. Venous thromboembolic events, however, were increased in women receiving raloxifene compared to women receiving placebo (relative risk 3.1; 95% CI [1.5–6.2]). This incidence of venous thromboembolic events was similar in frequency to that of patients receiving hormone replacement therapy or tamoxifen. Additional adverse events that were increased in women taking raloxifene included hot flashes, leg cramps, edema, and a flulike syndrome.

Interestingly, the incidence of breast cancer was reduced in both groups of women treated for 40 months with either dose of raloxifene (relative risk 0.3; 95% CI [0.2–0.6]) in the initial trial. With continued administration of raloxifene, it appears that the risk of breast cancer is significantly reduced with up to 8 years of treatment. In a large trial comparing raloxifene to tamoxifen both agents had similar effects to reduce the risk of invasive breast cancer in high-risk postmenopausal women selected for enrollment based on clinical risk factors for breast cancer.

In summary, raloxifene has modest positive effects on BMD and reduces vertebral, but not nonvertebral, fractures. It is a useful agent for younger postmenopausal women who have less severe osteoporosis and are at lower risk for hip fracture.

▷ Nasal Spray Calcitonin

Calcitonin, a 32-amino-acid peptide hormone, binds to receptors on osteoclasts, and this interaction inhibits osteoclast-mediated bone resorption. Calcitonin in the form of a nasal spray (200 units/d) is approved for the treatment of postmenopausal osteoporosis.

The PROOF (Prevent Recurrence of Osteoporotic Fractures) trial established the efficacy of nasal spray calcitonin by comparing it to placebo in 1255 postmenopausal women. All patients received 1000 mg elemental calcium and 400 international units vitamin D daily. After 5 years of therapy, nasal spray calcitonin (200 international units/d) induced 1.0–1.5% increases in lumbar spine BMD that were accompanied by a 33% reduction in new spinal fractures compared with placebo. Hip BMD and hip fractures were not significantly affected by therapy with calcitonin. Adverse events included nasal irritation (congestion, discharge, or sneezing). Calcitonin therefore has modest effects on spinal BMD and does not reduce hip fractures but has an excellent tolerability profile.

▷ Teriparatide

Teriparatide or parathyroid hormone (PTH) 1-34 is approved for the treatment of osteoporosis in postmenopausal women, men with osteoporosis, and patients with glucocorticoid-induced bone loss, especially those at high risk for fracture. PTH produces anabolic effects on the skeleton (ie, stimulates bone formation) when it is administered intermittently in low doses, while the chronic elevations of PTH, characteristic of primary hyperparathyroidism, are "catabolic" to bone, cause excessive resorption, and eventually increase fracture risk. Thus, PTH as a therapy for osteoporosis targets the narrow window between the anabolic and catabolic effects of PTH. Studies demonstrating the efficacy of PTH (1-34) in increasing BMD and reducing vertebral and nonvertebral fractures in postmenopausal women and the studies in men are described below.

A. Indications

1. Postmenopausal osteoporosis—The fracture prevention trial for teriparatide enrolled 1637 postmenopausal women with at least one moderate or two mild nontraumatic vertebral fractures and compared subcutaneous injections of teriparatide (20 mcg/d) with placebo. All participants took daily supplements of calcium (1000 mg) and vitamin D (400–1200 international units). After 21 months, teriparatide induced dramatic increases in spinal BMD (+9.7%) and modest but significant increases in femoral neck BMD (+2.8%).

Teriparatide reduced new vertebral fractures by 65% and all nonvertebral fractures combined (ie, hip, wrist, ankle, humerus, rib, and so forth) by 54%, but the number of hip fractures did not significantly differ in teriparatide- versus placebo-treated patients. New moderate or severe vertebral fractures were substantially reduced 78–90% in teriparatide- versus placebo-treated patients. Adverse events due to teriparatide included dizziness and leg cramps (both in <10% of patients). Hypercalcemia (defined as serum calcium >10.6 mg/dL) developed in 11% of patients receiving teriparatide, compared with 2% of patients in the placebo group. Ninety-five percent of these serum calcium values were <11.2 mg/dL and were managed by reducing calcium intake in most patients.

2. Male osteoporosis—In a study of teriparatide in men, 437 participants were enrolled with T-scores < −2 in the lumbar spine or hip. Their average age was 59, and approximately 50% had low serum free testosterone levels. Men were treated for 11 months with teriparatide or with placebo, and all patients received 1000 mg elemental calcium and 400–1200 international units vitamin D per day. This trial was prematurely terminated because ongoing toxicology studies in rats found an increased incidence of osteosarcomas (see below). At study termination, teriparatide (at 20 mcg/d subcutaneously) induced significant average increases in spinal BMD of +5.9%, in femoral neck BMD of +1.5%, and in total body BMD of +0.6%. Teriparatide was found to be effective in men regardless of their gonadal status, age, or baseline BMD values. The changes in BMD were impressive, given the short duration of the study, but the short duration and the limited number of participants rendered it underpowered to assess reduction in fractures.

3. Glucocorticoid-induced osteoporosis—An active comparator study of 428 men and women (aged 22–89) treated with long-term glucocorticoids (≥5 mg prednisone or its equivalent orally per day for 3 months or longer) compared the efficacy and safety of alendronate (10 mg/d orally) and teriparatide (20 mcg/d subcutaneously) in preserving bone mass and preventing fractures in this high-risk population. Approximately 75% of the patients enrolled had a rheumatologic disorder. After 18 months of therapy, teriparatide produced statistically greater increases in lumbar spine BMD [7.2 +/− 0.7% (teriparatide-treated) vs 3.4 +/− 0.7% (alendronate-treated)] and in total hip BMD [3.8 +/− 0.7% (teriparatide-treated vs 2.4 +/− 0.6% (alendronate-treated)] than daily alendronate. There were significantly less vertebral fractures in teriparatide-treated (0. 6%) vs alendronate-treated patients (6.1%). There were no significant differences in nonvertebral fractures in the two treatment arms of the study. There was a greater incidence of hypercalcemia-related adverse events in the study group treated with teriparatide.

B. Carcinogenic Effect of Teriparatide

Two of the above studies were terminated early due to results from standard carcinogenicity studies in rats showing that lifelong daily injections of high-dose teriparatide induced osteosclerosis and a markedly increased incidence of osteosarcomas (48% of rats treated with teriparatide [75 mcg/kg for 17 months]). The Food and Drug Administration has concluded that these findings do not preclude the use of teriparatide in humans but required a black box warning on the package insert to inform practitioners and patients of this result.

C. Guidelines for Use

Given the above findings plus the costs and inconvenience of daily subcutaneous injections, teriparatide is recommended to treat bone loss in the following groups: patients with severe osteoporosis (including those taking glucocorticoids), especially accompanied by fractures; patients intolerant of other therapies for osteoporosis; and patients who have not responded to other drugs for osteoporosis as evidenced by significant losses of BMD by DXA or by the development of fractures. Treatment is recommended not to exceed 2 years in duration and is approved for use in men and women. Teriparatide is *contraindicated* in growing children (with open epiphyses), patients with bone metastases or those who have had skeletal irradiation, and patients with Paget disease or an unexplained elevation in the alkaline phosphatase value.

Despite the above considerations, teriparatide holds promise for both building new bone and increasing the skeleton's biomechanical strength—outcomes that are highly desired to prevent ongoing osteoporotic fractures in high-risk patients. How should teriparatide be best used to treat osteoporosis? It is anticipated that 2 years of therapy with this agent will be followed by long-term therapy with antiresorptive drugs in an effort to maintain the gains in BMD achieved with this anabolic agent. While this idea is at present intuitively sound, the long-term efficacy of such regimens has been evaluated to only a limited extent as described below (see the section on combination and sequential regimens, below).

▶ Hormone Therapy

HT refers to the combination of estrogen and progestin while estrogen therapy (ET) involves the use of an estrogen preparation exclusively, typically only in patients who have had a hysterectomy. A variety of estrogen preparations have been used for the prevention and treatment of postmenopausal osteoporosis. Perhaps the most popular and best studied has been the combination of conjugated equine estrogens and medroxyprogesterone acetate in varying dosages. Studies like the PEPI (Postmenopausal Estrogen/Progestin Interventions) trial established the efficacy of various HT and ET regimens to prevent postmenopausal bone loss at the spine and hip, based on DXA measurements after 3 years of therapy. This and other trials did not address the antifracture benefit.

HT and ET were thought to reduce the risks of coronary heart disease and its complications, based on epidemiologic studies, and to have little or no effects on breast cancer. This view changed dramatically with the findings from the WHI. The WHI examined the risks and benefits of HT (0.625 mg conjugated equine estrogens and 2.5 mg medroxyprogesterone acetate per day) in 16,608 women in the primary prevention of several postmenopausal health outcomes. In 2002, this study reported a small but significant increased risk of invasive breast cancer in women receiving HT compared with those receiving placebo after 5.2 years (HR [hazard ratio] 1.26; 95% CI [1.00–1.59]) and a similarly small increase in coronary heart disease end points due to HT (HR 1.29; 95% CI [1.02–1.63]). Ironically, this study did show a reduction in hip fractures (HR 0.66; 95% CI [0.45–0.98]) due to HT.

In 2004, the results of the ET study in the WHI were reported. Of 10,739 postmenopausal women with prior hysterectomies, 5310 were randomized to ET (0.625 mg conjugated equine estrogens), and 5410 were treated with placebo for 6.8 years. Major clinical outcomes were an increased risk of stroke (HR 1.39; 95% CI [1.10–1.77]) and reduced risk of hip fractures (HR 0.61; 95% CI [0.41–0.91]). There was no increased risk of coronary heart disease, pulmonary embolism, or breast cancer.

The risk of fracture and changes in BMD were further examined in a subset of women in the HT trial in WHI. Total hip BMD increased by 3.7% after 3 years of therapy compared to 0.14% in the placebo group. The risk of all fractures was significantly reduced in women on HT (HR 0.76; 95% CI [0.69–0.83]) as were the risks of vertebral and lower arm/wrist fractures.

Despite the positive effects of HT on reducing fractures, the negative nonskeletal outcomes (cancer, cardiovascular events) have made HT undesirable for treating osteoporosis, given the availability of other options. Present recommendations are that HT be used for as short a time as possible after menopause, in the lowest possible doses, and mainly for the control of vasomotor symptoms.

▶ Anti-RANK-ligand Therapy

Over the last 10–15 years, a large body of molecular, cellular and preclinical studies has established the central importance of the RANK-L (receptor activator of nuclear factor kappa B ligand/RANK/OPG (osteoprotegerin) pathway in regulating the differentiation of cells in the osteoclast lineage and in the ability of mature osteoclasts to resorb bone. Preclinical studies strongly supported the approach of targeting RANK-L, a cytokine in the tumor necrosis factor superfamily, using denosumab, a monoclonal antibody that neutralizes this molecule essential to the formation and function of osteoclasts. Denosumab has been tested in several large clinical trials that have included postmenopausal women with osteoporosis, men with prostate cancer undergoing androgen deprivation therapy, and patients with various malignancies.

A. Indications

1. Postmenopausal osteoporosis—The phase 3 trial testing the safety and efficacy of RANK-L inhibition as a treatment for postmenopausal osteoporosis randomized 7868 women to subcutaneous placebo or denosumab injections (60 mg every 6 months) for 3 years. All patients were treated with either 400 or 800 international units vitamin D3 daily, based on their initial 25 hydroxyvitamin D level, and at least 1000 mg calcium daily. This multicenter international trial enrolled women between age 60 and 90 years with T scores of <–2.5 at the lumbar spine or total hip but >–4.0. Women were excluded if they had any severe clinical fracture or more than two moderate vertebral fractures. At randomization, women were on average 72-years-old with average BMD T-scores as follows: –2.8 (lumbar spine), –1.9 (total hip), and –2.2 (femoral neck). Prevalent vertebral fractures were noted in the initial baseline spine radiographs in 23–24% of patients enrolled. Thus, this was a moderately osteoporotic elderly population.

After 3 years of therapy with denosumab, BMD increased significantly in the lumbar spine by 9.2% (95% CI, 8.2–10.1) and in the total hip by 6.0% (95% CI, 5.2–6.7) compared to placebo. Markers of bone turnover were suppressed promptly post-injection with the denosumab. Treatment with denosumab was associated with statistically significant reductions in radiographic vertebral fractures by 68% (2.3% of denosumab- vs 7.2% of placebo-treated patients; $P < .001$); nonvertebral fractures by 20% (6.5% of denosumab- vs 8.0% of placebo-treated patients; $P = .01$), and hip fractures by 40% (0.7% of denosumab- vs 1.2% of placebo-treated patients; $P = .04$). New clinical vertebral fractures and multiple vertebral fractures were reduced by 69% and 61%, respectively, by denosumab vs placebo therapy ($P < .001$ for both). Adverse events were similar in the placebo- vs denosumab-treated groups for cardiovascular events, deaths, cancer, renal toxicity, or serious infections. There were no cases of osteonecrosis of the jaw. Eczema occurred at a greater frequency in denosumab- (3%) vs placebo-treated (1.7%) patients ($P < .001$). Although there were no differences in the overall rate of cellulitis reported as adverse events, there were more cases of cellulitis as a serious adverse event in denosumab-treated (N = 12) vs placebo-treated women (N = 1) (P = .002). The overall number of cases was small; however, this has led to increased surveillance for infection in general in patients who may be considered for therapy with this agent.

2. Male osteoporosis—The 3-year clinical trial testing denosumab in men recruited 1468 men receiving androgen deprivation therapy (bilateral orchiectomy or gonadotropin-releasing hormone agonist therapy) for nonmetastatic prostate cancer. Enrolled men were expected to be androgen-deprived for at least 12 months. Men were recruited if they were over 70 years of age or younger than 70 years of age with either a low BMD (T score <–1.0 at either the spine or hip sites) or a history of a fracture. In the full trial, men were on average 75 years of age on enrollment and had BMD scores indicating normal mineralization (lumbar spine and total hip) and mild osteopenia (femoral neck). Participants were treated with denosumab (60 mg every 6 months) or placebo for 36 months. BMD rose significantly at 24 and 36 months in denosumab compared to placebo-treated men achieving 6.7%, 4.8%, 3.9%, and 5.5% differences at the lumbar spine, total hip, femoral neck, and distal one third radius, respectively ($P < .001$ for all). These changes in BMD were associated with statistically significant reductions in new radiographic vertebral fractures assessed after 12, 24, and 36 months of treatment with denosumab with a cumulative reduction of 62% (relative risk, 0.38; 95% CI, 0.19–0.78; $P = .0006$) compared to placebo treatment. No statistically significant differences were seen in nonvertebral fractures between the denosumab- vs placebo-treated men over the 36 months of the trial. There were no differences in deaths, serious infections, renal toxicity, cancers or cardiovascular events in patients receiving denosumab vs placebo injections.

B. Guidelines for Use

Based on the findings from these and other studies, denosumab (dosing of 60 mg every 6 months by subcutaneous injection) was approved by the US Food and Drug Administration for the treatment of osteoporosis. The indications in the prescribing information include the following: postmenopausal women at high risk for fracture, men receiving androgen deprivation therapy for nonmetastatic cancer of the prostate, and women with breast cancer at high risk for fracture receiving adjuvant aromatase inhibitor therapy. In clinical practice, denosumab offers an advantage over bisphosphonates in that it is not contraindicated when renal function is impaired and is conveniently administered twice yearly by injection assuring full absorption of the active medication. Denosumab has been used in patients with rheumatic disorders receiving glucocorticoids but does

not have the specific indication for glucocorticoid-induced osteoporosis. Because of the potency of denosumab in suppressing bone turnover and the substantial amount of drug administered per dose, it is imperative that patients scheduled to receive the medication be treated with daily calcium (at least 1000 mg per day) and vitamin D supplements; 25 hydroxyvitamin D levels be checked prior to dosing and be sufficient. In addition, patients with renal dysfunction who have received the potent antiresorptive agent in small studies of short duration have demonstrated a greater tendency to hypocalcemia. Thus, calcium and vitamin D supplements remain a key component of therapy with denosumab.

▶ Combination & Sequential Regimens

A small number of trials have combined approved agents for the treatment of osteoporosis, either together or in sequence. In general, these studies are smaller than the pivotal trials that established the efficacy of individual therapies in the treatment of osteoporosis and prevention of fractures. The combination of two antiresorptive therapies typically achieves a small additional increase in BMD beyond that attained with either agent alone. None of the combination or sequential studies has had fracture reduction as an end point, and therefore a clear role for these approaches to prevent fractures is not yet established. Furthermore, costs and adverse events are potentially additive. There has been the additional concern that excessive blockade of resorption (with two antiresorptive agents) might produce such marked suppression of turnover as to impair the ability of bone to repair microdamage and microfractures and to respond to the normal forces acting on the remodeling process.

There is theoretical appeal for sequential regimens that first use anabolic agents like teriparatide to promote bone formation and then use antiresorptive drugs to maintain the bone mass gained. In this regard, the Parathyroid Hormone and Alendronate Study in postmenopausal women, compared alendronate (10 mg/d) and full-length PTH (PTH [1-84], 100 mcg/d) individually or in combination. There was no evidence of synergy when the agents were used concurrently; indeed at 1 year, the concurrent use of alendronate appeared to diminish bone formation. The second year of the study, however, showed that the gains in BMD achieved with PTH (1-84) alone for 12 months were not maintained unless PTH (1-84) was followed by alendronate. Similar conclusions were reached in a study of men using PTH (1-34) and alendronate. It appears that potent antiresorptive agents such as alendronate tend to blunt the "anabolic" effects of PTH when used concurrently but can maintain PTH-induced increases in BMD when used in a sequential or cyclic regimen. Not all antiresorptives behave in the same way. Raloxifene or HT in combination with PTH (1-34) did not blunt the anabolic actions of PTH (1-34). Currently, there are insufficient data to establish the superiority of one combination or sequence over another for the prevention of fractures.

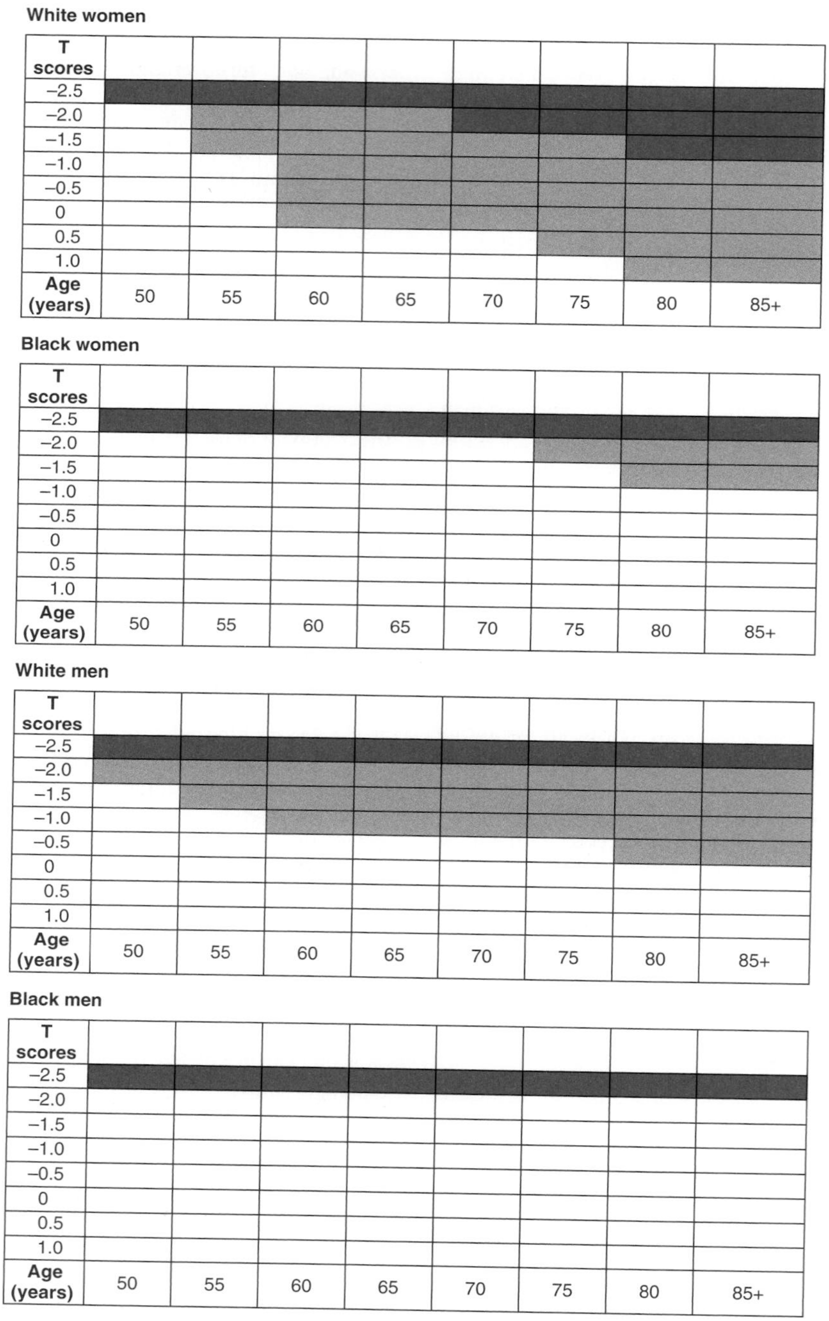

▲ **Figure 58–5.** Proposed assignment of fracture risk on the basis of clinical risk factors (age, gender, ethnicity, T scores) in patients (postmenopausal women and men >age 50) taking glucocorticoids shown as LOW (white), MEDIUM (light purple), and HIGH (dark purple) risk groups. Ten-year absolute risk of a major osteoporotic fracture derived from FRAX is considered to be approximately <10% (low), 10–20% (medium), and >20% (high) according to the panel of the American College of Rheumatology expert panels. (Adapted, with permission, from Grossman JM, et al. American College of Rheumatology 2010 recommendations for the prevention and treatment of glucocorticoid-induced osteoporosis. *Arthritis Care Res.* 2010;62:1515.)

MANAGEMENT OF GLUCOCORTICOID-INDUCED OSTEOPOROSIS

▶ Risk Assessment

The American College of Rheumatology's expert panels issued recommendations for the prevention and treatment of glucocorticoid-induced osteoporosis in 1996, 2001, and 2010. The 2010 recommendations were formulated not to include children, patients with transplants, or patients taking inhaled glucocorticoids. These recommendations were designed along the lines of clinical scenarios and organized clinical risk for fractures into three categories: high, medium, and low. The panel developed 48 patient risk factor combinations and profiles using the following risk factors: gender, age (55, 65, 75, 85), race/ethnicity (black and white), and femoral neck T-scores using the cut-points of 0, −1.0, −1.5, −2.0, and −2.5. Using FRAX, the expert panel calculated the two 10-year risk scores (major osteoporotic and hip fracture). All of the other FRAX risk factors were assumed to be negative in the simulations that were used. Other ethnicities were not considered because it was felt that their BMD values fell between white and black and the 48 scenarios offered sufficient complexity to inform the guidance for clinicians.

The panel recommended either the use of FRAX to calculate absolute fracture risk and grade it as low, medium, or high or to gauge risk for the patient in questions based on the scenarios described in the recommendations report (Figure 58–5). The 10-year risk of a major osteoporotic fracture (% calculated from FRAX) was used to define the risk categories along with other factors as follows: low (10% or less), medium (10–20%), and high (>20%, T-score of ≤ −2.5, or history of an osteoporotic fracture). The panel further noted that other clinical risk factors that they did not include in their models could shift/increase the risk in individual patients based on the judgment of the treating physician. Those risk factors included historical features (low body weight, parental history of hip fracture), lifestyle risk factors (excessive alcohol intake and smoking), and specific aspects of the therapy itself. Aspects related to the glucocorticoid therapy itself that they noted were higher daily doses, higher cumulative doses, and intravenous pulse therapy. These factors plus the observation that BMD is declining could all be used to shift the patient in question to the higher risk category.

▶ Therapeutic Options & Decision-making

The American College of Rheumatology panel divided their recommendations for management of skeletal health in patients treated with glucocorticoids into two broad groups: (1) postmenopausal women and men >age 50 years, and (2) premenopausal women and men <age 50 years. Once risk is assessed either through FRAX or their schema described above (see Figure 58–5) as low, medium, or high, then separate management algorithms were recommended to use to determine the need for treatment with specific medications for prevention and treatment of osteoporosis (Tables 58–10 and 58–11). These recommendations were put forward as guidance to clinicians managing patients taking glucocorticoids and were meant to be part of the decision-making process, factoring in other knowledge of the patient's overall skeletal risk profile including prevalent fragility fracture status.

TREATMENT FAILURES

An ominous clinical development in a patient already receiving treatment for osteoporosis is the occurrence of one or more fractures. Loss of BMD during therapy is also a cause for concern if the decrement in BMD exceeds the precision errors of DXA measurements.

Table 58–10. Approach to management of patients (postmenopausal women and men >age 50 years) who are expected to be treated with glucocorticoids for ≥3 months or for the times specified in the high risk group.[a]

Risk Category	Recommendations	
	If Glucocorticoid Dose is <7.5 mg/day Prednisone or Equivalent	If Glucocorticoid Dose is ≥7.5 mg/day Prednisone or Equivalent
Low	No drug therapy	Consider alendronate, risedronate, or zoledronic acid
Medium	Consider alendronate or risedronate	Consider alendronate, risedronate, or zoledronic acid
	If Glucocorticoid Dose is <5 mg/day Prednisone or Equivalent or ≤1 Month	If Glucocorticoid Dose is ≥5 mg/day Prednisone or Equivalent or for >1 Month
High	Consider alendronate, risedronate, or zoledronic acid	Consider alendronate, risedronate, zoledronic acid, or teriparatide

[a]The clinician should first determine risk (low, medium, high) according to the paradigm in Table 58–10 or by the FRAX algorithm and consider management below. Once management is determined, the patient should have routine monitoring of the skeletal response and other nutritional and lifestyle interventions as recommended in Table 58–3.
Modified, with permission, from Grossman JM, Gordon R, Ranganath VK, et al. American College of Rheumatology 2010 recommendations for the prevention and treatment of glucocorticoid-induced osteoporosis. *Arth Care Res.* 2010;62:1515.

Table 58–11. Approach to management of patients (postmenopausal women and men <age 50 years) who are expected to be treated with glucocorticoids for the times specified.[a]

Patient Group	Absense or Presence of Fragility Fractures		
	No Prevalent Fracture	Prevalent Fracture in Patients Receiving Glucocorticoid for 1–3 Months	Prevalent Fracture in Patients Receiving Glucocorticoid for >3 Months
Women of childbearing potential	No data for making recommendations	No consensus for making any recommendations	Alendronate, risedronate or teriparatide if ≥7.5 mg/d prednisone or equivalent If <7.5 mg/d prednisone or equivalent, no consensus for making recommendations
Women not of childbearing potential; men <age 50	No data for making recommendations	If ≥5 mg/d prednisone or equivalent, consider alendronate or risedronate If >7.5 mg/d prednisone or equivalent, consider zoledronic acid	Consider alendronate, risedronate, zoledronic acid, or teriparatide

[a]Once management is determined, the patient should have routine monitoring of the skeletal response and other nutritional and lifestyle interventions as recommended in *Table 58–3*.
Data from Grossman JM, Gordon R, Ranganath VK, et al. American College of Rheumatology 2010 recommendations for the prevention and treatment of glucocorticoid-induced osteoporosis. *Arth Care Res.* 2010;62:1515.

Noncompliance is a common explanation for treatment failure. Although the therapies discussed above (especially the bisphosphonates, teriparatide, and denosumab) are highly efficacious, no treatment strategy completely prevents all fractures. If noncompliance is not the explanation, then the clinician must decide whether the fracture was expected or unexpected in the context of the individual patient. The clinician must consider the length of therapy, underlying risk factors contributing to the patient's bone loss, baseline BMD values, the degree of trauma if any, and other medications and conditions that might exacerbate the fracture risk or bone loss. The clinician must also decide whether the initial work-up was sufficient and whether possible secondary causes were carefully considered and eliminated. On many occasions, especially in postmenopausal women, treatment failures prompt the first thorough investigation to exclude secondary causes of low BMD (eg, primary hyperparathyroidism, multiple myeloma, vitamin D deficiency, or celiac sprue). If the clinician is inexperienced with the evaluation of secondary osteoporosis or deciding whether BMD determinations indicate adequate responses to treatment, then this is an excellent time to refer a patient with fractures or ongoing bone loss while receiving therapy to a specialist (rheumatologist or endocrinologist) experienced in the care of patients with osteoporosis.

[American College of Rheumatology]
http://www.rheumatology.org/practice/clinical/guidelines/index.asp

Canalis E, Mazziotti G, Giustina A, Bilezikian JP. Glucocorticoid-induced osteoporosis: pathophysiology and therapy. *Osteo Int.* 2007;18:1319. [PMID: 17566815]

Compston J. Management of glucocorticoid-induced osteoporosis. *Nat Rev Rheumatol.* 2010;6:82. [PMID: 20125175]

Cummings S, San Martin J, McClung MR, et al. FREEDOM trial. Denosumab for prevention of fractures in postmenopausal women with osteoporosis. *N Engl J Med.* 2009;361:756. [PMID: 19671655]

Ebeling PR. Clinical practice. Osteoporosis in men. *N Engl J Med.* 2008;358:1474. [PMID: 18385499]

FRAX website:
https://www.sheffield.ac.uk/FRAX

Grossman JM, Gordon R, Ranganath VK, et al. American College of Rheumatology 2010 recommendations for the prevention and treatment of glucocorticoid-induced osteoporosis. *Arthritis Care Res.* 2010;62:1515. [PMID: 20662044]

Hodsman AB, Bauer DC, Dempster DW, et al. Parathyroid hormone and teriparatide for the treatment of osteoporosis: a review of the evidence and suggested guidelines for its use. *Endocr Rev.* 2005;26:688. [PMID: 15769903]

Holick MF, Siris ES, Binkley N, et al. Prevalence of Vitamin D inadequacy among postmenopausal North American women receiving osteoporosis therapy. *J Clin Endocrinol Metab.* 2005;90:3215. [PMID: 15797954]

Holick MF. Vitamin D deficiency. *N Engl J Med.* 2007;357:266. [PMID: 17634462]

Kanis JA. Diagnosis of osteoporosis and assessment of fracture risk. *Lancet.* 2002;359:1929. [PMID: 12057569]

Lewis CE, Ewing SK, Taylor BC, et al. Osteoporotic Fractures in Men (MrOS) Study Research Group. Predictors of non-spine fracture in elderly men: the MrOS study. *J Bone Miner Res.* 2007;22:211. [PMID: 17059373]

Medicare program; Medicare coverage of and payment for bone mass measurements—HCFA. Interim final rule with comment period. *Fed Regis.* 1998;63:34320. [PMID: 10180295]

National Osteoporosis Foundation. *Clinician's Guide to the Prevention and Treatment of Osteoporosis.* Accessed on www.nof.org (updated 1/2010).

National Institutes of Health Consensus Statement. Osteoporosis Prevention, Diagnosis, and Therapy, Office of the Director, 2000;17:5.

Orwoll ES, Bliziotes M. *Osteoporosis: Pathophysiology and Clinical Management.* Humana Press, 2003.

Rachner TD, Khosla S, Hofbauer LC. Osteoporosis: now and the future. *Lancet.* 2011;377:1276. [PMID: 21450337]

Recker RR, Lewiecki EM, Miller PD, Reiffel J. Safety of bisphosphonates in the treatment of osteoporosis. *Am J Med.* 2009;122 (2 Suppl):S22. [PMID: 19187809]

Rosen CJ. Postmenopausal osteoporosis. *N Engl J Med.* 2005;353:6. [PMID: 16093468]

Ross AC, Manson JE, Abrams SA, et al. The 2011 report on dietary reference intakes for calcium and vitamin D from the Institute of Medicine: what clinicians need to know. *J Clin Endocrinol Metabol.* 2011;96:53. [PMID: 21118827]

Saag KG, Shane E, Boonen S, et al. Teriparatide or alendronate in glucocorticoid-induced osteoporosis. *N Engl J Med.* 2007;357:2028. [PMID: 18003959]

Smith MR, Egerdie B, Toriz NH, et al. Denosumab HALT Prostate Cancer Study Group. Denosumab in men receiving androgen-deprivation therapy for prostate cancer. *N Engl J Med.* 2009;362:745. [PMID: 19671656]

[The American Society for Bone and Mineral Research] http://www.asbmr.org

US Preventive Services Task Force. Screening for osteoporosis: U.S. Preventive Services Task Force recommendation statement. *Ann Intern Med.* 2011;154:356. [PMID: 21242341]

Osteonecrosis

Lianne S. Gensler, MD

ESSENTIALS OF DIAGNOSIS

▶ Usually presents with pain upon weight-bearing and motion of the affected joint.

▶ The most common site is the femoral head, but the distal femur, ankles, shoulders, wrists and elbows may also be affected.

▶ There are many predisposing conditions but glucocorticoid therapy, alcohol abuse, and trauma account for the great majority of cases.

▶ MRI has sensitivity for early disease and can detect characteristic abnormalities before radiographic changes are apparent.

▶ General Considerations

Osteonecrosis results from impaired delivery of adequate oxygen to underlying bone. It typically affects the poorly vascularized fatty marrow and is characterized by areas of dead marrow and trabecular bone extending to the subchondral plate. Other terms frequently used for this condition are "ischemic necrosis," "avascular necrosis" and "aseptic necrosis." Osteochondritis dessicans and Kienböck disease are forms of osteonecrosis.

The femoral head is particularly susceptible to osteonecrosis. Typically, osteonecrosis of the femoral head develops in the anterolateral aspect just below the weight-bearing articular surface; this is the site of greatest mechanical stress. Once radiographic abnormalities are apparent, collapse of the femoral head is usually inevitable, at intervals ranging from weeks to years.

Osteonecrosis is not a discrete disease but represents the final common pathway of multiple conditions, most of which result in impaired blood supply to bone. Proposed mechanisms include occlusion of smaller arteries of the femoral head by lipid droplets, sickled red blood cells, or nitrogen bubbles from caisson disease. Alternatively, structural damage to the arterial or venous walls from trauma, vasculitis, radiation, or release of vasoactive substances may lead to ischemia. In some conditions, increased intraosseous pressure from enlargement of intramedullary fat cells or osteocytes may play a role. Through one or more of these pathways, osteonecrosis begins with interruption of the blood supply to bone; subsequently, the adjacent area becomes hyperemic, leading to demineralization, trabecular thinning and, if stressed, bony collapse. The process is usually progressive, resulting in joint destruction within 3–5 years if left untreated.

Elderly persons seem to be at decreased risk for developing osteonecrosis. In this age group, fat cells become smaller. The space between fat cells fills with a loose reticulum and mucoid fluid, resistant to ischemic necrosis. This is termed "gelatinous marrow," and even in the presence of increased intramedullary pressure, interstitial fluid is able to escape into the blood vessels, leaving the spaces free to absorb additional fluid.

The true prevalence of osteonecrosis is unknown, but it is estimated that there are approximately 10,000 to 20,000 new cases annually in the United States. Osteonecrosis is the underlying diagnosis in approximately 10% of all total hip replacements. For the most part, osteonecrosis affects the epiphyses of the long bones, such as the femoral and humeral heads, but other bones (eg, carpal and tarsal) can also be affected. The disease occurs more frequently in men than women, with the overall male to female ratio in the range of 8:1. The age distribution is wide, but most patients are younger than age 50 at the time of diagnosis. The average age of female cases exceeds that of males by almost 10 years.

▶ Causes

Osteonecrosis can develop in a variety of clinical settings (Table 59–1). Trauma, glucocorticoid use, and excessive alcohol intake account for more than 90% of adult cases in the United States.

Table 59–1. Conditions associated with osteonecrosis.

Trauma
    Fracture of the femoral neck
    Dislocation or fracture/dislocation of the hip
    Other
Glucocorticoid therapy
Excessive alcohol consumption
Dysbaric syndromes (caisson disease, divers' disease)
Sickle-cell disease
Gaucher disease
Radiation therapy
Systemic lupus erythematosus
Antiphospholipid antibody syndrome
Systemic vasculitis
Other connective tissue diseases
Pregnancy
Infection with HIV
Pancreatitis
Pancreatic cancer
Inherited thrombophilia (possible)

Trauma that results in the dislocation or fracture of the femoral neck, especially in the subcapital region, can interrupt the blood supply to the femoral head, leading to ischemia and osteonecrosis. Osteonecrosis can occur within 8 hours of traumatic disruption of the blood supply. The superior retinacular vessels and the nutrient artery can be damaged as they enter the femur. Intracapsular hematoma increases intracapsular pressure, which can cause tamponade of the joint capsule. The incidence of osteonecrosis in such cases, which is at least 30%, increases for badly displaced fractures, particularly in young adults. Intertrochanteric and extracapsular fractures of the femur rarely lead to osteonecrosis. Following hip dislocation, circulation is interrupted because of tears of the artery of the ligamentum teres. Tearing of the joint capsule compromises the vessels within the capsular reflections. Osteonecrosis following subcapital fractures of the femur may develop as late as 10 years following the fracture. Dislocation of the hip is much less common than hip fracture, but the incidence of osteonecrosis is quite high if reduction is delayed by more than 6 hours. A fracture of the wrist (scaphoid or lunate) is associated with an increased risk of osteonecrosis. Osteonecrosis of the lunate, known as Kienböck disease, may occur without an identifiable event.

Many studies have linked **glucocorticoid** use to the development of osteonecrosis. The incidence of osteonecrosis among patients treated with glucocorticoids is affected by the dose and duration of therapy with prolonged high doses (eg, prednisone >20 mg daily) conferring the greatest risk. The incidence of osteonecrosis is higher among patients treated with prednisone in whom a cushingoid appearance develops. In contrast, most studies have found that the risk is

low (<3%) among patients treated with doses of prednisone <15–20 mg daily. Osteonecrosis is a rare but recognized complication of Cushing syndrome due to pituitary or adrenal pathology.

Osteonecrosis develops in 3–30% of patients with **systemic lupus erythematosus (SLE)**. SLE is an independent risk factor for osteonecrosis, but patients who have taken glucocorticoids, particularly doses of prednisone consistently >20 mg daily, are at greatest risk. Osteonecrosis can develop in SLE patients within a relatively short time following the initiation of glucocorticoid therapy. A decrease in bone mineral density within the first year of glucocorticoid initiation may be a predictor of osteonecrosis. Risk factors for the development of osteonecrosis in SLE include use of cytotoxic drugs, black race, Raynaud phenomenon, antiphospholipid antibodies, and hyperlipidemia.

Osteonecrosis affects 4–25% of patients following **renal transplantation** and, in this setting, is often multifocal. The risk decreases following the introduction of cyclosporine, tacrolimus, and mycophenolate mofetil and consequent reduction in glucocorticoid dose. Apart from glucocorticoid dose, risk factors for osteonecrosis include acute rejection, delayed graft function, preexisting hyperparathyroidism, and osteopenia. Osteonecrosis occurs in other transplantation settings including hematopoietic transplantation where the sex of donor and recipient affects risk (female donor to female recipient carries the highest risk).

Excessive alcohol use and the development of osteonecrosis have been linked for decades. An elevated risk for regular drinkers and a clear dose-response relationship have been noted.

Osteonecrosis develops in about 50% of patients with **sickle cell disease** by age 35, likely due to the combined effects of sickled red blood cells and bone marrow hyperplasia. Concomitant α-thalassemia increases the risk, while elevated hemoglobin F appears to be protective.

Gaucher disease is an autosomal recessive disorder of glucocerebroside metabolism that leads to the accumulation of cerebroside-filled cells within the bone marrow. This may result in compression of the vasculature and subsequent osteonecrosis, which has been reported in 60% of patients with Gaucher disease.

In **dysbaric syndromes** such as **caisson disease** and **diver's disease** ("the bends"), decompression causes the formation of intravascular nitrogen bubbles that can occlude arterioles. Osteonecrosis can develop years after the exposure and is often multifocal. The pressure and number of decompressions are important risk factors.

Inherited thrombophilia may be a cause of osteonecrosis, but there is no consensus on this issue. There are conflicting data regarding the role of mutations in genes for proteins in the coagulation cascade and fibrinolytic pathways in the pathogenesis of osteonecrosis. Four reports suggested an increased prevalence of the factor V Leiden mutation in patients with osteonecrosis of the hip or knee compared with healthy controls, a finding that was not seen in another study.

Inherited osteonecrosis may be a potential cause of osteonecrosis as evidenced by mutations in the type II collagen gene variant (*COL2A1*), which has been found in several Chinese families with osteonecrosis.

Infection with the **HIV** may confer an increased risk of developing osteonecrosis of the femoral head. Additional risk factors in the HIV-infected population may be use of glucocorticoids, lipid-lowering drugs, testosterone, weight training, and anti-cardiolipin antibodies. Use of antiretroviral therapy does not appear to be an independent risk factor.

In patients with malignancy, use of **bisphosphonates** has been associated with osteonecrosis of the jaw, which presents as a nonhealing lesion of the socket following dental extraction.

▶ Clinical Findings

A. Symptoms and Signs

Most patients have had osteonecrosis for some time before the onset of symptoms, usually in the form of gradually worsening pain or aching in the affected joint during activity. In some instances, the pain begins abruptly. With hip involvement, the pain is usually felt in the groin. Many patients have bilateral involvement at the time of diagnosis.

Physical findings are nonspecific. In early stages of hip osteonecrosis, for example, decreased range of motion is related primarily to pain, particularly with forced internal rotation and abduction. Bone remodeling allows some patients to remain functional for years, despite limited range of motion. As the disease progresses, the pain increases, associated with stiffness and restricted range of motion of the involved joint. Limping is common late in the course of lower extremity disease. The time from onset of symptoms to development of end-stage joint varies widely, from months to years.

B. Imaging Studies

1. Radiography—Plain radiographs identify advanced disease but are less helpful in early stages. The evaluation for suspected osteonecrosis of the femoral head should begin with anteroposterior and frog-leg lateral radiographs. Lateral views are necessary to evaluate the superior portion of the femoral head, where subchondral abnormalities may be seen. The plain radiograph may remain normal for months after onset of symptoms; the earliest findings are mild density changes followed by sclerosis and cysts as the disease progresses (Figures 59–1 and 59–2). The pathognomonic crescent sign (subchondral radiolucency) is evidence of subchondral collapse. In later stages there is loss of sphericity or collapse of the femoral head. Eventually, joint space narrowing and degenerative changes in the acetabulum are apparent (Figure 59–3).

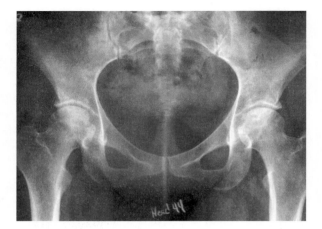

▲ **Figure 59–1.** Plain anteroposterior radiograph demonstrating features consistent with osteonecrosis of the femoral head. There is bilateral cystic change and sclerosis at the margins. There is a mottled increased density because of destruction of the bony trabecula. There is some evidence of collapse of the femoral head, as the joint space is not a smooth hemisphere.

2. Radionuclide bone scan—Technetium-99m bone scanning for the evaluation of suspected osteonecrosis has largely been supplanted by MRI. Bone scanning is limited by nonspecific findings. An exception is the characteristic (but unusual) "donut sign" or "cold in hot" image of decreased uptake observed within the center of an area of increased uptake.

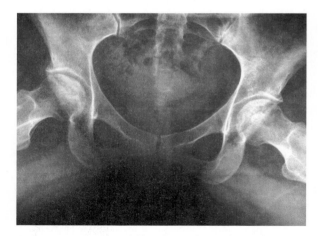

▲ **Figure 59–2.** Lateral/frog-leg radiography of the same patient shown in Figure 59–1, again demonstrating bilateral cystic change and sclerosis. There is some evidence of collapse of the femoral head, as the joint space is not a smooth hemisphere.

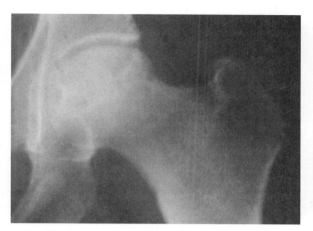

▲ **Figure 59–3.** Osteonecrosis of the femoral head. There is cystic change and sclerosis of the femoral head. There is evidence of collapse with irregular joint-space narrowing and loss of sphericity of the joint space.

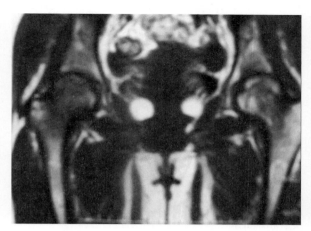

▲ **Figure 59–4.** Coronal magnetic resonance image demonstrates osteonecrosis bilaterally, with irregular shape of the femoral head, suggesting early collapse.

3. Computed tomography (CT)—CT images can display early sclerosis in the central part of the femoral head ("asterisk sign") and give an evaluation of the size of the sequestrum. Also, the anterior part, which is preferentially involved in osteonecrosis of the femoral head, is well demonstrated. In some cases, the slight anterior collapse is visible only on CT images.

4. MRI—In the early stages of osteonecrosis (eg, when plain radiographs are normal), MRI has the greatest sensitivity (91%) of the imaging techniques. In early osteonecrosis, MRI reveals an area of low-intensity signal in the medial aspect of the femoral head, particularly in the subchondral zone. A focal defect involving the anterosuperior aspect of the femoral head, but occasionally extending to the metaphysis, is the most common abnormality observed (96% of cases). The most characteristic image, seen in 60–80% of cases, is a margin of low signal on T1- and T2-weighted images (Figure 59–4). A second high intensity line appears on T2-weighted images (double-line sign) representing hypervascular granulation tissue and is considered pathognomonic for osteonecrosis.

Although MRI can identify a preclinical stage prior to onset of symptoms, caution should be exercised in interpreting MRI findings in asymptomatic patients. Treatment based on abnormal MRI findings alone in the absence of symptoms may result in overtreatment of some patients. The degree of femoral head involvement by MRI may predict progression to collapse.

C. Staging

Staging of osteonecrosis is usually based on radiologic and histologic features. There are several proposed systems of staging, based on the sequence of changes seen by radiography and by other investigative techniques. The Subcommittee of Nomenclature of the International Association on Bone Circulation and Bone Necrosis (ARCO: Association of Research Circulation Osseous) reassembled the various staging systems to establish an internationally accepted system of classification of the stages of osteonecrosis (Table 59–2). This standardized system is designed to enhance uniformity among comparative epidemiologic studies and to facilitate clinical trials of treatment strategies.

▶ Differential Diagnosis

At stages 3 and 4, radiographic findings are specific for osteonecrosis. If stage 5 and 6 is present at diagnosis, however, it is impossible to diagnose osteonecrosis as the cause of destruction of the hip, as virtually any cause of end-stage hip disease can produce the same radiographic appearance. The challenging differential diagnoses relate to stages 1 and 2. In stage 1, all diseases that may affect bone, cartilage, or synovial tissue must be considered as possible explanations for the joint pain. In stage 2, nonspecific bone lesions on radiographs should prompt MRI in patients at risk for osteonecrosis. Two entities in the differential diagnosis that can be difficult to distinguish from osteonecrosis clinically are transient osteoporosis of the hip, which typically occurs during pregnancy, and a subchondral fracture of the femoral head, which may be difficult to visualize on plain radiographs.

▶ Treatment

The management of osteonecrosis remains one of the most controversial topics in the orthopedic literature. The goal of

Table 59–2. Stages of osteonecrosis.

Stage 0
All diagnostic studies normal; diagnosis by histology, necrosis on biopsy. Thus, osteonecrosis can exist histologically without any associated clinical signs or symptoms.

Stage 1
Plain radiographs and computed tomography (CT) normal; radionuclide scan or MRI abnormal and biopsy positive, extent of involvement A, B, or C (less than 15%, 15–30%, and >30%, respectively). The patient may or may not be symptomatic at this stage.

Stage 2
A variety of radiographic abnormalities that are signs of eventual bone death are evident within the femoral head. These may include areas of linear sclerosis, focal mineralization, or cysts in the femoral head or neck. The femoral head, however, is still spherical, as evidenced on both anteroposterior and lateral radiographs and on the CT scan. There is no subchondral lucency or collapse; extent of involvement A, B, or C.

Stage 3
The femoral head has begun to fail mechanically. The radiolucent "crescent sign" appearing just beneath the subchondral end plate is the hallmark of this stage; it indicates collapse of the subchondral cancellous trabeculae. The spherical configuration of the articular surface remains intact. The crescent sign does not always develop as the femoral head progresses from earlier to later stages of involvement. Because the femoral head remains spherical, it should theoretically be possible to preserve its integrity by surgical measures that allow the necrotic and collapsed bone to be replaced by viable tissue. Extent of involvement A, B, or C.

Stage 4
The first sign of stage 4 is any evidence of flattening of the femoral head with joint space narrowing. This has important therapeutic implications because the hip has now progressed to the point at which the changes are irreversible. The collapse usually occurs in the anterolateral or superior weight-bearing region. The distinction between stage 2 and stage 4 is best demonstrated by CT scan, which is more sensitive than plain radiographs. Extent of involvement is quantitated A, B, or C as above, with further characterization by amount of depression (in millimeters).

Stage 5
Any or all of the preceding radiographic changes may be seen, and in addition there is a decrease in the joint space. In this situation, there is osteoarthritis secondary to the mechanical collapse of the femoral head, with sclerosis, cysts of the acetabulum, and occasionally marginal osteophytes.

Stage 6
Extensive destruction of the femoral head following the degenerative process.

Data from the Subcommittee on Nomenclature of the International Association on Bone Circulation and Bone Necrosis (ARCO: Association of Research Circulation Osseous.)

treatment is to preserve the native joint for as long as possible. There are four main therapeutic options:

- Conservative management.
- Joint replacement (eg, total hip arthroplasty).
- Core decompression with or without bone grafting.
- Osteotomy.

Conservative measures may be the only treatment needed for patients with stages 0 and 1 disease, although core decompression may provide some advantages in these cases. Total joint replacement in later-stage disease should be performed before total collapse of the femoral head occurs.

A. Conservative Therapy

Conservative treatment includes bed rest, partial weight-bearing with crutches, and weight-bearing as tolerated, in addition to nonsteroidal anti-inflammatory drugs or other analgesics, physical therapy to maintain muscle strength and prevent contractures, and assistive devices to facilitate ambulation. This approach is generally ineffective in halting the progression of disease. A meta-analysis looking at 21 studies of conservative therapy found slightly better results with no progression in 26% of patients.

Patients with stage 0, 1, or 2 osteonecrosis of non–weight-bearing joints may not require any intervention because they may have only mild to moderate pain, and minimal, tolerable functional limitation.

There is no consensus on the appropriate management of patients with asymptomatic osteonecrosis. Some experts have suggested that patients with lesions affecting less than 15% of the volume of the femoral head should be treated conservatively; those with lesions greater than 30% should be treated with elective total hip arthroplasty; and those with lesions of intermediate size (ie, between 15% and 30%) should be treated with either core decompression or osteotomy. Opinions on the optimal approach to certain osteonecrosis lesions, particularly those of intermediate severity and extent, vary from center to center.

B. Joint Replacement

Patients with persistent, intractable pain and progressive functional loss should be considered for arthroplasty. Ideally, this should be accomplished before total collapse of the femoral head occurs in patients with hip involvement. The usual treatment for late stage 3 or stage 4 disease has been total hip arthroplasty, but results have been inconsistent. Most studies suggest a worse prognosis in this disease than for others, with a higher rate of early failures compared with age-matched patients with other diagnoses. Possible reasons for the higher failure rate in patients with osteonecrosis include poor bone quality (size of necrotic area and degree of bone collapse), bilateral disease, and presence of an underlying condition.

C. Core Decompression

The failure of conservative management and the poor long-term survival of prosthetic devices in the early days of joint arthroplasty necessitated the development of other interventions aimed at preserving the femoral head and slowing or stopping the progression of osteonecrosis. The technique of core decompression was initially used as a diagnostic tool to measure bone marrow pressure and obtain biopsy specimens. It evolved into a treatment mode when it was observed that some patients had pain relief following the procedure. In the core decompression procedure, the orthopedist drills a hole through the femoral neck into the head of the femur.

The rationale for core decompression is to reduce intraosseous pressure, reestablish blood supply, and allow living bone adjacent to dead bone to contribute to the reparative process. Good to excellent results have been reported in most of patients with stages 1 and 2 osteonecrosis, and in a significant proportion of patients with stage 3 disease. The results of this technique are still controversial, and the best results vary from 34% to 95% in early stages, but they are always better than simply discontinuing weight-bearing.

D. Osteotomy

Osteotomy has also been used as a joint-sparing technique. The stated goal of this procedure is to remove the diseased section of the femoral head from the region of major weight-bearing, and to redistribute the weight-bearing forces to articular cartilage that is supported by healthy bone. Reports, largely in the European and Japanese literature, vary as to the efficacy of osteotomies for salvage of hips with stage 2 and 3 disease. All of these osteotomies require a period of restricted weight-bearing of 3 months to 1 year, and usually until there is radiographic evidence of healing of the osteotomy. One concern is that an osteotomy may complicate performance of a subsequent total hip arthroplasty. In later stage disease, when there is collapse of the femoral head, osteotomy may have better results than core decompression.

E. Bisphosphonates

Bisphosphonates (specifically alendronate) have been shown to decrease progression of the femoral head collapse in a controlled but not blinded study.

Based on available data, the following recommendations can be made for management of osteonecrosis of the femoral head:

- Asymptomatic lesions that involve less than 15% of the femoral head may resolve without surgical intervention and may therefore be treated conservatively.

- Asymptomatic lesions that involve more than 30% of the femoral head are likely to progress to collapse despite core decompression or osteotomy. Thus, these patients should be managed conservatively, in anticipation of the eventual need for total hip arthroplasty.

- In early stage 0 to 2 lesions in young, active patients, core decompression provides the best chance at preserving the femoral head.

- In later stage 2 lesions with cyst formation and stage 3 disease, osteotomy may be the best option.

- In stage 4 disease and in older sedentary patients with less severe disease, total hip replacement is the treatment of choice.

▶ Complications

Although the size and localization of the bone necrosis influence outcomes, the natural history of osteonecrosis is usually one of progressive disease leading to cortical collapse and joint dysfunction. Osteonecrosis can be a debilitating condition that leads to destruction of the hip in the third, fourth, or fifth decades of life. Early intervention, both surgical and nonsurgical, has improved outcomes, but still nearly 50% of cases of osteonecrosis of the femoral head require arthroplasty.

Aldridge JM 3rd, Urbaniak JR. Avascular necrosis of the femoral head: etiology, pathophysiology, classification, and current treatment guidelines. *Am J Orthop.* 2004;33:327. [PMID: 15344574]

Assouline-Dayan Y, Chang C, Greenspan A, Shoenfeld Y, Gershwin ME. Pathogenesis and natural history of osteonecrosis. *Semin Arthritis Rheum.* 2002;32:94. [PMID: 12430099]

Hamilton TW, Goodman SM, Figgie M. SAS Weekly Rounds: avascular necrosis. *HSS J.* 2009;5:99. [PMID: 19294340]

Jones LC, Hungerford DS. Osteonecrosis: etiology, diagnosis, and treatment. *Curr Opin Rheumatol.* 2004;16:443. [PMID: 15201609]

Miyanishi K, Kamo Y, Ihara H, Naka T, Hirakawa M, Sugioka Y. Risk factors for dysbaric osteonecrosis. *Rheumatology (Oxford).* 2006;45:855. [PMID: 16436490]

[National Osteonecrosis Foundation]
http://www.nonf.org

[The Center for Osteonecrosis Research and Education]
http://www.osteonecrosis.org

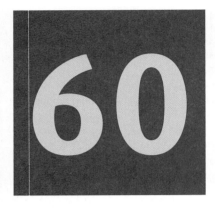

60

Paget Disease of Bone

Margaret Seton, MD

Paget disease of bone (PDB) is a remarkable disorder of aging bone. It was first described by Sir James Paget in 1877, in his paper entitled "On a Form of Chronic Inflammation of Bones (Osteitis Deformans)." In this sentinel paper, Paget catalogues the progressive deformity of bone that occurs over 26 years in an individual man, detailing the enlargement of his head, the settling of the skull over the spine, the evolving rigidity of the spine and bowing of the lower limbs. "The shape and habitual posture of the patient were thus made strange and peculiar." Paget attributed these skeletal changes to chronic inflammation of the affected bones, and called the disease osteitis deformans, writing "a better name may be given when more is known of it."

ESSENTIALS OF DIAGNOSIS

▶ Often asymptomatic; however, pain, early arthritis in proximal joints and bone fractures are common complications. Osteosarcomas develop in a small minority of patients.

▶ Accelerated bone remodeling results in enlarged, misshapen bone.

▶ Usually presents in persons older than 55 years.

▶ General Considerations

PDB is a focal disorder of bone remodeling that tends to present in individuals middle-aged or older. PDB is often associated with no other problem other than that due to progressive deformity of bone and is often asymptomatic. Treatment is effective and should be aimed at preventing disease progression as well as treating pain arising from pagetic bone.

▶ Pathophysiology & Epidemiology

Paget disease is a rich area of study, as genetic as well as environmental determinants are sought to explain the skeletal distribution and late onset of this disease. PDB affects males perhaps slightly more than females and exists as a familial disease with variable penetrance. It may also exist as a sporadic disease. It usually presents in persons older than 55, and does not occur in children. PDB is remarkable for the geographic clusters of disease as well.

Paget disease is presumed a disorder of the osteoclast, although it is clear that the bone marrow environment plays a critical role in permitting the accelerated bone turnover that characterizes this disease. In 2002, a consistent mutation in *SQSTM1* was identified in almost 50% of a Canadian cohort of patients with familial PDB, as well as in 16% of those with "sporadic disease." This mutation is often present on a shared haplotype, suggesting a founder effect. However, the predominance of the *SQSTM1* mutations present in the Canadian cohort is not found in other countries. How genes might interplay in the environment of aging bone disease or whether viruses or other environmental determinants may prove permissive to this focal disorder of bone is unknown.

▶ Clinical Findings

A. Symptoms and Signs

PDB is often asymptomatic, detected incidentally on a radiograph, or diagnosed in the course of evaluating an elevated serum alkaline phosphatase. It may be monostotic (one bone) or polyostotic (many bones). The process of accelerated bone remodeling that defines this disease results in enlarged, misshapen bone that softens and loses skeletal integrity. Pain, early arthritis at proximal joints, and fractures are a few salient symptoms of PDB, with deformity not infrequent in weight-bearing limbs. When PDB affects the skull, the overgrowth may lead to deafness, headache and, rarely, more serious neurologic impairment (such as dementia and apathy) as the bones thicken, vascular "steal" occurs, and basilar invagination develops.

In the spine, as in the skull, the enlargement of bone with encroachment of bony foramina results in pain, nerve impingement and, rarely, cauda equina syndrome. Despite increased fluxes of calcium into and out of bone, the measured serum calcium remains within normal limits, while the urinary calcium may show considerable variation. In patients with fracture, immobilization hypercalcemia may occur. Patients with PDB have an increased frequency of stones, and may manifest hyperparathyroidism. Vascular compromise, such as congestive heart failure, is rarely reported.

When pain presents in patients with PDB, it is usually a pattern of chronic pain seen in osteoarthritis associated with impairment of function. The older a patient gets, the more likely it is that pain is multifactorial in nature, driven by degenerative changes of joints proximal to a pagetic lesion, and compounded by osteoarthritis at other sites. At this stage, the following comorbidities complicate treatment: aging, hearing loss, visual impairment, and psychosocial elements of aging. Effective treatment depends on understanding these, and ensuring patients' expectations are reasonable. Hearing does not improve nor do radiographs ever "heal" completely.

Occasionally, the pain is focal, and associated with a pseudofracture on the convex surface of bone by radiographic imaging (Figure 60–1). This suggests an impending fracture, and should be treated urgently with orthopaedic consultation, no weight-bearing, and a bisphosphonate to diminish the vascularity of bone in anticipation of surgery. Emergency surgery for the "chalk stick" fracture (Figure 60–2) through a pagetic bone can be fraught with blood loss and carries with it a higher mortality.

B. Laboratory Findings

Suspicion for PDB may also be triggered by an elevated serum alkaline phosphatase. When the source of this enzyme is from bone, the elevated alkaline phosphatase marks the presence of excessive bone turnover characteristic of PDB. Other markers of bone formation and bone resorption may be elevated in patients with PDB, but they are unreliable predictors of the skeletal extent of disease and poor markers of response to therapy.

C. Imaging Studies and Special Tests

The diagnosis of PDB is confirmed by plain radiograph. Plain films demonstrate the local consequences of bony enlargement.

Curiously, the radiograph has a distinct pattern of beginning in subchondral bone and moving in one direction through that bone until the entire bone is affected. The process of accelerated bone remodeling leaves thickened cortices with tunneling evident in affected sites and a mixture of lytic and blastic lesions. Trabeculae are coarsened and the bone misshapen (Figure 60–1 and Figure 60–3). Unless there are bony bridges, pagetic bone will not cross into a new bone.

A bone scan is useful in documenting sites of disease throughout the skeleton. This tends to remain remarkably

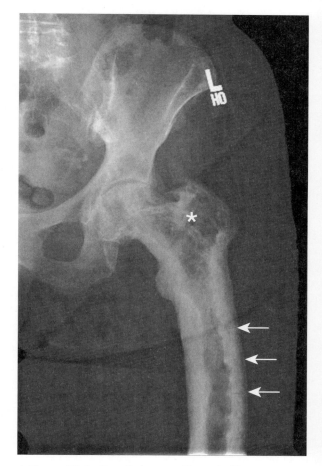

▲ **Figure 60–1.** Pagetic femur with cortical bone thickening, deformity, and pseudofractures marking the convex side of the bone (*arrows*). Note the accentuation of the trabecular markings, indicated by the asterisk (*).

stable throughout the course of a person's life; the reason for this is unknown.

A **biopsy** is needed in the following instances: presence of ivory vertebrae, a patient with prostate cancer has pelvic lesions, or younger patients with severe pain. Subtle lytic lesions can also elude radiographic diagnosis, as can the occurrence of PDB in patients where the disease is quite uncommon (India, Far East) and the diagnosis is one of exclusion. MRI or CT scanning can be useful to define the benign nature of the lesion, documenting intact cortical bone, accentuated trabeculae, and the presence of normal marrow fat. Osteosarcomas occasionally arise in pagetic bone, and the need to exclude this occurrence is another indication for bone biopsy in some patients.

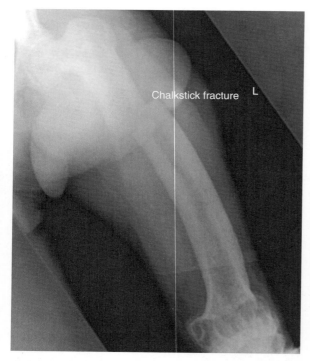

Chalkstick fracture   L

▲ **Figure 60–2.** Chalkstick fracture. This fracture occurred 2 weeks after the radiograph of the bowed femur depicted in Figure 60–3 was taken.

▶ Treatment

Prior to treatment, renal function must be assessed, and serum concentrations of calcium, phosphorus, magnesium, and vitamin D should be measured to ensure the absence of concurrent metabolic problems. Markers of bone formation and bone resorption are not required in the clinical management of patients with PDB.

Bisphosphonates have become the cornerstone of treatment for PDB. These medications prevent the long-term skeletal complications of this disorder and provide patients with a sustained biochemical remission. Treatment also eases many neurologic symptoms, relieves pain, and slows or perhaps halts disease progression. Despite effective treatment, however, the radiographs may remain unchanged.

The most effective treatment for PDB is probably zoledronate (5 mg administered intravenously once a year). The oral bisphosphonates alendronate and risedronate are also FDA-approved for the treatment of PDB. Adequate calcium and vitamin D are critical prior to treatment with bisphosphonates to ensure that clinically significant hypocalcemia does not occur.

In hospitalized patients or those receiving hospice care, calcitonin 50–100 international units subcutaneously every other evening can ease pain rapidly and effectively.

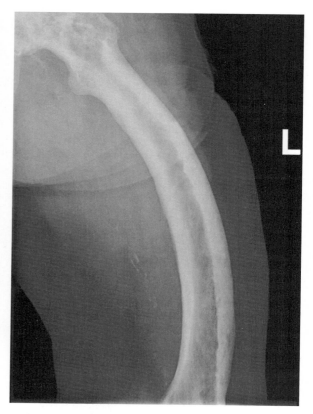

▲ **Figure 60–3.** Bowed pagetic femur. In this image, the entire left femur is affected by remodeling. The bone fractured 2 weeks after this image was taken.

One of the most remarkable findings with treatment of PDB is the occasional dramatic resolution of pain and the overlying erythema that may be present over pagetic bone as well as the reversal of neurologic compromise. Lytic lesions may heal and bone scans may normalize bone uptake. Over weeks to months, the markers of bone resorption should normalize, followed by markers of bone formation. Depending on the age of the patient, location of the pagetic lesions, and associated clinical and biochemical parameters, treatment may be given once or repeated periodically in the lifetime of an individual.

Hosking D, Lyles K, Brown JP, et al. Long-term control of bone turnover in Paget's disease with zoledronic acid and risedronate. *J Bone Miner Res.* 2007;22:142. [PMID: 17032148]

Morissette J, Laurin N, Brown JP. Sequestosome 1: mutation frequencies, haplotypes, and phenotypes in familial Paget's disease of bone. *J Bone Miner Res.* 2006;21 (Suppl 2):P38. [PMID: 17229007]

Paget SJ. On a Form of Chronic Inflammation of Bones (Osteitis Deformans). *Medical Chirulogical Transaction.* 1876; LX(read November 14th, 1978).

Common Rheumatologic Problems Encountered by the Hospitalist: Pearls & Myths

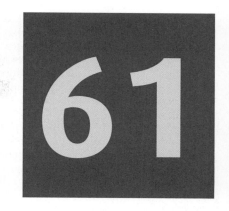

John H. Stone, MD, MPH

John B. Imboden, MD

David B. Hellmann, MD, MACP

▶ Clinical Problem: The Patient with an Active Rheumatic Disease

Pearl: Make sure the "punishment" fits the "crime."

Comment: One of the fundamental principles of rheumatology is to make certain that the intensity of treatment matches the severity of the disease. Pleuritis, arthralgia, and low-grade fever with systemic lupus erythematosus (SLE) will respond to 60 mg of prednisone given daily. But these manifestations will also respond generally to far less prednisone, eg, 10–20 mg daily, doses associated with a much lower risk of infection or other complications. In contrast, severe hemolytic anemia and glomerulonephritis in SLE may not respond to low-dose prednisone and often must be treated not only with high doses of prednisone but also additional agents.

▶ Clinical Problem: Supplemental Therapy for the Glucocorticoid-Treated Patient Who is Stressed by Serious Illness or Major Surgery

Myth: A normal cosyntropin stimulation test excludes adrenal insufficiency induced by glucocorticoid therapy.

Comment: The cosyntropin stimulation test determines the ability of the adrenal gland to produce cortisol in response to an exogenous corticotropin (adrenocorticotropic hormone, ACTH). However, the endogenous response to stress requires that all components of the hypothalamic-pituitary-adrenal axis be intact. Individuals treated currently with glucocorticoids and for many months after such therapy can have insufficiency of the central components of this axis (ie, normal adrenal response to exogenous ACTH but subnormal ability to produce ACTH endogenously).

Because tests of the central components of the axis are complex, most authorities recommend empiric hydrocortisone supplementation (100 mg three times daily) when these patients face major surgery or the stress of serious medical illness. Once the patient is beyond the perioperative period, the baseline prednisone dose can be resumed.

▶ Clinical Problem: Fever in the Patient with Rheumatic Disease: Underlying Disease or Superimposed Infection

Pearl: Rheumatoid arthritis rarely causes high-grade fever.

Comment: Although low-grade fevers in the range of 37.5°C often accompany active rheumatoid arthritis (RA), high-grade fevers are rare. Only 5% of cases manifest fever >38°C, and less than 1% have temperatures >38.3°C. Therefore, high-grade fever in a patient with well-established RA should prompt an investigation for an underlying cause (eg, infection) other than RA. In a patient with the new onset of inflammatory arthritis, the presence of high-grade fever is an argument against the diagnosis of RA or even a complication of RA, such as rheumatoid vasculitis (see Chapter 42). (See Chapter 4 for a discussion of the differential diagnosis of fever and arthritis).

Pearl: Flare of a single joint in a patient with RA signals serious concern about septic arthritis.

Comment: Most flares of RA are polyarticular. When signs of new, increased inflammation affect only one joint, infection should be strongly considered. The most common cause of septic arthritis in RA is *Staphylococcus aureus*. Absence of fever does not exclude infection because only 50% of patients with septic arthritis present with fever. In the patient who has RA with only one "active" joint, arthrocentesis should be performed to exclude infection before intensifying anti-inflammantory therapy.

Pearl: Always consider tuberculosis when a febrile illness develops in a patient treated with an anti–tumor necrosis factor agent.

Comment: Because tumor necrosis factor-α (TNF-α) is required for an intact host immune response to *Mycobacterium* tuberculosis, treatment with anti–TNF-α agents greatly increases the risk of tuberculosis. Although infliximab has been most closely associated with the greatest risk of tuberculosis in studies, the risk is likely a class effect shared by all anti–TNF-α agents. Most cases, caused by reactivation of infection, have developed within weeks of starting anti–TNF-α therapy. There is almost certainly an increased risk of disease from primary exposure as well, however.

In the setting of anti–TNF-α therapy, tuberculosis can be acute, is often disseminated or extrapulmonary, and has an atypical histopathology (TNF-α is required for granuloma formation). Anti–TNF-α therapy also carries an increased risk of infection with other intracellular pathogens, including *Listeria monocytogenes,* and fungi, such as *Histoplasma capsulatum* and *Coccidioides immitis.*

Pearl: When trying to distinguish between infection and active disease in a patient with SLE, the presence of rigors favors infection.

Comment: One of the great quandaries of hospital medicine for patients with SLE is determining whether an acute change is caused by infection or a flare of the disease. The presence of rigors *clearly* favors infection. Other clues may come from the complete blood count: many patients with SLE have a baseline tendency toward neutropenia (particularly lymphopenia) and thrombocytopenia. Elevations in either of these two blood counts raises the likelihood of infection.

Pearl: Fever that develops in a patient with SLE treated with high-dose glucocorticoids is due to infection until proven otherwise.

Comment: Infection is a leading cause of morbidity and mortality in SLE, particularly in the setting of immunosuppression with high-dose glucocorticoids. Although SLE itself can cause fever >39°C, fever due to SLE most often occurs in the setting of clinically active disease (particularly serositis) and usually responds to glucocorticoid therapy. Fever that develops *after* high-dose glucocorticoids have been started should be attributed to SLE only after a vigorous search for infectious causes, including opportunistic infections.

Pearl: When a patient with SLE remembers the precise hour that the disease "flared," the patient more likely has an acute infection.

Comment: Most flares of SLE develop over days or weeks. Infections tend to present more abruptly. Therefore, a patient who says, "my disease flared at 10 o'clock" probably has an infection.

Pearl: Apparent "flares" of rheumatic disease that occur while the patient is taking cyclophosphamide are almost always caused by a superimposed opportunistic infection rather than by activation of the underlying disease.

Comment: Over the last 25 years at one large medical center, not one patient transferred to that center because of "refractory vasculitis" has had active vasculitis: every one of the transferred patients has had an opportunistic infection.

▶ Clinical Problem: The Patient with Acute Monarthritis

Pearl: Acute monarthritis has three major causes: trauma, infection, and microcrystalline disease.

Comment: In the absence of trauma, acute monoarthritis usually means that the patient has an infection or has gout or pseudogout. Although crystal-induced arthritis is more common, it is critical not to overlook septic arthritis. Delay in the treatment of joint infections increases morbidity and mortality substantially.

Pearl: The wrist and knee are to pseudogout what the great toe and foot are to gout.

Comment: The most commonly affected joints in gout are the great toe and other sites of the foot. Pseudogout in contrast most commonly affects the wrist and the knee.

Pearl: Monarthritis of the knee is the most common articular manifestation of chronic Lyme arthritis.

Comment: In regions where *Ixodes* complex ticks and *Borrelia burgdorferi* are endemic, an individual with chronic, unexplained inflammation of the knee (synovial fluid negative for crystals and organisms) may have Lyme disease. Knee effusions due to Lyme disease can be intermittent.

Pearl: Arthrocentesis is the diagnostic procedure of choice for the patient with unexplained, acute monoarthritis.

Comment: Analysis of synovial fluid allows the physician to answer three questions: Is the joint inflamed? Is infection present? Is crystal disease present? The synovial fluid white blood cell (WBC) count is the best single discriminator between inflammatory (>2000 WBC/mcL) and noninflammatory (<2000 WBC/mcL) arthritis. In cases of nongonococcal septic arthritis, examination of synovial fluid by Gram staining has limited sensitivity (approximately 50%), but culture of the synovial fluid is positive in >90%. Polarized light microscopy is a sensitive and specific test for the presence of urate and calcium pyrophosphate dihydrate crystals in synovial fluid.

Myth: Synovial fluid should be tested for glucose level.

Comment: Synovial fluid glucose levels tend to be low when there is intense inflammation, especially when the joint is infected. The synovial fluid WBC count, however, is a far better measure of the severity of joint inflammation. The synovial fluid glucose level adds nothing to what is learned from the synovial fluid WBC count and should not be ordered. When the diagnosis is in question, synovial fluid should always be sent for the three Cs: cell count, culture, and crystals.

Myth: The serum uric acid is a reliable test for the presence or absence of gout in the patient with acute monarthritis.

Comment: The serum uric acid level neither establishes nor refutes the diagnosis of acute gout. Gout develops in most patients after years of hyperuricemia, but it is not uncommon for the serum uric acid level to fall to within the normal range at the time of an acute attack. Determining the serum uric acid has some value in that a low level makes gout quite unlikely. A high serum uric acid level increases the probability of gout but is not definitive; asymptomatic hyperuricemia is common and can be present in patients with acute arthritis unrelated to gout. The definitive test for the diagnosis of acute gout is demonstration of intracellular urate crystals in synovial fluid from the affected joint.

▶ Clinical Problem: The Patient with Acute Gout

Pearl: Gout has never killed a single patient. Not so its treatment.

Comment: Imprudent or improper use of gout therapies can be associated with a host of serious and even fatal complications. Gout should be treated, but treated wisely by informed clinicians mindful of the patient's entire clinical status. See the comments below on the potential dangers of specific gout treatments.

Myth: Intravenous colchicine is a first-line therapy for acute gout.

Comment: There is almost always a better option than intravenous colchicine for the treatment of gout. Intravenous colchicine can cause fatal bone marrow and multiorgan failure, particularly in patients who have renal insufficiency or liver disease or who have been taking oral colchicine. Because of its toxicity and the availability of safer alternatives (ie, nonsteroidal anti-inflammatory drugs [NSAIDs] and glucocorticoids), intravenous colchicine should be administered very rarely (if ever), and only by clinicians who are very familiar with its use.

Myth: Allopurinol is useful for the treatment of acute gout.

Comment: A common mistake in the treatment of acute gout is the failure to separate therapy of the acute arthritis from management of the chronically elevated serum uric acid. During a flare of gout, attention should focus on treating the acute arthritis with NSAIDs or glucocorticoids (see Chapter 44). In fact, the use of allopurinol in this setting may have a counterintuitive—and counterproductive—effect: by lowering serum uric acid abruptly, allopurinol may exacerbate the acute gout flare. Thus, initiation of allopurinol should be deferred until several weeks after resolution of the acute attack.

Pearl: Glucocorticoids are an effective treatment for acute gout in the patient with a contraindication to NSAIDs.

Comment: Glucocorticoids are an excellent therapeutic option for the gout patient who has a contraindication to NSAIDs (eg, renal insufficiency). When gout involves a readily accessible joint, an intra-articular glucocorticoid injection is a safe, rapidly effective treatment. For cases of polyarticular gout in which the injection of all involved joints is not possible, the efficacy of oral glucocorticoids (eg, prednisone 20–40 mg daily, tapered over 1–2 weeks)

is comparable to or greater than that of NSAIDs (and may have fewer side effects).

Because of the multiple comorbidities found in many hospitalized patients today, a short course of glucocorticoids (with close attention to the risk of hyperglycemia) is often the best approach to treating acute gout on the inpatient service.

Myth: Acute gout does not cause high fever.

Comment: Acute gout can present in myriad ways on the inpatient service. Polyarticular gout, which may develop after years of recurrent podagra, can mimic RA. Acute gout affecting many joints of one limb can mimic a stroke. Not infrequently, polyarticular gout can be associated with high fevers (ie, >39°C.) Septic arthritis or another infection should always be excluded in this setting, but in the end the explanation is often gout.

▶ Clinical Problem: Gout Prophylaxis

Pearl: Avoid using a dose of colchicine higher than one tablet (0.6 mg) per day in patients over the age of 65, especially if the serum creatinine is above 1.5 mg/dL.

Comment: Daily oral colchicine can rarely cause proximal muscle weakness (a neuromyopathy) that mimics polymyositis. Almost all the patients with this drug complication are older than the age of 60 and have decreased renal function. The dose of colchicine must be decreased in patients with kidney dysfunction.

Pearl: Avoid starting allopurinol in any patient taking azathioprine.

Comment: Allopurinol blocks the catabolism of azathioprine by xanthine oxidase, greatly augmenting the effect of this immunosuppressive agent. Failure to stop azathioprine or to reduce the daily dose dramatically (by at least 50%) can result in life-threatening cytopenia.

▶ Clinical Problem: The Patient with Nongonococcal Septic Arthritis

Pearl: Carefully examine all joints, particularly shoulders and hips, in a patient with suspected septic arthritis.

Comment: Nongonococcal septic arthritis is oligoarticular in approximately 15% of cases. Focus on an obviously inflamed joint (eg, a septic knee) can lead to the failure to appreciate infection of less visible joints, such as the shoulders and hips.

Pearl: Nongonococcal septic arthritis requires drainage.

Comment: Many physicians are surprised to learn that viable organisms can be obtained from a previously untapped septic joint despite 2 or more days of antibiotics. "Pus under pressure" prevents antibiotics from working effectively. Drainage is as important as antibiotics in the treatment of septic arthritis.

▶ Clinical Problem: The Diagnosis of Adult-Onset Still Disease

Pearl: Be skeptical of a "quotidian fever" when a patient is receiving antipyretics.

    Comment: The characteristic fever pattern of adult-onset Still disease is quotidian, with daily spikes, often >39°C, followed by spontaneous return of the temperature to normal. Administration of antipyretics, particularly on an "as needed" basis for fever, can convert a hectic fever into one with a quotidian pattern. The fever pattern should be observed in the absence of antipyretics when considering the diagnosis of adult-onset Still disease.

Myth: Marked elevations of the serum ferritin are specific for adult-onset Still disease.

    Comment: Although the majority of patients with active adult-onset Still disease have serum ferritin levels >3000 mg/mL, markedly elevated levels of serum ferritin are not specific for that disease and can be seen in other disorders, particularly hematologic malignancies.

Pearl: Atypical "adult-onset Still disease" is due to a paraneoplastic syndrome or infection until proven otherwise.

    Comment: The principle underlying this pearl is that an unusual manifestation of a common disease often is more likely than an atypical presentation of a rare disorder, such as adult-onset Still disease. Infections and malignancies, particularly lymphoproliferative disorders, can mimic many of the clinical features (fever, rash, lymphadenopathy, arthritis) and laboratory abnormalities of adult-onset Still disease. A hectic fever pattern, a rash that is intensely pruritic or that involves the face, or other clinical features atypical for adult-onset Still disease should prompt a rigorous search for an underlying malignancy or infection. The diagnosis of adult-onset Still disease—even in its most classic presentation—is always one of exclusion.

▶ Clinical Problem: Hypertension in a Patient with Scleroderma

Pearl: Elevated blood pressure in a patient with scleroderma may be an indication of incipient scleroderma renal crisis.

    Comment: Prior to the availability of angiotensin-converting enzyme inhibitors, the most common cause of death in patients with diffuse systemic sclerosis was scleroderma renal crisis. Scleroderma renal crisis occurs characteristically in diffuse (as opposed to limited) disease. Asymptomatic hypertension, particularly if documented to be new, may be a primary clue. Failure to recognize scleroderma renal crisis may lead to malignant hypertension with all of its attendant complications, renal failure, and a micro-angiopathic picture in the peripheral blood smear. On renal histopathology, scleroderma renal crisis is indistinguishable from thrombotic thrombocytopenic purpura. The cornerstone of therapy for scleroderma renal crisis is aggressive angiotensin-converting enzyme inhibition.

▶ Clinical Problem: The Patient with Giant Cell Arteritis

Pearl: Consider giant cell arteritis (GCA) in any adult over the age of 60 who has "above-the-neck" pain that cannot otherwise be explained.

    Comment: Headache, scalp tenderness, and jaw claudication are among the most common symptoms in patients with GCA. But GCA can also produce pain in other locations, including the tongue, the ear, the back of the neck, over the carotids, and along the jaw line. Thus, any pain above the neck that is not explained readily by trauma or some other cause should prompt consideration of GCA.

Pearl: Consider GCA in the differential diagnosis of the elderly patient with fever of unknown origin.

    Comment: GCA usually presents with symptoms referable to involvement of the cranial circulation (eg, headache, scalp tenderness, visual symptoms, and jaw claudication) but can cause fever without localizing signs or symptoms. Fever can be the sole clinical manifestation of the disease for weeks or months. Even in the absence of temporal artery abnormalities on physical examination, the diagnostic test of choice is temporal artery biopsy. If large-vessel disease (eg, subclavian or aortic involvement) is suspected on the basis of arm claudication or a diastolic murmur, magnetic resonance imaging/angiography of the great vessels may also be helpful.

Pearl: Among all GCA symptoms, jaw claudication is the most specific for that disease.

    Comment: Jaw claudication has a likelihood ratio of greater than 4 for the diagnosis of GCA, making it more likely than any other symptom to be associated with a temporal artery biopsy. The problem is that patients do not complain flagrantly about "jaw claudication." Further, unless prompted, they will not mention that they have pain in their jaw when they chew unless you specifically ask. The symptom of jaw claudication, which may present as facial pain or pressure felt soon after the initiation of chewing, must be actively elicited when taking the patient's history. In short, the clinician must be attuned to patients' describing synonyms for use of this phenomenon.

Myth: Glucocorticoid therapy for suspected GCA should be administered only after temporal artery biopsies have been obtained.

    Comment: Glucocorticoid therapy, which can prevent irreversible blindness and other feared complications of GCA, should be administered promptly when the diagnosis is considered. Glucocorticoid therapy does not interfere with histopathologic findings in the temporal arteries for at least 2 weeks. Start treatment, then get the biopsy (but don't fail to get the biopsy).

Pearl: GCA does not occur among individuals under the age of 50.

    Comment: This is a remarkably true statement. Among 1435 patients with biopsy-proven temporal arteritis, only two cases occurred in individuals younger than 50 years of age. It is possible that even those two patients did not have GCA but rather some other form of systemic vasculitis involving the temporal arteries (microscopic polyangiitis, granulomatosis with polyangiitis [formerly Wegener granulomatosis], and polyarteritis nodosa, for example, are known to do this).

Pearl: The addition of low-dose aspirin to glucocorticoid therapy may reduce the risk of blindness or stroke in patients with GCA.

Comment: A retrospective review of patients with GCA revealed that those receiving concomitant low-dose aspirin had a fivefold lower incidence of intracranial ischemic events compared to patients treated with glucocorticoids alone.

▶ Clinical Problem: The Patient with Suspected Primary Vasculitis

Pearl: Subacute bacterial endocarditis can cause palpable purpura, glomerulonephritis, and hypocomplementemia.

Comment: Chronic bacterial infections such as subacute bacterial endocarditis and chronic osteomyelitis can cause an immune-complex–mediated vasculitis. These diagnoses should always be considered in the differential diagnosis of a patient with small-vessel vasculitis.

Pearl: Consider cholesterol emboli syndrome when an elderly man with atherosclerotic disease develops "vasculitis."

Comment: Cholesterol emboli syndrome can be a remarkable mimic of vasculitis. Its diverse manifestations include peripheral emboli (often producing "blue toes"), livedo reticularis, cutaneous ulcers, acute kidney injury, elevated erythrocyte sedimentation rate, and eosinophilia. The syndrome, which typically develops days to weeks after an intravascular procedure (eg, cardiac catheterization) or the institution of anticoagulation therapy, is due to shedding of cholesterol emboli from destabilized atherosclerotic plaques.

Myth: Cold-induced symptoms dominate the clinical presentation of hepatitis C–associated cryoglobulinemia.

Comment: The cryoglobulins associated with hepatitis C (types II and III) are immune complexes that precipitate in the cold eg, several days at 4°C—not conditions that occur physiologically. Immune-complex–mediated disease accounts for the major clinical manifestations, such as palpable purpura and glomerulonephritis. In contrast, type I cryoglobulins (cryoprecipitating monoclonal gammopathies) can precipitate at temperatures achieved in the distal extremities, nose, ears, and elsewhere. Type I cryoglobulins often present with cold-induced symptoms.

Pearl: Suspect mixed cryoglobulinemia in a patient with a very low serum level of C4 and normal or near-normal level of C3.

Comment: Immune complexes in types II and III cryoglobulinemia activate the classical complement pathway leading to depletion of C4 and other early pathway components. In mixed cryoglobulinemia, the C4 level is usually disproportionately low compared to other complement components, even C3.

Myth: Patients with diffuse alveolar hemorrhage always have hemoptysis.

Comment: Diffuse alveolar hemorrhage is a life-threatening complication of vasculitis associated with antineutrophil cytoplasmic antibodies (ANCA), antiglomerular basement membrane disease, SLE, and other conditions. Classically, diffuse alveolar hemorrhage presents with hemoptysis, dyspnea, a fall in hematocrit, and the abrupt appearance of new infiltrates on chest radiography. Unfortunately, the presentation is highly variable, and hemoptysis, the clinical finding most suggestive of diffuse alveolar hemorrhage, is absent in up to one third of cases.

▶ Clinical Problem: Medical Complications of Levamisole-Adulterated Cocaine

Myth: The purpuric skin rash associated with levamisole-adulterated cocaine is due to a small-vessel vasculitis.

Comment: Exposure to levamisole, a prevalent adulterant in cocaine, can cause a distinctive syndrome of purpura and cutaneous necrosis affecting the extremities, ears, and cheeks. Purpura linked to levamisole is primarily due to a thrombotic microangiopathy that leads to extensive fibrin deposition within small dermal vessels. Although small-vessel vasculitis also can be present, vasculitis is a variable and relatively minor finding. The histopathology is in accord with the clinical appearance of the rash: retiform purpura, which is a manifestation of small vessel thrombosis, rather than the palpable purpura of small-vessel vasculitis. Patients with purpura induced by levamisole typically have IgM antibodies to phospholipid, lupus anticoagulants, and high titers of P-ANCA.

Pearl: Test for ANCA using indirect immunofluorescence, not just enzyme-linked immunosorbent assay (ELISA), when evaluating a patient for suspected purpura due to levamisole-adulterated cocaine.

Comment: There is discordance between results of testing for ANCA by indirect immunofluorescence assays and by ELISA in patients with levamisole-induced purpura. Exposure to levamisole can lead to autoantibodies directed against multiple neutrophil cytoplasmic antigens, such as elastase, cathepsin-G, and lactoferrin. In indirect immunofluorescence assays using fixed neutrophils, these autoantibodies produce very high titers of ANCA in a perinuclear pattern (P-ANCA). In contrast, ELISA testing for antibodies directed at myeloperoxidase or proteinase 3 is negative or detects only relatively low levels of reactivity.

▶ Clinical Problem: Gauging Disease Activity in Patients with ANCA-Associated Vasculitis

Myth: ANCA assays are useful in predicting disease flares in granulomatosis with polyangiitis (formerly Wegener granulomatosis).

Comment: Used properly, ANCA serologies may be invaluable in making the diagnosis of ANCA-associated vasculitis. Even so, significant numbers of patients with "ANCA-associated" vasculitis are ANCA negative. This is true for approximately 15% of patients with granulomatosis with polyangiitis (formerly Wegener granulomatosis) (and an even higher percentage of patients with limited disease), approximately 30% of those with microscopic polyangiitis, and 50% or more of those with eosinophilic granulomatosis with polyangiitis (the Churg-Strauss syndrome). Moreover, a number of studies have demonstrated that elevations in ANCA titers bear only a poor temporal correlation with disease activity. Specifically, given a significant rise in ANCA titer (either two- or fourfold, depending on the study), a disease flare may not present itself (if it presents at all) until 1 year or more after the ANCA elevation. Consequently, treatment decisions should never be predicated on ANCA titers.

Pearl: Arthritis is a common presentation of a flare in ANCA-associated vasculitis.

Comment: Perhaps because it improves so quickly after the institution of therapy, arthritis is a frequently overlooked sign of ANCA-associated vasculitis and a very common tip-off to disease flare. The arthritis commonly involves large joints in a migratory, asymmetric, oligoarticular pattern, one day involving a knee and an ankle, the next day a shoulder. Small joints may also be involved.

Pearl: Once renal involvement by granulomatosis with polyangiitis (formerly Wegener granulomatosis) begins, organ- or life-threatening disease may ensue swiftly.

Comment: Cases of granulomatosis with polyangiitis (formerly Wegener granulomatosis) "smoldering" in the upper respiratory tract for years (undiagnosed) are well documented in the literature. In many cases, the explanation for the chronic sinus dysfunction, nasal pain and bleeding, and other symptoms is understood only in retrospect, upon the occurrence of disease manifestations that threaten vital organs. Few diseases can cause renal deterioration as rapidly as granulomatosis with polyangiitis (formerly Wegener granulomatosis). Once the serum creatinine begins to rise in granulomatosis with polyangiitis (formerly Wegener granulomatosis), the disease often appears to accelerate substantially, with rapidly progressive glomerulonephritis, swift progression to renal failure, and the appearance of "disseminated" involvement (alveolar hemorrhage, mesenteric vasculitis, and so on). Thus, once the diagnosis of granulomatosis with polyangiitis (formerly Wegener granulomatosis) is considered, the evaluation must occur swiftly, especially if the patient has hematuria or an elevated serum creatinine.

▶ Clinical Problem: Evaluating Shortness of Breath in the Patient with ANCA-Associated Vasculitis

Pearl: Patients with granulomatosis with polyangiitis (formerly Wegener granulomatosis) are at substantially increased risk for deep venous thrombosis and pulmonary emboli.

Comment: In the Wegener Granulomatosis Etanercept Trial (WGET), 13 of the 180 patients had had venous thrombotic events prior to enrollment. During 228 person-years of prospective follow-up, venous thrombotic events occurred in 16 of the remaining 167 patients with no prior history of such events. The incidence rate of venous thrombotic events in granulomatosis with polyangiitis (formerly Wegener granulomatosis) was more than seven times higher than that of a comparable group of patients with SLE—a group known to have an increased thrombotic risk.

The etiology of venous thrombotic events in granulomatosis with polyangiitis (formerly Wegener granulomatosis), which is likely multifactorial, remains unclear. One possibility in addition to the debility, proteinuria, and other predisposing factors that may be associated with this disease is the fact that granulomatosis with polyangiitis (formerly Wegener granulomatosis) involves veins as well as arteries. It is conceivable that venous inflammation contributes in a major way to the elevated risk of venous thrombotic events in granulomatosis with polyangiitis (formerly Wegener granulomatosis). Vasculitic conditions related to granulomatosis with polyangiitis (formerly Wegener granulomatosis) such as microscopic polyangiitis and eosinophilic granulomatosis with polyangiitis (Churg-Strauss syndrome) are probably also associated with an increased risk of venous thrombotic events, although this has never been studied formally.

Pearl: Patients with either granulomatosis with polyangiitis (formerly Wegener granulomatosis) or relapsing polychondritis may have difficult airways.

Comment: The potential presence of subglottic stenosis is important to keep in mind among patients with granulomatosis with polyangiitis (formerly Wegener granulomatosis) or relapsing polychondritis, particularly those who may be undergoing bronchoscopy or elective intubation. Subglottic stenosis, a vasculitis complication that is peculiar to these two conditions, may lead to life-threatening narrowing of the airway just below the vocal cords. Passage of a bronchoscope or endotracheal tube may be difficult or impossible.

Pearl: The patient with inspiratory sounds most likely has subglottic stenosis and not asthma.

Comment: Asthma produces expiratory sounds; loud inspiratory sounds audible without the stethoscope are a sign of stridor, which in patients with granulomatosis with polyangiitis (formerly Wegener granulomatosis), is commonly caused by subglottic stenosis. Subglottic stenosis can usually be detected by observing patients as they talk: because of their upper airway narrowing, they must often pause slightly to suck in air before beginning a sentence.

▶ Clinical Problem: Treating Cryoglobulinemic Vasculitis Associated with Hepatitis C

Myth: The optimal therapy for hepatitis C–associated cryoglobulinemic vasculitis is always antiviral treatment.

Comment: Under ideal conditions, the treatment of vasculitis is directed against the underlying cause—in this case, hepatitis C. Currently, this means the combination of pegylated interferon and ribavirin. In the setting of severe, multiorgan system vasculitis, however, control of the underlying inflammation initially with anti-inflammatory therapies—glucocorticoids, cyclophosphamide, and even plasmapheresis—is recommended. In such situations, initial treatment with antiviral therapies alone may trigger a paradoxical worsening of the vasculitis through an unfavorable alteration of the antigen:antibody ratio. Initial treatment aimed at controlling the inflammatory response may prevent this complication. Following a couple of weeks of treatment with immunosuppressive agents, antiviral therapy may begin. Glucocorticoids and other therapies may be discontinued swiftly.

▶ Clinical Problem: Diagnosing Small-Vessel Cutaneous Vasculitis

Pearl: Direct immunofluorescence (DIF) should be performed on all skin biopsies performed to diagnose small-vessel vasculitis.

Comment: Hospitalists may have the opportunity to diagnose vasculitis by ordering skin biopsies. Full pathologic assessment of cutaneous vasculitis involves examination of a skin biopsy specimen by both light microscopy and DIF. DIF involves the testing of the skin biopsy sample for immunoglobulin, complement, and other immunoreactants. The presence of immunoreactants in the skin as well as their precise location (along the dermal epidermal border, around blood vessels, etc.) and pattern of deposition, reveals important characteristics about the underlying disease process. This information cannot be gleaned from the usual hematoxylin and eosin (H & E) stains examined by light microscopy; it requires DIF. The omission of DIF—an unfortunately common occurrence—wastes an opportunity to observe potentially valuable information and often leads to misdiagnoses (eg, the failure to distinguish Henoch-Schönlein purpura from a drug-induced vasculitis). DIF can only be performed on fresh skin biopsy samples, cannot be added on later, and therefore must be planned at the time of the biopsy. Insist that the dermatologist send skin biopsies for both H &E and DIF.

Perioperative Management of the Patient with Rheumatic Disease

C. Ronald MacKenzie, MD
Stephen A. Paget, MD

Since patients with rheumatic disease often require surgery, rheumatologists may be required to evaluate and care for patients in the perioperative setting. The goals of the preoperative medical consultation and perioperative management include the following: (1) identifying the nature, severity, and stability of all comorbid conditions affecting perioperative clinical decision-making; (2) optimizing treatment of all active medical problems; (3) assessing the risks associated with anesthesia and surgery; (4) anticipating, identifying, and managing postoperative complications; (5) educating patients and families about the perioperative experience; (6) motivating patients to adopt preoperative preventive practices (ie, smoking cessation, weight loss, medication compliance, and adherence to care plans preoperatively and postoperatively).

THE PREOPERATIVE EVALUATION

▶ History & Physical Examination

The needs of the patient in the perioperative setting depends on a number of considerations, notably age, functional capacity, comorbidity, the type of anesthesia to be used, and the surgery to be performed. A complete history and physical examination remains the bedrock of the evaluation because it provides the clinical context upon which informed management decisions can be made. Patients should be asked about their prior experience with surgery and anesthesia, and the presence, severity, and stability of all comorbid conditions should be established. All medications (including over-the-counter preparations, herbs, and supplements) as well as the use of tobacco, alcohol, and other drugs should be documented.

The preoperative examination should be thorough yet focused on patient characteristics that might adversely impact the patient's postoperative course. In addition to the vital signs, body mass index should be calculated because obesity is not only associated with various chronic diseases, it is a risk factor for surgery. Careful auscultation of the heart is important to rule out the presence of third and fourth heart sounds, which may indicate congestive heart failure. Further cardiac murmurs denote the presence of valvular heart disease, problems that may compromise cardiac function at times of physiologic stress (such as surgery). Obesity, large neck circumference, and hypertension predict obstructive sleep apnea, an important but underappreciated problem in the postoperative setting.

▶ Laboratory Studies

The benefit of preoperative laboratory testing has been examined in many studies and its benefit (or lack thereof) continues to be debated. When there are no clinical indications, laboratory studies rarely provide useful information. Thus, routine preoperative laboratory testing appears unnecessary for healthy patients undergoing minor procedures. Table 62–1 lists laboratory tests that may be considered for patients undergoing major surgical procedures.

▶ Assessment of Surgical Risk

While the history and physical examination remain the primary method for detecting conditions likely to affect surgical outcome, rating systems that are useful in identifying patients in whom postoperative complications are most likely to develop have been created.

The most widely used rating system is the American Society of Anesthesiologist (ASA) Physical Status Scale, which has a high correlation with the patient's postoperative course. This scale consists of 5 levels of risk, which are based on the presence of a systemic disturbance (Table 62–2). Although criticized for the vagueness of its criteria, the ASA classification has proven a highly durable and useful predictive tool.

For preoperative assessment of cardiac risk, a revision (Revised Cardiac Risk Index) of the original index

Table 62–1. Recommendations for laboratory testing before elective surgery.

Test	Incidence of Abnormalities that Influence Management	Positive Likelihood Ratio	Negative Likelihood Ratio	Indications
Hemoglobin	0.1%	3.3	0.90	Anticipated major blood loss or symptoms of anemia
White blood cell count	0.0%	0.0	1.00	Symptoms suggest infection, myeloproliferative disorder, or myelotoxic medications
Platelet count	0.0%	0.0	1.00	History of bleeding diathesis, myeloproliferative disorder, or myelotoxic medications
Prothrombin time	0.0%	0.0	1.01	History of bleeding diathesis, chronic liver disease, malnutrition, recent or long-term antibiotic use
Partial thromboplastin time	0.1%	1.7	0.86	History of bleeding diathesis
Electrolytes	1.8%	4.3	0.80	Known renal insufficiency, congestive heart failure, medications that affect electrolytes
Renal function	2.6%	3.3	0.81	Age >50 years, hypertension, cardiac disease, major surgery, medications that may affect renal function
Glucose	0.5%	1.6	0.85	Obesity or known diabetes
Liver function tests	0.1%			No indication. Consider albumin measurement for major surgery or chronic illness
Urinalysis	1.4%	1.7	0.97	No indication
Electrocardiogram	2.6%	1.6	0.96	Men >40 years, women >50 years, known CAD, diabetes, or hypertension
Chest radiograph	3.0%	2.5	0.72	Age >50 years, known cardiac or pulmonary disease, symptoms or examination suggest cardiac or pulmonary disease

CAD, coronary artery disease.
Modified, with permission, from Smetana GW, Macpherson DS. *Med Clin N Am.* 2003;87:7–40.

Table 62–2. American Society of Anesthesiologist physical status scale.

Level of Risk	Extent of Systemic Disease[a]
I	Absent (0.2%)
II	Mild (0.5%)
III	Severe/non-incapacitating (1.9%)
IV	Incapacitating/threat to life (4.9%)
V	Moribund/survival <24 h without surgery (NA) Emergency surgery (subdesignation E) doubles the risk

[a]Associated surgical mortality in parentheses.

of Goldman is now widely used (Table 62–3). One point is assigned for each of the 6 independent risk factors for major cardiac complications in patients undergoing non-cardiac surgery. The incidence of such complications in patients with 0, 1, 2, or 3 risk factors is 0.4%, 0.9%, 7%, and 11%, respectively.

The development of more global indicators of risk remains an important challenge. Holt and Silverman have proposed a resilience score for organ systems compromised by an underlying disease process. An overall resilience score for a given organ system is derived by adding the standard ASA score to a surgical complexity score (rate 1–5). The higher the score, the more likely that a given organ system will suffer injury or fail in the setting of a surgical stress.

Several broad themes relevant to perioperative care have emerged from other recent studies. First, the use of total joint arthroplasty has increased over time, as has the

Table 62–3. Revised cardiac risk index.

Each risk factor is assigned one point.
1. High-risk surgical procedures
   - Intraperitoneal
   - Intrathoracic
   - Suprainguinal vascular
2. History of ischemic heart disease
   - History of myocardial infarction
   - History of positive exercise test
   - Current complaint of chest pain considered secondary to myocardial ischemia
   - Use of nitrate therapy
   - ECG with pathological Q waves
3. History of congestive heart failure
   - History of congestive heart failure
   - Pulmonary edema
   - Paroxysmal nocturnal dyspnea
   - Bilateral rales or S3 gallop
   - Chest radiograph showing pulmonary vascular redistribution
4. History of cerebrovascular disease
   - History of transient ischemic attack or stroke
5. Preoperataive treatment with insulin
6. Preoperative serum creatinine >2.0 mg/dL

Risk of Major Cardiac Event		
Points	Class	Risk
0	I	0.4%
1	II	0.9%
2	III	6.6%
3 or more	IV	11%

"Major cardiac event" includes myocardial infarction, pulmonary edema, ventricular fibrillation, primary cardiac arrest, and complete heart block.
Data from: http://surgicalcriticalcare.net/Resources/revised_cardiac_risk_index.pdf
Lee TH, Marcantonio ER, Mangione CM, et al. Derivation of prospective validation of a simple index for prediction of cardiac risk of major noncardiac surgery. *Circulation.* 1999;10:1043.

prevalence of hypertension, diabetes mellitus, hypercholesterolemia, obesity, pulmonary disease, and coronary artery disease. Overall complication rates have decreased in spite of a decreasing length of stay except in the case of bilateral procedures. Indeed, among the population undergoing bilateral total joint arthroplasty, procedure-related complication rates were higher than unilateral procedures despite a younger average age and lower comorbidity burden. Mortality after total joint arthroplasty of the hip and knee were most strongly correlated with postoperative pulmonary embolism and stroke. Preoperative risk factors for in-hospital mortality were revision total joint arthroplasty, advanced age (>85 years), and the presence of specific comorbidities (predominately dementia, renal disease, and cerebrovascular disease).

▶ Anesthesia in Patients with Rheumatic Disease

Airway considerations, the site and anticipated duration of surgery, comorbidities, and the patient's emotional state are important determinants of the type of anesthesia to be used, as well as whether invasive monitoring will be required, and the length of time the patient will spend in the recovery room after surgery.

A. Type of Anesthesia

General and regional anesthesia are commonly used in the surgical treatment of patients with rheumatic disease. Although the debate concerning the relative superiority of these approaches remains unresolved, many surgical procedures, particularly orthopedic surgery, are well suited for regional anesthetic techniques. Regional anesthesia may reduce the incidence of major perioperative complications, including blood loss, deep venous thrombosis and pulmonary embolism, as well as postoperative respiratory events and death. Further, postoperative pain management, a significant problem for patients with a painful rheumatic disease, may be best managed with regional anesthetic approaches. Peripheral nerve blocks using longer acting anesthetics and infusion methods are another consideration since they provide both excellent intraoperative anesthesia and postoperative pain relief.

B. Monitoring Techniques

Patients undergoing major surgical procedures should have continuous electrocardiographic and pulse oximeter monitoring intraoperatively. Arterial line and Swan-Ganz catheter monitoring may be helpful in selected patients, particularly those with chronic cardiopulmonary disease. Such monitoring is also used in patients undergoing bilateral joint replacement surgery.

C. Postoperative Analgesia

A number of options exist for the control of postoperative pain, including the traditional intravenous or intramuscular routes versus the use of epidural analgesia. Patient-controlled analgesia via an epidural route of administration is an effective method of pain control after surgery and often facilitates postoperative physical therapy, which is important in the restoration of range of motion in patients undergoing orthopedic surgery. Parenterally administered nonsteroidal anti-inflammatory drugs are a useful alternative to traditional analgesia after surgery and can be used to reduce opioid requirements after major surgery. These drugs should not be given to patients with the common contraindications to nonsteroidal anti-inflammatory drugs, such as peptic ulcer and renal disease.

PERIOPERATIVE MANAGEMENT OF COMORBID MEDICAL CONDITIONS

1. Ischemic Heart Disease

Cardiovascular disease is the most investigated and well documented problem of perioperative medicine. Practical guidelines intended to guide physicians involved in the assessment and care of patients with cardiac disease are widely recognized and are updated regularly.

▶ Risk Assessment

With respect to the identification of the presence of preexisting cardiac disease, the predictive value of the routine clinical assessment, the history and physical examination, electrocardiogram, chest radiograph, supplemented by other noninvasive methodologies, is well established. In patients with ischemic heart disease, the postoperative risk is ultimately defined by the estimation of disease severity and stability in concert with age, functional capacity, comorbidity and type of surgery to be performed. A series of factors may predict postoperative myocardial infarction, congestive heart failure, and death after orthopedic surgery (Table 62–4).

The American College of Cardiology/American Heart Association Guidelines for the Perioperative Cardiovascular Evaluation for Noncardiac Surgery provides the most extensive discussion of the approach to the preoperative cardiac evaluation. In patients with high exercise tolerance, such testing provides little useful information. In patients with rheumatic disease, however, the evaluation of cardiac function preoperatively may be useful because the chronic illness often limits their activity thereby masking underlying significant cardiac dysfunction. Currently, it remains unclear whether one approach to stress testing is definitively superior to another. Indeed, all approaches may be reasonably good for preoperative risk assessment and which approach is chosen may be related more to the patient's physical capacity to participate in the stress induction and the local availability of such testing.

▶ Management Strategies

Strategies to reduce cardiac risk in noncardiac surgery may involve (1) medical therapy or invasive cardiac interventions performed preoperatively, (2) alterations in anesthetic technique, or (3) aggressive management of adverse hemodynamic developments before and after surgery. For the internist-rheumatologist who evaluates the patient preoperatively, the relevant approach includes medical management, specifically the use of β-blockers, antiplatelet agents, and statin therapy. Managing antiplatelet therapy in patients who have cardiac stents can be challenging (see below). On occasion, coronary revascularization prior to the noncardiac surgery is considered.

Theoretically, β-blockers can protect the heart in the perioperative period by improving myocardial oxygen balance by slowing the heart rate and reducing contractility. In addition, slowing of the heart rate improves diastolic filling while decreasing myocardial oxygen consumption. Studies on the impact of β-blocker use on perioperative morbidity and mortality have yielded conflicting results. In one study, patients with coronary artery disease or a significant risk factor profile were randomized to receive atenolol or placebo starting 7 days before surgery and continuing for 1 month after surgery. A significant reduction in cardiac events was noted postoperatively, a benefit that remained significant for 2 years. Some subsequent studies confirmed these results; however, a large randomized control trial showed that while prophylactic β-blockade significantly decreased the incidence of postoperative myocardial infarction, this benefit was negated by the higher incidence of death (3.1% vs 2.3%), stroke (1.0% vs 0.5%), clinically significant hypotension (15% vs 9.7%), and bradycardia (6.6% vs 2.4%). While controversy remains, the most prudent approach to the use of perioperative β-blockade is to use them only in selected circumstances, such as high-risk patients who currently take β-blockers.

Long-term aspirin therapy for the primary and secondary prevention of atherosclerotic cardiovascular disease is highly prevalent, and the use of aspirin and other antiplatelet agents

Table 62–4. Predictors of increased perioperative cardiac risk.

Major predictors
Recent myocardial infarction (<30 days)
Unstable or severe angina
Poorly compensated congestive heart failure
Significant arrhythmias
Severe valvular disease
Intermediate predictors
Mild angina
Prior myocardial infarction by history or pathologic Q waves
Compensated or prior congestive heart failure
Diabetes mellitus
Minor predictors
Advanced age
Abnormal ECG
Rhythm other than sinus
Low functional capacity
Prior stroke
Poorly controlled hypertension
Prior cardiac revascularization, currently asymptomatic

in the perioperative setting is commonplace. In the past, these agents were usually discontinued before surgery whenever possible because of their perceived bleeding risk. As the protective role of aspirin has been better appreciated, the practice of discontinuing aspirin prior to surgery has been called into question. A meta-analysis has demonstrated that aspirin withdrawal preceded up to 10% of all acute cardiovascular events and that while aspirin-related bleeding complications increased, the bleeding tended to be mild and of little significance (except in intracranial surgery and transurethral resection of the prostate). A related problem is the management of antiplatelet therapy in patients with intracoronary stents who are undergoing noncardiac surgery. Reports of perioperative stent thrombosis in patients who have discontinued antiplatelet therapy preoperatively have raised concern about the attendant risks. Such thrombosis is associated with high rates of myocardial infarction (up to 50%). Two major classes of stents are currently used: bare metal stents (BMS) and drug-eluting stents (DES). The latter contain drugs that prevent endothelialization of the stent and hence restenosis. Since antiplatelet agents (usually dual antiplatelet therapy) significantly reduce the incidence of stent thrombosis, the protective influence of such medication is important. Further, the risk of stent thrombosis varies with the type of stent used. The BMS have a lower risk of thrombosis than DES when antiplatelet therapy is discontinued. The heightened risk of thrombosis associated with DES is believed to persist for upwards of 1 year. According to a recent advisory statement, for patients who require surgery and have had a DES placed in the preceding 12 months, clopidogrel should not be discontinued for an elective procedure.

The statins have both lipid-lowering and anti-inflammatory activity, stabilizing coronary plaque, improving endothelial function, and inhibiting platelet aggregation. As a consequence of these benefits and a number of clinical trial suggesting a cardioprotective effect in the perioperative setting, statin therapy should be continued during the perioperative period.

While fewer patients with rheumatoid arthritis and spondyloarthropathies are undergoing orthopedic surgery due to modern treatment strategies, some patients require surgical intervention and their cardiovascular risks need to be appreciated. Rheumatoid arthritis results in premature development of atherosclerosis, myocardial infarction, and arterial stiffening. Congestive heart failure is likewise independently related to rheumatoid arthritis, possibly because of impaired left ventricular diastolic filling. Although effective control of disease activity may be beneficial in ameliorating vascular and myocardial disease, patients with severe disease are the most likely to have subclinical coronary disease. Like rheumatoid arthritis, systemic lupus erythematosus results in premature development of atherosclerosis, myocardial infarction, and arterial stiffening. Left ventricular hypertrophy develops in systemic lupus erythematosus unrelated to traditional stimuli to hypertrophy and may be due to inflammation-related arterial stiffening. All cyclooxygenase-2 selective and traditional nonsteroidal anti-inflammatory drugs increase the risk for ischemic heart disease and should be factored into the perioperative risk assessment.

2. Other Cardiovascular Conditions

The prevalence of hypertension in the perioperative setting is 20%. Its association with coronary artery disease secures it as a risk factor for adverse outcome after surgery. Indeed, it has been shown to be 1 of 5 independent predictors of postoperative myocardial ischemia and 1 of 3 predictors of postoperative mortality. Despite these associations, clinical experience suggests that the magnitude of risk conferred by blood pressure elevations alone appears small, and generally surgery need not be postponed in patients with mild to moderate elevations in blood pressure.

Dysfunction of the cardiac valves is a relatively common manifestation of the connective tissue diseases. There are the Libman-Sacks vegetations of systemic lupus erythematosus, regurgitation of the mitral valve in rheumatoid arthritis, and the aortic valve disease (particularly aortic insufficiency) that accompanies HLA-B27–associated spondyloarthropathies. In addition to these associations, there is the high prevalence of aortic and aortic valve involvement in the systemic vasculitides, including granulomatous disorders, systemic vasculitis, giant cell arteritis, and Takayasu arteritis. Along with perioperative prothrombotic issues, antiphospholipid antibodies in systemic lupus erythematosus are associated with mitral valve nodules and significant mitral regurgitation, possibly due to valvular endothelial cell activation.

Surgical risks in patients with valvular heart disease depend on the valve affected as well as the nature and severity of the valvular lesion. The greatest perioperative risk is associated with hemodynamically significant aortic stenosis, a relatively uncommon valvular lesion in the connective tissue diseases. Mitral valve disease and aortic insufficiency, unless severe, are well tolerated in the surgical setting. Therefore, patients with a significant cardiac murmur, especially if accompanied by signs or symptoms of left ventricular dysfunction, should undergo an echocardiographic assessment preoperatively, particularly if a major procedure is planned. Invasive hemodynamic monitoring perioperatively may also be indicated in patients at higher risk.

While cardiac arrhythmias and conduction system disease are frequently a marker for underlying cardiac or pulmonary disease, metabolic abnormalities, or drug toxicity, they are also more frequently seen in patients with the connective tissue diseases. This is especially true in scleroderma where myocardial fibrosis compromises the cardiac conduction system, resulting in heart block and other electrocardiographic abnormalities and arrhythmias. Therefore, when patients with this and other connective tissue diseases present preoperatively with conduction system problems such as high degrees of heart block or cardiac arrhythmias, the clinician should search for such conditions and institute corrective action, if possible, before surgery.

A common problem is the management of patients with chronic atrial fibrillation who receive long-term anticoagulation. In patients with chronic atrial fibrillation who do not have prosthetic valves or hypercoagulable states and who do not receive anticoagulation therapy, the risk of embolic stroke is low. Therefore, it is safe to temporarily discontinue warfarin preoperatively to allow for normalization of the prothrombin time and international normalized ratio (INR). Five days before surgery is generally sufficient and reinstitution on the night of surgery is safe and appropriate. Newer agents, including the direct thrombin inhibitors (dabigatran etexilate mesylate [Pradaxa]) as well as agents that inhibit Factor Xa (rivaroxaban [Xarelto]), will be increasingly seen in the preoperative setting. Based on a 17 hour half-life, Dabigatran should be stopped at least 2 days prior to surgery. Rivaroxaban, with its shorter (9 hour) half-life, should be stopped at least 1 full day before the procedure. Recent clinical trials focused on venous thrombosis prophylaxis suggest that both agents can started safely immediately after surgery. However, given their rapid onset of action, surgeons may prefer to wait until hemostasis has been achieved.

3. Pulmonary Disease

Postoperative pulmonary complications are frequent and important adverse events in the postoperative period. One large study (1055 patients) reported a 2.7% incidence of pulmonary complications in patients thought to be at low to moderate risk; patients in whom pulmonary complications developed had a significantly longer length of hospital stay (27.9 vs 4.5 days). Complications such as atelectasis, pneumonia, aspiration pneumonia, respiratory failure, and exacerbation of chronic obstructive pulmonary disease (COPD) may have more severe consequences than cardiac disease and have been shown to be more predictive of long-term mortality. Smoking is associated with a 1.4- to 4.3-fold risk of postoperative pulmonary complications. COPD is the most important patient-related factor predicting postoperative complications. Such patients have a 6–28% risk for the development of pulmonary complications after surgery. Patients with asthma are also at increased risk if the disease is not well controlled preoperatively. The increased prevalence of cardiovascular disease in these patients further heightens the perioperative risk of these patients.

Chronic pulmonary disease can be divided into three categories: asthma, obstructive lung disease, and restrictive lung disease. COPD (chronic bronchitis, emphysema) and asthma are the most prevalent and account for most of the pulmonary problems arising in the postoperative setting. Minor pulmonary complications (atelectasis, bronchitis) are increased in patients who smoke, who have a chronic cough, or have abnormal spirometry. The risk of severe postoperative pulmonary complications (pneumonia, respiratory failure) is increased mainly in patients with marked impairment in lung function (forced expiratory volume in 1 second [FEV_1] <1.5 L).

Restrictive lung disease, while generally less common, deserves mention owing to its prevalence in the connective tissue diseases. Defined by a symmetric decrease in FEV_1 and forced vital capacity (FVC), with a reduction in the total lung capacity (TLC), restrictive patterns of lung spirometry are characteristic of the functional abnormality seen in such conditions as rheumatoid arthritis, polymyositis/dermatomyositis, and systemic lupus erythematosus.

Patient- and procedure-related risk factors for postoperative pulmonary complications are recognized. Patient-related risk factors include age, existing COPD, cigarette use, congestive heart failure, comorbidities, functional capacity, obesity, sleep apnea, and cognitive impairment. In contrast, procedure-related risk factors include surgical site (increased complication rate in procedures near the diaphragm), duration of surgery, anesthetic technique, and emergency surgery. While attempts to develop a pulmonary predictive risk index similar to the Goldman Cardiac Risk index (or its descendants) have been unsuccessful, two complication-specific pulmonary risk indices have been published, one for the prediction of postoperative pneumonia and another for respiratory failure occurring after surgery.

Two other pulmonary-related conditions make important contributions to postoperative risk: sleep apnea and chronic pulmonary arterial hypertension (PAH). Sleep apnea syndrome is defined as ≥5 apneic events (airflow stops for ≥10 seconds despite continued respiratory effort) or ≥15/hour hypopneic events (airflow lessens >50% for ≥10 seconds) during a 7-hour sleep study. While three types sleep apnea are recognized (ie, obstructive, central, and mixed), it is the obstructive form that most often comes to light in the postoperative period. Typically, while morbidly obese patients with no documented history of the condition are observed in the recovery room, they demonstrate signs of upper airway obstruction, suggesting the presence of the condition. Other physical characteristics associated with obstructive sleep apnea include a neck circumference of 17 inches, craniofacial abnormalities affecting the airway, anatomic nasal obstruction, and tonsils touching in the midline. The preoperative interview is an efficient means of screening patients; the Berlin questionnaire, comprising 10 questions that pertain to risk factors for sleep apnea (snoring, wake time sleepiness/fatigue, hypertension), has been shown to be predictive of the condition. A number of management difficulties are present in patients with sleep apnea, including a difficult to manage airway; challenging intubation; and postoperative complications, such as hypoxemia, hypertension, atrial fibrillation, and heart failure.

PAH is also seen in the connective tissue diseases, a consequence of the pulmonary disease associated with such conditions as scleroderma and mixed connective tissue disease. In the surgical setting, PAH is an especially treacherous problem associated with a substantial mortality. A pathophysiologic state characterized by elevated right heart afterload, decreased venous return, reduced cardiac output and deficient oxygen saturation, PAH is categorized as primary (idiopathic) pulmonary hypertension or as secondary PAH arising as a consequence of left heart disease, hypoxic pulmonary disorders (for instance obstructive sleep apnea), or chronic thromboembolic phenomenon. Sustained elevations in pulmonary vascular resistance and pulmonary arterial pressure, coupled with impaired vascular reactivity, may result in systemic hypotension in the setting of anesthesia. The negative inotropic effects of some anesthetic agents may exacerbate this tendency precipitating right heart failure. Thus, the adverse consequences on the left side of the circulation (systemic hypotension) are further exacerbated by concomitant right-sided responses, the pulmonary vessels constrict in response to the resultant hypoxia thereby promoting the development of hypercarbia, acidosis, hypothermia, and the release of catecholamines, a cascade that may result in further hemodynamic deterioration and circulatory collapse. Although new medications (such as endothelin receptor antagonists and prostaglandins) can significantly decrease the pulmonary artery pressures, PAH is an important risk factor for adverse outcomes after surgery.

The degree of perioperative risk imposed by chronic pulmonary dysfunction is significantly influenced by the type of surgery to be performed. Patients with severe lung impairment can tolerate minor procedures, even under general anesthesia. The risk of pneumonia following major peripheral limb surgery (such as hip or knee surgery) is low, even in the patients with chronic lung disease. In contrast, intra-abdominal or intrathoracic procedures are associated with a high risk of atelectasis or pneumonia in patients, particularly in patients with severe COPD. Regional anesthesia for surgery on the extremities circumvents many of these problems with one important caveat. Interscalene block, frequently used in shoulder surgery, may transiently paralyze the ipsilateral diaphragm and reduce the FVC by 30–40%. Therefore, patients with lung disease undergoing shoulder surgery, in which interscalene block is being considered, should have pulmonary function studies performed preoperatively. In patients with severely impaired pulmonary function (FEV$_1$ <1 L), interscalene block should be avoided altogether. Patients with moderate COPD generally fare well with this anesthesia, especially if performed in the sitting position.

Patients using bronchodilators on a long-term basis should receive their standard dosage the night before surgery; bronchodilator therapy should be administered postoperatively usually by nebulizer. Incentive spirometry 10 times daily and early mobilization are helpful in the prevention of postoperative atelectasis.

4. Diabetes Mellitus

Diabetes is the most important endocrine disorder encountered in surgical patients and, in the postoperative setting, such patients should be regarded as at risk for complications including myocardial infarction, stroke, infection, and death. Patients who have diabetes mellitus with autonomic insufficiency (manifested by postural hypotension,

erectile dysfunction, nocturnal diarrhea) are at risk for sudden cardiopulmonary arrest postoperatively. Given the high prevalence of coronary artery disease, cardiovascular risk assessment is an important concern in diabetic patients; the management approach for diabetic patients is the same as that outlined earlier in the section concerning cardiovascular disease. Otherwise, the primary perioperative consideration is glycemic control.

The maintenance of good glycemic control in the surgical setting is often challenging. Because of a complex interplay of factors, the net effect of anesthesia and surgery is to drive the blood sugars higher. While the value of tight glycemic control in the perioperative setting has not been definitively established, 3 primary observations lend support to this practice. First, diabetes is a common clinical problem in surgical practice; it is estimated that 25% of diabetic patients will require surgery in the course of their lifetime. Second, many diabetic patients are at high risk in the surgical setting and efforts to reduce these risks are justified. Third, good glycemic control may reduce the rate of wound infection, vascular complications, and death in the perioperative setting.

At the preoperative evaluation, it is important to characterize the type of diabetes (type 1 or 2), determine the specifics of the patient's treatment (medications, timing of and adherence to therapy), and estimate the degree of glycemic control. The occurrence and frequency of hypoglycemia should also be ascertained. An understanding of the nature and magnitude of the type of surgery to be performed is also necessary.

In general, the goal of therapy is to maintain the glucose level between 150 mg/dL and 200 mg/dL during surgery in order to protect against hypoglycemia. Numerous regimens have been recommended to achieve this end; management approaches are dictated by the type and severity of the patient's diabetes. Regardless of the severity of the disease, however, management should be proactive as opposed to reactive. Whenever possible, diabetic patients should undergo surgery early in the day, thereby avoiding prolonged periods of fast on the day of surgery. For patients treated with oral agents, such medications are usually given on the day before surgery and then held in the early postoperative period. For insulin-dependent patients, the patient's usual insulin regimen should be continued. Patients with type 1 diabetes mellitus should take a fractional amount (one third to one-half their usual dosage) of their long-acting insulin on the morning of surgery. Patients with type 2 diabetes mellitus should take none to one third of their dosage, and those patients treated with an insulin pump should continue at their basal rate of insulin infusion.

In the early postoperative period, blood sugars may be difficult to control. Divided doses of intermediate-acting (twice daily) or short-acting insulin (usually 4–6 times/daily) can be supplemented by the subcutaneous administration according to a predetermined algorithm (ie, sliding scale). Continuous insulin infusions are occasionally used postoperatively in the patient with severe, brittle disease. This approach is maintained until the patient's oral intake is reestablished. Oral hypoglycemic agents can be resumed when the patient is eating.

5. Long-term Glucocorticoid Therapy

Since many patients with rheumatic disease take glucocorticoids, the management of the patient's glucocorticoid therapy in the perioperative setting is a common problem. Five to 7.5 mg daily of prednisone approximates the normal daily adrenal output of cortisol (30 mg). Patients believed to be at increased risk for adrenal insufficiency include (1) those currently taking >20 mg prednisone daily for >3 weeks, (2) those who have taken such doses for more than 2 weeks in the preceding year, and (3) those who are receiving replacement glucocorticoid therapy for known adrenal insufficiency. While surgery may produce sufficient "stress" to provoke adrenal insufficiency, surgeries vary in the amount of stress they produce and the circulating cortisol concentration usually normalize within 24–48 hours in most patients after surgery. Thus, supplementation should depend on the degree of stress (a function of the duration and severity of the surgical procedure) and the long-term daily glucocorticoid dose. Table 62–5 provides recommendations for perioperative glucocorticoid coverage according to the magnitude of the surgery to be performed.

6. Gastrointestinal Disease

Gastrointestinal problems may complicate the postoperative period and produce significant morbidity. Postoperative nausea and vomiting arises in 20–30% of patients after surgery and is perhaps the most frequently encountered management problem. Risk factors include female sex, use of opioids for postoperative pain, a history of motion sickness, or postoperative nausea and vomiting with prior surgery. The presence

of 0, 1, 2, 3, or 4 these risk factors is associated with an incidence of 10%, 21%, 39%, 61% or 79%, respectively. Nausea, abdominal distention and pain, and vomiting often herald the onset of more significant problems, specifically that of postoperative abdominal ileus.

The impairment of gastrointestinal motility after surgery is a common postoperative complication. Postoperative ileus is generally a self-limited condition lasting 3–5 days and is characterized by constipation, the accumulation of gas and fluids in the bowel with the development of abdominal distention and intolerance to enteral feeding. Perturbations in gastrointestinal motility after surgery result from a number of adverse influences arising after surgery. External risk factors include opioid analgesia and anesthesia, the fasting state, and the reintroduction of oral feeding. Internal or physiologic responses to surgery also play an important role and include increases in sympathetic tone, the hypothalamic release of corticotropin-releasing factor, and the release of nitric oxide each of which negatively influence gastrointestinal motility. In order to counteract these influences, careful consideration should be given to the optimal timing for the resumption of oral intake (both liquid and solid), and potent opioid therapy should be tapered and discontinued as quickly as possible. Early mobilization is also an effective preventive strategy. In more severe cases, medications that act on the autonomic nervous system (eg, bethanechol, carbachol, methacholine) or cholinesterase inhibitors (eg, neostigmine) may be required. Neostigmine is generally reserved for severe cases of adynamic ileus with massive dilatation of the colon in the absence of mechanical obstruction (Ogilvie syndrome), a highly threatening complication with an attendant mortality of 50%. For the motility problems arising as a consequence of postoperative opioid therapy, the *mu*-opioid-receptor antagonist methylnaltrexone may be useful in the postoperative setting. Last, a simple and novel preventive

Table 62–5. Recommendations for perioperative glucocorticoid coverage.

Surgical Stress	Target Hydrocortisone Equivalent	Preoperative Dose	Intraoperative Dose	Postoperative Dose[a]	Postoperative Dose Day 1[a]	Postoperative Dose Day 2[a]
Minor (eg, inguinal herniorrhaphy)	25 mg/d for 1 day	Usual daily dose	None[b]	None[b]	Usual daily dose[b]	
Moderate (eg, colon resection, total joint replacement, lower extremity revascularization)	50–75 mg/day for 1–2 days	Usual daily dose	50 mg hydrocortisone	20 mg hydrocortisone every 8 h	20 mg hydrocortisone every 8 h	
Major (eg, pancreatoduodenectomy, esophagectomy)	100–150 mg/d for 2–3 days	Usual daily dose	50 mg hydrocortisone	50 mg hydrocortisone every 8 h	50 mg hydrocortisone every 8 h	50 mg hydrocortisone every 8 h

[a]If postoperative complications occur, continued glucocorticoid administration will be necessary commiserate with the level of stress.
[b]If the postoperative course is uncomplicated, patients can resume their usual glucocorticoid dose on postoperative day 1.
Data from Salem M, Tainsh RE, Bromberg J, et al. Perioperative glucocorticoid coverage. A reassessment 42 years after emergence of a problem. *Ann Surg.* 1994;219:416–425.

approach is the use of chewing gum as a stimulant of gastrointestinal motility in the postoperative setting.

Other gastrointestinal conditions, such as intestinal volvulus (which is usually seen in patients with a history of abdominal surgery), diverticular disease (chronic disease may flare in the postoperative setting), and colon cancer, may present in the postoperative period. All 3 may mimic abdominal ileus. Another important consideration is the development of *Clostridium difficile*–induced colitis. As a result of an increasing prevalence of this organism in the population and the widespread colonization of hospitals, severe infectious colitis has been increasingly seen in the postoperative period. *C difficile*–induced colitis may be asymptomatic, present with diarrhea alone (without colitis), or as acute pseudomembranous colitis progressing to life-threatening toxic megacolon. Treatment requires aggressive fluid support and the institution of oral antibiotic therapy, either metronidazole (250 mg four times daily) or vancomycin (125 mg four times daily). Resistant cases have become more frequent. Surgery including total colectomy may be required in the most severe cases.

Peptic ulcer disease is a relatively common problem among patients with orthopedic or rheumatic disease because of long-term use of nonsteroidal anti-inflammatory agents and glucocorticoids. Should peptic ulcer disease become active after surgery, it poses a particular challenge in patients who require anticoagulation prophylaxis, such as those who have undergone total joint arthroplasty. Therefore, patients with a history of peptic ulcer disease, gastrointestinal bleeding, or active dyspepsia should receive a prophylactic proton pump inhibitor or H_2-blocker throughout the postoperative period. Elective surgery should be cancelled when there is an active peptic process. In patients at risk for the development of gastrointestinal bleeding after surgery, serial monitoring using stool guaiac tests are a satisfactory approach.

7. Genitourinary Conditions

Urinary catheters, which are frequently used in patients undergoing major surgery, should be removed as early as possible postoperatively. If the catheter is removed within 48 hours of surgery, urinary retention is avoided and the risk of urinary tract infection is small. There are simple questionnaires that are useful in predicting in whom postoperative urinary retention is likely to develop.

Prostatic hypertrophy leading to urinary obstruction is a common problem in men after surgery. In patients with significant chronic symptoms, urologic consultation should be obtained prior to surgery and therapy (including transurethral prostatectomy) instituted. In patients who have a predisposition for urinary retention and those with enlarged prostate glands and obstructive symptoms, treatment with terazosin and tamsulosin may be started before or at the time of surgery. In patients with a history of nephrolithiasis, dehydration should be rigorously avoided to help prevent acute renal colic.

8. Prevention of Postoperative Infection

Efforts to prevent and detect infectious processes before and after surgical procedures, such as total joint arthroplasty, are of utmost importance. The skin and urinary tract are sites of particular concern, and infection can be ruled out by a careful physical examination and routine preoperative urine culture. Dental consultation may be appropriate in patients with poor oral hygiene.

Prophylactic antibiotic therapy for total joint arthroplasty patients should begin <2 hours before surgery and continue for 24 hours. A recommended protocol involves cefazolin 1 g every 8 hours (total of three doses) or, in penicillin-allergic patients, vancomycin 1 g every 12 hours (total of two doses).

9. Neurologic Problems

▶ **Postoperative Delirium**

Acute confusional states frequently arise during the postoperative period, particularly in the elderly. Delirium is characterized by an alteration in the level of consciousness, a diminished ability to maintain and focus attention, hallucinations, delusions, and agitation. While its onset may occur during the day, it may become more severe at night (sundowning). The duration of delirium is unpredictable. Patients are at increased risk for the development of delirium after surgery due to a such risk factors as acute infections, drug (psychoactive, analgesia, anesthetic) and alcohol toxicity or withdrawal, dehydration, fluid/electrolyte/metabolic disturbances, and states of low perfusion (heart failure and shock). The incidence of this problem is high in some postoperative settings. For example, postoperative delirium reportedly developed in 37% of nondemented patients following hip fracture repair. The significance of this finding is underscored by the observation that among those who experienced delirium after surgery, frank dementia developed in 69% over a subsequent 5-year period of follow-up (compared with a 20% incidence in those without postoperative delirium). Further, patients with postoperative cognitive dysfunction at discharge have been reported to die within the first year after surgery.

Although usually a transient phenomenon, clinicians should focus on the detection and treatment of correctable causes of acute delirium arising postoperatively. These include metabolic disturbances (hyponatremia, hypoxemia) medications (which might be discontinued), infection, and various acute conditions (eg, respiratory failure, myocardial infarction, cardiac arrhythmias, congestive heart failure, pulmonary embolism, and fat embolism syndrome). Likewise, elderly patients and patients with underlying neurologic conditions (eg, parkinsonism) should be considered a high risk population. Formal neurologic consultation and work-up is generally unrevealing. The incidence of postoperative delirium can be reduced by proactive geriatric consultation.

Peripheral Nerve Injuries

Peripheral nerve injuries arise more often after upper and lower extremity surgery, most often a consequence of excessive traction on the nerve, direct compression on the nerve due to prolonged intraoperative positioning of the extremity or subsequently as a result of a cast. Early detection and intervention is critical to the ultimate outcome in these circumstances. Patients with antecedent neurologic disease (such as neuropathies associated with diabetes mellitus or spinal stenosis) are at increased risk for nerve injury.

10. Emotional/Psychiatric Problems

Patients living with a chronic rheumatic disease or disabling orthopedic condition may experience emotional difficulties due to chronic pain, disability, impaired social interactions and personal relationships, and constrained career opportunities. Because surgery is a significant life stress, such individuals may require additional emotional support perioperatively. Further, some patients may be taking or require antidepressant or anti-anxiolytic medication. In general, these medications may be continued throughout the perioperative period; however, monoamine oxidase inhibitors must be discontinued 10–14 days before surgery. Monoamine oxidase inhibitors may cause circulatory instability in patients receiving general anesthesia or certain opioids, especially meperidine.

POSTOPERATIVE MANAGEMENT OF COMPLICATIONS

1. Venous Thromboembolism

Prevention & Treatment

Venous thromboembolism following orthopedic surgery is the most studied postoperative complication. Pulmonary embolism remains an important cause of postoperative mortality. While treatment paradigms presented in the orthopedic surgery literature have focused on lower extremity arthroplasty, a recent study suggests that these treatment paradigms should also be considered after total shoulder arthroplasty, where the risk of thromboembolism may be higher than generally appreciated.

Virtually every surgery provokes a prothrombotic state. Thus, it is not whether prophylaxis is indicated but rather which approach should be used. After orthopedic surgery, a complicated balance exists between a possible life-threatening pulmonary embolus and the potential for postoperative bleeding. Numerous protocols have documented the effectiveness of starting a prevention regimen at the time of the procedure. Expeditious surgery reduces the risk of venous thrombosis as does the type of anesthesia. Epidural anesthesia reduces the risk of proximal deep venous thrombosis following total hip replacement by 2- to 3-fold and also reduces

the overall risk of venous thrombosis by at least 20%. Other intraoperative interventions, such as hypotensive anesthesia and intraoperative heparin administration, further reduce thrombogenesis. Mechanical methods of reducing risk of thromboembolism also have proven efficacy and include pneumatic compression boots, foot pumps, compression stockings, foot flexion/extension exercises, and early ambulation. These maneuvers are safe, effective, and do not increase the risk of bleeding.

The mainstay of prevention is prophylactic anticoagulation, which should begin immediately following surgery. Regimens include aspirin, warfarin (with a target INR of 2.0–2.5), low-molecular-weight heparin (LMWH) and recently the newer agents (dabigatran, rivaroxaban) have been shown in clinical trials to have equivalent efficacy to LMWH. Aspirin is also effective when combined with other modalities and continues to have its proponents, particularly in low-risk patients. A multimodal approach, relying on a combination of intraoperative modalities, postoperative mechanical devices, early ambulation, and low intensity postoperative anticoagulation, is preferred for the majority of patients by most experts and clinicians.

2. Fat Embolism Syndrome

The embolization of fat in the circulation is a well described complication of skeletal trauma and surgery, as well as procedures involving instrumentation of the femoral medullary canal. While it occurs in almost all patients who sustain hip or femoral fractures, the development of frank fat embolism syndrome occurs in relatively few; fat embolism syndrome develops in 1–3% of patients undergoing joint replacement surgery (particularly simultaneous bilateral procedures where it is presumably a "dose" effect) and in 5–10% of patients who have sustained multiple long bone fractures.

Clinical Findings

The signs and symptoms of fat embolism syndrome involve the respiratory, neurologic, hematologic, and cutaneous systems. Time of onset is variable. Hemodynamic instability may develop almost immediately (presaged by a rise in pulmonary artery pressure when the prosthesis is cemented) or insidiously over the first 2–3 days postoperatively. In the latter group, patients gradually become hypoxemic after surgery, may be hypotensive, and are often confused. Hematologic abnormalities, such as transient thrombocytopenia, are commonly seen. Respiratory signs are the most common manifestation of fat embolism syndrome. Mild to moderate hypoxemia and some radiographic changes (mainly bilateral alveolar infiltrates) develop in most patients. Acute respiratory distress syndrome (ARDS) develops in a minority of patients and requires aggressive supportive measures and intubation. Neurologic manifestations range from mild drowsiness to an acute confusional state to severe obtundation and coma, all consequences of the associated hypoxemia as well as the direct effect of the embolization of fat on the brain. The skin eruption, which is rare in the total joint arthroplasty patient, takes the form of a petechial rash involving the conjunctiva and oral mucosa and distributed over the folds of the neck and axillae. Retinal edema and hemorrhage are common.

▶ Treatment

Patients in whom fat embolism syndrome is suspected should be closely monitored; however, in most instances, the condition is generally clinically benign. Treatment is supportive and includes the administration of oxygen, the prevention of pulmonary hypertension by fluid restriction, and the use of diuretics and venodilators as well as pain management. Glucocorticoid therapy is not recommended. The condition resolves within 3–7 days in most patients, although the mortality rate remains in the 5–15% range in severe cases.

3. Antiphospholipid Syndrome

▶ Clinical Findings

Antiphospholipid syndrome consists of vascular thrombosis (or pregnancy-related morbidity) and arises as a consequence of the presence of antiphospholipid antibodies (aPL), usually the lupus anticoagulant or anticardiolipin antibodies. It occurs as a primary form or in association with an underlying connective tissue disease, most often systemic lupus erythematosus. Since patients with the antiphospholipid syndrome require long-term anticoagulation, perioperative management presents some challenges. The main challenge is balancing the patient's predisposition to thrombosis and the risk of postoperative bleeding.

▶ Treatment

When surgery is necessary, management should be guided by the following principles. First, conservative measures, including intermittent venous compression, should be used aggressively. Second, minimize the time anticoagulation is discontinued. Thus, for patients receiving long-term warfarin therapy, the medication should be stopped 3–4 days before surgery to allow the INR to normalize, while concomitant "bridging" therapy with LMWH is instituted at therapeutic dosages (1 mg/kg every 12 hours). LMWH should be continued until the night before surgery when it should be stopped. For many surgical procedures, particularly orthopedic surgery, warfarin can be restarted the night of the surgical procedure. If there is no contraindication, LMWH in prophylactic dosages (30 mg every 12 hours) can be restarted simultaneously with warfarin and maintained until a therapeutic INR has been achieved. It should be remembered that conventional dosages of these agents may result in "under coagulation" of patients with antiphospholipid syndrome and larger dosages, if feasible, may be considered necessary postoperatively, irrespective of the bleeding risk such therapy confers.

4. Hip Fracture

Hundreds of thousands of patients are hospitalized annually for treatment of a fractured hip, resulting in major costs to society, to patients, and to their families. Within the first year of fracture, 20% of elderly hip fracture patients die, compared with 9% of age-matched, non-fracture patients. Further, one sixth of those surviving 1 year after fracture are confined to long-term care facilities and another one third continue to require assistive devices or the help of others to manage their daily activities.

▶ Clinical Findings

Most hip fractures occur in frail, elderly women with osteoporosis who have fallen. Indeed, falls are the most common antecedent event and fractures are the most common serious fall-related injury. Risk factors for hip fracture include increasing age, poor general health, maternal history of hip fracture, a history of thyroid disease, poor depth perception, the use of psychoactive medication, sedentary lifestyle, and major life events.

The preoperative medical assessment and care of the patient with a fractured hip is very challenging. Because of the patient's age, frailty and functional compromise, existing comorbidities, and the poorer outcome when surgery is delayed, the opportunity to optimally evaluate and prepare such patients prior to surgery is limited and relies on general principles of perioperative care. Cardiac stress testing is not only difficult to perform in these cases, it is not helpful in this setting.

▶ Prognosis

Given the management challenges associated with patients who have sustained hip fracture, clinical pathways and other integrated co-management (medical-surgical) approaches have been reported both for hip fracture and total joint arthroplasty. The experience has been variable, although improvement in outcomes have been observed with such strategies in terms of length of stay, postoperative complications and mortality, readmission to hospital, and with respect to functional recovery. One study using proactive geriatric consultation reports a significant reduction in the incidence of postoperative delirium.

5. Cervical Spine Disease

▶ Clinical Findings & Treatment

Before a patient with advanced rheumatic disease undergoes surgery, cervical spine instability should be ruled out. In those patients with neck pain or crepitus on range of motion testing, radicular symptoms, or arm or leg weakness, flexion and extension radiographs should be obtained. Affected patients should wear a soft cervical collar to the operating room. When possible, epidural or spinal anesthesia should be used.

Additional problems arising from the rheumatoid disease process include involvement of the temporomandibular joint, which may limit jaw opening, and arthritis of the cricoarytenoid joints. Because these problems also may influence the choice of airway management, the anesthesiologist should be informed preoperatively about these manifestations of the disease process.

The converse situation arises in the patients with ankylosing spondylitis where the patient's rigid cervical spine may also present technical challenges for the anesthesiologist during intubation. Fiberoptic techniques are often used in this clinical setting.

6. Immunosuppressive/ Anti-Inflammatory Therapy

The potential contribution of glucocorticoids and other disease-modifying antirheumatic drugs (DMARDs) to the genesis of postoperative infection and wound dehiscence have been long recognized, although consensus pertaining to how to these medications should be managed in the perioperative setting has not been reached. The primary challenge is to achieve a balance between the control of the underlying disease while minimizing the risk of postoperative wound infection or breakdown. International study groups have recommended that anti-tumor necrosis factor agents should be discontinued for about 2–4 weeks. Some favor the 4-week interval for infliximab and adalimumab due to the longer half-lives of these agents. There is no information concerning postoperative infection and wound healing with the newer agents such as anakinra, rituximab, and abatacept. Recommendations similar to those of the other biologics will therefore have to suffice until more data can be gathered. Patient-related considerations should also be taken into account and influence decision-making. For example, in patients undergoing minor surgical procedures with an associated low risk of infection, the continuation of treatment through the perioperative period might be reasonable. However, even in this surgical setting, other patient-specific characteristics such as diabetes or prolonged glucocorticoid use would argue for an adherence to the above principles.

7. The Integument

As a result of long-term antirheumatic therapy (ie, glucocorticoids, immunosuppressive agents) or as a manifestation of the debilitating consequences of underlying rheumatic disease or orthopedic condition, skin integrity may be compromised before and after procedures in patients undergoing orthopedic surgery. In addition, delayed wound healing and a predisposition to infection may result from these influences.

The early institution of preventive measures to combat the development of decubitus ulcers (particularly of the heels and buttock region) is vital to an uncomplicated postoperative course.

8. The Eye

Patients taking long-term optic medication should have their eye drops instilled prior to surgery, especially if a prolonged procedure is anticipated. The one exception to this recommendation involves the use of phosphodiesterase inhibitors in the treatment of glaucoma. These agents may prolong the action of the neuromuscular blocker succinylcholine. This is particularly pertinent in patients with Sjögren syndrome who require artificial tears to prevent perioperative conjunctival injury.

Patients in the prone position are at risk for ocular injury secondary to external pressure. Patients with underlying vasculitis of the optic vessels are at particular risk for ischemic injury to the eye. Thus, the anesthesiologist must take particular care to position the patient carefully, avoiding excessive pressure on the eye and provide appropriate eye protection.

AAOS guidelines available at http://www.aaos.org/Research/guidelines/PE_guideline.pdf

Fleisher LA, Beckman JA, Brown KA, et al. ACC/AHA 2007 guidelines on perioperative cardiovascular evaluation and care for noncardiac surgery: a report of the American College of Cardiology/American Heart Association Task Force on Practice Guidelines. *J Am Coll Cardiol.* 2007;50:e242. [PMID: 17950140]

Goldman L, Caldera DL, Nussbaum SR, et al. Multifactorial index of cardiac risk in noncardiac surgical procedures. *N Engl J Med.* 1977;297:845. [PMID: 904659]

Holt NF, Silverman DG. Modeling perioperative risk: Can numbers speak louder than words? *Anesthesiol Clin.* 2006;24:427. [PMID: 17240601]

Lee HT, Marcantonio EF, Mangione CM, et al. Derivation and prospective validation of a simple index for prediction of cardiac risk of major noncardiac surgery. *Circulation.* 1999;10:1043. [PMID: 10477528]

MacKenzie CR. Perioperative Management of Rheumatoid Arthritis in Patients on Biologics. *Cont Topics in RA: Perioperative Management of Patients on Biologics.* 2008;2:2.

Monk TG, Weldon BC, Garvan CW, Dede DE, et al. Predictors of cognitive dysfunction after major noncardiac surgery. *Anesthesiology.* 2008;108:18. [PMID: 18156878]

Newman MF, Fleisher LA, Fink MP. *Perioperative Medicine: Managing for Outcome.* Philadelphia: Saunders Elsevier, 2008.

POISE Study Group; Devereaux PJ, Yang H, Yusuf S, et al. Effects of extended-release metoprolol succinate in patients undergoing non-cardiac surgery (POISE trial): a randomized controlled trial. *Lancet.* 2008;371:1839. [PMID: 18479744]

Smetana GW, Lawrence MD, Cornell JE. Preoperative pulmonary risk stratification for noncardiothoracic surgery: systematic review for the American College of Physicians. *Ann Intern Med.* 2006;144:581. [PMID: 16618956]

Smetana GW, Macpherson DS. The case against routine preoperative laboratory testing. *Med Clin North Am.* 2003;87:7. [PMID: 12575882]

Pulmonary Hypertension

Reda E. Girgis, MB, BCh

▶ Mean pulmonary artery pressure ≥25 mm Hg defines pulmonary hypertension.

▶ Values between 21 mm Hg and 24 mm Hg are considered borderline elevated.

▶ Pulmonary hypertension is classified as precapillary when the left heart filling pressure or pulmonary artery wedge pressure is ≤15 mm Hg.

▶ General Considerations

Pulmonary hypertension is among the most serious complications of rheumatic diseases. Pulmonary hypertension can be classified into one of five broad categories (Table 63–1). While rheumatic conditions can be associated with any classification of pulmonary hypertension (see Table 63–1), the most common category in which rheumatic conditions fall is pulmonary arterial hypertension—a pulmonary vasculopathy in the absence of left heart dysfunction, underlying parenchymal lung disease, thromboembolism, or other causes.

Connective tissue diseases accounted for one-quarter of all pulmonary arterial hypertension cases in REVEAL, a large US registry. Pulmonary arterial hypertension is particularly common in scleroderma or systemic sclerosis with a prevalence of 4–8%, and an estimated incidence of 0.61 cases per 100 patient years, accounting for 65% of connective tissue diseases associated with pulmonary arterial hypertension. In systemic sclerosis, pulmonary arterial hypertension typically occurs in older women (>80% female; mean age of 60 years) with limited scleroderma (up to 90%) and is more common among patients with late-onset systemic sclerosis. The average duration of systemic sclerosis prior to pulmonary arterial hypertension diagnosis varies from 4 to 14 years, but it can occur concomitant with or soon after disease onset.

The frequency of pulmonary arterial hypertension in other connective tissue diseases is not well characterized, but its occurrence is well recognized with lupus, representing 22% of all connective tissue disease–related pulmonary arterial hypertension, followed by rheumatoid arthritis at 9%. Features of systemic sclerosis are often present in such cases, ie, overlap syndrome or mixed connective tissue disease. In patients with lupus, the mean age at which pulmonary arterial hypertension is diagnosed is 46 years, and in the United States, most are nonwhite females.

Chronic interstitial lung disease is common in certain connective tissue diseases, particularly systemic sclerosis. Pulmonary hypertension complicates interstitial lung disease in about 30% of cases, depending on the extent of fibrosis. The combination of both pulmonary hypertension and interstitial lung disease portends a dramatically worse prognosis than either condition alone. In large series of systemic sclerosis patients undergoing evaluation for pulmonary hypertension, about one third of those with documented precapillary pulmonary hypertension had significant pulmonary fibrosis.

The most common type of pulmonary hypertension in the general population is that due to left heart disease, particularly nonsystolic left heart failure. Patients with rheumatic conditions may have left ventricular diastolic dysfunction associated with traditional cardiovascular risk factors or by virtue of direct cardiac involvement. Among patients with systemic sclerosis undergoing cardiac catheterization for suspected pulmonary arterial hypertension, 10–20% have elevated pulmonary artery wedge pressure indicative of left heart disease.

Chronic thromboembolic disease must be considered in any case of pulmonary hypertension, since surgical thromboendarterectomy can be curative. Antiphospholipid antibodies are present in 10% of such patients. Systemic vasculitides are rare causes of pulmonary hypertension, either due to direct vascular involvement or as a consequence of chronic parenchymal lung disease. In Takayasu arteritis, pulmonary hypertension has been noted in up to 12% of cases.

Table 63–1. Clinical classification of pulmonary hypertension.[a]

1. Pulmonary arterial hypertension
   1.1. Idiopathic
   1.2. Heritable
      1.2.1. BMPR2
      1.2.2. ALK1, endoglin
      1.2.3. Unknown
   1.3. Drug- and toxin-induced
   1.4. Associated with
      1.4.1. Connective tissue disease (eg, scleroderma)
      1.4.2. HIV infection
      1.4.3. Portal hypertension (eg, due to autoimmune hepatitis)
      1.4.4. Congenital heart disease
      1.4.5. Schistosomiasis
      1.4.6. Chronic hemolytic anemia
   1.5. Persistent pulmonary hypertension of the newborn
      1.5.1. Pulmonary veno-occlusive disease and pulmonary capillary hemangiomatosis (well described in scleroderma)
2. Pulmonary hypertension owing to left heart disease
   2.1. Systolic dysfunction
   2.2. Diastolic dysfunction
   2.3. Valvular disease
3. Pulmonary hypertension owing to lung disease or hypoxemia
   3.1. Chronic obstructive lung disease
   3.2. Interstitial lung disease (eg, associated with connective tissue diseases)
   3.3. Other pulmonary diseases with mixed restrictive and obstructive pattern
   3.4. Sleep-disordered breathing
   3.5. Alveolar hypoventilation disorders (eg, with neuromuscular disease)
   3.6. Chronic exposure to high altitude
   3.7. Developmental abnormalities
4. **Chronic thromboembolic pulmonary hypertension (eg, antiphospholipid antibody syndrome)**
5. Pulmonary hypertension with unclear multifactorial mechanisms
   5.1. Hematologic disorders: myeloproliferative disorders, splenectomy
   5.2. Systemic disorders: sarcoidosis, pulmonary Langerhans cell histiocytosis, lymphangioleiomyomatosis, neurofibromatosis, **vasculitis**
   5.3. Metabolic disorders: glycogen storage disease, Gaucher disease, thyroid disorders
   5.4. Others: tumoral obstruction, fibrosing mediastinitis, chronic renal failure on dialysis

[a]Bolded text indicate examples of pulmonary hypertension associated with rheumatologic diseases.
Data from World Health Organization Dana Point Conference, 2008.

A high degree of suspicion for the diagnosis is required, since symptoms of dyspnea and fatigue are often nonspecific. A comprehensive clinical testing algorithm is required to confirm the diagnosis, exclude other causes, and assess disease severity. Recent advances in the therapy of pulmonary arterial hypertension have improved the outlook considerably,

but mortality remains high. Collaboration with a pulmonary hypertension specialist is important to optimize long-term outcomes.

▶ Pathology & Pathophysiology

The pulmonary circulation is a low pressure, low resistance circuit designed to accommodate large changes in venous return with minimal increases in pressure. Over 50% of the vascular bed must be obstructed or destroyed before resting pulmonary artery pressure begins to rise. In pulmonary arterial hypertension, the site of obstruction is the small muscular pulmonary arteries and precapillary arterioles. Characteristic, although nonspecific, vascular lesions consist of concentric laminar and nonlaminar intimal fibrosis with lumenal obliteration (Figure 63–1) and eccentric intimal fibrosis, which may represent residua of thrombosis in situ. Medial hypertrophy and adventitial fibrosis may also be present to variable degrees. Plexiform lesions, which are complex glomerular-like sinusoidal channels lined by proliferating endothelial cells that may represent an attempt to bypass downstream obstruction or a precursor to concentric-obliterative lesions, are conspicuously rare or absent in systemic sclerosis-pulmonary arterial hypertension, compared with idiopathic pulmonary arterial hypertension. Another distinctive feature of systemic sclerosis-pulmonary arterial hypertension is the frequent occurrence of venous remodeling with features of pulmonary veno-occlusive disease. Focal perivascular accumulations of lymphocytes accompany the vascular lesions, but a true vasculitis is rare. With interstitial lung disease, vascular obliteration and destruction is

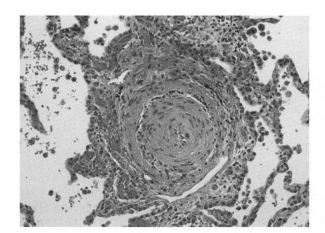

▲ **Figure 63–1.** Photomicrograph (H&E) demonstrating vascular obliteration by concentric laminar intimal proliferation in pulmonary arterial hypertension associated with scleroderma.

routinely present in areas of fibrosis, with normal vessels elsewhere. When severe pulmonary hypertension is present, diffuse vascular remodeling is typically observed in the lung.

Pulmonary vascular obstruction induces abnormalities in both gas exchange and cardiac function. Reduced pulmonary blood flow relative to ventilation leads to wasted ventilation or dead space physiology. As a result, minute ventilation must rise to avoid hypercapnia. Indeed, one of the earliest and characteristic findings of pulmonary vascular disease on cardiopulmonary exercise testing is an increase in dead space fraction and minute ventilation relative to carbon dioxide production with exercise. Obliteration of the capillary bed limits transit time with resultant exercise-induced hypoxemia. Resting oxygen desaturation suggests right-to-left shunting (either intrapulmonary due to opening of arteriovenous communications or cardiac related due to opening of a patent foramen ovale as a result of raised right atrial pressure) or the presence of low ventilation/perfusion ($\dot{V}/\dot{Q}$) units. The latter occurs in the setting of parenchymal lung disease (eg, interstitial lung disease). Superimposed pulmonary vascular disease dramatically worsens hypoxemia associated with $\dot{V}/\dot{Q}$ mismatching because the ability of the lung to redirect blood flow to better ventilated units is impaired.

Increased pulmonary vascular resistance initially induces concentric right ventricular hypertrophy to compensate for the increased afterload. This allows the cardiac output to be normal at rest and even with exercise early in the disease course. With progressive increases in pulmonary vascular resistance, the right ventricle begins to dilate, inducing a volume load due to tricuspid regurgitation, in addition to the pressure load. Stroke volume and ultimately cardiac output is unable to increase appropriately with exercise and begins to fall at rest. Right atrial pressure rises, leading to systemic vascular congestion. Massive dilatation of the right ventricle compromises left ventricular filling, further impairing cardiac performance. The dilated, hypertensive right ventricle has an increased oxygen demand. This, combined with low systemic blood pressure (resulting in reduced right coronary perfusion pressure gradient), creates a relative right ventricular ischemia that likely plays a role in the development of progressive right heart failure, the primary cause of death in pulmonary arterial hypertension.

► Clinical Findings

A. Symptoms and Signs

Dyspnea with activity is the most common complaint in pulmonary arterial hypertension and is the presenting symptom in most cases. The degree of functional limitation based on the New York Heart Association classification has important prognostic implications. Fatigue, chest pain, exertional syncope or near-syncope, palpitations, and leg edema are other frequent complaints. In systemic sclerosis, skin thickening may reduce the tendency for leg edema, and fluid may preferentially accumulate in the abdomen.

Pulmonary hypertension complicating interstitial lung disease is often heralded by abrupt worsening of dyspnea that had been previously stable for years and by an increase or new requirement for supplemental oxygen. Diffuse cutaneous involvement is present in over half of patients who have combined interstitial lung disease and pulmonary hypertension. Raynaud phenomenon and antiphospholipid antibodies (in the absence of thromboembolism) are more prevalent in lupus associated–pulmonary arterial hypertension compared with lupus patients without pulmonary arterial hypertension.

Physical examination findings of pulmonary hypertension include a left parasternal lift of right ventricular hypertrophy, an accentuated pulmonic component of the second heart sound, a holosystolic murmur of tricuspid insufficiency and a right ventricular gallop. Elevated jugular venous pressure, hepatomegaly, ascites, and lower extremity edema indicate right ventricular decompensation. Systemic hypertension suggests left ventricular diastolic dysfunction as the potential cause of pulmonary hypertension, whereas low blood pressure may signify right heart failure. Bibasilar crackles are often present with interstitial lung disease.

B. Initial Diagnostic Testing

A structured diagnostic approach is required to establish the correct diagnosis. Patients with symptoms and signs suggestive of pulmonary hypertension should undergo initial evaluation with a chest radiograph, pulmonary function testing, and Doppler echocardiography. The latter is a useful screening tool for pulmonary hypertension. It can demonstrate right heart enlargement (Figure 63–2) and right ventricular hypokinesis as well as provide an estimate of right ventricular

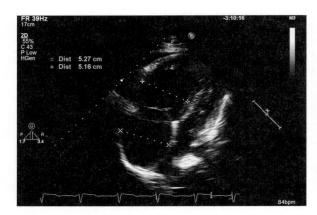

▲ **Figure 63–2.** Transthoracic echocardiogram, apical 4-chamber view in patient with severe pulmonary arterial hypertension. Note marked right atrial (RA) and right ventricular enlargement relative to the left heart chambers. PE denotes small pericardial effusion.

(and hence pulmonary artery) systolic pressure (RVSP) based on the modified Bernoulli equation where $RVSP = 4v^2 + $ right atrial pressure estimate, where v is the maximal tricuspid regurgitant velocity. The upper limit of normal for RVSP is 35 mm Hg and increases with age. However, RVSP estimates can be inaccurate, with both overestimations and underestimations of more than 10–20 mm Hg common. Another potential source of error is the right atrial pressure estimate. Many echocardiogram laboratories routinely add 10 mm Hg for right atrial pressure, whereas the normal right atrial pressure in the absence of right heart dysfunction is 3–5 mm Hg. As a result, the sensitivity and specificity of echocardiography using a cutoff RVSP of 40 mm Hg for detecting pulmonary hypertension confirmed by invasive hemodynamics can be as low as 75% and 60%, respectively. Thus, echocardiographic findings should not be solely relied upon to diagnose or exclude pulmonary hypertension but rather should be combined with other clinical features to ascertain the likelihood of pulmonary hypertension. Other echocardiographic findings suggestive of pulmonary hypertension include flattening of the interventricular septum and reduced pulmonary artery acceleration time. Doppler echocardiography also provides important information on left heart structure and function as a potential cause for pulmonary hypertension. Pericardial effusion is present in roughly one third of patients with pulmonary arterial hypertension-systemic sclerosis and is associated with increased mortality, likely reflecting increased right atrial pressure and right ventricular failure.

Expert consensus panels have recommended annual screening echocardiography in systemic sclerosis patients, irrespective of symptoms. Such a strategy has the potential to uncover mild pulmonary arterial hypertension that may be more responsive to therapy. However, the benefits and cost-effectiveness of this approach remain to be demonstrated. It is rare for a patient with pulmonary arterial hypertension to be truly asymptomatic unless physical activity is limited by other factors, eg, musculoskeletal conditions. Exercise echocardiography is currently being investigated as a potential screening method for pulmonary hypertension in systemic sclerosis.

A chest radiograph typically demonstrates cardiomegaly due to right heart enlargement and dilated central pulmonary arteries with significant pulmonary hypertension. The lung fields are clear in pulmonary arterial hypertension, whereas the presence of extensive reticular opacities signifies interstitial lung disease as the cause of pulmonary hypertension. Pulmonary vascular congestion and pleural effusions suggest left heart failure.

Pulmonary function testing is a key assessment in any patient with suspected pulmonary hypertension and in particular, those with connective tissue disease. Annual screening pulmonary function testing is recommended in systemic sclerosis. A reduced total lung capacity (TLC <80% predicted) or forced vital capacity (FVC) indicates a restrictive ventilatory defect as seen with interstitial lung disease, whereas a low forced expiratory volume in 1 second

over the (FEV_1/FVC <0.7) points to airflow limitation as in emphysema or bronchiolitis. Lung volumes and expiratory flow rates are normal or mildly reduced in pulmonary arterial hypertension. The diffusing capacity of the lung for carbon monoxide (DLCO) measures the rate of uptake of inspired CO by hemoglobin and reflects the capacity of the lung to transfer oxygen across the alveolar-capillary membrane. The determinants of DLCO are lung volume, distribution of ventilation, the diffusion properties of the membrane, the pulmonary capillary blood volume, and hemoglobin concentration. Both interstitial and pulmonary vascular diseases produce variable reductions in the membrane and capillary blood volume components. The DLCO is often severely decreased in pulmonary arterial hypertension associated with systemic sclerosis. In one series, a threshold of <50% of predicted had a specificity of 90% for pulmonary arterial hypertension in systemic sclerosis, but sensitivity was only 39%. In the setting of interstitial lung disease, the onset of pulmonary hypertension is often heralded by an abrupt decline in DLCO without an accompanying fall in lung volumes or radiographic progression of disease. In both pulmonary arterial hypertension and pulmonary hypertension combined with interstitial lung disease, the DLCO typically remains low after correcting for alveolar volume (DL/VA), also known as transfer coefficient or KCO. This ratio adjusts for reductions in DLCO due to low lung volume and heterogeneous ventilation. In another study, a DL/VA <70% of predicted had a sensitivity of 88% and specificity of 80% for the presence of pulmonary arterial hypertension in systemic sclerosis. Decreased diffusing capacity may also have utility in predicting the subsequent development of pulmonary arterial hypertension.

Circulating levels of brain natriuretic peptide (BNP) and N-terminal-proBNP are increasingly utilized as adjunctive tests in the evaluation of pulmonary hypertension. These markers of neurohormonal activation are released by ventricular myocardium in response to increased wall stress and have demonstrated modest correlations with measures of right ventricular dysfunction and mortality in pulmonary arterial hypertension. As a screening test for pulmonary arterial hypertension in systemic sclerosis, one study reported a sensitivity and specificity of 45% and 90%, respectively, for N-terminal-proBNP above a cut-off value of 239 pg/mL. BNP, which is not influenced by renal dysfunction, performed slightly better with a sensitivity of 60% and specificity of 87% at the optimal threshold of 64 pg/mL. Similarly, electrocardiography often demonstrates signs of right heart strain but lacks sufficient sensitivity to exclude pulmonary hypertension.

C. Additional Studies

Once pulmonary hypertension is suspected based on the initial assessment, additional testing is indicated. Screening for thromboembolic disease is mandatory if pulmonary hypertension is confirmed. Perfusion lung scanning is preferred as the initial modality because it avoids the need for intravenous contrast and may be more sensitive than spiral CT angiography. If one or more segmental perfusion defects are identified, further investigation with CT or pulmonary angiogram is indicated. High-resolution CT (HRCT) is useful to assess for the presence and extent of interstitial lung disease and other parenchymal pathologies.

Arterial blood gases should be obtained to exclude hypoxemia, since reliable pulse oximetry recordings can be difficult to obtain in the setting of digital ischemia. Hypercapnia indicates hypoventilation, which can be seen with diaphragmatic weakness in cases of myositis. $PaCO_2$ is typically normal or low in pulmonary arterial hypertension. An overnight polysomnogram should be considered if obstructive sleep apnea is suspected.

Pulmonary arterial hypertension is often associated with abnormal thyroid function, which can have a profound impact on cardiac function. Other causes of pulmonary arterial hypertension should be considered, including HIV and chronic liver disease. Hyponatremia and azotemia are strong prognostic markers in pulmonary arterial hypertension, reflecting right heart failure. Assessment of exercise capacity with a 6-minute walk distance is essential to gauge the severity of disease and as a baseline for comparison with serial measurements to monitor response to therapy.

D. Cardiac Catheterization

While noninvasive testing can suggest a diagnosis of pulmonary hypertension, right heart catheterization (RHC) is required to (1) confirm the presence of elevated pulmonary artery pressure, (2) exclude elevated left heart filling pressure as the cause, and (3) fully characterize the severity of disease. While severe elevations in Doppler estimated RVSP are likely to represent true pulmonary hypertension, more modest elevations (35–55 mm Hg) are not infrequently false-positives. Importantly, the false-negative rate of echocardiographic screening for pulmonary hypertension in connective tissue diseases is not well defined.

RHC is mandatory to confirm or exclude pulmonary hypertension because it can detect pulmonary arterial hypertension in a substantial proportion of patients who have systemic sclerosis and suspected pulmonary arterial hypertension (based on otherwise unexplained dyspnea or reduced DLCO). RHC is also required to measure the left heart filling pressure or pulmonary artery wedge pressure. Pulmonary hypertension is considered as being at least partly due to left heart disease if the pulmonary artery wedge pressure exceeds 15 mm Hg (normal: 8–12 mm Hg). Frequently, the elevated pulmonary artery wedge pressure is not accompanied by clear left heart abnormalities on echocardiogram. Careful attention to technical detail is often required to obtain a reliable and accurate wedge tracing. In rare cases, inability to wedge the catheter may require left heart catheterization to record left ventricular end-diastolic pressure.

Since prognosis in pulmonary arterial hypertension is mostly closely related to right ventricular function rather than pulmonary artery pressure, direct hemodynamic measurements of cardiac performance are critical in the assessment of disease severity. Cardiac output, stroke volume, right atrial pressure and mixed venous oxygen saturation have all been shown to predict survival in pulmonary arterial hypertension. None can be reliably estimated by echocardiography. Cardiac MRI may be a useful noninvasive modality to measure cardiac output as well as other indices of right ventricular function and structure but remains to be validated.

In experienced hands, RHC is safe and well-tolerated. The reported complication rate in pulmonary hypertension patients is 1.1%. Complications (eg, hematoma at puncture site or transient arrhythmia) are mostly mild to moderate in severity and resolve without intervention. Nevertheless, RHC is invasive and procedure-related mortality is about 1 in 2000.

In connective tissue disease patients, expert consensus guidelines recommend RHC when estimated RVSP is >50 mm Hg. RHC should be considered when RVSP is >36 mm Hg or if there is other echocardiographic evidence of pulmonary hypertension, eg, dilated right heart chambers, particularly in symptomatic individuals. Several large systemic sclerosis centers use the following as indications for RHC: (1) estimated RVSP >40 mm Hg, (2) DLCO <50% of predicted in the absence of pulmonary fibrosis, or (3) unexplained dyspnea. With this approach, 60% have normal resting hemodynamics at RHC.

In idiopathic pulmonary arterial hypertension, a vasodilator challenge with inhaled nitric oxide or other acute pulmonary vasodilator is indicated to assess the degree of vasoreactivity. Patients with significant reactivity (defined as a ≥10 mm Hg fall in mean pulmonary artery pressure to an absolute value ≤40 mm Hg with no change or increase in cardiac output) are likely to derive an excellent clinical response from high-dose calcium channel blocker therapy. Such an outcome is observed in 7% of patients with idiopathic pulmonary arterial hypertension. However, less than 1% of connective tissue disease patients with pulmonary arterial hypertension are long-term responders to calcium channel blocker therapy, and thus an acute vasodilator challenge is unlikely to be of clinical utility. It is not indicated in the setting of pulmonary hypertension associated with interstitial lung disease or left heart disease. Acute vasoreactivity is not predictive of the clinical response to the pulmonary arterial hypertension specific therapies described below.

The role of exercise challenge during RHC in the diagnosis of pulmonary arterial hypertension remains to be fully characterized. Many centers obtain hemodynamics during exercise in patients with suspected pulmonary arterial hypertension and normal resting mean pulmonary artery pressure. However, the significance of exercise-induced pulmonary hypertension is unknown. Moreover, the definition of an abnormal response is not clearly defined. Mean pulmonary artery pressure can reach up to 47 mm Hg during exercise in older healthy volunteers. In this regards, resting mean pulmonary artery pressure at the upper range of normal or borderline elevated between 18 mm Hg and 24 mm Hg have been associated with higher mean pulmonary artery pressure during exercise and with reduced 6-minute walk distance in systemic sclerosis. An abrupt rise in pulmonary artery wedge pressure during exercise may support left heart disease as the basis of pulmonary hypertension, particularly when resting pulmonary artery wedge pressure is in the borderline range of 13–15 mm Hg. The upper limit of normal rise in pulmonary artery wedge pressure is 20–25 mm Hg.

Differential Diagnosis

Anemia, thyroid dysfunction and other metabolic and systemic disorders need to be considered as potential causes of dyspnea and fatigue. Many pulmonary and cardiac diseases can share clinical features of pulmonary hypertension. Interstitial lung disease is the most common entity in the differential diagnosis, both as an alternate cause for symptoms of pulmonary hypertension and as the basis for pulmonary hypertension. HRCT findings of interstitial lung disease consist of reticular and ground-glass opacities with a basal and subpleural predominance and honeycombing in advanced cases. Pulmonary function tests demonstrate reduced lung volumes. Some degree of interstitial lung disease can be detected by HRCT in most patients with systemic sclerosis patients; thus, the distinction between pulmonary arterial hypertension and pulmonary hypertension associated with interstitial lung disease is arbitrary. Most clinical trials of pulmonary arterial hypertension therapies have defined the absence of significant interstitial lung disease (and hence defining pulmonary arterial hypertension) as a TLC >70% of predicted or a TLC between 60% and 70% with no more than mild changes on HRCT. However, extensive radiographic changes can occasionally be observed in patients with preserved lung volumes. On the other hand, lung volumes can be low from obesity or respiratory muscle weakness with no or minimal radiographic evidence of interstitial lung disease. A more accurate approach may be to begin with the HRCT. Extensive disease, defined as more than 30% of the lung involved, is associated with disease progression, whereas limited disease is defined as ≤10% of lung involvement as seen on HRCT. When HRCT is indeterminate (10–30% involvement), an FVC threshold of 70% predicted is used to distinguish between limited and extensive interstitial lung disease. The distinction is of more than academic importance. Combined pulmonary hypertension-interstitial lung disease is associated with dramatically worse outcomes than isolated pulmonary arterial hypertension in systemic sclerosis and therapies specific for pulmonary arterial hypertension have the potential to worsen gas exchange (see below).

Precapillary pulmonary hypertension in patients who have diffuse centrilobular ground-glass opacities, septal lines, and mediastinal lymphadenopathy demonstrated on HRCT raises the possibility of pulmonary veno-occlusive disease or pulmonary capillary hemangiomatosis, which can secondarily lead to compression of small pulmonary veins. Both entities have been well described in systemic sclerosis, and

significant hypoxemia is more common and more severe than in pulmonary arterial hypertension and may be refractory to supplemental oxygen therapy due to intrapulmonary shunting from alveolar edema. Pulmonary edema can be precipitated or exacerbated with vasodilator therapy.

Orthopnea, paroxysmal nocturnal dyspnea, and cardiovascular risk factors (such as systemic hypertension, diabetes mellitus, and coronary artery disease) point toward left heart disease as the basis for pulmonary hypertension. Left atrial enlargement, left ventricular hypertrophy, atrial fibrillation, and Doppler evidence of diastolic dysfunction also suggest left heart disease. Abnormalities in left ventricular diastolic function by echocardiography have been observed in 18% of systemic sclerosis patients. An overt restrictive cardiomyopathy can result from direct myocardial involvement. Left-sided valvular abnormalities, in particular aortic stenosis and mitral regurgitation, are also common underlying causes of pulmonary hypertension. Constrictive pericarditis should be considered in the setting of apparent right heart failure with no or mild pulmonary hypertension.

Treatment

A. General Measures

When an underlying condition is identified as the cause of pulmonary hypertension (eg, systemic blood pressure in left heart disease), efforts to optimize that condition should be pursued. Diuretics are extremely valuable in managing the systemic congestion of right heart failure and often lead to improvement in dyspnea. Care should be taken to avoid agents that can induce systemic hypotension (eg, intravenous anesthetic agents), since these agents are poorly tolerated in the setting of a dilated, failing right ventricle. In such cases, calcium channel blockers should be used sparingly for digital ischemia and better avoided if possible. As previously discussed, it is the exceedingly rare patient with connective tissue disease who is responsive to high-dose calcium channel blocker therapy for pulmonary arterial hypertension; this therapy should only be considered after acute vasoreactivity has been documented. Other negative inotropes, such as β-blockers, should also be avoided. Digoxin is preferable for initial rate control in atrial fibrillation or flutter. These arrhythmias are often poorly tolerated and should be dealt with aggressively to achieve resumption of sinus rhythm. Supplemental oxygen is prescribed for resting hypoxemia (PaO_2 <60 mm Hg). Ambulatory oxygen may be of symptomatic benefit when there is correctable desaturation with exercise. Physical activity should be encouraged as tolerated and formal pulmonary rehabilitation may be of considerable benefit.

Long-term oral anticoagulation is generally recommended in idiopathic pulmonary arterial hypertension based on limited data. However, no such data are available in pulmonary arterial hypertension associated with systemic sclerosis or other connective tissue diseases and these patients are at increased risk for gastrointestinal bleeding. Whether

Table 63–2. Currently available agents for pulmonary arterial hypertension.

Drug Name	Route	Dose/Frequency	Recommended for Functional Class	FDA Approval	Limitations/Drawbacks
Prostacyclin analogues					
Epoprostenol	Intravenous	Variable/Continuous	III–IV	1996	Delivery system
Treprostinil	Subcutaneous	Variable Continuous	III–IV	2002	Infusion site pain
Treprostinil	Intravenous	Variable/Continuous	III–IV	2004	Delivery system
Iloprost	Inhaled	5 mcg six to nine times daily	III–IV	2005	Frequent dosing
Treprostinil	Inhaled	Four times daily	III–IV	2009	Airway irritation
Endothelin receptor antagonists					
Bosentan	Oral	125 mg twice daily	II–IV	2001	Hepatoxicity
Ambrisentan	Oral	5–10 mg once daily	II–IV	2007	Fluid retention
Sitaxsentan	Oral	100 mg once daily	II–IV	Licensed in Europe (2006), Canada and Australia	Hepatoxicity
Phosphodiesterase-type 5 inhibitors					
Sildenafil	Oral	20–80 mg three times daily	II–IV	2005	Optimal long-term dose unknown
Tadalafil	Oral	40 mg once daily	II–IV	2009	Limited long-term data

anticoagulation should be used if antiphospholipid antibodies are present in the absence of thromboembolism is not known. Once chronic thromboembolic disease is identified, referral to a center experienced in thromboendarterectomy to assess surgical candidacy should not be delayed.

There have been anecdotal reports of clinical response to immunosuppressive therapy for pulmonary arterial hypertension associated with lupus and mixed connective tissue disease, but not with systemic sclerosis. In practice, such therapy is often used for other indications of disease activity and pulmonary arterial hypertension specific therapy is given concomitantly.

B. Specific Therapies for Pulmonary Arterial Hypertension

Currently available therapies for pulmonary arterial hypertension fall into one of three pharmacologic classes: prostacyclin analogues, endothelin-receptor antagonists (ETRA), and phosphodiesterase type 5 (PDE-5) inhibitors (Table 63–2). All these drugs have been shown to increase mean 6-minute walk distance as the primary outcome measure in short-term (12–16 weeks) randomized, controlled trials. Variable improvements in secondary outcomes have been observed, such as functional class, quality of life, and time to clinical worsening (typically defined as death, lung transplant, hospitalization for pulmonary arterial hypertension, need for additional therapy, or deterioration in functional class combined with a fall in 6-minute walk distance). Hemodynamic changes, when assessed, consist of a mean 10–25% increase in cardiac output

with smaller reductions in mean pulmonary artery pressure. Direct head-to-head comparison data between agents are sparse. For most pulmonary arterial hypertension patients with functional class II-III limitations, initial therapy with an oral agent from one of the two latter classes is appropriate. Continuous intravenous epoprostenol is recommended for functional class IV. Sequential combination therapy is often used when the clinical response to initial therapy is inadequate. Ideally, the treatment goals listed in Table 63–3 should be targeted, since these are associated with good long-term survival.

Table 63–3. Treatment goals in pulmonary arterial hypertension.

Parameter	Target Goal
NYHA functional class	Stable I-II
6-minute walk distance	>400 m or 75% of predicted
Clinical examination	Absence of signs of right heart failure
BNP or N-terminal-proBNP levels	Normal or near normal
Echocardiogram	No pericardial effusion; good right ventricular function
Hemodynamics	Normal right atrial pressure and cardiac output

BNP, brain natriuretic peptide; NYHA, New York Heart Association.

1. Phosphodiesterase type-5 inhibitors—PDE-5 inhibitors prevent the catabolism of cyclic guanosine monophosphate, the second messenger mediating most of the vascular effects of nitric oxide, such as vascular smooth muscle relaxation. Sildenafil is likely the most commonly prescribed drug for pulmonary arterial hypertension. The approved dose is 20 mg three times daily. Many clinicians escalate the dose up to 80 mg three times daily, but the effectiveness of this approach has not been demonstrated. Tadalafil is a long-acting, once daily PDE-5 inhibitor. Common, but usually self-limited, adverse effects include headache, flushing, gastrointestinal symptoms, and myalgia. The prescribing information for these agents contain warnings regarding sudden loss of vision (due to non–arteritic anterior ischemic optic neuropathy) and hearing, but the relationship of these rare occurrences to treatment is not determined. Minor visual disturbances consisting of color tinge, sensitivity to light, and blurred vision can occur with sildenafil due to inhibition of retinal PDE-6, which is not affected by tadalafil. Nasal congestion is a possible side effect with both PDE-5 inhibitors and ETRAs.

2. Endothelin receptor antagonists—The introduction of bosentan, a nonselective ETRA, blocking both the A and B receptors, marked a major advance in pulmonary arterial hypertension therapy, representing the first oral agent approved for this disease. The main adverse effect is a roughly 10% annual incidence of reversible elevations in hepatic transaminase levels requiring drug discontinuation in <5%. In an attempt to improve upon the efficacy of bosentan, ETRAs that selectively block the A receptor have been developed. The A receptor, localized to vascular smooth muscle, cardiomyocytes, and fibroblasts, is thought to mediate most of the vasculopathic effects of endothelin, whereas the B receptor, expressed predominantly on endothelial cells, is capable of inducing vasodilatation via release of prostacyclin and nitric oxide and is involved in clearance of circulating endothelin. However, this theoretical benefit of selective ETRA-A antagonism has not been substantiated in clinical trials and there are data to support a role for ETRA-B receptor activation in vascular smooth muscle and myofibroblast proliferation. Sitaxsentan, a highly selective ETR-A antagonist, was the first such compound to be tested in pulmonary arterial hypertension. Efficacy and safety have been comparable to effects observed with bosentan. Sitaxsentan is not approved by the US FDA, but it is licensed in Europe, Canada, and Australia.

Ambrisentan is a propanoic acid–based selective ETRA that is structurally distinct from bosentan and sitaxsentan, which are sulfonamide based. Efficacy in short-term clinical trials has been comparable to other oral agents in pulmonary arterial hypertension. Open label follow-up at 2 years has been reported and indicates sustained efficacy with clinical worsening in 28% of study participants. As anticipated by the different chemical structure and preclinical data, the frequency of elevated transaminase levels with ambrisentan has been considerably lower than that observed with other ETRAs, with an annual rate of ~2%, requiring discontinuation of drug in <1%. Nevertheless, given the experience with other ETRAs, monthly monitoring of liver function is currently mandated for all agents in this class. Peripheral edema and fluid retention also appear to be adverse effects common to this pharmacologic class, observed in 17% of patients treated with ambrisentan and in 8% of those treated with bosentan. The mechanisms are not clear and may involve increased capillary permeability from vasodilatation, renal sodium, and water retention or negative inotropic action on the myocardium. As a result, these drugs should be used cautiously in patients with overt right heart failure.

3. Prostacyclin analogues—Continuous intravenous epoprostenol is generally regarded as the gold standard therapy and is recommended as the first-line agent for patients with the most advanced symptoms. It is the only agent shown to reduce mortality in a 12-week, randomized, controlled study of idiopathic pulmonary arterial hypertension patients. The chief drawback of epoprostenol is related to its delivery system. It requires daily reconstitution and mixing of drug, maintaining the mixed drug under refrigeration or on ice, operation of a battery-operated pump and continuous infusion via a long-term central venous catheter. Beyond the inconvenience, catheter-related bloodstream infections and rebound pulmonary hypertension upon abrupt discontinuation are potentially life-threatening complications. Drug-related adverse effects, such as gastrointestinal and musculoskeletal complaints and a neuropathic type of lower extremity pain, can limit dosage.

To avoid the cumbersome nature of the intravenous delivery system, treprostinil, a prostacyclin analogue that is chemically stable at room temperature and is suitable for continuous subcutaneous administration was developed. While the subcutaneous delivery system offers several advantages over intravenous delivery, infusion site pain is extremely common and sufficiently severe to result in discontinuation in 23% of patients. Treprostinil can also be infused intravenously, where it still offers some advantages in terms of convenience over epoprostenol while avoiding local infusion site reactions; however, the risk of catheter-related bloodstream infections persists.

The inhaled route of prostanoid delivery offers an attractive alternative to continuous infusion. Inhaled iloprost and treprostinil have both been shown to have modest, but variable, efficacy when added to an oral pulmonary arterial hypertension regimen. They are associated with similar drug-related adverse effects, including cough, throat irritation, headache, flushing, and nausea. Oral prostacyclin analogues and receptor agonists are currently under investigation.

▶ **Complications**

The introduction of pulmonary arterial hypertension specific therapies has clearly had a beneficial impact on the natural history of these diseases. However, morbidity and mortality

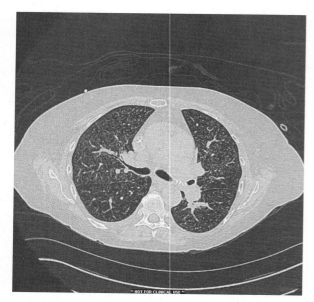

▲ **Figure 63–3.** High-resolution CT image of lung showing diffuse centrilobular ground-glass opacities and interlobular septal thickening. This patient had pulmonary arterial hypertension associated with scleroderma; the patient's dyspnea worsened and hypoxemia associated with the new development of these radiographic findings developed after the patient started therapy with intravenous epoprostenol. Autopsy revealed changes of pulmonary veno-occlusive disease.

remain high, and this is particularly true for connective tissue disease–related pulmonary arterial hypertension. A large UK registry reported a 3-year survival of only 47% in systemic sclerosis-pulmonary arterial hypertension, despite aggressive therapy. Survival was considerably better (75%) among lupus patients with pulmonary arterial hypertension. Large series of idiopathic pulmonary arterial hypertension studies reported 3-year survival rates ranging from 63% to 75%. The basis for the poor outcomes in systemic sclerosis is not clear and may include older age, more obliterative pulmonary vascular pathology, concomitant interstitial lung disease and comorbidity (including renal and intrinsic cardiac disease).

The efficacy and safety of these drugs has only been demonstrated in pulmonary arterial hypertension. Their off-label use in other types of pulmonary arterial hypertension has not been studied. In the setting of parenchymal lung disease, pulmonary vasodilators have the potential to worsen oxygenation by increasing blood flow to poorly ventilated units and intra-pulmonary shunting. Clinically significant deterioration in gas exchange has been observed with the use of pulmonary arterial hypertension specific therapy, particularly intravenous prostacyclins, in pulmonary hypertension associated with interstitial lung disease. The prognosis

in pulmonary hypertension combined with moderate-severe interstitial lung disease in systemic sclerosis is particularly grim with a 3-year survival of less than 30%. Worsening hypoxemia combined with new or increasing ground-glass opacities on HRCT suggests pulmonary veno-occlusive disease or pulmonary capillary hemangiomatosis, where increased pulmonary arterial inflow is impeded by venous obstruction (Figure 63–3). In the setting of left heart failure, these agents have the potential to exacerbate pulmonary congestion if the increased venous return to the left side cannot be accommodated. Intravenous epoprostenol increased mortality, and ETRAs were associated with increased hospitalizations and edema in left ventricular systolic failure.

Lung transplantation is a viable option in selected cases, although esophageal dysmotility and other comorbidities may complicate the posttransplantation course. Atrial septostomy is a rarely used, palliative intervention that can unload the right heart through creation of a right to left inter-atrial shunt. Several new pharmacologic targets are currently being investigated in pulmonary arterial hypertension, including tyrosine-kinase inhibitors, soluble guanylate cyclase stimulators, and serotonin receptor antagonists.

Avouac J, Airo P, Meune C, et al. Prevalence of pulmonary hypertension in systemic sclerosis in European Caucasians and metaanalysis of 5 studies. *J Rheumatol.* 2010;37:2290. [PMID: 20810505]

Cavagna L, Caporali R, Klersy C, et al. Comparison of brain natriuretic peptide (BNP) and NT-proBNP in screening for pulmonary arterial hypertension in patients with systemic sclerosis. *J Rheumatol.* 2010;37:2064. [PMID: 20634241]

Chung L, Liu J, Parsons L, et al. Characterization of connective tissue disease-associated pulmonary arterial hypertension the REVEAL: identifying systemic sclerosis as a unique phenotype. *Chest.* 2010;138:1383. [PMID: 20507945]

Condliffe R, Kiely DG, Peacock AJ, et al. Connective tissue disease-associated pulmonary arterial hypertension in the modern treatment era. *Am J Respir Crit Care Med.* 2009;179:151. [PMID: 18931333]

Hachulla E, de Groote P, Gressin V, et al. Itinér AIR-Sclérodermie Study Group. The three-year incidence of pulmonary arterial hypertension associated with systemic sclerosis in a multicenter nationwide longitudinal study in France. *Arthritis Rheum.* 2009;60:1831. [PMID: 19479881]

Le Pavec J, Humbert M, Mouthon L, Hassoun PM. Systemic sclerosis-associated pulmonary arterial hypertension. *Am J Respir Crit Care Med.* 2010;181:1285. [PMID: 20194816]

[Pulmonary Hypertension Association]
http://www.phassociation.org/

[Pulmonary Hypertension Page of MayoClinic.com]
http://www.mayoclinic.com/health/pulmonary-hypertension/DS00430

Task Force for Diagnosis and Treatment of Pulmonary Hypertension of European Society of Cardiology (ESC); European Respiratory Society (ERS); International Society of Heart and Lung Transplantation (ISHLT), Galie N, Hoeper MM, Humbert M, et al. Guidelines for the diagnosis and treatment of pulmonary hypertension. *Eur Respir J.* 2009; 34:1219. [PMID: 19749199]

Connective Tissue Disease–Associated Interstitial Lung Disease

64

Eunice J. Kim, MD
Harold R. Collard, MD

ESSENTIALS OF DIAGNOSIS

► Presents with nonspecific symptoms such as cough and dyspnea.

► Associated most often with rheumatoid arthritis, scleroderma, primary Sjögren syndrome, dermatomyositis, polymyositis, and mixed connective tissue disease; rarely with systemic lupus erythematosus.

► High-resolution computed tomography (HRCT) with thin-section images is the test of choice.

► Nonspecific interstitial pneumonia is the most common histopathologic pattern.

► Treatment with prednisone or immunomodulatory therapy (cyclophosphamide, mycophenolate mofetil, azathioprine) or both can be effective.

General Considerations

Interstitial lung disease (ILD) is a common pulmonary manifestation of systemic rheumatic diseases, including rheumatoid arthritis, scleroderma, the inflammatory myopathies, primary Sjögren syndrome, and mixed connective tissue disease. Collectively, these conditions are called **connective tissue disease–associated ILD.** Symptoms are nonspecific and include cough and dyspnea. ILD can be a significant cause of morbidity and mortality in this patient population, and early diagnosis is essential to help prevent progression of symptoms and decline in pulmonary function.

ILDs are generally categorized based on the underlying histopathologic pattern seen on surgical lung biopsy (Table 64–1). Patients with rheumatic diseases can manifest many of the histopathologic patterns seen in idiopathic cases of ILD, including usual interstitial pneumonia (UIP), nonspecific interstitial pneumonia (NSIP), organizing pneumonia, and lymphocytic interstitial pneumonia (LIP) (Table 64–2).

Although the diagnosis of connective tissue disease-associated ILD typically occurs after that of the rheumatic disease, ILD will present first in a certain proportion of patients. Thus, it is not only important to screen rheumatic disease patients for ILD, but the converse as well. Since there is no consensus approach to screening patients for the presence of ILD, obtaining a careful history and performing a physical examination targeting ILD is recommended in all patients with rheumatic disease. More specific testing should be reserved for those patients with signs or symptoms concerning for ILD or who are at high risk for its development (eg, scleroderma). A schematic approach to screening rheumatic patients for ILD is presented in Figure 64–1.

► Clinical Findings

A. History and Physical Examination

The clinician should screen patients for ILD by obtaining a detailed history and performing a physical examination. Patients with ILD often report symptoms of chronic dyspnea and cough as well as a change in exercise tolerance. Screening for occupational and environmental exposures, smoking history, and medications that could lead to pulmonary disease should also be performed. On physical examination, pulmonary auscultation may reveal inspiratory crackles, particularly in a basilar distribution. In addition, digital clubbing may be seen. Given that pulmonary hypertension is often seen in association with ILD, the clinician should also evaluate the patient for signs of right-sided heart failure, including an elevated jugular venous pressure and peripheral edema (see Chapter 63).

B. Imaging Studies

The chest radiograph is an inexpensive but insensitive way to evaluate for ILD. Affected patients may have a chest radiograph that demonstrates a bibasilar reticular pattern. However, because the chest radiograph lacks sensitivity,

Table 64-1. Key histopathologic and HRCT features of ILD patterns.

ILD Pattern	Histopathologic Features	HRCT Features
Nonspecific interstitial pneumonia	Homogeneous appearance Chronic inflammation or fibrosis Rare to no fibroblast foci	Peripheral, bibasilar distribution Predominant ground-glass attenuation Traction bronchiectasis and reticulation may be present Little or no honeycombing
Usual interstitial pneumonia	Areas of fibrotic lung next to normal lung ("temporal heterogeneity") Presence of fibroblast foci Fibrosis and architectural distortion, often with honeycombing	Peripheral, bibasilar distribution Traction bronchiectasis, reticulation and honeycombing Little to no ground-glass attenuation
Organizing pneumonia	Patchy distribution Organizing pneumonia (intralumenal fibrosis in distal airspaces) Preservation of lung architecture	Patchy areas of consolidation May be basilar predominant Ground-glass attenuation may be present
Lymphocytic interstitial pneumonia	Dense lymphoid infiltrate involving alveolar septa Lymphoid follicles may be present	Ground-glass attenuation Thin-walled cysts
Diffuse alveolar damage	Diffuse, homogeneous appearance Hyaline membranes Septal thickening due to fibrosis	Diffuse ground-glass attenuation and consolidation

HRCT, high-resolution computed tomography; ILD, interstitial lung disease.

particularly in early disease, it is recommended that an HRCT scan be performed in any patient with suspected ILD.

Advances in radiologic imaging have enhanced the ability to evaluate for ILD, especially with HRCT scans. Individual imaging centers may vary in how the HRCT protocol is performed. The recommended approach is to order an HRCT scan with 1-1.5 mm collimation (thin-section images) at 1-cm intervals. Prone imaging should be performed because atelectasis can develop in the dependent regions of the lung (ie, the posterior basal portions when supine) and mimic ILD. Lastly, air trapping is an important indicator of airways disease, and therefore expiratory imaging should also be included.

Because the approach to evaluating an HRCT scan is complex and involves looking for individual features of an ILD (eg, ground-glass opacities, reticulation, traction bronchiectasis, and honeycombing) as well as the underlying ILD histopathologic pattern (eg, NSIP, UIP) (see Table 64–1), a radiologist experienced in thoracic imaging should assess the HRCT scan. Usual interstitial pneumonia pattern is characterized by bibasilar, predominantly peripheral reticulation, traction bronchiectasis, and honeycombing (Figure 64–2). There is minimal to absent ground-glass opacities. Nonspecific interstitial pneumonia is suggested by the presence of ground-glass opacities and reticulation with little or no honeycombing (Figure 64–2). The predominant

Table 64-2. Histopathologic patterns of ILD found in the rheumatic diseases.

Rheumatic Disease	Histopathologic Pattern				
	Nonspecific Interstitial Pneumonia	Usual Interstitial Pneumonia	Organizing Pneumonia	Lymphocytic Interstitial Pneumonia	Diffuse Alveolar Damage
Inflammatory myopathies	++	+	+		+
Mixed connective tissue disease	++	+		+	
Rheumatoid arthritis	++	++	+		+
Sjögren syndrome	++	+	+	+	
Systemic lupus erythematosus	+	+		+	+
Scleroderma	++	+			
Undifferentiated connective tissue disease	++				

Key: ++, most common histopathologic pattern seen.

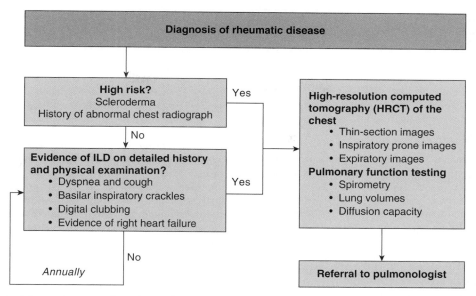

▲ **Figure 64–1.** Schematic approach to the evaluation of interstitial lung disease (ILD) in rheumatic disease.

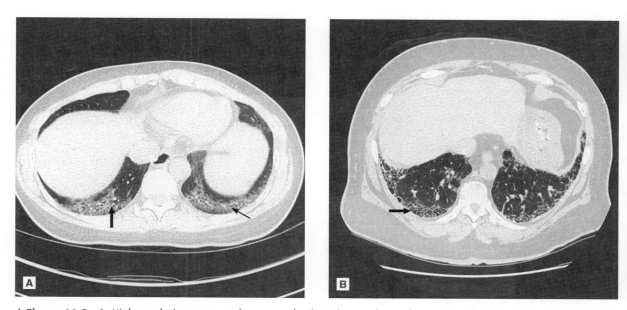

▲ **Figure 64–2. A:** High-resolution computed tomography (HRCT) scan shows the nonspecific interstitial pneumonia (NSIP) pattern in a patient with interstitial lung disease (ILD). Characteristic features include ground-glass attenuation (*thin arrow*) in a subpleural distribution. Traction bronchiectasis is also present (*thick arrow*). These findings were also seen on the corresponding prone imaging. Reticulation is also often seen in NSIP pattern. **B:** HRCT scan shows the usual interstitial pneumonia pattern in a patient with ILD. The scan demonstrates the typical bibasilar, peripheral distribution of traction bronchiectasis, reticulation and honeycombing (*thick arrow*). There is no ground-glass attenuation.

histopathologic pattern seen in association with systemic rheumatic diseases is NSIP.

C. Pulmonary Function Testing

All patients with a suspected ILD should undergo pulmonary function testing to characterize the degree of restriction and diffusing capacity impairment. In addition, pulmonary function tests are a relatively sensitive and noninvasive method for screening for ILD, particularly in rheumatic diseases known to have a high prevalence of ILD, such as scleroderma. The clinician should order complete pulmonary function tests, including spirometry, lung volume measurements, and diffusing capacity for carbon monoxide (DLco).

If an ILD is present, pulmonary function tests may demonstrate a restrictive lung process characterized by a reduction in the total lung capacity to <80% of predicted. Other findings suggestive of restriction include a decreased forced expiratory volume in 1 second (FEV_1) and forced vital capacity (FVC) with a preserved FEV_1/FVC ratio, a decreased vital capacity, and a decreased residual volume. There may also be evidence of abnormal gas exchange based on a reduction in the DLco. Occasionally, obstructive physiology can be seen in ILD, so a high index of suspicion should remain with any abnormality of pulmonary function.

D. Bronchoscopy

Bronchoscopy with bronchoalveolar lavage allows for the analysis of infection and inflammatory changes in alveolar fluid. Historically, it has been used for the diagnosis and staging of ILD. Bronchoalveolar lavage neutrophilia has been shown to correlate with worse outcomes in patients with scleroderma associated–ILD. However, bronchoalveolar lavage has little role in the diagnosis of ILD associated with systemic rheumatic diseases other than to evaluate for other causes of pulmonary disease, such as infection.

E. Lung Biopsy

In most centers, lung biopsy is rarely used in the diagnosis of ILD in systemic rheumatic disease. In general, in a patient with a known rheumatic disease, an HRCT demonstrating ILD is sufficient for the diagnosis if other causes of ILD (eg, drug or other exposures) can be excluded. At this time, it is unclear whether knowing the underlying histopathologic pattern (eg, NSIP vs UIP) imparts additional information in terms of clinical course or expected response to therapy. This is in contrast to idiopathic ILD, where the histopathologic pattern is an essential management consideration.

In the rare case that a tissue diagnosis is required, a surgical lung biopsy is the recommended method, generally by video-assisted thoracoscopic lung surgery. Transbronchial biopsies via a bronchoscopic approach are not recommended for the diagnosis of ILD given the small amount of tissue obtained and the inability of the pathologists to interpret the underlying histopathologic pattern.

▶ Differential Diagnosis

The differential diagnosis for a patient with a systemic rheumatic disease presenting with an ILD primarily includes medication, environmental, or occupational exposures. Careful history taking usually helps differentiate between the different etiologies. In cases where an alternative etiology is plausible, surgical lung biopsy should be considered.

Not uncommonly, ILD develops before a rheumatic disease is diagnosed. Pulmonologists should therefore carefully screen all ILD patients for signs and symptoms suggestive of a systemic rheumatic disease. There are no published guidelines on how best to screen these patients, but a reasonable approach includes serologic testing for commonly associated rheumatic conditions such as rheumatoid arthritis, primary Sjögren syndrome, scleroderma, and the inflammatory myopathies. Recent studies have demonstrated that a reasonable proportion of patients with an idiopathic ILD have detectable autoantibodies such as antinuclear antibody, antinucleolar antibodies (eg, Th/To), anti-cyclic citrullinated antibody, rheumatoid factor, and antisynthetase antibodies (eg, Jo-1, PL-12). It is unclear in what proportion of these patients a defined rheumatic disease eventually develops.

▶ Specific Systemic Rheumatic Diseases & ILD

A. Scleroderma

ILD is a common manifestation of scleroderma and is one of the diagnostic criteria for the disease. Up to 90% of patients with scleroderma have pulmonary involvement, of which about half is ILD. The presence of Scl-70 antibody increases the likelihood of ILD whereas the anticentromere antibody decreases the likelihood of ILD. In addition, black ethnicity and cardiac involvement (ie, pericardial effusion, arrhythmia, or cardiomyopathy) are associated with the development of ILD. Because of the high prevalence of ILD in scleroderma, it is generally recommended that all patients be aggressively screened for ILD.

NSIP is the most common histopathologic pattern seen in scleroderma-associated ILD, followed much less frequently by the UIP pattern. The corresponding HRCT findings of NSIP are typically seen and include ground-glass attenuation and reticular changes most pronounced at the bases and peripherally. Many patients respond to immunomodulatory treatment (see below). In addition, the results of the Scleroderma Lung Study, a multicenter, randomized control trial looking at the use of cyclophosphamide versus placebo, confirmed that many patients have relatively stable disease despite lack of therapy, making the decision about when to treat in early disease difficult.

B. Rheumatoid Arthritis

The prevalence of ILD in rheumatoid arthritis has been reported to anywhere between 4% and 68%, depending on the chosen method for screening (chest radiograph, HRCT, pulmonary function tests) and the population studied (symptomatic vs asymptomatic). By HRCT, ILD is diagnosed in approximately 20% of patients with rheumatoid arthritis, regardless of the presence of pulmonary symptoms. Studies have reported that risk factors for the development of ILD include male gender, smoking history, and possibly long-standing rheumatoid arthritis.

In contrast to the other systemic rheumatic diseases, rheumatoid arthritis typically demonstrates a UIP pattern. Other patterns seen include NSIP and organizing pneumonia. Rheumatoid arthritis can also involve the airways causing bronchiolitis, and upper lobe nodular disease has been described. There is growing data to suggest, that similar to the idiopathic ILDs, the presence of UIP pattern portends a worse survival. In addition, patients with rheumatoid arthritis and UIP pattern have a higher rate of acute exacerbation (ie, acute worsening of the ILD) compared to other systemic rheumatic diseases.

C. Idiopathic Inflammatory Myopathies

The reported prevalence of ILD in polymyositis and dermatomyositis varies greatly in the literature and may be as low as 5% or as high as 80% based on different published studies. The presence of an antisynthetase antibody increases the likelihood of developing ILD. NSIP pattern is the most common ILD pattern seen in myositis-associated ILD. Organizing pneumonia and UIP pattern are also seen.

Most patients with ILD associated with polymyositis or dermatomyositis have a chronic, indolent course. However, a small proportion of patients have a more acute, fulminant presentation with rapid onset of cough, shortness of breath and, often times, fever. This acute form of ILD is associated with an increased mortality rate as well as a diagnosis of amyopathic dermatomyositis. The histopathologic pattern seen in this acute form of ILD is diffuse alveolar damage, the same pattern seen in patients with the acute respiratory distress syndrome.

D. Undifferentiated Connective Tissue Disease

It is not uncommon for a patient to have ILD and concurrent signs of symptoms of a systemic rheumatic disease. If careful history taking, physical examination, and serologic analysis do not reveal a defined rheumatic disease, a patient may meet criteria for undifferentiated connective tissue disease. Of ILD patients with a diagnosis of undifferentiated connective tissue disease, the majority have NSIP pattern on lung biopsy. The natural history of this patient population appears to mirror that of idiopathic NSIP, with gradual progression over 5–10 years.

E. Mixed Connective Tissue Disease

ILD in mixed connective tissue disease has a prevalence of 18–67% based on studies using chest radiographs and HRCT, respectively. On HRCT, ground-glass opacities and reticulation are most commonly seen. The predominant histopathologic pattern is NSIP pattern. UIP pattern and LIP are also seen. Although specific prognostic information is not available, it has been reported that in a proportion of patients, ILD will progress to fibrosis if left untreated.

F. Primary Sjögren Syndrome

The prevalence of ILD in primary Sjögren syndrome ranges from 9% to 75%. The lung involvement in primary Sjögren syndrome involved both the interstitium and the small airways. Findings on HRCT scan include ground-glass opacities, reticulation, bronchiectasis, consolidation, micronodules, and cysts. Similar to other systemic rheumatic diseases, NSIP is the most common histopathologic pattern seen. Lymphocytic interstitial pneumonia is also associated with primary Sjögren syndrome. In LIP, lymphocytes proliferate and infiltrate the interstitium and alveoli of the lungs. Radiologically, LIP is characterized by ground-glass attenuation, centrilobular nodules, and thin-walled cysts. Other types of ILD seen in association with primary Sjögren syndrome include UIP pattern and organizing pneumonia. While few studies have looked at prognosis, it appears that the majority of patients with ILD and primary Sjögren syndrome have stabilization or improvement of pulmonary function tests with therapy.

G. Systemic Lupus Erythematosus

Although lung involvement is reported to occur in over 50% of patients with systemic lupus erythematosus, chronic ILD is uncommon. More typically, an acute pneumonitis (ie, acute lupus pneumonitis) is seen and may often be the presenting manifestation of systemic lupus erythematosus. Acute lupus pneumonitis is characterized by rapid onset of cough, dyspnea, tachypnea, and possibly fever. Chest imaging often demonstrates bilateral opacities, with corresponding histopathology revealing a diffuse alveolar damage pattern. From a clinical and radiologic perspective, it can be difficult to distinguish the findings seen in acute lupus pneumonitis from that of infection. Mortality is estimated at 50%.

In the rare case that a chronic ILD is identified in a patient with systemic lupus erythematosus, the most common ILD pattern seen is NSIP. UIP and LIP have also been reported.

▶ Treatment

Treatment of ILD in systemic rheumatic diseases is largely empiric. There are very few randomized, placebo-controlled clinical trials in this patient population. Most recently, the Scleroderma Lung Study compared the efficacy of oral cyclophosphamide given daily for 12 months with placebo in patients with ILD and scleroderma. This study found a modest benefit in the primary endpoint, change in percent predicted FVC at 12 months. Given the toxicities associated with cyclophosphamide, a second study comparing cyclophosphamide with mycophenolate mofetil is currently under way.

Beyond scleroderma, publications on treatment efficacy are mainly limited to case series, observational trials, and retrospective analysis. Generally, therapy should be considered for each individual, weighing the risks and benefits of using an immunomodulatory agent. In addition, therapeutic intervention is likely most beneficial earlier in the disease process, when symptoms and physiology are mildly to moderately impaired and before irreversible fibrosis has been established. Many pulmonologists recommend the initiation of a combination of glucocorticoids and an immunomodulatory agent, such as cyclophosphamide, mycophenolate mofetil, or azathioprine.

Therapeutic response may be defined as improvement in symptoms, chest imaging, or pulmonary physiology. Pulmonary function tests should be obtained every 3–6 months to assess for physiologic improvement. Treatment failure is defined by significant worsening of symptoms or gas exchange, a drop in FVC by 10% or more, or worsening of the HRCT findings.

There have been many case reports and series of other immunomodulatory agents that have been used in refractory cases of connective tissue disease–associated ILD. Depending on the underlying rheumatic disease, small studies have reported the use of cyclosporine, tacrolimus, and rituximab. Clearly, further studies are needed to determine the efficacy of these therapies in patients with ILD due to systemic rheumatic disease.

▶ Prognosis

In general, the prognosis of ILD associated with systemic rheumatic diseases is thought to be better than that of idiopathic ILD. This may be partially due to the fact that nonspecific interstitial pneumonia pattern is the predominant pattern seen in the systemic rheumatic diseases, whereas usual interstitial pneumonia pattern is more common in idiopathic cases (and has worse survival). As mentioned previously, it is unclear how the underlying histopathologic pattern influences response to therapy, physiologic decline, or survival in rheumatic disease.

American Thoracic Society; European Respiratory Society. American Thoracic Society/European Respiratory Society International Multidisciplinary Consensus Classification of the Idiopathic Interstitial Pneumonias. This joint statement of the American Thoracic Society (ATS), and the European Respiratory Society (ERS) was adopted by the ATS board of directors, June 2001 and by the ERS Executive Committee, June 2001. *Am J Respir Crit Care Med.* 2002;165:277. [PMID: 11790668]

Kinder BW, Collard HR, Koth L, et al. Idiopathic nonspecific interstitial pneumonia: lung manifestation of undifferentiated connective tissue disease? *Am J Respir Crit Care Med.* 2007;176:691. [PMID: 17556720]

Park JH, Kim DS, Park IN, et al. Prognosis of fibrotic interstitial pneumonia: idiopathic versus collagen vascular disease-related subtypes. *Am J Respir Crit Care Med.* 2007;175:705. [PMID: 17218621]

Tashkin DP, Elashoff R, Clements PJ, et al. Scleroderma Lung Study Research Group. Cyclophosphamide versus placebo in scleroderma lung disease. *N Engl J Med.* 2006;354:2655. [PMID: 16790698]

Musculoskeletal Magnetic Resonance Imaging

65

Susan V. Kattapuram, MD

Ravi S. Kamath, MD, PhD

Magnetic resonance imaging (MRI) relies on the intrinsic spin of protons, each of which has a magnetic moment. Protons tend to align their magnetic poles along the direction of a magnetic field. When protons are placed in a magnetic field, they can also absorb and then reemit electromagnetic radiation in the form of radiofrequency signals. Nuclei absorb energy from radiofrequency pulses and may resonate. This resonance induces orientation to the magnetic field; the required frequency of the pulse is determined by the strength of the magnetic field and the chemical properties of the target.

When the radiofrequency signal is removed, absorbed energy is released. This energy can be recorded as an electrical signal that can be used to create images, with the strength of the emitted radiowave corresponding to the signal intensity of a given area. This intensity depends on the concentration of protons and the longitudinal and transverse relaxation times, which in turn depend on the properties of water molecules within the given tissue.

Two relaxation times are important for MRI. The T1 (longitudinal) relaxation time describes the return of protons back to equilibrium after a radiofrequency pulse. The T2 (transverse) relaxation time describes the loss of phase coherence between individual protons immediately after the pulse. Different pulse sequences can be used to enhance the differences between T1 and T2, thus creating image contrast. Sequences with short repetition times (TR) (ie, <800 msec) and short echo times (TE) (ie, <30 msec) are termed **T1-weighted** and provide good anatomic detail. Sequences with long TR (>2000 msec) and TE (>60 msec) are termed **T2-weighted** and are useful for evaluating pathology. Sequences with intermediate TR (>1000 msec) and short TE (<30 msec) are termed **proton density sequences.** These provide good anatomic detail with maximal signal-to-noise ratios, at the cost of impaired tissue contrast. In musculoskeletal imaging, suppression of fat signal can often be useful for evaluating pathology. Thus, using the short tau inversion

recovery ("STIR") technique, the effects of prolonged T1 and T2 relaxation times are cumulative, leading to the suppression of fat signal ("fat saturation"). Fat saturation can also be performed using frequency-selective (chemical) techniques that improve spatial resolution.

Faster imaging techniques such as gradient-recalled echo (GRE) have become popular because they shorten imaging time. With GRE, pulse sequences are performed using variable flip angles of less than 90 degrees, which shortens imaging time since the low flip-angle radiofrequency pulses destroy only a portion of the longitudinal magnetization with each pulse cycle. In musculoskeletal imaging, GRE sequences are useful for imaging ligaments, tendons, and cartilage.

The musculoskeletal system is ideally suited for evaluation by MRI because different tissues demonstrate different signal intensities on T1- and T2-weighted images. For example, fat displays high signal on T1-weighted images and intermediate signal on T2-weighted images. Air, cortical bone, ligaments, tendons, and fibrocartilage demonstrate low signal on both T1- and T2-weighted images. Fluid displays intermediate signal on T1-weighted images and high signal on T2-weighted images. Traumatic, inflammatory, and infectious disorders are therefore evaluated effectively by MRI, since these conditions typically result in edema and associated hyperintensity on T2-weighted images. Figures 65–1 through 65–21 show MRI findings in various rheumatic conditions.

MR images can also be enhanced by intravenous administration of gadolinium in the form of Gd-DTPA, a paramagnetic compound that shortens the T1 and T2 relaxation times of tissues into which it extravasates, resulting in an increase in signal on T1-weighted images. Foci with increased vascular permeability, such as neoplasms or areas of inflammation or infection, therefore demonstrate increased signal, or enhancement, following the administration of intravenous gadolinium. Intra-articular administration of gadolinium

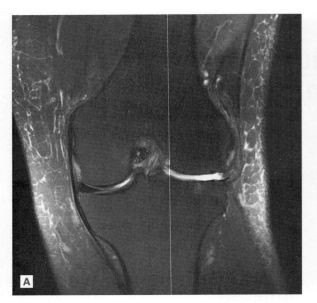
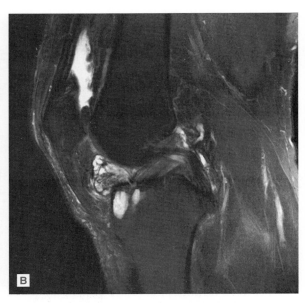

▲ **Figure 65–1.** Osteoarthritis of the knee. Coronal T2 fat saturated (**A**) images of the knee demonstrate absence of the lateral meniscus with adjacent full-thickness cartilage loss, cortical irregularity, marrow edema, and marginal osteophytes. Sagittal images (**B**) demonstrate a lobulated parameniscal cyst in Hoffa fat pad arising from the extensively torn lateral meniscus. A degenerative cyst is also seen underlying the insertion of the anterior cruciate ligament on the tibia.

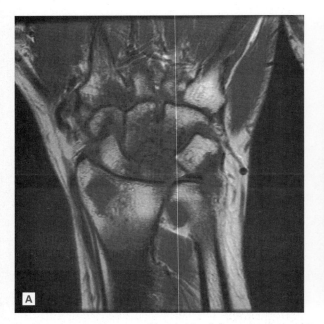
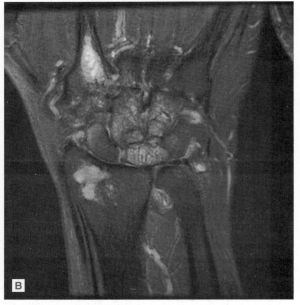

▲ **Figure 65–2.** Rheumatoid arthritis of the wrist. Coronal T1 (**A**), T2 fat saturated (**B**), and gradient-recalled echo (GRE)

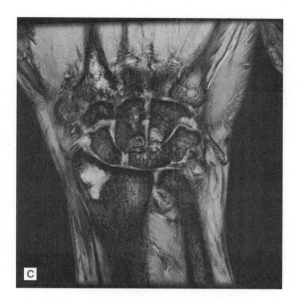

▲ **Figure 65–2.** (*Continued*) (**C**) images of the wrist demonstrate diffuse cartilage loss throughout the carpal bones with joint-space narrowing, intraosseous cysts, and extensive marrow edema. Small periarticular cortical erosions are seen in the lunate.

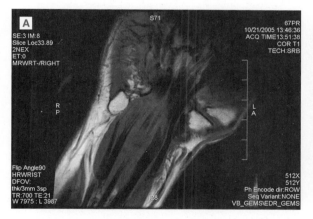

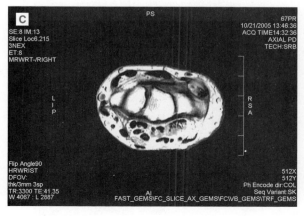

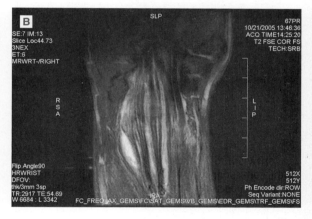

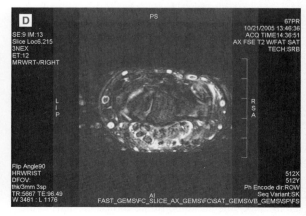

▲ **Figure 65–3.** Rheumatoid arthritis of the wrist. Coronal T1 (**A**) and T2 fat saturated (**B**) images and axial PD (**C**) and T2 fat saturated (**D**) images of the wrist demonstrate diffuse tenosynovitis involving the flexor tendons of the wrist.

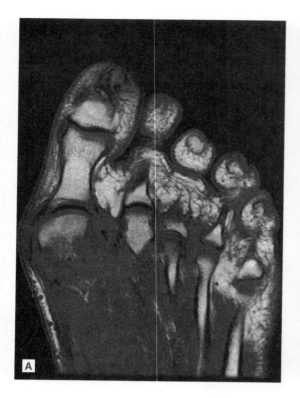

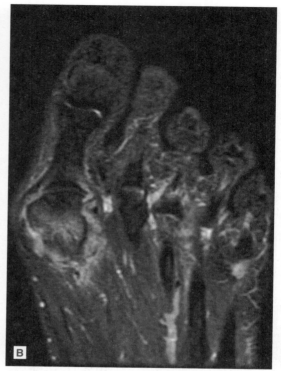

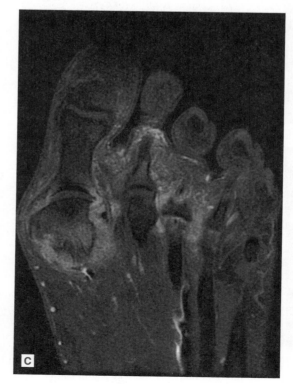

▲ **Figure 65–4.** Rheumatoid arthritis of the foot. Coronal T1 (**A**), T2 fat saturated (**B**), and T1 post-contrast fat saturated (**C**) images demonstrate cortical erosions in the distal first metatarsal with adjacent marrow edema, a joint effusion, and enhancing soft-tissue in the joint space.

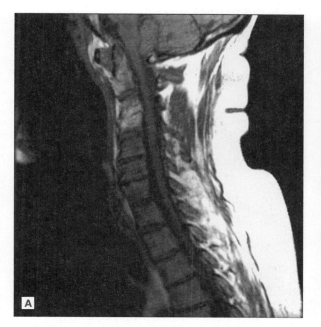

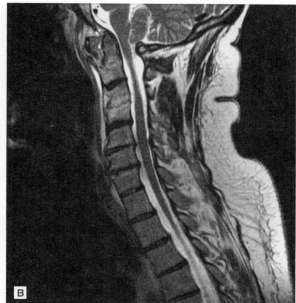

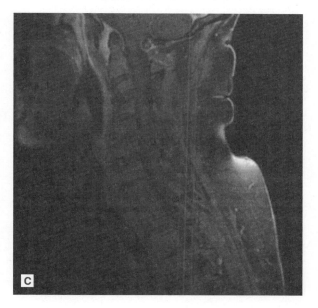

▲ **Figure 65–5.** Rheumatoid arthritis of the cervical spine. Coronal T1 (**A**), T2 (**B**), and T1 post-contrast fat saturated (**C**) images demonstrate abnormal enhancement of the soft-tissue surrounding the dens. There is superior displacement of the dens relative to the skull base and protrusion into the foramen magnum, consistent with basilar invagination. Abnormal marrow signal in the C2, C3, and C4 vertebral bodies is consistent with fatty replacement from chronic degenerative changes.

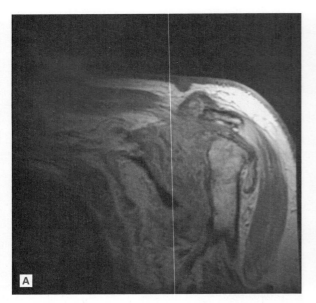
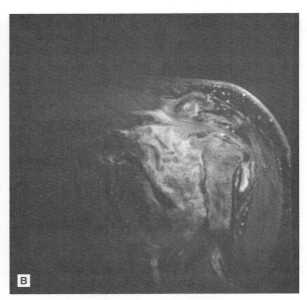

▲ **Figure 65–6.** Rheumatoid arthritis of the shoulder. Coronal T1 (**A**) and T2 fat saturated (**B**) images of the shoulder demonstrate end-stage changes from rheumatoid arthritis, including extensive bony destruction, a large joint effusion, and extensive synovitis with rice bodies.

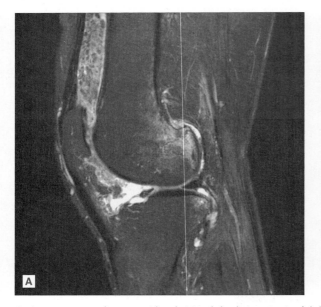
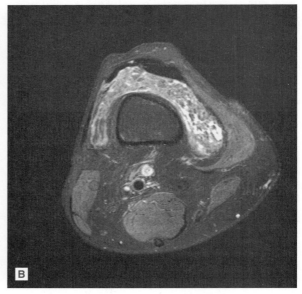

▲ **Figure 65–7.** Rheumatoid arthritis of the knee. Sagittal (**A**) and axial (**B**) T2 fat saturated images of the knee demonstrate a large joint effusion with extensive synovitis and rice bodies. Marrow edema in the posterior lateral femoral condyle and tibial plateau is also related to underlying rheumatoid arthritis.

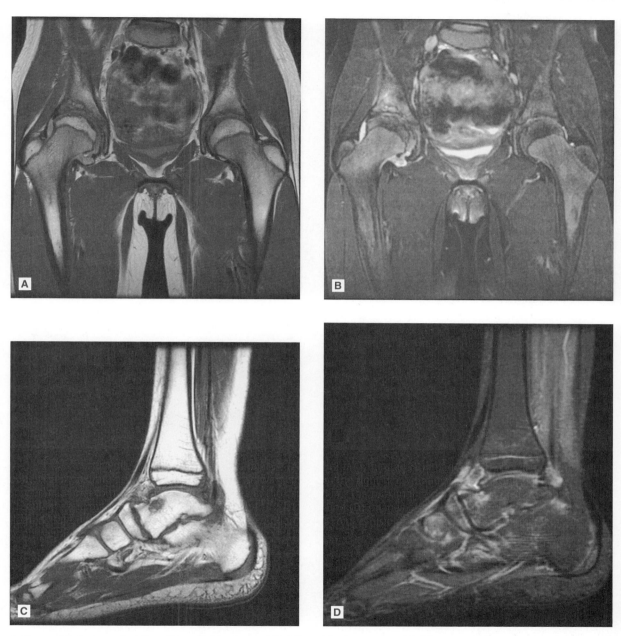

▲ **Figure 65–8.** Juvenile idiopathic arthritis. Coronal T1 (**A**) and T2 fat saturated (**B**) images of the pelvis in a pediatric patient demonstrate asymmetric joint-space narrowing involving the right hip with adjacent cortical irregularity, subchondral cyst formation, and marrow edema in the acetabulum. The proximal femur also demonstrates physeal irregularity and marrow edema. Sagittal T1 (**C**) and T2 fat saturated (**D**) images of the ankle in the same patient demonstrate diffuse joint-space narrowing, marrow edema, and joint effusion in the ankle and hindfoot. Note the open epiphyses in this pre-adolescent patient.

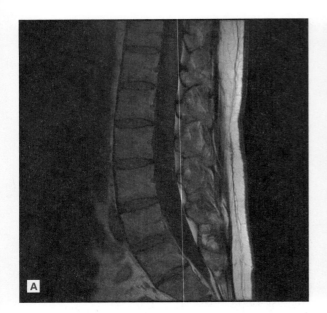

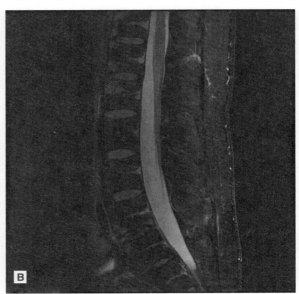

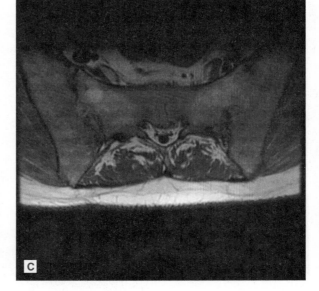

▲ **Figure 65–9.** Ankylosing spondylitis. Sagittal T1 (**A**) and STIR (**B**) images of the lumbar spine demonstrate focal marrow edema along the margins of the end plates, an early manifestation of so-called "shiny corners" that characterizes radiographs of the spines of some ankylosing spondylitis patients. An axial T1 image (**C**) of the sacrum demonstrates partial ankylosis of the sacroiliac joints.

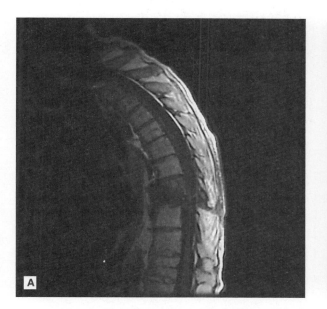

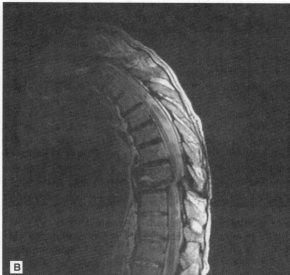

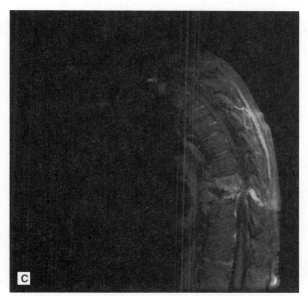

▲ **Figure 65–10.** Ankylosing spondylitis with Andersson lesion. Sagittal T1 (**A**), T2 (**B**), and T1 post-contrast fat saturated (**C**) images demonstrate fusion of the thoracic spine with syndesmophyte formation. There is a fracture in the midthoracic spine, termed an "Andersson lesion," with early pseudoarthrosis formation and resulting compromise of the central canal and cord compression. Edema and enhancement in the adjacent vertebral bodies likely reflect inflammation secondary to mechanical stress from the fracture.

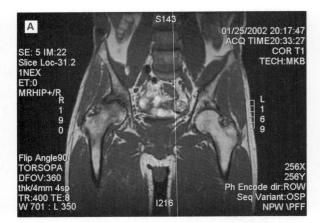

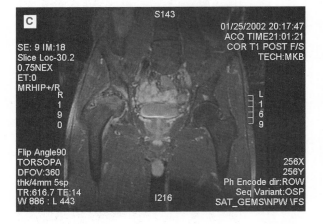

▲ Figure 65–11. Ankylosing spondylitis of the hip. Coronal T1 (**A**), STIR (**B**), and T1 post-contrast fat saturated (**C**) images demonstrate diffuse joint-space narrowing, periarticular erosions, adjacent marrow edema, and a small joint effusion.

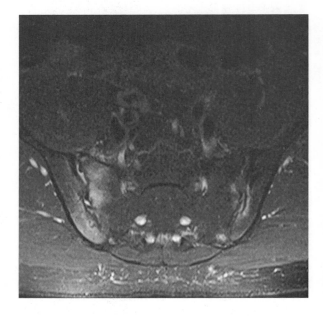

▲ Figure 65–12. Psoriasis of the sacroiliac joints. An axial image of the sacrum demonstrates bilateral asymmetric sacroiliitis.

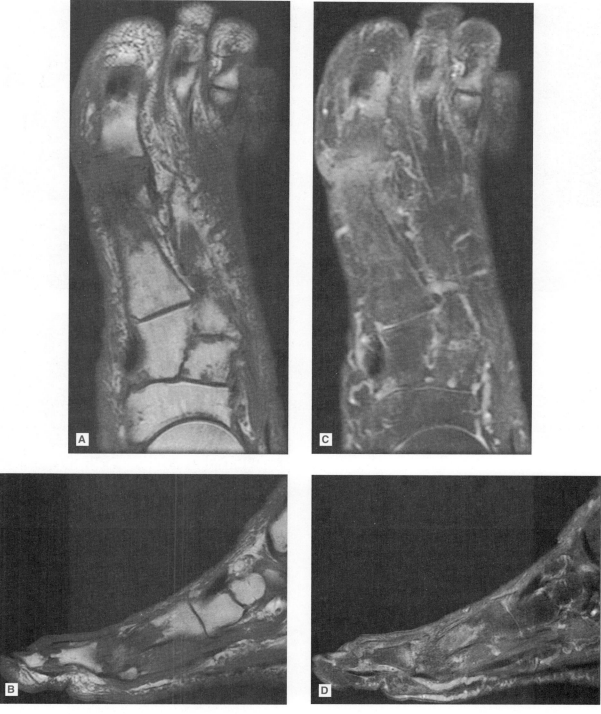

▲ **Figure 65–13.** Gout of the foot. Axial (**A**) and sagittal (**B**) T1 images and axial (**C**) and sagittal (**D**) T2 fat saturated images demonstrate sharply marginated periarticular erosions with overhanging edges, extensive adjacent marrow edema, and adjacent soft-tissue abnormality.

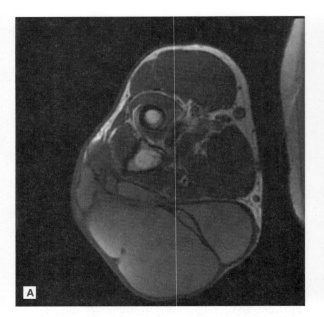

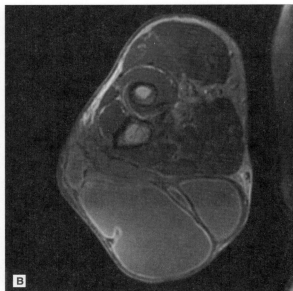

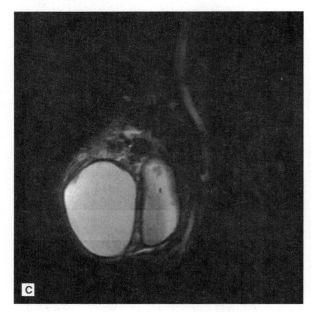

▲ **Figure 65–14.** Olecranon bursitis in the setting of gout. Axial T1 (**A**) and T1 post-contrast (**B**) images and a coronal (**C**) T2 fat saturated image of the elbow demonstrate a large, multiloculated fluid collection posterior to the olecranon with an irregular, enhancing wall and internal debris, consistent with olecranon bursitis in this patient with gout.

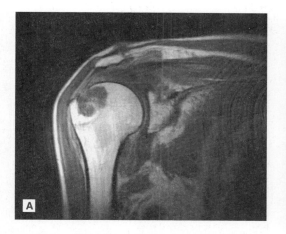

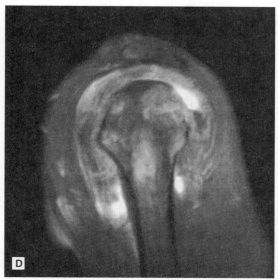

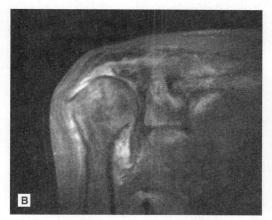

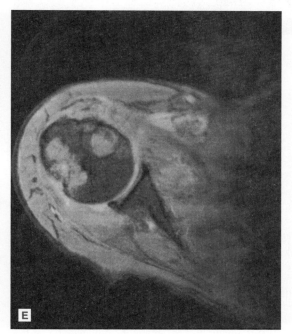

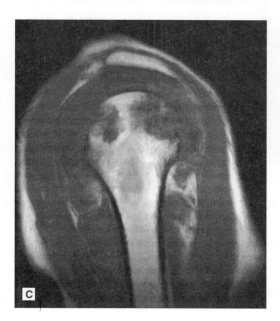

▲ **Figure 65–15.** Amyloid arthropathy. Coronal T1 (**A**) and T2 fat saturated (**B**) images, sagittal T1 (**C**) and T2 fat saturated (**D**) images, and an axial gradient-recalled echo (GRE) (**E**) image of the shoulder demonstrate distention of the joint with abnormal soft-tissue and large erosions extending into the humeral head. This patient with amyloid arthropathy also had an amyloid-associated cardiomyopathy in the setting of multiple myeloma.

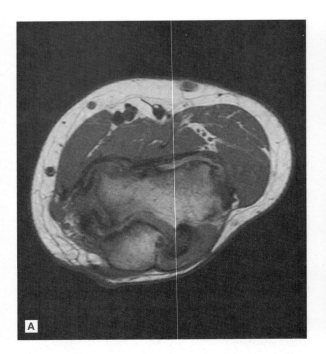

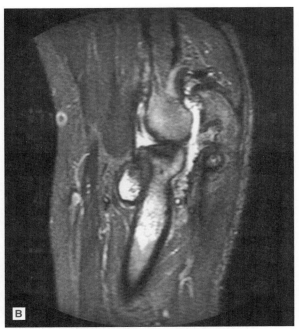

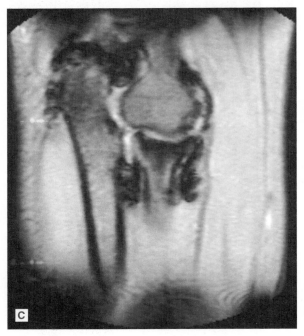

▲ **Figure 65–16.** Hemophilia of the elbow. Axial T1 (**A**), sagittal T2 (**B**), and coronal gradient-recalled echo (GRE) (**C**) images of the elbow demonstrate abnormal synovial thickening with diffuse T1 and T2 hypointensity, consistent with hemosiderin deposition that has resulted from recurrent intra-articular hemorrhage. Note the extensive "blooming" of the susceptibility artifact (dark signal) surrounding the paramagnetic hemosiderin on the GRE images (C). There are superimposed degenerative changes in the joint, with cartilage loss, cortical irregularity, and small erosions.

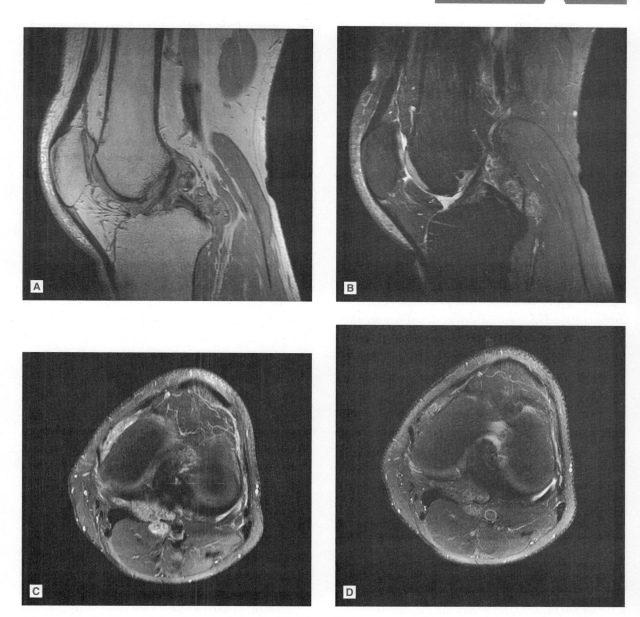

▲ **Figure 65–17.** Synovial chondromatosis. Sagittal T1 (**A**) and T2 fat saturated (**B**) images of the knee demonstrate multiple heterogeneously T2 hyperintense intra-articular masses in the posterior recess of the joint, consistent with cartilage. Axial T2 fat saturated (**C**) and T1 post-contrast fat saturated (**D**) demonstrate T2 hyperintense masses in the medial and posterior joint.

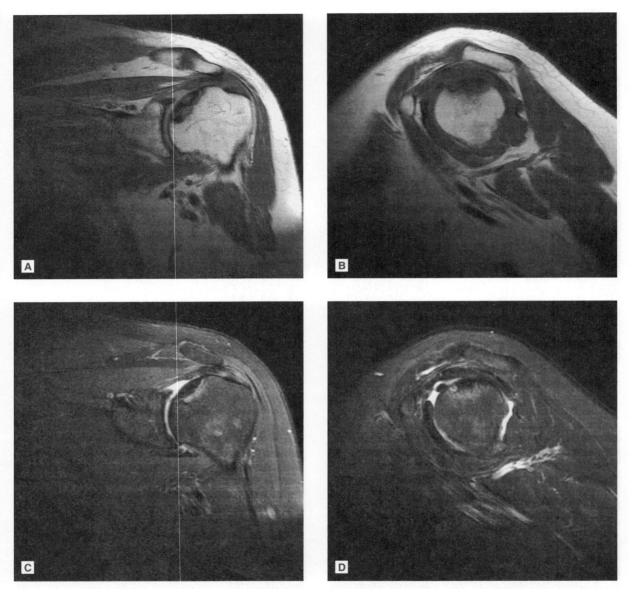

▲ **Figure 65–18.** Osteonecrosis of the shoulder. Coronal (**A**) and sagittal (**B**) T1 and coronal (**C**) and sagittal (**D**) T2 fat saturated images of the shoulder demonstrate a crescentic region of T1 and T2 hypointensity in the humeral head with a small amount of adjacent marrow edema, consistent with osteonecrosis in this patient who was previously taking long-term glucocorticoids.

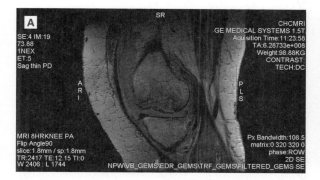

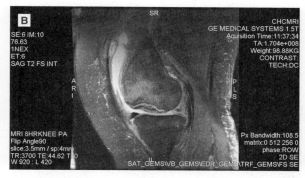

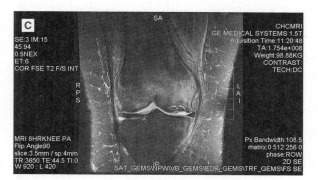

▲ **Figure 65–19.** Spontaneous osteonecrosis of the knee. Sagittal PD (**A**) and sagittal (**B**) and coronal (**C**) T2 fat saturated images of the knee demonstrate a mildly impacted subchondral fracture along the weight-bearing portion of the medial femoral condyle with extensive adjacent marrow edema. Although previously thought to result from venous occlusion, it is now more widely accepted that this disorder primarily results from an insufficiency-type osteoporotic fracture, which can result in secondary osteonecrosis.

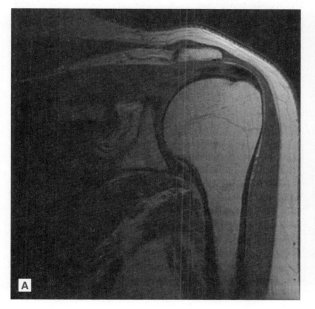

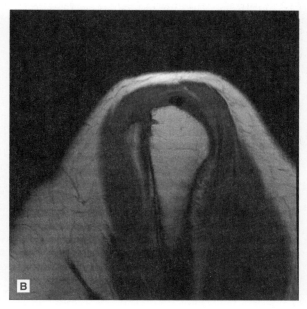

▲ **Figure 65–20.** Calcific tendinopathy. Coronal (**A**) and sagittal (**B**) T1 images, coronal

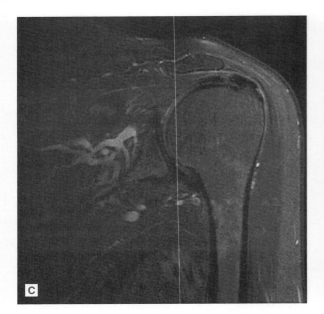

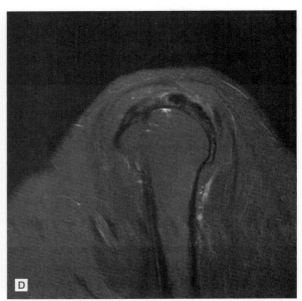

▲ **Figure 65–20.** (*Continued*) (**C**) and sagittal (**D**) T2 images, and an axial gradient-recalled echo (GRE) image of the shoulder (**E**) demonstrate a focus of T1 and T2 hypointensity within the distal supraspinatus tendon, consistent with hydroxyapatite deposition. Note that on the GRE image, there is "blooming" of susceptibility artifact (dark signal) surrounding the paramagnetic calcification.

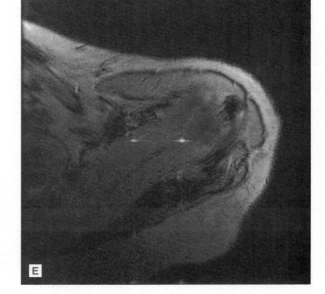

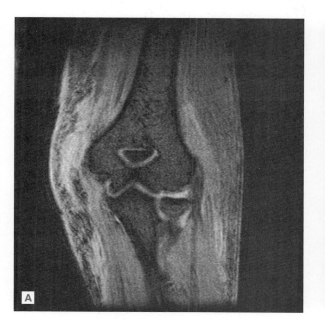

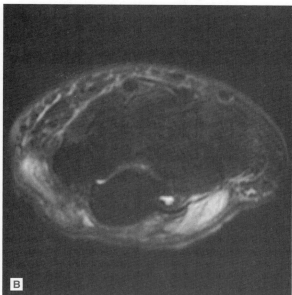

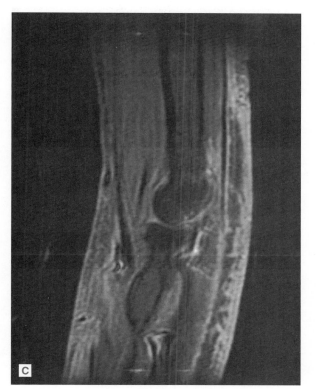

▲ **Figure 65–21.** Dermatomyositis. Coronal gradient-recalled echo (GRE) (**A**), axial T2 fat saturated (**B**), and sagittal T1 post-contrast fat saturated (**C**) images of the elbow demonstrate extensive subcutaneous edema and enhancement with skin thickening surrounding the elbow and fluid collections most pronounced posteriorly. Diffuse mild edema and enhancement is also seen throughout the visualized muscles.

for arthrography can also be used to evaluate for internal derangement of a joint.

Although MRI has many advantages over other imaging techniques for the evaluation of the musculoskeletal system, its utility is limited in certain instances. MRI is contraindicated, for example, in patients with cardiac pacemakers, neural stimulators, and some other implanted metallic devices. Claustrophobic patients are often unable to endure the tight confines of many MRI machines. Motion artifact that results from some patients' inability to hold still for any reason can render MRI data unreadable. This is a particular problem in the setting of the long scan times (eg, 30–60 minutes) required by some studies. Finally, some metallic objects that are safe for MRI nevertheless can create areas of signal void that obscure adjacent structures, and ferromagnetic objects can cause magnetic field distortion. These potential limitations of MRI must be understood in order to optimize the use of this technology.

Musculoskeletal Ultrasound

66

Dimitrios A. Pappas, MD

Musculoskeletal ultrasound (MSUS) imaging has been incorporated in the care of the rheumatologic patient for more than a decade in Europe. On the contrary, MSUS is a relatively recent addition in the diagnostic armamentarium of rheumatologists in the United States.

MSUS can significantly advance the diagnostic potential in rheumatology and improve the accuracy of musculoskeletal procedural interventions. The most experience with ultrasound stems from its applications in arthritic conditions. However, the diagnosis of a wide spectrum of rheumatologic conditions can be facilitated by its use.

ULTRASOUND TECHNOLOGY

Ultrasound machines consist of a processing unit and a transducer. Many models of different sizes and degrees of portability are available by various manufacturers. Ultrasound technology couples gray scale imaging and Doppler imaging to evaluate anatomic integrity and tissue inflammation.

▶ Gray Scale Imaging — The Echo Phenomenon

The human ear can perceive sound waves in frequencies between 20 Hz and 20,000 Hz. Sound waves above the hearing frequency are called ultrasounds.

The acquisition of ultrasound images is based on the echo phenomenon. A transducer attached to the ultrasound machine transmits ultrasound waves that "travel" through the tissues. Each tissue has different acoustic properties based on their consistency, compressibility, and density. Different acoustic properties translate into differences in the velocity with which ultrasound waves are transmitted through each particular tissue. Reflection at tissue interfaces generates

returning echoes that are collected by piezoelectric crystals in the transducer. The electric potentials generated at the piezoelectric crystals are then transformed to gray scale imaging displayed on a monitor.

The more echoes returned, the more "white" the tissues that generated the echoes will appear.

Structures without internal reflectors do not return any echoes, and this results in black areas in the ultrasound image. Such structures are fluid collections or tissues containing high concentrations of water such as the cartilage or joint effusions. These tissues are called **hypoechoic** in ultrasound terminology.

Structures that produce weaker ultrasound reflections generate low level echoes and correspond to dark gray areas in the ultrasound images. These structures are called **isoechoic** and include muscle, tendons, synovial tissue, and nerves (Figure 66–1).

Lastly, tissues with strong internal reflectors return strong echoes and generate bright gray or white areas in the ultrasound image. These structures are called **hyperechoic** and include bone, calcifications, and foreign bodies.

▶ The Doppler Phenomenon

Inflammation is associated with local hyperemia. Increased blood flow in synovitis (Figure 66–2 and Plate 50), tenosynovitis, and enthesitis (Figure 66–3) can be detected with the use of Doppler ultrasonography. The detection of blood flow locally is transformed to a color signal that is coupled with the gray image obtained as described above. The more intense the inflammation the more intense is the color signal. More details about the physics of the Doppler phenomenon are beyond the scope of this book.

Doppler sonography can permit differentiation between inflammatory and degenerative conditions, monitor the response to anti-inflammatory treatment, and detect mild

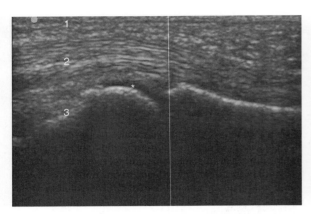

▲ **Figure 66–1.** A normal metacarpophalangeal joint. **Key:** 1, subcutaneous tissue; 2, extensor tendon; 3, metacarpal; *, metacarpal cartilage.

inflammation that may not be obvious or may be ambiguous with only gray scale imaging.

Advantages of MSUS

Most of the MSUS machines are portable. As opposed to MRI and plain radiography, ultrasound imaging can take place at bedside. This allows for immediate imaging at the time of the clinical evaluation and frequently obviates the need for referrals to radiology. MSUS allows dynamic evaluation of joints and also evaluation of multiple joints in one session depending on the needs of the clinical encounter. It is a low-cost procedure and there is no radiation exposure. Contraindications to other imaging modalities such as claustrophobia or metal implants do not apply to ultrasound imaging.

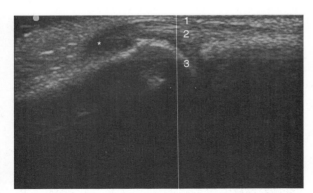

▲ **Figure 66–2.** Synovitis of metacarpophalangeal joint. **Key:** 1, subcutaneous tissue; 2, extensor tendon; 3, metacarpal; *, center of a hypoechoic collection corresponding to synovitis.

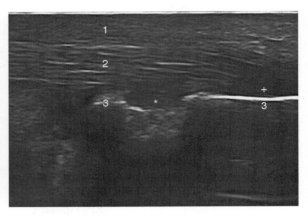

▲ **Figure 66–3.** Achilles tendon enthesitis. **Key:** 1, subcutaneous tissue; 2, Achilles tendon; 3, calcaneous; +, hypoechoic area at the enthesis of the Achilles tendon indicative of inflammation (decreased tendon echogenicity); *, the center of a discontinuation of the cortical surface of the calcaneous corresponding to an erosion.

Research has shown that patients with arthritis have lower expectations for their health and may compromise with a lower quality of life. Engaging the patient to actively participate in his or her treatment would potentially improve outcomes. Since ultrasound imaging is an interactive process performed by the treating rheumatologist, it allows the physician to share with the patient how inflammation responds to treatment, compare images acquired before and after initiation of therapy, or justify more aggressive treatment. This permits education, better collaboration with the patient, and possibly better patient outcomes.

APPLICATIONS OF MSUS

Applications in Rheumatoid Arthritis

Gray scale imaging allows the detection of inflammation within the joints by assessing the thickness of the synovium, the presence of fluid, and the synovial tissue compressibility. Doppler imaging may reveal the presence of low blood flow state and hyperemia associated with synovitis.

Ultrasound can detect synovitis early (Figure 66–2). Studies have shown superiority compared to clinical examination and equivalency compared to MRI. Ultrasound imaging may allow the detection of residual inflammation in patients otherwise—by physical examination or by traditional outcome measures—thought to be in remission. Erosions can also be detected at an earlier stage and with higher sensitivity compared to plain radiography.

MSUS joint examination is more time consuming compared to traditionally obtained joint counts by physical examination. Ongoing efforts are in place to validate the MSUS examination of lower joint counts in order to permit time efficient evaluation of patients in clinical practice and in research. MSUS obtained joint counts of few joints (as few as 7) have good correlation with higher (28 or 48) joint counts.

It is frequently challenging to predict which patients with early synovitis will proceed to develop persistent rheumatoid arthritis. Predictive models incorporating ultrasound imaging perform better in identifying patients in whom persistent inflammatory arthritis is going to develop and thus who requires disease modifying treatment.

Applications in Seronegative Spondyloarthropathies

Most experience in ultrasound imaging for seronegative spondyloarthropathies is derived from the evaluation of the peripheral skeleton and the detection of erosions and synovitis.

In addition, MSUS is sensitive and specific in detecting enthesitis. Enthesitis can be visualized in gray scale imaging as thickening of the tendons and decreased tendon echogenicity (Figure 66–3). Calcifications, insertion site erosions, or enthesophytes as well as increased Doppler signal are frequently seen.

Dactylitis can be detected as inflammation of the flexor digital tendon with or without adjacent joint synovitis. Gray scale, Doppler, and contrast enhancement–based ultrasound have been used in evaluating the axial skeleton and are capable to detect sacroiliitis.

Furthermore, characteristic sonographic changes in psoriatic skin involvement and onychopathy have been described. The extent and response to treatment of psoriatic plaque hyperemia and vascularity—as detected by power Doppler sonography—correlates well with relevant psoriasis outcome measures and with histologic changes.

Disease activity scoring systems are being developed incorporating MSUS imaging data to improve clinical practice and research in seronegative spondyloarthropathies.

Applications in Crystalline Disease

Ultrasonography appears to be useful in the diagnosis and management of patients with suspected or established crystalline disease. Compared to radiography, ultrasonography detects gouty erosions earlier. Ultrasound imaging can assist in differentiating tophi from rheumatoid nodules aiding in the differential diagnosis between rheumatoid arthritis and chronic polyarticular gouty arthritis, a diagnostic task which, at times, may be challenging.

Ultrasound imaging is useful in differentiating gout from pseudogout. Crystal deposition in gout is viewed

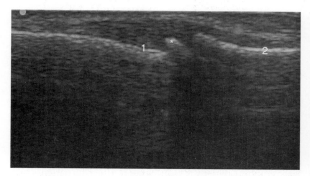

▲ **Figure 66–4.** Proximal interphalangeal joint osteoarthritis. **Key:** 1, proximal phalanx; 2, medial phalanx; *, osteophyte.

sonographically on the surface of the cartilage, while in pseudogout, it is detected as deeper depositions.

Applications in Osteoarthritis

The experience with MSUS in evaluating osteoarthritis is less substantial. Ultrasound can detect osteophytes, thinned cartilage (especially in large joints), effusions, and sometimes synovial thickening (Figure 66–4). However, ultrasonographic waves cannot penetrate the cortical surface, and as a result, subcortical cysts and marrow lesions cannot easily be visualized with MSUS.

In spite of these limitations, ultrasound has been proposed as a better modality to assess periarticular and intra-articular findings in knee osteoarthritis compared with radiography (Figure 66–5).

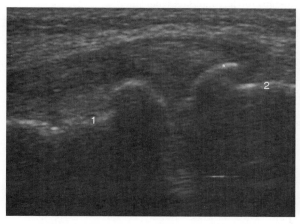

▲ **Figure 66–5.** Knee osteoarthritis. **Key:** 1, femur; 2, tibia; *, osteophyte.

Applications in Other Diseases

Ultrasound imaging has been applied in many other rheumatologic diseases. It is suggested that a characteristic sonographic appearance of salivary glands may help in diagnosing Sjögren syndrome and that salivary gland ultrasonography may be as sensitive as invasive sielography or even labial gland histology.

In giant cell arteritis, the temporal artery appears stenosed or occluded. Doppler sonography demonstrates a "halo" sign around the artery wall, probably corresponding to circumferential arterial wall thickening and edema. It has been suggested that a diagnosis may be established in patients who have a typical clinical presentation and a halo sign, obviating the need for a temporal artery biopsy.

Skin involvement in systemic sclerosis may be detected by ultrasound earlier and during the edematous phase preceding any obvious palpable thickening. Criteria to differentiate sclerodermatous skin involvement from other fibrotic entities and skin plaques have been proposed and have a high sensitivity and specificity.

Evaluation of superficial muscle inflammation in the myositides may add another diagnostic modality in detection and monitoring of myositis.

Digital artery ultrasound can assist in differentiation between primary and secondary Raynaud phenomenon and provide an estimation of the severity of the disease. Investigators have claimed that the same anatomic aspects seen with angiography of the hand can be viewed by ultrasound but in a more cost efficient and noninvasive way.

Sonography has been applied in studying peripheral nerve pathology. The most experience stems from evaluation of the median nerve for carpal tunnel syndrome. An increase in the cross-sectional area of the median nerve is considered accurate in diagnosing carpal tunnel syndrome. Ultrasound can also reveal reasons for nerve compression (such as synovitis) and also be used to guide glucocorticoid injections as a therapy for carpal tunnel syndrome.

Ultrasound is an invaluable tool in evaluation of shoulder pathology and in particular rotator cuff disease. The accuracy in detecting tendinopathy or tears is similar to MRI. In addition by allowing dynamic evaluation of the joint without involving radiation makes it the preferred method for shoulder evaluation not only by rheumatologist but also by some shoulder orthopedists.

ULTRASOUND GUIDED PROCEDURES

Ultrasound Guided Injections & Aspirations

Arthrocentesis for diagnostic purposes and intra-articular glucocorticoid injections are frequent procedures in rheumatology (Figures 66–6 and 66–7). A successful arthrocentesis

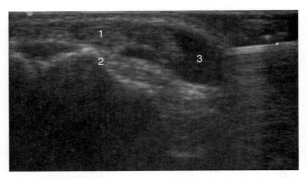

▲ **Figure 66–6.** Wrist arthrocentesis (transverse view of the wrist). Without ultrasound guidance this small collection would not be easily accessible. In addition, it would not be obvious that this is a collection within the tendon sheath and not within the joint per se. **Key:** 1, tendon; 2, cortical surface of bone; 3, hypoechoic collection adjacent to the tendon and contained within the tendon sheath; *, needle being advanced toward the fluid collection.

may help establish the diagnosis sparing the need for costly and time consuming diagnostic testing. An accurately placed glucocorticoid injection may offer immediate and longer lasting relief.

Effusions that are difficult to access may increase tissue trauma as well as the patient's discomfort during the procedure. Unsuccessful (dry) aspirations, especially of small joints or small effusions, is a common source of frustration for rheumatologists.

Accumulating evidence has established that glucocorticoid and viscosupplementation injections are significantly more accurate with real-time ultrasound guidance. For example, it has been shown that trainees performing guided injections are able to achieve better injection accuracy than experienced rheumatologists who perform blind (unguided) arthrocenteses.

Whether an improved accuracy translates to better long-term outcomes is a matter of debate. However, increasing evidence indicates that guided injections almost invariably result in less procedural pain and are more cost-effective compared with blind injections because guided injections may prolong the time to next injection.

A relatively recent study has shown that ultrasound imaging prior to any intra-articular injection may lead to change in the therapeutic plan. Up to 15% of intra-articular injections planned without ultrasound input may be cancelled when ultrasound imaging data are available. On the other hand, knowledge of ultrasound imaging findings may lead to a glucocorticoid injection or aspiration that would not take place otherwise.

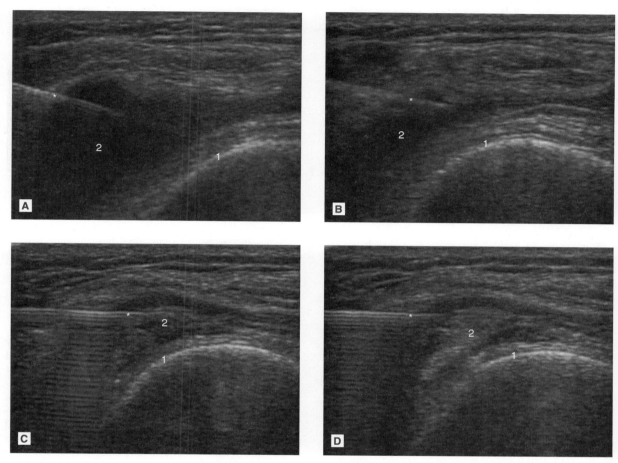

▲ **Figure 66–7.** Knee arthrocentesis and intra-articular glucocorticoid injection. **A** and **B:** A moderate amount of fluid is being aspirated through an arthrocentesis needle. The amount of fluid in panel B is considerably less than in panel A. **C:** A glucocorticoid injection has been started through a needle. **D:** The glucocorticoid injection has been completed. **Key:** 1, cortical surface of the femur; 2 (Panels A, B), hypoechoic collection corresponding to synovial fluid; 2 (Panels C, D), isoechoic collection corresponding to glucocorticoid injected into the joint; *, needle.

Backhaus M, Ohrndorf S, Kellner H, et al. Evaluation of a novel 7-joint ultrasound score in daily rheumatologic practice: a pilot project. *Arthritis Rheum.* 2009;61:1194. [PMID: 19714611]

Beggs I. Shoulder ultrasound. *Semin Ultrasound CT MR.* 2011;32:101. [PMID: 21414546]

Bode C, Taal E, Emons PA, Galetzka M, Rasker JJ, Van de Laar MA. Limited results of group self-management education for rheumatoid arthritis patients and their partners: explanations from the patient perspective. *Clin Rheumatol.* 2008;27:1523. [PMID: 18636308]

Brown AK, Quinn MA, Karim Z, et al. Presence of significant synovitis in rheumatoid arthritis patients with disease-modifying antirheumatic drug-induced clinical remission: evidence from an imaging study may explain structural progression. *Arthritis Rheum.* 2006;54:3761. [PMID: 17133543]

Checa A. Brief history parallel to the enthusiasm showed by rheumatologists at the American College of Rheumatology meeting for the musculoskeletal ultrasound. *Rheumatol Int.* 2011;31:117. [PMID: 20505941]

Cunnington J, Marshall N, Hide G, et al. A randomized, double-blind, controlled study of ultrasound-guided corticosteroid injection into the joint of patients with inflammatory arthritis. *Arthritis Rheum.* 2010;62:1862. [PMID: 20222114]

de Avila Fernandes E, Kubota ES, Sandim GB, Mitraud SA, Ferrari AJ, Fernandes AR. Ultrasound features of tophi in chronic tophaceous gout. *Skeletal Radiol.* 2011;40:309. [PMID: 20676636]

de Miguel E, Cobo T, Munoz-Fernandez S, et al. Validity of enthesis ultrasound assessment in spondyloarthropathy. *Ann Rheum Dis.* 2009;68:169. [PMID: 18390909]

Filer A, de Pablo P, Allen G, et al. Utility of ultrasound joint counts in the prediction of rheumatoid arthritis in patients with very early synovitis. *Ann Rheum Dis.* 2011;70:500. [PMID: 21115552]

Funck-Brentano T, Etchepare F, Joulin SJ, et al. Benefits of ultrasonography in the management of early arthritis: a cross-sectional study of baseline data from the ESPOIR cohort. *Rheumatology (Oxford).* 2009;48:1515. [PMID: 19755507]

Gutierrez M, De Angelis R, Bernardini ML, et al. Clinical, power Doppler sonography and histological assessment of the psoriatic plaque: short-term monitoring in patients treated with etanercept. *Br J Dermatol.* 2011;164:33. [PMID: 21070199]

Hesselstrand R, Scheja A, Wildt M, Akesson A. High-frequency ultrasound of skin involvement in systemic sclerosis reflects oedema, extension and severity in early disease. *Rheumatology (Oxford).* 2008;47:84. [PMID: 18077496]

Jain M, Samuels J. Musculoskeletal ultrasound in the diagnosis of rheumatic disease. *Bull NYU Hosp Jt Dis.* 2010;68:183. [PMID: 20969550]

Johnson CR, Chavez Chiang N, Delea S, et al. Sonographic guidance and the injection of the rheumatoid joint. *Arthritis Rheum (Abstract Supplement).* 2011;62(10):abstract 1055.

Kane D, Greaney T, Bresnihan B, Gibney R, FitzGerald O. Ultrasonography in the diagnosis and management of psoriatic dactylitis. *J Rheumatol.* 1999;26:1746. [PMID: 10451072]

Keen HI, Wakefield RJ, Grainger AJ, Hensor EM, Emery P, Conaghan PG. Can ultrasonography improve on radiographic assessment in osteoarthritis of the hands? A comparison between radiographic and ultrasonographic detected pathology. *Ann Rheum Dis.* 2008;67:1116. [PMID: 18037626]

Klauser AS, Halpern EJ, De Zordo T, et al. Carpal tunnel syndrome assessment with US: value of additional cross-sectional area measurements of the median nerve in patients versus healthy volunteers. *Radiology.* 2009;250:171. [PMID: 19037017]

Naredo E, D'Agostino MA, Conaghan PG, et al. Current state of musculoskeletal ultrasound training and implementation in Europe: results of a survey of experts and scientific societies. *Rheumatology (Oxford).* 2010;49:2438. [PMID: 20837495]

Olivieri I, Padula A, Scarano E, Scarpa R. Dactylitis or "sausage-shaped" digit. *J Rheumatol.* 2007;34:1217. [PMID: 17552053]

Schmidt WA. Technology Insight: the role of color and power Doppler ultrasonography in rheumatology. *Nat Clin Pract Rheumatol.* 2007;3:35. [PMID: 17203007]

Schmidt WA, Krause A, Schicke B, Wernicke D. Color Doppler ultrasonography of hand and finger arteries to differentiate primary from secondary forms of Raynaud's phenomenon. *J Rheumatol.* 2008;35:1591. [PMID: 18634148]

Takagi Y, Kimura Y, Nakamura H, Sasaki M, Eguchi K, Nakamura T. Salivary gland ultrasonography: can it be an alternative to sialography as an imaging modality for Sjogren's syndrome? *Ann Rheum Dis.* 2010;69:1321. [PMID: 20498211]

Unlu E, Pamuk ON, Cakir N. Color and duplex Doppler sonography to detect sacroiliitis and spinal inflammation in ankylosing spondylitis. Can this method reveal response to anti-tumor necrosis factor therapy? *J Rheumatol.* 2007;34:110. [PMID: 17216679]

Vlychou M, Koutroumpas A, Malizos K, Sakkas LI. Ultrasonographic evidence of inflammation is frequent in hands of patients with erosive osteoarthritis. *Osteoarthritis Cartilage.* 2009;17:1283. [PMID: 19447214]

Weber MA. Ultrasound in the inflammatory myopathies. *Ann N Y Acad Sci.* 2009;1154:159. [PMID: 19250237]

Wernicke D, Hess H, Gromnica-Ihle E, Krause A, Schmidt WA. Ultrasonography of salivary glands—a highly specific imaging procedure for diagnosis of Sjogren's syndrome. *J Rheumatol.* 2008;35:285. [PMID: 18203316]

Ocular Inflammatory Diseases for Rheumatologists

67

James T. Rosenbaum, MD

The distance from the surface of the eye to the optic nerve is only about 2.5 cm, but within that short distance, an incredible diversity of tissue resides and almost any portion of that tissue could become inflamed. A rheumatologist should have a working knowledge of uveitis, keratitis, scleritis, episcleritis, conjunctivitis, optic neuritis, anterior ischemic optic neuropathy, dry eye, and orbital inflammation because rheumatologic diseases can be associated with inflammation in each of these areas and because managing a patient with one of these problems may require systemic immunosuppression, a form of treatment that is outside the expertise of the vast majority of ophthalmologists.

UVEITIS

ESSENTIALS OF DIAGNOSIS

▶ Divided into anterior, intermediate, and posterior forms. Different disease entities are associated with different forms of uveitis.

▶ Panuveitis, the occurrence of anterior, intermediate, and posterior uveitis in the same patient, is particularly characteristic of Behçet disease and sarcoidosis.

▶ Management strategies vary according to whether the uveitis is anterior, intermediate, or posterior.

▶ General Considerations

The uvea—the middle layer of the eye—includes the iris, ciliary body, and choroid. Anatomic subsets of uveitis can be defined: anterior uveitis (or iritis); iridocyclitis, when the ciliary body is inflamed along with the iris; intermediate uveitis (inflammation in the vitreous humor); posterior uveitis (involvement of the choroid or retina); and panuveitis, when the iris, vitreous, and retina all show evidence

of inflammation. Uveitis can also be classified by etiology (Tables 67–1 and 67–2). A rheumatologist is usually essential in treating inflammation that is confined to the uveal tract or part of a systemic disease involving the uveal tract.

▶ Clinical Findings

Uveitis has a variety of complications including cataract, glaucoma, posterior synechiae, macular edema, and retinal vasculitis. In an unpublished series, retinal vasculitis (Plate 51) was detected in one of every seven patients with uveitis, but retinal vasculitis does not have the same therapeutic implication as systemic vasculitis and patients with retinal vasculitis rarely have a systemic disease.

▶ Treatment

Many patients with uveal inflammation can be treated with topical medications or by periocular or intraocular injections of glucocorticoids. Many ophthalmologists feel comfortable prescribing a short course of oral glucocorticoids. Glucocorticoid-sparing medications are generally indicated if the condition is not infectious or malignant, has not responded to local ophthalmic treatments listed earlier in this paragraph either due to lack of efficacy or lack of tolerance, and interferes with activities of daily living.

Commonly chosen glucocorticoid-sparing medications include methotrexate, azathioprine, mycophenolate mofetil, and cyclosporine. A calcineurin antagonist such as cyclosporine or tacrolimus can be combined with an antimetabolite, offering greater efficacy than either medication alone but also posing greater risk. Although some groups advocate the use of an alkylating agent such as cyclophosphamide or chlorambucil, the author rarely uses medications in this class to treat uveitis.

The underlying diagnosis often plays a minor role in the selection of therapy. For example, about 30% of patients with uveitis in a referral clinic are labeled as having idiopathic

Table 67–1. Causes of uveitis.

Infections such as herpes simplex, herpes zoster, or toxoplasmosis
Syndromes confined to the eye such as pars planitis, sympathetic ophthalmia, or birdshot retinochoroidopathy
Masquerade syndromes such as lymphoma, leukemia, or retinal degeneration
Systemic immunologic disease as listed in Table 67-2

disease, meaning that no specific etiology could be determined and it is presumably immune-mediated. Patients with idiopathic uveitis are often treated the same as a patient with sarcoid-associated uveitis or a patient with birdshot chorioretinopathy (Plate 52). A discussion about the nuances of therapy for specific forms of uveitis is beyond the scope of this chapter. However, methotrexate is used preferentially for children with juvenile idiopathic arthritis based on the experience using this medication in childhood. Vogt-Koyanagi-Harada syndrome (a form of uveitis characterized by bilateral anterior and posterior uveitis with serous retinal detachments and often eighth nerve disease and sterile meningitis) is generally treated with more sustained, relatively high-dose prednisone compared to other forms of uveitis. Behçet disease is especially responsive to infliximab, a drug that is sometimes instituted relatively soon in the approach to a patient with this diagnosis.

Although several oral or parenteral treatments for uveitis are currently undergoing clinical trials, no systemic immunomodulatory therapy has been approved. Of the biologic therapies, monoclonal antibodies to tumor necrosis factor (TNF) are the most widely used. Despite the lack of randomized, comparative efficacy data, the TNF therapies that are based on either chimeric or humanized monoclonal antibodies

Table 67–2. Systemic immunologic diseases commonly associated with uveitis.

Ankylosing spondylitis
Behçet disease
Drug reactions (eg, rifabutin)
Familial granulomatous synovitis with uveitis
Inflammatory bowel disease
Interstitial nephritis
Juvenile idiopathic arthritis
Multiple sclerosis
Neonatal-onset multisystem inflammatory disease
Psoriatic arthritis
Reactive arthritis
Relapsing polychondritis
Sarcoidosis
Systemic lupus erythematosus
Vasculitis, especially Kawasaki syndrome and Cogan syndrome
Vogt-Koyanagi-Harada syndrome

(eg, infliximab or adalimumab) are more consistently effective for eye disease than is etanercept, a soluble fusion protein. One prospective series using infliximab to treat various forms of uveitis found a 77% early response rate as well as a surprisingly high rate of toxicity. For example, drug-induced lupus develop in nearly 10% of the participants. Despite the efficacy, 52% of the initial participants did not continue infliximab therapy beyond 1 year.

Both infliximab and adalimumab are useful for patients with uveitis associated with juvenile idiopathic arthritis and an inadequate response to methotrexate. These children are more likely to experience sustained benefit with adalimumab rather than infliximab.

Uveitis, common among patients with ankylosing spondylitis, usually manifests itself as recurrent, unilateral, anterior disease (acute anterior uveitis). Several TNF inhibitors as well as sulfasalazine and possibly nonsteroidal anti-inflammatory drugs reduce the frequency of episodes of acute anterior uveitis in this setting. Paradoxically, TNF inhibition (especially etanercept use) sometimes appears to trigger uveitis.

SCLERITIS

ESSENTIALS OF DIAGNOSIS

▶ Erythema or a deep purplish hue of the sclera and intense pain are hallmarks of scleritis.

▶ There is a spectrum of disease severity, but scleritis can pose a vision-threatening complication of rheumatic diseases, particularly rheumatoid arthritis and granulomatosis with polyangiitis (GPA; formerly Wegener granulomatosis.)

▶ Clinical Findings & Treatment

Most patients with scleritis have a very painful and persistent redness that can affect visual acuity or could result in complications such as uveitis or glaucoma. Approximately 40% of patients with scleritis have a systemic disease (see Table 67–3). The two most common systemic illnesses are rheumatoid arthritis or GPA. Patients with GPA who have scleritis often have disease that is confined to the region above the clavicle and are at lower risk for pulmonary or renal disease. (However, the ocular disease alone often justifies treatment for severe disease.) Different forms of scleritis may have distinctive pathways involved in their pathogenesis, but most forms of scleritis are regarded as localized forms of vasculitis. A minority of patients with scleritis respond to oral nonsteroidal anti-inflammatory drugs but most require oral glucocorticoids and either an antimetabolite or an alkylating agent (such as cyclophosphamide). A positive assay for antineutrophil cytoplasmic antibodies

Table 67–3. Systemic diseases associated with scleritis.

Granulomatosis with polyangiitis (formerly Wegener granulomatosis), especially limited forms
Rheumatoid arthritis
Inflammatory bowel disease
Relapsing polychondritis
Polyarteritis nodosa, Cogan syndrome, giant cell arteritis, and additional forms of vasculitis
Behçet disease
Sarcoidosis
Systemic lupus erythematosus
Spondyloarthritis

(ANCA) in a patient with scleritis generally identifies a patient with more severe, sight-threatening disease.

Scleritis in association with rheumatoid arthritis could be a manifestation of a rheumatoid nodule in the sclera. This results in a condition known as scleromalacia perforans. A necrotizing scleritis also occurs in patients with rheumatoid arthritis (Plate 53), especially in those who have long-standing disease with nodules, vasculitic neuropathy, or pleuropericarditis. Management of the underlying joint disease as with a biologic generally helps control the disease in the sclera. Similarly, the scleritis that is associated with a systemic disease, such as inflammatory bowel disease or relapsing polychondritis, may respond to the treatment of the underlying condition.

Although scleritis is a vasculitis, most patients do not require an alkylating drug for control of the inflammation. Uncontrolled, preliminary data support the use of rituximab to treat patients with scleritis who have not responded to glucocorticoids and at least one antimetabolite.

KERATITIS

 ESSENTIALS OF DIAGNOSIS

▶ The most severe form of this condition, termed "P.U.K." (peripheral ulcerative keratitis) by ophthalmologists, can lead to vision loss within days through a syndrome known as "corneal melt." Rheumatoid arthritis and GPA are the rheumatic conditions most likely to be associated with P.U.K.

▶ "Non-syphilitic interstitial keratitis" is a buzzword for the most common ocular manifestation of Cogan syndrome.

▶ Clinical Findings & Treatment

Corneal inflammation in the form of peripheral ulcerative keratitis is a classic manifestation of a systemic vasculitis.

Other synonyms for this condition include corneal melt or marginal keratolysis. It usually occurs in association with scleritis at the margin of the cornea, which is contiguous with the sclera. Corneal thinning could lead to a perforation of the eye, and thus, it is a potential cause of blindness. Topical therapy and surgery should obviously be guided by an ophthalmologist. In patients with rheumatoid arthritis, the corneal disease usually responds to treatment of the synovial disease. Patients in whom a corneal melt develops as a component of a systemic vasculitis usually experience improvement in the eye disease when the systemic disease is adequately treated.

A Mooren ulcer resembles a corneal melt but it develops in the absence of scleritis or a systemic illness. The condition is too rare to have been studied with randomized controlled treatment trials, but anecdotes and small series support the use of immunosuppression, including infliximab, to treat this condition.

OCULAR CICATRICIAL PEMPHIGOID (OCP)

 ESSENTIALS OF DIAGNOSIS

▶ Cicatricial pemphigoid is an autoimmune blistering disease that can be associated with lesions in the oral mucosa and respiratory tract, in addition to involving the eye.

▶ Clinical Findings

This rare disease of the elderly is considered to be an autoimmune disease in which inflammation is directed against antigens, such as β_4 integrin, in the basement membrane of the ocular mucosa. Bullous lesions can develop elsewhere, particularly the mouth. Ocular symptoms of OCP include redness and irritation. The eyelid inverts (entropion) so that eyelashes scrape against the corneal surface, and these must be mechanically removed. An adhesion known as a symblepharon forms between the mucosal surface of the lower eyelid and the globe itself (Plate 54). The disease progresses slowly but frequently leads to bilateral blindness as the cornea opacifies and becomes neovascularized. Rarely, an adverse reaction to topical medications could cause similar symptoms, but the immunohistology showing immunoglobulin deposition along the basement membrane of the conjunctiva is unique to OCP.

▶ Treatment

Most practitioners treat OCP initially with dapsone. Mycophenolate mofetil has become popular as an antimetabolite for those who do not respond to dapsone. The traditional gold standard for therapy is oral cyclophosphamide. Recent uncontrolled trials have indicated the potential for successful treatment with intravenous immunoglobulin or rituximab or both.

DYSFUNCTIONAL TEAR FILM SYNDROME

ESSENTIALS OF DIAGNOSIS

▶ A clinical entity that can result from several disease-related pathways, leading to disease of the meibomian glands or dysfunction of goblet cells.

▶ Clinical Findings & Treatment

The tear film is complex and includes an oil layer made primarily by meibomian glands, an aqueous layer produced by the lacrimal gland, and mucins coming predominantly from goblet cells and epithelial cells. The lacrimal gland is a principal target of an autoimmune response in primary Sjögren syndrome. Dysfunctional tears, however, could result from disease of the meibomian glands such as blepharitis or dysfunction of goblet cells. Thus, patients who have blepharitis resulting from seborrhea may have symptoms of ocular redness and scratchiness that mimic the symptoms of lacrimal gland dysfunction. Furthermore, lacrimal gland dysfunction has many causes including aging, alcoholism, diabetes, Sjögren syndrome, sarcoidosis, IgG4-related disease, and HIV infection. A wide spectrum of medications can contribute to ocular dryness. Accordingly, dysfunctional tear syndrome is sometimes but not always the result of primary or secondary Sjögren syndrome.

A detailed discussion of the treatment of dry eye is beyond the scope of this chapter. However, the following principles may prove helpful:

1. Use artificial tears liberally. If tears are needed more than twice per day, avoid the use of preservatives that may be harmful to the corneal epithelium. Any artificial tear that "gets the red out" contains medication that contributes to dryness.

2. Minimize the use of oral medications that have an anticholinergic effect.

3. Encourage patients to rest their eyes or blink frequently, especially during tasks such as reading, driving, or using a computer. Blinking helps lubricate the ocular surface and is reduced during activities such as computer use.

4. Be sure that the house and work environment are humidified. Tears evaporate faster in a dry environment.

5. Consider the use of punctal occlusion to minimize drainage of tears.

ORBITAL INFLAMMATORY DISEASE

ESSENTIALS OF DIAGNOSIS

▶ A syndrome composed of several different diseases characterized by distinct histopathologies, generally leading to proptosis, often to pain, and occasionally to vision loss through pressure on the optic nerve or its blood supply.

▶ Multiple retrobulbar or ocular adnexal structures can be involved, including the extraocular muscles ("orbital myositis"), lacrimal gland, and retrobulbar space.

▶ Clinical Findings

Many structures within the orbit, including extraocular muscle, fat, and the lacrimal gland, may become inflamed. Symptoms from orbital inflammation include pain, proptosis, and diplopia. Vision loss can result if the optic nerve is compressed.

Proptosis or exophthalmos can result from thyroid orbitopathy, lacrimal gland inflammation, infections, metastatic disease and other tumors, lymphoma, histiocytosis, and a condition sometimes called nonspecific orbital inflammation (which was previously known as orbital pseudotumor). Imaging by MRI or CT scan, laboratory testing such as thyroid antibodies, and physical examination findings may help distinguish these causes, although biopsy is sometimes required.

▶ Treatment

Orbital inflammatory disease is frequently treated with a high dose of oral glucocorticoids. Excellent success with antimetabolites such as glucocorticoid-sparing drugs has been reported. More recently, rituximab is emerging as a promising modality in those patients who do not respond to both glucocorticoid and antimetabolite therapy. A significant proportion of patients with orbital inflammatory disease appear to have IgG$_4$-related disease, a condition that seems to be exquisitely responsive to B cell depletion.

CANCER-ASSOCIATED RETINOPATHY

ESSENTIALS OF DIAGNOSIS

▶ A poorly understood "autoimmune retinopathy" that occurs in association with some malignancies.

Clinical Findings

Visual loss can occur as a rare paraneoplastic syndrome. The immune response can be directed against a variety of different antigens, but recoverin and enolase are the two targets that have been implicated most convincingly. A similar autoimmune retinopathy can also occur in the absence of malignancy.

The diagnosis is usually made by a thorough, dilated ophthalmic examination that fails to show an alternative cause for visual loss, the demonstration of antiretinal antibodies (which, unfortunately, are also found in other retinal diseases and sometimes in healthy controls), and characteristic findings on electroretinography.

Treatment

Autoimmune retinopathy is usually treated by immunosuppression. Some experts consider intravenous immunoglobulin the gold standard, but the evidence is anecdotal. Rituximab is a potential therapeutic option that has not been studied in detail.

GLUCOCORTICOID-RESPONSIVE OPTIC NEUROPATHY

 ESSENTIALS OF DIAGNOSIS

▶ Disease of the optic nerve(s) that does not appear to occur on the basis of demyelination and is therefore distinct from multiple sclerosis and optic neuritis and sensitive to treatment with glucocorticoids.

▶ Devic syndrome (neuromyelitis optica, NMO) refers to the combination of optic neuritis and transverse myelitis.

Clinical Findings & Treatment

The most common immune-mediated cause of optic nerve disease is multiple sclerosis due to demyelination. Glucocorticoid-responsive optic neuropathy is another cause of optic nerve disease, although much less common. This diagnosis is usually made by a neuro-ophthalmologist who identifies a patient with an optic neuritis that cannot be ascribed to a demyelinating disease. Such a patient will not have brain lesions detectable on MRI that suggest multiple sclerosis. Unlike the optic neuropathy associated with multiple sclerosis, the process is often active bilaterally. Moreover, in contrast to the optic neuropathy of multiple sclerosis, glucocorticoid-responsive optic neuropathy improves with oral glucocorticoids. Optic neuropathy is well-known to occur in several immune-mediated diseases, including systemic lupus erythematosus and sarcoidosis.

Devic syndrome or neuromyelitis optica (NMO) refers to the combination of optic neuritis and transverse myelitis. This disease is associated with antibodies to aquaporin 4. The transverse myelitis typically involves the spinal cord over the length of at least two vertebral bodies. Patients with immune-mediated diseases may be at increased risk for NMO.

Antimetabolites can reduce the need for glucocorticoid therapy in patients with glucocorticoid-responsive optic neuropathy. An alkylating drug such as cyclophosphamide is likely to be more effective than an antimetabolite. One anecdotal report indicated a favorable response to intravenous immunoglobulin.

OPHTHALMIC DISEASE DUE TO MEDICATIONS USED TO TREAT RHEUMATIC DISEASE

Some eye disease in patients with rheumatologic disease is related to treatment rather than to the underlying inflammatory process. Examples include retinopathy secondary to antimalarials; posterior subcapsular cataracts, central serous retinopathy, or glaucoma from glucocorticoids; iritis or scleritis from intravenous bisphosphonate therapy; and infections secondary to immunosuppression.

Galor A, Thorne JE. Scleritis and peripheral ulcerative keratitis. *Rheum Dis Clin North Am.* 2007;33:835. [PMID: 18037120]

Kirzhner M, Jakobiec FA. Ocular cicatricial pemphigoid: a review of clinical features, immunopathology, differential diagnosis, and current management. *Semin Ophthalmol.* 2011;26:270. [PMID: 21958173]

Schmidt J, Pulido JS, Matteson EL. Ocular manifestations of systemic disease: antineutrophil cytoplasmic antibody-associated vasculitis. *Curr Opin Ophthalmol.* 2011;22:489. [PMID: 21918443]

Thornton IL, Rizzo JF, Cestari DM. Neuromyelitis optica: a review. *Semin Ophthalmol.* 2011;26:337. [PMID: 21958184]

68

Sensorineural Hearing Loss (Immune-mediated Inner Ear Disease)

John H. Stone, MD, MPH

Howard W. Francis, MD, MBA

ESSENTIALS OF DIAGNOSIS

- ► When sensorineural hearing loss occurs in the context of an inflammatory condition, it is referred to most appropriately as immune-mediated inner ear disease (IMIED).
- ► May be associated with disturbances of balance as well as hearing loss because the inner ear mediates vestibular function as well as hearing.
- ► May occur as a primary inner ear problem or as a complication of a recognized inflammatory condition such as Cogan syndrome, granulomatosis with polyangiitis (formerly Wegener granulomatosis), giant cell arteritis, Sjögren syndrome, and others.
- ► Symptoms include tinnitus, vertigo, nausea, and difficulties with two issues related to hearing: acuity and speech discrimination.

► General Considerations

Sensorineural hearing loss (SNHL) is an idiopathic inflammatory disorder, either secondary to a known autoimmune disease or occurring as a primary form of disease limited to the ear. The anatomy of the inner ear is shown in Figure 68–1. SNHL is a common feature of some primary forms of vasculitis (eg, Cogan syndrome, granulomatosis with polyangiitis (formerly Wegener granulomatosis), giant cell arteritis). SNHL also occasionally occurs in association with systemic autoimmune disorders, such as systemic lupus erythematosus (SLE) and Sjögren syndrome. Finally, SNHL may represent an organ-specific inflammatory process confined to the inner ear. Injury to the stria vascularis associated with antibody deposition around vessels and vascular occlusion observed in temporal bone specimens is likely to impair the metabolic processes that support hearing transduction. Because hearing loss is often not the sole feature of this syndrome—vertigo, tinnitus, and a sense of aural fullness often

occur as well—and because the symptoms respond frequently to immunosuppression, **immune-mediated inner ear disease** (IMIED) is the preferred term for this disorder when symptoms and signs are confined entirely to the ear. Devastating disabilities including profound deafness and severe vestibular dysfunction are potential sequelae of IMIED. Yet, if diagnosed promptly, IMIED is amenable to treatment. Unfortunately, the prognosis is difficult to gauge except in the setting of profound, sustained SNHL, in which case significant recovery of hearing is unlikely.

Several characteristics distinguish IMIED from other syndromes of inner ear dysfunction. First, its time course is relatively rapid. IMIED is analogous to rapidly progressive glomerulonephritis in that inner ear inflammation progresses to severe, irreversible damage within 3 months of onset (and often much more quickly). With IMIED, in fact, the complete loss of hearing within a week or two of symptom onset is not unusual. Second, IMIED is usually bilateral to some degree, albeit the left and right sides may be affected asymmetrically and asynchronously. Typically, weeks or months separate involvement of the two sides, but the interval may be as long as a year or more. Finally, although some cases of IMIED are marked by precipitous, irretrievable losses of inner ear function, others demonstrate fluctuating symptom patterns over a period of several months. Recurrent bouts of SNHL often lead to consistent decrements in hearing capabilities, causing profound hearing deficits in many patients over time.

Although IMIED usually occurs in middle-aged individuals, the syndrome has been described in young children and also in the elderly. Two thirds of the patients with IMIED are women.

► Clinical Findings

A. Symptoms and Signs

1. Hearing—Hearing loss in IMIED may take two forms. First, patients may complain primarily of diminished hearing *acuity* (the ability to perceive sound). Crude assessments of

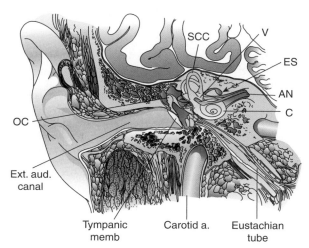

▲ **Figure 68–1.** Anatomy of the temporal bone and audiovestibular apparatus. AN, auditory nerve; C, cochlea; ES, endolymphatic sac; OC, ossicular chain; SCC, semicircular canals; V, vestibule. (© 2000 John H. Stone, Md, MPH.)

hearing sensitivity using the mechanical sounds of a watch, the dial-tone of a telephone, or the rubbing of fingers, are inadequate to detect subtle but clinically significant deficits in hearing acuity. Second, patients may also note decreased *discrimination* (the ability to distinguish individual words). Communication problems arising from poor word discrimination often constitute the chief complaint. Patients with significant deficits in word discrimination are able to hear the sound of a voice on the telephone, but fail to understand what is being said. They also have difficulty participating in conversations conducted amid background noise. Understanding conversations in crowded rooms or restaurants is particularly problematic.

Otoscopy is usually normal in IMIED, even among patients with profound SNHL. In patients with SNHL secondary to granulomatosis with polyangiitis, otoscopy may reveal findings consistent with otitis media caused by granulomatous inflammation within the middle ear cavity, tympanic membrane clouding, or even rupture.

In granulomatosis with polyangiitis, conductive hearing loss caused by middle ear disease is more common than SNHL, but SNHL occurs with a frequency that is probably underrecognized because of failure to obtain audiologic testing in all patients. Conductive hearing loss in granulomatosis with polyangiitis results from a variety of mechanisms, including opacification of the middle ear cleft with fluid or discontinuity of the ossicular ear chain. In contrast, the ischemic sequelae of vasculitis are believed responsible for SNHL. Both vasculitis of the vasa nervorum and compression of the VIIth cranial nerve by granulomatous inflammation as it courses through the middle ear can cause peripheral facial nerve paralysis.

Two simple physical examination tests are useful in distinguishing SNHL from conductive hearing loss: the Weber test and the Rinne test. In the **Weber test,** a vibrating 512 Hz tuning fork is placed on an upper incisor tooth or mid-forehead. The tone will sound louder in the ipsilateral ear if conductive hearing loss is present, and in the contralateral ear if SNHL is present. The test can be repeated for higher frequencies. In the **Rinne test,** a vibrating 512 Hz tuning fork is first placed 3 cm from the opening of the ear and then in contact with the mastoid bone. A comparison is made between the loudness of the tone generated in air and that on the bone. A conductive hearing loss of at least 30 dB is suggested when bone conduction exceeds air conduction in loudness. A normal Rinne test (air conduction >bone conduction) in an ear to which the Weber has lateralized, suggests SNHL in that ear.

2. Balance—Otolaryngologists and neurologists, who should become involved in patients' care if SNHL is suspected, should be expert at evaluating patients' vestibulo-ocular reflexes (VORs). Other tests, including audiometric testing and electronystagmography, are also essential components of the work-up.

Evaluations of the VORs consist of assessments for nystagmus in response to repetitive head shaking, and for gaze stability during rapid lateral rotation of the head. By detecting head movement, the inner ear provides afferent input to the VOR upon which the central nervous system depends for accuracy in the compensatory saccadic movements of the eyes. Disturbance of the inner ear's role in maintaining a stable image on the retina leads to a perception of dizziness, which is worsened by head movement and relieved at rest. The rapid changes in afferent input to the central nervous system associated with IMIED lead to VOR decompensation, an inability to maintain a stable retinal image, and a persistent illusion of movement known as vertigo.

The acute phase of vertigo resolves to motion-induced dizziness through central compensation after days to weeks. In the acute phase of vestibular decompensation, spontaneous nystagmus may be seen when visual fixation is suppressed (eg, in the dark or behind Frensel lenses). The VOR can be assessed for each ear separately at the bedside by asking the patient to fix her eyes on the examiner's nose while the examiner quickly turns the patient's head 30 degrees toward the ear in question. Normal VORs generate smooth, accurate compensatory ocular saccades. In contrast, abnormal VORs are associated with under- or overshooting of the eye movements, followed by a corrective saccade.

A feeling of perpetual motion known as oscillopsia is a disabling consequence of bilateral VOR loss. The presence of oscillopsia and bilateral vestibular hypofunction can be detected by comparing visual acuity with the Snellen chart while the head is at rest versus during head shaking. A difference in visual acuity of 3 or more lines is an indication of peripheral vestibular dysfunction. Larger decrements are expected in bilateral disease.

Electronystagmography provides objective measure and comparison between ears of peripheral vestibular function, more specifically the lateral semicircular canal. The vestibular electromyographic potential measured in the sternocleidomastoid muscle in response to stimulation of the saccule by low frequency sound assesses another component of peripheral vestibular function.

3. Eyes—Cogan syndrome, described in detail in Chapter 42, can be associated with virtually any form of ocular inflammation, including orbital pseudotumor, scleritis, and uveitis. The most characteristic ocular manifestation of Cogan syndrome, however, is interstitial keratitis. Granulomatosis with polyangiitis (see Chapter 32) also has a host of potential ocular complications. Diplopia, amaurosis fugax, and anterior ischemic optic neuropathy are common manifestations of giant cell arteritis. Aside from secondary sicca symptoms, the most common eye problem in SLE (see Chapters 21 and 22) is retinopathy, which may be associated with either retinal vasculitis or a clotting diathesis, such as that associated with antiphospholipid antibodies. Keratoconjunctivitis sicca is a hallmark of Sjögren syndrome (see Chapter 26).

B. Laboratory Findings

The results of routine laboratory test in IMIED are usually unremarkable. There is typically no indication, for example, of a systemic inflammatory response; acute phase reactants are usually normal. The measurement of several types of autoantibodies is highly appropriate, however, in the search for an underlying cause of SNHL that might have alternative treatment indications. Autoantibodies relevant to the assessment of a patient with SNHL are shown in Table 68–1.

C. Imaging Studies

Magnetic resonance imaging studies are essential to exclude tumors of the cerebellopontine angle.

Table 68–1. Autoantibodies and other assays appropriate to the evaluation of sensorineural hearing loss.

Anti-nuclear antibody
Anti-Ro antibody
Anti-La antibody
dsDNA antibody
Serum C3 and C4
Antineutrophil cytoplasmic antibody (ANCA)
FTA-ABS
Lyme serology
Antibodies to HSP-70 (68-kD antigen)
Routine blood and urine tests to exclude signs of systemic disease: complete blood count, serum chemistries, urinalysis with microscopy

FTA-ABS, fluorescent treponemal antibody absorption test.

D. Special Tests

1. Audiogram and electronystagmogram—Formal hearing tests should be performed on any patient with a complaint of hearing loss. The audiogram (Figure 68–2A) is a graphic representation of the lowest volume at which individual tones ranging from 250 Hz to 8000 Hz can be distinguished. An audiogram from a patient with classic SNHL is depicted in Figure 68–2B. The **reception threshold** measures the lowest volume at which speech is heard. The **discrimination score** measures the ability to discriminate words. Electronystagmography measures ocular movement in response to various stimuli, including warm and cold caloric stimulation of the ears. This test assesses the functional strength and symmetry of the VORs in response to input from both ears. Audiometry and electronystagmography testing may confirm clinical impressions of inner ear dysfunction and quantify the degree of organ involvement.

2. Serologic testing for antibodies to the 68 kD antigen—The impact of early diagnosis and treatment on long-term hearing prognosis in patients with IMIED has prompted the search for specific markers of inner ear inflammation. The sera of patients with rapidly progressive bilateral SNHL contain antibodies that react with a variety of antigens from human and bovine inner ears. However, antibodies to cochlear-specific antigens have low specificities for rapidly progressive SNHL. In contrast, antibodies to a non-organ specific protein, a 68-kD antigen found in the inner ear, kidney, brain, and other organs of non-human species (eg, cows), appear to have relatively high specificity for IMIED in humans. In a group of 72 patients with rapidly progressive bilateral SNHL, investigators found that 58% of participants possessed antibodies to the 68-kD antigen, compared to only 2% of normal participants and none of the participants with otosclerosis or Cogan syndrome ($P < .01$). This test may therefore be useful in helping establish the diagnosis of IMIED if the clinical scenario is compatible, but the test characteristics (sensitivity, specificity, positive, and negative predictive values) remain to be established firmly in the context of day-to-day practice.

▶ Differential Diagnosis

Because the treatments for various inner ear disorders vary dramatically according to cause, precise distinction between etiologies is critical. Table 68–2 depicts the major disease categories that require exclusion in the work-up of patients with possible IMIED. The etiologies of inner ear dysfunction may differ in several respects: (1) their rates of progression; (2) their degrees of symmetry; and (3) and their relative effects on hearing and balance. The etiologies may be divided into six major categories: aging, trauma, tumors, infections, ototoxic drugs, and finally, cases presumed to be immunologic in nature.

Slowly progressive, symmetric loss of high frequency hearing without vestibular symptoms distinguishes hearing

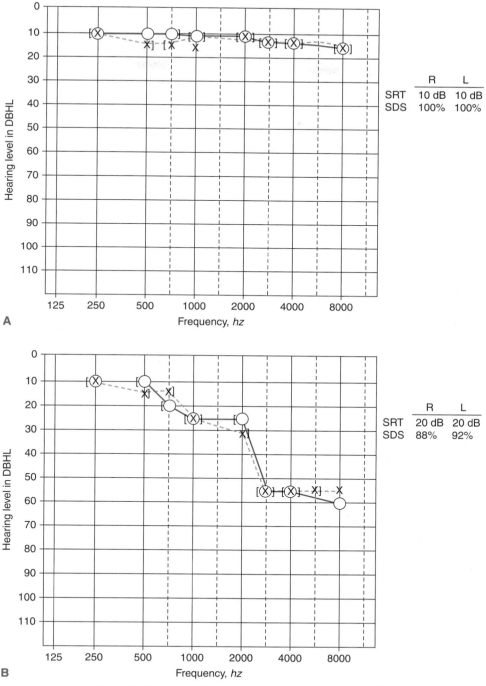

▲ **Figure 68–2.** Audiogram. **A:** Normal bilateral hearing. **B:** Symmetric high-frequency hearing loss in a patient with IMIED. Bone conduction thresholds (R = [and L =]) are measures of auditory function of the cochlea and proximal neural pathway, whereas air conduction thresholds (R = circle, L = X) measure function of the entire auditory system. SRT, speech reception threshold; SDS, speech discrimination score. (© 2000 Lippincott Williams & Wilkins.)

Table 68–2. Differential diagnosis of sensorineural hearing loss.

Time Course	Associated Disorders and Medications	Vestibular Symptoms	Distinguishing Features
Slowly progressive (>3 months to years)	Meniere syndrome	+	Episodic vertigo, unilateral hearing loss, tinnitus, aural fullness
	Presbycusis	−	Symmetric high frequency hearing loss
	Latent or tertiary syphilis	+/−	+ FTA-ABS, +/− RPR
	Acoustic neuroma	+/−	Unilateral hearing loss, tinnitus; enhancing lesion on MRI
Intermediate (days – 3 months)	**IMIED**	+/−	
	Primary		See text
	Secondary (vasculitis, connective tissue disorder)		Signs and symptoms of systemic inflammatory disorders
	Drugs		
	Aminoglycosides	+	Chronic dysequilibrium; signs of bilateral vestibular hypofunction (eg, oscillopsia)
	Antimalarials		
	Loop diuretics		
	NSAIDs		
	Lyme disease	+/−	Exposure risk Positive *Borrelia burgdorferi* serology
	Latent or tertiary syphilis	+/−	+ FTA-ABS, +/− RPR
	Acoustic neuroma	+/−	Unilateral hearing loss, tinnitus; enhancing lesion on MRI
Sudden (hours to days)	Acoustic trauma	−	Recent intense noise exposure
	Barotrauma	+/−	Recent deep sea diving, barotrauma
	Perilymph fistula	+	Otolaryngology evaluation
	Viral/bacterial labyrinthitis	+	Acute vertigo and/or hearing loss
	Early or secondary syphilis	+	+ FTA-ABS, + RPR
	Acoustic neuroma	+/−	Unilateral hearing loss, tinnitus; enhancing lesion on MRI

FTA-ABS, fluorescent treponemal antibody absorption test; IMIED, immune-mediated inner ear disease; MRI, magnetic resonance imaging; NSAIDs, nonsteroidal anti-inflammatory drugs; RPR, rapid plasma regain.

loss due to aging and chronic noise exposure from IMIED. In addition, rapidly progressive hearing loss and dysequilibrium due to ototoxic drugs, sudden acoustic trauma, or barotrauma can be excluded by taking a careful history. Meniere syndrome, a symptom complex of gradual, fluctuating hearing loss punctuated by episodes of vertigo, tinnitus, and aural fullness, is a common sequela to many causes of inner ear inflammation, including IMIED. In the absence of identifiable causes, the syndrome is termed **Meniere disease.**

Time course is the principal criterion for distinguishing Meniere disease from IMIED. In Meniere disease, hearing loss occurs over a period of several years, rather than the weeks or months characteristic of IMIED. Meniere disease is also usually limited to one ear, but delayed involvement of the contralateral ear occurs in approximately one third of cases. Because IMIED is more likely to respond to the early institution of aggressive immunosuppression, distinguishing between these two disorders is critical.

Other causes of rapid changes in auditory and balance function are difficult to distinguish from IMIED by history alone. For example, tumors that compress the eighth cranial nerve (eg, schwannomas at the cerebellopontine angle) cause asymmetric hearing loss with variable rates of progression,

ranging from days to years. MRI with gadolinium is essential to exclude such tumors. Rapid increases in intracranial or middle ear pressures (eg, as induced by trauma or a forceful Valsalva maneuver) may lead to a breach in the bony capsule of the inner ear. This condition, known as a perilymph fistula, produces rapid unilateral hearing loss accompanied by vertigo. Patients with perilymph fistulas are candidates for prompt surgical repair.

Bacterial and viral causes of inner ear dysfunction, including meningitis, may lead to swift, dramatic, irreversible hearing loss. These must be excluded quickly with appropriate cultures and serologies. Table 68–2 includes a partial list of infections associated with inner ear disease. Syphilis deserves special emphasis because of the many similarities between otosyphilis and IMIED. Syphilitic complications span the entire spectrum of inner ear disease, ranging from the sudden onset of hearing loss and vertigo associated with secondary syphilis to the gradual hearing loss associated with latent and tertiary stages of disease (sometimes accompanied by Meniere syndrome). Specific treponemal tests, eg, the fluorescent treponemal antibody absorption (FTA-ABS) assay, are indicated in all patients with unexplained hearing loss. Non-treponemal tests such as the rapid plasma reagin (RPR) have unacceptably high false-negative rates in latent and tertiary infection. Susac syndrome is a poorly understood disease entity, marked by encephalopathy, branch retinal artery occlusion, and SNHL.

Treatment

In the absence of significant numbers of rigorous, controlled studies, the treatment approach for IMIED is based largely on anecdotal experience, case series, and inference from the treatment of related conditions. Because of the devastating nature of severely impaired hearing and vestibular function, IMIED should be regarded in the same fashion as any other threat to vital organ mediated by an immunologic injury. In such conditions, aggressive immunosuppression—glucocorticoids and, in most cases, a cytotoxic agent—may halt the inflammatory response and prevent permanent organ damage. In contrast, failure to treat these disorders promptly leads to substantial, irreversible organ dysfunction within a brief time.

Numerous case reports and small case series demonstrate the responsiveness of IMIED to immunosuppression in its early stages, including recovery of vestibular function. In steroid-responsive cases, intratympanic glucocorticoids offer an alternative to systemic therapy with the potential of maintaining function with serial treatments. The authors' approach to the treatment of IMIED is guided by the concept that if IMIED is worth treating (ie, if significant inner ear function appears recoverable), it is worth treating aggressively. Thus, in the setting of rapidly progressive SNHL, treatment with 1 mg/kg/d of prednisone, not to exceed 80 mg/day, is instituted. If there is significant improvement in auditory and vestibular function within 2 weeks, prednisone is continued at this dosage for a total of 1 month, and then tapered to discontinuation over an 2 additional months. In patients with recurrent disease, some maintenance prednisone (eg, 5–10 mg/d) may be prudent. Intratympanic glucocorticoid therapy is administered serially to maintain initial benefit in response to a glucocorticoid pulse in patients who cannot tolerate prolonged therapy because of side effects or are losing benefit during or following the taper. A variety of concentrations have been suggested although the authors currently use buffered dexamethasone (12 mg/mL) which is injected into the middle ear where it remains for 30 minutes with the patient supine, and is then suctioned.

If hearing and balance deteriorate despite prednisone or do not improve significantly within the 2 weeks of treatment, cyclophosphamide (2 mg/kg/d) can be added to the regimen. Cyclophosphamide can also be considered if patients do not maintain audiovestibular gains during their prednisone tapers. Because of the potential toxicities of cyclophosphamide, treatment beyond 4–6 months is not advised. Rather, if a convincing treatment response has been established, switching to another immunosuppressive agent (eg, methotrexate, up to 25 mg/week; azathioprine, 2 mg/kg/d; or

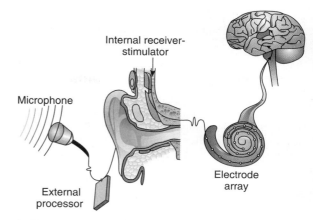

▲ **Figure 68–3.** Cochlear implant. (Reproduced, with permission, from Niparko JK, Kirk KI, Mellon NK, et al. *Cochlear Implants: Principles and Practices.* Lippincott Williams & Wilkins; 2000.)

mycophenolate mofetil, up to 1500 mg twice daily) is recommended after this time. At present, there are no data regarding the use of biologic agents to make firm recommendations on treatment with these medications.

Unless active disease in other organ systems justifies continuation of significant immunosuppression, the maintenance of such therapy after irreversible organ damage (ie, profound hearing loss) has occurred places patients at risk for treatment complications with little potential benefit. In the setting of profound hearing disturbances despite aggressive immunosuppression, the hearing that a patient may derive from a cochlear implant (Figure 68–3) may render this the most appropriate course of action. Consequently, if patients have not demonstrated a response by the end of 3 months of therapy, the medications should be discontinued.

The treatment of SNHL associated with granulomatosis with polyangiitis, Cogan syndrome, and other primary disorders are discussed in their appropriate chapters.

Prognosis

Seropositivity for antibodies to the 68-kD antigen may correlate with both active disease and the likelihood of a treatment response. One study found that antibodies against the 68-kD antigen were significantly more common in patients with rapidly progressive SNHL of less than 3 months duration compared with patients whose hearing loss had been present for more than 3 months. Compared to patients who did not have antibodies to the 68-KD antigen, seropositive patients were also more likely to respond to glucocorticoid therapy. These observations support an association between antibodies to the 68-kD antigen and the early stages of IMIED. Other studies of antibodies directed against this antigen, however, have been significantly less conclusive about its relevance to IMIED.

Hearing & Vestibular Rehabilitation

All patients with functionally significant bilateral hearing loss should be supplied with appropriate hearing aids. When speech discrimination remains poor in both ears despite maximal medical therapy and the use of powerful hearing aids, the patient may be a candidate for cochlear implantation. Cochlear implants process and deliver sound to the auditory nerve in the form of encoded electrical signals, increasing both hearing acuity and speech understanding.

For patients with dizziness due to a significant loss of peripheral vestibular function, compensation by the central nervous system is effectively enhanced through a program of vestibular rehabilitation. Such programs, administered by appropriately trained physical therapists, promote a variety of strategies to maintain balance and minimize fall risk. In the treatment of dizziness, long-term use of vestibular suppressant drugs (eg, meclizine) should be avoided because they impede the development of central compensation mechanisms.

Aftab S, Semaan MT, Murray GS, Megerian CA. Cochlear implantation outcomes in patients with autoimmune and immune-mediated inner ear disease. *Otol Neurotol.* 2010; 31:1337. [PMID: 20729775]

Calzada AP, Balaker AE, Ishiyama G, Lopez IA, Ishiyama A. Temporal bone histopathology and immunoglobulin deposition in Sjögren's syndrome. *Otol Neurotol.* 2012;33:258. [PMID: 22215450]

Francis HW, Makary C, Halpin C, Crane BT, Merchant SN. Temporal bone findings in a case of Susac's syndrome. *Otol Neurotol.* 2011;32:1198. [PMID: 21897318]

Hu A, Parnes LS. Intratympanic steroids for inner ear disorders: a review. *Audiol Neurootol.* 2009;14:373. [PMID: 19923807]

Moscicki RA, San Martin JE, Quintero CH, Rauch SD, Nadol JB Jr, Bloch KJ. Serum antibody to inner ear proteins in patients with progressive hearing loss. Correlation with disease activity and response to corticosteroid treatment. *JAMA.* 1994;272:611. [PMID: 8057517]

Quaranta N, Bartoli R, Giagnotti F, DiCuonzo F, Quaranta A. Cochlear implants in systemic autoimmune vasculitis syndromes. *Acta Otolaryngol Suppl.* 2002;(548):44. [PMID: 12211357]

Shepard NT, Telian SA, Erman AB. Vestibular and balance rehabilitation: Program essentials. In: *Cummings Otolaryngology-Head and Neck Surgery,* 5th edition. Flint PA et al. Editor, Mosby Elsevier, Philadelphia; 2010:2372–79.

[The Johns Hopkins Vasculitis Center]
    http://vasculitis.med.jhu.edu

Pregnancy & Rheumatic Diseases

69

Megan E. B. Clowse, MD, MPH

Bernadette C. Siaton, MD

Patients with rheumatic disease commonly have questions regarding conception, pregnancy, and breast-feeding, as well as using medication during all of these phases. In this chapter, these issues are discussed in the context of rheumatoid arthritis (RA), systemic lupus erythematosus (SLE), the antiphospholipid syndrome, scleroderma, and the systemic vasculitides Takayasu arteritis and antineutrophil cytoplasmic antibodies (ANCA)-associated vasculitis. The use of individual medications is also discussed.

RHEUMATOID ARTHRITIS

The classic teaching that RA improves during pregnancy and worsens in the postpartum period has been confirmed in several studies. For reasons that remain incompletely understood, pregnancy ameliorates RA activity in many women, even after the cessation of medications.

ESSENTIALS OF DIAGNOSIS

▶ Most pregnant patients with RA report improvement in joint pain and swelling during pregnancy.

▶ Clinical improvement is often more pronounced in patients with moderate-high disease activity compared to those with low disease activity.

▶ RA generally returns to its prior state of activity postpartum.

▶ Pathophysiology

The mechanisms for improvement of disease in RA patients during pregnancy likely involve several mechanisms. HLA disparities, hormonal fluctuations, and changes in innate immunity have all been studied. Higher maternal-fetal incompatibility in HLA class II alloantigens has been associated with good pregnancy outcomes and improvement of clinical disease. Such findings suggest that greater recognition of the fetal allograft by the maternal immune system leads to more tolerance of maternal autoantigens.

Regulatory T Cells (T_{reg}) are involved in the pathogenesis of RA. These cells promote tolerance both by suppressing the activity of effector T-cells and dendritic cells, and by producing anti-inflammatory cytokines such as interleukin (IL)-10 and tumor growth factor (TGF)-β. In nonpregnant RA patients, T_{reg} activity is impaired, but during pregnancy, these T_{reg} cells regain some activity, thus promoting an anti-inflammatory environment. Other alterations in immunity such as a down-regulation of Th1 cells and subsequent shift toward Th2 responses may also contribute to clinical improvement.

▶ Pregnancy Effects on Disease

Up to three quarters of pregnant patients with RA report improvement in joint pain, joint swelling, and total number of joints involved. The average rate of remission in the third trimester nears 30%. Clinical improvement is more pronounced in patients with moderate-high disease activity than in patients with low disease activity. Disease response in previous pregnancies predicts clinical responses for subsequent pregnancies. RA often returns to its prior state of activity postpartum.

▶ Effect of Disease Activity on Fetus

Although the data regarding pregnancy morbidity in the literature are mixed, consensus favors mildly increased rates of premature birth, preeclampsia or hypertensive disorders, and lower birth weights. Disease activity in the third trimester has been associated with lower birth weight. Prednisone use during pregnancy is associated with a higher likelihood of preterm delivery (before 37 weeks).

SYSTEMIC LUPUS ERYTHEMATOSUS

SLE is a multisystem autoimmune disease with a predisposition for females of reproductive age. Fertility is not affected by the disease; however, treatment with immunosuppressive drugs, such as cyclophosphamide, may result in premature ovarian failure and reduced fertility rates. SLE itself is not a contraindication to pregnancy, with the exception of active severe lupus nephritis or pulmonary hypertension. Women with SLE have an increased risk of disease flare and adverse pregnancy outcomes. Pregnancy outcomes are affected by a number of factors, including disease status at the time of conception, presence of renal disease, and the presence of antiphospholipid antibodies, anti-Ro/SSA, and anti-La/SSB antibodies. In order to optimize pregnancy outcomes, medications should be altered to decrease the risk of teratogenicity but maintain disease quiescence, and pregnancy should be delayed until the disease has been well controlled for 6 months. Antenatal care should be provided in tandem with rheumatology and high-risk obstetrics. Regular rheumatology follow-up visits should be scheduled for every 4–6 weeks; the interval should be adjusted based on clinical status.

ESSENTIALS OF DIAGNOSIS

▶ Disease status at the time of conception strongly influences pregnancy outcomes.
▶ Lupus flares are usually mild and accompanied by skin and joint disease.
▶ Patients are at risk for thrombosis as well as infectious and hematologic complications.

▶ Effects of Pregnancy on Disease Activity

Lupus flares are more common during pregnancy and in the puerperium. Flares are usually mild and accompanied by skin and joint disease. Serious flares, manifested by central nervous system dysfunction, nephritis, hematologic abnormalities, or vasculitis, occur in up to 20% of patients who experience disease exacerbations during or after pregnancy. Due to the natural disease course of SLE, rates of pregestational diabetes, hypertension, pulmonary hypertension, renal failure, and thrombophilia are higher in SLE patients compared with healthy women.

Pregnancy itself is a prothrombotic state and the risk of thrombosis is significantly increased in SLE patients, with a relative risk approximately 35 times higher than that of healthy women. Pregnant patients with SLE are also at higher risk for infectious complications (such as pneumonia and sepsis) and hematologic complications (including thrombocytopenia, anemia, hemorrhage, and increased transfusion requirements).

▶ Effect of Disease on Fetus

Disease status at the time of conception strongly influences pregnancy outcomes. In the Johns Hopkins lupus cohort, a prospective study divided women into two groups: low disease activity and high disease activity, based on the clinician's estimate of activity. Results showed that having highly active SLE prior to conception led to a four-fold increase in pregnancy loss. Risk factors for poor pregnancy outcomes in lupus can be remembered by the PATH acronym: proteinuria, antiphospholipid syndrome, thrombocytopenia, and hypertension. The presence of any of these four risk factors during the first trimester of pregnancy is associated with at 30–40% risk of pregnancy loss.

A. Nephritis and Pregnancy

Patients with both a history of lupus nephritis and currently active lupus nephritis have worse outcomes, often due to hypertension or worsening renal disease. Mild flares of renal disease are not uncommon; however, progression to irreversible renal damage may occur in a small percentage of patients. Lupus nephritis may be difficult to discern from preeclampsia or pregnancy-induced hypertension. Key elements in distinguishing between lupus nephritis and pregnancy-induced hypertension are the timing of the symptoms prior to the third trimester, the finding of an active urine sediment, and the presence of SLE activity in other organs. Compared with women who do not have active lupus nephritis at the time of conception, those with active renal disease are 4 times more likely to develop pregnancy-induced hypertension and more than 1.5 times likely to have adverse fetal outcomes.

B. Fetal Morbidity and SLE

Disease activity during pregnancy strongly influences obstetric outcomes. Rates of spontaneous abortion, preterm birth, stillbirth, intrauterine growth restriction (IUGR), bleeding complications, and neonatal morbidity are increased compared with healthy controls. The risk of preeclampsia is up to 22%, 3-fold higher than expected and eclampsia is 0.5%, 4-fold higher than expected.

C. Neonatal SLE

Neonatal SLE is an autoimmune disease associated with the presence of anti-Ro/SSA and anti-La/SSB antibodies. All women should be screened for the presence of these antibodies early in pregnancy to identify patients at risk. The incidence of congenital heart block is about 2%, with a recurrence rate of around 10–20% in subsequent pregnancies. Heart block results from the deposition of antibodies into the cardiac conduction system, leading to local inflammation and irreversible damage to the atrioventricular node. This condition develops between 18 and 30 weeks gestation. Case reports support the reversal or halting of first and second degree block with dexamethasone 4 mg/d, but complete heart block is irreversible. Repeated fetal echocardiography can be performed to detect early cardiac block allowing a potential window for therapeutic intervention.

Annular polycyclic skin plaques are the most common manifestation of neonatal SLE, occurring in up to 15% of exposed infants. The lesions appear on the face and scalp after sun or UV exposure within the first 3–5 months of life. Disappearance of this rash coincides with disappearance of serum antibodies. The hematologic and hepatobiliary systems are less commonly affected and effects are generally transient.

ANTIPHOSPHOLIPID SYNDROME

ESSENTIALS OF DIAGNOSIS

► The inherently hypercoagulable state associated with pregnancy can be heightened in patients with the antiphospholipid syndrome, with potentially dire consequences for both the mother and fetus.

► The diagnosis of antiphospholipid syndrome is a strong contraindication to pregnancy.

► Background & Clinical Manifestations

Antiphospholipid antibodies (aPL) bind negatively charged phospholipids, leading to thrombosis and recurrent fetal loss. The antiphospholipid syndrome is defined by at least one clinical event, such as vascular thrombosis or pregnancy morbidity, in combination with the presence of one or more of the following antibodies: lupus anticoagulant, anti-β_2-glycoprotein I (β_2GPI), or anticardiolipin (aCL) antibodies. The antiphospholipid syndrome may be accompanied by thrombocytopenia.

β_2GPI is a primary autoantigen in antiphospholipid syndrome that plays a role in anticoagulation by inhibiting platelet adhesion and activation of protein C and mediates binding to endothelial cells, monocytes, trophoblast, and neuronal cells. Inhibition of β_2GPI results in thrombosis and fetal loss. Anti-β_2GPI antibodies induce tissue factor release, which has negative effects on both the trophoblast and placenta and leads to thrombosis and fetal loss by affecting trophoblast differentiation and implantation.

► Complications

Pregnancy itself is a hypercoagulable state with a risk of venous thrombosis that is elevated up to 6-fold at baseline. The risk of thrombosis and resulting morbidity is further increased in the presence of antiphospholipid syndrome. Pregnancy morbidity associated with antiphospholipid syndrome includes recurrent miscarriage, stillbirth, IUGR, decreased birth weight, premature birth, and placental insufficiency or placental infarction. The rate of IUGR ranges from 11% to 20%, and rates of fetal loss range between 6% and 28%.

Maternal morbidity includes the hemolytic anemia, elevated liver enzymes, and low platelet (HELLP) syndrome, catastrophic antiphospholipid syndrome, hypertension, preeclampsia, eclampsia, and thrombosis. HELLP syndrome may occur in primary or secondary antiphospholipid syndrome. It may be the initial manifestation of antiphospholipid syndrome in some patients. HELLP syndrome is estimated to occur in 0.01–0.2% of the general population, with a higher incidence of 10–12% in pregnancies affected by antiphospholipid syndrome. HELLP in antiphospholipid syndrome may occur earlier during pregnancy when compared with pregnancies in the general population. Most cases of HELLP are associated with preeclampsia or eclampsia.

► Treatment

Women with antiphospholipid syndrome and previous thrombosis should receive lifelong anticoagulation, and this should be continued throughout pregnancy. Warfarin is teratogenic and should be avoided. Low-dose aspirin is the mainstay of treatment. Live birth rates of women with antiphospholipid syndrome who were treated with low-dose aspirin alone have been reported anywhere between 42% and 80% in the literature. Data supporting the use of combination therapy of low-dose aspirin and either unfractionated heparin or low-molecular-weight heparin are mixed. Both unfractionated heparin and low-molecular-weight heparin may be used in pregnancy, but low-molecular-weight heparin is typically preferred over heparin due to ease of dosing, lower risk of osteoporosis, and ease of laboratory follow up. Prednisone use has fallen out of favor due to increased pregnancy complications.

There are no formal guidelines regarding thromboprophylaxis in women who have aPL without prior clinical complication such as pregnancy morbidity or thrombosis. These patients are considered high-risk, and low-dose aspirin should be used.

SYSTEMIC SCLEROSIS (SCLERODERMA)

ESSENTIALS OF DIAGNOSIS

► Pregnancy outcomes in systemic sclerosis depend primarily on the extent of major organ dysfunction at baseline, particularly on the severity of cardiopulmonary and renal involvement.

General Considerations

In the past, women with systemic sclerosis were advised to avoid pregnancy because of the potential for poor maternal and fetal outcomes. Actual pregnancy outcomes, however, are better than expected and can be improved through planning and effective disease management.

Clinical Findings

Raynaud phenomenon often improves during pregnancy secondary to increased cardiac output. Gastroesophageal reflux disease worsens, but this is common in all pregnancies. Women who have had systemic sclerosis symptoms for less than 4 years, who have diffuse cutaneous systemic sclerosis, and who have antibodies to either topoisomerase or RNA polymerase III are at higher risk for aggressive disease. Women with systemic sclerosis are approximately 4 times more likely to have hypertensive disorders during pregnancy, including preeclampsia, than women who do not have systemic sclerosis. There is also an increased likelihood of preterm birth as well as newborns being small for gestational age.

The most dangerous complication of pregnancy in systemic sclerosis is scleroderma renal crisis, which can be difficult to distinguish from preeclampsia because both present with proteinuria and hypertension.

Treatment

Preeclampsia improves with delivery of the infant. Angiotensin-converting enzyme inhibitors are potentially teratogenic and normally contraindicated during pregnancy, but use of these medications must be considered during scleroderma renal crisis to save the mother's life.

TAKAYASU ARTERITIS

Takayasu arteritis, a form of large-vessel vasculitis, affects women of childbearing age and involves the aorta, its branches, and the pulmonary arteries. The most commonly observed complications include hypertension, preeclampsia, and IUGR. Disease does not typically flare during pregnancy, but caution with regard to pregnancy is advised in several settings: the presence of aortic aneurysms and the presence of renal or intrarenal arterial stenoses. Circulation should be monitored closely during childbirth as blood pressure readings may be inaccurate if vascular narrowings are present in the subclavian and femoral arteries. Catheter angiography with direct measurement of the central aortic pressures is necessary in some cases to obtain accurate blood pressure measurements.

ANCA-ASSOCIATED VASCULITIS

Granulomatosis with polyangiitis (formerly Wegener granulomatosis) is a vasculitis that affects the lungs, respiratory tract, and kidneys, among other organs. Related diseases include microscopic polyangiitis and eosinophilic granulomatosis with polyangiitis (the Churg-Strauss syndrome). All three of these conditions are associated to varying degrees with ANCA. Reported pregnancy outcomes vary among patients with these conditions. Many patients do well during and after pregnancy, particularly if disease management has been optimized prior to conception. There are no well-established relationships between pregnancy and disease flare. Patients with ANCA-associated vasculitis and histories of renal disease should be monitored particularly carefully during pregnancy.

MEDICATIONS IN PREGNANCY & BREASTFEEDING

The disease-modifying antirheumatic drugs (DMARDs) and biologic agents used to treat rheumatologic diseases have risks, including immunosuppression, increased risk of malignancy and infection, infertility, and hypersensitivity reactions. Treatment of rheumatologic disease during pregnancy requires carefully weighing the risks and benefits to both mother and fetus of medication continuation. Continued use may prevent disease flare and maintain disease stability, thus improving the likelihood for the birth of a live infant at full term. However, this comes at the potential expense of toxicity to the fetus or newborn. Proper education regarding the risks and benefits of continued use is paramount. Close follow-up and surveillance for adverse effects is warranted.

Table 69–1 categorizes the commonly used rheumatic disease medications according to whether they are considered low-, medium-, or high-risk in pregnancy, or whether their risk profile is poorly defined. Table 69–2 shows the US Food and Drug Administration classification.

Nonsteroidal Anti-inflammatory Drugs (NSAIDs)

NSAIDs should be avoided around the time of conception and in the early first trimester, as well as in the late third trimester. NSAID use around the time of conception has been associated with increased risk of miscarriage but is not associated with congenital malformations. During the second half of pregnancy, NSAIDs cross the placenta and enter the fetal circulation, which may have deleterious effects. Fetal and neonatal renal function can be affected, and NSAIDs promote oligohydramnios as a result of restricted fetal blood flow. After gestational week 20, there is a dose-related association between NSAID use and the constriction and premature closure of the ductus arteriosus. As a result, all NSAIDs except low-dose aspirin should be withdrawn prior to the third trimester. The use of NSAIDs late in pregnancy may lengthen labor via prostaglandin inhibition. In addition, NSAID use during parturition increases the risk of hemorrhage, and use late in pregnancy may lead to pulmonary hypertension in the newborn.

Table 69–1. Commonly used medications categorized by risk.[a]

Low Risk	Medium Risk	High Risk	Unknown Safety
Hydroxychloroquine (C)	TNF inhibitors (B)	Leflunomide (X)	Abatacept (C)
Sulfasalazine (B)	Azathioprine (D)	Methotrexate (X)	Rituximab (C)
Low-dose aspirin (B)	6-Mercaptopurine (D)	Cyclophosphamide (D)	Tocilizumab (C)
Low-molecular-weight heparin (B)	Cyclosporine (C)	Mycophenolate mofetil (D)	
Heparin (B)	Glucocorticoids (B)	Warfarin (X)	
Intravenous immunoglobulin (C)	NSAIDs (B)		
	Lepirudin (B)		
	Fondaparinux (B)		

[a]See Table 69–2 for explanation of parenthetical letters.
NSAIDs, nonsteroidal anti-inflammatory drugs.

Low-dose aspirin is safe during pregnancy and decreases rates of preeclampsia, preterm birth, and other adverse pregnancy outcomes. Most NSAIDs are excreted in small quantities into breastmilk. Ibuprofen is considered the safest option due to a low level of excretion into the breastmilk and its shorter half-life.

Anticoagulants

Warfarin is teratogenic and contraindicated in pregnancy because it freely crosses the placenta and may cause abortion, stillbirth, and congenital anomalies. Warfarin should be stopped prior to conception, and unfractionated heparin or low-molecular-weight heparin should be started. Women may resume warfarin postpartum, since very small amounts are secreted into breastmilk. Mothers should monitor infants for petechiae or bruising. Animal studies show excretion of

drug into breastmilk in rats. There are no formal recommendations regarding safety with breastfeeding.

Glucocorticoids

Glucocorticoids are associated with an increased risk of cleft lip and palate, although this risk is extremely low (approximately 2 of 1000 births). Pregnancy-specific complications include premature rupture of membranes (PROM), preterm birth, and IUGR. Less than 10% of active nonfluorinated glucocorticoid (prednisone, prednisolone) crosses the placenta and reaches the fetus. Prophylactic prednisone should not be administered during pregnancy; however, prednisone is an effective and relatively safe treatment for disease activity during pregnancy. The goal should be to keep the prednisone at the lowest effective dose.

Fluorinated glucocorticoids (betamethasone and dexamethasone) are poorly metabolized by the placenta, allowing a higher percentage of these glucocorticoids to reach the fetus. Single courses of fluorinated glucocorticoids are approved for use in pregnant women with risk of preterm delivery, since it has reduced risk of death, respiratory distress syndrome, and cerebral hemorrhage. They are also administered when early congenital heart block has been identified in an effort to prevent evolution to complete heart block. Patients on high-dose glucocorticoid therapy should receive stress-doses at time of delivery. The infant should be monitored for signs of adrenal insufficiency after delivery. Breastfeeding is allowed at doses of less than 40 mg. Mothers should delay breastfeeding for 4 hours if doses greater than 20 mg are used.

Antimalarials

Hydroxychloroquine is not associated with congenital malformations. It is considered safe if used at recommended doses and should be continued throughout pregnancy to prevent disease flares. Discontinuation of hydroxychloroquine was associated with more active disease and increased rates of flare as well as higher doses of prednisone use. Antimalarials are considered safe in breastfeeding.

Table 69–2. Evidence classification established by the US Food and Drug Administration.

Category	Definition
A	Human studies show no risk to fetus Very small possibility of harm
B	No risk in animal studies, no human studies Animal studies do not show harm
C	Adverse effect seen in animal studies No controlled human or animal studies Drugs should be given only if the potential benefits outweigh risk
D	Adverse effect seen in human studies Use in pregnancy may be acceptable despite the risk for life-threatening situation or serious disease
X	Adverse effect in animal or human studies Contraindicated in pregnancy

Source: Food and Drug Administration. *Federal Register*. 1980; 44:37434–37467.

Sulfasalazine

Sulfasalazine is not associated with increased risk of congenital abnormalities at doses less than 2 g/d. Sulfasalazine does not affect fertility in women but transiently affects fertility in men. Folate supplementation is recommended for concomitant use with sulfasalazine. Pregnant women with inflammatory bowel disease (IBD) who used sulfasalazine with or without glucocorticoids had similar fetal morbidity and mortality to both untreated IBD pregnancies and the general population. Breastfeeding is permitted, except in premature infants or infants with hyperbilirubinemia or glucose 6-phosphate dehydrogenase deficiency.

Leflunomide

Leflunomide is teratogenic and contraindicated in pregnancy. It should be withdrawn prior to pregnancy, and cholestyramine should be given to increase elimination. Rates of major structural defects are approximately 5% among leflunomide-exposed mothers (if treated with cholestyramine when pregnancy is discovered), compared with approximately 4% among nonexposed and healthy control groups.

Azathioprine & 6-Mercaptorpurine

Animal studies using supra-therapeutic doses have induced central nervous system and skeletal defects in exposed offspring. Both azathioprine and 6-mercaptopurine and their inactive metabolite, thiouric acid, cross the placenta. However, outcomes of human studies are encouraging. Rates of congenital malformation among children born to women exposed to azathioprine during pregnancy have been estimated to be 4% in some studies – similar to the background rate – but azathioprine use is associated with shorter gestations. Other studies have failed to confirm the association with preterm birth. The risk of defects appears to be higher with use in the first trimester. Fertility is not affected by azathioprine use.

If the use of azathioprine is believed necessary to maintain disease stability during pregnancy, doses should be limited to 2 mg/kg/d whenever possible. Case reports suggest that breastfeeding is relatively safe.

Methotrexate

Methotrexate is contraindicated in pregnancy because it can lead to congenital anomalies of the central nervous system, the cranium, limbs, and palate. It has been associated with growth retardation. Under ideal circumstances, methotrexate is stopped 3 months prior to conception and folic acid supplementation is used throughout pregnancy. First-trimester methotrexate exposure in 101 pregnant women led to live births in 66% of the women, miscarriages in 23%, elective abortions in 18%, and minor neonatal malformations in 5%. However, there was insufficient evidence to conclude that the disparity in miscarriage rate was due to methotrexate exposure alone. Fertility is not affected by methotrexate use. Breastfeeding is not recommended for mothers taking methotrexate.

Cyclophosphamide

Cyclophosphamide is not recommended during pregnancy. The medication causes structural abnormalities in the fetus when given in the first trimester, including abnormalities of the craniofacial structures, ears, limbs, and organs. It also causes growth retardation and developmental delay during childhood. Although structural abnormalities are not observed with exposure in the second and third trimester, growth restriction, defects in neurologic development, and impaired hematopoiesis have been observed.

Exposure to cyclophosphamide prior to pregnancy is not associated with congenital abnormalities or increased rates of miscarriage. However, cyclophosphamide impairs fertility in a dose- and age-dependent manner. Concomitant use of gonadotrophin-releasing hormone agonists has been shown to preserve gonadal function in women during cyclophosphamide therapy. Women should delay pregnancy for 3 months after completion of therapy. Breastfeeding is not recommended for women receiving cyclophosphamide.

Cyclosporine A

Cyclosporine A may be used during pregnancy at low doses. The rates of congenital abnormalities in patients using cyclosporine A are not different than the general population. Maternal blood pressure and renal function should be monitored during therapy. Breastfeeding is not recommended.

Mycophenolate Mofetil

Mycophenolate mofetil is contraindicated during pregnancy. Women should stop mycophenolate mofetil a minimum of 6 weeks prior to pregnancy (3 months ideal). Animal studies have shown birth defects in offspring, affecting the central nervous system as well as the cardiovascular and renal systems. Reports from the National Transplantation Pregnancy Registry show a 45.5% risk of first trimester pregnancy loss and 22% congenital malformation, including major ear malformation and abnormalities of the lung, heart, gastrointestinal tract, and kidneys. Breastfeeding is not recommended.

Biologics

A. TNF Inhibitors

The data are limited on use during pregnancy, but TNF inhibitors appear to be safe. Use of TNF inhibitors does not appear to increase the risk of infection. Attempts should be made to discontinue anti-TNF therapy prior to pregnancy. Many women tolerate a drug holiday; however, TNF inhibitors may be continued throughout pregnancy if needed to control disease.

The use of infliximab and etanercept during pregnancy is not associated with increased rates of miscarriage, prematurity, or congenital malformations. Data from the US Food and Drug Administration suggest an association with TNF and VACTERL (vertebral, anal, cardiac, trachea-esophageal, renal, and limb) abnormalities, but supportive evidence for this is weak. In the OTIS (Organization of Teratology Information Specialists) registry, babies of women exposed to TNF inhibitors during pregnancy were noted to be small for gestational age and have lower mean birth weights. However, these rates were not different from those of disease controls, and it is possible that the effects observed are attributable to the underlying disease rather than the use of TNF inhibitors. Breastfeeding appears to be relatively safe, although these data are compiled from case reports. Very minimal, if any, amounts of the drug appear to be excreted in breast milk. Children exposed to breast milk during maternal treatment with TNF inhibitors had normal growth and development.

B. Abatacept

There is a paucity of data regarding the use of abatacept in pregnancy. Contraception should be used for 10 weeks after discontinuation of its use. This medication should not be used during pregnancy or breastfeeding.

C. Rituximab

Data regarding rituximab use during pregnancy are scarce. Rituximab should be stopped prior to pregnancy, and conception should be delayed until the patient has confirmation of negative serum levels. Rituximab appears to cross the placenta and may have immunosuppressive effects on the newborn, particularly if exposure occurs in the second or third trimester. However, case reports of exposure during pregnancy have been associated with good outcomes.

Clowse ME, Jamison M, Myers E, James AH. A national study of the complications of lupus in pregnancy. *Am J Obstet Gynecol.* 2008;199:127. [PMID: 18456233]

Clowse ME, Magder LS, Witter F, Petri M. Early risk factors for pregnancy loss in lupus. *Obstet Gynecol.* 2006;107:293. [PMID: 16449114]

Clowse ME, Magder LS, Witter F, Petri M. The impact of increased lupus activity on obstetric outcomes. *Arthritis Rheum.* 2005;52:514. [PMID: 15692988]

Friedman DM, Kim MY, Copel JA, Llanos C, Davis C, Buyon JP. Prospective evaluation of fetuses with autoimmune-associated congenital heart block followed in the PR Interval and Dexamethasone Evaluation (PRIDE) Study. *Am J Cardiol.* 2009;103:1102. [PMID: 19361597]

Llanos C, Izmirly PM, Katholi M, et al. Recurrence rates of cardiac manifestations associated with neonatal lupus and maternal/fetal risk factors. *Arthritis Rheum.* 2009;60:3091. [PMID: 19790064]

Petri M. The Hopkins Lupus Pregnancy Center: ten key issues in management. *Rheum Dis Clin North Am.* 2007;33:227. [PMID: 17499704]

Somers EC, Marder W, Christman GM, Ognenovski V, McCune WJ. Use of a gonadotropin-releasing hormone analog for protection against premature ovarian failure during cyclophosphamide therapy in women with severe lupus. *Arthritis Rheum.* 2005;52:2761. [PMID: 16142702]

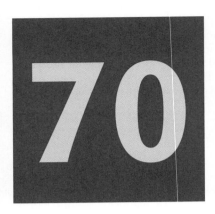

Complex Regional Pain Syndromes (Reflex Sympathetic Dystrophy) & Posttraumatic Neuralgia

Anne Louise Oaklander, MD, PhD

ESSENTIALS OF DIAGNOSIS

► Consider when limb injury causes unexpectedly severe or prolonged distal pain.

► The complex regional pain syndrome (CRPS) diagnosis also requires regional microvascular dysfunction (edema or abnormal skin color or temperature).

► Posttraumatic neuralgia (PTN) does not require microvascular dysfunction.

► CRPS often devolves through PTN as it heals.

► Variably present symptoms not required for the diagnosis of CRPS include disordered movement, sweating, and posture (eg, dystonia).

► Symptoms can be mild and transient, moderate, or severe and prolonged. Severe and prolonged symptoms are uncommon. Cases that are not associated with trauma may have an internal cause that requires attention. Such cases comprise a minority of CRPS cases.

▶ General Considerations

The cardinal symptom of CRPS is chronic pain (neuralgia) in a region influenced by one or more damaged nerves. Full CRPS usually only develops in limbs because of their circulatory constraints; PTN can develop anywhere. Onset is usually immediate or within days of the injury. Nerve damage can be disproportionate to the visible injury, such as when routine venipuncture for phlebotomy or insertion of an intravenous catheter transects nerve twigs that encircle blood vessels. Approximately 80% of CRPS patients are female. The median age at onset is approximately 40, and the condition is rare in young children and the elderly. Contrary to widespread belief, most CRPS patients and virtually all children with this disorder recover spontaneously. Patients with prolonged or severe illnesses are uncommon and in many cases

have complicating endogenous factors that impede healing (eg, smoking).

Different names have been used in the past for CRPS, depending on whether or not nerve injury was evident. **Causalgia** was first described in wounded Civil War soldiers with major nerve injuries. **Reflex sympathetic dystrophy** (RSD) described patients with seemingly trivial injuries without overt nerve damage. Other names included **algodystrophy** and **Sudeck atrophy**. In 1994, these terminologies were renamed **CRPS types I** (RSD) and **II** (causalgia). However, the use of this divided nomenclature is fading because later studies found subtle nerve injuries in CRPS I/RSD; the concept of "sympathetically maintained pain" is also fading, since it had little clinical utility. CRPS may be a complex form of PTN that involves neurogenic inflammation as well as pain. Both CRPS and PTN trigger extensive abnormalities of neural processing in the spinal cord and brain, including emotion and learning; fortunately, these seem to reverse during recovery. CRPS/PTN often spreads beyond classic single-nerve territories. These were mapped from myelinated motor and sensory axons, but CRPS/PTN primarily involves the thinly myelinated (A-delta) and C-fibers that often have far larger receptive fields and innervate bone and blood vessels outside the traditional nerve-map areas. Their axon terminals can couple electrically to adjacent neurons. Thus, injured axons can influence uninjured neighbors within nerve trunks, roots, and the spinal cord, explaining how tiny lesions can trigger regional dysfunction.

There is new appreciation of other contributors to the symptoms, including tissue ischemia likely initiated or maintained by malfunctioning microvessels. Neurogenic inflammation further recruits immunocytes to the area that perpetuate and extend inflammation and injury. Patients' intrinsic biology seems to influence the development and persistence of symptoms even more than does the inciting injury. New epidemiologic data link CRPS with asthma and other hypersensitivity syndromes, and perhaps even with autoimmunity.

Table 70–1. Iatrogenic nerve injuries that can cause CRPS and PTN.

Medical Procedure	Location of Worst Pain	Nerve Damaged
Third molar extraction	Mandible	Alveolar nerves of mandible
Lymph node surgery in neck	Behind ear	Greater auricular nerve
Breast surgery (mastectomy, lumpectomy, axillary node dissection)	Upper inner arm	Intercostobrachial nerve
Thoracotomy or chest tube	Unilateral thoracic dermatome	Intercostal nerves
Carpal tunnel release	Thenar eminience (base of thumb)	Palmar cutaneous branch of median nerve
Venipuncture at antecubital fossa or cephalic–basilic vein	Medial or lateral inner forearm	Medial or lateral antebrachial cutaneous nerves
Venipuncture on back of hand	Back of hand	Radial nerve
Herniorrhaphy	Genitals, inguinal crease	Ilioinguinal or genitofemoral nerve
Endovascular catheterization via femoral artery	Anterior thigh	Femoral nerve
Arthroscopic or open surgery of knee	Lower anterior knee, knee joint, medial lower leg	Infrapatellar branch of saphenous nerve
Casting or compression below knee	Outer lower leg, dorsum of foot	Peroneal nerve
Saphenous vein stripping	Medial lower leg, arch of foot (variable)	Descending branch of saphenous nerve

CRPS, complex regional pain syndrome; PTN, posttraumatic neuralgia.

Prevention

Accidental injuries, including fractures, sprains, and strains, are the most common cause of CRPS/PTN. About half occur on the job, and some trigger lawsuits. Medical (iatrogenic) injuries are a close second. It may not be the actual sprain that initiates CRPS, but the arthroscopy or casting used to treat it. The best prevention is to avoid unnecessary medical procedures and to remember that CRPS/PTN may possibly develop after any procedure involving cutting or punctures (Table 70–1). Tight casts are another well-documented cause. Limb edema, whether from the injury or from early CRPS, can create a compartment syndrome under a cast. Too many patients report being unable to get a constricting cast urgently removed. Early CRPS responds better to treatment than established cases, so any suggestion of early CRPS requires prompt evaluation and treatment.

Clinical Findings

A. Symptoms and Signs

The 1994 consensus definition developed by the International Association for the Study of Pain (Table 70–2) needs updating. More rigorous definitions have been proposed for research use.

1. Pain—The characteristics of neuropathic pain typically vary over time and gradually resolve. Many patients report allodynia, meaning that innocuous stimuli such as light touch are perceived as painful. Hyperalgesia refers to excessive pain after a painful stimulus, such as pinprick. Other types of pain

are present even without any stimulus, including a deep, diffuse aching or sharp, shooting pains. The pain epicenter is usually distal to the site of injury, reflecting involvement of nerves, blood vessels, and sometimes bone. Disuse (eg,

Table 70–2. Diagnostic criteria established by the International Association for the Study of Pain (IASP).

CRPS-I (Reflex Sympathetic Dystrophy)
1. The presence of an initiating noxious event, or a cause of immobilization.
2. Continuing pain, allodynia, or hyperalgesia with which the pain is disproportionate to any inciting event.
3. Evidence at some time of edema, changes in skin blood flow, or abnormal sudomotor activity in the region of pain.
4. This diagnosis is excluded by the existence of conditions that would otherwise account for the degree of pain and dysfunction.
Note: Criteria 2-4 must be satisfied.

CRPS-II (Causalgia)
5. The presence of continuing pain, allodynia, or hyperalgesia after a nerve injury, not necessarily limited to the distribution of the injured nerve.
6. Evidence at some time of edema, changes in skin blood flow, or abnormal sudomotor activity in the region of pain.
7. This diagnosis is excluded by the existence of conditions that would otherwise account for the degree of pain and dysfunction.
Note: All three criteria must be satisfied.

CRPS, complex regional pain syndrome.
Data from Merskey H, Bogduk N. *Classification of chronic pain: Descriptions of chronic pain syndromes and definitions of pain terms,* 2nd edition. Seattle: IASP Press, 1994.

adhesive capsulitis of the shoulder) and deconditioning can contribute. Pain characteristics can guide selection of pain medications. Many patients report worsening of their pain in cold weather and may need more pain medication during cold seasons.

2. Microvascular dysregulation causing focal swelling and color and temperature changes—These objective signs distinguish CRPS from PTN. Color and temperature changes can indicate cutaneous hypoperfusion (cool and pale) or hyperperfusion (red and hot) (Plate 55). These can alternate due to microvascular hypersensitivity to circulating catecholamines. Edema is common (Plate 56). Disuse and limb dependency can contribute. Dysregulated higher brain function can also cause delusions of edema, just as a lip numbed by dental anesthesia can falsely feel swollen.

3. Sensory loss—This can be primary, due to the underlying nerve injury, or secondary due to tissue ischemia (Plate 56). The hallmark of neuropathic pain is colocalization of pain with an area of sensory loss. CRPS most often arises after subtle, partial nerve injuries and sensation may be relatively preserved.

4. Disorders of movement—These are common although not required for diagnosis. Motor axon injury can cause weakness, muscle atrophy, and fasciculations but lead more often to slowed, clumsy movements, sometimes accompanied by intermittent muscle spasms. Range of motion can become reduced from disuse (Plate 56). Less than 10% of patients have dystonia, a sustained abnormal posture that can lead to contractures that require orthopedic treatment.

5. Disorders of sweating, hair growth, and skin appearance (trophic changes)—These symptoms are also not required for diagnosis, but they are common in severe cases. Patients are more likely to notice areas of excess rather than reduced sweating, but patches of both can be present, or they can alternate at different times. Skin that has lost its normal innervation can become thin, shiny, lose hair follicles, and be vulnerable to injury. If allodynia prevents regular washing, the skin develops a scaly appearance because of the accumulation of squamous cells.

6. Bone and joint resorption—Bone metabolism is regulated by small-fibers, and nerve injury can increase osteoclast activity and decrease bone density that may already be threatened by disuse. Regional osteopenia can cause pathologic fractures, and excess bone resorption can be independently painful. Nasal calcitonin or bisphosphonates can help.

B. Laboratory Findings, Imaging Studies, & Special Tests

No diagnostic blood or imaging tests are specific for CRPS or PTN. CT or MRI sometimes reveals corroborating edema of bone marrow, joints, or soft-tissues, and 3-phase bone scan can reveal the bony hypermetabolism discussed above.

However, normal studies do not exclude the diagnosis, which is a clinical one (Table 70–2). Electrodiagnostic testing (electromyography and nerve conduction study) should be considered in severe or prolonged cases. Abnormal results can help localize a suspected nerve injury, but these tests are insensitive to conduction in small-fibers, so normal results do not exclude a small-fiber predominant nerve injury. Special MRI studies can be requested to evaluate the health and continuity of a specific nerve (MR neurography). Localizing causal nerve injuries becomes important if surgical exploration or nerve stimulation is considered, and verifying an objective nerve injury can help improve physician motivation and insurance coverage for patients lacking a clear cause for chronic pain.

▶ Differential Diagnosis

CRPS and PTN symptoms are prolonged versions of the normal injury response. It is, therefore, worth considering the many causes of chronic limb injury and inflammation, including osteomyelitis and focal arthritides (such as gout). Arterial or venous occlusion (eg, deep venous thrombosis) can produce limb pain and swelling, and vascular ultrasound is often appropriate in acute cases. Rare cases without known trauma may reflect internal causes of nerve damage or irritation (eg, nerve entrapment, infection, infarction, tumor, or vascular malformation). As these may require specific treatment, neurologic consultation is recommended.

CRPS is invoked too often in circumstances where the diagnosis is implausible. This is particularly true when the situation involves symptoms of gradual onset or worsening, bilateral or widespread pain, and no injury. These suggest generalized nerve damage (polyneuropathy) such as from diabetes, which classically presents with bilateral foot pain or 4-limb "stocking and glove" neuralgia unrelated to any trauma.

▶ Complications

By definition, PTN and CRPS are complications of injury. In severe cases, affected limbs can become ischemic, infected, and ulcerated; very rarely, amputation is required. Amputation is ineffective for pain relief in CRPS/PTN, and good medical care should prevent the need for it. Desperate patients may seek unproven and potentially harmful treatments, so good communication and identifying evidence-supported treatment options is important. Many patients with unremitting severe pain consider suicide. Thus, severe CRPS/PTN should always inspire compassion and urgent medical attention.

▶ Treatment
A. Early CRPS/PTN

These cases are most likely to respond to treatment. Early intervention may prevent a downward spiral of pain and disability. Remobilization and rehabilitation are the most important treatments. Patients may require physical and occupational therapy, aggressive management of pain, and treatment of comorbidities (such as depression). Remobilization can improve circulation to affected limb to speed healing, and reduce maladaptive brain plasticity triggered by disuse. Several trials show efficacy of glucocorticoids and some data support the use of free radical scavengers, including vitamin C. Given their safety and low cost, nonsteroidal anti-inflammatory drugs are worth considering even though they have not been subjected to rigorous trials in this condition. Although sympathetic or somatic nerve blocks–a traditional CRPS treatment may temporarily improve limb perfusion, their cost and potential adverse effects (including nerve damage) argue against routine use. Moreover, meta-analyses have failed to demonstrate long-term benefit from this procedure.

B. Treatment of Pain

The bulk of pain is neuropathic – caused by injury to nociceptive axons. In the absence of high-quality evidence from treatment trials involving patients with CRPS or PTN, recommendations must come from trials in related conditions, such as postherpetic neuralgia. Evidence-based guidelines identify several initial options, including the secondary tricyclic amines (nortriptyline, desipramine), serotonin/norepinephrine reuptake inhibitors (venlafaxine, duloxetine), calcium channel $\alpha_2\delta$ ligands (gabapentin, pregabalin), and topical lidocaine. Opioid analgesics and tramadol are reasonable options to consider in patients with severe, uncontrolled pain. Limb ischemia should prompt consideration of medications such as calcium-channel blockers.

C. Treatment of Dystonia

This requires additional treatment, although many cases are intractable. Muscle relaxants such as cyclobenzaprine or diazepam may help transiently but usually fail to provide long-term benefit. Anticholinergic drugs as trihexyphenidyl, benztropine, or ethopropazine are often limited by central and peripheral side effects. The most effective oral agent is often baclofen, which augments GABA-B transmission. Intrathecal administration of baclofen through an implanted pump may be considered for those patients who response is limited due to adverse effects. Injection of botulinum toxin into affected muscles is often effective, but each injection only lasts about 3 months. Because of the expense and effort, it is only practical for small regions.

D. Surgical Treatment

The need to consider internal sources (eg, nerve entrapment, infection, tumor, or vascular malformation) has been commented upon, particularly for patients with spontaneous onset in the absence of identifiable trauma and those who do not recover within a reasonable time period. Precise localization is required before recommending surgical

exploration or biopsy. If medical management has been ineffective and surgical exploration not indicated, evidence supports consideration of implanted bipolar neural stimulators. These can be implanted at various locations, including the proximal portion of an injured nerve, spinal cord, motor cortex, and deep within the brain. Stimulation of the dorsal columns of the spinal cord is most common because a temporary lead can be placed through a spinal needle to allow a trial before permanent implantation. Completely external (transcranial) magnetic or direct-current stimulation of the motor cortex is effective for neuropathic pain, particularly affecting the hand, but treatments need to be repeated to maintain benefit so a long-term role has yet to be defined.

E. Emerging Medical Treatments

Preliminary evidence supports the use of ketamine infusions for CRPS. Ketamine is toxic and a drug of abuse, so caution is indicated. Emerging data highlight a potential autoimmune contribution to CRPS, and in 2010, a small but well-designed randomized trial found modest benefit of intravenous immunoglobulin (IVIG). Given the expense of this therapy, IVIG is not likely to become widely used. A large trial of lenalidomide, a safer and more potent analogue of thalidomide, was completed in patients with CRPS but not published. Local injection of botulinum toxin type A, which inhibits release of glutamate and substance P from nociceptive nerve endings, is effective in PTN independent of its effects on muscle tone. Ziconotide, a conotoxin administered intrathecally for refractory neuropathic pain, has preliminary case support. There is emerging support for cannabinoids in neuropathic pain, whereas the NMDA (N-methyl-D-aspartate) antagonists, dextromethorphan, memantine, and riluzole, have generally been ineffective.

▶ Prognosis

Epidemiologic study shows that most patients recover spontaneously and that the prognosis is particularly good in children. Recovery within 1 year after an injury leading to CRPS is a reasonable expectation. Early diagnosis, remobilization, and pain relief are essential. Barriers to the healing of nerves and blood vessels, including tobacco use, excess alcohol, hyperglycemia or diabetes, cardiovascular impediments, malnutrition, and subclinical polyneuropathy, may require treatment.

de Mos M, de Bruijn AG, Huygen FJ, Dieleman JP, Stricker BH, Sturkenboom MC. The incidence of complex regional pain syndrome: a population-based study. *Pain.* 2007;129:12. [PMID: 17084977]

Dworkin RH, O'Connor AB, Audette J, et al. Recommendations for the pharmacological management of neuropathic pain: an overview and literature update. *Mayo Clin Proc.* 2010;85:S3. [PMID: 20194146]

Goebel A, Baranowski A, Maurer K, Ghiai A, McCabe C, Ambler G. Intravenous immunoglobulin treatment of the complex regional pain syndrome: a randomized trial. *Ann Intern Med.* 2010;152:152. [PMID: 20124231]

Lebel A, Becerra L, Wallin D, et al. fMRI reveals distinct CNS processing during symptomatic and recovered complex regional pain syndrome in children. *Brain.* 2008;131:1854. [PMID: 18567621]

Oaklander AL, Fields HL. Is reflex sympathetic dystrophy/complex regional pain syndrome type I a small-fiber neuropathy? *Ann Neurol.* 2009;65:629. [PMID: 19557864]

Ranoux D, Attal N, Morain F, Bouhassira D. Botulinum toxin type A induces direct analgesic effects in chronic neuropathic pain. *Ann Neurol.* 2008;64:274. [PMID: 18546285]

Schwartzman RJ, Alexander GM, Grothusen JR, Paylor T, Reichenberger E, Perreault M. Outpatient intravenous ketamine for the treatment of complex regional pain syndrome: a double-blind placebo controlled study. *Pain.* 2009;147:107. [PMID: 19783371]

IgG4-Related Disease

71

John H. Stone, MD, MPH

ESSENTIALS OF DIAGNOSIS

- ▶ IgG4-related disease (IgG4-RD) is a potentially multi-organ disease with highly characteristic pathology findings and immunostaining characteristics across involved tissues.

- ▶ Organ system involvement may be confined to single organs but in many cases evolves over months to years to involve multiple organs in either a sequential or simultaneous fashion.

- ▶ Commonly involved organs include the salivary glands (submandibular, parotid); the orbits and lacrimal glands; the thyroid gland; the lymph nodes; the thoracic and abdominal aorta; the mediastinum, retroperitoneum, and mesentery; the lungs, biliary tree, pancreas, and kidneys.

- ▶ IgG4-RD has also been reported in the pachymeninges, the skin, and the prostate gland.

- ▶ Serum IgG4 concentrations are elevated in most patients (approximately 70%). One explanation for the finding of normal serum IgG4 concentrations may be the prozone phenomenon, a spuriously low result reported sometimes when the analyte (IgG4) is actually present at exceptionally high concentrations. This problem may be circumvented by diluting test samples sufficiently.

- ▶ Serum IgG4 concentrations sometimes correlate with disease activity.

- ▶ Histopathologic hallmarks: lymphoplasmacytic tissue infiltrate, storiform fibrosis, obliterative phlebitis, germinal center formation, and mild to modest tissue eosinophilia.

- ▶ Immunostaining characteristics: A high percentage of plasma cells stain positively for IgG4.

▶ General Considerations

IgG4-RD is a systemic fibroinflammatory condition recognized in the first decade of this century and now identified increasingly across a wide array of organ systems. The condition is characterized by a tendency to form tumefactive lesions; a dense lymphoplasmacytic infiltrate rich in IgG4-positive plasma cells; storiform fibrosis; and, often but not always, elevated serum IgG4 concentrations. The first organ within the spectrum of IgG4-RD to be linked with elevations in serum IgG4 concentrations was the pancreas. Pancreatic involvement by IgG4-RD is now termed type 1 autoimmune pancreatitis. In 2003, extrapancreatic manifestations were identified in patients with this pancreatic disease, and IgG4-RD has now been described in virtually every organ system: the biliary tree, salivary glands, periorbital tissues, kidneys, lungs, lymph nodes, meninges, aorta, breast, prostate, thyroid, pericardium, and skin. The histopathologic features bear striking similarities across organs. In 2011, recommendations for the nomenclature of individual organ system manifestations were put forth following an international symposium on this condition.

One consequence of the recognition of IgG4-RD is that many medical conditions once viewed as separate conditions isolated to single organs are now acknowledged to be part of the IgG4-RD spectrum. Examples of this include "Mikulicz syndrome," "Küttner tumor," and Riedel thyroiditis. In addition, IgG4-RD also accounts for substantial percentages of diseases characterized by the presence of pseudotumors or fibrotic lesions of previously unclear etiologies. IgG4-RD is responsible for significant proportions of cases of orbital pseudotumors, retroperitoneal fibrosis, and sclerosing mesenteritis, among other cases of inflammation within organs that until recently has been considered to be of obscure origin.

The etiology of IgG4-RD remains unknown. There is no definitive evidence for a link with autoimmunity. Many patients have overlaps with allergic conditions, such as asthma and allergic rhinitis. Few population-based studies of IgG4-RD have been performed and the disease epidemiology remains poorly described, but certain striking demographic features are evident. Cases in children are rare but described. Approximately 60–80% of patients are males older than the age of 50, but some variations on these demographic features occur in the different organs affected by IgG4-RD. For example, in the case of IgG4-RD affecting the organs of the head and neck, women appear to be affected as frequently as men. Much remains unknown about the behavior of IgG4 in vivo and the nature of its role in IgG4-RD (primary or secondary) remains to be fully defined.

▶ Clinical Findings

A. Symptoms and Signs

The major symptoms and differential diagnoses of each organ lesion are summarized in Table 71–1. IgG4-RD usually presents subacutely and most patients are not constitutionally ill, but a minority of patients have strong clinical manifestations of systemic inflammation at diagnosis, eg, fevers and elevations of acute phase reactants. IgG4-RD is often identified through findings observed unexpectedly by the radiologist or pathologist.

IgG4-RD sometimes remains confined to one organ, eg, the salivary or lacrimal glands, for many years. However, some patients have major clinical disease in one organ but less obvious or even subclinical involvement in other organs. As an example, although patients with autoimmune pancreatitis generally have pancreatic dysfunction as a major clinical manifestation, careful scrutiny by physical examination, urinalysis, cross-sectional imaging, positron emission tomography (PET) scanning, or other evaluations may unveil disease in the lungs, kidneys, lymph nodes, or other organs.

Table 71–1. Differential diagnosis of IgG4-related disease.

Systemic autoimmune conditions and vasculitides
Sjögren syndrome
Granulomatosis with polyangiitis (formerly Wegener granulomatosis)
Eosinophilic granulomatosis with polyangiitis (Churg-Strauss syndrome)
Giant cell arteritis/giant cell aortitis
Takayasu arteritis
Granulomatous disorders
Sarcoidosis
Fungal infections (histoplasmosis, blastomycosis, coccidioidomycosis)
Malignancies
Lymphoma, particularly MALT lymphoma
Multicentric Castleman disease
Adenocarcinoma of the pancreas
Renal cell carcinoma
Bronchoalveolar carcinoma of the lung

Multi-organ disease may be evident at diagnosis but can also evolve metachronously, over months to years. Spontaneous improvement, sometimes leading to at least temporary clinical resolution in certain organ system manifestations, can occur.

Tumefactive lesions and allergic disease are common manifestations of IgG4-RD. IgG4-RD account for a variable proportion of tumorous swellings in organs such as the orbits, salivary and lacrimal glands, lungs, kidneys, and other organs. One series and other clinical experience indicate, for example, that 25–50% of orbital pseudotumors fall within the spectrum of IgG4-RD. Allergic features such as atopy, eczema, asthma, and modest peripheral eosinophilia also accompany IgG4-RD in up to 40% of patients.

The clinical manifestations of each of the commonly involved organs are discussed below.

1. Salivary glands—Both the submandibular and parotid glands can be affected by IgG4-RD. The disease has a particular predilection to involve the submandibular glands bilaterally and in isolation (Plate 57), a point that frequently helps distinguish it from Sjögren syndrome. The usual symptom at presentation is glandular swelling, with variable degrees of discomfort and tenderness that range from mild to substantial. Xerostomia often results from chronic sclerosing sialadenitis but this is less frequent than in Sjögren syndrome. The entity once known as "Mikulicz disease," used nonspecifically to designate swelling of the submandibular, parotid, and lacrimal glands that was not associated with cancer, is probably more accurately called IgG4-RD in most cases.

2. Lacrimal gland and orbital disease—Many cases of "idiopathic" orbital pseudotumor in the past, including those involving the lacrimal gland (Plate 58), have not been subjected to biopsy. Even if biopsied, IgG4 staining has seldom been performed. Consequently, the frequency with which IgG4-RD affects the orbit has been overlooked until recently. Substantial proptosis can result from IgG4-RD involvement of the orbit, even in the setting of lacrimal disease alone. Such proptosis is one of several manifestations through which IgG4-RD mimics granulomatosis with polyangiitis (formerly Wegener granulomatosis). Orbital disease associated with IgG4-RD occasionally extends into the sinuses or the cavernous sinus, and disease originating from those sites can also affect the orbit. Vision loss can ensue if the blood supply to the optic nerve is disrupted by the mass effect.

3. Thyroid gland—Riedel thyroiditis, a disorder associated with fibrosis and woody enlargement of the thyroid gland, was of obscure etiology until recently when the link between this condition and IgG4-RD was ascertained. Riedel thyroiditis has been known for decades to occur in association with fibrotic lesions in other organs, eg, the lacrimal glands, retroperitoneum, and mediastinum, in the context of an entity labeled "multifocal fibrosclerosis." IgG4-RD now appears to account for the majority of such cases.

4. Lymph nodes—IgG4-RD can be associated with tender or nontender lymphadenopathy, with or without other organ manifestations of the disease. The diagnosis of IgG4-RD is difficult to make on the basis of a lymph node biopsy alone, as lymph nodes seldom undergo the degree of "storiform fibrosis" (see Special Tests, Biopsy, below) observed in other organs.

5. Thoracic aorta—IgG4-RD appears to cause approximately 10% of cases of "idiopathic" ascending aortitis, and is known to lead to complications such as aneurysm and dissection. Primary branch involvement of the thoracic aorta is less common than in other causes of large-vessel vasculitis, eg, Takayasu arteritis or giant cell aortitis.

6. Abdominal aorta and retroperitoneal fibrosis—The abdominal aorta can also be involved by the syndrome of "inflammatory abdominal aortic aneurysm," which overlaps to a large degree with retroperitoneal fibrosis and perianeurysmal fibrosis under a larger heading of chronic periaortitis.

7. Fibrosing mediastinitis and sclerosing mesenteritis—These two conditions are rare entities that also have other causes (eg, histoplasmosis in the setting of fibrosing mediastinitis). However, small case series now document the relatively high frequency with which biopsies from patients with these disorders demonstrate the typical histopathologic and immunohistochemical staining patterns of IgG4-RD.

8. Lungs—The pulmonary lesions of IgG4-RD remain rather poorly described but several small series have identified a remarkable diversity of clinical and radiologic presentations, making it clear that IgG4-RD can mimic many disorders with lung features. In some patients, lung lesions due to IgG4-related pulmonary disease are asymptomatic and are only diagnosed during broader work-up designed to exclude systemic causes of IgG4-RD manifestations in other organs. However, cough and dyspnea can also be presenting symptoms in patients with IgG4-RD. The diverse radiologic manifestations of IgG4-RD in the lung are described below.

9. Biliary tree—For years it was recognized that a subset of patients with "primary sclerosing cholangitis" had disease that was responsive to glucocorticoids. Histopathologic evaluations of liver biopsies in such patients, interpreted now in the light of IgG4-RD, reveal IgG4-related cholangitis, characterized by lymphoplasmacytic infiltrates surrounding the bile ducts, and high IgG4/total IgG ratio among plasma cells in the lesions, storiform fibrosis, obliterative phlebitis, and modest tissue eosinophilia, all hallmarks of IgG4-RD. The distinction of IgG4-related sclerosing cholangitis from primary sclerosing cholangitis is crucial because of the differential responses to therapy that are characteristic of these separate conditions.

10. Pancreas—Type 1 autoimmune pancreatitis is the paradigm of organ involvement in IgG4-RD. In the setting of pancreatic masses, patients often have painless jaundice. As a result, many patients have undergone Whipple procedures for presumed adenocarcinoma of the pancreas. The classic demographic profile of such patients—middle-aged to elderly men—facilitates misdiagnosis in this setting because such a demographic profile is also typical of pancreatic cancer. In addition to icterus, patients may also have nonspecific abdominal pain, anorexia, weight loss, and features of IgG4-RD in extrapancreatic organs that may be overlooked. The radiologic features of type 1 autoimmune pancreatitis are discussed below. Type 1 autoimmune pancreatitis must be differentiated from type 2 disease, a condition with which it shares some clinical features but also vital pathologic distinctions.

11. Kidneys—Renal disease in IgG4-RD has two major clinical presentations: mass-like lesions that can mimic renal cell carcinoma and tubulointerstitial nephritis. A small number of cases to date have also been documented to have membranous glomerulonephritis (occurring simultaneously with tubulointerstitial disease), but the antibody specificity in such cases of glomerular disease appears to be different from that associated with idiopathic membranoproliferative glomerulonephritis. The mass lesions in IgG4-related kidney disease can be multiple and bilateral, and biopsy typically reveals tubulointerstitial nephritis. Laboratory findings in this setting are subnephrotic range proteinuria and mild to moderate hypocomplementemia of the third and fourth components of complement. The hypocomplementemia is consistent with the detection of immune complexes within the kidney by both immunofluorescence and electron microscopy. Azotemia occurs in a minority of patients and end-stage renal disease has been reported.

12. Other—IgG4-RD has also been described in the pachymeninges, skin, prostate gland, pericardium, and middle ear. Bone-destructive lesions have been reported in the middle ear in some patients, mimicking granulomatosis with polyangiitis (formerly Wegener granulomatosis), chronic infection, and malignancy.

B. Laboratory Findings

1. Serum IgG4 concentration—Most patients with IgG4-RD have elevated serum IgG4 concentrations, but the range varies widely. Approximately 30% of patients have normal serum IgG4 concentrations despite classic pathologic findings of IgG4-RD. One explanation for this finding in some patients is the prozone effect—a laboratory error (spuriously low result) induced by failure of the laboratory to perform a sufficient number of dilutions of the sample in the setting of a large quantity of analyte. Extremely limited data exist regarding the test characteristics of serum IgG4 concentrations in patients with potential IgG4-RD, and some of these data are confounded by clinical misclassification or laboratory error or both.

Monitoring IgG4 concentrations during glucocorticoid treatment yields unreliable data on disease activity. In most patients who have elevated IgG4 concentrations at baseline, glucocorticoid therapy lowered serum levels. In others, serum concentrations normalized. However, serum IgG4 concentrations remain abnormal in most. Patients can achieve clinical remissions without serum IgG4 concentrations normalizing and may relapse despite having normal serum IgG4 measurements. At the present time, the usefulness of serial serum IgG4 concentrations as a gauge of disease activity must be individualized for each patient.

2. Inflammatory markers—Several patterns of acute phase reactant levels are observed in IgG4-RD. Only a small percentage (approximately 10%) have striking elevations of both the erythrocyte sedimentation rate (ESR) and the C-reactive protein (CRP). It is more common, however, for both of these measurements to be normal. Because the ESR is often affected by the level of hypergammaglobulinemia, another common pattern observed is a moderate to high elevation of the ESR in the setting of a normal CRP. Neither the ESR nor the CRP appears to be a reliable biomarker across the spectrum of disease activity in IgG4-RD.

3. Eosinophilia—Mild to moderate peripheral eosinophilia is a common finding in the blood of patients with IgG4-RD, just as eosinophilia is frequently present within the tissue of affected organs. Peripheral eosinophilias of 20% of the total white blood cell count are typical of IgG4-RD.

4. Complement levels—Mild hypocomplementemia of both the third and fourth components of complement can be detected in IgG4-RD, particularly in those patients with renal disease. Presumably this finding is indicative of immune complex deposition within the kidney and other organs, although additional studies of this phenomenon and the nature of immune complexes detectable at sides of disease are required.

5. Urinalysis—Subnephrotic range proteinuria is typical of the tubulointerstitial disease of IgG4-RD.

C. Imaging Studies

1. Radiography—Chest radiographs are often the route through which unsuspected pulmonary disease is identified. However, other imaging studies of the lungs are more useful in delineating the nature and extent of pulmonary involvement in IgG4-RD.

2. Computed tomography (CT)—CT scans are useful in three major settings in IgG4-RD: pulmonary disease, pancreatic disease, and renal disease.

a. Pulmonary disease—CT scans have identified a number of pleuropulmonary lesions that are characteristic of IgG4-RD. These include nodules, ground-glass opacities, interstitial lesions leading sometimes to honeycombing, thickening of the bronchovascular bundle, and pleural thickening. These radiologic lesions may mimic many forms of rheumatologic, oncologic, or infectious disease (see Table 71–1).

b. Pancreatic disease—Abdominal CT scans may reveal a "sausage-shaped" pancreas, sometimes accompanied by an echogenic halo of surrounding edema. The pancreas is typically diffusely enlarged. The classic radiologic presentation in the proper clinical setting is strongly suggestive of type 1 (IgG4-related) autoimmune pancreatitis, but biopsy is essential in atypical presentations to exclude pancreatic carcinoma.

c. Renal disease—A high percentage of patients with type 1 (IgG4-related) autoimmune pancreatitis have IgG4-related kidney disease as well. Diffusely enlarged kidneys may be evident, and pseudotumors may resemble renal cell carcinoma strongly. IgG4-related pseudotumors within the kidney typically have a hypoattenuated appearance on CT.

3. Positron emission tomography (PET)—Total body PET imaging appears to be a sensitive modality for defining the extent of disease in IgG4-RD. Additional studies are required to define its sensitivity to change following treatment and its role as an outcome measure in studies of this disease.

4. Magnetic resonance imaging (MRI)—MRI is most useful in the evaluation of patients with the two most common neurologic manifestations of IgG4-RD: namely, pachymeningitis and hypophysitis. MRI can also identify perineural encasement by IgG4-related inflammation that may be symptomatic or asymptomatic.

D. Special Tests

The crux of an IgG4-RD diagnosis is the nature of the histopathologic findings in a biopsy from an affected organ. Misdiagnoses of IgG4-RD result if excessive emphasis is placed on moderate serum concentration elevations of IgG4 or overreliance on the finding of IgG4-positive plasma cells in tissue.

A key morphologic feature of IgG4-RD is a dense lymphoplasmacytic infiltrate that is organized in a storiform pattern (Plates 59 and 60). "Storiform" refers to a matted, irregularly whorled pattern of fibrosis. The fibrosis appears to swirl past cellular elements of the tissues as water flowing by rocks in a stream. Other histopathologic hallmarks are obliterative phlebitis, a mild to moderate eosinophil infiltrate, and the presence of germinal centers. The inflammatory lesion frequently forms a tumefactive mass that is associated with tissue destruction.

Some histopathologic findings are distinctly unusual in IgG4-RD, and their presence should conjure other potential diagnoses. Such findings include necrosis, granulomatous inflammation, and significant collections of neutrophilic inflammation.

The histologic appearance of IgG4-RD is highly characteristic and essential to the diagnosis, but this may be clinched by the findings of immunostaining studies. The ratio of IgG4-positive plasma cells to the total number of plasma cells within tissue (ie, the IgG4/total IgG ratio) is usually high (0.4 to 0.8 or higher). Such high ratios are particularly remarkable when one considers that in normal individuals IgG4 comprises approximately 4% of the circulating immunoglobulin pool. Among patients with IgG4-RD whose tissues are biopsied at stages of advanced fibrosis, as is true of many patients with retroperitoneal fibrosis, for example, the link to IgG4-RD may be more difficult to establish because of smaller overall numbers of plasma cells. However, the IgG4:total IgG ratio remains high in that setting.

Both clinicians and pathologists must bear in mind that IgG4-positive cells are found in a wide variety of inflammatory infiltrates and that the detection of significant numbers of IgG4-positive plasma cells is not diagnostic of IgG4-RD. However, a diffuse IgG4-positive plasma cell infiltrate with more than 30 IgG4-positive cells/HPF and an IgG4:IgG ratio greater than 50% provides compelling evidence of IgG4-RD, particularly in conjunction with the appropriate histopathologic appearance.

The inflammatory infiltrate is composed of an admixture of T- and B-lymphocytes. Whereas B cells are typically organized in germinal centers, the T cells are distributed diffusely throughout the lesion. All immunoglobulin subclasses may be represented within involved tissue, but IgG4 predominates. Clonality studies are required to exclude these malignancies.

Differential Diagnosis

The differential diagnosis of IgG4-RD is shown in Table 71–1.

Treatment

IgG4-RD can lead to serious organ dysfunction and failure. Consequently, vital organ involvement such as that affecting the biliary tree, aorta, or retroperitoneum must be identified quickly and treated aggressively. On the other hand, not all disease manifestations require immediate treatment. For example, IgG4-related lymphadenopathy is often indolent and asymptomatic. Watchful waiting is therefore prudent in some cases.

Glucocorticoids are typically the first line of therapy. One approach pioneered in Japan for the treatment of type 1 (IgG4-related) autoimmune pancreatitis involves the use of prednisone, 0.6 mg/kg/d for 2–4 weeks followed by a taper over 3–6 months to 5 mg/d, and then continued at a dose between 2.5 mg/d and 5.0 mg/d for up to 3 years. Disease relapses are common despite the use of maintenance glucocorticoids, however. Another approach has been to discontinue glucocorticoids entirely within 3 months. Glucocorticoids appear to be effective (initially, at least) in the majority of IgG4-RD patients, but disease flares are common. The true role of potentially steroid-sparing agents (such as azathioprine, mycophenolate mofetil, and methotrexate),

if any, remains unclear. Their efficacy has never been tested in clinical trials, and observational studies suggest that their efficacy is limited. For patients with recurrent or refractory disease, B-cell depletion with rituximab appears to be a useful approach. Swift clinical responses have been observed with a striking targeting of the serum IgG4 level, accompanied by clinical improvement within weeks.

Complications

IgG4-RD often causes major tissue damage and can lead to organ failure but generally does so subacutely. Nevertheless, a subset of patients appear to have more fulminant disease, with progression to serious organ damage over a period of weeks. Destructive bone lesions in the sinuses, head, and middle ear spaces that mimic granulomatous polyangiitis (formerly Wegener granulomatosis) occur in a small number of patients, but less aggressive lesions are the rule in most. In other organs, untreated IgG4-related cholangitis can lead to hepatic failure within months, and IgG4-related aortitis can cause aneurysms and dissections. Substantial renal dysfunction and even renal failure can ensue from IgG4-related tubulointerstitial disease. The ability to identify patients at risk for lesions that are swiftly destructive of involved tissues is presently suboptimal. Early diagnosis, comprehensive evaluations, and close follow-up are essential to ensuring good outcomes in this disease that is usually highly treatable.

When to Refer

The number of subspecialists who are conversant on the topic of this emerging disease is growing yet remains small. It is important that patients be evaluated by clinicians who are familiar with this condition and willing to educate themselves further on the nuances of the disease. Evaluation of tissue biopsies by pathologists skilled in the diagnosis of this disease is also crucial to the establishment of the correct diagnosis.

Deshpande V, Zen Y, Ferry JA, et al. Consensus Statement on the Pathology of IgG4-related disease. *Mod Pathol.* 2012; in press.

Khosroshahi A, Carruthers MD, Deshpande V, Unizony S, Bloch D, Stone JH. Rituximab for the treatment of IgG4-related disease: Lessons from 10 consecutive patients. *Medicine (Baltimore).* 2012;91:57. [PMID: 22210556]

Khosroshahi A, Stone JH. A clinical overview of IgG4-related disease. *Curr Opin Rheumatol.* 2011;23:57. [PMID: 21124086]

Khosroshahi A, Stone JH. IgG4-related systemic disease: the age of discovery. *Curr Opin Rheumatol.* 2011;23:72. [PMID: 21124088]

Stone JH, Khosroshahi A, Deshpande V, et al. IgG4-Related Disease: Recommendations for the Nomenclature of this Condition and its Individual Organ System Manifestations. *Arthritis Rheum.* (in press).

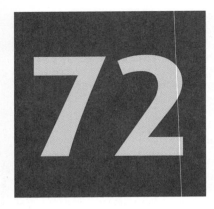

Common Injuries from Running

Calvin R. Brown Jr., MD

Approximately 11 million people in the United States run more than 100 days per year. Recreational exercise is attractive because it improves the quality of life and increases longevity. Runners note a range of salutary effects, from improved cardiopulmonary capacity to enhanced mental health, less depression and anxiety, and a greater sense of tranquility.

Regular exercise enhances sleep patterns; promotes a stronger and more stable musculoskeletal system; and results in decreases in disability, hypertension, diabetes, cancer, stroke, and osteoporosis. Runners report increased appetite and healthier weight, a desirable combination. Except for walking, running may be the most easily accessible and least expensive form of regular exercise.

However, there are important health concerns that develop as a consequence of running as well. These include the risk of sudden death, musculoskeletal injuries, and potentially deleterious effects on joints. Approximately 45–70% of runners will experience musculoskeletal injuries each year.

Risk Factors

Repetitive use, rather than a single traumatic event, causes the majority of running injuries. Table 72–1 lists the 10 most common injuries seen in one clinic and is representative of reports from other large series. Risk factors for running injuries include history of a previous injury, competitive running, high weekly mileage (>25 miles per week), and abrupt increases in the intensity or duration of training. Injuries are more likely to occur when the runner's shoes are worn down, leading to the recommendation that shoes be replaced every 6 months or after 400 miles of use.

Stretching is of particular interest because runners frequently report performing better and feeling better after stretching. However, a large controlled trial of stretching as taught by an Olympic marathon coach showed no difference in injury type or frequency between the intervention and control groups. Thus, the well-entrenched lore of stretching and running does not have evidence-based support.

Similarly, there is little or no evidence to support proposed links between running injuries and age, gender, body mass, hill running, running on hard surfaces, time of year, and time of day.

Physical Examination

The physical examination of an injured runner should not only focus on the area of pain but should also include an examination of adjacent joints, alignment, and flexibility. Approximately 20–40% of running injuries can be related to structural abnormalities. The foot must dissipate 110 tons of force for every mile run, and alignment abnormalities of the foot are associated with increased frequency of injury. A high-arched foot (pes cavus) is rigid and tends to transmit impact up the leg. A flat foot (pes planus) leads to excessive pronation of the foot during running, which in turn increases stress on the medial structures of the ankle, shin, and knee. Orthotics may be helpful for either type of structural abnormality.

Hamstring and calf flexibility can be assessed with the runner in the supine position on the examining table, the femur at 90 degrees to the table, and the foot at 90 degrees to the tibia. The physician should be able to passively extend the knee to within 15 degrees of full extension. Although there is little evidence that stretching prevents running injuries, stretching may be of therapeutic value for the injured runner with limited flexibility.

Shoe Evaluation

The athletic shoe industry is a $13 billion-per-year industry that sells more than 350 million pairs of shoes annually. Sports shoes, particularly running shoes, have penetrated into every facet of mainstream America. They have become a fashion statement, and even convey some of us to work. Consequently, the use of athletic shoes for casual and fashion wear has had a large influence on their appearance and

Table 72–1. The 10 most common running injuries.

Medical Diagnosis	Percentage	n
Patellar pain syndrome	25.8	468
Stress fractures	13.2	239
Achilles tendinitis	6.0	109
Plantar fasciitis	4.7	85
Patellar tendinitis	4.5	81
Iliotibial band syndrome	4.3	78
Metatarsalgia	3.2	58
Tibial stress syndrome	2.6	47
Tibialis posterior tendinitis	2.5	45
Peroneus tendinitis	1.9	34
Total	68.7	1224

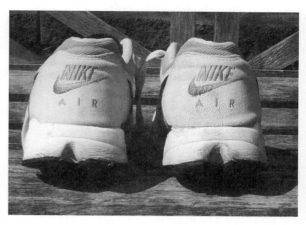

▲ **Figure 72–1.** Shoe wear. The upper of the left shoe tilts toward the inside, a finding indicative of overpronation.

features. Fortunately, podiatric biomechanical thought and technology have sunk deeply into the psyche of the industry and buying public. Terms such as pronation, stability, and motion control are now widely used in the description and rankings of running shoes.

Today's running shoes are designed with an eye toward accommodating various types and shapes of feet. Shoes are made that allow for differences between men and women, light-and heavyweight runners, pronated and supinated (under-pronated) feet, and narrow and wide feet. Increasingly sports-specific shoes meet the diverse needs of different sports, and even different running conditions such as trail running and racing on various surfaces.

Evaluation of an injured runner should always include examination of a well-used pair of running shoes, so patients coming to a new visit should be advised to bring a pair with them as part of the evaluation. Most important is to examine shoe tilt by looking at shoes from the rear at eye level. Do not pay attention to the heel or outsole wear, but rather look at the angle of the upper (the top part of the shoe that the foot fits into) relative to perpendicular. If the upper is tilting, bent or smashed toward the inside of the foot, overpronation is occurring (Figure 72–1). If the upper has no tilt, the biomechanics are normal or neutral. Finally, if the upper is tilting or bent toward the outside of the foot, the biomechanics are those of supination, also known as underpronation.

Current thinking is that runners with excessive pronation need a shoe that has more rearfoot control but can have a bit less shock absorption. These shoes are described as "motion control" shoes, and employ dual-density midsoles and medial posts to control excessive pronation. Neutral runners can use a shoe without this technology, saving both cost and weight. These are referred to, somewhat confusingly, as "stability" shoes. People with a high-arched (cavus) foot need more cushioning because of the rigid nature of their foot. These

are more obviously referred to as "cushioned" shoes. Some general principles of shoe fitting for all running athletes are outlined in Table 72–2.

PATELLOFEMORAL PAIN SYNDROME

ESSENTIALS OF DIAGNOSIS

► Insidious onset of anterior knee pain.
► Compression of patella during contraction of the quadriceps causes pain.

Table 72–2. Athletic shoe fitting: advice for patients.

1. Buy shoes for the specific sport for which you intend to use them.
2. Shop at a reputable store with a knowledgeable staff.
3. Bring the socks you plan to wear with the new athletic shoes.
4. Bring your orthotic or other inserts with you to try on shoes.
5. Allow for one fingers's width (about 3/8 inch) at the front of the shoe in front of the big toe. Running shoes should fit bigger than casual shoes.
6. Make certain that the shoe flexes only where the toes bend, which should also be the widest part of the shoe.
7. Check the inside and outside of the shoe for defects. The shoe should sit level when checked on a flat surface.
8. Check your shoes often for wear such as (a) the outsole worn to the midsole, (b) the heel counter tilted inward (valgus) or outward (varus), (c) the forefoot upper shifted medially or laterally. Replace shoes every 400 miles, even in the absence of notable wear.
9. For a listing of shoes that have been evaluated, visit the website of the American Academy of Podiatric Sports Medicine at www.aapsm.org.

General Considerations

The most common injury in runners, and probably the most common cause of knee pain in all active individuals, is the patellofemoral or anterior knee pain syndrome. Individuals with this syndrome usually experience the insidious onset of poorly localized pain on the anterior surface of the knee. Pain is worse when arising from a seated position, particularly after sitting for several minutes (the "theater sign") and when walking up or, more commonly, down stairs.

Clinical Findings

On physical examination, the Q angle between the femur and tibia should be measured (see Chapter 12). An angle greater than 16 degrees is associated with a higher incidence of patellofemoral pain syndrome. Compression of the patella causes pain, particularly when the quadriceps muscle is contracted simultaneously. The "patellar inhibition sign" is performed by compressing the patella against the femur with the leg extended and then asking the patient to isometrically contract the quadriceps, causing loading of the patellofemoral joint. This maneuver should reproduce the patient's knee pain.

STRESS FRACTURES

ESSENTIALS OF DIAGNOSIS

▶ Local tenderness of bone in lower extremity.
▶ Tibia and fibula most commonly involved.

Clinical Findings

A stress fracture is an incomplete fracture that results from repetitive strain on the bone rather than a single traumatic episode. Stress fractures occur in all sports that require repetitive running and jumping but are far more common in long-distance runners than in any other athletes. The vast majority occurs in people who are running more than 20 miles per week. Continued, repetitive stress overcomes the normal remodeling response of bone, leading to trabecular micro-fractures. The tibia and fibula are most commonly involved (Figure 72–2). Displacement of stress fractures is rare except for femoral neck fractures, which also carry the risk of avascular necrosis.

In most patients, the diagnosis of a stress fracture should be made on the clinical history. Any running athlete who complains of pain localized to a bone in the lower extremity

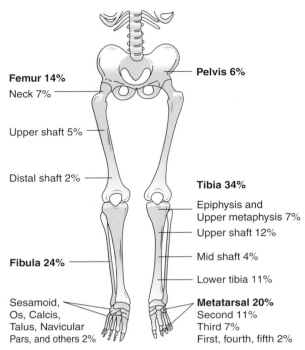

Figure 72–2. Stress fractures resulting from failure of bone remodeling.

Femur 14%
Neck 7%
Upper shaft 5%
Distal shaft 2%
Pelvis 6%
Tibia 34%
Epiphysis and Upper metaphysis 7%
Upper shaft 12%
Mid shaft 4%
Lower tibia 11%
Fibula 24%
Sesamoid, Os, Calcis, Talus, Navicular Pars, and others 2%
Metatarsal 20%
Second 11%
Third 7%
First, fourth, fifth 2%

should be considered to have a stress fracture. If local tenderness over the bone is found, further work-up should include radiographs or bone scan. MRI is expensive but can be used in rare instances when the lesion on bone scan is indistinct (Figure 72–3).

Treatment

Several general rules apply to the treatment of stress fractures regardless of their location. Nonsteroidal anti-inflammatory drugs usually control pain. The patient must significantly decrease or stop running to reduce the excess strain that is causing the stress fracture. During this rest phase of treatment, alternative exercise possibilities include swimming, biking, and the use of a stair-climber or elliptical trainer. This hiatus offers an excellent chance to increase muscle mass and strength and thereby avoid further stress fractures. When local tenderness has disappeared, a final radiograph can be obtained, and running activities can be gradually reintroduced. At this point one has to know the previous running history and must be certain that the return to running is gradual.

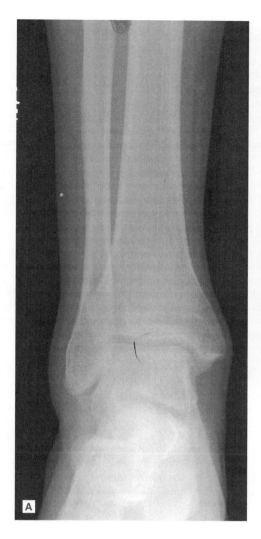

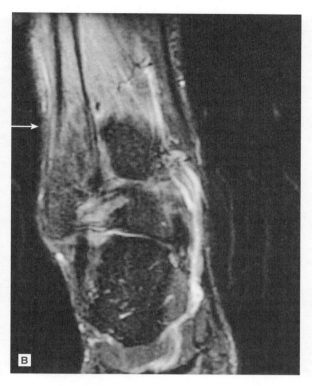

▲ **Figure 72–3.** Detection of early stress fracture using MRI. **A:** The initial radiograph shows no abnormality. **B:** The fat suppression MRI shows increased signal in the fibula at the area indicated by arrow, indicative of bone injury.

MEDIAL TIBIAL STRESS SYNDROME (SHIN SPLINTS)

 ESSENTIALS OF DIAGNOSIS

▶ Diffuse, nagging pain over tibia while running.

▶ Tibial stress fracture should be considered when pain persists after running.

▶ Clinical Findings & Treatment

Persons with medial tibial stress syndrome complain of diffuse, nagging pain over the tibia that worsens with running. If the pain persists after running and is noted with routine ambulation, the diagnosis of a tibial stress fracture should be suspected. Medial tibial stress syndrome is common in beginning runners. The pathophysiology is thought to be inflammation of the anterior and posterior calf musculature and periostitis of the tibia. Treatment consists of a break from full or vigorous training, correction of any misalignment, and substituted aerobic activities to prevent deconditioning.

ACHILLES TENDINITIS

 ESSENTIALS OF DIAGNOSIS

▶ Palpation along tendon elicits pain.

▶ Fusiform swelling may be present.

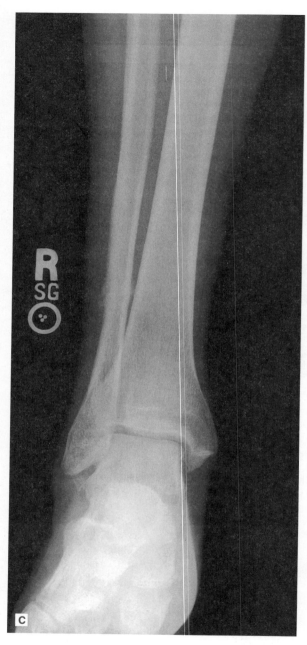

▲ Figure 72–3. (*Continued*) **C:** The follow-up radiograph 1 month later confirms periosteal bone reaction indicative of stress fracture.

General Considerations

Runners and jumping athletes may complain of pain in the substance of the Achilles tendon, which connects the soleus and the gastrocnemius muscles to the calcaneus. A relatively avascular or "watershed" area in the Achilles tendon approximately 4–5 cm proximal to its insertion is a factor in its vulnerability to injury and rupture. Diverse factors are thought to incite overuse injuries of the Achilles tendon, including running on hard surfaces, abrupt increases in mileage or training intensity, and shoe design. Fortunately, the latter has been addressed in contemporary running shoes. A person with a high-arched foot may also be at increased risk for Achilles tendinitis and rupture.

Clinical Findings

Clinically, fusiform swelling with or without warmth may be evident along the Achilles tendon. Crepitation may be present with motion. Palpation along the tendon elicits pain. To test integrity of the Achilles tendon, the calf should be squeezed with the foot held in dorsiflexion (the Thompson squeeze test); this maneuver results in a modest amount of plantar flexion if the tendon is intact.

Treatment

Treatment of Achilles tendinitis consists of reduction of activities, anti-inflammatory medication, heel lifts or orthotics, and gentle stretching. Once the Achilles tendon is no longer tender to palpation and the athlete has restored his or her flexibility, slow progressive return to activity is permitted. There have been reports of iatrogenic Achilles tendon rupture secondary to inadvertent intratendinous glucocorticoid injection, and thus injection should be avoided.

PLANTAR FASCIITIS

ESSENTIALS OF DIAGNOSIS

▶ Heel pain exacerbated by weight bearing and dorsiflexion of toes.

▶ Tenderness along the plantar fascia and at its insertion onto the calcaneus.

Clinical Findings

Plantar fasciitis typically occurs over the midportion of the plantar fascia and is usually exacerbated by standing after a period of inactivity, dorsiflexion of the toes, and direct pressure over the fascia. Lateral squeeze of the heel also precipitates pain. Individuals with chronic plantar fascial pain have microtears and partial rupture of the plantar fascia near its origin. In the case of rupture, a gap in the tendon is often palpable.

▶ Treatment

Treatment consists of ice, anti-inflammatory drugs, and physical therapy to increase heel and Achilles flexibility in order to relieve stress and tension on the plantar fascia. Orthotics may be useful.

PATELLAR TENDINITIS

ESSENTIALS OF DIAGNOSIS

▶ Pain localized to inferior pole of patella.

▶ Swelling not usually present.

▶ General Considerations

Patellar tendinitis is often referred to as "jumper's knee" because of its common association with jumping sports, such as basketball. However, it can occur in any running sport, which can be thought of as a series of one-legged-jumps. Abnormal foot biomechanics and running up hills are cited as aggravating factors.

▶ Clinical Findings

Pain is localized to the inferior pole of the patella, and swelling is generally not present. Knee range of motion is within normal limits. Affected persons feel a sensation of the knee giving way with hard jumping. On examination, tenderness is felt directly on the lower tip of the patella. Radiographs are normal, but bone scans may be positive at the inferior pole of the patella, and MRI may show chronic tendinopathy.

▶ Treatment

Unfortunately, patellar tendinitis is often chronic, taking many months to a year for complete healing. Nonsteroidal anti-inflammatory drugs are helpful, as are exercises to stretch and strengthen leg muscles. In some cases, surgery is needed to remove scarred portions of the tendon. Long-term restriction of jumping may be required for 1 or 2 years. Patellar tendinitis can affect the long-term playing ability of jumping athletes, such as volleyball or basketball players and long-distance runners.

ILIOTIBIAL BAND SYNDROME

ESSENTIALS OF DIAGNOSIS

▶ Pain localized to lateral aspect of femoral condyle.

▶ May radiate up the thigh to the hip.

▶ Clinical Findings

Iliotibial band syndrome is an overuse condition that is common in runners and cyclists and is characterized by an ache or burning sensation of the lateral aspect of the knee during or after activity. It is thought to be due to local friction of the tendon band as it rubs over the lateral femoral condyle. Clinically, pain symptoms are localized to the lateral aspect of the femoral condyle and may radiate up the side of the thigh to the hip. Motion of the knee is normal, but tightness and snapping may be perceived. Apart from well-localized tenderness, the knee examination is normal. Radiographs generally are normal, and MRI is not indicated.

▶ Treatment

Progressive healing is the rule with iliotibial band syndrome. The athlete can continue moderate activities during this condition. Treatment consists of local icing both before and after activities, and frequent regular stretching of the lateral hip muscles and iliotibial band.

METATARSALGIA

ESSENTIALS OF DIAGNOSIS

▶ Synovitis and capsulitis most common causes.

▶ Second metatarsophalangeal joint most commonly involved.

▶ General Considerations

Metatarsalgia, which is more a description than a diagnosis, refers to a syndrome of pain in one or more metatarsophalangeal (MTP) joints due to a variety of causes, including capsulitis and synovitis, degenerative arthritis, neuroma, synovial cyst, and stress fracture. Synovitis and capsulitis are probably the most common causes. Although any of the MTP joints can be affected, the second MTP joint is the most commonly involved.

Biomechanical factors such as a hypermobile first MTP joint accompanied by a long second metatarsal can result in second MTP synovitis. Anterior ankle impingement may cause diffuse forefoot pain. Plantar fat pad atrophy and plantar flexion of the metatarsal may also cause MTP joint synovitis.

▶ Clinical Findings

Physical findings associated with MTP joint synovitis include swelling and pain with manipulation of the joint. Vertical subluxation of the toe places pressure on the plantar capsule, eliciting pain.

▶ Treatment

Treatment is almost always conservative and is generally successful. Ice massage and anti-inflammatory medications reduce swelling and pain. Orthotics with metatarsal relief padding reduce stress on the joint and can be of great help. In resistant cases, an intra-articular injection is indicated. This should be done judiciously because repeated injections may be destructive to the ligamentous capsular support of the joint. Surgery, in the form of synovectomy and metatarsal osteotomy, is rarely necessary.

Browning KH, Donley BG. Evaluation and management of common running injuries. *Cleve Clin J Med.* 2000;67:511. [PMID: 10902242]

[Medline Plus—A service of the US National Library of Medicine] http://www.nlm.nih.gov/medlineplus/sportsinjuries.html

[The American Academy of Podiatric Sports Medicine] www.aapsm.org

van Gent RN, Siem D, van Middelkoop M, van Os AG, Bierma-Zeinstra SMA, Koes BW. Incidence and determinants of lower extremity running injuries in long distance runners: a systematic review. *Br J Sports Med.* 2007;41:469. [PMID: 17473005]

Selected Topics in Neurology for the Rheumatologist

73

Richard Rosenbaum, MD

CNS SYNDROMES OF SYSTEMIC LUPUS ERYTHEMATOSUS

ESSENTIALS OF DIAGNOSIS

▶ According to the American College of Rheumatology, the following are central nervous system (CNS) manifestations of systemic lupus erythematosus (SLE):

- Acute confusional state.
- Anxiety disorder.
- Aseptic meningitis.
- Cerebrovascular disease.
- Cognitive dysfunction.
- Demyelinating disease.
- Headache.
- Mood disorder.
- Movement disorder (chorea).
- Myelopathy.
- Psychosis.
- Seizure disorder.

▶ General Considerations

The general term "neuropsychiatric lupus" is being superseded by the understanding that lupus can affect the nervous system in diverse ways, each with distinctive clinical findings, pathogenesis, prognosis, and treatment. The American College of Rheumatology distinguished 12 central neurologic manifestations of SLE. Neurologists subdivide these in greater detail, noting, for example, many different mechanisms and localizations of strokes or seizures. Neurologic manifestations of lupus often occur early in the disease. The CNS syndromes discussed below

are presented in approximate order of prevalence; however, prevalences are inexact due to variations of definition and clinical sampling. Patients with SLE are also at risk for peripheral nervous system disease (Table 73–1).

1. Cognitive Dysfunction & Acute Confusional State

▶ Clinical Findings

Cognitive dysfunction, especially in domains such as visual or verbal memory, attention, executive function, and psychomotor speed, is the most common neuropsychiatric aspect of lupus. These disturbances can range from subtle to severe. Prevalence figures vary greatly, depending on diagnostic criteria and extent of psychometric testing. Mild cognitive dysfunction typically waxes and wanes without clear correlation to other aspects of disease activity. Patients with antiphospholipid antibodies have increased risk of developing cognitive dysfunction.

Severe cognitive dysfunction, including acute confusional states or delirium, affects only a small percentage of lupus patients and can overlap with other neuropsychiatric aspects of lupus, such as psychosis and affective disorders. Patients with these more severe neuropsychiatric presentations usually have serum and cerebrospinal fluid (CSF) antibodies against the NR2-NMDA receptor. These antibodies are probably not solely responsible for the mental changes because titers often remain elevated in the CSF months after symptoms have resolved. Moreover, these antibodies are less likely to be elevated in lupus patients with focal neurologic syndromes. Other autoantibodies, such as those directed against antiribosomal P, can occur in patients with neurologic manifestations of lupus, but none is particularly helpful in diagnosing whether or not a patient has lupus or if new neurologic findings are due to SLE or other etiology.

In 50% or more of patient with lupus, brain MRI shows T2-bright lesions in the white matter. These lesions can be present in patients without clinical CNS disease. However,

Table 73–1. Peripheral nervous system manifestation of systemic lupus erythematosus.

Acute inflammatory demyelinating polyneuropathy
Autonomic disorder
Mononeuropathy, single or multiplex
Myasthenia gravis
Cranial neuropathy
Plexopathy
Polyneuropathy

Data from the American College of Rheumatology, 1999.

the lesions are more common among patients with cognitive impairment, seizures, hypertension, or antiphospholipid antibodies, and become more common as the disease progresses.

Differential Diagnosis

Patients with severe cognitive dysfunction merit laboratory testing for alternative metabolic causes, brain imaging, electroencephalography, and lumbar puncture. Cognitive dysfunction in SLE is sometimes a reflection of other neurologic effects of lupus, such as strokes or seizures. The differential diagnosis includes medication effects and other metabolic disturbances, hypertensive or uremic encephalopathy, and opportunistic infections.

Treatment

Most instances of mild cognitive dysfunction need no specific treatment. Cognitive behavioral therapies may help. Once other treatable systemic causes are excluded, patients with severe confusional states including psychosis can be treated with acute immunosuppression, usually starting with intravenous high-dose glucocorticoids.

2. Headache

Clinical Findings

Recurrent tension or migraine headaches affect more than half of patients with lupus. However, there is no distinctive severe intractable "lupus headache", and whether headache is more common in patients in lupus than in the general population is debatable. Most recurrent headaches in patients with lupus do not require extensive imaging or other neurologic investigations.

Differential Diagnosis

Important causes of headache include stroke, meningitis, posterior reversible leukoencephalopathy, and pseudotumor cerebri. When a patient with lupus has a new type of headache or other warning signs (such as fever, seizures, an altered mental status, or focal neurologic findings), a thoughtful and thorough evaluation is required.

Treatment

Tension and migraine headaches in patients with lupus can be treated by avoiding precipitating factors, using analgesics or triptans for acute attacks, and considering migraine prophylactic drugs for patients with frequent and disabling headaches. These are the same tactics used for such complaints in patients without lupus. Headache alone is not due to active inflammation and is not an indication for immunosuppressive therapies.

3. Mood & Anxiety Disorders

Clinical Findings

Patients with lupus have an increased incidence of anxiety, depression, and even mania compared with age and gender matched controls. Perhaps one-fifth of patients with lupus have an episode of major depression during the course of their illness.

Differential Diagnosis

Affect can also be influenced by the severity of illness, medications (eg, glucocorticoids and anticonvulsants), or other manifestations of disease, such as depression or a complication of stroke.

Treatment

The treatment of affective disorders in SLE differs little from that of the general treatment of these conditions. Small studies have suggested that cognitive behavioral therapy can ameliorate depression, anxiety, and cognitive dysfunction.

4. Seizure Disorder

Clinical Findings

Seizures or psychosis are the only two neuropsychiatric syndromes that are included among the American College of Rheumatology classification criteria for lupus. Nearly one-tenth of patients with lupus have a seizure sometime during the course of their lives. The seizures can take a variety of forms (eg, focal or generalized, single or recurrent).

Differential Diagnosis

Every patient with SLE and seizures needs careful evaluation for type and cause of seizure, including an electroencephalogram and MRI of the brain, and an evaluation for potential metabolic causes. Seizures can accompany a number of other lupus manifestations, such as strokes, other focal brain lesions, psychosis, uremia, hypertensive encephalopathy, or posterior reversible leukoencephalopathy. Seizures can be caused by electrolyte disturbances or opportunistic CNS infections. Patients with elevated antiphospholipid or anti-Smith antibodies have increased risk of seizures.

▶ Treatment

Seizures in patients with lupus are treated with the same anticonvulsants used in epilepsy of other causes. Seizures are not an indication for increased immunosuppression unless brain imaging or examinations of the CSF demonstrate evidence of brain inflammation.

5. Psychosis

▶ Clinical Findings

Psychosis affects only a small percentage of lupus patients. The psychosis presents as delusions, often paranoid, and hallucinations, more often auditory than visual or olfactory. Lupus psychosis most often occurs within the first year of presentation of the disease, accompanied by other systemic manifestations of disease activity and by affective or cognitive changes.

▶ Differential Diagnosis

Lupus psychosis must be distinguished from psychosis caused by glucocorticoids, other drugs, or metabolic disturbances. Patients with glucocorticoid-induced psychosis are usually taking more than 40 mg daily of prednisone (or equivalent dose of other glucocorticoids), often have had a recent increase in glucocorticoid dose, and are more likely than patients with lupus psychosis to be alert, cognitively intact, and free of other active neurologic complications (such as seizures).

▶ Treatment

Patients with lupus psychosis need aggressive immunosuppressive therapy, usually starting with high-dose glucocorticoids (eg, intravenous methylprednisolone). They also commonly need treatment with typical or atypical antipsychotic drugs until the immunosuppression becomes effective.

▶ Prognosis

Most patients with lupus psychosis have excellent psychiatric recovery within months of increasing or beginning immunosuppressive treatment. Many patients are able to stop taking antipsychotic medication but continue taking immunosuppressive agents, which are titrated according to other lupus manifestations. A minority of patients have a recurrent episode of psychosis, which can occur many years after the first episode.

6. Cerebrovascular Disease

▶ Clinical Findings & Differential Diagnosis

The timing and focal clinical signs of stroke in lupus are similar to those of cerebrovascular accidents in the general population. Most strokes in patients with lupus are due to atherosclerosis or hypertensive cardiovascular disease. Patients who have antiphospholipid antibodies have an important additional risk factor for thrombotic strokes. Strokes due to Libman-Sacks endocarditis are much less common, and those caused by true cerebral vasculitis are quite rare.

▶ Treatment

The treatment of acute stroke in patients with lupus is similar to that of stroke in the general population. Stroke is not an indication for immunosuppression except in the rare instances of CNS vasculitis. Because of their general increased stroke risk, patients with lupus should be attentive to primary stroke prevention: avoiding smoking; controlling blood pressure, diabetes, and lipids; and taking low-dose aspirin if not contraindicated by other factors. These measures are also important for secondary stroke prevention. Oral anticoagulation with warfarin is reserved for patients with cardiogenic causes of embolic stroke or for those with antiphospholipid antibodies. The optimal international normalized ratio (INR) during warfarin therapy in patients with antiphospholipid antibodies is controversial; some experts favor an INR of 2.0–3.0, while others favor an INR of 3.0–4.0.

7. Aseptic Meningitis

▶ Clinical Findings

Aseptic meningitis presents with fever, headache, or stiff neck and is diagnosed by the finding of a CSF pleocytosis. The pleocytosis is usually mononuclear, and cultures are negative. Aseptic meningitis develops in less than 1% of patients with SLE.

▶ Differential Diagnosis

Patients with meningitis must have CSF cultures and serology to exclude opportunistic or other infectious causes of meningitis. Nonsteroidal anti-inflammatory drugs can also cause aseptic meningitis, and therefore constitute a potential confounder in patients with SLE.

▶ Treatment & Prognosis

The aseptic meningitis of lupus usually resolves spontaneously without specific treatment.

8. Movement Disorder

Clinical Findings

Chorea is the most common movement disorder that complicates lupus, affecting about 1% of patients. It can be unilateral or bilateral and occur early or late in the disease. Chorea is sensitive to levels of female hormones; the incidence is increased in women during menses, during pregnancy, and in those who take oral contraceptives. Hence, lupus is a risk factor for the development of chorea gravidarum. Patients with lupus and chorea often have antiphospholipid antibodies, but the chorea is not due to antibody-associated thrombosis. MRI usually does not implicate any focal lesion in this setting and is typically normal in the absence of other baseline neuropathology related to SLE or comorbid conditions. Other movement disorders, such as reversible parkinsonism, can also occur as a manifestation of lupus.

Differential Diagnosis

The differential diagnosis of chorea in patients with lupus includes Huntington disease, rheumatic fever, and medications.

Treatment & Prognosis

Typically, lupus chorea progresses over weeks, then resolves. There is no proof that immunosuppression aids recovery. Antidopaminergic drugs, such as haloperidol or tetrabenazine, might help suppress choreiform movements.

9. Myelopathy

Clinical Findings

Myelopathy develops in about 1% of patients with SLE. In the setting of SLE, myelopathy can be so severe that is causes quadriplegia or it can be significantly milder, leading to ascending paresthesia. The site of spinal cord pathology can be anywhere cephalad to the level indicated by the sensory findings. The posterior column modalities of vibration sense and proprioception are sometimes relatively spared. MRI of the spinal cord typically shows a lesion within the spinal cord, bright on T2-weighted images, sometimes enhancing. This lesion is characteristically "longitudinally extensive," meaning that it includes multiple spinal segments. CSF usually shows pleocytosis and elevated protein. Some patients have acute flaccid paralysis and urinary retention, often associated with systemic findings of fever, nausea, and vomiting. Other patients have spasticity and hyperreflexia. This group is more likely to have antiphospholipid antibodies or antibodies directed against aquaporin 4. Antibodies to aquaporin 4 are associated with the condition known as neuromyelitis optica.

Differential Diagnosis

Every patient with myelopathy needs imaging of the entire spinal cord, usually with MRI, to exclude a compressive lesion and to evaluate the extent and number of lesions within the spinal cord. The most common causes of inflammatory myelitis are multiple sclerosis and infectious or postinfectious transverse myelitis. Longitudinally extensive lesions can also be seen in isolated neuromyelitis optica and in the myelopathy that can occur in Sjögren syndrome. Paraneoplastic myelopathy is rare. Anterior spinal artery ischemic stroke can cause an acute myelopathy that spares posterior column function; this is typically atherosclerotic or embolic but rarely can be due to vasculitis. The most common metabolic causes of myelopathy are vitamin B_{12} or copper deficiencies. Epidural lipomatosis is an unusual cause of spinal cord compression in patients taking glucocorticoids.

Treatment

Acute myelopathy in SLE is an indication for aggressive anti-inflammatory treatment, usually starting with high-dose glucocorticoids. Therapies such as plasmapheresis, intravenous immune globulin, cyclophosphamide, and rituximab are used frequently if glucocorticoids are ineffective or even from the outset of treatment. In this uncommon condition with variable prognosis, definitive data on the optimal treatment strategy are lacking.

Prognosis

Patients who have myelopathy with flaccid paralysis are at high risk for permanent paresis and urinary catheter dependence. Patients in whom spasticity is present are more likely to recover but are at risk for attacks of either optic neuritis or recurrent myelitis, particularly if they have antibodies to aquaporin 4.

10. Demyelinating Syndromes

Clinical Findings

The American College of Rheumatology lists demyelinating syndromes among the neuropsychiatric lupus syndromes. However, there is little evidence that SLE actually causes CNS demyelination. The coincident occurrence of lupus and multiple sclerosis, the paradigmatic demyelinating disease, probably occurs more often than predicted by chance alone. However, a number of clinical observations compare SLE with multiple sclerosis. Both can cause relapsing-remitting neurologic syndromes. Both can cause multiple lesions on MRI brain scan. Both can cause CSF changes. The oligoclonal bands found in the CSF of 90% of patients with multiple sclerosis are also present in a small percentage of patients with CNS syndromes secondary to SLE.

Optic neuritis, a common manifestation of multiple sclerosis, affects perhaps 1% of patients with lupus, and less than 1% of patients with optic neuritis have lupus. Patients with lupus can have recurrent or bilateral optic neuritis and episodic myelitis. Neuromyelitis optica (Devic disease), once considered a form of multiple sclerosis, is now recognized as a distinct syndrome characterized by antibodies to aquaporin-4 and longitudinally extensive spinal cord lesions. Patients with lupus and optic neuritis often have Devic disease.

Appenzeller S, Vasconcelos Faria A, Li LM, Costallat LT, Cendes F. Quantitative magnetic resonance imaging analyses and clinical significance of hyperintense white matter lesions in systemic lupus erythematosus patients. *Ann Neurol.* 2008;64:635. [PMID: 19107986]

Arinuma Y, Yanagida T, Hirohata S. Association of cerebrospinal fluid anti-NR2 glutamate receptor antibodies with diffuse neuropsychiatric systemic lupus erythematosus. *Arthritis Rheum.* 2008;58:1130. [PMID: 18383393]

Bachen EA, Chesney MA, Criswell LA. Prevalence of mood and anxiety disorders in women with systemic lupus erythematosus. *Arthritis Rheum.* 2009;61:822. [PMID: 19479699]

Baizabal-Carvallo JF, Delgadillo-Marquez G, Estanol B, Garcia-Ramos G. Clinical characteristics and outcomes of the meningitides in systemic lupus erythematosus. *Eur Neurol.* 2009;61:143. [PMID: 19092250]

Birnbaum J, Petri M, Thompson R, Izbudak I, Kerr D. Distinct subtypes of myelitis in systemic lupus erythematosus. *Arthritis Rheum.* 2009;60:3378. [PMID: 19877037]

Mitsikostas DD, Sfikakis PP, Goadsby PJ. A meta-analysis for headache in systemic lupus erythematosus: the evidence and the myth. *Brain.* 2004;127:1200. [PMID: 15047589]

Navarrete-Navarrete N, Peralta-Ramirez MI, Sabio-Sanchez JM, et al. Efficacy of cognitive behavioural therapy for the treatment of chronic stress in patients with lupus erythematosus: a randomized controlled trial. *Psychother Psychosom.* 2010;79:107. [PMID: 20090397]

Pego-Reigosa JM, Isenberg DA. Psychosis due to systemic lupus erythematosus: characteristics and long-term outcome of this rare manifestation of the disease. *Rheumatology (Oxford).* 2008;47:1498. [PMID: 18658205]

SENSORY NEURONOPATHY IN SJÖGREN SYNDROME

 ESSENTIALS OF DIAGNOSIS

▶ Sensory neuronopathy impairs all sensory modalities.

▶ Sensory loss is asymmetric, often including face, trunk, or proximal limbs.

▶ Symptoms evolve subacutely or chronically.

▶ Autonomic nerve fibers are often involved.

Table 73–2. Neurologic syndromes reported in patients with Sjögren syndrome.

Focal CNS syndromes	Hemiparesis
	Hemisensory dysfunction
	Focal seizures
	Movement disorders
	Optic neuritis
	Brainstem disorders
	Cerebellar dysfunction
	Myelopathy
Nonfocal CNS syndromes	Diffuse encephalopathy
	Aseptic meningitis or encephalitis
	Generalized seizures
	Neuropsychiatric disorders
	Dementia
Peripheral nervous system syndromes	Distal sensory or sensorimotor neuropathy
	Sensory neuronopathy
	Autonomic neuropathy
	Entrapment neuropathy
	Mononeuritis multiplex
	Chronic inflammatory demyelinating polyneuropathy
	Myopathies
	Myasthenia gravis

▶ General Considerations

Sjögren syndrome can be associated with myriad neurologic syndromes (Table 73–2). Sensory neuronopathy can occur in a number of patterns in Sjögren syndrome and affects only a minority of patients. However, its symptoms are distinctive and can present before the sicca features of the disease become evident.

▶ Clinical Findings

Sensory neuronopathy can cause pain, paresthesia, or severe disturbance of all sensory modalities. The sensory loss is often asymmetric on the face, trunk, or limbs (proximal or distal) and can develop in less than a month or progress over years. Joint position sense impairment can be severe, leading to a disabling sensory ataxia. Tendon reflexes are often lost when a limb is involved. Patients can have focal autonomic neuropathies, hearing loss, or ventilatory dysfunction. Motor function is preserved, yet patients may perceive that they are weak.

Nerve conduction studies demonstrate absent or low amplitude sensory nerve action potentials, but motor conduction and electromyography needle examinations are normal. Spinal cord MRI may show T2-bright signal in the posterior columns. The pathologic basis is inflammation of dorsal root ganglia with T cell infiltrates, including perivascular infiltrates but not necrotizing vasculitis. The autonomic findings may be caused by similar inflammation in autonomic ganglia. The diagnosis of Sjögren syndrome can be supported by the presence of sicca symptoms, the finding of autoantibodies directed against the Ro or La antigens, and by abnormal minor salivary gland biopsy. As noted, the neurologic symptoms of dorsal root ganglionopathy may occur in the absence of sicca symptoms.

Differential Diagnosis

Paraneoplastic syndromes and medications such as cisplatin and high-dose pyridoxine can also cause sensory neuropathies. The majority of patients with paraneoplastic syndromes associated with dorsal root ganglionopathy have antibodies against anti-Hu in their serum.

Treatment & Prognosis

Approximately half of patients with Sjögren syndrome who have dorsal root ganglionopathy stabilize or improve with immunosuppressive therapies. Neuropathic pain may be approached with medication such as gabapentin, pregabalin, tricyclic antidepressants, or duloxetine.

Chad D, Stone JH, Gupta R. Case records of the Massachusetts General Hospital. Case 14-2011. A woman with asymmetric sensory loss and paresthesias. *N Engl J Med.* 2011;364:1856. [PMID: 21561352]

VASCULITIC NEUROPATHY

ESSENTIALS OF DIAGNOSIS

▶ Vasculitic neuropathy usually presents as acute painful mononeuropathy or mononeuritis multiplex.

▶ Vasculitic neuropathy sometimes causes a distal symmetric sensorimotor neuropathy.

General Considerations

Vasculitic neuropathy can occur as part of a systemic vasculitis (Table 73–3) but may also be nonsystemic, limited to nerve and muscle.

Clinical Findings

The classic presentation of vasculitic neuropathy is one or more painful mononeuropathies, evolving acutely, causing motor and sensory deficits. Large nerves are usually affected proximally due to nerve infarcts caused by vasculitis of epineural vasa nervorum. Leg nerves (such as the peroneal, posterior tibial, and femoral nerves) are affected more often than are nerves to the upper extremity. Electromyogram shows

Table 73–3. Causes of vasculitic neuropathy.

Nonsystemic Vasculitic Neuropathy	Associated Rheumatic Condition
Primary vasculitides	Microscopic polyangiitis Eosinophilic granulomatosis with polyangiitis (Churg-Strauss syndrome) Polyarteritis nodosa Granulomatosis with polyangiitis (formerly Wegener granulomatosis) Cryoglobulinemia Small-vessel vasculitis Giant cell arteritis
Vasculitis secondary to connective tissue disease	Rheumatoid arthritis Sjögren syndrome Systemic lupus erythematosus Sarcoidosis
Vasculitis secondary to infection	
Paraneoplastic vasculitis	
Vasculitis in diabetes mellitus	

evidence of axonal neuropathy with decreased amplitudes of sensory nerve and compound muscle action potentials, and low normal or mildly decreased nerve conduction velocities. Findings on electromyography needle examination that implicate a neuropathic process include fibrillations, positive sharp waves, motor units of increased amplitude and duration, and decreased number of motor units.

The diagnosis of vasculitic neuropathy is proven by biopsy showing necrotizing vasculitis of epineurial, endoneurial, or muscle arterioles. The vasculitis involves only a fraction of the vasa nervorum. Thus, a normal nerve biopsy does not disprove the diagnosis. The diagnostic yield is heightened by performing a biopsy of the highly vascular muscle tissue adjacent to the peripheral nerve at the same time.

Differential Diagnosis

Table 73–4 shows other causes of multiple mononeuropathies. The differential diagnosis of symmetric distal axonal neuropathies is even more extensive, including common neuropathies like those due to diabetes mellitus; prediabetic glucose intolerance; alcohol, toxic, metabolic, or nutritional factors; paraproteinemia; and familial and paraneoplastic neuropathies.

Treatment

Glucocorticoids are the preferred first treatment of vasculitic neuropathies. Prednisone is started at doses of 1 mg/kg/d, sometimes preceded by "pulse" intravenous glucocorticoid treatment. Cyclophosphamide is often added if the neuropathy is severe or if it is indicated for concomitant systemic

Table 73–4. Causes of multiple mononeuropathies other than vasculitis.

Multiple compression neuropathies
Multifocal motor neuropathy with conduction block and other
   asymmetric immune-mediated neuropathies
Infectious neuropathies, eg, leprosy, herpes zoster, Lyme borreliosis,
   HIV, CMV, and trichinosis
Vasculopathic neuropathies due to injection drug abuse
Ischemic neuropathies due to such causes as cholesterol emboli,
   sickle cell disease, or hyperviscosity
Neuropathies due hemorrhagic diatheses
Neuropathies in eosinophilic myalgia or hypereosinophilic syndromes
Neuropathies due to lymphatoid granulomatosis
Neoplastic nerve invasion
Multiple nerve tumors, as in neurofibromatosis
Neuropathies due to amyloidosis
Porphyric neuropathy
A minority of toxic neuropathies; examples include neuropathies in
   toxic oil syndrome, after jellyfish stings, or in lead intoxication
Neuropathies caused by multifocal trauma

Adopted, with permission, from Donofrio.

vasculitis. Various other immunosuppressants have also been used. A few patients with nonsystemic vasculitic neuropathy are observed, rather than treated, if the neuropathy has been stable for a number of months and the nerve biopsy does not show active vasculitis.

▶ Prognosis

Nerves infarcted by vasculitis may recover slowly or incompletely. However, treatment of vasculitic neuropathy can usually prevent progression of neuropathy and can lead to some neurologic improvement. The prognosis of patients with systemic vasculitis is usually more dependent on the non-neuropathic aspects of their illnesses.

Collins MP, Dyck PJ, Gronseth GS, et al. Peripheral Nerve Society. Peripheral Nerve Society Guideline on the classification, diagnosis, investigation, and immunosuppressive therapy of non-systemic vasculitic neuropathy: executive summary. *J Peripher Nerv Syst.* 2010;15:176. [PMID: 21040139]

RADICULOPATHY OR MYELOPATHY DUE TO SPONDYLOSIS

ESSENTIALS OF DIAGNOSIS

▶ Cervical radiculopathic pain can be dysesthetic in a dermatomal pattern or deep, achy, and poorly localized over upper thorax, shoulder, or arm. Neck pain, loss of neck range of motion, and headache are common additional symptoms.

▶ Lumbar radiculopathic pain from L5 or S1 roots produces sciatica. Compression of higher lumbar roots can cause anterior thigh pain.

▶ Radiculopathies can cause myotomal weakness, dermatomal sensory changes, and focal depression of tendon reflexes, but neurologic examination can be normal despite marked pain. Nerve stretch or compression tests, such as the straight leg raise and Spurling sign (reproduction of pain by neck rotation or extension to the side of the pain), are helpful.

▶ Cervical spondylotic myelopathy can cause weakness in any limb, leg spasticity, sensory changes on limbs or trunk, and sphincter dysfunction.

▶ Stenosis of the lumbar spinal canal can cause neurogenic intermittent claudication but leads to abnormal neurologic examination only when severe.

▶ General Considerations

Spondylosis, encompassing osteoarthritis of facet joints and degeneration of the intervertebral disks, is a universal aspect of aging. The annual incidence of cervical radiculopathies is about 1 per 1000, with a peak risk in the early 50s. Cervical spondylotic myelopathy is less common than radiculopathy but is the most common type of myelopathy in older adults. Most people have an episode of low back pain sometime in their lives and about 1 in 20 has chronic low back pain but only about 1 in 100 has serious lumbar radiculopathy. Thoracic spondylotic radiculopathies or myelopathies are much less common.

▶ Clinical Findings

Cervical radiculopathy typically presents with sudden or gradual appearance of radiculopathic pain, usually accompanied by neck pain and loss of neck range of motion. Headache may also by present. Spurling sign is a relatively specific but insensitive sign. Some patients report pain relief with gentle cervical traction or when they raise the painful arm above their heads.

   The most commonly involved nerve root is C7, exiting between the C6 and C7 vertebral bodies. C7 radiculopathy can cause weakness, particularly in triceps and pronators teres. The weakness of monoradiculopathy is usually mild because most muscles are innervated by multiple roots. The triceps reflex may be depressed. C7 dermatomal sensory findings are classically in the middle finger, but often patients have paresthesia on other parts of the arm. The second most commonly involved nerve root is C6, which can cause depression of the biceps reflex or weakness in muscles with C5 and C6 innervation, like deltoid, infraspinatus, and biceps. The classic C6 dermatomal area is the thumb, index finger, and lateral hand. Patients can have very painful radiculopathies with a complete normal neurologic examination.

Acute sciatica, unilateral leg pain radiating into the buttock and lateral or posterior thigh, is the typical symptom of L5 or S1 radiculopathy. Not all sciatica is due to radiculopathy; nerve root compression is more likely if the pain radiates beyond the knee. Patients commonly also have low back pain. L5 radiculopathy, usually due to L4–L5 disk herniation, typically causes medial foot and hallux pain and paresthesia; the most sensitive neurologic sign for L5 dysfunction is weakness of hallux extension. S1 nerve root compression, usually due to L5–S1 herniation, typically causes lateral foot pain and paresthesia; the most sensitive sign for S1 dysfunction is a depressed Achilles tendon reflex. Many patients with painful radiculopathy have no objective neurologic deficit; in these patients, reproducing pain with nerve stretch tests such as the straight leg raise helps separate radiculopathic from non-radiculopathic sciatica.

Most patients with clinical radiculopathies do not need imaging, unless they have had recent trauma, there is suspicion of infection or malignancy, or there is significant motor or sphincter dysfunction. When patients have not improved after 4–6 weeks of conservative therapy (or earlier if they have intractable pain or significant weakness), nerve roots are best imaged with an MRI scan. Occasionally, a CT myelogram provides additional detail. The imaging studies always need to be interpreted in clinical context because patients usually have multilevel spondylosis, most of which is asymptomatic. Electromyography has low sensitivity for mild radiculopathy, but in complex cases, it can be helpful for localizing the level of nerve root involvement and checking for alternative diagnoses (eg, mononeuropathies or plexopathies).

Cervical spondylotic myelopathy usually develops gradually, often without pain, but can progress stepwise or be worsened by trauma. Neurologic changes can include leg spasticity, arm weakness or clumsiness, and limb or trunk sensory changes. Sphincter dysfunction can occur but is rarely the first neurologic deficit. Lhermitte sign, which is the presence of trunk or leg paresthesia induced by neck flexion, can occur with cervical myelopathy of any cause. MRI or CT scans of the cervical spine of patients with cervical spondylotic myelopathy show focal stenoses of the spinal canal and compressions of the spinal cord. On T2-weighted MRI images, the compressed cord can have focal brightness. However, the extent of neurologic dysfunction correlates imperfectly with the degree of cord compression.

Neurogenic intermittent claudication is discomfort anywhere in the legs or buttocks, with or without paresthesia, elicited by walking, standing straight, or lumbar extension, and relieved within minutes by stopping walking, sitting, or bending forward. The most common cause is lumbar canal stenosis. Patients with neurogenic claudication usually have a normal neurologic examination of the legs and normal straight leg raising tests. If they do have objective signs of cauda equina dysfunction, they need more immediate surgical decompression.

Differential Diagnosis

Radiculopathy can be caused by other pathology of the spine including metastatic disease, epidural abscess, nerve root tumor, syringomyelia, and myelitis. Herpes zoster can cause radiculopathic pain and occasionally causes myotomal weakness. Orthopedic conditions often cause limb pain, so shoulder disease must be separated from C5 or C6 radiculopathy and hip and knee disease from sciatica. Neuralgic amyotrophy (Parsonage-Turner syndrome or acute brachial plexitis) presents with acute severe arm pain followed by focal weakness; lumbosacral radiculoplexopathies, especially in diabetics, can cause leg pain and focal neurologic deficits. Mononeuropathies such as carpal tunnel syndrome, ulnar neuropathy, peroneal neuropathy, and sciatic neuropathy often merit consideration.

Every patient with cervical radiculopathy needs clinical evaluation to exclude cervical myelopathy, which if present warrants early neck imaging.

Causes of myelopathy other than cervical spondylotic myelopathy are described above in the section on SLE.

Treatment & Prognosis

Most patients with cervical or lumbar radiculopathy improve in 6–8 weeks with nonsurgical therapies. For cervical radiculopathies, a soft cervical collar or cervical traction may be helpful. Bed rest, if needed for acute sciatica, should be as brief as possible. Nonsteroidal anti-inflammatory drugs or physical or manipulative therapies may be effective in symptom relief. When symptoms persist for more than 6 weeks, surgical decompression (cervical anterior discectomy or posterior laminectomy or lumbar laminectomy) usually gives relief. Earlier surgery is occasionally indicated for patients with significant weakness or intractable pain. Epidural glucocorticoid injections may give transient relief of symptoms but have no proven long-term value. There is no class I evidence proving the best treatment approach.

Decompressive surgery is a common treatment for cervical spondylotic myelopathy; however, which patients with mild myelopathy can avoid surgery and the optimal surgical approach are unproven.

Neurogenic intermittent claudication can cause tolerable symptoms for years or improve over time. Patients can adjust walking and standing habits, perhaps stooping slightly with a cane. When pain is intractable or neurologic deficits appear, laminectomies of the stenosed segments of the spinal canal usually improve leg pain and stabilize or improve neurologic deficit.

Katz JN, Harris MB. Clinical practice. Lumbar spinal stenosis. *N Engl J Med.* 2008;358:818. [PMID: 18287604]

Nikolaidis I, Fouyas IP, Sandercock PA, Statham PF. Surgery for cervical radiculopathy or myelopathy. *Cochrane Database Syst Rev.* 2010;(1)CD001466. [PMID: 20091520]

CAUDA EQUINA SYNDROME WITH ANKYLOSING SPONDYLITIS

ESSENTIALS OF DIAGNOSIS

▶ Lumbar oligoradiculopathy can develop insidiously and present with a combination of radicular pain, sensory loss, weakness, tendon reflex loss, and rectal or urinary sphincter dysfunction in patients with long-term ankylosing spondylitis.

▶ The cause is lumbar dural ectasia, visible by MRI or CT scan.

▶ General Considerations & Clinical Findings

Cauda equina syndrome, manifest by dysfunction of multiple lumbar and sacral nerve roots, develops slowly but progressively in a few patients with chronic ankylosing spondylitis. Early symptoms can include leg pain, sensory disturbance, or loss of sphincter control. Over time, leg weakness, atrophy, sensory loss, and loss of leg tendon reflexes develop. The diagnosis is confirmed when lumbar MRI or CT shows lumbar thecal diverticula, arising from the posterior lumbosacral arachnoid and sometimes eroding bone.

▶ Differential Diagnosis

The differential diagnosis of cauda equina syndrome includes various causes of nerve root compression, including degenerative stenoses, vertebral and epidural metastases, or epidural infections, nerve root tumors, autoimmune polyradiculitis (eg, Guillain-Barre syndrome), and infections (eg, cytomegalovirus or herpes zoster infection). Acute cauda equina syndrome is an emergency that needs immediate lumbar imaging to check for indications for surgical nerve root decompression. Most cases of cauda equina syndrome in patients with ankylosing spondylitis are slowly progressive but must have lumbar imaging to excluding alternative treatable diagnoses. Dural ectasia can also occur in Marfan syndrome, Ehlers-Danlos syndrome, or neurofibromatosis I, but the ectasia in these conditions arises from the anterior thecal sac.

▶ Treatment & Prognosis

There is limited experience treating the cauda equina syndrome, and treatment is often unsuccessful. Perhaps surgical decompression or lumboperitoneal shunting helps some patients. Treatment with glucocorticoids seems ineffective, but infliximab has been reported to be helpful in some anecdotal cases. Progression slows in some patients without treatment.

Liu CC, Lin YC, Lo CP, Chang TP. Cauda equina syndrome and dural ectasia: rare manifestations in chronic ankylosing spondylitis. *Br J Radiol.* 2011;84:e123. [PMID: 21606066]

ATLANTOAXIAL JOINT DISEASE IN RHEUMATOID ARTHRITIS

ESSENTIALS OF DIAGNOSIS

▶ In patients with rheumatoid arthritis, subluxation at the atlantoaxial joint is a common asymptomatic finding on cervical imaging studies.

▶ Atlantoaxial subluxation can cause head or neck pain.

▶ Neurologic effects of atlantoaxial subluxation range from asymptomatic hyperreflexia to more severe spinal cord or lower brainstem damage.

▶ General Considerations

Atlantoaxial subluxation can develop early in patients with rheumatoid arthritis but becomes more common and more severe as the disease progresses. Successful disease-modifying therapies decrease the incidence of this complication. Anterior atlantoaxial subluxation is more common than posterior, vertical, and lateral subluxations. Patients with rheumatoid arthritis usually also have lower cervical spondylosis.

▶ Clinical Findings

Many patients with atlantoaxial subluxation are asymptomatic. In these patients, the subluxation is best detected by lateral cervical radiographs with flexion and extension views. The normal distance between the anterior portion of the ring of C1 and the odontoid should be 3 mm or less. Most patients with advanced rheumatoid arthritis have occipital headache or neck pain, but symptoms correlate imperfectly with presence or extent of atlantoaxial subluxation. When atlantoaxial subluxation causes myelopathy, the most subtle sign is tendon hyperreflexia in the arms or legs. Loss of arm or leg strength is less common but can be difficult to evaluate in patients with peripheral joint pain and deformities. Sensory loss, sphincter dysfunction, and extensor plantar reflexes are more serious myelopathic findings.

Vertical atlantoaxial joint subluxation can lead to brainstem compression, with neurologic effects ranging from hyperreflexia to quadriplegia. Other neurologic syndromes caused by vertical subluxation include trigeminal sensory loss, vertigo, impaired eye movement, drop attacks, hydrocephalus, and sleep apnea.

Radiologic anterior separation of the atlantoaxial joint correlates imperfectly with presence or absence of neurologic compression. The posterior atlanto-dental interval and sagittal canal diameter at C1 are somewhat better predictors of compression. A number of radiologic parameters on plain radiographs, eg, McGregor line, Ranawat distance, and the Redlund-Johnell index, are indicators of vertical subluxation. However, MRI scans of the cervical spine and posterior fossa provide much better visualization of cord and brainstem relationships. This is because plain radiographs generally underestimate the extent of the rheumatoid pannus, which can contribute to compression.

Differential Diagnosis

Atlantoaxial subluxation can also occur with a variety of congenital anomalies. It occurs in patients with Down syndrome. Other causes include ankylosing spondylitis, trauma, osteomyelitis, local neoplasms, and bone conditions (such as vitamin D–resistant rickets).

Atlantoaxial subluxation is the most common cause of myelopathy in patients with rheumatoid arthritis; however, other causes of myelopathy in these patients include lower cervical cord compression; rare causes are cord compression by rheumatoid pachymeningitis or by a rheumatoid nodule, thoracic disk disease, transverse myelitis due to medications or to rheumatoid vasculitis, or syringomyelia.

Complications

Rheumatoid atlantoaxial disease can cause quadriplegia or deadly brainstem compressions. Many patients with rheumatoid arthritis need lateral radiographs of the atlantoaxial joint prior to general anesthesia, so that the anesthesiologist can plan the safest mode of intubation and neck protection.

Treatment

Surgical stabilization of the atlantoaxial joint is clearly indicated for patients with atlantoaxial instability in whom neurologic deficits develop. However, indications for surgery for neck pain, asymptomatic subluxation, or mild hyperreflexia are controversial. Patients who have pain without neurologic deficits may palliate pain with a cervical collar, but this does not prevent progression to neurologic compression syndromes.

Prognosis

In patients with rheumatoid arthritis, atlantoaxial joint subluxation is a progressive condition that needs radiologic and neurologic follow-up. Most patients who undergo surgery for neurologic deficits have persistent deficits after surgery. After successful surgical stabilization of the atlantoaxial joint, patients have low risk of subluxations lower in the cervical spine.

Krauss WE, Bledsoe JM, Clarke MJ, Nottmeier EW, Pichelmann MA. Rheumatoid arthritis of the craniovertebral junction. *Neurosurgery.* 2010;66:83. [PMID: 20173532]

Complementary & Alternative Therapies

74

Anan Haija, MD

Sharon L. Kolasinski, MD

Most patients with chronic rheumatic diseases seek adjunctive care outside the medical mainstream. Although patients usually maintain relationships with medical physicians and take prescription medications, most will add some form of complementary and alternative therapy at some point during the course of their illness. Patient choices reflect their cultural and ethnic background, their financial resources, the availability of alternative providers, and their perception and satisfaction with conventional medicine. Not all interventions have been studied in a scientifically rigorous manner, but well-designed clinical trials continue to be published in a wide range of areas relevant to patients with rheumatic diseases.

Definition

Complementary and alternative medicine (CAM) has been defined as a group of diverse medical and health care systems, practices, and products that are not generally considered part of conventional medicine. With the recognition of its widespread use and the provision of services like acupuncture within academic medical centers, however, defining the limits of alternative medicine has become more difficult. The National Center for Complementary and Alternative Medicine (NCCAM), established by Congress in 1998 as one of the centers within the National Institutes of Health (NIH), has revised its categorization of CAM therapies into (1) natural products (herbal medicines, vitamins, minerals, dietary supplements, probiotics); (2) mind-body medicine (meditation, yoga, acupuncture, deep-breathing exercises, guided imagery, hypnotherapy, progressive relaxation, qi gong, tai chi); (3) manipulative and body-based practices (spinal manipulation, massage therapy); (4) movement therapies (Feldenkrais method, Alexander technique, Pilates, Rolfing Structural Integration, Trager psychophysical integration); (5) practices of traditional healers (Native American practices); (6) energy medicine (magnet therapy,

light therapy, Reiki, healing touch); and (7) whole medical systems (Ayurvedic medicine, traditional Chinese medicine). Furthermore, with the increasing number of randomized controlled trials examining these therapies, practitioners have a growing body of resources with which to evaluate the usefulness of CAM therapies, provide advice to patients, and consider incorporating CAM into standard treatment plans.

Epidemiology

Epidemiologic evidence from the 2007 National Health Interview Survey suggests that about 38% of the general public seek alternative care in a given year. Demographic data show that patients who use CAM are more likely to be older than age 65, have some college education, be in higher income brackets, and are less likely to be a member of a racial or ethnic minority. Patients with rheumatic disease who seek alternative care, however, use CAM more frequently and are more demographically diverse. Use correlates with pain and, for instance, over 90% of patients with diagnoses such as fibromyalgia may seek alternative care. Similarly, a variety of ethnic and racial groups and the elderly with musculoskeletal complaints have higher rates of CAM use than average American populations. Furthermore, recent data show that patients are considerably more likely to discuss their CAM use with their physician than they were in the past.

Quality & Safety Issues

Practitioners have a responsibility to help inform patients regarding their choices of alternative therapies, particularly where medical data exist. One of the most important sources of information is the NCCAM website (http://nccam.nih.gov/), particularly since it maintains an updated summary of references to studies supported by NCCAM funding. However, in this diverse and wide-ranging field, data may be lacking on a specific product or practice and patients often hold strong beliefs that alternative products are effective and safe.

Efforts to study aspects of traditional Chinese and Ayurvedic medicine and many herbal therapies have been hampered by the passage of the Dietary Supplement and Health Education Act by the US Congress in 1994. This legislation permitted the classification of numerous over-the-counter products with pharmacologic activity as dietary supplements. Dietary supplements are regulated like food. As such, they are exempted from the safety and efficacy requirements that must be met by prescription drugs. In fact, this legislation mandated that the US Food and Drug Administration (USFDA) assume the burden of proof when a product is considered for removal from the market as unsafe. Furthermore, consumers may make certain assumptions about testing, quality, and efficacy since the Dietary Supplement and Health Education Act permits labeling claims regarding "structure and function" that may suggest to the consumer that the products being sold have been proven to have health benefits. However, a manufacturer does not have to prove the safety and effectiveness of a dietary supplement before it is marketed. Dietary supplements do not need approval from USFDA before they are marketed. A manufacturer is permitted to say that a dietary supplement addresses a nutrient deficiency, supports health, or is linked to a particular body function (eg, immunity), if there is research to support the claim. Such a claim must be followed by the words "This statement has not been evaluated by the U.S. Food and Drug Administration (FDA). This product is not intended to diagnose, treat, cure, or prevent any disease." Manufacturers are expected to follow certain "good manufacturing practices" to ensure that dietary supplements are processed consistently and meet quality standards. Requirements for Good Manufacturing Practices went into effect in 2008 for large manufacturers and have been phased in for small manufacturers through 2010.

Recently, a number of safety considerations concerning herbal remedies were reviewed. A variety of herbs may themselves have toxic side effects (Table 74–1). They may also have important interactions with prescription medications. Garlic and gingko may increase bleeding risk in patients taking warfarin, whereas ginseng may reduce the ability of warfarin to lead to appropriate anticoagulation. St. John's wort may reduce the plasma levels of numerous medications, including antidepressants, antiretroviral agents, oral contraceptives, and immunosuppressive drugs. Thus, even if a patient is not taking an herbal product to address arthritis symptoms, he or she should be questioned about all over-the-counter product use since medication interactions may be significant.

Adulterants and contaminants in herbal preparations have been reported, including heavy metals, microorganisms and their toxins, and pesticides. Unsuspected botanicals other than those identified on the label may be present. One such case involved contamination of a weight loss preparation with the root of *Aristolochia fangchi*, resulting in interstitial renal fibrosis, renal failure, and in some persons, urothelial carcinoma. Pharmaceuticals may be present

Table 74–1. Potential adverse effects of herbal remedies and their major constituents.

Cardiotoxicity
Aconite root tuber
Herbs rich in cardioactive glycosides
Herbs rich in colchicine
Leigongteng
Licorice root
Ma huang
Pokeweed leaf or root
Scotch broom
Squirting cucumber
Hepatotoxicity
Certain herbs rich in anthranoids
Certain herbs rich in protoberberine alkaloids
Chaparral leaf or stem
Germander spp.
Green tea leaf
Herbs rich in coumarin
Herbs rich in podophyllotoxin
Herbs rich in toxic pyrrolizidine alkaloids
Impila root
Kava rhizome
Kombucha
Ma huang
Pennyroyal oil
Skullcap
Soy phytoestrogens
Neurotoxicity, convulsions
Aconite root tuber
Alocasia macrorrhiza root tuber
Artemisia spp. rich in santonin
Essential oils rich in ascaridole
Essential oils rich in thujone
Gingko seed or leaf
Herbs rich in colchicine
Herbs rich in podophyllotoxin
Indian tobacco herb
Kava rhizome
Ma huang
Nux vomica
Pennyroyal oil
Star fruit
Yellow jessamine rhizome
Renal toxicity
β-Aescin (saponin mixture from horse chestnut leaf)
Cape aloes
Cat's claw
Certain essential oils
Chaparral leaf or stem
Chinese yew
Herbs rich in aristolochic acid
Impila root
Jering fruit
Squirting cucumber
Star fruit

Used, with permission, from De Smet PA. Herbal remedies. *N Engl J Med.* 2003;347:2046.

Table 74–2. US FDA warnings and safety information on dietary supplements.

Year	Dietary Supplement	Action	Area of Concern
1999	Triax Metabolic Accelerator	Consumer warning	Thyroid hormone leading to myocardial infarction and cerebrovascular accidents
2000	St John's wort	Public health advisory	Interaction with indinavir, others
2001	Weight loss preparation contaminated by *Aristolochia fangchi*	Statement issued	Interstitial renal fibrosis, renal failure, urothelial carcinoma
2001	Comfrey	Advisory to industry to remove from market	Hepatotoxicity
2001	LipoKinetix	Consumer advisory, letter to health care professionals, letter to distributors	Hepatotoxicity
2002	Chaso (Jianfei) diet capsules, Chaso Genpi	Consumer warning	Contamination with fenfluramine
2002	Kava	Consumer advisory, letter to health care professionals	Hepatotoxicity
2002	PC SPES	Consumer warning	Contamination with warfarin, estrogen
2004	Androstenedione	Industry warning	Altered secondary sexual characteristics, carcinogenesis
2004	Ephedrine alkaloids	Declared by federal rule to be adulterated under the Federal Food, Drug and Cosmetic Act	Myocardial infarction, cerebrovascular accidents, seizure, psychosis, death
2007	Red yeast rice	Consumer warning	Contamination with lovastatin
2009	Colloidal silver	Consumer advisory	Argyria (permanent skin discoloration)

as well. A number of reports have detailed the presence of glucocorticoids and nonsteroidal anti-inflammatory drugs (NSAIDs) in herbal arthritis preparations, with resultant side effects including gastrointestinal bleeding and hepatotoxicity. Contamination of other herbal products with warfarin, estrogen, fenfluramine, and glyburide has been reported.

To date, the USFDA has issued specific warnings about a number of alternative products (Table 74–2) but has only banned those containing ephedrine alkaloids.

Ephedrine alkaloids were found to present an unreasonable risk under ordinary conditions of use, including myocardial infarction, cerebrovascular accident, seizure and death, after numerous reports of toxicity and an extensive review of the literature, as well as congressional hearings on these agents. For a complete list of all FDA announcements regarding dietary supplements, go to http://nccam.nih.gov/news/alerts/.

In November 2004, the USFDA announced three initiatives to further implement the Dietary Supplement and Health Education Act: formulating a regulatory strategy that will improve the evidenciary basis for USFDA actions with regard to dietary supplements by working collaboratively with the NIH and federal regulatory bodies; holding a public meeting for discussion of issues arising from the regulation of dietary supplements; and formulating a draft document detailing the amount and type of evidence that should be used to substantiate "structure function claims." On December 15, 2010, the USFDA took new steps aimed at

protecting consumers from harmful products that are marketed as dietary supplements and that contain undeclared or deceptively labeled ingredients. USFDA found that these products are often promoted for weight loss, sexual enhancement, and bodybuilding. The new steps include (1) sending a letter from Commissioner of Food and Drugs Margaret A. Hamburg to the dietary supplement industry emphasizing its legal obligation and responsibilities to prevent tainted products from reaching the US market; (2) implementing a new rapid public notification system (RSS Feed) on its website to more quickly warn consumers about these products; and (3) implementing a mechanism for industry to alert USFDA about potentially tainted products and about the firms that make them. The USFDA encourages the reporting of adverse events by consumers, physicians, and manufacturers via their web site (www.fda.gov/medwatch) or telephone (consumers: 1-800-MEDWATCH; physicians: 1-800-FDA-1088).

The American College of Rheumatology revised its position statement on the use of CAM therapies in August 2008. The American College of Rheumatology acknowledges that CAM use is widespread among patients with rheumatic diseases. It notes that all therapies must meet the same rigorous standards of scientific scrutiny using scientific methods and that those proven safe and effective can be integrated into the therapeutic armamentarium. It further suggests that rheumatologists should be informed about CAM therapies and be able to knowledgeably discuss them with their patients. Many studies show that little discussion about CAM occurs

Table 74–3. Obtaining and providing information about CAM therapies.

Questions for patients

1. Are you taking any vitamins, supplements, or herbal remedies? If so, which ones?
2. How much are you taking of each? How often do you take each? How long have you been taking each?
3. What are the symptoms you want to treat?
4. Do you have a prescription medication for the same symptoms? If so, are you still taking it?
5. Have you noticed any improvement or worsening of symptoms since taking the remedy?

Information for patients

1. Natural does not always mean safe.
2. Commercial availability does not guarantee safety and efficacy. Manufacturers are not legally required to back their claims with scientific studies.
3. The quantity and quality of active ingredients may vary from product to product and from time to time in the same product.
4. Herbal products are not regulated like prescription drugs, and contamination can occur.
5. Supplements or remedies may interact with prescribed medication or with each other with possible serious consequences.
6. Some products are safe for short-term use but long-term studies with appropriate controls are generally lacking.
7. Infants, children, pregnant women, women trying to conceive, and the elderly should not use any CAM therapy without medical supervision.

CAM, complementary and alternative medicine.
Reproduced, with permission, from Kolasinski SL. Complementary and alternative therapies for rheumatic disease. *Hosp Pract.* 2001;36:31.

in the office visit setting, however. Several authors have offered advice to physicians on what information should be discussed in order to facilitate the dialogue, particularly when patients are using herbal products (Table 74–3). Additional suggestions for both patients and practitioners to address this subject are given on the NCCAM website.

Barnes PM, Bloom B, Nahin RL. Complementary and Alternative Medicine Use Among Adults and Children: United States, 2007. *National Health Statistics Reports.* No. 12, December 10, 2008. [http://nccam.nih.gov/news/2008/nhsr12.pdf]

De Smet PA. Herbal remedies. *N Engl J Med.* 2003;347:2046. [PMID: 12490687]

Ernst E, ed. *The Desktop Guide to Complementary and Alternative Medicine. An Evidence-Based Approach.* Mosby, 2001.

Peng CC, Glassman PA, Trilli LE, Hayes-Hunter J, Good CB. Incidence and severity of potential drug-dietary supplement interactions in primary care patients: an exploratory study of 2 outpatient practices. *Arch Intern Med.* 2004;164:630. [PMID: 15037491]

Wu CH, Wang CC, Kennedy J. Changes in herb and dietary supplement use in the US adult population: a comparison of the 2002 and 2007 National Health Interview Surveys. *Clin Ther.* 2011;33:1749. [PMID: 22030445]

HERBAL MEDICINES

▶ Avocado/Soybean Unsaponifiables

A popular treatment for osteoarthritis (OA) in Europe, avocado/soybean unsaponifiables is an extract of oils in a one third avocado to two thirds soybean mixture. A large body of in vitro and animal data suggest that this mixture possesses anti-inflammatory actions. A prospective, randomized, double-blind, placebo-controlled multicenter clinical trial of patients with knee and hip OA showed promising results. After 6 months of treatment with 300 mg of the extract, patients experienced significant reductions in pain and functional disability. Many required less NSAIDs. No significant side effects were reported. Patients with hip OA seemed to benefit more than those with knee OA. Avocado/soybean unsaponifiables may achieve these benefits through structural effects on cartilage, as suggested by a subsequent study. This 2-year trial showed that avocado/soybean unsaponifiables may reduce cartilage loss in patients with hip OA and advanced joint-space narrowing at baseline. A more recent, 6-month head-to-head comparison with chondroitin showed avocado/soybean unsaponifiables to be as effective in reducing pain and the need for rescue medication; however, the trial design without a placebo arm fails to address the potential that the results could be explained by simple regression to the mean. This product has become available in the United States but the utility of the product to alter the course of OA has yet to be confirmed.

▶ Capsaicin

The American College of Rheumatology Subcommittee on Osteoarthritis 2000 and the European League Against Rheumatism 2009 Guidelines identify topical capsaicin cream as an option for treatment of OA symptoms. It may be used as an adjunct to systemic therapy or as monotherapy in those who wish to avoid oral medications. The cream should be applied four times daily. It initially results in a burning sensation but judicious and repeated use lessens the severity of the burning, which rarely results in discontinuation of therapy.

Capsaicin is one of a number of pharmacologically active substances found in the *Capsicum* red pepper. It is known to initially induce the release of the neurotransmitter substance P from skin sensory C fibers when applied topically. Repeated application leads to specific blockade of transport and de novo synthesis of substance P, resulting in desensitization to pain by raising the pain threshold. A number of randomized trials have suggested that capsaicin is useful in the treatment of neurogenic pain, including the pain of diabetic neuropathy, as well as low back pain and pain due to OA. A randomized, double-blind, parallel-group, placebo-controlled trial used instillation of capsaicin 15 mg or placebo vehicle into the surgical site following total knee arthroplasty prior to wound closure and results from the first 14 patients were recently reported. Pain scores did not differ between the groups tested but opioid use was reduced during the first 72 hours postoperatively and range of motion was increased at 14 days postoperatively in those who had received capsaicin.

Ginger

Extracts of members of the Zingiberaceae family have been used in Chinese traditional medicine and Ayurvedic tradition for millennia. Over 100 species have been tested and a number have been found to have anti-inflammatory effects, including inhibition of the actions of cyclooxygenase and lipoxygenase, synthesis of leukotrienes, and rat paw edema in an animal model of inflammation. Like other herbal products, what is labeled ginger is pharmacologically complex and may contain salicylate (though in amounts that are not thought to account for all of its anti-inflammatory effect), gingeroles, β-carotene, capsaicin, caffeic acid, and curcumin.

Fifty-six patients in Copenhagen with radiographically verified OA of the knee participated in a study in which they received either a ginger extract (Eurovita Extract 33, 170 mg orally three times a day), ibuprofen 400 mg orally three times a day, or placebo in each of three treatment periods of 3 weeks each. Overall, the investigators could demonstrate no differences between ginger and placebo. A larger multicenter study included 247 patients with radiographically confirmed knee OA. Participants were required to have visual analogue scores between 40 mm and 70 mm on a 100-mm scale for pain on standing during the 24 hours preceding the baseline visit. They received either placebo or ginger extract (Eurovita Extract 77, 255 mg orally twice daily) for 6 weeks in this double-blind, randomized trial. Patients in both placebo- and ginger-treated groups had improvement in pain on standing, but the ginger group had a higher percentage of responders (63% vs 50%), a greater degree of response on average (8.1 mm more in the ginger group), and a greater percentage of participants with large responses. Pain after walking and overall functioning measured by the Western Ontario and McMaster Universities OA composite index (WOMAC) were also significantly improved in the ginger group. Gastrointestinal side effects (eructation, dyspepsia, and nausea) were more common in the ginger group (45% vs 16%), but none were serious. The investigators concluded that ginger has efficacy for pain management in knee OA, but that a future dose-finding study would be of benefit as would long-term investigation of side effects. However, subsequent systematic reviews of the use of ginger for pain relief have concluded that evidence remains weak for its efficacy. Furthermore, a study of a ginger-based Ayurvedic preparation found no efficacy in the treatment of OA.

Thundergod Vine

Extracts of *Tripterygium wilfordii* Hook F, or thundergod vine, have been used in traditional Chinese medicine to treat a variety of autoimmune and inflammatory disorders, including rheumatoid arthritis, systemic lupus erythematosus (SLE), ankylosing spondylitis, psoriasis, and idiopathic

IgA nephropathy. Traditional use dates back centuries, and while the Chinese literature has been uncontrolled, it does represent observations made on thousands of patients for time periods as long as a decade. Laboratory data suggest that active ingredients include triptolide and tripdiolide and that these substances inhibit in vitro inflammation, delayed-type hypersensitivity reactions, and primary antibody responses.

Uncontrolled reports from China on a total of about 250 patients have shown that thundergod vine can be of benefit in treating SLE. Subjects have experienced improvements in fatigue, arthralgias, fever, skin rash, lymphadenopathy, hepatomegaly, and laboratory abnormalities including proteinuria, renal function, thrombocytopenia, and the presence of antinuclear antibodies. Reports have suggested that glucocorticoid doses can be reduced, and sometimes, eliminated.

The Chinese experience with thundergod vine has also been considerable with rheumatoid arthritis patients. An early placebo-controlled trial of 70 patients with rheumatoid arthritis had a crossover design. The majority of patients improved in parameters of disease activity and laboratory abnormalities. Peripheral blood mononuclear cells from those receiving active treatment produced less IgM rheumatoid factor than cells from placebo-treated persons. Adverse effects gleaned from the Chinese experience include dry mouth, loss of appetite, nausea or vomiting, abdominal pain, diarrhea, leukopenia, thrombocytopenia, rash, skin pigmentation changes, and amenorrhea.

The safety and efficacy of the herb have been examined in a randomized, double-blind, sulfasalazine-controlled trial of patients with rheumatoid arthritis seen at the National Institutes of Health and at the University of Texas. While 121 patients entered the trial, data from only 62 patients were assessed at 24 weeks. Of the group receiving the herb, 65% achieved a 20% improvement in symptoms as established by the American College of Rheumatology response criteria, while only 32.8% of the sulfasalazine-treated group responded to the same extent.

Chopra A, Saluja M, Tillu G, et al. A Randomized Controlled Exploratory Evaluation of Standardized Ayurvedic Formulations in Symptomatic Osteoarthritis Knees: A Government of India NMITLI Project. *Evid Based Complement Alternat Med.* 2011;2011:724291. [PMID: 20981160]

De Silva V, El-Metwally A, Ernst E, Lewith G, Macfarlane GJ; Arthritis Research UK Working Group on Complementary and Alternative Medicines. Evidence for the efficacy of complementary and alternative medicines in the management of osteoarthritis: a systemic review. *Rheumatology.* 2011;50:911. [PMID: 21169345]

Goldbach-Mansky R, Wilson M, Fleischmann R, et al. Comparison of *Tripterygium wilfordii* Hook F versus sulfasalazine in the treatment of rheumatoid arthritis: a randomized trial. *Ann Intern Med.* 2009;151:229. [PMID: 19687490]

Hartrick CT, Pestano C, Carlson N, Hartrick S. Capsaicin instillation for postoperative pain following total knee arthroplasty: a preliminary report of a randomized, double-blind, parallel-group, placebo-controlled, multicentre trial. *Clin Drug Investig.* 2011;31:877. [PMID: 21971213]

Pavelka K, Coste P, Geher P, Krejci G. Efficacy and safety of piascledine 300 versus chondroitin sulfate in a 6 months treatment plus 2 months observation in patients with osteoarthritis of the knee. *Clin Rheumatol*. 2010;29:659. [PMID: 20179981]

Recommendations for the medical management of osteoarthritis of the hip and knee; 2000 update. American College of Rheumatology Subcommittee on Osteoarthritis Guidelines. *Arthritis Rheum*. 2000;43:1905. [PMID: 11014340]

DIETARY SUPPLEMENTS

▶ Dehydroepiandrosterone

Wild Mexican yam is a natural source of diosgenin, an inactive prohormone of dehydroepiandrosterone (DHEA). However, wild yam products do not contain DHEA and require chemical treatment to yield usable hormone. DHEA is widely available without prescription in pharmacies and health food stores. However, before passage of the Dietary Supplement and Health Education Act, DHEA was considered a drug and was banned from over-the-counter sales since the 1980s. DHEA is a weak androgen and increases testosterone and estrogen levels; it also alters cytokine production.

The following observations have fueled interest in DHEA as a treatment for SLE: (1) there is a striking female predominance among SLE patients; (2) there are low circulating levels of DHEA in lupus patients; and (3) DHEA is beneficial in a mouse model of lupus. Several human trials have been published and offer intriguing findings.

A double-blind, randomized trial monitored 191 patients with SLE for 7–9 months. The investigators found that a significantly greater proportion of persons who took oral DHEA (at the 200-mg/d dose but not at the 100-mg/d dose) were able to reduce their prednisone dose to ≤7.5 mg/d orally and sustain disease quiescence for 2 months than were those persons receiving placebo. However, differences between groups were small. Forty-one percent of the placebo-treated group responded, compared with 44% of the low-dose DHEA group and 51% of the higher-dose group. Furthermore, 65% of those with SLE disease activity index scores of 0 or 1 were responders and the percentage of responders decreased progressively and rapidly as baseline scores increased. The most common side effect was acne, occurring in twice as many DHEA-treated patients as those receiving placebo. High-density lipoprotein cholesterol and C3 levels were reduced, and serum levels of testosterone and estrogen were increased.

A second multicenter, randomized, double-blind, placebo-controlled trial was published later in 2002 that monitored 120 female patients with SLE in Taiwan. Participants took either placebo or 200 mg/d of oral DHEA for 6 months. These investigators found no difference between the clinical status of patients in the two groups as measured by the systemic lupus activity measure or SLE disease activity index. However, the number of disease flares was significantly lower in the DHEA group, and this group had a significant improvement in the patient global assessment. Serious adverse events were mostly characterized as disease flares and were increased in the placebo group. Increased levels of testosterone and increased incidence of acne were noted in the DHEA group. C3 and C4 levels also declined in the DHEA group in this study.

A subsequent follow-up report of 293 patients receiving prasterone 200 mg/d or placebo for up to 12 months showed a small but statistically significant difference between groups. Those who took prasterone more frequently demonstrated improvement or stabilization of symptoms of lupus without clinical deterioration. Acne developed in one third of prasterone-treated patients and hirsutism developed in 16%, but few patients withdrew from the trial as a result.

In two randomized controlled trials done in primary Sjögren syndrome patients, administration of DHEA did not show any efficacy in a variety of outcomes, including general fatigue, depressive mood, mental well-being, physical functioning, pain, sicca complaints and disease activity parameters.

A small pilot study confirmed reductions in low-density lipoprotein cholesterol and showed a trend toward impairment of endothelial function in 13 lupus patients treated in a double-blind, placebo-controlled, 22-week crossover trial. There was no difference in lupus activity with DHEA treatment in this trial. Questions remain about the possible contribution of this hormone to risk of myocardial infarction or cerebrovascular accidents due to accelerated atherogenesis, altered cholesterol profile, or increased insulin resistance. In addition, concern has been raised because consequent elevations in sex hormones levels could result in increases in breast, ovarian, uterine, and prostate cancer risk.

▶ Glucosamine Sulfate & Chondroitin Sulfate

Glucosamine sulfate and chondroitin sulfate are the most commonly used over-the-counter alternative therapy for arthritis. Their tremendous popularity in the United States results in part from the 1997 best-selling book, *The Arthritis Cure,* by Jason Theodosakis, MD, and its subsequent revision. Dr. Theodosakis drew on decades of use and study in Europe in making his recommendations. While not a cure, glucosamine and chondroitin are of interest because they occur naturally in connective tissue, and are, therefore, intrinsically appealing as "nutraceuticals" for OA. In vitro work suggests a multitude of potential mechanisms, including inhibitory effects on cartilage-damaging agents like lysosomal enzymes, oxygen free radicals, matrix metalloproteinases, and aggrecanase, as well as dose-dependent increases in proteoglycan synthesis.

Glucosamine is available in a sulfate and a hydrochloride form, but studies have been carried out most often with the sulfate form. Most studies have been small and short in duration. Meta-analyses suggest that an analgesic benefit can be obtained from an oral dose of 1500 mg/d in a majority of those who take it. The effect is similar in magnitude to that of NSAIDs but is delayed in onset. The duration of the analgesic benefit is not known.

Controversy remains concerning the interpretation of two long-term studies of glucosamine because they suggested that glucosamine could halt radiographic progression of OA. In a 3-year Belgian trial, 212 patients received either 500 mg of oral glucosamine sulfate three times daily or placebo. Radiographs obtained at baseline and at 1 and 3 years of follow-up suggested that no radiographic progression occurred in those taking glucosamine while those receiving placebo had 0.34 mm joint-space narrowing detectable after 3 years. However, the radiographic technique used and its ability to detect the very small differences noted have been questioned. Nonetheless, a 3-year study of 202 OA patients seen at the Prague Institute of Rheumatology had similar results: those who took glucosamine had no radiographic progression while those taking placebo lost 0.35 mm of joint space after 3 years. Both studies have reported a reduction in the rate of joint replacement surgery needed for those who took glucosamine at 5-year follow-up. Trials suggest that chondroitin has analgesic benefit in OA as well. An oral dose of 1200 mg/d has generally been used. Studies of chondroitin have been subject to the same criticisms as those of glucosamine; namely, they involve small numbers of participants and are of short duration, in addition to often being industry-sponsored.

Recently, the Glucosamine/Chondroitin Arthritis Intervention Trial (GAIT) was done in a double-blinded, placebo-controlled method. This trial included 572 patients with knee OA who satisfied radiographic criteria (Kellgren/Lawrence) grade 2 or grade 3 and joint space width of at least 2 mm at baseline. The primary outcome was the mean change in joint space width from baseline. Patients were randomized to receive glucosamine, 500 mg three times daily; chondroitin sulfate, 400 mg three times daily; a combination of both; celecoxib; or placebo of both. At 2 years, no treatment achieved a predefined threshold of clinically important difference in joint space width loss compared with placebo. However, knees with K/L grade 2 radiographic OA appeared to have the greatest potential for modification by these treatments.

Many had hoped that more definitive answers on the efficacy of glucosamine and chondroitin would emerge when the 2006 NIH-sponsored GAIT was completed and published. This 5-armed multicenter, double-blind, placebo- and celecoxib-controlled study randomly assigned patients with symptomatic knee osteoarthritis to receive 1500 mg of glucosamine daily, 1200 mg of chondroitin sulfate daily, both glucosamine and chondroitin sulfate, 200 mg of celecoxib daily, or placebo for 24 weeks. Overall, glucosamine and chondroitin sulfate were not significantly better than placebo in reducing knee pain by 20 percent. Some have suggested the finding that for patients with moderate-to-severe pain at baseline, the rate of response was significantly higher with combined glucosamine and chondroitin therapy than with placebo (79.2% vs 54.3%, $P = .002$) has clinical significance.

However, most analysts note that the placebo response rate of 60% in this trial was so high as to make the results uninterpretable. Furthermore, evaluation of GAIT follow-up data published in 2010 showed no efficacy at 2 years. Proponents and detractors of the use of glucosamine and chondroitin continue to debate the merits of these dietary supplements as subsequent reanalysis of data and additional small studies continue to appear hinting at potential clinical and radiologic benefits.

The side-effect profiles of glucosamine and chondroitin have been indistinguishable from those of placebo in many of the short-term studies that have been carried out. Occasionally, gastrointestinal intolerance leads to discontinued use.

▶ Methylsulfonylmethane

Methylsulfonylmethane (MSM) is a commonly used ingredient in over-the-counter topical and oral preparations for the treatment of a wide variety of conditions, including musculoskeletal pain, inflammation, asthma, allergies, headaches, cancer prevention, gastrointestinal complaints, and parasitic infections. Despite considerable popularity and millions of dollars in sales annually, few data support its use as an arthritis treatment. MSM is naturally present in a variety of foods including grains, meat, eggs, and fish, as well as raw broccoli, peppers, brussels sprouts, onions, and cabbage. When taken as a dietary supplement, doses of 1000–6000 mg/d are generally recommended.

MSM is a metabolite of dimethyl sulfoxide (DMSO), which was itself popular as a topical arthritis treatment throughout the last century. However, the pungent odor and occasional skin irritation associated with use of DMSO have likely contributed to its decline and the increase in popularity of MSM. Until recently, few toxicologic data were available on MSM. A study in rats showed no toxicity from a dose 5–7 times higher than the recommended human dose given as a single gavage dose nor from long-term use of a 1.5-g/kg dose over 90 days.

One randomized, double-blinded, placebo-controlled trial was conducted; 50 patients with symptomatic osteoarthritis were enrolled in an outpatient medical center. Patients were randomized to receive 3 g of MSM twice daily or placebo, for a total of 6 weeks. MSM produced significant decreased in WOMAC pain and physical function impairment; MSM also produced improvement in performing activities of daily living when compared to placebo on the SF-36 evaluation.

Evidence that MSM is of benefit in arthritis treatment is largely anecdotal and published in the lay press. Celebrity endorsements and a best-selling volume by two physician proponents have enhanced public awareness of this substance. However, a 2009 systematic analysis of the available trials evaluating DMSO and MSM has concluded that no statistically or clinically significant effects have been demonstrated for these products. A 2011 study evaluating a combination of MSM and boswellic acids was no better than placebo in affecting the pain visual analogue scale and the Lesquesne Index.

Omega-3 Fatty Acids

The most frequently used over-the-counter dietary supplement for all indications is fish oil. Omega-3 fatty acids have been well documented to have a range of in vitro and in vivo effects of relevance to the treatment of rheumatic diseases, including antagonism of the production of proinflammatory and prothrombotic eicosanoids, suppression of production of proinflammatory cytokines, and reduction of cartilage-degrading enzymes. Omega-3 fatty acids are most readily available via the consumption of fish oil which contains both eicosapentaenoic acid and docosahexaenoic acid. Eicosapentaenoic acid competitively inhibits utilization of arachidonic acid and becomes a substrate for the production of alternative products of the cyclooxygenase and 5-lipoxygenase pathways. Thromboxane A_3 and prostacyclin I_3 are increased, resulting in decreased platelet aggregation, and leukotriene B_4 is decreased, presumably an important mechanism in reducing inflammation. A considerable number of short-term clinical trials performed over the last two decades have suggested efficacy in the treatment of rheumatoid arthritis. When given a daily dose of 3 g of omega-3 fatty acids, investigators have confirmed a reduction in morning stiffness, in the number of tender joints, and in the dose of NSAIDs required. Concomitant reduction in the level of interleukin-1 has been reported but fish oil has not been demonstrated to act as a disease-modifying agent in rheumatoid arthritis.

The clinical status of patients with SLE may also be affected by ingestion of fish oil. Murine models have suggested that consumption of an omega-3 fatty acid–rich diet could reduce autoantibody and inflammatory cytokine production and result in a prolonged lifespan in lupus-prone mice. A number of small, short-term trials in humans suggested improvements might occur but rigorous outcome measures were not generally used. A recent 6-month trial compared the status of lupus patients who received fish oil or placebo olive oil with or without copper supplements using the systemic lupus activity measure. Significant improvements of systemic lupus activity measure scores were noted at 6 months, as was an overall sense of well-being, but no detectable difference was found in weight, blood pressure measurements, blood counts, blood chemistry, erythrocyte sedimentation rate, complement levels, or levels of antibodies to double-stranded DNA or anticardiolipin.

Considerable interest continues in the use of fish oil supplementation in the treatment of OA, despite the fact that OA is generally thought of as a noninflammatory condition. Potential mechanisms for benefit include the in vitro demonstration that exposure to omega-3 fatty acids, but not other fatty acids, reduced, in a dose-dependent manner, the endogenous and interleukin-1–induced release of proteoglycan metabolites from the articular cartilage explants,

abolished endogenous aggrecanase and collagenase proteolytic activities, and reduced of mRNA expression for metalloproteinases and inflammatory cytokines. Relatively increased dietary content of omega-3 fatty acids has been associated with a reduction in predictors of knee pain and cartilage loss in OA in one epidemiologic study that correlated MRI findings with diet.

Vitamins

Vitamins are among the most popular and readily accessible supplements that patients might choose to treat their arthritis symptoms. There are a number of possible mechanisms through which vitamins could be of benefit, particularly in the pathogenesis of OA; however, in general, clinical trials have not borne out the promise of a significant clinical impact of these presumably readily available, nontoxic supplements. It is hypothesized, for example, that oxidative stress could be a major contributor to the progression of OA and antioxidant vitamins like C and E might, therefore, have a role in slowing progression. Framingham data were analyzed for a relationship between knee OA and intake of vitamins B_1, B_6, C, E, β-carotene, niacin, and folate as assessed by food frequency questionnaire. Six hundred forty participants were available for analysis and incident and progressive OA developed in 81 and 68 knees, respectively. The investigators found a threefold reduction in risk of OA progression for the middle and highest tertiles of vitamin C intake. This finding correlated predominantly with a reduced risk of cartilage loss. Interestingly, those with high vitamin C intake also had a reduced risk of developing knee pain. A less consistent reduction in risk of OA progression was also seen for β-carotene and vitamin E. A 2011 analysis of self reported vitamin C usage in 1023 individuals in the Clearwater Osteoarthritis Study suggested that vitamin C supplementation reduced the risk of incident OA by 11% but had no effect on progression. In contrast, a recent long-term prospective trial of vitamin E supplementation in patients with osteoarthritis of the knee failed to demonstrate efficacy.

A recent prospective cohort study to evaluate the effects of vitamin C supplementation on incident and progressive knee osteoarthritis was done, although this study did not show any evidence to support a protective role of vitamin C in the progression of knee OA. The data did suggest, however, that vitamin C supplementation may be beneficial in preventing knee OA.

The current concept of OA as a disease not just of articular cartilage, but also of the subchondral bone has contributed to interest in vitamin D as a potential modulator of OA incidence and progression. Vitamin D plays an important role in bone mineralization, proteoglycan synthesis by chondrocytes, and reduction of degradative matrix metalloproteinases, all of which could be protective from OA progression. A 1996 study analyzing Framingham data was the first to suggest that vitamin D intake could have an impact on OA progression. The investigators analyzed 788 normal and 126 osteoarthritic knees and found that the risk of radiographic progression of prevalent OA at baseline was markedly increased in those in the middle and lower tertiles for both intake and serum levels of vitamin D. The Study of Osteoporotic Fractures also appeared to support the notion that vitamin D might have an effect on cartilage metabolism with the finding that low serum 25-hydroxyvitamin D levels were associated with a threefold increase in the incidence of hip OA measured by radiographic joint-space narrowing but not osteophyte formation. However, 2007 Framingham data indicated that there was no relationship between radiographic OA and vitamin D levels. Furthermore, a 2011 report on 805 Finnish participants in a national health examination survey with a mean 22 year long follow-up showed that the development of OA was not associated with serum 25(OH) vitamin D levels. Rather, the authors demonstrated that the season of the year during which blood was drawn to measure the level of vitamin D was a potent effect modifier.

Vitamin D has also recently received considerable attention because of its potential to influence autoimmune disease. Vitamin D receptors have been identified in mononuclear cells, dendritic cells, antigen-presenting cells, as well as activated B lymphocytes and CD4+ T cells. The ubiquity of receptors has been hypothesized to suggest a regulatory role for vitamin D in the immune response. To date, results have been conflicting. Women's Health Initiative data suggest that high exposure to vitamin D may increase rheumatoid arthritis incidence. However, Nurses' Health Study data fail to demonstrate a relationship between vitamin D levels and the risk of developing rheumatoid arthritis or SLE. Nonetheless, numerous studies from around the world demonstrate the very common finding of vitamin D deficiency in many different disease populations, including those with autoimmune disease. Some studies have correlated lower levels of 25(OH) vitamin D with rheumatoid arthritis disease activity and increased levels with reductions in musculoskeletal pain. However, others have noted the significant limitations of the epidemiologic data amassed so far and have cautioned against the use of excessive supplementation. In a large cohort study, 1248 participants were monitored in a prospective manner; at baseline, vitamin D intake, bone mineral density, and 25-hydroxy vitamin D serum levels were measured. After a mean follow-up of 6.5 years, participants with low dietary vitamin D intake had an increased progression or knee radiographic OA. In persons with low baseline bone mineral density, vitamin D status seems to influence the incidence and progression of knee OA.

Bergink AP, Uitterlinden AG, Van Leeuwen JP, et al. Vitamin D status, bone mineral density, and the development of radiographic osteoarthritis of the knee: The Rotterdam Study. *J Clin Rheumatol.* 2009;15:230. [PMID: 19654490]

Bhangle S, Kolasinski SL. Fish oil in rheumatic diseases. *Rheum Dis Clin North Am.* 2011;37:77. [PMID: 21220087]

Brien S, Prescott P, Lewith G. Meta-analysis of the Related Nutritional Supplements Dimethyl Sulfoxide and Methylsulfonylmethane in the Treatment of Osteoarthritis of the Knee. *Evid Based Complement Alternat Med.* 2009 May 27. [Epub ahead of print] [PMID: 19474240]

Clegg DO, Reda DJ, Harris CL, et al. Glucosamine, chondroitin sulfate, and the two in combination for painful knee osteoarthritis. *N Engl J Med.* 2006;354:795. [PMID: 16495392]

Costenbader KH, Feskanich D, Holmes M, Karlson EW, Benito-Garcia E. Vitamin D intake and risks of systemic lupus erythematosus and rheumatoid arthritis in women. *Ann Rheum Dis.* 2008;67:530. [PMID: 17666449]

Duffy EM, Meenagh GK, McMillan SA, et al. The clinical effect of dietary supplementation with omega-3 fish oils and/or copper in systemic lupus erythematosus. *J Rheumatol.* 2004;31:1551. [PMID: 15290734]

Felson DT, Niu J, Clancy M, et al. Low levels of vitamin D and worsening of knee osteoarthritis: results of two longitudinal studies. *Arthritis Rheum.* 2007;56:129. [PMID: 17195215]

Harari M, Dramsdahl E, Shany S, et al. Increased vitamin D serum levels correlate with clinical improvement of rheumatic diseases after Dead Sea climatotherapy. *Isr Med Assoc J.* 2011;13:212. [PMID: 21598808]

Hartkamp A, Geenen R, Godaert GL, et al. Effect of dehydroepiandrosterone administration on fatigue, well-being, and functioning in women with primary Sjögren syndrome: a randomised controlled trial. *Ann Rheum Dis.* 2008;67:91. [PMID: 17545193]

Kim LS, Axelrod LJ, Howard P, Buratovich N, Waters RF. Efficacy of methylsulfonylmethane (MSM) in osteoarthritis pain of the knee: a pilot clinical trial. *Osteoarthritis Cartilage.* 2006;14:286. [PMID: 16309928]

Konstari S, Paananen M, Heliövaara M, et al. Association of 25-hydroxyvitamin D with the incidence of knee and hip osteoarthritis: a 22-year follow-up study. *Scand J Rheumatol.* 2012;41:124. [PMID: 22043944]

Marder W, Somers EC, Kaplan MJ, Anderson MR, Lewis EE, McCune WJ. Effects of prasterone (dehydroepiandrosterone) on markers of cardiovascular risk and bone turnover in premenopausal women with systemic lupus erythematosus: a pilot study. *Lupus.* 2010;19:1229. [PMID: 20530522]

National Center for Complimentary and Alternative Medicine. The NIH Glucosamine/Chondroitin Arthritis Intervention Trial (GAIT). *J Pain Palliat Care Pharmacother.* 2008;22:39. [PMID: 19062354]

Peregoy J, Wilder FV. The effects of vitamin C supplementation on incident and progressive knee osteoarthritis: a longitudinal study. *Public Health Nutr.* 2011;14:709. [PMID: 20707943]

Virkki LM, Porola P, Forsblad-d'Elia H, Valtysdottir S, Solovieva SA, Konttinen VT. Dehydroepiandrosterone (DHEA) substitution treatment for severe fatigue in DHEA-deficient patients with primary Sjögren's syndrome. *Arthritis Care Res (Hoboken).* 2010;62:118. [PMID: 20191499]

Welsh P, Peters MJ, Sattar N. Is vitamin D in rheumatoid arthritis a magic bullet or a mirage? The need to improve the evidence base prior to calls for supplementation. *Arthritis Rheum.* 2011;63:1763. [PMID: 21400480]

Zold E, Szodoray P, Gaal J, et al. Vitamin D deficiency in undifferentiated connective tissue disease. *Arthritis Res Ther.* 2008;10:R123. [PMID: 18928561]

Zwerina K, Baum W, Axmann R, et al. Vitamin D receptor regulates TNF-mediated arthritis. *Ann Rheum Dis.* 2011;70:1122. [PMID: 21415051]

PHYSICAL INTERVENTIONS

► Acupuncture

Acupuncture is the centuries-old practice of inserting needles into predetermined locations. In the traditional Chinese explanation for the efficacy of acupuncture, the movement of chi, or vital energy, along channels called meridians is influenced by the placement of the needles. An imbalance in the flow of chi can be redressed by certain needle placements, depending on the ailment being treated, and may improve health and well-being. In the Western medical tradition, it is recognized that one explanation, although incomplete, of the efficacy of acupuncture may be that needle placement stimulates the production of endogenous opioids. Inadequate understanding of the mechanism of action of acupuncture, however, is not as much of an impediment to systematic study as is the very nature of the intervention. Deciding what an appropriate control is (Can an intervention that does not use needles provide adequate control? Where should control needles be placed? How many? For how long?) has an important bearing on interpretation and comparison of trials. Regardless of the availability of scientific appraisal of acupuncture, about 1 million consumers in the United States seek treatment each year.

Recently, a few blinded randomized trials have been done to assess the efficacy of acupuncture. A study was done that blindly randomized patients with symptomatic knee OA, to two groups (each with 34 patients). One group received acupuncture and the other non-penetrating sham acupuncture; patients who received acupuncture had an improved WOMAC pain score, however, the improvement was short-term only.

Another single blinded study was done in 193 outpatients with OA of the knee. Participants were randomized into four groups: placebo, diclofenac, electroacupuncture and combined electroacupuncture and diclofenac. There was a significant improvement in WOMAC pain index between the combined and placebo group; there was also an improvement in the visual analogue scale between the electroacupuncture group and the placebo group as well as the electroacupuncture group compared to the diclofenac group. Another randomized, controlled, single-blinded trial compared 97 patients split into two groups: one received diclofenac and acupuncture and the other received diclofenac and placebo acupuncture. The WOMAC index presented a greater reduction in the intervention group than in the control group. The same was observed in the pain visual analogue scale. One acupuncture trial randomized 44 patients with rheumatoid arthritis to receive electroacupuncture or autogenic training for 6 weeks. There was a significant improvement in the acupuncture group in the mean weekly pain intensity, disease activity score 28, use of pain medications, pain disability index, clinical global impression, and pro-inflammatory cytokine levels. On the other hand, two larger studies showed different results. One study compared acupuncture with sham acupuncture. Acupuncture was not shown to be superior to sham acupuncture with outcomes targeting pain and WOMAC index. The study involved 455 patients and 72 controls. Acupuncturists were trained to interact in one of two communication styles, high or neutral expectations, and patients were randomized to one of three style groups, waiting list, high, or neutral, and nested within style. The other study was a randomized controlled trial, that included three groups of patients: group one included 116 patients who received advice about OA and exercise program; the second group included 117 patients who received advice, exercise, and true acupuncture; and the last group included 119 patients who received exercise, advice, and non-penetrating acupuncture. Outcomes included WOMAC index; function; pain intensity; unpleasantness of pain at 2 weeks, 6 weeks, 6 months, and 12 months. The addition of acupuncture to advice and exercise for OA of the knee delivered by physiotherapists provided no significant additional improvement in pain scores. One shared weakness in these studies is sample size in addition to study lengths. Encouraging results though should motivate the design of new, large, prospective randomized controlled trials.

No individual trials have been adequately designed to address the efficacy of acupuncture in pain control in rheumatic diseases. However, a huge number of trials have been performed for a wide variety of painful conditions over many decades using many different types of controls. At least eight Cochrane reviews of acupuncture trials for pain have been performed.

The most recent Cochrane Database Systematic Review of acupuncture for OA involved 16 trials with 3498 participants, most with knee OA. The authors predefined thresholds for clinical relevance in outcome measure and were not able to demonstrate that the studies met them even though the short-term improvements in pain and function reported were statistically significant. In addition, when they restricted their analysis to sham-controlled trials using shams judged most likely to adequately blind participants to treatment assignment (which were also the same shams judged most likely to have physiologic activity), pooled short-term benefits of acupuncture were smaller and non-significant. The authors believe that what little benefit was shown was likely the result of placebo effect due to incomplete blinding. Wait list-controlled trials showed greater improvements due to acupuncture than sham-controlled trials. Acupuncture as an adjuvant to an exercise-based physiotherapy program did not result in any greater improvements than the exercise program alone.

Acupuncture has been used in several trials as a therapy for the pain of fibromyalgia. A systematic review identified seven randomized, controlled trials that treated 385 patients over a mean of nine acupuncture treatments. There was a great variability of the methodologic quality of the studies evaluated. The investigators found that when ascertainment bias and lack of blinding were minimized, acupuncture was less likely to be found to be of analgesic benefit. For instance, trials with individual selection of acupuncture points, with electrostimulation and less than 10 sessions had significant effects on pain at post-treatment, but not studies with standardized selection of acupuncture points, manual stimulation, and more than 10 sessions. Furthermore, no studies supported a role for acupuncture in mitigating fatigue, sleep disturbance, or poor functioning.

Few trials have addressed the use of acupuncture in rheumatoid arthritis. A systematic review of eight available studies in which 536 participants were treated showed that six demonstrated reductions in pain but not stiffness. Though reductions in erythrocyte sedimentation rate were demonstrated in five studies, the mean change was a fall of only 3.9 mm/h. Evidence was judged to be conflicting in the placebo-controlled trials.

Despite the fact that trials in patients with rheumatic diseases have affirmed the safety of acupuncture, occasional adverse events due to acupuncture have been documented and include rare instances of pneumothorax, cardiac tamponade, spinal injuries, septic complications, and hepatitis C. However, a considerable amount of evidence supports the safety of acupuncture. A survey was conducted of preceptors and interns at a Japanese national medical facility at which about 60% of the patients undergo acupuncture. Results were compiled over 55,000 acupuncture treatments, and 64 adverse events were identified. The most frequent was failure to remove the needle after the procedure was completed. Almost as common were dizziness, discomfort, and perspiration thought to be associated with a transient vasovagal episode. Less common side effects were burn injuries due to moxibustion, ecchymoses, and needling site reactions. A systematic review of the literature revealed a similar safety record. Nine prospective surveys encompassing over 250,000 acupuncture treatments were reviewed. Minor side effects were common. These included pain at the site of needling and pain due to aggravation of the presenting condition that occurred in up to half of those undergoing acupuncture. Postprocedure fatigue was noted in up to about 40%; an unusual feeling of relaxation (characterized by some as necessary for efficacy) was seen in over 80%. Minor bleeding was seen in up to about 40% as well. Fainting was reported in less than 0.2%. Serious side effects reported included two cases of pneumothorax and two cases in which needles needed to be retrieved surgically after they fractured.

Tai Chi

Tai chi is a centuries-old Chinese form of conditioning exercise based in martial arts traditions and consisting of slow, flowing movements, relaxation, and deep breathing. The aim of the practice is balance of mind and body by stimulating chi. Tai chi involves cognitive, cardiovascular, and musculoskeletal responses that evoke physiologic and psychological changes including maximum oxygen consumption, muscular strength, and flexibility. Early studies encouraged enthusiasm for tai chi as an intervention for geriatric patients since these small trials suggested that improvements in balance and fall prevention could follow training in tai chi. A study of 72 patients with OA showed that a 12-week program held

three times weekly improved WOMAC scores for pain and function. On physical fitness testing, subjects demonstrated enhanced balance and abdominal muscle strength. A more recent trial of 40 subjects with a mean age of 65 and a mean body mass index of 30 also noted improvements in pain and function for this group with knee OA. Sixty minutes of tai chi twice weekly for 12 weeks was associated with increased improvements in WOMAC scores, as well as chair stand time and measures of self-efficacy and depression. No serious side effects of tai chi have been reported. In a randomized clinical trial of 152 older patients with chronic and symptomatic hip and knee OA, investigators found that when compared with a waiting list control group, both hydrotherapy and tai chi classes groups provided large sustained improvements both at 12 weeks. Another study was done to evaluate 41 adults with knee OA. This was a tai chi program that is 6 weeks long, followed by 6 weeks of home tai chi. Compared to baseline, the tai chi group showed significant improvements in mean overall knee pain, maximum knee pain, and WOMAC subscales of physical function and stiffness.

In a study of 40 individuals with symptomatic knee OA, patients were randomly assigned to 60 minutes of tai chi group or to an attention control group, both for 12 weeks. The primary outcome was the WOMAC pain score at 12 weeks. The tai chi group showed a significantly better improvement in WOMAC pain, physical function, self-efficacy, depression, and health-related quality of life for knee OA.

One single-blinded study compared the classic Yang-style tai chi with a control intervention consisting of wellness education and stretching in patients with fibromyalgia patients. This study, although small, did show significant improvement in Fibromyalgia Impact Questionnaire score, and the Short-Form Health Survey (SF-36). This result is very exciting and merits a long-term study in a larger sample.

The role of tai chi in patients with rheumatoid arthritis has not been studied extensively. One trial randomized 20 patients to tai chi or attention control in twice-weekly sessions for 12 weeks. At 12 weeks, 50% of patients randomized to tai chi achieved an ACR 20 response compared with 0% in the control group. The tai chi group had a greater improvement in the disability index, vitality subscale of the Medical Outcome Study short form 36, and the depression index. There are no large double-blinded placebo-controlled trials of tai chi in rheumatoid arthritis, although the results of this study should encourage such trial.

Yoga

Yoga derives from a more than 2000-year-old Indian tradition based on eight branches of practice, including postures (asanas), breathing, and meditation. The aim of hatha yoga, or the practice of asanas, is to prepare the practitioner for the spiritual experience of purifying the body. The ultimate goal of this practice is the achievement of harmony in body, mind, and spirit. A number of studies have attempted to quantify physiologic effects of yoga and found reductions in oxygen consumption, minute ventilation, and heart rate after exercise in persons participating in regular yoga practice.

Small studies have suggested that yoga may be efficacious for a variety of musculoskeletal conditions, but all studies to date have methodologic limitations that reduce their generalizability. Nonetheless, the trials that have been carried out support a role for yoga in reducing pain and increasing function. Persons with carpal tunnel syndrome participated in an 8-week yoga program and had significant improvements in grip strength and pain. A study of the effects of a 10-week course of yoga for symptoms of OA of the hands showed reductions in finger joint tenderness and range of motion and hand pain during activity. A more recent trial has suggested that yoga represents an exercise alternative for even obese patients with OA of the knee who are not regular exercisers. Reductions in pain and functional disability using WOMAC scores were demonstrated in a group who completed an 8-week yoga program.

A study to examine whether the physical function in women with rheumatoid arthritis can be altered through a yoga intervention included sixteen independently living, postmenopausal women with rheumatoid arthritis. The group participated in three 75-minute yoga classes a week over a 10-week period. Results showed significantly decreased Health Assessment Questionnaire (HAQ) disability index, decreased perception of pain and depression, and improved balance.

An ongoing study is evaluating the use of yoga in rheumatoid arthritis patients. This study is comparing 70 patients who are split into two groups: one is randomized to receive a 6 week yoga program and the other group is randomized to a 6-week wait-list control condition. The second group will participate in the yoga program following completion the first arm of the study. Data will be collected quantitatively using questionnaires and markers of disease activity, and qualitatively using semi-structured interviews. No serious side effects have been reported in the trials assessing yoga for musculoskeletal complaints. There have been rare reports of reversible compression neuropathy after 6 hours of kneeling and very rare instances of vertebral and basilar artery occlusion after neck standing and prolonged flexion of the cervical spine. There is also a report of isolated rupture of the lateral collateral ligament during yoga practice.

Bernateck M, Becker M, Schwake C, et al. Adjuvant auricular electroacupuncture and autogenic training in rheumatoid arthritis: a randomized controlled trial. Auricular acupuncture and autogenic training in rheumatoid arthritis. *Forsch Komplementmed.* 2008;15:187. [PMID: 18787327]

Bosch PR, Traustadóttir T, Howard P, Matt KS. Functional and physiological effects of yoga in women with rheumatoid arthritis: a pilot study. *Altern Ther Health Med.* 2009;15:24. [PMID: 19623830]

Brismée JM, Paige RL, Chyu MC, et al. Group and home-based tai chi in elderly subjects with knee osteoarthritis: a randomized controlled trial. *Clin Rehabil.* 2007;21:99. [PMID: 17264104]

Ernst E, White AR. Prospective studies of the safety of acupuncture. A systematic review. *Am J Med.* 2001;110:481. [PMID: 11331060]

Evans S, Cousins L, Tsao JC, Subramanian S, Sternlieb B, Zeltzer LK. A randomized controlled trial examining Iyengar yoga for young adults with rheumatoid arthritis: a study protocol. *Trials.* 2011;12:19. [PMID: 21255431]

Foster NE, Thomas E, Barlas P, et al. Acupuncture as an adjunct to exercise based physiotherapy for osteoarthritis of the knee: randomised controlled trial. *BMJ.* 2007;335:436. [PMID: 17699546]

Fransen M, Nairn L, Winstanley J, Lam P, Edmonds J. Physical activity for osteoarthritis management: a randomized controlled trial evaluating hydrotherapy or Tai Chi classes. *Arthritis Rheum.* 2007;57:407. [PMID: 17443749]

Jubb RW, Tukmachi ES, Jones PW, Dempsey E, Waterhouse L, Brailsford S. A blinded randomised trial of acupuncture (manual and electroacupuncture) compared with a non-penetrating sham for the symptoms of osteoarthritis of the knee. *Acupunct Med.* 2008;26:69. [PMID: 18591906]

Kim JY, Won JE, Jeong SH, et al. Acute hepatitis C in Korea: different modes of infection, high rate of spontaneous recovery, and low rate of seroconversion. *J Med Virol.* 2011;83:1195. [PMID: 21567423]

Kolasinski SL. Acupuncture for arthritis. *Altern Med Alert.* 2002;5:37.

Kolasinski SL, Garfinkel M, Tsai AG, Matz W, Van Dyke A, Schumacher HR. Iyengar yoga for the treatment of symptoms of osteoarthritis of the knees: a pilot study. *J Altern Complement Med.* 2005;11:689. [PMID: 16131293]

Langhorst J, Klose P, Musial F, Irnich D, Häuser W. Efficacy of acupuncture in fibromyalgia syndrome—a systematic review with a meta-analysis of controlled clinical trials. *Rheumatology (Oxford).* 2010;49:778. [PMID: 20100789]

Manheimer E, Cheng K, Linde K, et al. Acupuncture for peripheral joint osteoarthritis. *Cochrane Database Syst Rev.* 2010;(1):CD001977. [PMID: 20091527]

Patel SC, Parker DA. Isolated rupture of the lateral collateral ligament during yoga practice: a case report. *J Orthop Surg (Hong Kong).* 2008;16:378. [PMID: 19126911]

Sangdee C, Teekachunhatean S, Sananpanich K, et al. Electroacupuncture versus diclofenac in symptomatic treatment of osteoarthritis of the knee: a randomized controlled trial. *BMC Complement Altern Med.* 2002;2:3. [PMID: 11914160]

Suarez-Almazor ME, Looney C, Liu Y, et al. A randomized controlled trial of acupuncture for osteoarthritis of the knee: effects of patient-provider communication. *Arthritis Care Res (Hoboken).* 2010;62:1229. [PMID: 20506122]

Vas J, Méndez C, Perea-Milla E, et al. Acupuncture as a complementary therapy to the pharmacological treatment of osteoarthritis of the knee: randomised controlled trial. *BMJ.* 2004;329:1216. [PMID: 15494348]

Wang C. Tai Chi improves pain and functional status in adults with rheumatoid arthritis: results of a pilot single-blinded randomized controlled trial. *Med Sport Sci.* 2008;52:218. [PMID: 18487901]

Wang C, de Pablo P, Chen X, Schmid C, McAlindon T. Acupuncture for pain relief in patients with rheumatoid arthritis: a systematic review. *Arthritis Rheum.* 2008;59:1249. [PMID: 18759255]

Wang C, Schmid CH, Hibberd PL, et al. Tai Chi is effective in treating knee osteoarthritis: a randomized controlled trial. *Arthritis Rheum.* 2009;61:1545. [PMID: 19877092]

Wang C, Schmid CH, Rones R, et al. A randomized trial of tai chi for fibromyalgia. *N Engl J Med.* 2010;363:743. [PMID: 20818876]

Index

Note: Page numbers followed by *f* or *t* indicate figures or tables, respectively.